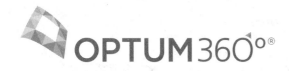

Urology/ Nephrology

A comprehensive illustrated guide to coding and reimbursement

2021

optum360coding.com

Publisher's Notice

Coding Companion for Urology/Nephrology is designed to be an authoritative source of information about coding and reimbursement issues affecting urological and nephrology procedures. Every effort has been made to verify accuracy and all information is believed reliable at the time of publication. Absolute accuracy cannot be guaranteed, however. This publication is made available with the understanding that the publisher is not engaged in rendering legal or other services that require a professional license.

American Medical Association Notice

CPT © 2020 American Medical Association. All rights reserved.

Fee schedules, relative value units, conversion factors and/or related components are not assigned by the AMA, are not part of CPT, and the AMA is not recommending their use. The AMA does not directly or indirectly practice medicine or dispense medical services. The AMA assumes no liability for data contained or not contained herein.

CPT is a registered trademark of the American Medical Association.

The responsibility for the content of any "National Correct Coding Policy" included in this product is with the Centers for Medicare and Medicaid Services and no endorsement by the AMA is intended or should be implied. The AMA disclaims responsibility for any consequences or liability attributable to or related to any use, nonuse or interpretation of information contained in this product.

Our Commitment to Accuracy

Optum360 is committed to producing accurate and reliable materials.

To report corrections, please email accuracy@optum.com. You can also reach customer service by calling 1.800.464.3649, option 1.

Copyright

Property of Optum360, LLC. Optum360 and the Optum360 logo are trademarks of Optum360, LLC. All other brand or product names are trademarks or registered trademarks of their respective owner.

© 2020 Optum360, LLC. All rights reserved.

Made in the USA

ISBN 978-1-62254-608-4

Acknowledgments

Marianne Randall, CPC, *Product Manager*

Stacy Perry, *Manager, Desktop Publishing*

Jacqueline Petersen, BS, RHIA, CHDA, CPC, *Subject Matter Expert*

Anita Schmidt, BS, RHIA, AHIMA-approved ICD-10-CM/PCS Trainer, *Subject Matter Expert*

Tracy Betzler, *Senior Desktop Publishing Specialist*

Hope M. Dunn, *Senior Desktop Publishing Specialist*

Katie Russell, *Desktop Publishing Specialist*

Kimberli Turner, *Editor*

Subject Matter Experts

Jacqueline Petersen, BS, RHIA, CHDA, CPC

Ms. Petersen has more than 25 years of experience in the health care profession. She has served as Senior Clinical Product Research Analyst with Optum360 developing business requirements for edits to support correct coding and reimbursement for claims processing applications. Her experience includes development of data-driven and system rules for both professional and facility claims and in-depth analysis of claims data inclusive of ICD-10-CM, CPT, HCPCS, and modifiers. Her background also includes consulting work for Optum, serving as a SME, providing coding and reimbursement education to internal and external clients. Ms. Petersen is a member of the American Academy of Professional Coders (AAPC), and the American Health Information Management Association (AHIMA).

Anita Schmidt, BS, RHIA, AHIMA-approved ICD-10-CM/PCS Trainer

Ms. Schmidt has expertise in ICD-10-CM/PCS, DRG, and CPT with more than 15 years' experience in coding in multiple settings, including inpatient, observation, and same-day surgery. Her experience includes analysis of medical record documentation, assignment of ICD-10-CM and PCS codes, and DRG validation. She has conducted training for ICD-10-CM/PCS and electronic health record. She has also collaborated with clinical documentation specialists to identify documentation needs and potential areas for physician education. Most recently she has been developing content for resource and educational products related to ICD-10-CM, ICD-10-PCS, DRG, and CPT. Ms. Schmidt is an AHIMA-approved ICD-10-CM/PCS trainer and is an active member of the American Health Information Management Association (AHIMA) and the Minnesota Health Information Management Association (MHIMA).

Contents

Getting Started with Coding Companion

Coding Companion for Urology/Nephrology is designed to be a guide to the specialty procedures classified in the CPT® book. It is structured to help coders understand procedures and translate physician narrative into correct CPT codes by combining many clinical resources into one, easy-to-use source book.

The book also allows coders to validate the intended code selection by providing an easy-to-understand explanation of the procedure and associated conditions or indications for performing the various procedures. As a result, data quality and reimbursement will be improved by providing code-specific clinical information and helpful tips regarding the coding of procedures.

CPT Codes

For ease of use, evaluation and management codes related to Urology/Nephrology are listed first in the *Coding Companion*. All other CPT codes in *Coding Companion* are listed in ascending numeric order. Included in the code set are all surgery, radiology, laboratory, and medicine codes pertinent to the specialty. Each CPT code is followed by its official CPT code description.

Resequencing of CPT Codes

The American Medical Association (AMA) employs a resequenced numbering methodology. According to the AMA, there are instances where a new code is needed within an existing grouping of codes, but an unused code number is not available to keep the range sequential. In the instance where the existing codes were not changed or had only minimal changes, the AMA assigned a code out of numeric sequence with the other related codes being grouped together. The resequenced codes and their descriptions have been placed with their related codes, out of numeric sequence.

CPT codes within the Optum360 *Coding Companion* series display in their resequenced order. Resequenced codes are enclosed in brackets for easy identification.

ICD-10-CM

Overall, the 10th revision goes into greater clinical detail than did ICD-9-CM and addresses information about previously classified diseases, as well as those diseases discovered since the last revision. Conditions are grouped with general epidemiological purposes and the evaluation of health care in mind. New features have been added, and conditions have been reorganized, although the format and conventions of the classification remain unchanged for the most part.

Detailed Code Information

One or more columns are dedicated to each procedure or service or to a series of similar procedures/services. Following the specific CPT code and its narrative, is a combination of features. A sample is shown on page ii. The black boxes with numbers in them correspond to the information on the pages following the sample.

Appendix Codes and Descriptions

Some CPT codes are presented in a less comprehensive format in the appendix. The CPT codes appropriate to the specialty are included in the appendix with the official CPT code description. The codes are presented in numeric order, and each code is followed by an easy-to-understand lay description of the procedure.

The codes in the appendix are presented in the following order:

- HCPCS
- Surgery
- Radiology
- Pathology and Laboratory
- Medicine Services
- Category III

Category II codes are not published in this book. Refer to the CPT book for code descriptions.

CCI Edit Updates

The *Coding Companion* series includes the list of codes from the official Centers for Medicare and Medicaid Services' National Correct Coding Policy Manual for Part B Medicare Contractors that are considered to be an integral part of the comprehensive code or mutually exclusive of it and should not be reported separately. The codes in the Correct Coding Initiative (CCI) section are from version 26.3, the most current version available at press time. The CCI edits are located in a section at the back of the book. Optum360 maintains a website to accompany the Coding Companions series and posts updated CCI edits on this website so that current information is available before the next edition. The website address is http://www.optum360coding.com/ProductUpdates/. The 2021 edition password is: **SPECIALTY21**. Log in each quarter to ensure you receive the most current updates. An email reminder will also be sent to you to let you know when the updates are available.

Index

A comprehensive index is provided for easy access to the codes. The index entries have several axes. A code can be looked up by its procedural name or by the diagnoses commonly associated with it. Codes are also indexed anatomically. For example:

69501   Transmastoid antrotomy (simple mastoidectomy)

could be found in the index under the following main terms:

Antrotomy
   Transmastoid, 69501

OR

Excision
   Mastoid
   Simple, 69501

General Guidelines

Providers

The AMA advises coders that while a particular service or procedure may be assigned to a specific section, it is not limited to use only by that specialty group (see paragraphs two and three under "Instructions for Use of the CPT Codebook" on page xiv of the CPT Book). Additionally, the procedures and services listed throughout the book are for use by any qualified physician or other qualified health care professional or entity (e.g., hospitals, laboratories, or home health agencies). Keep in mind that there may be other policies or guidance that can affect who may report a specific service.

Supplies

Some payers may allow physicians to separately report drugs and other supplies when reporting the place of service as office or other nonfacility setting. Drugs and supplies are to be reported by the facility only when performed in a facility setting.

Professional and Technical Component

Radiology and some pathology codes often have a technical and a professional component. When physicians do not own their own equipment and send their patients to outside testing facilities, they should append modifier 26 to the procedural code to indicate they performed only the professional component.

CPT © 2020 American Medical Association. All Rights Reserved.

36415-36416

36415   Collection of venous blood by venipuncture
36416   Collection of capillary blood specimen (eg, finger, heel, ear stick)

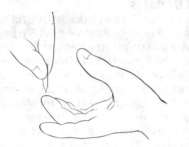

Capillary blood is collected.
The specimen is typically collected by finger stick

Explanation

A needle is inserted into the skin over a vein to puncture the blood vessel and withdraw blood for venous collection in 36415. In 36416, a prick is made into the finger, heel, or ear and capillary blood that pools at the puncture site is collected in a pipette. In either case, the blood is used for diagnostic study and no catheter is placed.

Coding Tips

These procedures do not include laboratory analysis. If a specimen is transported to an outside laboratory, report 99000 for handling or conveyance. For venipuncture, younger than 3 years of age, femoral or jugular vein, see 36400; scalp or other vein, see 36405–36406. For venipuncture, age 3 years or older, for non-routine diagnostic or therapeutic purposes, necessitating the skill of a physician or other qualified healthcare professional, see 36410. Do not append modifier 63 to 36415 as the description or nature of the procedure includes infants up to 4 kg. Medicare and some payers may require HCPCS Level II code G0471 to report this service when provided in an FQHC.

ICD-10-CM Diagnostic Codes

The application of this code is too broad to adequately present ICD-10-CM diagnostic code links here. Refer to your ICD-10-CM book.

Associated HCPCS Codes

G0471   Collection of venous blood by venipuncture or urine sample by catheterization from an individual in a skilled nursing facility (SNF) or by a laboratory on behalf of a home health agency (HHA)

AMA: 36415 2019,Aug,8; 2018,Jan,8; 2017,Jan,8; 2016,Jan,13; 201___,___,6; 2014,May,4; 2014,Jan,11

Relative Value Units/Medicare Edits

Non-Facility RVU	Work	PE	MP	Total
36415	0.0	0.0	0.0	0.0
36416	0.0	0.0	0.0	0.0
Facility RVU	**Work**	**PE**	**MP**	**Total**
36415	0.0	0.0	0.0	0.0
36416	0.0	0.0	0.0	0.0

	FUD	Status	MUE	Modifiers				IOM Reference
36415	N/A	X	2(3)	N/A	N/A	N/A	N/A	None
36416	N/A	B	0(3)	N/A	N/A	N/A	N/A	

* with documentation

Terms To Know

blood vessel. Tubular channel consisting of arteries, veins, and capillaries that transports blood throughout the body.

capillary. Tiny, minute blood vessel that connects the arterioles (smallest arteries) and the venules (smallest veins) and acts as a semipermeable membrane between the blood and the tissue fluid.

catheter. Flexible tube inserted into an area of the body for introducing or withdrawing fluid.

diagnostic. Examination or procedure to which the patient is subjected, or which is performed on materials derived from a hospital outpatient, to obtain information to aid in the assessment of a medical condition or the identification of a disease. Among these examinations and tests are diagnostic laboratory services such as hematology and chemistry, diagnostic x-rays, isotope studies, EKGs, pulmonary function studies, thyroid function tests, psychological tests, and other given to determine the nature and severity of an ailment or injury.

pipette. Small, narrow glass or plastic tube with both ends open used for measuring or transferring liquids.

specimen. Tissue cells or sample of fluid taken for analysis, pathologic examination, and diagnosis.

venipuncture. Piercing a vein through the skin by a needle and syringe or sharp-ended cannula or catheter to draw blood, start an intravenous infusion, instill medication, or inject another substance such as radiopaque dye.

venous. Relating to the veins.

© 2020 Optum360, LLC

CPT © 2020 American Medical Association. All Rights Reserved.

1. CPT Codes and Descriptions

This edition of *Coding Companion* is updated with CPT codes for year 2021.

The following icons are used in *Coding Companion*:

● This CPT code is new for 2021.

▲ This CPT code description is revised for 2021.

+ This CPT code is an add-on code.

Add-on codes are not subject to multiple procedure rules, reimbursement reduction, or appending modifier 50 or 51. Add-on codes describe additional intraservice work associated with the primary procedure performed by the same physician on the same date of service and are not reported as stand-alone procedures. Add-on codes for procedures performed on bilateral structures are reported by listing the add-on code twice.

★ This CPT code is identified by CPT as appropriate for telemedicine services.

The Centers for Medicare and Medicaid Services (CMS) have identified additional services that may be performed via telehealth. Due to the COVID-19 public health emergency (PHE), some services have been designated as temporarily appropriate for telehealth. These CMS approved services are identified in the coding tips where appropriate. Most payers require telehealth/telemedicine to be reported with place of service 02 Telehealth and modifier 95 appended. If specialized equipment is used at the originating site, HCPCS Level II code Q3014 may be reported. Individual payers should be contacted for additional or different guidelines regarding telehealth/telemedicine services. Documentation should include the type of technology used for the treatment in addition to the patient evaluation, treatment, and consents.

[ ] CPT codes enclosed in brackets are resequenced and may not appear in numerical order.

2. Illustrations

The illustrations that accompany the *Coding Companion* series provide coders a better understanding of the medical procedures referenced by the codes and data. The graphics offer coders a visual link between the technical language of the operative report and the cryptic descriptions accompanying the codes. Although most pages will have an illustration, there will be some pages that do not.

3. Explanation

Every CPT code or series of similar codes is presented with its official CPT code description. However, sometimes these descriptions do not provide the coder with sufficient information to make a proper code selection. In *Coding Companion*, an easy-to-understand step-by-step clinical description of the procedure is provided. Technical language that might be used by the physician is included and defined. *Coding Companion* describes the most common method of performing each procedure.

4. Coding Tips

Coding tips provide information on how the code should be used, provides related CPT codes, and offers help concerning common billing errors, modifier usage, and anesthesia. This information comes from consultants and subject matter experts at Optum360 and from the coding guidelines provided in the CPT book and by the Centers for Medicare and Medicaid Services (CMS).

5. ICD-10-CM Diagnostic Codes

ICD-10-CM diagnostic codes listed are common diagnoses or reasons the procedure may be necessary. This list in most cases is inclusive to the specialty. Please note that in some instances the ICD-10-CM codes for only one side of the body (right) have been listed with the CPT code. The associated ICD-10-CM codes for the other side and/or bilateral may also be appropriate. Codes that refer to the right or left are identified with the ☑ icon to alert the user to

check for laterality. In some cases, not every possible code is listed and the ICD-10-CM book should be referenced for other valid codes.

6. Associated HCPCS Codes

Medicare and some other payers require the use of HCPCS Level II codes and not CPT codes when reporting certain services. The HCPCS codes and their description are displayed in this field. If there is not a HCPCS code for this service, this field will not be displayed.

HCPCS codes are current as of time of print. Updated HCPCS codes will be posted at https://www.optum360coding.com/ProductUpdates/. The 2021 edition password is **SPECIALTY21**.

7. AMA References

The AMA references for *CPT Assistant* are listed by CPT code, with the most recent reference listed first. Generally only the last six years of references are listed.

8. Relative Value Units/Medicare Edits

Medicare edits are provided for most codes. These Medicare edits were current as of November 2020.

The 2021 Medicare edits were not available at the time this book went to press. Updated 2021 values will be posted at https://www.optum360coding.com/ProductUpdates/. The 2021 edition password is **SPECIALTY21**.

Relative Value Units

In a resource based relative value scale (RBRVS), services are ranked based on the relative costs of the resources required to provide those services as opposed to the average fee for the service, or average prevailing Medicare charge. The Medicare RBRVS defines three distinct components affecting the value of each service or procedure:

- Physician work component, reflecting the physician's time and skill
- Practice expense (PE) component, reflecting the physician's rent, staff, supplies, equipment, and other overhead
- Malpractice (MP) component, reflecting the relative risk or liability associated with the service
- Total RVUs are a sum of the work, PE, and MP RVUs

There are two groups of RVUs listed for each CPT code. The first RVU group is for facilities (Facility RVU), which includes services provided in hospitals, ambulatory surgical centers, or skilled nursing facilities. The second RVU group is for nonfacilities (Non-Facility RVU), which represents services provided in physician offices, patient's homes, or other nonhospital settings. The appendix includes RVU components for facility and non-facility. Because no values have been established by CMS for the Category III codes, no relative value unit/grids are identified. Refer to the RBRVS tool or guide for the RVUs when the technical (modifier TC) or professional (modifier26) component of a procedure is provided.

Medicare Follow-Up Days (FUD)

Information on the Medicare global period is provided here. The global period is the time following a surgery during which routine care by the physician is considered postoperative and included in the surgical fee. Office visits or other routine care related to the original surgery cannot be separately reported if they occur during the global period.

Status

The Medicare status indicates if the service is separately payable by Medicare. The Medicare RBRVS includes:

A Active code—separate payment may be made

B Bundled code—payment is bundled into other service

C Carrier priced—individual carrier will price the code

I Not valid—Medicare uses another code for this service

N   Non-covered—service is not covered by Medicare

R   Restricted—special coverage instructions apply

T   Paid as only service—These codes are paid only if there are no other services payable under the PFS billed on the same date by the same practitioner. If any other services payable under the PFS are billed on the same date by the same practitioner, these services are bundled into the service(s) for which payment is made.

X   Statutory exclusion—no RVUs or payment

Medically Unlikely Edits

This column provides the maximum number of units allowed by Medicare. However, it is also important to note that not every code has a Medically Unlikely Edit (MUE) available. Medicare has assigned some MUE values that are not publicly available. If there is no information in the MUE column for a particular code, this doesn't mean that there is no MUE. It may simply mean that CMS has not released information on that MUE. Watch the remittance advice for possible details on MUE denials related to those codes. If there is not a published MUE, a dash will display in the field.

An additional component of the MUE edit is the MUE Adjudication Indicator (MAI). This edit is the result of an audit by the Office of the Inspector General (OIG) that identified inappropriate billing practices that bypassed the MUE edits. These included inappropriate reporting of bilateral services and split billing.

There are three MUE Adjudication Indicators.

- 1 Line Edit
- 2 Date of Service Edit: Policy
- 3 Date of Service Edit: Clinical

The MUE will be listed following the MAI value. For example code 11446 has a MUE value of 2 and a MAI value of 3. This will display in the MUE field as "2(3)."

Modifiers

Medicare identifies some modifiers that are required or appropriate to report with the CPT code. When the modifiers are not appropriate, it will be indicated with N/A. Four modifiers are included.

51   Multiple Procedure
Medicare and other payers reduce the reimbursement of second and subsequent procedures performed at the same session to 50 percent of the allowable. For endoscopic procedures, the reimbursement is reduced by the value of the endoscopic base code.

50   Bilateral Procedures
This modifier is used to identify when the same procedure is performed bilaterally. Medicare requires one line with modifier 50 and the reimbursement is 50 percent of the allowable. Other payers may require two lines and will reduce the second procedure.

62*   Two Surgeons
Medicare identifies procedures that may be performed by co-surgeons. The reimbursement is split between both providers. Both surgeons must report the same code when using this modifier.

80*   Assistant Surgeon
An assistant surgeon is allowed if modifier 80 is listed. Reimbursement is usually 20 percent of the allowable. For Medicare it is 16 percent to account for the patient's co-pay amount.

* with documentation

Modifiers 62 and 80 may require supporting documentation to justify the co- or assistant surgeon.

Medicare Official Regulatory Information

Medicare official regulatory information provides official regulatory guidelines. Also known as the CMS Online Manual System, the Internet-only Manuals (IOM) contain official CMS information pertaining to program issuances, instructions, policies, and procedures based on statutes, regulations, guidelines, models, and directives. Optum360 has provided the reference for the surgery codes. The full text of guidelines can be found online at http://www.cms.gov/Regulations-and-Guidance/Guidance/Manuals/.

9.   Terms to Know

Some codes are accompanied by general information pertinent to the procedure, labeled "Terms to Know." This information is not critical to code selection, but is a useful supplement to coders hoping to expand their knowledge of the specialty.

99202-99205

▲★99202 Office or other outpatient visit for the evaluation and management of a new patient, which requires a medically appropriate history and/or examination and straightforward medical decision making. When using time for code selection, 15-29 minutes of total time is spent on the date of the encounter.

▲★99203 Office or other outpatient visit for the evaluation and management of a new patient, which requires a medically appropriate history and/or examination and low level of medical decision making. When using time for code selection, 30-44 minutes of total time is spent on the date of the encounter.

▲★99204 Office or other outpatient visit for the evaluation and management of a new patient, which requires a medically appropriate history and/or examination and moderate level of medical decision making. When using time for code selection, 45-59 minutes of total time is spent on the date of the encounter.

▲★99205 Office or other outpatient visit for the evaluation and management of a new patient, which requires a medically appropriate history and/or examination and high level of medical decision making. When using time for code selection, 60-74 minutes of total time is spent on the date of the encounter.

Explanation

Providers report these codes for new patients being seen in the doctor's office, a multispecialty group clinic, or other outpatient environment. All require a medically appropriate history and/or examination. Code selection is based on the level of medical decision making (MDM) or total time personally spent by the physician and/or other qualified health care professional(s) on the date of the encounter. Factors to be considered in MDM include the number/complexity of problems addressed during the encounter, amount and complexity of data requiring review and analysis, and the risk of complications and/or morbidity or mortality associated with patient management. The most basic service is represented by 99202, which entails straightforward MDM. If time is used for code selection, 15 to 29 minutes of total time is spent on the day of encounter. Report 99203 for a visit requiring a low level of MDM or 30 to 44 minutes of total time; 99204 for a visit requiring a moderate level of MDM or 45 to 59 minutes of total time; and 99205 for a visit requiring a high level of MDM or 60 to 74 minutes of total time.

Coding Tips

These codes are used to report office or other outpatient services for a new patient. A medically appropriate history and physical examination, as determined by the treating provider, should be documented. The level of history and physical examination are no longer used when determining the level of service. Codes should be selected based upon the CPT revised 2021 Medical Decision Making table. Alternately, time alone may be used to select the appropriate level of service. Total time for reporting these services includes face-to-face and non-face-to-face time personally spent by the physician or other qualified health care professional on the date of the encounter. For office or other outpatient services for an established patient, see 99211-99215. For observation care services, see 99217-99226. For patients admitted and discharged from observation or inpatient status on the same date, see 99234-99236. Telemedicine services may be reported by the performing provider by adding modifier 95 to these procedure codes. Services at the origination site are reported with HCPCS Level II code Q3014.

ICD-10-CM Diagnostic Codes

The application of this code is too broad to adequately present ICD-10-CM diagnostic code links here. Refer to your ICD-10-CM book.

AMA: **99202** 2020,Sep,3; 2020,Sep,14; 2020,May,3; 2020,Jun,3; 2020,Jan,3; 2020,Feb,3; 2019,Oct,10; 2019,Jan,3; 2019,Feb,3; 2018,Sep,14; 2018,Mar,7; 2018,Jan,8; 2018,Apr,9; 2018,Apr,10; 2017,Jun,6; 2017,Jan,8; 2017,Aug,3; 2016,Sep,6; 2016,Mar,10; 2016,Jan,7; 2016,Jan,13; 2016,Dec,11; 2015,Oct,3; 2015,Jan,16; 2015,Jan,12; 2015,Dec,3; 2014,Oct,8; 2014,Oct,3; 2014,Nov,14; 2014,Jan,11; 2014,Aug,3 **99203** 2020,Sep,3; 2020,Sep,14; 2020,May,3; 2020,Jun,3; 2020,Jan,3; 2020,Feb,3; 2019,Oct,10; 2019,Jan,3; 2019,Feb,3; 2018,Sep,14; 2018,Mar,7; 2018,Jan,8; 2018,Apr,10; 2018,Apr,9; 2017,Jun,6; 2017,Jan,8; 2017,Aug,3; 2016,Sep,6; 2016,Mar,10; 2016,Jan,7; 2016,Jan,13; 2016,Dec,11; 2015,Oct,3; 2015,Jan,12; 2015,Jan,16; 2015,Dec,3; 2014,Oct,3; 2014,Oct,8; 2014,Nov,14; 2014,Jan,11; 2014,Aug,3 **99204** 2020,Sep,14; 2020,Sep,3; 2020,May,3; 2020,Jun,3; 2020,Jan,3; 2020,Feb,3; 2019,Oct,10; 2019,Jan,3; 2019,Feb,3; 2018,Sep,14; 2018,Mar,7; 2018,Jan,8; 2018,Apr,9; 2018,Apr,10; 2017,Jun,6; 2017,Jan,8; 2017,Aug,3; 2016,Sep,6; 2016,Mar,10; 2016,Jan,13; 2016,Jan,7; 2016,Dec,11; 2015,Oct,3; 2015,Jan,12; 2015,Jan,16; 2015,Dec,3; 2014,Oct,3; 2014,Oct,8; 2014,Nov,14; 2014,Jan,11; 2014,Aug,3 **99205** 2020,Sep,3; 2020,Sep,14; 2020,May,3; 2020,Jun,3; 2020,Jan,3; 2020,Feb,3; 2019,Oct,10; 2019,Jan,3; 2019,Feb,3; 2018,Sep,14; 2018,Mar,7; 2018,Jan,8; 2018,Apr,10; 2018,Apr,9; 2017,Jun,6; 2017,Jan,8; 2017,Aug,3; 2016,Sep,6; 2016,Mar,10; 2016,Jan,7; 2016,Jan,13; 2016,Dec,11; 2015,Oct,3; 2015,Jan,12; 2015,Jan,16; 2015,Dec,3; 2014,Oct,8; 2014,Oct,3; 2014,Nov,14; 2014,Jan,11; 2014,Aug,3

Relative Value Units/Medicare Edits

Non-Facility RVU	Work	PE	MP	Total
99202	0.93	1.12	0.09	2.14
99203	1.42	1.48	0.13	3.03
99204	2.43	1.98	0.22	4.63
99205	3.17	2.4	0.28	5.85
Facility RVU	Work	PE	MP	Total
99202	0.93	0.41	0.09	1.43
99203	1.42	0.59	0.13	2.14
99204	2.43	1.01	0.22	3.66
99205	3.17	1.33	0.28	4.78

	FUD	Status	MUE	Modifiers				IOM Reference
99202	N/A	A	1(2)	N/A	N/A	N/A	80*	None
99203	N/A	A	1(2)	N/A	N/A	N/A	80*	
99204	N/A	A	1(2)	N/A	N/A	N/A	80*	
99205	N/A	A	1(2)	N/A	N/A	N/A	80*	

* with documentation

Terms To Know

new patient. Patient who is receiving face-to-face care from a provider/qualified health care professional or another physician/qualified health care professional of the exact same specialty and subspecialty who belongs to the same group practice for the first time in three years. For OPPS hospitals, a patient who has not been registered as an inpatient or outpatient, including off-campus provider based clinic or emergency department, within the past three years.

99211-99215

▲ **99211** Office or other outpatient visit for the evaluation and management of an established patient, that may not require the presence of a physician or other qualified health care professional. Usually, the presenting problem(s) are minimal.

▲★**99212** Office or other outpatient visit for the evaluation and management of an established patient, which requires a medically appropriate history and/or examination and straightforward medical decision making. When using time for code selection, 10-19 minutes of total time is spent on the date of the encounter.

▲★**99213** Office or other outpatient visit for the evaluation and management of an established patient, which requires a medically appropriate history and/or examination and low level of medical decision making. When using time for code selection, 20-29 minutes of total time is spent on the date of the encounter.

▲★**99214** Office or other outpatient visit for the evaluation and management of an established patient, which requires a medically appropriate history and/or examination and moderate level of medical decision making. When using time for code selection, 30-39 minutes of total time is spent on the date of the encounter.

▲★**99215** Office or other outpatient visit for the evaluation and management of an established patient, which requires a medically appropriate history and/or examination and high level of medical decision making. When using time for code selection, 40-54 minutes of total time is spent on the date of the encounter.

Explanation

Providers report these codes for established patients being seen in the doctor's office, a multispecialty group clinic, or other outpatient environment. All require a medically appropriate history and/or examination excluding the most basic service represented by 99211 that describes an encounter in which the presenting problems are typically minimal and may not require the presence of a physician or other qualified health care professional. For the remainder of codes within this range, code selection is based on the level of medical decision making (MDM) or total time personally spent by the physician and/or other qualified health care professional(s) on the date of the encounter. Factors to be considered in MDM include the number/complexity of problems addressed during the encounter, amount and complexity of data requiring review and analysis, and the risk of complications and/or morbidity or mortality associated with patient management. Report 99212 for a visit that entails straightforward MDM. If time is used for code selection, 10 to 19 minutes of total time is spent on the day of encounter. Report 99213 for a visit requiring a low level of MDM or 20 to 29 minutes of total time; 99214 for a moderate level of MDM or 30 to 39 minutes of total time; and 99215 for a high level of MDM or 40 to 54 minutes of total time.

Coding Tips

These codes are used to report office or other outpatient services for an established patient. A medically appropriate history and physical examination, as determined by the treating provider, should be documented. The level of history and physical examination are no longer used when determining the level of service. Codes should be selected based upon the CPT revised 2021 Medical Decision Making table. Alternately, time alone may be used to select the appropriate level of service. Total time for reporting these services includes face-to-face and non-face-to-face time personally spent by the physician or other qualified health care professional on the date of the encounter. Code

99211 does not require the presence of a physician or other qualified health care professional. For office or other outpatient services for a new patient, see 99202-99205. For observation care services, see 99217-99226. For patients admitted and discharged from observation or inpatient status on the same date, see 99234-99236. Medicare has identified 99211 as a telehealth/telemedicine service. Commercial payers should be contacted regarding their coverage guidelines. Telemedicine services may be reported by the performing provider by adding modifier 95 to these procedure codes. Services at the origination site are reported with HCPCS Level II code Q3014.

ICD-10-CM Diagnostic Codes

The application of this code is too broad to adequately present ICD-10-CM diagnostic code links here. Refer to your ICD-10-CM book.

AMA: **99211** 2020,Sep,14; 2020,Sep,3; 2020,May,3; 2020,Jun,3; 2020,Jan,3; 2020,Feb,3; 2019,Oct,10; 2019,Jan,3; 2019,Feb,3; 2018,Sep,14; 2018,Mar,7; 2018,Jan,8; 2018,Apr,10; 2018,Apr,9; 2017,Mar,10; 2017,Jun,6; 2017,Jan,8; 2017,Aug,3; 2016,Sep,6; 2016,Mar,10; 2016,Jan,13; 2016,Jan,7; 2016,Dec,11; 2015,Oct,3; 2015,Jan,12; 2015,Jan,16; 2015,Dec,3; 2014,Oct,8; 2014,Oct,3; 2014,Nov,14; 2014,Mar,13; 2014,Jan,11; 2014,Aug,3 **99212** 2020,Sep,14; 2020,Sep,3; 2020,May,3; 2020,Jun,3; 2020,Jan,3; 2020,Feb,3; 2019,Oct,10; 2019,Jan,3; 2019,Feb,3; 2018,Sep,14; 2018,Mar,7; 2018,Jan,8; 2018,Apr,9; 2018,Apr,10; 2017,Oct,5; 2017,Jun,6; 2017,Jan,8; 2017,Aug,3; 2016,Sep,6; 2016,Mar,10; 2016,Jan,13; 2016,Jan,7; 2016,Dec,11; 2015,Oct,3; 2015,Jan,16; 2015,Jan,12; 2015,Dec,3; 2014,Oct,8; 2014,Oct,3; 2014,Nov,14; 2014,Jan,11; 2014,Aug,3 **99213** 2020,Sep,3; 2020,Sep,14; 2020,May,3; 2020,Jun,3; 2020,Jan,3; 2020,Feb,3; 2019,Oct,10; 2019,Jan,3; 2019,Feb,3; 2018,Sep,14; 2018,Mar,7; 2018,Jan,8; 2018,Apr,10; 2018,Apr,9; 2017,Jun,6; 2017,Jan,8; 2017,Aug,3; 2016,Sep,6; 2016,Mar,10; 2016,Jan,7; 2016,Jan,13; 2016,Dec,11; 2015,Oct,3; 2015,Jan,12; 2015,Jan,16; 2015,Dec,3; 2014,Oct,3; 2014,Oct,8; 2014,Nov,14; 2014,Jan,11; 2014,Aug,3 **99214** 2020,Sep,14; 2020,Sep,3; 2020,May,3; 2020,Jun,3; 2020,Jan,3; 2020,Feb,3; 2019,Oct,10; 2019,Jan,3; 2019,Feb,3; 2018,Sep,14; 2018,Mar,7; 2018,Jan,8; 2018,Apr,9; 2018,Apr,10; 2017,Jun,6; 2017,Jan,8; 2017,Aug,3; 2016,Sep,6; 2016,Mar,10; 2016,Jan,13; 2016,Jan,7; 2016,Dec,11; 2015,Oct,3; 2015,Jan,16; 2015,Jan,12; 2015,Dec,3; 2014,Oct,8; 2014,Oct,3; 2014,Nov,14; 2014,Jan,11; 2014,Aug,3 **99215** 2020,Sep,3; 2020,Sep,14; 2020,May,3; 2020,Jun,3; 2020,Jan,3; 2020,Feb,3; 2019,Oct,10; 2019,Jan,3; 2019,Feb,3; 2018,Sep,14; 2018,Mar,7; 2018,Jan,8; 2018,Apr,9; 2018,Apr,10; 2017,Jun,6; 2017,Jan,8; 2017,Aug,3; 2016,Sep,6; 2016,Mar,10; 2016,Jan,13; 2016,Jan,7; 2016,Dec,11; 2015,Oct,3; 2015,Jan,12; 2015,Jan,16; 2015,Dec,3; 2014,Oct,3; 2014,Oct,8; 2014,Nov,14; 2014,Jan,11; 2014,Aug,3

Relative Value Units/Medicare Edits

Non-Facility RVU	Work	PE	MP	Total
99211	0.18	0.46	0.01	0.65
99212	0.48	0.75	0.05	1.28
99213	0.97	1.06	0.08	2.11
99214	1.5	1.45	0.11	3.06
99215	2.11	1.85	0.15	4.11
Facility RVU	Work	PE	MP	Total
99211	0.18	0.07	0.01	0.26
99212	0.48	0.2	0.05	0.73
99213	0.97	0.4	0.08	1.45
99214	1.5	0.62	0.11	2.23
99215	2.11	0.89	0.15	3.15

	FUD	Status	MUE	Modifiers				IOM Reference
99211	N/A	A	1(3)	N/A	N/A	N/A	80*	None
99212	N/A	A	2(3)	N/A	N/A	N/A	80*	
99213	N/A	A	2(3)	N/A	N/A	N/A	80*	
99214	N/A	A	2(3)	N/A	N/A	N/A	80*	
99215	N/A	A	1(3)	N/A	N/A	N/A	80*	

* with documentation

Terms To Know

established patient. Patient who has received professional services in a face-to-face setting within the last three years from the same physician/qualified health care professional or another physician/qualified health care professional of the exact same specialty and subspecialty who belongs to the same group practice. If the patient is seen by a physician/qualified health care professional who is covering for another physician/qualified health care professional, the patient will be considered the same as if seen by the physician/qualified health care professional who is unavailable.

non-physician practitioner. Health care services rendered by physician assistants (PA), nurse practitioners (NP), advance practice nurses (APN), certified nurse specialists (CNS), certified registered nurse anesthetists (CRNA), and certified nurse midwifes (CNM).

other qualified health care professional. Individual who is qualified by education, training, licensure/regulation, and facility privileging to perform a professional service within his or her scope of practice and independently (or as incident-to) report the professional service without requiring physician supervision. Payers may state exemptions in writing or state and local regulations may not follow this definition for performance of some services. Always refer to any relevant plan policies and federal and/or state laws to determine who may perform and report services.

99217

99217   Observation care discharge day management (This code is to be utilized to report all services provided to a patient on discharge from outpatient hospital "observation status" if the discharge is on other than the initial date of "observation status." To report services to a patient designated as "observation status" or "inpatient status" and discharged on the same date, use the codes for Observation or Inpatient Care Services [including Admission and Discharge Services, 99234-99236 as appropriate.])

Explanation

This code describes the final processes associated with discharging a patient from outpatient hospital observation status and includes a patient exam, a discussion about the hospital stay, instructions for ongoing care, as well as preparing the medical discharge records. Report this code only when the patient has been discharged from observation services on a date other than the initial date of observation care. There are no key components or time estimates associated with this service.

Coding Tips

This code is used to report hospital outpatient observation discharge services. This code includes patient examination, discharge and follow-up care instructions, and preparation of all medical records. Time is not a factor when selecting this E/M service. For patients admitted and discharged from observation or inpatient status on the same date, see 99234-99236; for hospital inpatient discharge services, see 99238-99239. Medicare has provisionally identified this code as a telehealth/telemedicine service. Current Medicare coverage guidelines should be reviewed. Commercial payers should be contacted regarding their coverage guidelines. Telemedicine services may be reported by the performing provider by adding modifier 95 to this procedure code. Services at the origination site are reported with HCPCS Level II code Q3014.

ICD-10-CM Diagnostic Codes

The application of this code is too broad to adequately present ICD-10-CM diagnostic code links here. Refer to your ICD-10-CM book.

AMA: 99217 2019,Jul,10; 2018,Jan,8; 2017,Jun,6; 2017,Jan,8; 2017,Aug,3; 2016,Jan,13; 2016,Jan,7; 2016,Dec,11; 2015,Jan,16; 2015,Dec,3; 2014,Oct,8; 2014,Nov,14; 2014,Jan,11

Relative Value Units/Medicare Edits

Non-Facility RVU	Work	PE	MP	Total
99217	1.28	0.68	0.09	2.05
Facility RVU	Work	PE	MP	Total
99217	1.28	0.68	0.09	2.05

	FUD	Status	MUE	Modifiers				IOM Reference
99217	N/A	A	1(2)	N/A	N/A	N/A	80*	100-04,11,40.1.3; 100-04,12,30.6.4; 100-04,12,30.6.8; 100-04,12,100; 100-04,32,130.1

* with documentation

CPT © 2020 American Medical Association. All Rights Reserved.   ● New   ▲ Revised   + Add On   ★ Telemedicine   AMA: CPT Assist   [Resequenced]   ☑ Laterality   © 2020 Optum360, LLC

99218-99220

99218 Initial observation care, per day, for the evaluation and management of a patient which requires these 3 key components: A detailed or comprehensive history; A detailed or comprehensive examination; and Medical decision making that is straightforward or of low complexity. Counseling and/or coordination of care with other physicians, other qualified health care professionals, or agencies are provided consistent with the nature of the problem(s) and the patient's and/or family's needs. Usually, the problem(s) requiring admission to outpatient hospital "observation status" are of low severity. Typically, 30 minutes are spent at the bedside and on the patient's hospital floor or unit.

99219 Initial observation care, per day, for the evaluation and management of a patient, which requires these 3 key components: A comprehensive history; A comprehensive examination; and Medical decision making of moderate complexity. Counseling and/or coordination of care with other physicians, other qualified health care professionals, or agencies are provided consistent with the nature of the problem(s) and the patient's and/or family's needs. Usually, the problem(s) requiring admission to outpatient hospital "observation status" are of moderate severity. Typically, 50 minutes are spent at the bedside and on the patient's hospital floor or unit.

99220 Initial observation care, per day, for the evaluation and management of a patient, which requires these 3 key components: A comprehensive history; A comprehensive examination; and Medical decision making of high complexity. Counseling and/or coordination of care with other physicians, other qualified health care professionals, or agencies are provided consistent with the nature of the problem(s) and the patient's and/or family's needs. Usually, the problem(s) requiring admission to outpatient hospital "observation status" are of high severity. Typically, 70 minutes are spent at the bedside and on the patient's hospital floor or unit.

Explanation

Initial hospital observation service codes describe the first visit of the patient's admission for hospital outpatient observation care by the supervising qualified clinician. Hospital outpatient observation status includes the supervision of the care plan for observation as well as periodic reassessments. The patient is not required to be physically located in a designated observation area within a hospital; however, if such an area is utilized, these codes should be reported. When a patient is admitted to observation status during the course of another encounter from a different site of service, such as the physician's office, a nursing home, or the emergency department, all of the E/M services rendered by the supervising clinician as part of the observation status are considered part of the initial observation care services when they are performed on the same day; the level of initial observation code reported by the clinician should incorporate the other services related to the hospital outpatient observation admission that were provided in any other sites of services as well as those provided in the actual observation setting. Codes are reported per day and do not differentiate between new or established patients. Under the initial observation care category, there are three levels represented by 99218, 99219, and 99220. These levels require all three key components to be documented. The lowest level of care within this category, 99218, requires a detailed or comprehensive history and exam as well as straightforward or low complexity medical decision making (MDM) with approximately 30 minutes time being spent at the patient's bedside and on the patient's floor or unit. For the mid-level and highest level observation care codes, a comprehensive history and examination are required. Medical decision making is the differentiating factor for these two levels. For moderate complexity, report 99219. For observation care requiring MDM of high complexity, report 99220. The clinician

typically spends 50 (99219) to 70 (99220) minutes at the patient's bedside or on the unit accordingly.

Coding Tips

These codes are used to report initial hospital outpatient observation services. All three key components (history, exam, and medical decision making) must be met or exceeded for the level of service selected. Time may be used to select the level of service when counseling and coordination of care are documented as at least half of the time spent face-to-face with the patient. All evaluation and management services provided by the clinician leading up to the initiation of the observation status are part of the patient's initial observation care when performed on the same date of service. The designation of "observation status" refers to the initiation of observation care and not to a specific area of the facility. CPT guidelines indicate these services are reported only by the admitting/supervising provider; all other providers should report 99224-99226 or 99241-99245. Medicare and some payers may allow providers of different specialties to report initial hospital services and require the admitting/supervising provider to append modifier AI. For observation discharge on a different date of service than the admission, see 99217. For patients admitted and discharged from observation or inpatient status on the same date, see 99234-99236. Medicare has provisionally identified these codes as telehealth/telemedicine services. Current Medicare coverage guidelines should be reviewed. Commercial payers should be contacted regarding their coverage guidelines. Telemedicine services may be reported by the performing provider by adding modifier 95 to these procedure codes. Services at the origination site are reported with HCPCS Level II code Q3014.

ICD-10-CM Diagnostic Codes

The application of this code is too broad to adequately present ICD-10-CM diagnostic code links here. Refer to your ICD-10-CM book.

AMA: 99218 2020,Sep,3; 2019,Jul,10; 2018,Jan,8; 2018,Dec,8; 2018,Dec,8; 2017,Jun,6; 2017,Jan,8; 2017,Aug,3; 2016,Jan,13; 2016,Jan,7; 2016,Dec,11; 2015,Mar,3; 2015,Jul,3; 2015,Jan,16; 2015,Dec,3; 2014,Oct,8; 2014,Nov,14; 2014,Jan,11 **99219** 2020,Sep,3; 2019,Jul,10; 2018,Jan,8; 2018,Dec,8; 2018,Dec,8; 2017,Jun,6; 2017,Jan,8; 2017,Aug,3; 2016,Jan,13; 2016,Jan,7; 2016,Dec,11; 2015,Jul,3; 2015,Jan,16; 2015,Dec,3; 2014,Oct,8; 2014,Nov,14; 2014,Jan,11 **99220** 2020,Sep,3; 2019,Jul,10; 2018,Jan,8; 2018,Dec,8; 2018,Dec,8; 2017,Jun,6; 2017,Jan,8; 2017,Aug,3; 2016,Jan,13; 2016,Jan,7; 2016,Dec,11; 2015,Jul,3; 2015,Jan,16; 2015,Dec,3; 2014,Oct,8; 2014,Nov,14; 2014,Jan,11

Relative Value Units/Medicare Edits

Non-Facility RVU	Work	PE	MP	Total
99218	1.92	0.74	0.16	2.82
99219	2.6	1.05	0.18	3.83
99220	3.56	1.4	0.26	5.22
Facility RVU	**Work**	**PE**	**MP**	**Total**
99218	1.92	0.74	0.16	2.82
99219	2.6	1.05	0.18	3.83
99220	3.56	1.4	0.26	5.22

	FUD	Status	MUE	Modifiers				IOM Reference
99218	N/A	A	1(2)	N/A	N/A	N/A	80*	100-04,12,100
99219	N/A	A	1(2)	N/A	N/A	N/A	80*	
99220	N/A	A	1(2)	N/A	N/A	N/A	80*	

* with documentation

© 2020 Optum360, LLC   **N** Newborn: 0   **P** Pediatric: 0-17   **M** Maternity: 9-64   **A** Adult: 15-124   ♂ Male Only   ♀ Female Only   CPT © 2020 American Medical Association. All Rights Reserved.

[99224, 99225, 99226]

99224   Subsequent observation care, per day, for the evaluation and management of a patient, which requires at least 2 of these 3 key components: Problem focused interval history; Problem focused examination; Medical decision making that is straightforward or of low complexity. Counseling and/or coordination of care with other physicians, other qualified health care professionals, or agencies are provided consistent with the nature of the problem(s) and the patient's and/or family's needs. Usually, the patient is stable, recovering, or improving. Typically, 15 minutes are spent at the bedside and on the patient's hospital floor or unit.

99225   Subsequent observation care, per day, for the evaluation and management of a patient, which requires at least 2 of these 3 key components: An expanded problem focused interval history; An expanded problem focused examination; Medical decision making of moderate complexity. Counseling and/or coordination of care with other physicians, other qualified health care professionals, or agencies are provided consistent with the nature of the problem(s) and the patient's and/or family's needs. Usually, the patient is responding inadequately to therapy or has developed a minor complication. Typically, 25 minutes are spent at the bedside and on the patient's hospital floor or unit.

99226   Subsequent observation care, per day, for the evaluation and management of a patient, which requires at least 2 of these 3 key components: A detailed interval history; A detailed examination; Medical decision making of high complexity. Counseling and/or coordination of care with other physicians, other qualified health care professionals, or agencies are provided consistent with the nature of the problem(s) and the patient's and/or family's needs. Usually, the patient is unstable or has developed a significant complication or a significant new problem. Typically, 35 minutes are spent at the bedside and on the patient's hospital floor or unit.

Explanation

Subsequent hospital observation service codes describe visits that occur after the first encounter of the patient's admission for observation care by the supervising qualified clinician. Observation status includes supervision of the care plan for observation as well as periodic reassessments. The patient is not required to be physically located in a designated observation area within a hospital; however, if such an area is utilized, these codes are reported. Codes are reported per day and, as with the initial observation care codes, do not differentiate between new or established patients. Under the subsequent observation care category, there are three levels represented by resequenced codes 99224, 99225, and 99226. All three of these levels require at least two out of the three key components to be documented. The lowest level of care, 99224, describes a problem-focused interval history as well as a problem-focused examination with straightforward or low complexity medical decision making and involves approximately 15 minutes of time by the provider at the patient's bedside or on the unit. For mid-level observation care code 99225, an expanded problem-focused history and examination are required with moderate medical decision making. Time associated with this level usually involves 25 minutes at the bedside or on the patient's floor. The third and highest level of follow-up observation care, 99226, requires a detailed history and exam as well as medical decision making of high complexity; the provider typically spends around 35 minutes with the patient or on the unit. All three levels of subsequent observation care involve the clinician reviewing the patient's medical record, results from diagnostic studies, as well as any changes to the patient's status such as the condition, response to treatments, or changes in health history since the last assessment.

Coding Tips

These codes are used to report subsequent hospital outpatient observation services. Two of the three key components (history, exam, and medical decision making) must be met or exceeded for the level of service selected. Time may be used to select the level of service when counseling and coordination of care are documented as at least half of the time spent face-to-face with the patient. Subsequent hospital outpatient observation care services include review of the medical record, including all diagnostic studies, as well as changes noted in the patient's condition and response to treatment since the last evaluation. The designation of "observation status" refers to the initiation of observation care and not to a specific area of the facility. For initial observation care, see 99218-99220; for observation discharge on a different date of service than the admission, see 99217. For patients admitted and discharged from observation or inpatient status on the same date, see 99234-99236. Medicare has provisionally identified these codes as telehealth/telemedicine services. Current Medicare coverage guidelines should be reviewed. Commercial payers should be contacted regarding their coverage guidelines. Telemedicine services may be reported by the performing provider by adding modifier 95 to these procedure codes. Services at the origination site are reported with HCPCS Level II code Q3014.

ICD-10-CM Diagnostic Codes

The application of this code is too broad to adequately present ICD-10-CM diagnostic code links here. Refer to your ICD-10-CM book.

AMA: **99224** 2020,Sep,3; 2019,Jul,10; 2018,Jan,8; 2017,Jun,6; 2017,Jan,8; 2017,Aug,3; 2016,Jan,13; 2016,Jan,7; 2016,Dec,11; 2015,Jan,16; 2015,Dec,3; 2014,Oct,8; 2014,Nov,14; 2014,Jan,11 **99225** 2020,Sep,3; 2019,Jul,10; 2018,Jan,8; 2017,Jun,6; 2017,Jan,8; 2017,Aug,3; 2016,Jan,13; 2016,Jan,7; 2016,Dec,11; 2015,Jan,16; 2015,Dec,3; 2014,Oct,8; 2014,Nov,14; 2014,Jan,11 **99226** 2020,Sep,3; 2019,Jul,10; 2018,Jan,8; 2017,Jun,6; 2017,Jan,8; 2017,Aug,3; 2016,Jan,13; 2016,Jan,7; 2016,Dec,11; 2015,Jan,16; 2015,Dec,3; 2014,Oct,8; 2014,Nov,14; 2014,Jan,11

Relative Value Units/Medicare Edits

Non-Facility RVU	Work	PE	MP	Total
99224	0.76	0.3	0.06	1.12
99225	1.39	0.57	0.09	2.05
99226	2.0	0.82	0.13	2.95
Facility RVU	**Work**	**PE**	**MP**	**Total**
99224	0.76	0.3	0.06	1.12
99225	1.39	0.57	0.09	2.05
99226	2.0	0.82	0.13	2.95

	FUD	Status	MUE	Modifiers				IOM Reference
99224	N/A	A	1(2)	N/A	N/A	N/A	80*	None
99225	N/A	A	1(2)	N/A	N/A	N/A	80*	
99226	N/A	A	1(2)	N/A	N/A	N/A	80*	

* with documentation

Terms To Know

observation patient. Patient who needs to be monitored and assessed for inpatient admission or referral to another site for care.

CPT © 2020 American Medical Association. All Rights Reserved.   ● New   ▲ Revised   + Add On   ★ Telemedicine   AMA: CPT Assist   [Resequenced]   ☑ Laterality   © 2020 Optum360, LLC

99221-99223

99221   Initial hospital care, per day, for the evaluation and management of a patient, which requires these 3 key components: A detailed or comprehensive history; A detailed or comprehensive examination; and Medical decision making that is straightforward or of low complexity. Counseling and/or coordination of care with other physicians, other qualified health care professionals, or agencies are provided consistent with the nature of the problem(s) and the patient's and/or family's needs. Usually, the problem(s) requiring admission are of low severity. Typically, 30 minutes are spent at the bedside and on the patient's hospital floor or unit.

99222   Initial hospital care, per day, for the evaluation and management of a patient, which requires these 3 key components: A comprehensive history; A comprehensive examination; and Medical decision making of moderate complexity. Counseling and/or coordination of care with other physicians, other qualified health care professionals, or agencies are provided consistent with the nature of the problem(s) and the patient's and/or family's needs. Usually, the problem(s) requiring admission are of moderate severity. Typically, 50 minutes are spent at the bedside and on the patient's hospital floor or unit.

99223   Initial hospital care, per day, for the evaluation and management of a patient, which requires these 3 key components: A comprehensive history; A comprehensive examination; and Medical decision making of high complexity. Counseling and/or coordination of care with other physicians, other qualified health care professionals, or agencies are provided consistent with the nature of the problem(s) and the patient's and/or family's needs. Usually, the problem(s) requiring admission are of high severity. Typically, 70 minutes are spent at the bedside and on the patient's hospital floor or unit.

Explanation

Initial hospital inpatient service codes describe the first encounter with the patient by the admitting physician or qualified clinician. For initial encounters by a physician other than the admitting physician, see the initial inpatient consultation codes or subsequent inpatient care codes. When the patient is admitted to the hospital under inpatient status during the course of another encounter from a different site of service, such as the physician's office, a nursing home, or the emergency department, all of the E/M services rendered by the supervising clinician as part of the inpatient admission status are considered part of the initial inpatient care services when they are performed on the same day. The level of initial inpatient care reported by the clinician should incorporate the other services related to the hospital admission that were provided in any other sites of services as well as those provided in the actual inpatient setting. Codes are reported per day and do not differentiate between new or established patients. Under the initial inpatient care category, there are three levels represented by 99221, 99222, and 99223. All of these levels require all three key components, history, exam, and medical decision-making (MDM), to be documented. The lowest level of care within this category, 99221, requires a detailed or comprehensive history and exam as well as straightforward or low complexity medical decision-making with approximately 30 minutes time being spent at the patient's bedside and on the patient's floor or unit. For the mid-level and highest level initial inpatient care codes, a comprehensive history and examination are required. MDM is the differentiating factor for these two levels; for moderate complexity, report 99222 and for initial inpatient care requiring MDM of high complexity, report 99223. The clinician typically spends 50 (99222) to 70 (99223) minutes at the patient's bedside or on the unit accordingly. Note that these codes include services provided to patients in a "partial hospital" setting.

Coding Tips

These codes are used to report initial hospital inpatient services. All three key components (history, exam, and medical decision making) must be met or exceeded for the level of service selected. Time may be used to select the level of service when counseling and coordination of care are documented as at least half of the floor/unit time spent with the patient. Evaluation and management services provided by the clinician leading up to the initiation of observation status or inpatient admission are considered to be part of the patient's initial hospital care when performed on the same date of service. Codes may be selected based upon the 1995 or the 1997 Evaluation and Management Guidelines. CPT guidelines indicate these services are reported only by the admitting/supervising provider; all other providers should report 99231-99233 or 99251-99255. Medicare and some payers may allow providers of different specialties to report initial hospital services and require the admitting/supervising provider to append modifier AI. For subsequent inpatient care, see 99231-99233. For discharge from an inpatient stay on a different date of service than the admission, see 99238-99239. For patients admitted and discharged from observation or inpatient status on the same date, see 99234-99236. Medicare has provisionally identified these codes as telehealth/telemedicine services. Current Medicare coverage guidelines should be reviewed. Commercial payers should be contacted regarding their coverage guidelines. Telemedicine services may be reported by the performing provider by adding modifier 95 to these procedure codes. Services at the origination site are reported with HCPCS Level II code Q3014.

ICD-10-CM Diagnostic Codes

The application of this code is too broad to adequately present ICD-10-CM diagnostic code links here. Refer to your ICD-10-CM book.

AMA: **99221** 2020,Sep,3; 2018,Jan,8; 2018,Dec,8; 2018,Dec,8; 2017,Jun,6; 2017,Jan,8; 2017,Aug,3; 2016,Mar,10; 2016,Jan,13; 2016,Jan,7; 2016,Dec,11; 2015,Jul,3; 2015,Jan,16; 2015,Dec,3; 2015,Dec,18; 2014,Oct,8; 2014,Nov,14; 2014,Jan,11 **99222** 2020,Sep,3; 2018,Jan,8; 2018,Dec,8; 2018,Dec,8; 2017,Jun,6; 2017,Jan,8; 2017,Aug,3; 2016,Mar,10; 2016,Jan,13; 2016,Jan,7; 2016,Dec,11; 2015,Mar,3; 2015,Jul,3; 2015,Jan,16; 2015,Dec,3; 2015,Dec,18; 2014,Oct,8; 2014,Nov,14; 2014,Jan,11 **99223** 2020,Sep,3; 2018,Jan,8; 2018,Dec,8; 2018,Dec,8; 2017,Jun,6; 2017,Jan,8; 2017,Aug,3; 2016,Mar,10; 2016,Jan,13; 2016,Jan,7; 2016,Dec,11; 2015,Jul,3; 2015,Jan,16; 2015,Dec,3; 2015,Dec,18; 2014,Oct,8; 2014,Nov,14; 2014,Jan,11

Relative Value Units/Medicare Edits

Non-Facility RVU	Work	PE	MP	Total
99221	1.92	0.77	0.19	2.88
99222	2.61	1.06	0.22	3.89
99223	3.86	1.57	0.28	5.71
Facility RVU	Work	PE	MP	Total
99221	1.92	0.77	0.19	2.88
99222	2.61	1.06	0.22	3.89
99223	3.86	1.57	0.28	5.71

	FUD	Status	MUE	Modifiers				IOM Reference
99221	N/A	A	1(3)	N/A	N/A	N/A	80*	100-04,12,30.6.4;
99222	N/A	A	1(3)	N/A	N/A	N/A	80*	100-04,12,30.6.9;
99223	N/A	A	1(3)	N/A	N/A	N/A	80*	100-04,12,30.6.9.1;
								100-04,12,30.6.15.1;
								100-04,12,100

* with documentation

99231-99233

★99231 Subsequent hospital care, per day, for the evaluation and management of a patient, which requires at least 2 of these 3 key components: A problem focused interval history; A problem focused examination; Medical decision making that is straightforward or of low complexity. Counseling and/or coordination of care with other physicians, other qualified health care professionals, or agencies are provided consistent with the nature of the problem(s) and the patient's and/or family's needs. Usually, the patient is stable, recovering or improving. Typically, 15 minutes are spent at the bedside and on the patient's hospital floor or unit.

★99232 Subsequent hospital care, per day, for the evaluation and management of a patient, which requires at least 2 of these 3 key components: An expanded problem focused interval history; An expanded problem focused examination; Medical decision making of moderate complexity. Counseling and/or coordination of care with other physicians, other qualified health care professionals, or agencies are provided consistent with the nature of the problem(s) and the patient's and/or family's needs. Usually, the patient is responding inadequately to therapy or has developed a minor complication. Typically, 25 minutes are spent at the bedside and on the patient's hospital floor or unit.

★99233 Subsequent hospital care, per day, for the evaluation and management of a patient, which requires at least 2 of these 3 key components: A detailed interval history; A detailed examination; Medical decision making of high complexity. Counseling and/or coordination of care with other physicians, other qualified health care professionals, or agencies are provided consistent with the nature of the problem(s) and the patient's and/or family's needs. Usually, the patient is unstable or has developed a significant complication or a significant new problem. Typically, 35 minutes are spent at the bedside and on the patient's hospital floor or unit.

Explanation

Subsequent hospital inpatient service codes describe visits that occur after the first encounter of the patient's inpatient hospital admission by the supervising physician or qualified clinician. Codes are reported per day and do not differentiate between new or established patients. Under the subsequent inpatient care category, there are three levels represented by 99231, 99232, and 99233. All of these levels require at least two out of the three key components—history, exam, and medical decision making—to be documented. The lowest level of care within this category, 99231, describes a problem-focused interval history as well as a problem-focused examination with straightforward or low complexity medical decision making and involves approximately 15 minutes of time by the provider at the patient's bedside or on the unit. For the mid-level subsequent inpatient care code, 99232, an expanded problem-focused history and examination are required with moderate medical decision making. Time associated with this level usually involves 25 minutes at the bedside or on the patient's floor. The third and highest level of subsequent inpatient care, 99233, requires a detailed history and exam as well as medical decision making of high complexity. For this level of care, the provider typically spends around 35 minutes with the patient or on the unit. All three levels of subsequent inpatient care involve the clinician reviewing the patient's medical record, results from diagnostic studies, as well as any changes to the patient's status such as physical condition, response to treatments, or changes in health history since the last assessment.

Coding Tips

These codes are used to report subsequent hospital inpatient services. Two of the three key components (history, exam, and medical decision making) must be met or exceeded for the level of service selected. Time may be used to select the level of service when counseling and coordination of care are documented as at least half of the floor/unit time spent with the patient. Codes may be selected based upon the 1995 or the 1997 Evaluation and Management Guidelines. Subsequent inpatient care services include review of the medical record, including all diagnostic studies, as well as changes noted in the patient's condition and response to treatment since the last evaluation. For initial inpatient care, see 99221-99223. For discharge from an inpatient stay on a different date of service than the admission, see 99238-99239. For patients admitted and discharged from observation or inpatient status on the same date, see 99234-99236. Telemedicine services may be reported by the performing provider by adding modifier 95 to these procedure codes. Services at the origination site are reported with HCPCS Level II code Q3014.

ICD-10-CM Diagnostic Codes

The application of this code is too broad to adequately present ICD-10-CM diagnostic code links here. Refer to your ICD-10-CM book.

AMA: **99231** 2020,Sep,3; 2018,Jan,8; 2018,Dec,8; 2018,Dec,8; 2017,Jun,6; 2017,Jan,8; 2017,Aug,3; 2016,Jan,7; 2016,Jan,13; 2016,Dec,11; 2015,Jul,3; 2015,Jan,16; 2015,Dec,3; 2014,Oct,8; 2014,Nov,14; 2014,May,4; 2014,Jan,11 **99232** 2020,Sep,3; 2018,Jan,8; 2018,Dec,8; 2018,Dec,8; 2017,Jun,6; 2017,Jan,8; 2017,Aug,3; 2016,Oct,8; 2016,Jan,7; 2016,Jan,13; 2016,Dec,11; 2015,Jul,3; 2015,Jan,16; 2015,Dec,3; 2014,Oct,8; 2014,Nov,14; 2014,Jan,11 **99233** 2020,Sep,3; 2018,Jan,8; 2018,Dec,8; 2018,Dec,8; 2017,Jun,6; 2017,Jan,8; 2017,Aug,3; 2016,Oct,8; 2016,Jan,7; 2016,Jan,13; 2016,Dec,11; 2015,Jul,3; 2015,Jan,16; 2015,Dec,3; 2014,Nov,14; 2014,May,4; 2014,Jan,11

Relative Value Units/Medicare Edits

Non-Facility RVU	Work	PE	MP	Total
99231	0.76	0.29	0.06	1.11
99232	1.39	0.56	0.09	2.04
99233	2.0	0.81	0.13	2.94
Facility RVU	Work	PE	MP	Total
99231	0.76	0.29	0.06	1.11
99232	1.39	0.56	0.09	2.04
99233	2.0	0.81	0.13	2.94

	FUD	Status	MUE	Modifiers				IOM Reference
99231	N/A	A	1(3)	N/A	N/A	N/A	80*	100-04,12,30.6.9.2;
99232	N/A	A	1(3)	N/A	N/A	N/A	80*	100-04,12,100
99233	N/A	A	1(3)	N/A	N/A	N/A	80*	

* with documentation

Terms To Know

inpatient. Time period in which a patient is housed in a hospital or facility offering medical, surgical, and/or psychiatric services, usually without interruption.

interval history. History documenting what has occurred in a given area since the last visit, usually associated with subsequent hospital, nursing home, rest home, and home visit services.

subsequent care. All evaluation and instructions for care rendered subsequent to the inpatient admission by the admitting provider and all other providers.

CPT © 2020 American Medical Association. All Rights Reserved. ● New ▲ Revised + Add On ★ Telemedicine AMA: CPT Assist [Resequenced] ☑ Laterality © 2020 Optum360, LLC

99234-99236

99234 Observation or inpatient hospital care, for the evaluation and management of a patient including admission and discharge on the same date, which requires these 3 key components: A detailed or comprehensive history; A detailed or comprehensive examination; and Medical decision making that is straightforward or of low complexity. Counseling and/or coordination of care with other physicians, other qualified health care professionals, or agencies are provided consistent with the nature of the problem(s) and the patient's and/or family's needs. Usually the presenting problem(s) requiring admission are of low severity. Typically, 40 minutes are spent at the bedside and on the patient's hospital floor or unit.

99235 Observation or inpatient hospital care, for the evaluation and management of a patient including admission and discharge on the same date, which requires these 3 key components: A comprehensive history; A comprehensive examination; and Medical decision making of moderate complexity. Counseling and/or coordination of care with other physicians, other qualified health care professionals, or agencies are provided consistent with the nature of the problem(s) and the patient's and/or family's needs. Usually the presenting problem(s) requiring admission are of moderate severity. Typically, 50 minutes are spent at the bedside and on the patient's hospital floor or unit.

99236 Observation or inpatient hospital care, for the evaluation and management of a patient including admission and discharge on the same date, which requires these 3 key components: A comprehensive history; A comprehensive examination; and Medical decision making of high complexity. Counseling and/or coordination of care with other physicians, other qualified health care professionals, or agencies are provided consistent with the nature of the problem(s) and the patient's and/or family's needs. Usually the presenting problem(s) requiring admission are of high severity. Typically, 55 minutes are spent at the bedside and on the patient's hospital floor or unit.

Explanation

Hospital observation or inpatient care service in cases where the patient is admitted and discharged on the same date of service by the supervising or qualified clinician is reported with 99234-99236. Observation status includes the supervision of the care plan for observation, as well as the periodic reassessments. The patient is not required to be physically located in a designated observation area within a hospital; however, if such an area is utilized, these codes should be reported. When a patient is admitted to the hospital from observation status on the same date of service, the clinician should only report the appropriate level of initial hospital care code. The level of care reported should reflect all of the other services from the observation status services the clinician rendered to the patient on the same date of service, as well as those provided in the actual inpatient setting. Codes do not differentiate between new or established patients. Under this care category, there are three levels represented by 99234, 99235, and 99236. All of these levels require all three key components (history, exam, and medical decision-making [MDM]) to be documented. The lowest level of care within this category, 99234, requires a detailed or comprehensive history and exam, as well as straightforward medical decision-making or that of low complexity with approximately 40 minutes time being spent at the patient's bedside and on the patient's floor or unit. For the mid-level and highest level observation or inpatient care codes, a comprehensive history and examination are required. Medical decision-making is the differentiating factor for these two levels; for moderate complexity, report 99235 and for observation or inpatient care requiring MDM of high complexity, report 99236. The clinician typically spends 50 (99235) to 55 (99236) minutes at the patient's bedside or on the unit

accordingly. Note that these codes should be reported only when the patient has been admitted and discharged on the same date of service.

Coding Tips

These codes are used to report observation or initial hospital services for the patient admitted and discharged on the same date of service. All three key components (history, exam, and medical decision making) must be met or exceeded for the level of service selected. Evaluation and management services provided by the clinician leading up to the initiation of observation status or inpatient admission are considered to be part of the patient's initial hospital care when performed on the same date of service. The designation of "observation status" refers to the initiation of observation care and not to a specific area of the facility. For patients admitted to observation status, initial care, see 99218-99220; subsequent observation care, see 99224-99226; for observation discharge on a different date of service than the admission, see 99217. For initial inpatient care, see 99221-99223; subsequent inpatient care, see 99231-99233. For discharge from an inpatient stay on a different date of service than the admission, see 99238-99239. Medicare has provisionally identified these codes as telehealth/telemedicine services. Current Medicare coverage guidelines should be reviewed. Commercial payers should be contacted regarding their coverage guidelines. Telemedicine services may be reported by the performing provider by adding modifier 95 to these procedure codes. Services at the origination site are reported with HCPCS Level II code Q3014.

ICD-10-CM Diagnostic Codes

The application of this code is too broad to adequately present ICD-10-CM diagnostic code links here. Refer to your ICD-10-CM book.

AMA: **99234** 2020,Sep,3; 2018,Jan,8; 2018,Dec,8; 2018,Dec,8; 2018,Apr,10; 2017,Jun,6; 2017,Jan,8; 2017,Aug,3; 2016,Jan,13; 2016,Dec,11; 2015,Jul,3; 2015,Jan,16; 2014,Oct,8; 2014,Jan,11 **99235** 2020,Sep,3; 2018,Jan,8; 2018,Dec,8; 2018,Dec,8; 2018,Apr,10; 2017,Jun,6; 2017,Jan,8; 2017,Aug,3; 2016,Jan,13; 2016,Dec,11; 2015,Jul,3; 2015,Jan,16; 2014,Oct,8; 2014,Jan,11 **99236** 2020,Sep,3; 2018,Jan,8; 2018,Dec,8; 2018,Dec,8; 2018,Apr,10; 2017,Jun,6; 2017,Jan,8; 2017,Aug,3; 2016,Jan,13; 2016,Dec,11; 2015,Jul,3; 2015,Jan,16; 2014,Oct,8; 2014,Jan,11

Relative Value Units/Medicare Edits

Non-Facility RVU	Work	PE	MP	Total
99234	2.56	1.0	0.21	3.77
99235	3.24	1.3	0.23	4.77
99236	4.2	1.64	0.3	6.14
Facility RVU	Work	PE	MP	Total
99234	2.56	1.0	0.21	3.77
99235	3.24	1.3	0.23	4.77
99236	4.2	1.64	0.3	6.14

	FUD	Status	MUE	Modifiers				IOM Reference
99234	N/A	A	1(3)	N/A	N/A	N/A	80*	100-04,12,30.6.4;
99235	N/A	A	1(3)	N/A	N/A	N/A	80*	100-04,12,30.6.9;
99236	N/A	A	1(3)	N/A	N/A	N/A	80*	100-04,12,30.6.9.1; 100-04,12,30.6.9.2; 100-04,12,100

* with documentation

99238-99239

99238   Hospital discharge day management; 30 minutes or less
99239   more than 30 minutes

Explanation

Hospital discharge services are time-based codes that, when reported, describe the amount of time spent by the qualified clinician during all final steps involved in the discharge of a patient from the hospital on a date that differs from the date of admission, including the last patient exam, discussing the hospital stay, instructions for ongoing care as it relates to all pertinent caregivers, as well as preparing the medical discharge records, prescriptions, and/or referrals as applicable. Time reported should be for the total duration of time spent by the provider even when the time spent on that date is not continuous. For a hospital discharge duration of 30 minutes or less, report 99238; for a duration of greater than 30 minutes, report 99239. There are no key components associated with these services.

Coding Tips

These codes are used to report all discharge day services for the hospital inpatient, including patient examination, discharge and follow-up care instructions, and preparation of all medical records. These are time-based codes and time spent with the patient must be documented in the medical record. For observation discharge on a different date of service than the admission, see 99217. For patients admitted and discharged from observation or inpatient status on the same date, see 99234-99236. Medicare has provisionally identified these codes as telehealth/telemedicine services. Current Medicare coverage guidelines should be reviewed. Commercial payers should be contacted regarding their coverage guidelines. Telemedicine services may be reported by the performing provider by adding modifier 95 to these procedure codes. Services at the origination site are reported with HCPCS Level II code Q3014.

ICD-10-CM Diagnostic Codes

The application of this code is too broad to adequately present ICD-10-CM diagnostic code links here. Refer to your ICD-10-CM book.

AMA: 99238 2018,Jan,8; 2018,Dec,8; 2018,Dec,8; 2017,Jun,6; 2017,Jan,8; 2017,Aug,3; 2016,Jan,13; 2016,Dec,11; 2015,Jan,16; 2014,Oct,8; 2014,Jan,11
99239 2018,Jan,8; 2018,Dec,8; 2018,Dec,8; 2017,Jun,6; 2017,Jan,8; 2017,Aug,3; 2016,Jan,13; 2016,Dec,11; 2015,Jan,16; 2014,Oct,8; 2014,Jan,11

Relative Value Units/Medicare Edits

Non-Facility RVU	Work	PE	MP	Total
99238	1.28	0.69	0.09	2.06
99239	1.9	1.0	0.12	3.02
Facility RVU	**Work**	**PE**	**MP**	**Total**
99238	1.28	0.69	0.09	2.06
99239	1.9	1.0	0.12	3.02

	FUD	Status	MUE	Modifiers				IOM Reference
99238	N/A	A	1(3)	N/A	N/A	N/A	80*	100-04,12,30.6.4;
99239	N/A	A	1(3)	N/A	N/A	N/A	80*	100-04,12,30.6.9;
								100-04,12,30.6.9.1;
								100-04,12,30.6.9.2;
								100-04,12,100

* with documentation

99241-99245

★99241 Office consultation for a new or established patient, which requires these 3 key components: A problem focused history; A problem focused examination; and Straightforward medical decision making. Counseling and/or coordination of care with other physicians, other qualified health care professionals, or agencies are provided consistent with the nature of the problem(s) and the patient's and/or family's needs. Usually, the presenting problem(s) are self limited or minor. Typically, 15 minutes are spent face-to-face with the patient and/or family.

★99242 Office consultation for a new or established patient, which requires these 3 key components: An expanded problem focused history; An expanded problem focused examination; and Straightforward medical decision making. Counseling and/or coordination of care with other physicians, other qualified health care professionals, or agencies are provided consistent with the nature of the problem(s) and the patient's and/or family's needs. Usually, the presenting problem(s) are of low severity. Typically, 30 minutes are spent face-to-face with the patient and/or family.

★99243 Office consultation for a new or established patient, which requires these 3 key components: A detailed history; A detailed examination; and Medical decision making of low complexity. Counseling and/or coordination of care with other physicians, other qualified health care professionals, or agencies are provided consistent with the nature of the problem(s) and the patient's and/or family's needs. Usually, the presenting problem(s) are of moderate severity. Typically, 40 minutes are spent face-to-face with the patient and/or family.

★99244 Office consultation for a new or established patient, which requires these 3 key components: A comprehensive history; A comprehensive examination; and Medical decision making of moderate complexity. Counseling and/or coordination of care with other physicians, other qualified health care professionals, or agencies are provided consistent with the nature of the problem(s) and the patient's and/or family's needs. Usually, the presenting problem(s) are of moderate to high severity. Typically, 60 minutes are spent face-to-face with the patient and/or family.

★99245 Office consultation for a new or established patient, which requires these 3 key components: A comprehensive history; A comprehensive examination; and Medical decision making of high complexity. Counseling and/or coordination of care with other physicians, other qualified health care professionals, or agencies are provided consistent with the nature of the problem(s) and the patient's and/or family's needs. Usually, the presenting problem(s) are of moderate to high severity. Typically, 80 minutes are spent face-to-face with the patient and/or family.

Explanation

Office and other outpatient consultation service codes describe encounters where another qualified clinician's advice or opinion regarding diagnosis and treatment or determination to accept transfer of care of a patient is rendered at the request of the primary treating provider. Consultations may also be requested by another appropriate source; for example, a third-party payer may request a second opinion. The request for a consultation must be documented in the medical record, as well as a written report of the consultation findings. During the course of a consultation, the physician consultant can initiate diagnostic or therapeutic services at the same encounter or at a follow-up visit. Other separately reportable procedures or services performed in conjunction with the consultation may be reported separately. Codes do not differentiate between new or established patients. Services are reported based on meeting all three key components (history, exam, and medical decision-making [MDM]) within each level of service. The most basic service, 99241, describes a problem-focused history and exam with straightforward medical decision-making encompassing approximately 15 minutes of face-to-face time with the patient and/or family discussing a minor or self-limiting complaint. The mid-level services describe problems involving an expanded problem focused history and exam or a detailed history and exam as represented by 99242 and 99243, respectively. Medical decision-making for 99242 is the same as for a level one visit (straightforward) and is designated as low complexity for the level three service (99243). At these levels of service, the encounter can involve face-to-face time of 30 (99242) to 40 (99243) minutes involving minimal to low severity concerns. The last two levels of service in this category represent moderate to high-severity problems and both services involve comprehensive history and examination components. The differentiating factor between the two levels is the medical decision-making; code 99244 involves moderate complexity MDM and approximately 60 minutes of face-to-face time with the patient and/or family, while the highest level of service in this category, 99245, involves MDM of high complexity and approximately 80 minutes of face-to-face time.

Coding Tips

These codes are used to report consultations in the office or outpatient setting. All three key components (history, exam, and medical decision making) must be met or exceeded for the level of service selected. Time may be used to select the level of service when counseling and coordination of care are documented as at least half of the time spent face-to-face with the patient. Codes may be selected based upon the 1995 or the 1997 Evaluation and Management Guidelines. Consultation codes are not covered by Medicare and some payers. Report new or established outpatient E/M codes for consultation services. Consultation services should not be reported when the care and management of a problem or condition is assumed prior to the initial examination of the patient. In these situations, the appropriate initial or subsequent evaluation and management service should be reported. For office or other outpatient services for a new patient, see 99202-99205; for an established patient, see 99211-99215. For inpatient consultation services, see 99251-99255. Telemedicine services may be reported by the performing provider by adding modifier 95 to these procedure codes. Services at the origination site are reported with HCPCS Level II code Q3014.

ICD-10-CM Diagnostic Codes

The application of this code is too broad to adequately present ICD-10-CM diagnostic code links here. Refer to your ICD-10-CM book.

AMA: 99241 2020,Sep,3; 2018,Mar,7; 2018,Jan,8; 2018,Apr,9; 2018,Apr,10; 2017,Jun,6; 2017,Jan,8; 2017,Aug,3; 2016,Sep,6; 2016,Jan,13; 2016,Jan,7; 2016,Dec,11; 2015,Jan,12; 2015,Jan,16; 2014,Sep,13; 2014,Oct,8; 2014,Nov,14; 2014,Jan,11; 2014,Aug,3 **99242** 2020,Sep,3; 2018,Mar,7; 2018,Jan,8; 2018,Apr,9; 2018,Apr,10; 2017,Jun,6; 2017,Jun,8; 2017,Jan,8; 2017,Aug,3; 2016,Sep,6; 2016,Jan,13; 2016,Jan,7; 2016,Dec,11; 2015,Jan,12; 2015,Jan,16; 2014,Sep,13; 2014,Oct,8; 2014,Nov,14; 2014,Jan,11; 2014,Aug,3 **99243** 2020,Sep,3; 2018,Mar,7; 2018,Jan,8; 2018,Apr,9; 2018,Apr,10; 2017,Jun,6; 2017,Jan,8; 2017,Aug,3; 2016,Sep,6; 2016,Jan,13; 2016,Jan,7; 2016,Dec,11; 2015,Jan,12; 2015,Jan,16; 2014,Sep,13; 2014,Oct,8; 2014,Nov,14; 2014,Jan,11; 2014,Aug,3 **99244** 2020,Sep,3; 2018,Mar,7; 2018,Jan,8; 2018,Apr,9; 2018,Apr,10; 2017,Jun,6; 2017,Jan,8; 2017,Aug,3; 2016,Sep,6; 2016,Jan,13; 2016,Jan,7; 2016,Dec,11; 2015,Jan,12; 2015,Jan,16; 2014,Sep,13; 2014,Oct,8; 2014,Nov,14; 2014,Jan,11; 2014,Aug,3 **99245** 2020,Sep,3; 2018,Mar,7; 2018,Jan,8; 2018,Apr,9; 2018,Apr,10; 2017,Jun,6; 2017,Jan,8; 2017,Aug,3; 2016,Sep,6; 2016,Jan,13; 2016,Jan,7; 2016,Dec,11; 2015,Jan,16; 2015,Jan,12; 2014,Sep,13; 2014,Oct,8; 2014,Nov,14; 2014,Jan,11; 2014,Aug,3

Relative Value Units/Medicare Edits

Non-Facility RVU	Work	PE	MP	Total
99241	0.64	0.66	0.05	1.35
99242	1.34	1.1	0.11	2.55
99243	1.88	1.46	0.15	3.49
99244	3.02	1.96	0.25	5.23
99245	3.77	2.3	0.3	6.37
Facility RVU	Work	PE	MP	Total
99241	0.64	0.24	0.05	0.93
99242	1.34	0.51	0.11	1.96
99243	1.88	0.71	0.15	2.74
99244	3.02	1.14	0.25	4.41
99245	3.77	1.38	0.3	5.45

	FUD	Status	MUE	Modifiers				IOM Reference
99241	N/A	I	0(3)	N/A	N/A	N/A	N/A	100-04,4,160;
99242	N/A	I	0(3)	N/A	N/A	N/A	N/A	100-04,12,30.6.4;
99243	N/A	I	0(3)	N/A	N/A	N/A	N/A	100-04,12,30.6.10;
99244	N/A	I	0(3)	N/A	N/A	N/A	N/A	100-04,12,30.6.15.1;
99245	N/A	I	0(3)	N/A	N/A	N/A	N/A	100-04,12,100

* with documentation

Terms To Know

consultation. Advice or opinion regarding diagnosis and treatment or determination to accept transfer of care of a patient rendered by a medical professional at the request of the primary care provider.

Medicare. Federally funded program authorized as part of the Social Security Act that provides for health care services for people age 65 or older, people with disabilities, and people with end-stage renal disease (ESRD).

outpatient. Person who has not been admitted as an inpatient but who is registered on the hospital or CAH records as an outpatient and receives services (rather than supplies alone) directly from the hospital or CAH. (Code of Federal Regulations, section 410.2.)

99251-99255

★**99251** Inpatient consultation for a new or established patient, which requires these 3 key components: A problem focused history; A problem focused examination; and Straightforward medical decision making. Counseling and/or coordination of care with other physicians, other qualified health care professionals, or agencies are provided consistent with the nature of the problem(s) and the patient's and/or family's needs. Usually, the presenting problem(s) are self limited or minor. Typically, 20 minutes are spent at the bedside and on the patient's hospital floor or unit.

★**99252** Inpatient consultation for a new or established patient, which requires these 3 key components: An expanded problem focused history; An expanded problem focused examination; and Straightforward medical decision making. Counseling and/or coordination of care with other physicians, other qualified health care professionals, or agencies are provided consistent with the nature of the problem(s) and the patient's and/or family's needs. Usually, the presenting problem(s) are of low severity. Typically, 40 minutes are spent at the bedside and on the patient's hospital floor or unit.

★**99253** Inpatient consultation for a new or established patient, which requires these 3 key components: A detailed history; A detailed examination; and Medical decision making of low complexity. Counseling and/or coordination of care with other physicians, other qualified health care professionals, or agencies are provided consistent with the nature of the problem(s) and the patient's and/or family's needs. Usually, the presenting problem(s) are of moderate severity. Typically, 55 minutes are spent at the bedside and on the patient's hospital floor or unit.

★**99254** Inpatient consultation for a new or established patient, which requires these 3 key components: A comprehensive history; A comprehensive examination; and Medical decision making of moderate complexity. Counseling and/or coordination of care with other physicians, other qualified health care professionals, or agencies are provided consistent with the nature of the problem(s) and the patient's and/or family's needs. Usually, the presenting problem(s) are of moderate to high severity. Typically, 80 minutes are spent at the bedside and on the patient's hospital floor or unit.

★**99255** Inpatient consultation for a new or established patient, which requires these 3 key components: A comprehensive history; A comprehensive examination; and Medical decision making of high complexity. Counseling and/or coordination of care with other physicians, other qualified health care professionals, or agencies are provided consistent with the nature of the problem(s) and the patient's and/or family's needs. Usually, the presenting problem(s) are of moderate to high severity. Typically, 110 minutes are spent at the bedside and on the patient's hospital floor or unit.

Explanation

Inpatient consultation service codes describe encounters with patients admitted to the hospital, residing in nursing facilities, or to patients in a partial hospital setting where another qualified clinician's advice or opinion regarding diagnosis and treatment or determination to accept transfer of care of a patient is rendered at the request of the primary treating provider. The request for a consultation must be documented in the patient's medical record, as well as a written report of the findings of the consultation to the primary treating physician. During the course of a consultation, the physician consultant can initiate diagnostic or therapeutic services at the same encounter or at a follow-up visit. Other procedures or services performed in conjunction with the consultation may be reported separately. Codes do not differentiate between new or established patients and only one inpatient consultation services code should be reported per admission. Services are reported based on meeting all three key components (history, exam, and medical decision-making [MDM]) within each level of service. The most basic service, as represented by 99251, describes a problem focused history and exam with straightforward medical decision-making for a minor or self-limiting complaint encompassing approximately 20 minutes of time at the patient's bedside or on the unit. The mid-level services describe problems involving an expanded problem focused history and exam or a detailed history and exam as represented by 99252 and 99253, respectively. Medical decision-making for 99252 is the same (straightforward) as for a level one visit (99251) and is designated as low complexity for the level three service (99253). At these levels of service, the encounter can involve time at the patient's bedside or on the unit of 40 (99252) to 55 (99253) minutes involving minimal to low severity concerns. The last two levels of service in this category represent moderate to high-severity problems and both services involve comprehensive history and examination components. The differentiating factor between the two levels is the medical decision-making. Code 99254 involves moderate complexity MDM and approximately 80 minutes of time at the patient's bedside or on the unit, while the highest level of service in this category, 99255, involves MDM of high complexity and approximately 110 minutes at the patient's bedside or on the unit.

Coding Tips

These codes are used to report consultations in the inpatient setting. All three key components (history, exam, and medical decision making) must be met or exceeded for the level of service selected. Time may be used to select the level of service when counseling and coordination of care are documented as at least half of the time spent face-to-face with the patient. Consultation codes are not covered by Medicare and some payers. Report new or established inpatient E/M codes for consultation services. Consultation services should not be reported when the care and management of a problem or condition is assumed prior to the initial examination of the patient. In these situations, the appropriate initial or subsequent evaluation and management service should be reported. Do not report an inpatient and outpatient consultation when both are related to the same inpatient admission. For initial hospital care services, see 99221-99223; for subsequent hospital care services, see 99231-99233. For office or other outpatient consultation services, see 99241-99245. Telemedicine services may be reported by the performing provider by adding modifier 95 to these procedure codes. Services at the origination site are reported with HCPCS Level II code Q3014.

ICD-10-CM Diagnostic Codes

The application of this code is too broad to adequately present ICD-10-CM diagnostic code links here. Refer to your ICD-10-CM book.

AMA: **99251** 2020,Sep,3; 2018,Jan,8; 2017,Jun,6; 2017,Jan,8; 2017,Aug,3; 2016,Jan,7; 2016,Jan,13; 2016,Dec,11; 2015,Jan,16; 2014,Oct,8; 2014,Nov,14; 2014,Jan,11 **99252** 2020,Sep,3; 2018,Jan,8; 2017,Jun,6; 2017,Jan,8; 2017,Aug,3; 2016,Jan,7; 2016,Jan,13; 2016,Dec,11; 2015,Jan,16; 2014,Oct,8; 2014,Nov,14; 2014,Jan,11 **99253** 2020,Sep,3; 2018,Jan,8; 2017,Jun,6; 2017,Jan,8; 2017,Aug,3; 2016,Jan,13; 2016,Jan,7; 2016,Dec,11; 2015,Jan,16; 2014,Oct,8; 2014,Nov,14; 2014,Jan,11 **99254** 2020,Sep,3; 2018,Jan,8; 2017,Jun,6; 2017,Jan,8; 2017,Aug,3; 2016,Jan,13; 2016,Jan,7; 2016,Dec,11; 2015,Jan,16; 2014,Oct,8; 2014,Nov,14; 2014,Jan,11 **99255** 2020,Sep,3; 2018,Jan,8; 2017,Jun,6; 2017,Jan,8; 2017,Aug,3; 2016,Jan,13; 2016,Jan,7; 2016,Dec,11; 2015,Jan,16; 2014,Oct,8; 2014,Nov,14; 2014,Jan,11

Relative Value Units/Medicare Edits

Non-Facility RVU	Work	PE	MP	Total
99251	1.0	0.32	0.09	1.41
99252	1.5	0.52	0.11	2.13
99253	2.27	0.84	0.18	3.29
99254	3.29	1.23	0.27	4.79
99255	4.0	1.44	0.32	5.76
Facility RVU	Work	PE	MP	Total
99251	1.0	0.32	0.09	1.41
99252	1.5	0.52	0.11	2.13
99253	2.27	0.84	0.18	3.29
99254	3.29	1.23	0.27	4.79
99255	4.0	1.44	0.32	5.76

	FUD	Status	MUE	Modifiers				IOM Reference
99251	N/A	I	0(3)	N/A	N/A	N/A	N/A	100-04,12,30.6.4;
99252	N/A	I	0(3)	N/A	N/A	N/A	N/A	100-04,12,30.6.10;
99253	N/A	I	0(3)	N/A	N/A	N/A	N/A	100-04,12,100
99254	N/A	I	0(3)	N/A	N/A	N/A	N/A	
99255	N/A	I	0(3)	N/A	N/A	N/A	N/A	

* with documentation

Terms To Know

consultation. Advice or opinion regarding diagnosis and treatment or determination to accept transfer of care of a patient rendered by a medical professional at the request of the primary care provider.

inpatient. Time period in which a patient is housed in a hospital or facility offering medical, surgical, and/or psychiatric services, usually without interruption.

medical decision making. Consideration of the differential diagnoses, the amount and/or complexity of data reviewed and considered (medical records, test results, correspondence from previous treating physicians, etc.), current diagnostic studies ordered, and treatment or management options and risk (complications of the patient's condition, the potential for complications, continued morbidity, risk of mortality, any comorbidities associated with the patient's disease process).

99281-99285

99281 Emergency department visit for the evaluation and management of a patient, which requires these 3 key components: A problem focused history; A problem focused examination; and Straightforward medical decision making. Counseling and/or coordination of care with other physicians, other qualified health care professionals, or agencies are provided consistent with the nature of the problem(s) and the patient's and/or family's needs. Usually, the presenting problem(s) are self limited or minor.

99282 Emergency department visit for the evaluation and management of a patient, which requires these 3 key components: An expanded problem focused history; An expanded problem focused examination; and Medical decision making of low complexity. Counseling and/or coordination of care with other physicians, other qualified health care professionals, or agencies are provided consistent with the nature of the problem(s) and the patient's and/or family's needs. Usually, the presenting problem(s) are of low to moderate severity.

99283 Emergency department visit for the evaluation and management of a patient, which requires these 3 key components: An expanded problem focused history; An expanded problem focused examination; and Medical decision making of moderate complexity. Counseling and/or coordination of care with other physicians, other qualified health care professionals, or agencies are provided consistent with the nature of the problem(s) and the patient's and/or family's needs. Usually, the presenting problem(s) are of moderate severity.

99284 Emergency department visit for the evaluation and management of a patient, which requires these 3 key components: A detailed history; A detailed examination; and Medical decision making of moderate complexity. Counseling and/or coordination of care with other physicians, other qualified health care professionals, or agencies are provided consistent with the nature of the problem(s) and the patient's and/or family's needs. Usually, the presenting problem(s) are of high severity, and require urgent evaluation by the physician, or other qualified health care professionals but do not pose an immediate significant threat to life or physiologic function.

99285 Emergency department visit for the evaluation and management of a patient, which requires these 3 key components within the constraints imposed by the urgency of the patient's clinical condition and/or mental status: A comprehensive history; A comprehensive examination; and Medical decision making of high complexity. Counseling and/or coordination of care with other physicians, other qualified health care professionals, or agencies are provided consistent with the nature of the problem(s) and the patient's and/or family's needs. Usually, the presenting problem(s) are of high severity and pose an immediate significant threat to life or physiologic function.

Explanation

Emergency department services codes describe E/M services provided to patients in the emergency department (ED). ED codes are typically reported per day and do not differentiate between new or established patients. Under the emergency department services category, there are five levels represented by 99281-99285. All levels require the three key components (history, exam, and medical decision-making [MDM]) to be documented. The lowest level of care, 99281, requires a problem-focused history and exam with straightforward medical decision-making involving a minor or self-limiting complaint. Mid-level services describe an expanded problem-focused history and exam with MDM of low or moderate complexity as represented by 99282 and 99283, respectively. At these levels of service, the encounter typically addresses low to moderate severity health concerns. The last two levels of service in this

© 2020 Optum360, LLC   N Newborn: 0   P Pediatric: 0-17   M Maternity: 9-64   A Adult: 15-124   ♂ Male Only   ♀ Female Only   CPT © 2020 American Medical Association. All Rights Reserved.

category represent high-severity problems. Code 99284 describes a high-severity health concern that does not pose an immediate threat to life or physiologic function; a detailed history and exam in conjunction with moderate complexity MDM are required for reporting this level of service. The highest level of service, 99285, requires a comprehensive history and examination with high complexity MDM for high-severity health issues that pose an immediate threat to the life or physiologic function of the patient. Time is not listed as a component in the code descriptors for emergency department services as these types of services are provided based on the varying intensity of the patient's condition and may involve emergency providers caring for several patients over an extended period of time involving multiple encounters, making it difficult for the clinician to accurately detail the amount of time spent face-to-face with the patient.

Coding Tips

These codes are used to report emergency department services for the new or established patient. All three key components (history, exam, and medical decision making) must be met or exceeded for the level of service selected. Time is not a factor when selecting this E/M service. An emergency department is typically described as an organized hospital-based facility available 24 hours a day, providing unscheduled episodic services to patients in need of urgent medical attention. For critical care services provided in the emergency department, see 99291-99292. For observation care services provided to a patient located in the emergency department, see 99217-99220. For patients admitted and discharged from observation or inpatient status on the same date, see 99234-99236. Report place of service code 23 for services provided in the hospital emergency room. Medicare has provisionally identified these codes as telehealth/telemedicine services. Current Medicare coverage guidelines should be reviewed. Commercial payers should be contacted regarding their coverage guidelines. Telemedicine services may be reported by the performing provider by adding modifier 95 to these procedure codes. Services at the origination site are reported with HCPCS Level II code Q3014.

ICD-10-CM Diagnostic Codes

The application of this code is too broad to adequately present ICD-10-CM diagnostic code links here. Refer to your ICD-10-CM book.

AMA: 99281 2020,Jul,13; 2019,Jul,10; 2018,Jan,8; 2017,Jun,6; 2017,Jan,8; 2017,Aug,3; 2016,Jan,13; 2016,Jan,7; 2015,Jan,12; 2015,Jan,16; 2014,Oct,8; 2014,Nov,14; 2014,Jan,11 **99282** 2020,Jul,13; 2019,Jul,10; 2018,Jan,8; 2017,Jun,6; 2017,Jan,8; 2017,Aug,3; 2016,Jan,13; 2016,Jan,7; 2015,Jan,16; 2015,Jan,12; 2014,Oct,8; 2014,Nov,14; 2014,Jan,11 **99283** 2020,Jul,13; 2019,Jul,10; 2018,Jan,8; 2017,Jun,6; 2017,Jan,8; 2017,Aug,3; 2016,Jan,13; 2016,Jan,7; 2015,Jan,16; 2015,Jan,12; 2014,Oct,8; 2014,Nov,14; 2014,Jan,11 **99284** 2020,Jul,13; 2019,Jul,10; 2018,Jan,8; 2017,Jun,6; 2017,Jan,8; 2017,Aug,3; 2016,Jan,13; 2016,Jan,7; 2015,Jan,12; 2015,Jan,16; 2014,Oct,8; 2014,Nov,14; 2014,Jan,11 **99285** 2020,Jul,13; 2020,Jan,12; 2019,Jul,10; 2018,Jan,8; 2017,Jun,6; 2017,Jan,8; 2017,Aug,3; 2016,Jan,13; 2016,Jan,7; 2015,Jan,16; 2015,Jan,12; 2014,Oct,8; 2014,Nov,14; 2014,Jan,11

Relative Value Units/Medicare Edits

Non-Facility RVU	Work	PE	MP	Total
99281	0.48	0.11	0.05	0.64
99282	0.93	0.21	0.09	1.23
99283	1.42	0.29	0.13	1.84
99284	2.6	0.51	0.27	3.38
99285	3.8	0.71	0.4	4.91
Facility RVU	Work	PE	MP	Total
99281	0.48	0.11	0.05	0.64
99282	0.93	0.21	0.09	1.23
99283	1.42	0.29	0.13	1.84
99284	2.6	0.51	0.27	3.38
99285	3.8	0.71	0.4	4.91

	FUD	Status	MUE	Modifiers				IOM Reference
99281	N/A	A	1(3)	N/A	N/A	N/A	80*	100-04,4,160;
99282	N/A	A	1(3)	N/A	N/A	N/A	80*	100-04,12,30.6.4;
99283	N/A	A	1(3)	N/A	N/A	N/A	80*	100-04,12,30.6.11;
99284	N/A	A	1(3)	N/A	N/A	N/A	80*	100-04,12,100
99285	N/A	A	1(3)	N/A	N/A	N/A	80*	

* with documentation

Terms To Know

emergency. Serious medical condition or symptom (including severe pain) resulting from injury, sickness, or mental illness that arises suddenly and requires immediate care and treatment, generally received within 24 hours of onset, to avoid jeopardy to the life, limb, or health of a covered person.

emergency department. Organized hospital-based facility for the provision of unscheduled episodic services to patients who present for immediate medical attention. The facility must be available 24 hours a day.

99291-99292

	99291	Critical care, evaluation and management of the critically ill or critically injured patient; first 30-74 minutes
+	99292	each additional 30 minutes (List separately in addition to code for primary service)

Explanation

Critical care services are reported by a physician or other qualified health care provider for critically ill or injured patients. Critical illnesses or injuries are defined as those with impairment to one or more vital organ systems with an increased risk of rapid or imminent health deterioration. Critical care services require direct patient/provider involvement with highly complex decision making in order to evaluate, control, and support vital systems functions to treat one or more vital organ system failures and/or to avoid further decline of the patient's condition. Vital organ system failure includes, but is not limited to, failure of the central nervous, circulatory, or respiratory systems; kidneys; liver; shock; and other metabolic processes. Generally, critical care services necessitate the interpretation of many physiologic parameters and/or other applications of advanced technology as available in a critical care unit, pediatric intensive care unit, respiratory care unit, in an emergency facility, patient room or other hospital department; however, in emergent situations, critical care may be provided where these elements are not available. Critical care may be provided so long as the patient's condition continues to warrant the level of care according to the criteria described. Care provided to patients residing in a critical care unit but not fitting the criteria for critical care is reported using other E/M codes, as appropriate. These codes are time based codes, meaning the total time spent must be documented and includes direct patient care bedside or time spent on the patient's floor or unit (reviewing laboratory results or imaging studies and discussing the patient's care with medical staff, time spent with family members, caregivers, or other surrogate decision makers to gather information on the patient's medical history, reviewing the patient's condition or prognosis, and discussing various treatment options or limitations of treatment), as long as the clinician is immediately available and not providing services to any other patient during the same time period. Time spent outside of the patient's unit or floor, including telephone calls, caregiver discussions, or time spent in actions that do not directly contribute to the patient's care rendered in the critical unit are not reported as critical care. Report these codes for attendance of the patient during transport for patients 24 months of age or older to or from a facility. Code 99291 represents the first 30 to 74 minutes of critical care and is reported once per day. Additional time beyond the first 74 minutes is reported in 30 minute increments with 99292.

Coding Tips

These codes are used to report critical care services. These are time-based services and the total time spent providing critical care must be documented in the medical record. All time spent providing critical care on the same date of service is added together and does not need to be contiguous. Time is reported for practitioner time spent in care of the critically ill or injured patient at the patient's bedside and on the floor/unit. Time spent off the patient unit, even if related to patient care, is not counted. Do not report critical care for patients who may be in the critical care unit but are not currently critically ill. The following services are considered inclusive to the critical care codes when reported by the clinician: interpretation of cardiac output measurements, chest x-rays, pulse oximetry, blood gases, collection and interpretation of physiologic data, computer data such as ECGs, gastric intubation, vascular access, and ventilation management. Code 99291 is reported once per day. Code 99292 is reported in addition to code 99291. Medicare and some other payers may allow 99292 to be reported alone when critical care is reported by another physician of the same group and specialty the same date as another provider reporting 99291. For care of the critically ill neonate, see 99468-99469;

for patients 29 days through 24 months, see 99471-99472; and for patients 2 through 5 years, see 99475-99476. Medicare has provisionally identified these codes as telehealth/telemedicine services. Current Medicare coverage guidelines should be reviewed. Commercial payers should be contacted regarding their coverage guidelines. Telemedicine services may be reported by the performing provider by adding modifier 95 to these procedure codes. Services at the origination site are reported with HCPCS Level II code Q3014.

ICD-10-CM Diagnostic Codes

The application of this code is too broad to adequately present ICD-10-CM diagnostic code links here. Refer to your ICD-10-CM book.

AMA: 99291 2020,Jan,12; 2020,Feb,7; 2019,Jul,10; 2019,Dec,14; 2019,Aug,8; 2018,Jun,9; 2018,Jan,8; 2018,Dec,8; 2018,Dec,8; 2017,Jun,6; 2017,Jan,8; 2017,Aug,3; 2016,Oct,8; 2016,May,3; 2016,Jan,13; 2016,Aug,9; 2015,Jul,3; 2015,Jan,16; 2015,Feb,10; 2014,Oct,8; 2014,Oct,14; 2014,May,4; 2014,Jan,11; 2014,Aug,5 **99292** 2020,Feb,7; 2019,Jul,10; 2019,Dec,14; 2019,Aug,8; 2018,Jun,9; 2018,Jan,8; 2018,Dec,8; 2018,Dec,8; 2017,Jun,6; 2017,Jan,8; 2017,Aug,3; 2016,May,3; 2016,Jan,13; 2016,Aug,9; 2015,Jul,3; 2015,Jan,16; 2015,Feb,10; 2014,Oct,8; 2014,Oct,14; 2014,May,4; 2014,Jan,11; 2014,Aug,5

Relative Value Units/Medicare Edits

Non-Facility RVU	Work	PE	MP	Total
99291	4.5	2.99	0.4	7.89
99292	2.25	1.03	0.21	3.49
Facility RVU	**Work**	**PE**	**MP**	**Total**
99291	4.5	1.38	0.4	6.28
99292	2.25	0.7	0.21	3.16

	FUD	Status	MUE	Modifiers				IOM Reference
99291	N/A	A	1(2)	N/A	N/A	N/A	80*	100-04,4,160;
99292	N/A	A	8(3)	N/A	N/A	N/A	80*	100-04,12,30.6.9; 100-04,12,100

* with documentation

Terms To Know

critical care. Treatment of critically ill patients in a variety of medical emergencies that requires the constant attendance of the physician (e.g., cardiac arrest, shock, bleeding, respiratory failure, postoperative complications, critically ill neonate).

documentation. Physician's written or transcribed notations about a patient encounter, including a detailed operative report or written notes about a routine encounter. Source documentation must be the treating provider's own account of the encounter and may be transcribed from dictation, dictated by the physician into voice recognition software, or be hand- or typewritten. A signature or authentication accompanies each entry.

monitoring. Recording of events; keep track, regulate, or control patient activities and record findings.

99304-99306

99304 Initial nursing facility care, per day, for the evaluation and management of a patient, which requires these 3 key components: A detailed or comprehensive history; A detailed or comprehensive examination; and Medical decision making that is straightforward or of low complexity. Counseling and/or coordination of care with other physicians, other qualified health care professionals, or agencies are provided consistent with the nature of the problem(s) and the patient's and/or family's needs. Usually, the problem(s) requiring admission are of low severity. Typically, 25 minutes are spent at the bedside and on the patient's facility floor or unit.

99305 Initial nursing facility care, per day, for the evaluation and management of a patient, which requires these 3 key components: A comprehensive history; A comprehensive examination; and Medical decision making of moderate complexity. Counseling and/or coordination of care with other physicians, other qualified health care professionals, or agencies are provided consistent with the nature of the problem(s) and the patient's and/or family's needs. Usually, the problem(s) requiring admission are of moderate severity. Typically, 35 minutes are spent at the bedside and on the patient's facility floor or unit.

99306 Initial nursing facility care, per day, for the evaluation and management of a patient, which requires these 3 key components: A comprehensive history; A comprehensive examination; and Medical decision making of high complexity. Counseling and/or coordination of care with other physicians, other qualified health care professionals, or agencies are provided consistent with the nature of the problem(s) and the patient's and/or family's needs. Usually, the problem(s) requiring admission are of high severity. Typically, 45 minutes are spent at the bedside and on the patient's facility floor or unit.

Explanation

Initial nursing facility service codes describe the first encounter with the patient by the admitting physician to nursing facilities, formerly referred to as skilled nursing facilities (SNF), intermediate care facilities (ICF), or long term care facilities (LTCF). These facilities provide specialized care to its residents, such as convalescent, rehabilitative, or long-term care. These codes are also reported for services rendered to patients in a psychiatric residential treatment center (a 24-hour live-in facility, a standalone facility, or separate part of a psychiatric facility), staffed with medical professionals in a structured therapeutic environment. When the patient is admitted to the nursing facility during the course of another encounter from a different site of service, such as the physician's office or the emergency department, all of the E/M services rendered by the supervising clinician are considered part of the initial nursing facility care services when performed on the same day and the level of care reported for that date is inclusive of these services. Physician services may also include information necessary to complete the Resident Assessment Instrument (RAI). Every RAI is comprised of the Minimum Data Set (MDS), Resident Assessment Protocols (RAP), and the utilization guidelines. Initial nursing facility codes do not differentiate between new or established patients. Under the initial nursing facility care category, there are three levels represented by 99304, 99305, and 99306. All of these levels require all three key components (history, exam, and medical decision-making [MDM]) to be documented. The lowest level of care within this category, 99304, requires a detailed or comprehensive history and exam, as well as straightforward medical decision-making or that of low severity with approximately 25 minutes being spent at the patient's bedside and on the patient's floor or unit. The midlevel and highest level initial nursing facility care codes require a comprehensive history and examination. Medical decision-making is the differentiating factor for these two levels; for moderate complexity, report 99305, and for initial

nursing facility care requiring MDM of high complexity, report 99306. The clinician typically spends 35 (99305) to 45 (99306) minutes at the patient's bedside or on the unit accordingly.

Coding Tips

These codes are used to report the initial encounter in the nursing facility setting or psychiatric residential treatment center. All three key components (history, exam, and medical decision making) must be met or exceeded for the level of service selected. Time may be used to select the level of service when counseling and coordination of care are documented as at least half of the floor/unit time spent with the patient. CPT guidelines indicate these services are reported only by the admitting/supervising provider; all other providers should report 99307-99310 or 99251-99255. Medicare and some payers may allow providers of different specialties to report initial nursing facility services and require the admitting/supervising provider to append modifier AI. All evaluation and management services provided in other settings (e.g., office, emergency department) leading up to the nursing facility admission are part of the patient's initial nursing facility admission when performed on the same date of service and should be reflected in the code selection. These codes are used to report the initial evaluation of a patient including the Resident Assessment Instrument (RAI). The major components of the RAI include the Minimum Data Set (MDS), a screening and assessment tool, the Resident Assessment Protocols (RAPs) that identify potential problems, and follow-up assessment guidelines. Hospital inpatient or observation discharge services may be reported separately when performed on the same date of service. For care plan oversight services provided to nursing facility residents, see 99379-99380. For subsequent nursing facility care services, see 99307-99310. For nursing facility discharge services, see 99315-99316. Medicare has provisionally identified these codes as telehealth/telemedicine services. Current Medicare coverage guidelines should be reviewed. Commercial payers should be contacted regarding their coverage guidelines. Telemedicine services may be reported by the performing provider by adding modifier 95 to these procedure codes. Services at the origination site are reported with HCPCS Level II code Q3014.

ICD-10-CM Diagnostic Codes

The application of this code is too broad to adequately present ICD-10-CM diagnostic code links here. Refer to your ICD-10-CM book.

AMA: 99304 2020,Sep,3; 2018,Jan,8; 2017,Jun,6; 2017,Jan,8; 2017,Aug,3; 2016,Jan,13; 2016,Jan,7; 2016,Dec,11; 2015,Jan,16; 2014,Oct,8; 2014,Nov,14; 2014,Jan,11 **99305** 2020,Sep,3; 2018,Jan,8; 2017,Jun,6; 2017,Jan,8; 2017,Aug,3; 2016,Jan,7; 2016,Jan,13; 2016,Dec,11; 2015,Jan,16; 2014,Oct,8; 2014,Nov,14; 2014,Jan,11 **99306** 2020,Sep,3; 2018,Jan,8; 2017,Jun,6; 2017,Jan,8; 2017,Aug,3; 2016,Jan,13; 2016,Jan,7; 2016,Dec,11; 2015,Jan,16; 2014,Oct,8; 2014,Nov,14; 2014,Jan,11

Relative Value Units/Medicare Edits

Non-Facility RVU	Work	PE	MP	Total
99304	1.64	0.8	0.11	2.55
99305	2.35	1.17	0.13	3.65
99306	3.06	1.46	0.19	4.71
Facility RVU	**Work**	**PE**	**MP**	**Total**
99304	1.64	0.8	0.11	2.55
99305	2.35	1.17	0.13	3.65
99306	3.06	1.46	0.19	4.71

	FUD	Status	MUE	Modifiers				IOM Reference
99304	N/A	A	1(2)	N/A	N/A	N/A	80*	100-04,12,30.6.4;
99305	N/A	A	1(2)	N/A	N/A	N/A	80*	100-04,12,30.6.13
99306	N/A	A	1(2)	N/A	N/A	N/A	80*	

* with documentation

Terms To Know

coordination of care. Care provided concurrently with counseling that includes treatment instructions to the patient or caregiver; special accommodations for home, work, school, vacation, or other locations; coordination with other providers and agencies; and living arrangements.

nursing facility. Services provided to inpatients of a skilled nursing facility, intermediate care facility, long-term care facility, or psychiatric residential treatment center that provides convalescent, rehabilitative, or long-term care of patients.

rehabilitation. Restoration of physical and mental functions to allow the usual daily activities of life.

99307-99310

★**99307** Subsequent nursing facility care, per day, for the evaluation and management of a patient, which requires at least 2 of these 3 key components: A problem focused interval history; A problem focused examination; Straightforward medical decision making. Counseling and/or coordination of care with other physicians, other qualified health care professionals, or agencies are provided consistent with the nature of the problem(s) and the patient's and/or family's needs. Usually, the patient is stable, recovering, or improving. Typically, 10 minutes are spent at the bedside and on the patient's facility floor or unit.

★**99308** Subsequent nursing facility care, per day, for the evaluation and management of a patient, which requires at least 2 of these 3 key components: An expanded problem focused interval history; An expanded problem focused examination; Medical decision making of low complexity. Counseling and/or coordination of care with other physicians, other qualified health care professionals, or agencies are provided consistent with the nature of the problem(s) and the patient's and/or family's needs. Usually, the patient is responding inadequately to therapy or has developed a minor complication. Typically, 15 minutes are spent at the bedside and on the patient's facility floor or unit.

★**99309** Subsequent nursing facility care, per day, for the evaluation and management of a patient, which requires at least 2 of these 3 key components: A detailed interval history; A detailed examination; Medical decision making of moderate complexity. Counseling and/or coordination of care with other physicians, other qualified health care professionals, or agencies are provided consistent with the nature of the problem(s) and the patient's and/or family's needs. Usually, the patient has developed a significant complication or a significant new problem. Typically, 25 minutes are spent at the bedside and on the patient's facility floor or unit.

★**99310** Subsequent nursing facility care, per day, for the evaluation and management of a patient, which requires at least 2 of these 3 key components: A comprehensive interval history; A comprehensive examination; Medical decision making of high complexity. Counseling and/or coordination of care with other physicians, other qualified health care professionals, or agencies are provided consistent with the nature of the problem(s) and the patient's and/or family's needs. The patient may be unstable or may have developed a significant new problem requiring immediate physician attention. Typically, 35 minutes are spent at the bedside and on the patient's facility floor or unit.

Explanation

Subsequent nursing facility care services codes describe visits that occur after the first encounter of the patient's nursing facility admission by the supervising qualified clinician. Codes are reported per day and do not differentiate between new or established patients. Under the subsequent nursing facility care category, there are four levels of service represented by 99307, 99308, 99309, and 99310. Each level requires at least two out of the three key components—history, exam, and medical decision making—to be documented. The lowest level of care within this category, 99307, describes a problem-focused interval history as well as a problem-focused examination with straightforward medical decision making involving approximately 10 minutes of time by the provider at the patient's bedside or on the unit. For the mid-level subsequent nursing facility care code, 99308, an expanded problem-focused history and examination are required with low complexity medical decision making. Time associated with this level usually involves 15 minutes at the bedside or on the patient's floor. The third level of follow-up nursing facility care, 99309, requires a detailed history and exam as well as medical decision making of moderate complexity; for this level of care, the provider typically spends approximately 25 minutes at the bedside or on the patient's floor or unit. The fourth and highest level of nursing facility care is reported with 99310 and requires a comprehensive history and examination with high complexity medical decision making. The provider generally spends 35 minutes at the patient's bedside or on the unit or floor. All four levels of subsequent nursing facility care involve the clinician reviewing the patient's medical record, results from diagnostic studies, as well as any changes to the patient's status such as physical condition, response to treatments, or changes in health history since the last assessment.

Coding Tips

These codes are used to report the subsequent encounters in the nursing facility setting or psychiatric residential treatment center. Two of the three key components (history, exam, and medical decision making) must be met or exceeded for the level of service selected. Time may be used to select the level of service when counseling and coordination of care are documented as at least half of the floor/unit time spent with the patient. Codes may be selected based upon the 1995 or the 1997 Evaluation and Management Guidelines. Subsequent nursing facility services include review of the medical record, including all diagnostic studies, as well as changes noted in the patient's condition and response to treatment since the last evaluation. For care plan oversight services provided to nursing facility residents, see 99379-99380. For initial nursing facility care services, see 99304-99306; for nursing facility discharge services, see 99315-99316. Report place of service (POS) code 31 for the skilled nursing facility; report POS code 32 for the nursing facility; and report POS code 56 for the psychiatric residential treatment center. Telemedicine services may be reported by the performing provider by adding modifier 95 to these procedure codes. Services at the origination site are reported with HCPCS Level II code Q3014.

ICD-10-CM Diagnostic Codes

The application of this code is too broad to adequately present ICD-10-CM diagnostic code links here. Refer to your ICD-10-CM book.

AMA: **99307** 2020,Sep,3; 2018,Jan,8; 2017,Jun,6; 2017,Jan,8; 2017,Aug,3; 2016,Jan,13; 2016,Jan,7; 2016,Dec,11; 2015,Jan,16; 2014,Oct,8; 2014,Nov,14; 2014,Jan,11 **99308** 2020,Sep,3; 2018,Jan,8; 2017,Jun,6; 2017,Jan,8; 2017,Aug,3; 2016,Jan,13; 2016,Jan,7; 2016,Dec,11; 2015,Jan,16; 2014,Oct,8; 2014,Nov,14; 2014,Jan,11 **99309** 2020,Sep,3; 2018,Jan,8; 2017,Jun,6; 2017,Jan,8; 2017,Aug,3; 2016,Jan,13; 2016,Jan,7; 2016,Dec,11; 2015,Jan,16; 2014,Oct,8; 2014,Nov,14; 2014,Jan,11 **99310** 2020,Sep,3; 2018,Jan,8; 2017,Jun,6; 2017,Jan,8; 2017,Aug,3; 2016,Jan,7; 2016,Jan,13; 2016,Dec,11; 2015,Jan,16; 2014,Oct,8; 2014,Nov,14; 2014,Jan,11

Relative Value Units/Medicare Edits

Non-Facility RVU	Work	PE	MP	Total
99307	0.76	0.43	0.05	1.24
99308	1.16	0.71	0.08	1.95
99309	1.55	0.93	0.09	2.57
99310	2.35	1.31	0.13	3.79
Facility RVU	Work	PE	MP	Total
99307	0.76	0.43	0.05	1.24
99308	1.16	0.71	0.08	1.95
99309	1.55	0.93	0.09	2.57
99310	2.35	1.31	0.13	3.79

	FUD	Status	MUE	Modifiers				IOM Reference
99307	N/A	A	1(2)	N/A	N/A	N/A	80*	None
99308	N/A	A	1(2)	N/A	N/A	N/A	80*	
99309	N/A	A	1(2)	N/A	N/A	N/A	80*	
99310	N/A	A	1(2)	N/A	N/A	N/A	80*	

* with documentation

Terms To Know

coordination of care. Care provided concurrently with counseling that includes treatment instructions to the patient or caregiver; special accommodations for home, work, school, vacation, or other locations; coordination with other providers and agencies; and living arrangements.

nursing facility. Services provided to inpatients of a skilled nursing facility, intermediate care facility, long-term care facility, or psychiatric residential treatment center that provides convalescent, rehabilitative, or long-term care of patients.

other qualified health care professional. Individual who is qualified by education, training, licensure/regulation, and facility privileging to perform a professional service within his or her scope of practice and independently (or as incident-to) report the professional service without requiring physician supervision. Payers may state exemptions in writing or state and local regulations may not follow this definition for performance of some services. Always refer to any relevant plan policies and federal and/or state laws to determine who may perform and report services.

99315-99316

99315   Nursing facility discharge day management; 30 minutes or less
99316   more than 30 minutes

Explanation

Nursing facility discharge services are time-based codes that describe the amount of time spent by the clinician during all final steps involved in the discharge of a patient from the nursing facility, including the last patient exam, discussing the nursing facility stay, instructions for ongoing care as it relates to all pertinent caregivers, and preparing the medical discharge records, prescriptions, and/or referrals as applicable. Time reported should be for the total duration of time spent by the provider even when the time spent on that date is not continuous. For a nursing facility discharge duration of 30 minutes or less, report 99315; for a duration of greater than 30 minutes, report 99316. These codes are reported following initial and subsequent nursing facility care codes 99304-99306 and 99307-99310.

Coding Tips

These codes are used to report all discharge day services for the nursing facility resident. These codes include patient examination, follow-up care instructions to appropriate caregivers, prescriptions, referrals, and preparation of all medical records. These are time-based codes and floor unit time spent caring for the patient must be documented in the medical record. All time spent providing discharge services on the same date of service is added together and does not need to be contiguous. For initial nursing facility care services, see 99304-99306; for subsequent nursing facility care services, see 99307-99310. Report place of service (POS) code 31 for the skilled nursing facility; report POS code 32 for the nursing facility; and report POS code 56 for the psychiatric residential treatment center. Medicare has provisionally identified these codes as telehealth/telemedicine services. Current Medicare coverage guidelines should be reviewed. Commercial payers should be contacted regarding their coverage guidelines. Telemedicine services may be reported by the performing provider by adding modifier 95 to these procedure codes. Services at the origination site are reported with HCPCS Level II code Q3014.

ICD-10-CM Diagnostic Codes

The application of this code is too broad to adequately present ICD-10-CM diagnostic code links here. Refer to your ICD-10-CM book.

AMA: **99315** 2018,Jan,8; 2017,Jun,6; 2017,Jan,8; 2017,Aug,3; 2016,Jan,13; 2016,Jan,7; 2016,Dec,11; 2015,Jan,16; 2014,Oct,8; 2014,Nov,14; 2014,Jan,11 **99316** 2018,Jan,8; 2017,Jun,6; 2017,Jan,8; 2017,Aug,3; 2016,Jan,13; 2016,Jan,7; 2016,Dec,11; 2015,Jan,16; 2014,Oct,8; 2014,Nov,14; 2014,Jan,11

Relative Value Units/Medicare Edits

Non-Facility RVU	Work	PE	MP	Total
99315	1.28	0.7	0.09	2.07
99316	1.9	0.96	0.11	2.97
Facility RVU	Work	PE	MP	Total
99315	1.28	0.7	0.09	2.07
99316	1.9	0.96	0.11	2.97

	FUD	Status	MUE	Modifiers				IOM Reference
99315	N/A	A	1(2)	N/A	N/A	N/A	80*	100-04,12,30.6.4;
99316	N/A	A	1(2)	N/A	N/A	N/A	80*	100-04,12,30.6.13; 100-04,12,100

* with documentation

99318

99318   Evaluation and management of a patient involving an annual nursing facility assessment, which requires these 3 key components: A detailed interval history; A comprehensive examination; and Medical decision making that is of low to moderate complexity. Counseling and/or coordination of care with other physicians, other qualified health care professionals, or agencies are provided consistent with the nature of the problem(s) and the patient's and/or family's needs. Usually, the patient is stable, recovering, or improving. Typically, 30 minutes are spent at the bedside and on the patient's facility floor or unit.

Explanation

This code describes a yearly nursing facility evaluation and does not differentiate between new or established patients. This level of care requires a detailed interval history, as well as a comprehensive examination and low to moderate medical decision making. The clinician spends approximately 30 minutes at the patient's bedside or on the unit. Generally speaking, the patient's condition would be described in the documentation as stable, improving, or recovering.

Coding Tips

This code is used to report the annual evaluation of a nursing facility patient, including the Resident Assessment Instrument (RAI). The major components of the RAI include the Minimum Data Set (MDS), a screening and assessment tool, the Resident Assessment Protocols (RAPs) that identify potential problems, and follow-up assessment guidelines. Physicians play a primary role in the resident assessment and medical plan of care. Do not report 99318 in addition to 99304-99316 for the same date of service. Report place of service (POS) code 31 for the skilled nursing facility; report POS code 32 for the nursing facility.

ICD-10-CM Diagnostic Codes

The application of this code is too broad to adequately present ICD-10-CM diagnostic code links here. Refer to your ICD-10-CM book.

AMA: **99318** 2018,Jan,8; 2017,Jun,6; 2017,Jan,8; 2017,Aug,3; 2016,Jan,13; 2016,Jan,7; 2016,Dec,11; 2015,Jan,16; 2014,Oct,8; 2014,Nov,14; 2014,Jan,11

Relative Value Units/Medicare Edits

Non-Facility RVU	Work	PE	MP	Total
99318	1.71	0.89	0.11	2.71
Facility RVU	Work	PE	MP	Total
99318	1.71	0.89	0.11	2.71

	FUD	Status	MUE	Modifiers				IOM Reference
99318	N/A	A	1(2)	N/A	N/A	N/A	80*	100-04,12,30.6.4; 100-04,12,30.6.9; 100-04,12,30.6.13; 100-04,12,30.6.15.1

* with documentation

99324-99328

99324 Domiciliary or rest home visit for the evaluation and management of a new patient, which requires these 3 key components: A problem focused history; A problem focused examination; and Straightforward medical decision making. Counseling and/or coordination of care with other physicians, other qualified health care professionals, or agencies are provided consistent with the nature of the problem(s) and the patient's and/or family's needs. Usually, the presenting problem(s) are of low severity. Typically, 20 minutes are spent with the patient and/or family or caregiver.

99325 Domiciliary or rest home visit for the evaluation and management of a new patient, which requires these 3 key components: An expanded problem focused history; An expanded problem focused examination; and Medical decision making of low complexity. Counseling and/or coordination of care with other physicians, other qualified health care professionals, or agencies are provided consistent with the nature of the problem(s) and the patient's and/or family's needs. Usually, the presenting problem(s) are of moderate severity. Typically, 30 minutes are spent with the patient and/or family or caregiver.

99326 Domiciliary or rest home visit for the evaluation and management of a new patient, which requires these 3 key components: A detailed history; A detailed examination; and Medical decision making of moderate complexity. Counseling and/or coordination of care with other physicians, other qualified health care professionals, or agencies are provided consistent with the nature of the problem(s) and the patient's and/or family's needs. Usually, the presenting problem(s) are of moderate to high severity. Typically, 45 minutes are spent with the patient and/or family or caregiver.

99327 Domiciliary or rest home visit for the evaluation and management of a new patient, which requires these 3 key components: A comprehensive history; A comprehensive examination; and Medical decision making of moderate complexity. Counseling and/or coordination of care with other physicians, other qualified health care professionals, or agencies are provided consistent with the nature of the problem(s) and the patient's and/or family's needs. Usually, the presenting problem(s) are of high severity. Typically, 60 minutes are spent with the patient and/or family or caregiver.

99328 Domiciliary or rest home visit for the evaluation and management of a new patient, which requires these 3 key components: A comprehensive history; A comprehensive examination; and Medical decision making of high complexity. Counseling and/or coordination of care with other physicians, other qualified health care professionals, or agencies are provided consistent with the nature of the problem(s) and the patient's and/or family's needs. Usually, the patient is unstable or has developed a significant new problem requiring immediate physician attention. Typically, 75 minutes are spent with the patient and/or family or caregiver.

Explanation

Providers report domiciliary, rest home, or custodial care services codes for E/M services rendered to new patients residing in a facility, usually long-term, that offers room and board as well as other personal assistance services. These codes may also be reported for patients residing in an assisted living facility. Services are reported based on meeting all three key components—history, exam, and medical decision making (MDM)—within each level of service. The most basic service, 99324, describes a problem focused history and exam with straightforward medical decision making for low severity problems encompassing approximately 20 minutes of time with the patient and/or family or caregiver. Mid-level services require an expanded problem focused

history and exam or a detailed history and exam, represented by 99325 and 99326, respectively. Medical decision making for 99325 is designated as low complexity; moderate complexity for 99326. At these levels of service, the encounter can involve physician time spent with the patient and/or family or caregiver of 30 (99325) to 45 minutes (99326). The last two levels of service in this category require documenting comprehensive history and examination components. The differentiating factor between the two levels is the medical decision making; 99327 involves moderate complexity MDM and approximately 60 minutes of time with the patient and/or family or caregiver for high severity problems, while the highest level of service in this category, 99328, involves MDM of high complexity and 75 minutes of time with the patient and/or family or caregiver as a result of the patient being unstable or having developed a significant, new problem necessitating the immediate attention of the clinician.

Coding Tips

These codes are used to report services provided in a domiciliary setting for a new patient, including services provided in a group home, assisted living facility, intermediate care, or custodial care facilities. All three key components (history, exam, and medical decision making) must be met or exceeded for the level of service selected. Time may be used to select the level of service when counseling and coordination of care are documented as at least half of the time spent face-to-face with the patient. Codes may be selected based upon the 1995 or the 1997 Evaluation and Management Guidelines. These services are reported by the admitting/supervising provider; all other providers should report other E/M services. For care plan oversight services provided to a patient residing in a domiciliary facility under the care of a hospice agency, see 99377-99378; for a home health agency, see 99374-99375. For care plan oversight services provided to a patient under home, domiciliary, or rest home (assisted living) care, see 99339-99340. Medicare has provisionally identified these codes as telehealth/telemedicine services. Current Medicare coverage guidelines should be reviewed. Commercial payers should be contacted regarding their coverage guidelines. Telemedicine services may be reported by the performing provider by adding modifier 95 to these procedure codes. Services at the origination site are reported with HCPCS Level II code Q3014.

ICD-10-CM Diagnostic Codes

The application of this code is too broad to adequately present ICD-10-CM diagnostic code links here. Refer to your ICD-10-CM book.

AMA: 99324 2020,Sep,3; 2018,Jan,8; 2018,Apr,9; 2017,Jun,6; 2017,Jan,8; 2017,Aug,3; 2016,Jan,13; 2016,Jan,7; 2016,Dec,11; 2015,Jan,16; 2014,Oct,8; 2014,Oct,3; 2014,Nov,14; 2014,Jan,11 **99325** 2020,Sep,3; 2018,Jan,8; 2018,Apr,9; 2017,Jun,6; 2017,Jan,8; 2017,Aug,3; 2016,Jan,13; 2016,Jan,7; 2016,Dec,11; 2015,Jan,16; 2014,Oct,8; 2014,Oct,3; 2014,Nov,14; 2014,Jan,11 **99326** 2020,Sep,3; 2018,Jan,8; 2018,Apr,9; 2017,Jun,6; 2017,Jan,8; 2017,Aug,3; 2016,Jan,7; 2016,Jan,13; 2016,Dec,11; 2015,Jan,16; 2014,Oct,8; 2014,Oct,3; 2014,Nov,14; 2014,Jan,11 **99327** 2020,Sep,3; 2018,Jan,8; 2018,Apr,9; 2017,Jun,6; 2017,Jan,8; 2017,Aug,3; 2016,Jan,13; 2016,Jan,7; 2016,Dec,11; 2015,Jan,16; 2014,Oct,8; 2014,Oct,3; 2014,Nov,14; 2014,Jan,11 **99328** 2020,Sep,3; 2018,Jan,8; 2018,Apr,9; 2017,Jun,6; 2017,Jan,8; 2017,Aug,3; 2016,Jan,13; 2016,Jan,7; 2016,Dec,11; 2015,Jan,16; 2014,Oct,8; 2014,Oct,3; 2014,Nov,14; 2014,Jan,11

Relative Value Units/Medicare Edits

Non-Facility RVU	Work	PE	MP	Total
99324	1.01	0.48	0.05	1.54
99325	1.52	0.64	0.08	2.24
99326	2.63	1.14	0.13	3.9
99327	3.46	1.59	0.19	5.24
99328	4.09	1.86	0.25	6.2
Facility RVU	Work	PE	MP	Total
99324	1.01	0.48	0.05	1.54
99325	1.52	0.64	0.08	2.24
99326	2.63	1.14	0.13	3.9
99327	3.46	1.59	0.19	5.24
99328	4.09	1.86	0.25	6.2

	FUD	Status	MUE	Modifiers				IOM Reference
99324	N/A	A	1(2)	N/A	N/A	N/A	80*	100-04,12,30.6.4;
99325	N/A	A	1(2)	N/A	N/A	N/A	80*	100-04,12,30.6.14
99326	N/A	A	1(2)	N/A	N/A	N/A	80*	
99327	N/A	A	1(2)	N/A	N/A	N/A	80*	
99328	N/A	A	1(2)	N/A	N/A	N/A	80*	

* with documentation

Terms To Know

domiciliary. Facility, such as an assisted living, group home, custodial care, or an intermediate care facility, that provides room and board on a long-term basis and may include personal assistance services.

initial. First stage in a series of events.

key components. Three components of history, examination, and medical decision making are considered the keys to selecting the correct level of E/M codes. In most cases, all three components must be addressed in the documentation. However, in established, subsequent, and follow-up categories, only two of the three must be met or exceeded for a given code.

new patient. Patient who is receiving face-to-face care from a provider/qualified health care professional or another physician/qualified health care professional of the exact same specialty and subspecialty who belongs to the same group practice for the first time in three years. For OPPS hospitals, a patient who has not been registered as an inpatient or outpatient, including off-campus provider based clinic or emergency department, within the past three years.

99334-99337

99334 Domiciliary or rest home visit for the evaluation and management of an established patient, which requires at least 2 of these 3 key components: A problem focused interval history; A problem focused examination; Straightforward medical decision making. Counseling and/or coordination of care with other physicians, other qualified health care professionals, or agencies are provided consistent with the nature of the problem(s) and the patient's and/or family's needs. Usually, the presenting problem(s) are self-limited or minor. Typically, 15 minutes are spent with the patient and/or family or caregiver.

99335 Domiciliary or rest home visit for the evaluation and management of an established patient, which requires at least 2 of these 3 key components: An expanded problem focused interval history; An expanded problem focused examination; Medical decision making of low complexity. Counseling and/or coordination of care with other physicians, other qualified health care professionals, or agencies are provided consistent with the nature of the problem(s) and the patient's and/or family's needs. Usually, the presenting problem(s) are of low to moderate severity. Typically, 25 minutes are spent with the patient and/or family or caregiver.

99336 Domiciliary or rest home visit for the evaluation and management of an established patient, which requires at least 2 of these 3 key components: A detailed interval history; A detailed examination; Medical decision making of moderate complexity. Counseling and/or coordination of care with other physicians, other qualified health care professionals, or agencies are provided consistent with the nature of the problem(s) and the patient's and/or family's needs. Usually, the presenting problem(s) are of moderate to high severity. Typically, 40 minutes are spent with the patient and/or family or caregiver.

99337 Domiciliary or rest home visit for the evaluation and management of an established patient, which requires at least 2 of these 3 key components: A comprehensive interval history; A comprehensive examination; Medical decision making of moderate to high complexity. Counseling and/or coordination of care with other physicians, other qualified health care professionals, or agencies are provided consistent with the nature of the problem(s) and the patient's and/or family's needs. Usually, the presenting problem(s) are of moderate to high severity. The patient may be unstable or may have developed a significant new problem requiring immediate physician attention. Typically, 60 minutes are spent with the patient and/or family or caregiver.

Explanation

Providers report domiciliary, rest home, or custodial care services codes for E/M services rendered to established patients residing in a facility, usually long-term, that offers room and board, as well as other personal assistance services. These codes may also be reported for patients residing in an assisted living facility. Services in this category are reported based on meeting at least two of the three key components (history, exam, and medical decision-making [MDM]) within each level of service. The most basic service, 99334, describes a problem-focused interval history and problem-focused exam with straightforward medical decision-making for problems considered minimal and generally involves approximately 15 minutes of time with the patient and/or family or caregiver. Mid-level services require an expanded problem focused history and exam or a detailed history and exam as represented by 99335 and 99336, respectively. Medical decision-making for 99335 is designated as low complexity; moderate complexity for 99336. At these levels of service, the encounter can involve clinician time spent with the patient and/or family or caregiver of 25 (99335) to 40 minutes (99336) for problems

© 2020 Optum360, LLC   **N Newborn: 0**   **P Pediatric: 0-17**   **M Maternity: 9-64**   **A Adult: 15-124**   ♂ **Male Only**   ♀ **Female Only**   CPT © 2020 American Medical Association. All Rights Reserved.

considered to be of a low to moderate or moderate to high severity. The last level of service in this category, 99337, consists of a comprehensive history and examination, as well as MDM of moderate to high complexity. The clinician can expect to spend approximately 60 minutes duration with the patient and/or family or caregiver for moderate to high-severity problems as a result of the patient being unstable or having developed a significant, new problem necessitating the immediate attention of the provider.

Coding Tips

These codes are used to report services provided in a domiciliary setting for an established patient, including services provided in a group home, assisted living facility, intermediate care, or custodial care facilities. Two of the three key components (history, exam, and medical decision making) must be met or exceeded for the level of service selected. Time may be used to select the level of service when counseling and coordination of care are documented as at least half of the time spent face-to-face with the patient. Codes may be selected based upon the 1995 or the 1997 Evaluation and Management Guidelines. For care plan oversight services provided to a patient residing in a domiciliary facility under the care of a hospice agency, see 99377-99378; provided under the care of a home health agency, see 99374-99375. For care plan oversight services provided to a patient under home, domiciliary, or rest home (assisted living) care, see 99339-99340. Medicare has provisionally identified these codes as telehealth/telemedicine services. Current Medicare coverage guidelines should be reviewed. Commercial payers should be contacted regarding their coverage guidelines. Telemedicine services may be reported by the performing provider by adding modifier 95 to these procedure codes. Services at the origination site are reported with HCPCS Level II code Q3014.

ICD-10-CM Diagnostic Codes

The application of this code is too broad to adequately present ICD-10-CM diagnostic code links here. Refer to your ICD-10-CM book.

AMA: 99334 2020,Sep,3; 2018,Jan,8; 2018,Apr,9; 2017,Jun,6; 2017,Jan,8; 2017,Aug,3; 2016,Jan,13; 2016,Jan,7; 2016,Dec,11; 2015,Jan,16; 2014,Oct,8; 2014,Oct,3; 2014,Nov,14; 2014,Jan,11 **99335** 2020,Sep,3; 2018,Jan,8; 2018,Apr,9; 2017,Jun,6; 2017,Jan,8; 2017,Aug,3; 2016,Jan,13; 2016,Jan,7; 2016,Dec,11; 2015,Jan,16; 2014,Oct,8; 2014,Oct,3; 2014,Nov,14; 2014,Jan,11 **99336** 2020,Sep,3; 2018,Jan,8; 2018,Apr,9; 2017,Jun,6; 2017,Jan,8; 2017,Aug,3; 2016,Jan,13; 2016,Jan,7; 2016,Dec,11; 2015,Jan,16; 2014,Oct,8; 2014,Oct,3; 2014,Nov,14; 2014,Jan,11 **99337** 2020,Sep,3; 2018,Jan,8; 2018,Apr,9; 2017,Jun,6; 2017,Jan,8; 2017,Aug,3; 2016,Jan,13; 2016,Jan,7; 2016,Dec,11; 2015,Jan,16; 2014,Oct,8; 2014,Oct,3; 2014,Nov,14; 2014,Jan,11

Relative Value Units/Medicare Edits

Non-Facility RVU	Work	PE	MP	Total
99334	1.07	0.57	0.06	1.7
99335	1.72	0.88	0.09	2.69
99336	2.46	1.21	0.13	3.8
99337	3.58	1.68	0.22	5.48
Facility RVU	Work	PE	MP	Total
99334	1.07	0.57	0.06	1.7
99335	1.72	0.88	0.09	2.69
99336	2.46	1.21	0.13	3.8
99337	3.58	1.68	0.22	5.48

	FUD	Status	MUE	Modifiers				IOM Reference
99334	N/A	A	1(3)	N/A	N/A	N/A	80*	None
99335	N/A	A	1(3)	N/A	N/A	N/A	80*	
99336	N/A	A	1(3)	N/A	N/A	N/A	80*	
99337	N/A	A	1(3)	N/A	N/A	N/A	80*	

* with documentation

Terms To Know

domiciliary. Facility, such as an assisted living, group home, custodial care, or an intermediate care facility, that provides room and board on a long-term basis and may include personal assistance services.

established patient. Patient who has received professional services in a face-to-face setting within the last three years from the same physician/qualified health care professional or another physician/qualified health care professional of the exact same specialty and subspecialty who belongs to the same group practice. If the patient is seen by a physician/qualified health care professional who is covering for another physician/qualified health care professional, the patient will be considered the same as if seen by the physician/qualified health care professional who is unavailable.

99341-99345

99341 Home visit for the evaluation and management of a new patient, which requires these 3 key components: A problem focused history; A problem focused examination; and Straightforward medical decision making. Counseling and/or coordination of care with other physicians, other qualified health care professionals, or agencies are provided consistent with the nature of the problem(s) and the patient's and/or family's needs. Usually, the presenting problem(s) are of low severity. Typically, 20 minutes are spent face-to-face with the patient and/or family.

99342 Home visit for the evaluation and management of a new patient, which requires these 3 key components: An expanded problem focused history; An expanded problem focused examination; and Medical decision making of low complexity. Counseling and/or coordination of care with other physicians, other qualified health care professionals, or agencies are provided consistent with the nature of the problem(s) and the patient's and/or family's needs. Usually, the presenting problem(s) are of moderate severity. Typically, 30 minutes are spent face-to-face with the patient and/or family.

99343 Home visit for the evaluation and management of a new patient, which requires these 3 key components: A detailed history; A detailed examination; and Medical decision making of moderate complexity. Counseling and/or coordination of care with other physicians, other qualified health care professionals, or agencies are provided consistent with the nature of the problem(s) and the patient's and/or family's needs. Usually, the presenting problem(s) are of moderate to high severity. Typically, 45 minutes are spent face-to-face with the patient and/or family.

99344 Home visit for the evaluation and management of a new patient, which requires these 3 key components: A comprehensive history; A comprehensive examination; and Medical decision making of moderate complexity. Counseling and/or coordination of care with other physicians, other qualified health care professionals, or agencies are provided consistent with the nature of the problem(s) and the patient's and/or family's needs. Usually, the presenting problem(s) are of high severity. Typically, 60 minutes are spent face-to-face with the patient and/or family.

99345 Home visit for the evaluation and management of a new patient, which requires these 3 key components: A comprehensive history; A comprehensive examination; and Medical decision making of high complexity. Counseling and/or coordination of care with other physicians, other qualified health care professionals, or agencies are provided consistent with the nature of the problem(s) and the patient's and/or family's needs. Usually, the patient is unstable or has developed a significant new problem requiring immediate physician attention. Typically, 75 minutes are spent face-to-face with the patient and/or family.

Explanation

Home services codes are reported by providers for E/M services rendered to new patients residing in a personal residence. Services are reported based on meeting all three key components (history, exam, and medical decision-making [MDM]) within each level of service. The most basic service, 99341, describes a problem-focused history and exam with straightforward medical decision-making for low severity problems encompassing approximately 20 minutes of time with the patient and/or family or caregiver. Mid-level services require an expanded problem-focused history and exam or a detailed history and exam as represented by 99342 and 99343, respectively. Medical decision-making for 99342 is designated as low complexity; moderate complexity for 99343. At these levels of service, the encounter can involve face-to-face time spent with the patient and/or family or caregiver of 30 (99342) to 45 minutes (99343). The last two levels of service in this category require documenting comprehensive history and examination components. The differentiating factor between the two levels is the MDM: 99344 involves moderate complexity MDM and approximately 60 minutes of face-to-face time with the patient and/or family or caregiver for high-severity problems, while the highest level of service in this category, 99345, involves MDM of high complexity and 75 minutes of face-to-face time with the patient and/or family or caregiver as a result of the patient being unstable or having developed a significant, new problem necessitating the immediate attention of the clinician.

Coding Tips

These codes are used to report evaluation and management services provided in a private residence, temporary lodging, or short-term accommodation such as a hotel, campground, hostel, or cruise ship for a new patient. All three key components (history, exam, and medical decision making) must be met or exceeded for the level of service selected. Time may be used to select the level of service when counseling and coordination of care are documented as at least half of the time spent face-to-face with the patient. For commercial payers, consider assigning the appropriate consultation code instead of these codes when an opinion or advice about a specific problem has been requested by another qualified provider. Consultation codes are not covered by Medicare and some payers. Report the appropriate new or established outpatient E/M code for consultation services. For care plan oversight provided in the home under the care of a hospice agency, see 99377-99378; provided under the care of a home health agency, see 99374-99375. For care plan oversight services provided to a patient under home, domiciliary, or rest home (assisted living) care, see 99339-99340. Report place of service (POS) code 12 for services rendered in a private residence. Medicare has provisionally identified these codes as telehealth/telemedicine services. Current Medicare coverage guidelines should be reviewed. Commercial payers should be contacted regarding their coverage guidelines. Telemedicine services may be reported by the performing provider by adding modifier 95 to these procedure codes. Services at the origination site are reported with HCPCS Level II code Q3014.

ICD-10-CM Diagnostic Codes

The application of this code is too broad to adequately present ICD-10-CM diagnostic code links here. Refer to your ICD-10-CM book.

AMA: **99341** 2020,Sep,3; 2018,Jan,8; 2018,Apr,9; 2017,Jun,6; 2017,Jan,8; 2017,Aug,3; 2016,Jan,13; 2016,Jan,7; 2016,Dec,11; 2015,Jan,16; 2014,Oct,8; 2014,Oct,3; 2014,Nov,14; 2014,Jan,11 **99342** 2020,Sep,3; 2018,Jan,8; 2018,Apr,9; 2017,Jun,6; 2017,Jan,8; 2017,Aug,3; 2016,Jan,13; 2016,Jan,7; 2016,Dec,11; 2015,Jan,16; 2014,Oct,8; 2014,Oct,3; 2014,Nov,14; 2014,Jan,11 **99343** 2020,Sep,3; 2018,Jan,8; 2018,Apr,9; 2017,Jun,6; 2017,Jan,8; 2017,Aug,3; 2016,Jan,13; 2016,Jan,7; 2016,Dec,11; 2015,Jan,16; 2014,Oct,8; 2014,Oct,3; 2014,Nov,14; 2014,Jan,11 **99344** 2020,Sep,3; 2018,Jan,8; 2018,Apr,9; 2017,Jun,6; 2017,Jan,8; 2017,Aug,3; 2016,Jan,13; 2016,Jan,7; 2016,Dec,11; 2015,Jan,16; 2014,Oct,8; 2014,Oct,3; 2014,Nov,14; 2014,Jan,11 **99345** 2020,Sep,3; 2018,Jan,8; 2018,Apr,9; 2017,Jun,6; 2017,Jan,8; 2017,Aug,3; 2016,Jan,13; 2016,Jan,7; 2016,Dec,11; 2015,Jan,16; 2014,Oct,8; 2014,Oct,3; 2014,Nov,14; 2014,Jan,11

Relative Value Units/Medicare Edits

Non-Facility RVU	Work	PE	MP	Total
99341	1.01	0.48	0.05	1.54
99342	1.52	0.61	0.08	2.21
99343	2.53	0.97	0.13	3.63
99344	3.38	1.55	0.22	5.15
99345	4.09	1.9	0.28	6.27
Facility RVU	Work	PE	MP	Total
99341	1.01	0.48	0.05	1.54
99342	1.52	0.61	0.08	2.21
99343	2.53	0.97	0.13	3.63
99344	3.38	1.55	0.22	5.15
99345	4.09	1.9	0.28	6.27

	FUD	Status	MUE	Modifiers				IOM Reference
99341	N/A	A	1(2)	N/A	N/A	N/A	80*	100-04,12,30.6.4;
99342	N/A	A	1(2)	N/A	N/A	N/A	80*	100-04,12,30.6.14;
99343	N/A	A	1(2)	N/A	N/A	N/A	80*	100-04,12,30.6.14.1;
99344	N/A	A	1(2)	N/A	N/A	N/A	80*	100-04,12,30.6.15.1
99345	N/A	A	1(2)	N/A	N/A	N/A	80*	

* with documentation

Terms To Know

new patient. Patient who is receiving face-to-face care from a provider/qualified health care professional or another physician/qualified health care professional of the exact same specialty and subspecialty who belongs to the same group practice for the first time in three years. For OPPS hospitals, a patient who has not been registered as an inpatient or outpatient, including off-campus provider based clinic or emergency department, within the past three years.

other qualified health care professional. Individual who is qualified by education, training, licensure/regulation, and facility privileging to perform a professional service within his or her scope of practice and independently (or as incident-to) report the professional service without requiring physician supervision. Payers may state exemptions in writing or state and local regulations may not follow this definition for performance of some services. Always refer to any relevant plan policies and federal and/or state laws to determine who may perform and report services.

99347-99350

99347 Home visit for the evaluation and management of an established patient, which requires at least 2 of these 3 key components: A problem focused interval history; A problem focused examination; Straightforward medical decision making. Counseling and/or coordination of care with other physicians, other qualified health care professionals, or agencies are provided consistent with the nature of the problem(s) and the patient's and/or family's needs. Usually, the presenting problem(s) are self limited or minor. Typically, 15 minutes are spent face-to-face with the patient and/or family.

99348 Home visit for the evaluation and management of an established patient, which requires at least 2 of these 3 key components: An expanded problem focused interval history; An expanded problem focused examination; Medical decision making of low complexity. Counseling and/or coordination of care with other physicians, other qualified health care professionals, or agencies are provided consistent with the nature of the problem(s) and the patient's and/or family's needs. Usually, the presenting problem(s) are of low to moderate severity. Typically, 25 minutes are spent face-to-face with the patient and/or family.

99349 Home visit for the evaluation and management of an established patient, which requires at least 2 of these 3 key components: A detailed interval history; A detailed examination; Medical decision making of moderate complexity. Counseling and/or coordination of care with other physicians, other qualified health care professionals, or agencies are provided consistent with the nature of the problem(s) and the patient's and/or family's needs. Usually, the presenting problem(s) are moderate to high severity. Typically, 40 minutes are spent face-to-face with the patient and/or family.

99350 Home visit for the evaluation and management of an established patient, which requires at least 2 of these 3 key components: A comprehensive interval history; A comprehensive examination; Medical decision making of moderate to high complexity. Counseling and/or coordination of care with other physicians, other qualified health care professionals, or agencies are provided consistent with the nature of the problem(s) and the patient's and/or family's needs. Usually, the presenting problem(s) are of moderate to high severity. The patient may be unstable or may have developed a significant new problem requiring immediate physician attention. Typically, 60 minutes are spent face-to-face with the patient and/or family.

Explanation

Home services codes are reported by providers for E/M services rendered to established patients residing in a personal residence. Services are reported based on meeting two out of the three key components—history, exam, and medical decision making (MDM)—within each level of service. The most basic service, 99347, describes a problem focused history and exam with straightforward medical decision making for problems that are self-limiting or minor encompassing approximately 15 minutes of face-to-face time with the patient and/or family or caregiver. Mid-level services require an expanded problem focused history and exam or a detailed history and exam as represented by 99348 and 99349, respectively. Medical decision making for 99348 is designated as low complexity; moderate complexity for 99349. At these levels of service, the encounter can involve face-to-face time spent with the patient and/or family or caregiver of 25 (99348) to 40 minutes (99349) for low to moderate or moderate to high severity problems. The last level of service in this category, 99350, consists of a comprehensive history and examination as well as medical decision making of moderate to high complexity. The clinician can expect to spend approximately 60 minutes face-to-face duration with the patient and/or family or caregiver for moderate to high severity problems as a result of the patient being unstable or having developed a significant, new problem necessitating the immediate attention of the clinician.

Coding Tips

These codes are used to report evaluation and management services provided in a private residence for an established patient. Two of the three key components (history, exam, and medical decision making) must be met or exceeded for the level of service selected. Time may be used to select the level of service when counseling and coordination of care are documented as at least half of the time spent face-to-face with the patient. For commercial payers, consider assigning the appropriate consultation code instead of these codes when an opinion or advice about a specific problem has been requested by another qualified provider. Consultation codes are not covered by Medicare and some payers. Report new or established outpatient E/M codes for consultation services. For care plan oversight provided in the home under the care of a hospice agency, see 99377-99378; provided under the care of a home health agency, see 99374-99375. For care plan oversight services provided to a patient under home, domiciliary, or rest home (assisted living) care, see 99339-99340. Report place of service (POS) code 12 for services rendered in a private residence. Medicare has provisionally identified these codes as telehealth/telemedicine services. Current Medicare coverage guidelines should be reviewed. Commercial payers should be contacted regarding their coverage guidelines. Telemedicine services may be reported by the performing provider by adding modifier 95 to these procedure codes. Services at the origination site are reported with HCPCS Level II code Q3014.

ICD-10-CM Diagnostic Codes

The application of this code is too broad to adequately present ICD-10-CM diagnostic code links here. Refer to your ICD-10-CM book.

AMA: **99347** 2020,Sep,3; 2018,Jan,8; 2018,Apr,9; 2017,Jun,6; 2017,Jan,8; 2017,Aug,3; 2016,Jan,13; 2016,Jan,7; 2016,Dec,11; 2015,Jan,16; 2014,Oct,8; 2014,Oct,3; 2014,Nov,14; 2014,Jan,11 **99348** 2020,Sep,3; 2018,Jan,8; 2018,Apr,9; 2017,Jun,6; 2017,Jan,8; 2017,Aug,3; 2016,Jan,13; 2016,Jan,7; 2016,Dec,11; 2015,Jan,16; 2014,Oct,8; 2014,Oct,3; 2014,Nov,14; 2014,Jan,11 **99349** 2020,Sep,3; 2018,Jan,8; 2018,Apr,9; 2017,Jun,6; 2017,Jan,8; 2017,Aug,3; 2016,Jan,13; 2016,Jan,7; 2016,Dec,11; 2015,Jan,16; 2014,Oct,3; 2014,Oct,8; 2014,Nov,14; 2014,Jan,11 **99350** 2020,Sep,3; 2018,Jan,8; 2018,Apr,9; 2017,Jun,6; 2017,Jan,8; 2017,Aug,3; 2016,Jan,7; 2016,Jan,13; 2016,Dec,11; 2015,Jan,16; 2014,Oct,3; 2014,Oct,8; 2014,Nov,14; 2014,Jan,11

Relative Value Units/Medicare Edits

Non-Facility RVU	Work	PE	MP	Total
99347	1.0	0.49	0.05	1.54
99348	1.56	0.72	0.09	2.37
99349	2.33	1.17	0.13	3.63
99350	3.28	1.56	0.22	5.06
Facility RVU	Work	PE	MP	Total
99347	1.0	0.49	0.05	1.54
99348	1.56	0.72	0.09	2.37
99349	2.33	1.17	0.13	3.63
99350	3.28	1.56	0.22	5.06

	FUD	Status	MUE	Modifiers				IOM Reference
99347	N/A	A	1(3)	N/A	N/A	N/A	80*	None
99348	N/A	A	1(3)	N/A	N/A	N/A	80*	
99349	N/A	A	1(3)	N/A	N/A	N/A	80*	
99350	N/A	A	1(3)	N/A	N/A	N/A	80*	

* with documentation

Terms To Know

established patient. Patient who has received professional services in a face-to-face setting within the last three years from the same physician/qualified health care professional or another physician/qualified health care professional of the exact same specialty and subspecialty who belongs to the same group practice. If the patient is seen by a physician/qualified health care professional who is covering for another physician/qualified health care professional, the patient will be considered the same as if seen by the physician/qualified health care professional who is unavailable.

medical decision making. Consideration of the differential diagnoses, the amount and/or complexity of data reviewed and considered (medical records, test results, correspondence from previous treating physicians, etc.), current diagnostic studies ordered, and treatment or management options and risk (complications of the patient's condition, the potential for complications, continued morbidity, risk of mortality, any comorbidities associated with the patient's disease process).

99354-99359

+▲★99354 Prolonged service(s) in the outpatient setting requiring direct patient contact beyond the time of the usual service; first hour (List separately in addition to code for outpatient Evaluation and Management or psychotherapy service, except with office or other outpatient services [99202, 99203, 99204, 99205, 99212, 99213, 99214, 99215])

+▲★99355   each additional 30 minutes (List separately in addition to code for prolonged service)

+▲ 99356 Prolonged service in the inpatient or observation setting, requiring unit/floor time beyond the usual service; first hour (List separately in addition to code for inpatient or observation Evaluation and Management service)

+ 99357   each additional 30 minutes (List separately in addition to code for prolonged service)

99358 Prolonged evaluation and management service before and/or after direct patient care; first hour

+ 99359   each additional 30 minutes (List separately in addition to code for prolonged service)

Explanation

Prolonged services involve face-to-face patient contact or psychotherapy services beyond the typical service time and should only be reported once per day. Direct patient contact also includes additional non-face-to-face time, such as time spent on the patient's floor or unit in the hospital or nursing facility setting. For prolonged services rendered in the outpatient setting for the first hour, report 99354; for each additional 30 minutes, report 99355. For prolonged services rendered in the inpatient or observation setting for the first hour, report 99356; for each additional 30 minutes, report 99357. Codes should be reported using the total duration of face-to-face time spent by the clinician on the date of service even when the time spent is not continuous. Report prolonged service without direct patient contact with 99358-99359.

Coding Tips

These codes are used to report prolonged services, with direct patient contact (99354-99357) or without direct patient contact (99358-99359) beyond the usual service. These are time-based codes and time spent with the patient must be documented in the medical record. Codes 99354-99357 are only reported in addition to other time-based E/M services. Time spent on other separately reported services excluding the E/M service should not be counted toward the prolonged service time. Code selection is based on whether the service is provided in the outpatient setting or an inpatient or observation setting. For prolonged services provided by a physician or other qualified health care professional with or without direct patient contact in the office or other outpatient setting (i.e., 99205 or 99215), see 99417. For prolonged services provided by a physician or other qualified health care professional involving total time spent at the patient's bedside and on the floor/unit in the hospital or nursing facility, see 99356-99357. For prolonged services provided by a physician or other qualified health care professional without face-to-face contact or unit/floor time, see 99358-99359. Codes 99358-99359 may be reported on a different date of service than the primary service and do not require the primary service to have an established time. Prolonged service of less than 30 minutes should not be reported separately. Report 99354, 99356, and 99358 only once per day for the initial hour of prolonged service care; for each additional 30-minute block of time beyond the initial hour, see 99355, 99357, and 99359. For prolonged services provided by clinical staff, see 99415-99416. Do not report 99354-99355 with 99202-99205, 99212-99215, or 99415-99417. Report 99354 in addition to 90837, 90847, 99241-99245, 99324-99337, 99341-99350, and 99483. Report 99355 in addition to 99354. Report 99356 in addition to 90837, 90847, 99218-99220, 99221-99223,

99224-99226, 99231-99233, 99234-99236, 99251-99255, and 99304-99310. Report 99357 in addition to 99356. Do not report 99358-99359 on the same date of service as 99202-99205, 99212-99215, or 99417. Do not report 99358 or 99359 for time spent performing the following E/M or monitoring services: 93792-93793, 99339, 99340, 99374-99380, 99366-99368, 99421-99423, 99446-99449, 99451-99452, or 99491. Report 99359 in addition to 99358. Medicare has identified 99356 and 99357 as telehealth/telemedicine services. Commercial payers should be contacted regarding their coverage guidelines. Telemedicine services may be reported by the performing provider by adding modifier 95 to 99354-99357. Services at the origination site are reported with HCPCS Level II code Q3014.

ICD-10-CM Diagnostic Codes

This/these CPT code(s) are add-on code(s). See the primary procedure code that this code is performed with for your ICD-10-CM code selections.

AMA: **99354** 2020,Sep,3; 2020,Feb,3; 2019,Oct,10; 2019,Jun,7; 2018,Jan,8; 2017,Jan,8; 2016,Jan,13; 2016,Dec,11; 2015,Oct,3; 2015,Oct,9; 2015,Jan,16; 2014,Oct,8; 2014,Jun,14; 2014,Jan,11; 2014,Apr,6 **99355** 2020,Sep,3; 2020,Feb,3; 2019,Oct,10; 2019,Jun,7; 2018,Jan,8; 2017,Jan,8; 2016,Jan,13; 2016,Dec,11; 2015,Oct,3; 2015,Oct,9; 2015,Jan,16; 2014,Oct,8; 2014,Jun,14; 2014,Jan,11; 2014,Apr,6 **99356** 2020,Sep,3; 2019,Jun,7; 2018,Jan,8; 2017,Jan,8; 2016,Jan,13; 2016,Dec,11; 2015,Oct,3; 2015,Oct,9; 2015,Jan,16; 2014,Oct,8; 2014,Jun,14; 2014,Jan,11; 2014,Apr,6 **99357** 2020,Sep,3; 2019,Jun,7; 2018,Jan,8; 2017,Jan,8; 2016,Jan,13; 2016,Dec,11; 2015,Oct,3; 2015,Oct,9; 2015,Jan,16; 2014,Oct,8; 2014,Jun,14; 2014,Jan,11; 2014,Apr,6 **99358** 2020,Sep,3; 2020,Feb,3; 2019,Jun,7; 2019,Jan,13; 2018,Oct,9; 2018,Jan,8; 2017,Jan,8; 2016,Jan,13; 2015,Jan,16; 2014,Oct,3; 2014,Oct,8; 2014,Jan,11 **99359** 2020,Sep,3; 2020,Feb,3; 2019,Jun,7; 2019,Jan,13; 2018,Oct,9; 2018,Jan,8; 2017,Jan,8; 2016,Jan,13; 2015,Jan,16; 2014,Oct,3; 2014,Oct,8; 2014,Jan,11

Relative Value Units/Medicare Edits

Non-Facility RVU	Work	PE	MP	Total
99354	2.33	1.18	0.15	3.66
99355	1.77	0.9	0.11	2.78
99356	1.71	0.79	0.11	2.61
99357	1.71	0.81	0.11	2.63
99358	2.1	0.92	0.13	3.15
99359	1.0	0.46	0.08	1.54
Facility RVU	**Work**	**PE**	**MP**	**Total**
99354	2.33	0.96	0.15	3.44
99355	1.77	0.71	0.11	2.59
99356	1.71	0.79	0.11	2.61
99357	1.71	0.81	0.11	2.63
99358	2.1	0.92	0.13	3.15
99359	1.0	0.46	0.08	1.54

	FUD	Status	MUE	Modifiers				IOM Reference
99354	N/A	A	1(2)	N/A	N/A	N/A	80*	100-04,11,40.1.3; 100-04,12,30.6.4; 100-04,12,30.6.13; 100-04,12,30.6.14; 100-04,12,30.6.15.1; 100-04,12,30.6.15.2; 100-04,12,100
99355	N/A	A	4(3)	N/A	N/A	N/A	80*	
99356	N/A	A	1(2)	N/A	N/A	N/A	80*	
99357	N/A	A	4(3)	N/A	N/A	N/A	80*	
99358	N/A	A	1(2)	N/A	N/A	N/A	80*	
99359	N/A	A	2(3)	N/A	N/A	N/A	80*	

* with documentation

[99415, 99416]

+▲ **99415** Prolonged clinical staff service (the service beyond the highest time in the range of total time of the service) during an evaluation and management service in the office or outpatient setting, direct patient contact with physician supervision; first hour (List separately in addition to code for outpatient Evaluation and Management service)

+▲ **99416** Prolonged clinical staff service (the service beyond the highest time in the range of total time of the service) during an evaluation and management service in the office or outpatient setting, direct patient contact with physician supervision; each additional 30 minutes (List separately in addition to code for prolonged service)

Explanation

Prolonged clinical staff services are reported with resequenced codes that were added to describe special situations in which the physician's staff provided assistance to a patient beyond the usual time associated with circumstances requiring observation of the patient, such as in cases where the patient was administered a new medication or inhaled drug requiring monitoring to ensure patient safety in the office or outpatient setting. Such cases do not necessitate the clinician being face-to-face with the patient throughout the entire time period; observation and monitoring of the patient can be performed by a member of the clinician's staff under the provider's supervision. Report these codes in conjunction with the designated E/M service code along with any other service provided at the same encounter. Codes in this category should report the total amount of face-to-face time spent with the patient by the clinical staff on the same date of service even if the time is not continuous; time spent rendering other separately reportable services other than the E/M service do not count toward the prolonged services time. The highest total time in the time ranges of the code descriptions is used in defining when prolonged services time should begin. Report the first hour of prolonged services on a given date with 99415; for each additional 30 minutes of prolonged services, report 99416.

Coding Tips

These codes are used to report prolonged face-to-face services beyond the highest total time indicated in the code description provided by the clinical staff in the office or outpatient setting. These are time-based codes and time spent with the patient must be documented in the medical record. Time spent on other separately reported services excluding the E/M service should not be counted toward the prolonged service time. These codes are reported in addition to the other E/M service provided on the same date of service. A provider must be available to provide direct supervision of the clinical staff. Report 99415 only once per day for the initial hour of prolonged service care; for each additional 30-minute block of time beyond the initial hour, see 99416. Prolonged service of less than 30 minutes should not be reported separately. For prolonged services with or without direct patient contact provided by the physician or other qualified health care provider in the office or other outpatient setting, see 99417. Do not report 99415-99416 with 99354, 99355, or 99417. Report 99415 in addition to 99202-99205 and 99212-99215. Report 99416 in addition to 99415.

ICD-10-CM Diagnostic Codes

This/these CPT code(s) are add-on code(s). See the primary procedure code that this code is performed with for your ICD-10-CM code selections.

AMA: **99415** 2020,Sep,3; 2020,Feb,3; 2019,Oct,10; 2018,Jan,8; 2017,Jan,8; 2016,Mar,8; 2016,Jan,13; 2016,Feb,13; 2015,Oct,3 **99416** 2020,Sep,3; 2020,Feb,3;

2019,Oct,10; 2018,Jan,8; 2017,Jan,8; 2016,Mar,8; 2016,Jan,13; 2016,Feb,13; 2015,Oct,3

Relative Value Units/Medicare Edits

Non-Facility RVU	Work	PE	MP	Total
99415	0.0	0.27	0.01	0.28
99416	0.0	0.12	0.0	0.12
Facility RVU	Work	PE	MP	Total
99415	0.0	0.27	0.01	0.28
99416	0.0	0.12	0.0	0.12

	FUD	Status	MUE	Modifiers				IOM Reference
99415	N/A	A	1(2)	N/A	N/A	N/A	80*	None
99416	N/A	A	3(3)	N/A	N/A	N/A	80*	

* with documentation

Terms To Know

clinical staff. Someone who works for, or under, the direction of a physician or qualified health care professional and does not bill services separately. The person may be licensed or regulated to help the physician perform specific duties.

direct supervision. Situation in which the physician must be present in the office suite and immediately available to provide assistance and direction throughout a given procedure. The physician is not, however, required to be present in the room when the procedure is performed.

face to face. Interaction between two parties, usually provider and patient, that occurs in the physical presence of each other.

[99417]

+●★99417 Prolonged office or other outpatient evaluation and management service(s) beyond the minimum required time of the primary procedure which has been selected using total time, requiring total time with or without direct patient contact beyond the usual service, on the date of the primary service, each 15 minutes of total time (List separately in addition to codes 99205, 99215 for office or other outpatient Evaluation and Management services)

Explanation

Code 99417 reports prolonged total time (time with and without direct patient contact combined) that is provided by the physician or other qualified health care professional on the date of an office visit or other outpatient service. This code is assigned only when the code for the primary E/M service has been selected based solely on total time, and only after exceeding by 15 minutes the minimum time that is required to report the highest-level service. For example, when reporting an established patient encounter (99215), code 99417 would not be reported until at least 15 minutes of time beyond 40 minutes has been accumulated (i.e., 55 minutes) on the day of the encounter.

Coding Tips

This code reports prolonged service time by the physician or other qualified health care professional provided on the same date as 99205 or 99215. The prolonged time may be with or without direct patient contact. This service is reported only when time was the criteria used to select code 99205 or 99215 and the time exceeds the minimum time required to report these levels of service by at least 15 minutes. Code 99417 may be reported once for each additional 15 minutes spent providing prolonged services. Time performing other reportable services is not counted as prolonged service. Prolonged services provided on a date other than the date of the face-to-face encounter may be reported with 99358-99359. Prolonged services provided by clinical staff are reported with 99415-99416. Do not report 99417 with 99354-99355, 99358-99359, or 99415-99416. Telemedicine services may be reported by the performing provider by adding modifier 95 to this procedure code. Services at the origination site are reported with HCPCS Level II code Q3014.

ICD-10-CM Diagnostic Codes

The application of this code is too broad to adequately present ICD-10-CM diagnostic code links here. Refer to your ICD-10-CM book.

Relative Value Units/Medicare Edits

Non-Facility RVU	Work	PE	MP	Total
99417				
Facility RVU	**Work**	**PE**	**MP**	**Total**
99417				

	FUD	Status	MUE	Modifiers				IOM Reference
99417	N/A		-	N/A	N/A	N/A	N/A	None

* with documentation

Terms To Know

prolonged physician services. Extended pre- or post-service care provided to a patient whose condition requires services beyond the usual.

99406-99409

★99406 Smoking and tobacco use cessation counseling visit; intermediate, greater than 3 minutes up to 10 minutes
★99407   intensive, greater than 10 minutes
★99408 Alcohol and/or substance (other than tobacco) abuse structured screening (eg, AUDIT, DAST), and brief intervention (SBI) services; 15 to 30 minutes
★99409   greater than 30 minutes

Explanation

Individual behavior change intervention services are counseling and/or intervention services directed at high-risk behaviors such as tobacco, alcohol, and substance abuse. These services can be reported as treatment of the condition or in relation to the condition that has the potential of causing illness or injury. Additionally, the encounter uses validated instruments to determine the patient's opinion related to behavior change and providing input on a plan to change behavior with appropriate actions and motivation. Report 99406 for smoking and tobacco cessation counseling requiring three to 10 minutes of time and 99407 for counseling requiring more than ten minutes. Report 99408 for alcohol and/or substance abuse screening utilizing such instruments as AUDIT, DAST, and intervention services requiring 15 to 30 minutes; for more than 30 minutes, report 99409.

Coding Tips

These codes are used to report interventional counseling services provided to patients to promote behavioral change when the behavior is considered an illness itself or to change the behavior before it results in an illness. These are time-based codes and time spent with the patient must be documented in the medical record. When documentation supports that a significant, separately identifiable problem-oriented evaluation and management (E/M) service is rendered, the appropriate code for the E/M service may be reported separately. Append modifier 25 to the service code selected to indicate that a separately identifiable E/M service was provided on the same date of service as the counseling service. Codes 99408 and 99409 should only be reported for the initial screening and brief intervention. Do not report 99407 in addition to 99406. Do not report 99409 in addition to 99408. Do not report 99408 or 99409 in addition to 96160-96161. Do not report 96156-96159 or 96164-96171 in addition to 99406-99409 on the same date of service. For preventive medicine counseling provided to an individual, see 99401-99404. For preventive medicine counseling provided in a group setting, see 99411-99412. Telemedicine services may be reported by the performing provider by adding modifier 95 to these procedure codes. Services at the origination site are reported with HCPCS Level II code Q3014.

ICD-10-CM Diagnostic Codes

Z71.41	Alcohol abuse counseling and surveillance of alcoholic
Z71.42	Counseling for family member of alcoholic
Z71.6	Tobacco abuse counseling
Z72.0	Tobacco use

AMA: **99406** 2020,Sep,14; 2020,Aug,3; 2018,Jan,8; 2017,Nov,3; 2017,Jan,8; 2016,Mar,8; 2016,Jan,13; 2015,Jan,16; 2014,Oct,8; 2014,Jan,11 **99407** 2020,Aug,3; 2018,Jan,8; 2017,Nov,3; 2017,Jan,8; 2016,Mar,8; 2016,Jan,13; 2015,Jan,16; 2014,Oct,8; 2014,Jan,11 **99408** 2020,Aug,3; 2018,Jan,8; 2017,Nov,3; 2017,Jan,8; 2016,Nov,5; 2016,Mar,8; 2016,Jan,13; 2015,Jan,16; 2014,Oct,8; 2014,Jan,11 **99409** 2020,Aug,3; 2018,Jan,8; 2017,Nov,3; 2017,Jan,8; 2016,Nov,5; 2016,Mar,8; 2016,Jan,13; 2015,Jan,16; 2014,Oct,8; 2014,Jan,11

Relative Value Units/Medicare Edits

Non-Facility RVU	Work	PE	MP	Total
99406	0.24	0.17	0.02	0.43
99407	0.5	0.27	0.05	0.82
99408	0.65	0.32	0.05	1.02
99409	1.3	0.57	0.11	1.98
Facility RVU	Work	PE	MP	Total
99406	0.24	0.09	0.02	0.35
99407	0.5	0.19	0.05	0.74
99408	0.65	0.25	0.05	0.95
99409	1.3	0.5	0.11	1.91

	FUD	Status	MUE	Modifiers				IOM Reference
99406	N/A	A	1(2)	N/A	N/A	N/A	80*	None
99407	N/A	A	1(2)	N/A	N/A	N/A	80*	
99408	N/A	N	0(3)	N/A	N/A	N/A	N/A	
99409	N/A	N	0(3)	N/A	N/A	N/A	N/A	

* with documentation

Terms To Know

AUDIT. Alcohol use disorder identification test.

behavior management. Education and modification techniques or methodologies aimed at helping a patient change undesirable habits or behaviors.

counseling. Discussion with a patient and/or family concerning one or more of the following areas: diagnostic results, impressions, and/or recommended diagnostic studies; prognosis; risks and benefits of management (treatment) options; instructions for management (treatment) and/or follow-up; importance of compliance with chosen management (treatment) options; risk factor reduction; and patient and family education.

DAST. Drug abuse screening test.

intervention. Purposeful interaction of the physical therapist with the patient and, when appropriate, with other individuals involved in patient care, using various physical therapy procedures and techniques to produce changes in the condition.

99441-99443

99441 Telephone evaluation and management service by a physician or other qualified health care professional who may report evaluation and management services provided to an established patient, parent, or guardian not originating from a related E/M service provided within the previous 7 days nor leading to an E/M service or procedure within the next 24 hours or soonest available appointment; 5-10 minutes of medical discussion

99442 11-20 minutes of medical discussion

99443 21-30 minutes of medical discussion

Explanation

Telephone services are non-face-to-face encounters originating from the established patient for evaluation or management of a problem provided by a qualified clinician. The problem may not be related to an E/M encounter that occurred within the previous seven days nor can the problem lead to an E/M encounter or other service within the following 24 hours or next available in-office appointment opening. Report 99441 for services lasting five to 10 minutes; 99442 for services lasting 11 to 20 minutes; and 99443 for calls lasting 21 to 30 minutes.

Coding Tips

These codes are used to report non-face-to-face patient services initiated by an established patient via the telephone. These are time-based codes and time spent with the patient must be documented in the medical record. These codes should not be reported if the provider decides to see the patient within 24 hours or by the next available urgent visit appointment, or if the provider performed a related E/M service within the previous seven days or the call is initiated within a postoperative period. Medicare and other payers may not reimburse separately for these services. Check with the specific payer to determine coverage. Do not report 99441-99443 when the same provider has reported 99421-99423 for the same problem in the previous seven days. For nonphysician telephone medical services, see 98966-98968. Do not report these services when performed concurrently with other billable services, such as 99339-99340, 99374-99380, 99487-99489, or 99495-99496. Do not report these services for INR monitoring when reporting 93792 or 93793. Medicare has provisionally identified these codes as telehealth/telemedicine services. Current Medicare coverage guidelines should be reviewed. Commercial payers should be contacted regarding their coverage guidelines. Telemedicine services may be reported by the performing provider by adding modifier 95 to these procedure codes. Services at the origination site are reported with HCPCS Level II code Q3014.

ICD-10-CM Diagnostic Codes

The application of this code is too broad to adequately present ICD-10-CM diagnostic code links here. Refer to your ICD-10-CM book.

AMA: 99441 2020,Jul,1; 2019,Mar,8; 2018,Mar,7; 2018,Jan,8; 2017,Jan,8; 2016,Jan,13; 2015,Jan,16; 2014,Oct,8; 2014,Oct,3; 2014,Jan,11 **99442** 2020,Jul,1; 2019,Mar,8; 2018,Mar,7; 2018,Jan,8; 2017,Jan,8; 2016,Jan,13; 2015,Jan,16; 2014,Oct,3; 2014,Oct,8; 2014,Jan,11 **99443** 2020,Jul,1; 2019,Mar,8; 2018,Mar,7; 2018,Jan,8; 2017,Jan,8; 2016,Jan,13; 2015,Jan,16; 2014,Oct,3; 2014,Oct,8; 2014,Jan,11

Relative Value Units/Medicare Edits

Non-Facility RVU	Work	PE	MP	Total
99441	0.48	0.75	0.05	1.28
99442	0.97	1.06	0.08	2.11
99443	1.5	1.45	0.11	3.06
Facility RVU	Work	PE	MP	Total
99441	0.48	0.2	0.05	0.73
99442	0.97	0.4	0.08	1.45
99443	1.5	0.62	0.11	2.23

	FUD	Status	MUE	Modifiers				IOM Reference
99441	N/A	A	1(2)	N/A	N/A	N/A	80*	None
99442	N/A	A	1(2)	N/A	N/A	N/A	80*	
99443	N/A	A	1(2)	N/A	N/A	N/A	80*	

* with documentation

Terms To Know

established patient. Patient who has received professional services in a face-to-face setting within the last three years from the same physician/qualified health care professional or another physician/qualified health care professional of the exact same specialty and subspecialty who belongs to the same group practice. If the patient is seen by a physician/qualified health care professional who is covering for another physician/qualified health care professional, the patient will be considered the same as if seen by the physician/qualified health care professional who is unavailable.

other qualified health care professional. Individual who is qualified by education, training, licensure/regulation, and facility privileging to perform a professional service within his or her scope of practice and independently (or as incident-to) report the professional service without requiring physician supervision. Payers may state exemptions in writing or state and local regulations may not follow this definition for performance of some services. Always refer to any relevant plan policies and federal and/or state laws to determine who may perform and report services.

E/M Services

[99421, 99422, 99423]

99421 Online digital evaluation and management service, for an established patient, for up to 7 days, cumulative time during the 7 days; 5-10 minutes

99422 Online digital evaluation and management service, for an established patient, for up to 7 days, cumulative time during the 7 days; 11-20 minutes

99423 Online digital evaluation and management service, for an established patient, for up to 7 days, cumulative time during the 7 days; 21 or more minutes

Explanation

Online medical evaluation services are non-face-to-face encounters originating from the established patient to the physician or other qualified health care professional for evaluation or management of a problem utilizing internet resources. The service includes all communication, prescription, and laboratory orders with permanent storage in the patient's medical record. The service may include more than one provider responding to the same patient and is only reportable once during seven days for the same encounter. Do not report these codes if the online patient request is related to an E/M service that occurred within the previous seven days or within the global period following a procedure. Report 99421 if the cumulative time during the seven-day period is five to 10 minutes; 99422 for 11 to 20 minutes; and 99423 for 21 or more minutes.

Coding Tips

These codes are used to report non-face-to-face patient services initiated by an established patient via an on-line inquiry. Providers must provide a timely response to the inquiry and the encounter must be stored permanently to report this service. These services are reported once in a seven-day period and are reported for the cumulative time devoted to the service over the seven days. Cumulative time of less than five minutes should not be reported. A new/unrelated problem initiated within seven days of a previous E/M visit that addresses a different problem may be reported separately. Medicare and other payers may not reimburse separately for these services. Check with the specific payer to determine coverage. For nonphysician on-line medical services, see 98970, 98971, and 98972. Do not report these services when performed concurrently with other billable services, such as 99202-99205, 99212-99215, 99241-99245, or when using the following codes for the same communication: 99091, 99339-99340, 99374-99380, or 99487-99489. Do not report these services for INR monitoring when reporting 93792 or 93793.

ICD-10-CM Diagnostic Codes

The application of this code is too broad to adequately present ICD-10-CM diagnostic code links here. Refer to your ICD-10-CM book.

AMA: **99421** 2020,Jan,3 **99422** 2020,Jan,3 **99423** 2020,Jan,3

Relative Value Units/Medicare Edits

Non-Facility RVU	Work	PE	MP	Total
99421	0.25	0.16	0.02	0.43
99422	0.5	0.31	0.05	0.86
99423	0.8	0.51	0.08	1.39
Facility RVU	Work	PE	MP	Total
99421	0.25	0.1	0.02	0.37
99422	0.5	0.21	0.05	0.76
99423	0.8	0.33	0.08	1.21

	FUD	Status	MUE	Modifiers				IOM Reference
99421	N/A	A	1(2)	N/A	N/A	N/A	80*	None
99422	N/A	A	1(2)	N/A	N/A	N/A	80*	
99423	N/A	A	1(2)	N/A	N/A	N/A	80*	

* with documentation

Terms To Know

established patient. Patient who has received professional services in a face-to-face setting within the last three years from the same physician/qualified health care professional or another physician/qualified health care professional of the exact same specialty and subspecialty who belongs to the same group practice. If the patient is seen by a physician/qualified health care professional who is covering for another physician/qualified health care professional, the patient will be considered the same as if seen by the physician/qualified health care professional who is unavailable.

evaluation. Dynamic process in which the clinician makes clinical judgments based on data gathered during the examination.

99487-99489 [99439, 99490, 99491]

▲ **99490** Chronic care management services with the following required elements: multiple (two or more) chronic conditions expected to last at least 12 months, or until the death of the patient, chronic conditions place the patient at significant risk of death, acute exacerbation/decompensation, or functional decline, comprehensive care plan established, implemented, revised, or monitored; first 20 minutes of clinical staff time directed by a physician or other qualified health care professional, per calendar month.

+● **99439** Chronic care management services with the following required elements: multiple (two or more) chronic conditions expected to last at least 12 months, or until the death of the patient, chronic conditions place the patient at significant risk of death, acute exacerbation/decompensation, or functional decline, comprehensive care plan established, implemented, revised, or monitored; each additional 20 minutes of clinical staff time directed by a physician or other qualified health care professional, per calendar month (List separately in addition to code for primary procedure)

99491 Chronic care management services, provided personally by a physician or other qualified health care professional, at least 30 minutes of physician or other qualified health care professional time, per calendar month, with the following required elements: multiple (two or more) chronic conditions expected to last at least 12 months, or until the death of the patient; chronic conditions place the patient at significant risk of death, acute exacerbation/decompensation, or functional decline; comprehensive care plan established, implemented, revised, or monitored

▲ **99487** Complex chronic care management services with the following required elements: multiple (two or more) chronic conditions expected to last at least 12 months, or until the death of the patient, chronic conditions place the patient at significant risk of death, acute exacerbation/decompensation, or functional decline, comprehensive care plan established, implemented, revised, or monitored, moderate or high complexity medical decision making; first 60 minutes of clinical staff time directed by a physician or other qualified health care professional, per calendar month.

+▲ **99489** each additional 30 minutes of clinical staff time directed by a physician or other qualified health care professional, per calendar month (List separately in addition to code for primary procedure)

Explanation

Care management services are defined as the management and support services rendered by clinical staff under the supervision of a qualified clinician for patients living in a personal residence, domiciliary, rest home, or assisted living facility. Some components of care management services include, but are not limited to, creating, implementing, altering, or monitoring a care plan; coordinating with other professionals and/or agencies; and providing education to the patient or caregiver on the patient's medical condition, care plan, and prognosis. The clinician is also responsible for the oversight of those services, as well as for the patient's other medical conditions, psychosocial needs, and normal activities of daily living (ADL). Care plans address all of the patient's health issues and are based on a thorough evaluation involving assessment of the patient's physical, mental, cognitive, social, and functional health, as well as an environmental review, and are revised as necessary. Codes may only be reported by the clinician who has the role of care manager with a particular patient for that one-month period. Time spent face-to-face or non-face-to-face with clinical staff communicating with the patient, family, caregivers, other health care professionals, and agencies revising, documenting, and putting into action the care plan or teaching the patient self-management skills or techniques may be used to determine the care management staff time for that one-month time period. Time with clinical staff is reported only when there are two or more staff members meeting regarding the specific patient. Additionally, time with clinical staff should not be counted if the clinician has reported an E/M service for that same date. Generally, services provided by clinical staff involve such activities as ongoing review of the patient's status, including reviewing laboratory or other test results that are not reported as part of an E/M service, evaluating whether the patient is following the treatment regime, and medication management. Chronic care management services are represented by resequenced codes 99490, 99439, and 99491 and describe services provided to patients with medical and/or psychosocial needs that necessitate creating, implementing, changing, or monitoring the care plan. Typically, patients receiving this care have a minimum of two and possibly more chronic ongoing or episodic health conditions that are anticipated to last at least one year or until the patient expires and put the patient at increased risk of death, exacerbation, or functional decline. Code 99490 should be reported once per calendar month for the first 20 minutes of clinical staff time when directed by a physician or other qualified health care professional; for each additional 20 minutes, report 99439. Code 99439 should not be reported more than twice per calendar month. Code 99491 is also reported monthly and represents at least 30 minutes of the physician or other qualified health care professional involved with care management activities. Complex chronic care management services represented by 99487 and add-on code 99489 differ from chronic care management in that the adult patient generally has at least two or more complex chronic conditions being treated by three or more prescription medications and generally receives other types of interventions including physical or occupational therapy; pediatric patients usually receive three or more interventions that may include medications, nutritional support, or respiratory therapy. Complex chronic care management services consist of problems that require medical decision making of moderate or high complexity. Report 99487 when approximately one hour of clinical staff time overseen by a clinician is rendered during a single calendar month. Report 99489 for each additional 30 minutes.

Coding Tips

These codes are used to report care management services provided by the clinical staff under the direction of a qualified health care professional to a patient residing at home or in an assisted living facility, domiciliary, or rest home. These are time-based codes and total time spent performing care management services during the calendar month should be documented in the patient record. Do not report these codes if all elements listed in the code description are not performed. If the physician provides face-to-face E/M visits in the same calendar month, these visits may be reported separately. Do not count clinical staff time for a particular day if the physician reports an E/M service on that day. Codes 99487-99489 and 99490-99491 may only be reported once per calendar month by the provider that assumes the care management role for the patient. Code 99489 should only be reported in addition to 99487. Do not report 99490 if less than 20 minutes of chronic care management is provided in the calendar month. Code 99439 should be reported with 99490 for each additional 20 minutes of clinical staff time provided. This code should not be reported more than twice per 30-day period. Report 99491 when more than 30 minutes of chronic care management is provided by the physician or other qualified health care provider in the same calendar month. Do not report 99439 or 99490 with 99491 during the same calendar month; do not report

any of the three with 99487 or 99489. Do not report 99487 if less than 60 minutes of complex chronic care management is provided in a calendar month. Do not report 99489 if less than 30 minutes of additional time beyond the first 60 minutes of complex chronic care is provided. Do not report these codes in addition to 90951-90970 for ESRD services or in the postoperative period of a reported surgery. Do not report these codes in addition to 99339-99340, 99374-99380, or 99605-99607 in the same calendar month. Do not report 99439, 99487, 99489, 99490, or 99491 for service time reported with 93792-93793, 98960-98962, 98966-98968, 99071, 99078, 99080, 99091, 99358-99359, 99366-99368, 99421-99423, or 99441-99443. Do not report 99439 or 99490 with 98970-98972 or 99605-99607 for the same time period. In addition, do not report 99487 with 98969 for the same time period. For psychiatric care management services, see 99492-99494.

ICD-10-CM Diagnostic Codes

The application of this code is too broad to adequately present ICD-10-CM diagnostic code links here. Refer to your ICD-10-CM book.

AMA: 99487 2020,Feb,7; 2020,Apr,5; 2019,Jan,6; 2018,Oct,9; 2018,Mar,5; 2018,Mar,7; 2018,Jul,12; 2018,Jan,8; 2018,Feb,7; 2018,Apr,9; 2017,Jan,8; 2017,Apr,9; 2016,Jan,13; 2015,Jan,16; 2014,Oct,3; 2014,Oct,8; 2014,Jun,3; 2014,Jan,11; 2014,Feb,3 **99489** 2020,Feb,7; 2020,Apr,5; 2019,Jan,6; 2018,Oct,9; 2018,Mar,7; 2018,Mar,5; 2018,Jul,12; 2018,Jan,8; 2018,Feb,7; 2018,Apr,9; 2017,Jan,8; 2017,Apr,9; 2016,Jan,13; 2015,Jan,16; 2014,Oct,3; 2014,Oct,8; 2014,Jun,3; 2014,Jan,11 **99490** 2020,Feb,7; 2020,Apr,5; 2019,Jan,6; 2018,Oct,9; 2018,Mar,5; 2018,Mar,7; 2018,Jul,12; 2018,Jan,8; 2018,Feb,7; 2018,Apr,9; 2017,Jan,8; 2016,Jan,13; 2015,Jan,16; 2015,Feb,3; 2014,Oct,3 **99491** 2020,Apr,5

Relative Value Units/Medicare Edits

Non-Facility RVU	Work	PE	MP	Total
99490	0.61	0.51	0.05	1.17
99439				
99491	1.45	0.79	0.09	2.33
99487	1.0	1.5	0.06	2.56
99489	0.5	0.71	0.03	1.24
Facility RVU	Work	PE	MP	Total
99490	0.61	0.25	0.05	0.91
99439				
99491	1.45	0.79	0.09	2.33
99487	1.0	0.42	0.06	1.48
99489	0.5	0.2	0.03	0.73

	FUD	Status	MUE	Modifiers				IOM Reference
99490	N/A	A	1(2)	N/A	N/A	N/A	80*	None
99439	N/A		-	N/A	N/A	N/A	N/A	
99491	N/A	A	1(2)	N/A	N/A	N/A	80*	
99487	N/A	A	1(2)	N/A	N/A	N/A	80*	
99489	N/A	A	10(3)	N/A	N/A	N/A	80*	

* with documentation

99495-99496

★**99495** Transitional Care Management Services with the following required elements: Communication (direct contact, telephone, electronic) with the patient and/or caregiver within 2 business days of discharge Medical decision making of at least moderate complexity during the service period Face-to-face visit, within 14 calendar days of discharge

★**99496** Transitional Care Management Services with the following required elements: Communication (direct contact, telephone, electronic) with the patient and/or caregiver within 2 business days of discharge Medical decision making of high complexity during the service period Face-to-face visit, within 7 calendar days of discharge

Explanation

Transitional care management services are reported for patients requiring moderate to high complex medical decision making who are transitioning from an inpatient facility to a home or community type setting, such as a domiciliary or assisted living facility. The start date is the day of discharge from the inpatient setting and lasts through the following 29 days. These services include one face-to-face encounter in addition to other services performed within the specific timeframe by licensed clinical staff. These services are provided under direct qualified clinician supervision and may include communication with family and care givers, evaluation of treatment and medication, education on resources with assistance to available care, and review of discharge information, follow-up appointments, and interaction with other qualified health care professionals. To report these services, the initial direct contact (includes telephone/electronic) must occur within two days of discharge with review of medication regimen by the date of the initial face-to-face encounter. The date of the direct contact and medical decision making drives the code selection. Report 99495 when MDM is at least moderate complexity in addition to the face-to-face encounter within 14 days of hospital discharge. Report 99496 when MDM is high complexity in addition to the face-to-face encounter within seven days of hospital discharge.

Coding Tips

These codes are used to report services provided to a new or established patient whose medical or psychological issues necessitate a moderate or high level of medical decision making while transitioning from an inpatient facility, partial hospital, observation status, or skilled nursing facility to an assisted living facility, home, domiciliary, or rest home. Transitional care management (TCM) services require a face-to-face visit, initial patient contact, and medication reconciliation all within a specific timeframe. Do not report these codes if all elements listed in the code description are not performed. These codes may only be reported one time within 30 days of discharge and by only one provider. Code 99495 requires the face-to-face visit within 14 calendar days of discharge. Code 99496 requires one face-to-face visit within seven calendar days of discharge. If the physician or other qualified health care professional provides more than one face-to-face E/M visit within the 30 days, these visits may be reported separately. Do not report 99495 or 99496 in addition to 93792 or 93793. Do not report these codes when reporting 99441-99443 or 99497-99498. Telemedicine services may be reported by the performing provider by adding modifier 95 to these procedure codes. Services at the origination site are reported with HCPCS Level II code Q3014.

ICD-10-CM Diagnostic Codes

The application of this code is too broad to adequately present ICD-10-CM diagnostic code links here. Refer to your ICD-10-CM book.

AMA: **99495** 2020,Jan,3; 2020,Feb,7; 2019,Jan,6; 2018,Mar,7; 2018,Mar,5; 2018,Jul,12; 2018,Jan,8; 2018,Feb,7; 2018,Apr,9; 2017,Jan,8; 2016,Jan,13; 2015,Jan,16; 2014,Oct,8; 2014,Oct,3; 2014,Mar,13; 2014,Jan,11 **99496** 2020,Jan,3; 2020,Feb,7; 2019,Jan,6; 2018,Mar,7; 2018,Mar,5; 2018,Jul,12; 2018,Jan,8; 2018,Feb,7; 2018,Apr,9; 2017,Jan,8; 2016,Jan,13; 2015,Jan,16; 2014,Oct,3; 2014,Oct,8; 2014,Mar,13; 2014,Jan,11

Relative Value Units/Medicare Edits

Non-Facility RVU	Work	PE	MP	Total
99495	2.36	2.71	0.13	5.2
99496	3.1	3.58	0.19	6.87
Facility RVU	**Work**	**PE**	**MP**	**Total**
99495	2.36	0.99	0.13	3.48
99496	3.1	1.3	0.19	4.59

	FUD	Status	MUE	Modifiers				IOM Reference
99495	N/A	A	1(2)	N/A	N/A	N/A	80*	None
99496	N/A	A	1(2)	N/A	N/A	N/A	80*	

* with documentation

Terms To Know

coordination of care. Care provided concurrently with counseling that includes treatment instructions to the patient or caregiver; special accommodations for home, work, school, vacation, or other locations; coordination with other providers and agencies; and living arrangements.

domiciliary. Facility, such as an assisted living, group home, custodial care, or an intermediate care facility, that provides room and board on a long-term basis and may include personal assistance services.

face to face. Interaction between two parties, usually provider and patient, that occurs in the physical presence of each other.

medical decision making. Consideration of the differential diagnoses, the amount and/or complexity of data reviewed and considered (medical records, test results, correspondence from previous treating physicians, etc.), current diagnostic studies ordered, and treatment or management options and risk (complications of the patient's condition, the potential for complications, continued morbidity, risk of mortality, any comorbidities associated with the patient's disease process).

99497-99498

99497 Advance care planning including the explanation and discussion of advance directives such as standard forms (with completion of such forms, when performed), by the physician or other qualified health care professional; first 30 minutes, face-to-face with the patient, family member(s), and/or surrogate

+ 99498 each additional 30 minutes (List separately in addition to code for primary procedure)

Explanation

Advance care planning services are reported for the discussion and explanation of advanced directives by a qualified clinician. These services are time-based services that do not involve any active management of problems during the course of the face-to-face service between the provider and a patient, family member, or surrogate and may be reported on the same day as another E/M service. Report 99497 for the first 30 minutes of advance care planning and 99498 for each additional 30 minutes.

Coding Tips

These codes are used to report counseling and discussion of advance care directives face-to-face with the patient, family member, or surrogate. An advance directive document appointing an agent and/or recording of the wishes of the patient's medical treatment should be recorded in the medical record. These codes may be reported separately when performed on the same day as another E/M service. Use 99498 in addition to 99497. These codes may be reported in addition to the following E/M codes when performed on the same date of service: 99202-99215, 99217-99226, 99231-99236, 99238-99239, 99241-99245, 99251-99255, 99281-99285, 99304-99310, 99315-99316, 99318, 99324-99328, 99334-99337, 99341-99345, 99347-99350, 99381-99397, and 99495-99496. Do not report these codes when reporting 99291-99292, 99468-99469, 99471-99472, 99475-99480, or 99483 on the same date of service. Medicare has identified these codes as telehealth/telemedicine services. Commercial payers should be contacted regarding their coverage guidelines.

ICD-10-CM Diagnostic Codes

The application of this code is too broad to adequately present ICD-10-CM diagnostic code links here. Refer to your ICD-10-CM book.

AMA: 99497 2018,Jan,8; 2018,Apr,9; 2017,Jan,8; 2016,Jan,13; 2016,Feb,7; 2015,Jan,16; 2014,Dec,11 **99498** 2018,Jan,8; 2018,Apr,9; 2017,Jan,8; 2016,Jan,13; 2016,Feb,7; 2015,Jan,16; 2014,Dec,11

Relative Value Units/Medicare Edits

Non-Facility RVU	Work	PE	MP	Total
99497	1.5	0.82	0.09	2.41
99498	1.4	0.62	0.09	2.11
Facility RVU	Work	PE	MP	Total
99497	1.5	0.64	0.09	2.23
99498	1.4	0.61	0.09	2.1

	FUD	Status	MUE	Modifiers				IOM Reference
99497	N/A	A	1(2)	N/A	N/A	N/A	80*	None
99498	N/A	A	3(3)	N/A	N/A	N/A	80*	

* with documentation

10021 [10004, 10005, 10006, 10007, 10008, 10009, 10010, 10011, 10012]

	10021	Fine needle aspiration biopsy, without imaging guidance; first lesion
+	**10004**	Fine needle aspiration biopsy, without imaging guidance; each additional lesion (List separately in addition to code for primary procedure)
	10005	Fine needle aspiration biopsy, including ultrasound guidance; first lesion
+	**10006**	Fine needle aspiration biopsy, including ultrasound guidance; each additional lesion (List separately in addition to code for primary procedure)
	10007	Fine needle aspiration biopsy, including fluoroscopic guidance; first lesion
+	**10008**	Fine needle aspiration biopsy, including fluoroscopic guidance; each additional lesion (List separately in addition to code for primary procedure)
	10009	Fine needle aspiration biopsy, including CT guidance; first lesion
+	**10010**	Fine needle aspiration biopsy, including CT guidance; each additional lesion (List separately in addition to code for primary procedure)
	10011	Fine needle aspiration biopsy, including MR guidance; first lesion
+	**10012**	Fine needle aspiration biopsy, including MR guidance; each additional lesion (List separately in addition to code for primary procedure)

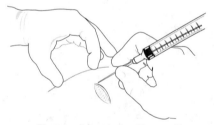

Fine needle aspiration biopsy with
or without imaging guidance

Explanation

Fine needle aspiration (FNA) is a diagnostic percutaneous procedure that uses a fine gauge needle (often 22 or 25 gauge) and a syringe to sample fluid from a cyst or remove clusters of cells from a solid mass. The skin is cleansed. If a lump can be felt, the radiologist or surgeon guides a needle into the area by palpating the lump. If the lump is non-palpable, the FNA procedure is performed using ultrasound, fluoroscopy, computed tomography (CT), or MR imaging with the patient positioned according to the area of concern. Ultrasonography-guided aspiration biopsy involves inserting an aspiration catheter needle device through the accessory channel port of the echoendoscope; the needle is placed into the area to be sampled under endoscopic ultrasonographic guidance. After the needle is placed into the region of the lesion, a vacuum is created and multiple in and out needle motions are performed. Several needle insertions are usually required to ensure that an adequate tissue sample is taken. In fluoroscopic guidance, intermittent

fluoroscopy guides the advancement of the needle. CT image guidance allows computer-assisted targeting of the area to be sampled. At the completion of the procedure, the needle is withdrawn and a small bandage is placed over the area. MR image guidance involves the use of a magnetic field, radiowaves, and computer-assisted targeting to identify the area for biopsy without the use of ionizing radiation. Report 10021 for fine needle aspiration of the initial lesion performed without imaging guidance; for each subsequent lesion, report 10004. Report 10005 for FNA of the first lesion using ultrasound guidance; for each additional lesion, report 10006. Report 10007 for FNA of the first lesion using fluoroscopy; for each additional lesion, report 10008. Report 10009 for FNA of the first lesion utilizing CT imaging; for each subsequent lesion, report 10010. Report 10011 when MR imaging is used for the initial lesion; for each additional lesion, report 10012.

Coding Tips

When these procedures are performed with another separately identifiable procedure, the highest dollar value code is listed as the primary procedure and subsequent procedures are appended with modifier 51. When FNA biopsy and core needle biopsies are performed during the same session on separate lesions using a different imaging source, both the core needle biopsy and the imaging guidance are reported separately using modifier 59. Report 10004 in addition to 10021; 10006 in addition to 10005; 10008 in addition to 10007; 10010 in addition to 10009; and 10012 in addition to 10011. Do not report 10004 or 10021 with 10005-10012. Imaging guidance codes 76942, 77002, 77012, and 77021 should not be reported separately. For evaluation of fine needle aspirate, see 88172–88173 and 88177. For percutaneous needle biopsy, abdominal or retroperitoneal mass, see 49180; kidney, see 50200; testis, see 54500; and epididymis, see 54800. For percutaneous image-guided fluid collection drainage of soft tissue via catheter, see 10030.

ICD-10-CM Diagnostic Codes

A36.83	Diphtheritic polyneuritis
A36.84	Diphtheritic tubulo-interstitial nephropathy
A52.76	Other genitourinary symptomatic late syphilis
C61	Malignant neoplasm of prostate ♂
C62.01	Malignant neoplasm of undescended right testis ♂ ☑
C62.02	Malignant neoplasm of undescended left testis ♂ ☑
C62.11	Malignant neoplasm of descended right testis ♂ ☑
C62.12	Malignant neoplasm of descended left testis ♂ ☑
C63.01	Malignant neoplasm of right epididymis ♂ ☑
C63.02	Malignant neoplasm of left epididymis ♂ ☑
C65.1	Malignant neoplasm of right renal pelvis ☑
C65.2	Malignant neoplasm of left renal pelvis ☑
C79.82	Secondary malignant neoplasm of genital organs
D07.5	Carcinoma in situ of prostate ♂
D07.61	Carcinoma in situ of scrotum ♂
D07.69	Carcinoma in situ of other male genital organs ♂
D09.19	Carcinoma in situ of other urinary organs
D17.6	Benign lipomatous neoplasm of spermatic cord ♂
D17.71	Benign lipomatous neoplasm of kidney
D17.72	Benign lipomatous neoplasm of other genitourinary organ
D29.1	Benign neoplasm of prostate ♂
D29.21	Benign neoplasm of right testis ♂ ☑
D29.22	Benign neoplasm of left testis ♂ ☑
D29.31	Benign neoplasm of right epididymis ♂ ☑
D29.32	Benign neoplasm of left epididymis ♂ ☑
D30.11	Benign neoplasm of right renal pelvis ☑

D30.12	Benign neoplasm of left renal pelvis ☑	
D40.0	Neoplasm of uncertain behavior of prostate ♂	
D40.11	Neoplasm of uncertain behavior of right testis ♂ ☑	
D40.12	Neoplasm of uncertain behavior of left testis ♂ ☑	
D41.01	Neoplasm of uncertain behavior of right kidney ☑	
D41.02	Neoplasm of uncertain behavior of left kidney ☑	
D41.11	Neoplasm of uncertain behavior of right renal pelvis ☑	
D41.12	Neoplasm of uncertain behavior of left renal pelvis ☑	
D41.21	Neoplasm of uncertain behavior of right ureter ☑	
D41.22	Neoplasm of uncertain behavior of left ureter ☑	
E29.1	Testicular hypofunction ♂	
L02.215	Cutaneous abscess of perineum	
L03.314	Cellulitis of groin	
L03.315	Cellulitis of perineum	
L03.324	Acute lymphangitis of groin	
L03.325	Acute lymphangitis of perineum	
M35.04	Sicca syndrome with tubulo-interstitial nephropathy	
N17.0	Acute kidney failure with tubular necrosis	
N17.1	Acute kidney failure with acute cortical necrosis	
N17.2	Acute kidney failure with medullary necrosis	
N18.1	Chronic kidney disease, stage 1	
N18.2	Chronic kidney disease, stage 2 (mild)	
N18.31	Chronic kidney disease, stage 3a	
N18.32	Chronic kidney disease, stage 3b	
N18.4	Chronic kidney disease, stage 4 (severe)	
N18.5	Chronic kidney disease, stage 5	
N18.6	End stage renal disease	
N25.0	Renal osteodystrophy	
N28.1	Cyst of kidney, acquired	
N41.0	Acute prostatitis 🅰 ♂	
N41.1	Chronic prostatitis 🅰 ♂	
N41.2	Abscess of prostate 🅰 ♂	
N41.3	Prostatocystitis 🅰 ♂	
N41.4	Granulomatous prostatitis 🅰 ♂	
N41.8	Other inflammatory diseases of prostate 🅰 ♂	
N42.0	Calculus of prostate 🅰 ♂	
N42.1	Congestion and hemorrhage of prostate 🅰 ♂	
N42.81	Prostatodynia syndrome 🅰 ♂	
N42.82	Prostatosis syndrome 🅰 ♂	
R59.0	Localized enlarged lymph nodes	
R59.1	Generalized enlarged lymph nodes	
R93.811	Abnormal radiologic findings on diagnostic imaging of right testicle ♂ ☑	
R93.812	Abnormal radiologic findings on diagnostic imaging of left testicle ♂ ☑	
R93.813	Abnormal radiologic findings on diagnostic imaging of testicles, bilateral ♂ ☑	
R97.21	Rising PSA following treatment for malignant neoplasm of prostate 🅰 ♂	
T86.11	Kidney transplant rejection	
T86.12	Kidney transplant failure	
T86.13	Kidney transplant infection	

AMA: **10004** 2019,Feb,8; 2019,Apr,4 **10005** 2019,May,10; 2019,Feb,8; 2019,Apr,4 **10006** 2019,Feb,8; 2019,Apr,4 **10007** 2019,Feb,8; 2019,Apr,4 **10008** 2019,Feb,8; 2019,Apr,4 **10009** 2019,Feb,8; 2019,Apr,4 **10010** 2019,Feb,8; 2019,Apr,4 **10011** 2019,Feb,8; 2019,Apr,4 **10012** 2019,Feb,8; 2019,Apr,4 **10021** 2019,May,10; 2019,Feb,8; 2019,Apr,4; 2018,Jan,8; 2017,Jan,8; 2016,Jan,13; 2015,Jan,16; 2014,Jan,11

Relative Value Units/Medicare Edits

Non-Facility RVU	Work	PE	MP	Total
10021	1.03	1.64	0.13	2.8
10004	0.8	0.57	0.11	1.48
10005	1.46	2.08	0.13	3.67
10006	1.0	0.61	0.09	1.7
10007	1.81	6.44	0.18	8.43
10008	1.18	3.49	0.12	4.79
10009	2.26	10.84	0.22	13.32
10010	1.65	6.22	0.15	8.02
10011	0.0	0.0	0.0	0.0
10012	0.0	0.0	0.0	0.0
Facility RVU	**Work**	**PE**	**MP**	**Total**
10021	1.03	0.44	0.13	1.6
10004	0.8	0.34	0.11	1.25
10005	1.46	0.48	0.13	2.07
10006	1.0	0.33	0.09	1.42
10007	1.81	0.7	0.18	2.69
10008	1.18	0.46	0.12	1.76
10009	2.26	0.8	0.22	3.28
10010	1.65	0.58	0.15	2.38
10011	0.0	0.0	0.0	0.0
10012	0.0	0.0	0.0	0.0

	FUD	Status	MUE	Modifiers				IOM Reference
10021	N/A	A	1(2)	51	N/A	N/A	80*	100-04,13,80.1; 100-04,13,80.2
10004	N/A	A	3(3)	N/A	N/A	N/A	80*	
10005	N/A	A	1(2)	51	N/A	N/A	80*	
10006	N/A	A	3(3)	N/A	N/A	N/A	80*	
10007	N/A	A	1(2)	51	N/A	N/A	80*	
10008	N/A	A	2(3)	N/A	N/A	N/A	80*	
10009	N/A	A	1(2)	51	N/A	N/A	80*	
10010	N/A	A	3(3)	N/A	N/A	N/A	80*	
10011	N/A	C	1(2)	51	N/A	N/A	80*	
10012	N/A	C	3(3)	N/A	N/A	N/A	80*	

* with documentation

Terms To Know

fine needle aspiration. 22- or 25-gauge needle attached to a syringe is inserted into a lesion/tissue and a few cells are aspirated for biopsy and diagnostic study. Aspiration is also used to remove fluid from a benign cyst.

imaging. Radiologic means of producing pictures for clinical study of the internal structures and functions of the body, such as x-ray, ultrasound, magnetic resonance, or positron emission tomography.

10030

10030 Image-guided fluid collection drainage by catheter (eg, abscess, hematoma, seroma, lymphocele, cyst), soft tissue (eg, extremity, abdominal wall, neck), percutaneous

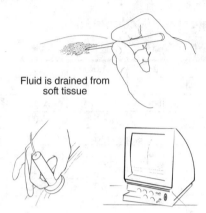

Fluid is drained from soft tissue

A transducer is passed over the site and the results are viewed on a monitor

Explanation

A fluid collection in the soft tissue, such as a hematoma, seroma, abscess, lymphocele, or cyst, is drained using a catheter. The area over the abnormal tissue is cleansed and local anesthesia is administered. Imaging is performed to assist in the insertion of a needle or guidewire into the fluid collection. Small tissue samples may be collected from the site for pathological examination. A catheter is inserted to drain and collect the fluid for analysis. More imaging may be performed to ensure hemostasis. In some cases, the catheter may be attached to a drainage system to allow for further drainage over the course of days. Once the fluid has completely drained, the catheter is removed. A bandage is applied. Report 10030 for each fluid collection drained using a separate catheter.

Coding Tips

Report 10030 once per individual collection drained with a separate catheter. Do not report 10030 with imaging codes 75989, 76942, 77002–77003, 77012, or 77021. For percutaneous or transvaginal/transrectal, image-guided fluid collection of the visceral, peritoneal, or retroperitoneal areas, see 49405–49407.

ICD-10-CM Diagnostic Codes

L02.211	Cutaneous abscess of abdominal wall
L02.214	Cutaneous abscess of groin
L02.215	Cutaneous abscess of perineum
L02.818	Cutaneous abscess of other sites
L05.01	Pilonidal cyst with abscess
L05.02	Pilonidal sinus with abscess
L72.0	Epidermal cyst
L72.2	Steatocystoma multiplex
L72.3	Sebaceous cyst
L72.8	Other follicular cysts of the skin and subcutaneous tissue
L76.22	Postprocedural hemorrhage of skin and subcutaneous tissue following other procedure
L76.32	Postprocedural hematoma of skin and subcutaneous tissue following other procedure
L76.34	Postprocedural seroma of skin and subcutaneous tissue following other procedure
M72.8	Other fibroblastic disorders
M79.81	Nontraumatic hematoma of soft tissue
M96.831	Postprocedural hemorrhage of a musculoskeletal structure following other procedure
T79.2XXA	Traumatic secondary and recurrent hemorrhage and seroma, initial encounter
T81.41XA	Infection following a procedure, superficial incisional surgical site, initial encounter
T81.42XA	Infection following a procedure, deep incisional surgical site, initial encounter

AMA: **10030** 2019,Apr,4; 2018,Jan,8; 2017,Jan,8; 2017,Aug,9; 2016,Jan,13; 2015,Jan,16; 2014,May,3; 2014,May,9

Relative Value Units/Medicare Edits

Non-Facility RVU	Work	PE	MP	Total
10030	2.75	14.52	0.26	17.53
Facility RVU	**Work**	**PE**	**MP**	**Total**
10030	2.75	0.97	0.26	3.98

	FUD	Status	MUE	Modifiers				IOM Reference
10030	0	A	2(3)	51	N/A	N/A	80*	None

* with documentation

Terms To Know

catheter. Flexible tube inserted into an area of the body for introducing or withdrawing fluid.

drainage. Releasing, taking, or letting out fluids and/or gases from a body part.

guidewire. Flexible metal instrument designed to lead another instrument in its proper course.

hemostasis. Interruption of blood flow or the cessation or arrest of bleeding.

imaging. Radiologic means of producing pictures for clinical study of the internal structures and functions of the body, such as x-ray, ultrasound, magnetic resonance, or positron emission tomography.

percutaneous. Through the skin.

soft tissue. Nonepithelial tissues outside of the skeleton.

specimen. Tissue cells or sample of fluid taken for analysis, pathologic examination, and diagnosis.

transducer. Apparatus that transfers or translates one type of energy into another, such as converting pressure to an electrical signal.

10180

10180   Incision and drainage, complex, postoperative wound infection

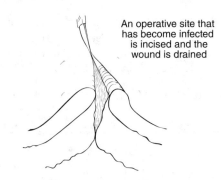

An operative site that has become infected is incised and the wound is drained

The procedure is considered complex in nature

Explanation

This procedure treats an infected postoperative wound. A more complex than usual incision and drainage procedure is necessary to remove the fluid and allow the surgical wound to heal. The physician first removes the surgical sutures or staples and/or makes additional incisions into the skin. The wound is drained of infected fluid. Any necrotic tissue is removed from the surgical site and the wound is irrigated. The wound may be sutured closed or packed open with gauze to allow additional drainage. If closed, the surgical site may have suction or latex drains placed into the wound. If packed open, the wound may be sutured again during a later procedure.

Coding Tips

Drain placement is included in this procedure and should not be reported separately. For incision and drainage of a hematoma, seroma, or fluid collection, see 10140. For simple secondary closure of a surgical wound, see 12020–12021. For extensive or complicated secondary closure of a surgical wound or dehiscence, see 13160. Supplies used when providing this procedure may be reported with the appropriate HCPCS Level II code(s). Surgical trays, A4550, are not separately reimbursed by Medicare; however, other third-party payers may cover them. Check with the specific payer to determine coverage.

ICD-10-CM Diagnostic Codes

A48.52	Wound botulism
K68.11	Postprocedural retroperitoneal abscess
T81.41XA	Infection following a procedure, superficial incisional surgical site, initial encounter
T81.42XA	Infection following a procedure, deep incisional surgical site, initial encounter
T81.49XA	Infection following a procedure, other surgical site, initial encounter

AMA: 10180 2018,Jan,8; 2017,Jan,8; 2016,Jan,13; 2015,Jan,16; 2014,Nov,5; 2014,Jan,11

Relative Value Units/Medicare Edits

Non-Facility RVU	Work	PE	MP	Total
10180	2.3	4.51	0.49	7.3
Facility RVU	**Work**	**PE**	**MP**	**Total**
10180	2.3	2.32	0.49	5.11

	FUD	Status	MUE	Modifiers			IOM Reference
10180	10	A	2(3)	51	N/A	N/A	N/A	None

* with documentation

Terms To Know

classification of surgical wounds. Surgical wounds fall into four categories that determine treatment methods and outcomes: *1)* Clean wound: No inflammation or contamination; treatment performed with no break in sterile technique; no alimentary, respiratory, or genitourinary tracts involved in the surgery; infection rate = up to 5 percent. *2)* Clean-contaminated wound: No inflammation; treatment performed with minor break in surgical technique; no unusual contamination resulting when alimentary, respiratory, genitourinary, or oropharyngeal cavity is entered; infection rate = up to 11 percent. *3)* Contaminated wound: Less than four hours old with acute, nonpurulent inflammation; treatment performed with major break in surgical technique; gross contamination resulting from the gastrointestinal tract; infection rate = up to 20 percent. *4)* Dirty and infected wound: More than four hours old with existing infection, inflammation, abscess, and nonsterile conditions due to perforated viscus, fecal contamination, necrotic tissue, or foreign body; infection rate = up to 40 percent.

dehiscence. Complication of healing in which the surgical wound ruptures or bursts open, superficially or through multiple layers.

drain. Device that creates a channel to allow fluid from a cavity, wound, or infected area to exit the body.

hematoma. Tumor-like collection of blood in some part of the body caused by a break in a blood vessel wall, usually as a result of trauma.

infection. Presence of microorganisms in body tissues that may result in cellular damage.

necrotic. Pathological condition of death occurring in a group of cells or tissues within a living part or organism.

packing. Material placed into a cavity or wound, such as gels, gauze, pads, and sponges.

seroma. Swelling caused by the collection of serum, or clear fluid, in the tissues.

CPT © 2020 American Medical Association. All Rights Reserved.   ● New   ▲ Revised   + Add On   ★ Telemedicine   AMA: CPT Assist   [Resequenced]   ☑ Laterality   © 2020 Optum360, LLC

11004-11006

11004 Debridement of skin, subcutaneous tissue, muscle and fascia for necrotizing soft tissue infection; external genitalia and perineum
11005 abdominal wall, with or without fascial closure
11006 external genitalia, perineum and abdominal wall, with or without fascial closure

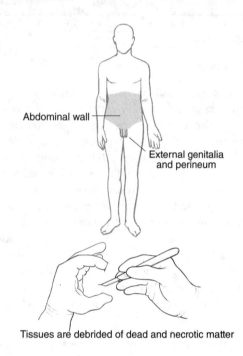

Abdominal wall

External genitalia and perineum

Tissues are debrided of dead and necrotic matter

Explanation

Debridement is carried out for a severe type of tissue infection that causes gangrenous changes, systemic disease, and tissue death. These types of infections are caused by virulent strains of bacteria, such as "flesh-eating" streptococcus, and affect the skin, subcutaneous fat, fascia, and muscle tissue. Surgery is performed immediately upon diagnosis to open and drain the infected area and excise the dead or necrotic tissue. Report 11004 for surgical debridement of necrotic soft tissue of the external genitalia and perineum; 11005 for the abdominal wall, with or without repair of the abdominal fascia; and 11006 for both areas, with or without repair of the abdominal fascia.

Coding Tips

This type of debridement is done on high-risk patients who have a life-threatening infection such as Fournier's gangrene. Necrosis is often caused by infection from a combination of dangerously virulent micro-organisms. Fistulas, herniations, and organ destruction may occur, requiring an extensive level of repair and possible organ removal or transplantation. Tissue flaps or skin grafting are reported separately when used for repair or closure. Orchiectomy is reported with 54520, when performed. For testicular transplantation, if performed, see 54680. Removal of prosthetic material or mesh from the abdominal wall is reported with 11008.

ICD-10-CM Diagnostic Codes

A48.0	Gas gangrene
I96	Gangrene, not elsewhere classified
M72.6	Necrotizing fasciitis
N49.3	Fournier gangrene ♂
N76.89	Other specified inflammation of vagina and vulva ♀

T81.41XA	Infection following a procedure, superficial incisional surgical site, initial encounter
T81.42XA	Infection following a procedure, deep incisional surgical site, initial encounter

AMA: **11004** 2019,Nov,14; 2018,Jan,8; 2018,Feb,10; 2017,Jan,8; 2016,Jan,13; 2015,Jan,16; 2014,Jan,11 **11005** 2019,Nov,14; 2018,Jan,8; 2018,Feb,10; 2017,Jan,8; 2016,Jan,13; 2015,Jan,16; 2014,Jan,11 **11006** 2019,Nov,14; 2018,Jan,8; 2017,Jan,8; 2016,Jan,13; 2015,Jan,16; 2014,Jan,11

Relative Value Units/Medicare Edits

Non-Facility RVU	Work	PE	MP	Total
11004	10.8	3.9	1.98	16.68
11005	14.24	5.24	3.24	22.72
11006	13.1	4.77	2.62	20.49
Facility RVU	**Work**	**PE**	**MP**	**Total**
11004	10.8	3.9	1.98	16.68
11005	14.24	5.24	3.24	22.72
11006	13.1	4.77	2.62	20.49

	FUD	Status	MUE	Modifiers				IOM Reference
11004	0	A	1(2)	51	N/A	N/A	N/A	None
11005	0	A	1(2)	N/A	N/A	N/A	80*	
11006	0	A	1(2)	51	N/A	N/A	N/A	

* with documentation

Terms To Know

debridement. Removal of dead or contaminated tissue and foreign matter from a wound.

Fournier's gangrene. Necrotizing fasciitis of the scrotum, penis, or male perineum, caused by enteric, anaerobic, or gram-positive bacteria.

gangrene. Death of tissue, usually resulting from a loss of vascular supply, followed by a bacterial attack or onset of disease.

microorganism. Microscopic organisms, including bacteria, fungi, and protozoa.

necrotic. Pathological condition of death occurring in a group of cells or tissues within a living part or organism.

soft tissue. Nonepithelial tissues outside of the skeleton that includes subcutaneous adipose tissue, fibrous tissue, fascia, muscles, blood and lymph vessels, and peripheral nervous system tissue.

11008

+ **11008** Removal of prosthetic material or mesh, abdominal wall for infection (eg, for chronic or recurrent mesh infection or necrotizing soft tissue infection) (List separately in addition to code for primary procedure)

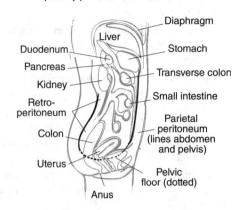

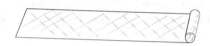

Synthetic material (commonly mesh) is often used to repair surgically created defects in the abdominal wall. The mesh provides support and structure for the healing process

Explanation

The physician removes prosthetic material or mesh previously placed in the abdominal wall. This may be done due to the presence of a chronic infection, a necrotizing soft tissue infection, or a recurrent mesh infection. Surgery is performed immediately after diagnosis and usually under general anesthesia. The skin is incised and the tissue dissected exposing the prosthetic material. Debridement of the tissue adjacent to or incorporated in the mesh may be performed with instruments or irrigation. Unincorporated or infected areas of the mesh are excised and removed with any remaining areas of infection or necrotic tissue. Incorporated mesh that is not infected may be left in the wound. The area is irrigated and the wound is sutured.

Coding Tips

Report 11008 in addition to 10180 and 11004–11006. When mesh is used for the closure, report 49568. Skin grafts or flaps may be reported separately when performed for closure at the same session as 11008. Do not report 11008 with 11000–11001 or 11010–11044.

ICD-10-CM Diagnostic Codes

This/these CPT code(s) are add-on code(s). See the primary procedure code that this code is performed with for your ICD-10-CM code selections.

AMA: **11008** 2019,Jan,14; 2018,Jan,8; 2017,Jan,8; 2016,Jan,13; 2015,Jan,16; 2014,Jan,11

Relative Value Units/Medicare Edits

Non-Facility RVU	Work	PE	MP	Total
11008	5.0	1.83	1.16	7.99
Facility RVU	Work	PE	MP	Total
11008	5.0	1.83	1.16	7.99

	FUD	Status	MUE	Modifiers				IOM Reference
11008	N/A	A	1(2)	N/A	N/A	N/A	80*	None

* with documentation

Terms To Know

chronic. Persistent, continuing, or recurring.

dissect. Cut apart or separate tissue for surgical purposes or for visual or microscopic study.

excise. Remove or cut out.

gangrene. Death of tissue, usually resulting from a loss of vascular supply, followed by a bacterial attack or onset of disease.

infection. Presence of microorganisms in body tissues that may result in cellular damage.

irrigate. Washing out, lavage.

mesh. Synthetic fabric used as a prosthetic patch in hernia repair.

necrotic. Pathological condition of death occurring in a group of cells or tissues within a living part or organism.

prosthesis. Man-made substitute for a missing body part.

soft tissue. Nonepithelial tissues outside of the skeleton that includes subcutaneous adipose tissue, fibrous tissue, fascia, muscles, blood and lymph vessels, and peripheral nervous system tissue.

12001-12007

12001 Simple repair of superficial wounds of scalp, neck, axillae, external genitalia, trunk and/or extremities (including hands and feet); 2.5 cm or less
12002 2.6 cm to 7.5 cm
12004 7.6 cm to 12.5 cm
12005 12.6 cm to 20.0 cm
12006 20.1 cm to 30.0 cm
12007 over 30.0 cm

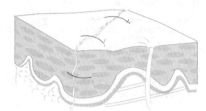

Example of a simple closure involving only one skin layer, the epidermis

Explanation

The physician performs wound closure of superficial lacerations of the scalp, neck, axillae, external genitalia, trunk, or extremities using sutures, staples, tissue adhesives, or a combination of these materials. A local anesthetic is injected around the wound and it is cleansed, explored, and often irrigated with a saline solution. The physician performs a simple, one-layer repair of the epidermis, dermis, or subcutaneous tissues. For multiple wounds of the same complexity and in the same anatomical area, the length of all wounds sutured is summed and reported as one total length. Report 12001 for a total length of 2.5 cm or less; 12002 for 2.6 cm to 7.5 cm; 12004 for 7.6 cm to 12.5 cm; 12005 for 12.6 cm to 20 cm; 12006 for 20.1 cm to 30 cm; and 12007 if the total length is greater than 30 cm.

Coding Tips

Wounds treated with tissue glue or staples qualify as a simple repair even if they are not closed with sutures. Intermediate repair is used when layered closure of one or more of the deeper layers of subcutaneous tissue and superficial fascia, in addition to the skin, require closure. Intermediate repair is also reported for single-layer closure of heavily contaminated wounds that require extensive cleaning or removal of particulate matter. To report extensive debridement of soft tissue and/or bone, not associated with open fracture(s) and/or dislocation(s), resulting from penetrating and/or blunt trauma, see 11042–11047. For wound care closure by tissue adhesive(s) only, see HCPCS Level II code G0168. Surgical trays, A4550, are not separately reimbursed by Medicare; however, other third-party payers may cover them. Check with the specific payer to determine coverage.

ICD-10-CM Diagnostic Codes

S30.810A	Abrasion of lower back and pelvis, initial encounter
S30.811A	Abrasion of abdominal wall, initial encounter
S30.812A	Abrasion of penis, initial encounter ♂
S30.813A	Abrasion of scrotum and testes, initial encounter ♂
S30.814A	Abrasion of vagina and vulva, initial encounter ♀
S31.010A	Laceration without foreign body of lower back and pelvis without penetration into retroperitoneum, initial encounter
S31.030A	Puncture wound without foreign body of lower back and pelvis without penetration into retroperitoneum, initial encounter
S31.050A	Open bite of lower back and pelvis without penetration into retroperitoneum, initial encounter
S31.110A	Laceration without foreign body of abdominal wall, right upper quadrant without penetration into peritoneal cavity, initial encounter ☑
S31.111A	Laceration without foreign body of abdominal wall, left upper quadrant without penetration into peritoneal cavity, initial encounter ☑
S31.112A	Laceration without foreign body of abdominal wall, epigastric region without penetration into peritoneal cavity, initial encounter
S31.113A	Laceration without foreign body of abdominal wall, right lower quadrant without penetration into peritoneal cavity, initial encounter ☑
S31.114A	Laceration without foreign body of abdominal wall, left lower quadrant without penetration into peritoneal cavity, initial encounter ☑
S31.115A	Laceration without foreign body of abdominal wall, periumbilic region without penetration into peritoneal cavity, initial encounter
S31.130A	Puncture wound of abdominal wall without foreign body, right upper quadrant without penetration into peritoneal cavity, initial encounter ☑
S31.131A	Puncture wound of abdominal wall without foreign body, left upper quadrant without penetration into peritoneal cavity, initial encounter ☑
S31.132A	Puncture wound of abdominal wall without foreign body, epigastric region without penetration into peritoneal cavity, initial encounter
S31.133A	Puncture wound of abdominal wall without foreign body, right lower quadrant without penetration into peritoneal cavity, initial encounter ☑
S31.134A	Puncture wound of abdominal wall without foreign body, left lower quadrant without penetration into peritoneal cavity, initial encounter ☑
S31.135A	Puncture wound of abdominal wall without foreign body, periumbilic region without penetration into peritoneal cavity, initial encounter
S31.150A	Open bite of abdominal wall, right upper quadrant without penetration into peritoneal cavity, initial encounter ☑
S31.151A	Open bite of abdominal wall, left upper quadrant without penetration into peritoneal cavity, initial encounter ☑
S31.152A	Open bite of abdominal wall, epigastric region without penetration into peritoneal cavity, initial encounter
S31.153A	Open bite of abdominal wall, right lower quadrant without penetration into peritoneal cavity, initial encounter ☑
S31.154A	Open bite of abdominal wall, left lower quadrant without penetration into peritoneal cavity, initial encounter ☑
S31.155A	Open bite of abdominal wall, periumbilic region without penetration into peritoneal cavity, initial encounter
S31.21XA	Laceration without foreign body of penis, initial encounter ♂
S31.23XA	Puncture wound without foreign body of penis, initial encounter ♂
S31.25XA	Open bite of penis, initial encounter ♂
S31.31XA	Laceration without foreign body of scrotum and testes, initial encounter ♂
S31.33XA	Puncture wound without foreign body of scrotum and testes, initial encounter ♂

Integumentary

S31.35XA	Open bite of scrotum and testes, initial encounter ♂
S31.41XA	Laceration without foreign body of vagina and vulva, initial encounter ♀
S31.43XA	Puncture wound without foreign body of vagina and vulva, initial encounter ♀
S31.45XA	Open bite of vagina and vulva, initial encounter ♀

Associated HCPCS Codes

| G0168 | Wound closure utilizing tissue adhesive(s) only |

AMA: 12001 2018,Sep,7; 2018,Jan,8; 2017,Jan,8; 2017,Dec,14; 2016,Jan,13; 2015,Jan,16; 2014,Jan,11 **12002** 2018,Sep,7; 2018,Jan,8; 2017,Jan,8; 2016,Jan,13; 2015,Jan,16; 2014,Oct,14; 2014,Jan,11 **12004** 2018,Sep,7; 2018,Jan,8; 2017,Jan,8; 2016,Jan,13; 2015,Jan,16; 2014,Jan,11 **12005** 2018,Sep,7; 2018,Jan,8; 2017,Jan,8; 2016,Jan,13; 2015,Jan,16; 2014,Jan,11 **12006** 2018,Sep,7; 2018,Jan,8; 2017,Jan,8; 2016,Jan,13; 2015,Jan,16; 2014,Jan,11 **12007** 2018,Sep,7; 2018,Jan,8; 2017,Jan,8; 2016,Jan,13; 2015,Jan,16; 2014,Jan,11

Relative Value Units/Medicare Edits

Non-Facility RVU	Work	PE	MP	Total
12001	0.84	1.59	0.15	2.58
12002	1.14	1.8	0.22	3.16
12004	1.44	1.98	0.27	3.69
12005	1.97	2.53	0.38	4.88
12006	2.39	2.91	0.46	5.76
12007	2.9	3.14	.54	6.58
Facility RVU	**Work**	**PE**	**MP**	**Total**
12001	0.84	0.31	0.15	1.3
12002	1.14	0.37	0.22	1.73
12004	1.44	0.44	0.27	2.15
12005	1.97	0.45	0.38	2.8
12006	2.39	0.58	0.46	3.43
12007	2.9	0.79	0.54	4.23

	FUD	Status	MUE	Modifiers				IOM Reference
12001	0	A	1(2)	51	N/A	N/A	N/A	None
12002	0	A	1(2)	51	N/A	N/A	N/A	
12004	0	A	1(2)	51	N/A	N/A	N/A	
12005	0	A	1(2)	51	N/A	N/A	N/A	
12006	0	A	1(2)	51	N/A	N/A	N/A	
12007	0	A	1(2)	51	N/A	62*	N/A	

* with documentation

Terms To Know

laceration. Tearing injury; a torn, ragged-edged wound.

repair. Surgical closure of a wound. The wound may be a result of injury/trauma or it may be a surgically created defect. Repairs are divided into three categories: simple, intermediate, and complex.

superficial. On the skin surface or near the surface of any involved structure or field of interest.

12020-12021

| 12020 | Treatment of superficial wound dehiscence; simple closure |
| 12021 | with packing |

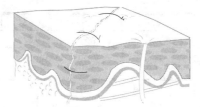

Example of a simple closure involving only one skin layer

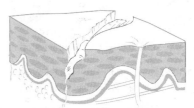

Example of a wound left open with packing due to infection

Explanation

There has been a breakdown of the healing skin either before or after suture removal. The skin margins have opened. The physician cleanses the wound with irrigation and antimicrobial solutions. The skin margins may be trimmed to initiate bleeding surfaces. Report 12020 if the wound is sutured in a single layer. Report 12021 if the wound is left open and packed with gauze strips due to the presence of infection. This allows infection to drain from the wound and the skin closure will be delayed until the infection is resolved.

Coding Tips

For extensive or complicated secondary wound closure, see 13160. For wound closure by tissue adhesive(s) only, see HCPCS Level II code G0168. To report extensive debridement of soft tissue and/or bone, not associated with open fracture(s) and/or dislocation(s), resulting from penetrating and/or blunt trauma, see 11042–11047. Surgical trays, A4550, are not separately reimbursed by Medicare; however, other third-party payers may cover them. Check with the specific payer to determine coverage.

ICD-10-CM Diagnostic Codes

| T81.32XA | Disruption of internal operation (surgical) wound, not elsewhere classified, initial encounter |
| T81.33XA | Disruption of traumatic injury wound repair, initial encounter |

Associated HCPCS Codes

| G0168 | Wound closure utilizing tissue adhesive(s) only |

AMA: 12020 2019,Nov,3; 2018,Jan,8; 2017,Jan,8; 2016,Jan,13; 2015,Jan,16; 2014,Jan,11 **12021** 2019,Nov,3; 2018,Jan,8; 2017,Jan,8; 2016,Jan,13; 2015,Jan,16; 2014,Jan,11

Relative Value Units/Medicare Edits

Non-Facility RVU	Work	PE	MP	Total
12020	2.67	5.31	0.43	8.41
12021	1.89	2.69	0.32	4.9
Facility RVU	**Work**	**PE**	**MP**	**Total**
12020	2.67	2.33	0.43	5.43
12021	1.89	1.8	0.32	4.01

	FUD	Status	MUE	Modifiers			IOM Reference
12020	10	A	2(3)	51	N/A	N/A	N/A	None
12021	10	A	3(3)	51	N/A	N/A	N/A	

* with documentation

Terms To Know

closure. Repairing an incision or wound by suture or other means.

dehiscence. Complication of healing in which the surgical wound ruptures or bursts open, superficially or through multiple layers.

drain. Device that creates a channel to allow fluid from a cavity, wound, or infected area to exit the body.

infection. Presence of microorganisms in body tissues that may result in cellular damage.

irrigation. To wash out or cleanse a body cavity, wound, or tissue with water or other fluid.

margin. Boundary, edge, or border, as of a surface or structure.

packing. Material placed into a cavity or wound, such as gels, gauze, pads, and sponges.

superficial. On the skin surface or near the surface of any involved structure or field of interest.

wound repair. Surgical closure of a wound is divided into three categories: simple, intermediate, and complex. *simple repair:* Surgical closure of a superficial wound, requiring single layer suturing of the skin epidermis, dermis, or subcutaneous tissue. *intermediate repair:* Surgical closure of a wound requiring closure of one or more of the deeper subcutaneous tissue and non-muscle fascia layers in addition to suturing the skin; contaminated wounds with single layer closure that need extensive cleaning or foreign body removal. *complex repair:* Repair of wounds requiring more than layered closure (debridement, scar revision, stents, retention sutures).

12041-12047

12041	Repair, intermediate, wounds of neck, hands, feet and/or external genitalia; 2.5 cm or less
12042	2.6 cm to 7.5 cm
12044	7.6 cm to 12.5 cm
12045	12.6 cm to 20.0 cm
12046	20.1 cm to 30.0 cm
12047	over 30.0 cm

Layered suturing

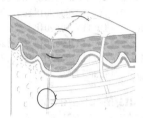

The laceration(s) are deep and require layered closure

Explanation

The physician performs a repair of a wound located on the external genitalia. A local anesthetic is injected around the laceration, and the wound is cleansed, explored, and often irrigated with a saline solution. Due to deeper or more complex lacerations, deep subcutaneous or layered suturing techniques are required. The physician closes tissue layers under the skin with dissolvable sutures before suturing the skin. Extensive cleaning or removal of foreign matter from a heavily contaminated wound that is closed with a single layer may also be reported as an intermediate repair. With multiple wounds of the same complexity and in the same anatomical area, the length of all wounds sutured is summed and reported as one total length. Report 12041 for a total length of 2.5 cm or less; 12042 for 2.6 cm to 7.5 cm; 12044 for 7.6 cm to 12.5 cm; 12045 for 12.6 cm to 20 cm; 12046 for 20.1 cm to 30 cm; and 12047 if the total length is greater than 30 cm.

Coding Tips

Intermediate repair is used when layered closure of one or more of the deeper layers of subcutaneous tissue and superficial fascia, in addition to the skin, require closure. Intermediate repair is also reported for single-layer closure of heavily contaminated wounds that require extensive cleaning or removal of particulate matter. For simple (nonlayered) closure of the neck, hands, feet, and/or external genitalia, see 12001–12007. For complex repairs, see 13131–13133. For wound closure by tissue adhesive(s) only, see HCPCS Level II code G0168.

ICD-10-CM Diagnostic Codes

C51.0	Malignant neoplasm of labium majus ♀
C51.1	Malignant neoplasm of labium minus ♀
C60.0	Malignant neoplasm of prepuce ♂
C60.1	Malignant neoplasm of glans penis ♂
C60.2	Malignant neoplasm of body of penis ♂
C60.8	Malignant neoplasm of overlapping sites of penis ♂
C63.2	Malignant neoplasm of scrotum ♂
C63.7	Malignant neoplasm of other specified male genital organs ♂
C63.8	Malignant neoplasm of overlapping sites of male genital organs ♂
C79.2	Secondary malignant neoplasm of skin

Integumentary

C79.82	Secondary malignant neoplasm of genital organs	
D07.1	Carcinoma in situ of vulva ♀	
D07.2	Carcinoma in situ of vagina ♀	
D07.39	Carcinoma in situ of other female genital organs ♀	
D07.4	Carcinoma in situ of penis ♂	
D07.61	Carcinoma in situ of scrotum ♂	
D07.69	Carcinoma in situ of other male genital organs ♂	
D18.01	Hemangioma of skin and subcutaneous tissue	
D28.0	Benign neoplasm of vulva ♀	
D29.0	Benign neoplasm of penis ♂	
D29.4	Benign neoplasm of scrotum ♂	
D48.5	Neoplasm of uncertain behavior of skin	
I78.1	Nevus, non-neoplastic	
S31.21XA	Laceration without foreign body of penis, initial encounter ♂	
S31.23XA	Puncture wound without foreign body of penis, initial encounter ♂	
S31.25XA	Open bite of penis, initial encounter ♂	
S31.31XA	Laceration without foreign body of scrotum and testes, initial encounter ♂	
S31.32XA	Laceration with foreign body of scrotum and testes, initial encounter ♂	
S31.33XA	Puncture wound without foreign body of scrotum and testes, initial encounter ♂	
S31.34XA	Puncture wound with foreign body of scrotum and testes, initial encounter ♂	
S31.35XA	Open bite of scrotum and testes, initial encounter ♂	
S31.41XA	Laceration without foreign body of vagina and vulva, initial encounter ♀	
S31.42XA	Laceration with foreign body of vagina and vulva, initial encounter ♀	
S31.43XA	Puncture wound without foreign body of vagina and vulva, initial encounter ♀	
S31.44XA	Puncture wound with foreign body of vagina and vulva, initial encounter ♀	
S31.45XA	Open bite of vagina and vulva, initial encounter ♀	
S38.231A	Complete traumatic amputation of scrotum and testis, initial encounter ♂	
S38.232A	Partial traumatic amputation of scrotum and testis, initial encounter ♂	

Associated HCPCS Codes

G0168	Wound closure utilizing tissue adhesive(s) only

AMA: 12041 2019,Nov,3; 2018,Sep,7; 2018,Jan,8; 2017,Jan,8; 2016,Jan,13; 2015,Jan,16; 2014,Jan,11 **12042** 2019,Nov,3; 2018,Sep,7; 2018,Jan,8; 2017,Jan,8; 2016,Jan,13; 2015,Jan,16; 2014,Jan,11 **12044** 2019,Nov,3; 2018,Sep,7; 2018,Jan,8; 2017,Jan,8; 2016,Jan,13; 2015,Jan,16; 2014,Jan,11 **12045** 2019,Nov,3; 2018,Sep,7; 2018,Jan,8; 2017,Jan,8; 2016,Jan,13; 2015,Jan,16; 2014,Jan,11 **12046** 2019,Nov,3; 2018,Sep,7; 2018,Jan,8; 2017,Jan,8; 2016,Jan,13; 2015,Jan,16; 2014,Jan,11 **12047** 2019,Nov,3; 2018,Sep,7; 2018,Jan,8; 2017,Jan,8; 2016,Jan,13; 2015,Jan,16; 2014,Jan,11

Relative Value Units/Medicare Edits

Non-Facility RVU	Work	PE	MP	Total
12041	2.1	4.82	0.27	7.19
12042	2.79	5.44	0.31	8.54
12044	3.19	6.95	0.46	10.6
12045	3.75	7.24	0.64	11.63
12046	4.3	8.71	1.04	14.05
12047	4.95	9.27	1.21	15.43
Facility RVU	Work	PE	MP	Total
12041	2.1	1.85	0.27	4.22
12042	2.79	2.54	0.31	5.64
12044	3.19	2.51	0.46	6.16
12045	3.75	3.37	0.64	7.76
12046	4.3	3.74	1.04	9.08
12047	4.95	3.97	1.21	10.13

	FUD	Status	MUE	Modifiers				IOM Reference
12041	10	A	1(2)	51	N/A	N/A	N/A	None
12042	10	A	1(2)	51	N/A	N/A	N/A	
12044	10	A	1(2)	51	N/A	N/A	N/A	
12045	10	A	1(2)	51	N/A	N/A	N/A	
12046	10	A	1(2)	51	N/A	N/A	80*	
12047	10	A	1(2)	51	N/A	62*	80	

* with documentation

Terms To Know

closure. Repairing an incision or wound by suture or other means.

intermediate repair. *1)* Surgical closure of a wound requiring closure of one or more of the deeper subcutaneous tissue and non-muscle fascia layers in addition to the skin. *2)* Contaminated wounds with single layer closure that need extensive cleaning or foreign body removal. *3)* Wounds with limited undermining less than the width of the wound.

laceration. Tearing injury; a torn, ragged-edged wound.

repair. Surgical closure of a wound. The wound may be a result of injury/trauma or it may be a surgically created defect. Repairs are divided into three categories: simple, intermediate, and complex.

subcutaneous tissue. Sheet or wide band of adipose (fat) and areolar connective tissue in two layers attached to the dermis.

wound. Injury to living tissue often involving a cut or break in the skin.

Integumentary

13131, 13132-13133

13131 Repair, complex, forehead, cheeks, chin, mouth, neck, axillae, genitalia, hands and/or feet; 1.1 cm to 2.5 cm

13132 2.6 cm to 7.5 cm

+ **13133** each additional 5 cm or less (List separately in addition to code for primary procedure)

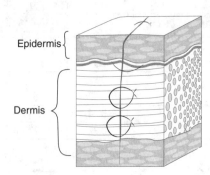

Epidermis

Dermis

Schematic of complex layered suturing
of torn or deeply lacerated tissue

Explanation

The physician repairs wounds located on the genitalia. The physician performs complex, layered suturing of torn, crushed, or deeply lacerated tissue. The physician debrides the wound by removing foreign material or damaged tissue. Irrigation of the wound is performed and antimicrobial solutions are used to decontaminate and cleanse the wound. The physician may trim skin margins with a scalpel or scissors to allow for proper closure. The wound is closed in layers. The physician may perform scar revision, which creates a complex defect requiring repair. Stents or retention sutures may also be used in complex repair of a wound. Reconstructive procedures, such as utilization of local flaps, may be required and are reported separately. Report 13131 for wounds 1.1 cm to 2.5 cm; 13132 for 2.6 cm to 7.5 cm; and 13133 for each additional 5 cm or less.

Coding Tips

Report 13133 in addition to 13132. These procedures include the repair of wounds requiring more than layered closure, such as extensive undermining, stents, or retention sutures. They may also include creation of the defect and necessary preparation for repairs or the debridement and repair of complicated lacerations or avulsions. When multiple wounds are repaired, the lengths of all wounds in the same classification are added together and reported with one code. For wounds of 1.0 cm or less, report simple or intermediate repairs.

ICD-10-CM Diagnostic Codes

C60.0	Malignant neoplasm of prepuce ♂
C60.1	Malignant neoplasm of glans penis ♂
C60.2	Malignant neoplasm of body of penis ♂
C60.8	Malignant neoplasm of overlapping sites of penis ♂
C63.2	Malignant neoplasm of scrotum ♂
C63.7	Malignant neoplasm of other specified male genital organs ♂
C63.8	Malignant neoplasm of overlapping sites of male genital organs ♂
C79.82	Secondary malignant neoplasm of genital organs
D07.1	Carcinoma in situ of vulva ♀
D07.2	Carcinoma in situ of vagina ♀
D07.39	Carcinoma in situ of other female genital organs ♀
D07.4	Carcinoma in situ of penis ♂
D07.61	Carcinoma in situ of scrotum ♂
D07.69	Carcinoma in situ of other male genital organs ♂
D28.0	Benign neoplasm of vulva ♀
D29.0	Benign neoplasm of penis ♂
D29.4	Benign neoplasm of scrotum ♂
D39.8	Neoplasm of uncertain behavior of other specified female genital organs ♀
D40.8	Neoplasm of uncertain behavior of other specified male genital organs ♂
N90.811	Female genital mutilation Type I status ♀
N90.812	Female genital mutilation Type II status ♀
N90.813	Female genital mutilation Type III status ♀
N90.818	Other female genital mutilation status ♀
S31.21XA	Laceration without foreign body of penis, initial encounter ♂
S31.22XA	Laceration with foreign body of penis, initial encounter ♂
S31.23XA	Puncture wound without foreign body of penis, initial encounter ♂
S31.24XA	Puncture wound with foreign body of penis, initial encounter ♂
S31.25XA	Open bite of penis, initial encounter ♂
S31.31XA	Laceration without foreign body of scrotum and testes, initial encounter ♂
S31.32XA	Laceration with foreign body of scrotum and testes, initial encounter ♂
S31.33XA	Puncture wound without foreign body of scrotum and testes, initial encounter ♂
S31.34XA	Puncture wound with foreign body of scrotum and testes, initial encounter ♂
S31.35XA	Open bite of scrotum and testes, initial encounter ♂
S31.41XA	Laceration without foreign body of vagina and vulva, initial encounter ♀
S31.42XA	Laceration with foreign body of vagina and vulva, initial encounter ♀
S31.43XA	Puncture wound without foreign body of vagina and vulva, initial encounter ♀
S31.44XA	Puncture wound with foreign body of vagina and vulva, initial encounter ♀
S31.45XA	Open bite of vagina and vulva, initial encounter ♀
S38.211A	Complete traumatic amputation of female external genital organs, initial encounter ♀
S38.212A	Partial traumatic amputation of female external genital organs, initial encounter ♀
S38.221A	Complete traumatic amputation of penis, initial encounter ♂
S38.222A	Partial traumatic amputation of penis, initial encounter ♂
S38.231A	Complete traumatic amputation of scrotum and testis, initial encounter ♂
S38.232A	Partial traumatic amputation of scrotum and testis, initial encounter ♂

AMA: **13131** 2019,Nov,3; 2018,Sep,7; 2018,Jan,8; 2017,Jan,8; 2017,Apr,9; 2016,Jan,13; 2015,Jan,16; 2014,Jan,11 **13132** 2019,Nov,3; 2018,Sep,7; 2018,Jan,8; 2017,Jan,8; 2017,Apr,9; 2016,Jan,13; 2015,Jan,16; 2014,Oct,14; 2014,Jan,11 **13133** 2019,Nov,3; 2018,Sep,7; 2018,Jan,8; 2017,Jan,8; 2017,Apr,9; 2016,Jan,13; 2015,Jan,16; 2014,Jan,11

© 2020 Optum360, LLC   **N** Newborn: 0   **P** Pediatric: 0-17   **M** Maternity: 9-64   **A** Adult: 15-124   ♂ Male Only   ♀ Female Only   CPT © 2020 American Medical Association. All Rights Reserved.

Integumentary

Relative Value Units/Medicare Edits

Non-Facility RVU	Work	PE	MP	Total
13131	3.73	6.95	0.43	11.11
13132	4.78	8.3	0.51	13.59
13133	2.19	2.52	0.27	4.98
Facility RVU	Work	PE	MP	Total
13131	3.73	2.88	0.43	7.04
13132	4.78	3.52	0.51	8.81
13133	2.19	1.23	0.27	3.69

	FUD	Status	MUE	Modifiers				IOM Reference
13131	10	A	1(2)	51	N/A	N/A	N/A	None
13132	10	A	1(2)	51	N/A	N/A	N/A	
13133	N/A	A	7(3)	N/A	N/A	N/A	N/A	

* with documentation

Terms To Know

complex repair. Surgical closure of a wound requiring more than layered closure of the deeper subcutaneous tissue and fascia.

debridement. Removal of dead or contaminated tissue and foreign matter from a wound.

defect. Imperfection, flaw, or absence.

flap. Mass of flesh and skin partially excised from its location but retaining its blood supply that is moved to another site to repair adjacent or distant defects.

irrigation. To wash out or cleanse a body cavity, wound, or tissue with water or other fluid.

laceration. Tearing injury; a torn, ragged-edged wound.

margin. Boundary, edge, or border, as of a surface or structure.

reconstruction. Recreating, restoring, or rebuilding a body part or organ.

retention suture. Secondary stitching that bridges the primary suture, providing support for the primary repair. A plastic or rubber bolster may be placed over the primary repair and under the retention sutures.

tissue. Group of similar cells with a similar function that form definite structures and organs. Tissue types include epithelial tissue, muscle tissue, connective tissue, and nervous tissue.

wound. Injury to living tissue often involving a cut or break in the skin.

13160

13160   Secondary closure of surgical wound or dehiscence, extensive or complicated

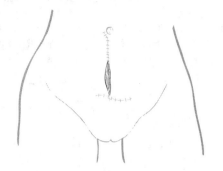

An extensive or complicated dehiscence or surgical wound is treated and closed secondarily

Explanation

The physician secondarily repairs a surgical skin closure after an infectious breakdown of the healing skin. After resolution of the infection, the wound is now ready for closure. The physician uses a scalpel to excise granulation and scar tissue. Skin margins are trimmed to bleeding edges. The wound is sutured in several layers.

Coding Tips

For simple closure of secondary wound dehiscence, see 12020; with packing, see 12021. If incision and drainage of a hematoma, seroma, or fluid collection is performed, see 10140. Do not report 13160 with 11960. Supplies used when providing this procedure may be reported with the appropriate HCPCS Level II code. Check with the specific payer to determine coverage. Surgical trays, A4550, are not separately reimbursed by Medicare; however, other third-party payers may cover them. Check with the specific payer to determine coverage.

ICD-10-CM Diagnostic Codes

T81.30XA	Disruption of wound, unspecified, initial encounter
T81.31XA	Disruption of external operation (surgical) wound, not elsewhere classified, initial encounter
T81.32XA	Disruption of internal operation (surgical) wound, not elsewhere classified, initial encounter
Z48.1	Encounter for planned postprocedural wound closure

AMA: 13160 2019,Nov,3; 2018,Jan,8; 2017,Jan,8; 2016,Jan,13; 2015,Jan,16; 2014,Jan,11

Relative Value Units/Medicare Edits

Non-Facility RVU	Work	PE	MP	Total
13160	12.04	8.89	2.06	22.99
Facility RVU	Work	PE	MP	Total
13160	12.04	8.89	2.06	22.99

	FUD	Status	MUE	Modifiers			IOM Reference
13160	90	A	2(3)	51	N/A	N/A	N/A	None

* with documentation

CPT © 2020 American Medical Association. All Rights Reserved.   ● New   ▲ Revised   + Add On   ★ Telemedicine   AMA: CPT Assist   [Resequenced]   ☑ Laterality   © 2020 Optum360, LLC

15002-15003

15002 Surgical preparation or creation of recipient site by excision of open wounds, burn eschar, or scar (including subcutaneous tissues), or incisional release of scar contracture, trunk, arms, legs; first 100 sq cm or 1% of body area of infants and children

+ 15003 each additional 100 sq cm, or part thereof, or each additional 1% of body area of infants and children (List separately in addition to code for primary procedure)

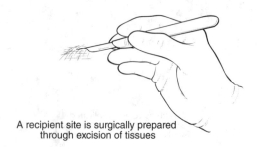

A recipient site is surgically prepared through excision of tissues

Explanation

The physician prepares tissue to receive a free skin graft needed to close or repair a defect. Skin, subcutaneous tissue, scars, burn eschar, and lesions are excised to provide a healthy, vascular tissue bed (where new vessels have been formed) onto which a skin graft will be placed. Alternatively, the physician may prepare tissue by incising or excising a scar contracture that is causing excessive tightening of the skin. Simple debridement of granulations or of recent avulsion is included. Report 15002 for the first 100 sq cm or 1 percent of body area of infants and children for grafts of the trunk arms and legs. Report 15003 for each additional 100 sq cm (or part thereof) of graft area or each additional 1 percent of surface body area in infants and children within the same areas.

Coding Tips

Report 15003 in addition to 15002. These procedures are for preparation or creation of the recipient site only and should be reported with the appropriate skin graft/replacement codes, see 15050–15261 and 15271–15278. For linear scar revision, see 13100–13153. Surgical trays, A4550, are not separately reimbursed by Medicare; however, other third-party payers may cover them. Check with the specific payer to determine coverage.

ICD-10-CM Diagnostic Codes

C43.59	Malignant melanoma of other part of trunk
C44.519	Basal cell carcinoma of skin of other part of trunk
C44.529	Squamous cell carcinoma of skin of other part of trunk
C44.599	Other specified malignant neoplasm of skin of other part of trunk
C4A.59	Merkel cell carcinoma of other part of trunk
D03.59	Melanoma in situ of other part of trunk
D04.5	Carcinoma in situ of skin of trunk
D22.5	Melanocytic nevi of trunk
S31.010A	Laceration without foreign body of lower back and pelvis without penetration into retroperitoneum, initial encounter
S31.020A	Laceration with foreign body of lower back and pelvis without penetration into retroperitoneum, initial encounter
S31.030A	Puncture wound without foreign body of lower back and pelvis without penetration into retroperitoneum, initial encounter
S31.040A	Puncture wound with foreign body of lower back and pelvis without penetration into retroperitoneum, initial encounter
S31.050A	Open bite of lower back and pelvis without penetration into retroperitoneum, initial encounter
S31.113A	Laceration without foreign body of abdominal wall, right lower quadrant without penetration into peritoneal cavity, initial encounter ☑
S31.114A	Laceration without foreign body of abdominal wall, left lower quadrant without penetration into peritoneal cavity, initial encounter ☑
S31.115A	Laceration without foreign body of abdominal wall, periumbilic region without penetration into peritoneal cavity, initial encounter
S31.123A	Laceration of abdominal wall with foreign body, right lower quadrant without penetration into peritoneal cavity, initial encounter ☑
S31.124A	Laceration of abdominal wall with foreign body, left lower quadrant without penetration into peritoneal cavity, initial encounter ☑
S31.125A	Laceration of abdominal wall with foreign body, periumbilic region without penetration into peritoneal cavity, initial encounter
S31.133A	Puncture wound of abdominal wall without foreign body, right lower quadrant without penetration into peritoneal cavity, initial encounter ☑
S31.134A	Puncture wound of abdominal wall without foreign body, left lower quadrant without penetration into peritoneal cavity, initial encounter ☑
S31.135A	Puncture wound of abdominal wall without foreign body, periumbilic region without penetration into peritoneal cavity, initial encounter
S31.143A	Puncture wound of abdominal wall with foreign body, right lower quadrant without penetration into peritoneal cavity, initial encounter ☑
S31.144A	Puncture wound of abdominal wall with foreign body, left lower quadrant without penetration into peritoneal cavity, initial encounter ☑
S31.145A	Puncture wound of abdominal wall with foreign body, periumbilic region without penetration into peritoneal cavity, initial encounter
S31.153A	Open bite of abdominal wall, right lower quadrant without penetration into peritoneal cavity, initial encounter ☑
S31.154A	Open bite of abdominal wall, left lower quadrant without penetration into peritoneal cavity, initial encounter ☑
S31.155A	Open bite of abdominal wall, periumbilic region without penetration into peritoneal cavity, initial encounter
S38.3XXA	Transection (partial) of abdomen, initial encounter
S39.021A	Laceration of muscle, fascia and tendon of abdomen, initial encounter
S39.023A	Laceration of muscle, fascia and tendon of pelvis, initial encounter
T21.32XA	Burn of third degree of abdominal wall, initial encounter
T21.39XA	Burn of third degree of other site of trunk, initial encounter
T21.72XA	Corrosion of third degree of abdominal wall, initial encounter
T21.79XA	Corrosion of third degree of other site of trunk, initial encounter

AMA: **15002** 2019,Nov,3; 2018,Jan,8; 2017,Jan,8; 2016,Jan,13; 2015,Jan,16; 2014,Mar,12; 2014,Jan,11 **15003** 2019,Nov,3; 2018,Jan,8; 2017,Jan,8; 2016,Jan,13; 2015,Jan,16; 2014,Mar,12; 2014,Jan,11

Integumentary

Relative Value Units/Medicare Edits

Non-Facility RVU	Work	PE	MP	Total
15002	3.65	5.75	0.64	10.04
15003	0.8	1.12	0.16	2.08
Facility RVU	**Work**	**PE**	**MP**	**Total**
15002	3.65	2.16	0.64	6.45
15003	0.8	0.36	0.16	1.32

	FUD	Status	MUE	Modifiers				IOM Reference
15002	0	A	1(2)	N/A	N/A	N/A	80*	None
15003	N/A	A	60(3)	N/A	N/A	N/A	80*	

* with documentation

Terms To Know

avulsion. Forcible tearing away of a part, by surgical means or traumatic injury.

contracture. Shortening of muscle or connective tissue.

debridement. Removal of dead or contaminated tissue and foreign matter from a wound.

defect. Imperfection, flaw, or absence.

eschar. Leathery slough produced by burns.

excise. Remove or cut out.

free graft. Unattached piece of skin and tissue moved to another part of the body and sutured into place to repair a defect.

granulation. Formation of small, bead-like masses of cytoplasm or granules on the surface of healing wounds of an organ, membrane, or tissue.

incise. To cut open or into.

lesion. Area of damaged tissue that has lost continuity or function, due to disease or trauma.

scar tissue. Fibrous connective tissue that forms around a wounded area or injury, composed mainly of fibroblasts or collagenous fibers.

subcutaneous tissue. Sheet or wide band of adipose (fat) and areolar connective tissue in two layers attached to the dermis.

15004-15005

15004   Surgical preparation or creation of recipient site by excision of open wounds, burn eschar, or scar (including subcutaneous tissues), or incisional release of scar contracture, face, scalp, eyelids, mouth, neck, ears, orbits, genitalia, hands, feet and/or multiple digits; first 100 sq cm or 1% of body area of infants and children

+   15005   each additional 100 sq cm, or part thereof, or each additional 1% of body area of infants and children (List separately in addition to code for primary procedure)

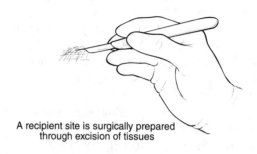

A recipient site is surgically prepared through excision of tissues

Explanation

The physician prepares tissue to receive a free skin graft needed to close or repair a defect. Skin, subcutaneous tissue, scars, burn eschar, and lesions are excised to provide a healthy, vascular tissue bed (where new vessels have been formed) onto which a skin graft will be placed. Alternatively, the physician may prepare tissue by incising or excising a scar contracture that is causing excessive tightening of the skin. Simple debridement of granulations or of recent avulsion is included. Report 15004 for the first 100 sq cm or 1 percent of body area in infants and children of the genitalia. Report 15005 for each additional 100 sq cm (or part thereof) or each additional 1 percent of body area in infants and children.

Coding Tips

Report 15005 in addition to 15004. These procedures are for preparation or creation of the recipient site only and should be reported with the appropriate skin graft/replacement codes, see 15050–15261 and 15271–15278. Surgical trays, A4550, are not separately reimbursed by Medicare; however, other third-party payers may cover them. Check with the specific payer to determine coverage.

ICD-10-CM Diagnostic Codes

C51.0	Malignant neoplasm of labium majus ♀
C51.1	Malignant neoplasm of labium minus ♀
C51.2	Malignant neoplasm of clitoris ♀
C51.8	Malignant neoplasm of overlapping sites of vulva ♀
C52	Malignant neoplasm of vagina ♀
C57.7	Malignant neoplasm of other specified female genital organs ♀
C57.8	Malignant neoplasm of overlapping sites of female genital organs ♀
C60.0	Malignant neoplasm of prepuce ♂
C60.2	Malignant neoplasm of body of penis ♂
C60.8	Malignant neoplasm of overlapping sites of penis ♂
C63.2	Malignant neoplasm of scrotum ♂
C63.7	Malignant neoplasm of other specified male genital organs ♂
C63.8	Malignant neoplasm of overlapping sites of male genital organs ♂

CPT © 2020 American Medical Association. All Rights Reserved.   ● New   ▲ Revised   + Add On   ★ Telemedicine   AMA: CPT Assist   [Resequenced]   ☑ Laterality   © 2020 Optum360, LLC

Integumentary

S31.21XA	Laceration without foreign body of penis, initial encounter ♂
S31.22XA	Laceration with foreign body of penis, initial encounter ♂
S31.23XA	Puncture wound without foreign body of penis, initial encounter ♂
S31.24XA	Puncture wound with foreign body of penis, initial encounter ♂
S31.25XA	Open bite of penis, initial encounter ♂
S31.31XA	Laceration without foreign body of scrotum and testes, initial encounter ♂
S31.32XA	Laceration with foreign body of scrotum and testes, initial encounter ♂
S31.33XA	Puncture wound without foreign body of scrotum and testes, initial encounter ♂
S31.34XA	Puncture wound with foreign body of scrotum and testes, initial encounter ♂
S31.35XA	Open bite of scrotum and testes, initial encounter ♂
S31.41XA	Laceration without foreign body of vagina and vulva, initial encounter ♀
S31.42XA	Laceration with foreign body of vagina and vulva, initial encounter ♀
S31.43XA	Puncture wound without foreign body of vagina and vulva, initial encounter ♀
S31.44XA	Puncture wound with foreign body of vagina and vulva, initial encounter ♀
S31.45XA	Open bite of vagina and vulva, initial encounter ♀
S38.211A	Complete traumatic amputation of female external genital organs, initial encounter ♀
S38.212A	Partial traumatic amputation of female external genital organs, initial encounter ♀
S38.221A	Complete traumatic amputation of penis, initial encounter ♂
S38.222A	Partial traumatic amputation of penis, initial encounter ♂
S38.231A	Complete traumatic amputation of scrotum and testis, initial encounter ♂
S38.232A	Partial traumatic amputation of scrotum and testis, initial encounter ♂
S39.848A	Other specified injuries of external genitals, initial encounter
T21.36XA	Burn of third degree of male genital region, initial encounter ♂
T21.37XA	Burn of third degree of female genital region, initial encounter ♀
T21.76XA	Corrosion of third degree of male genital region, initial encounter ♂
T21.77XA	Corrosion of third degree of female genital region, initial encounter ♀

AMA: **15004** 2019,Nov,3; 2018,Jan,8; 2017,Jan,8; 2016,Jan,13; 2015,Jan,16; 2014,Mar,12; 2014,Jan,11 **15005** 2019,Nov,3; 2018,Jan,8; 2017,Jan,8; 2016,Jan,13; 2015,Jan,16; 2014,Mar,12; 2014,Jan,11

Relative Value Units/Medicare Edits

Non-Facility RVU	Work	PE	MP	Total
15004	4.58	6.24	0.62	11.44
15005	1.6	1.58	0.32	3.5
Facility RVU	Work	PE	MP	Total
15004	4.58	2.45	0.62	7.65
15005	1.6	0.74	0.32	2.66

	FUD	Status	MUE	Modifiers				IOM Reference
15004	0	A	1(2)	N/A	N/A	N/A	80*	None
15005	N/A	A	19(3)	N/A	N/A	N/A	80*	

* with documentation

Terms To Know

debridement. Removal of dead or contaminated tissue and foreign matter from a wound.

eschar. Leathery slough produced by burns.

graft. Tissue implant from another part of the body or another person.

scar tissue. Fibrous connective tissue that forms around a wounded area or injury, composed mainly of fibroblasts or collagenous fibers.

wound. Injury to living tissue often involving a cut or break in the skin.

15120-15121

15120 Split-thickness autograft, face, scalp, eyelids, mouth, neck, ears, orbits, genitalia, hands, feet, and/or multiple digits; first 100 sq cm or less, or 1% of body area of infants and children (except 15050)

+ 15121 each additional 100 sq cm, or each additional 1% of body area of infants and children, or part thereof (List separately in addition to code for primary procedure)

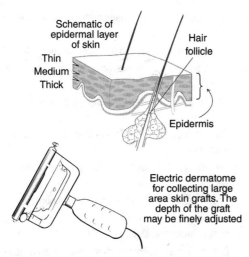

Schematic of epidermal layer of skin
Thin
Medium
Thick
Hair follicle
Epidermis

Electric dermatome for collecting large area skin grafts. The depth of the graft may be finely adjusted

A split thickness skin graft is harvested and applied

Explanation

The physician takes a split-thickness skin autograft from one area of the body and grafts it to an area needing repair. This procedure is performed when direct wound closure or adjacent tissue transfer is not possible. The physician harvests a split-thickness skin graft with a dermatome. The epidermis or top layer of skin is taken, along with a small portion of the dermis or bottom layer of the skin. This graft is sutured or stapled onto the recipient area of the genitalia. Report 15120 for the first 100 sq cm or less in adults or children age 10 or over or 1 percent of the total body area of infants and children younger than age 10. Report 15121 for each additional 100 sq cm and each additional 1 percent of total body area of infants and children.

Coding Tips

Report 15121 in addition to 15120. Preparation of the recipient site is reported separately, see 15004–15005. Repair of the donor site requiring skin grafts or local flaps is added as an additional procedure. Local anesthesia is included in these services. However, these procedures may be performed under general anesthesia, depending on the age and/or condition of the patient. Surgical trays, A4550, are not separately reimbursed by Medicare; however, other third-party payers may cover them. Check with the specific payer to determine coverage.

ICD-10-CM Diagnostic Codes

C51.0	Malignant neoplasm of labium majus ♀
C51.1	Malignant neoplasm of labium minus ♀
C51.2	Malignant neoplasm of clitoris ♀
C51.8	Malignant neoplasm of overlapping sites of vulva ♀
C52	Malignant neoplasm of vagina ♀
C57.7	Malignant neoplasm of other specified female genital organs ♀
C57.8	Malignant neoplasm of overlapping sites of female genital organs ♀

C60.0	Malignant neoplasm of prepuce ♂
C60.2	Malignant neoplasm of body of penis ♂
C60.8	Malignant neoplasm of overlapping sites of penis ♂
C63.2	Malignant neoplasm of scrotum ♂
C63.7	Malignant neoplasm of other specified male genital organs ♂
C63.8	Malignant neoplasm of overlapping sites of male genital organs ♂
S31.21XA	Laceration without foreign body of penis, initial encounter ♂
S31.23XA	Puncture wound without foreign body of penis, initial encounter ♂
S31.25XA	Open bite of penis, initial encounter ♂
S31.31XA	Laceration without foreign body of scrotum and testes, initial encounter ♂
S31.33XA	Puncture wound without foreign body of scrotum and testes, initial encounter ♂
S31.35XA	Open bite of scrotum and testes, initial encounter ♂
S31.41XA	Laceration without foreign body of vagina and vulva, initial encounter ♀
S31.43XA	Puncture wound without foreign body of vagina and vulva, initial encounter ♀
S31.45XA	Open bite of vagina and vulva, initial encounter ♀
S39.848A	Other specified injuries of external genitals, initial encounter

AMA: 15120 2018,Jan,8; 2017,Jan,8; 2016,Jun,8; 2016,Jan,13; 2015,Jan,16; 2014,Jan,11 **15121** 2018,Jan,8; 2017,Jan,8; 2016,Jun,8; 2016,Jan,13; 2015,Jan,16; 2014,Jan,11

Relative Value Units/Medicare Edits

Non-Facility RVU	Work	PE	MP	Total
15120	10.15	12.6	1.61	24.36
15121	2.0	3.66	0.39	6.05
Facility RVU	**Work**	**PE**	**MP**	**Total**
15120	10.15	8.19	1.61	19.95
15121	2.0	1.51	0.39	3.9

	FUD	Status	MUE	Modifiers				IOM Reference
15120	90	A	1(2)	51	N/A	N/A	N/A	None
15121	N/A	A	8(3)	N/A	N/A	62*	N/A	

* with documentation

Terms To Know

autograft. Any tissue harvested from one anatomical site of a person and grafted to another anatomical site of the same person. Most commonly, blood vessels, skin, tendons, fascia, and bone are used as autografts.

dermis. Skin layer found under the epidermis that contains a papillary upper layer and the deep reticular layer of collagen, vascular bed, and nerves.

epidermis. Outermost, nonvascular layer of skin that contains four to five differentiated layers depending on its body location: stratum corneum, lucidum, granulosum, spinosum, and basale.

graft. Tissue implant from another part of the body or another person.

split thickness skin graft. Graft using the epidermis and part of the dermis.

15240-15241

15240 Full thickness graft, free, including direct closure of donor site, forehead, cheeks, chin, mouth, neck, axillae, genitalia, hands, and/or feet; 20 sq cm or less

+ 15241 each additional 20 sq cm, or part thereof (List separately in addition to code for primary procedure)

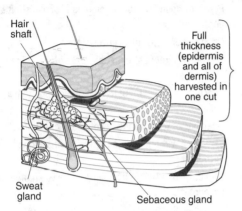

Hair shaft

Full thickness (epidermis and all of dermis) harvested in one cut

Sweat gland

Sebaceous gland

Explanation

The physician harvests a full-thickness skin graft from one area of the body and grafts it to an area on the genitalia needing repair. A full-thickness skin graft consists of the superficial and deeper layers of skin (epidermis and dermis). The resulting surgical wound at the donor site is closed by lifting the remaining skin edges and placing sutures to close directly. Residual adipose tissue is removed from the underside of the graft. The graft is sutured onto the wound bed to cover a defect of no more than 20 sq cm. Report 15241 for each additional 20 sq cm or part thereof.

Coding Tips

Report 15241 in addition to 15240. Preparation of the recipient site is reported separately, see 15002–15005. Repair of the donor site requiring a skin graft or local flaps is to be added as an additional procedure.

ICD-10-CM Diagnostic Codes

C51.0	Malignant neoplasm of labium majus ♀
C51.1	Malignant neoplasm of labium minus ♀
C51.2	Malignant neoplasm of clitoris ♀
C51.8	Malignant neoplasm of overlapping sites of vulva ♀
C52	Malignant neoplasm of vagina ♀
C57.7	Malignant neoplasm of other specified female genital organs ♀
C57.8	Malignant neoplasm of overlapping sites of female genital organs ♀
C60.0	Malignant neoplasm of prepuce ♂
C60.2	Malignant neoplasm of body of penis ♂
C60.8	Malignant neoplasm of overlapping sites of penis ♂
C63.2	Malignant neoplasm of scrotum ♂
C63.7	Malignant neoplasm of other specified male genital organs ♂
C63.8	Malignant neoplasm of overlapping sites of male genital organs ♂
S31.21XA	Laceration without foreign body of penis, initial encounter ♂
S31.22XA	Laceration with foreign body of penis, initial encounter ♂

S31.23XA	Puncture wound without foreign body of penis, initial encounter ♂
S31.24XA	Puncture wound with foreign body of penis, initial encounter ♂
S31.25XA	Open bite of penis, initial encounter ♂
S31.31XA	Laceration without foreign body of scrotum and testes, initial encounter ♂
S31.32XA	Laceration with foreign body of scrotum and testes, initial encounter ♂
S31.33XA	Puncture wound without foreign body of scrotum and testes, initial encounter ♂
S31.34XA	Puncture wound with foreign body of scrotum and testes, initial encounter ♂
S31.35XA	Open bite of scrotum and testes, initial encounter ♂
S31.41XA	Laceration without foreign body of vagina and vulva, initial encounter ♀
S31.42XA	Laceration with foreign body of vagina and vulva, initial encounter ♀
S31.43XA	Puncture wound without foreign body of vagina and vulva, initial encounter ♀
S31.44XA	Puncture wound with foreign body of vagina and vulva, initial encounter ♀
S31.45XA	Open bite of vagina and vulva, initial encounter ♀
S38.211A	Complete traumatic amputation of female external genital organs, initial encounter ♀
S38.212A	Partial traumatic amputation of female external genital organs, initial encounter ♀
S38.221A	Complete traumatic amputation of penis, initial encounter ♂
S38.222A	Partial traumatic amputation of penis, initial encounter ♂
S38.231A	Complete traumatic amputation of scrotum and testis, initial encounter ♂
S38.232A	Partial traumatic amputation of scrotum and testis, initial encounter ♂
S39.848A	Other specified injuries of external genitals, initial encounter
T21.36XA	Burn of third degree of male genital region, initial encounter ♂
T21.37XA	Burn of third degree of female genital region, initial encounter ♀
T21.76XA	Corrosion of third degree of male genital region, initial encounter ♂
T21.77XA	Corrosion of third degree of female genital region, initial encounter ♀

AMA: 15240 2018,Jan,8; 2017,Jan,8; 2016,Jun,8; 2016,Jan,13; 2015,Jan,16; 2014,Jan,11 **15241** 2018,Jan,8; 2017,Jan,8; 2016,Jun,8; 2016,Jan,13; 2015,Jan,16; 2014,Jan,11

Relative Value Units/Medicare Edits

Non-Facility RVU	Work	PE	MP	Total
15240	10.41	14.78	1.34	26.53
15241	1.86	3.04	0.28	5.18
Facility RVU	**Work**	**PE**	**MP**	**Total**
15240	10.41	10.99	1.34	22.74
15241	1.86	1.01	0.28	3.15

	FUD	Status	MUE	Modifiers				IOM Reference
15240	90	A	1(2)	51	N/A	N/A	N/A	None
15241	N/A	A	9(3)	N/A	N/A	N/A	N/A	

* with documentation

Integumentary

17270-17276

17270 Destruction, malignant lesion (eg, laser surgery, electrosurgery, cryosurgery, chemosurgery, surgical curettement), scalp, neck, hands, feet, genitalia; lesion diameter 0.5 cm or less

17271 lesion diameter 0.6 to 1.0 cm

17272 lesion diameter 1.1 to 2.0 cm

17273 lesion diameter 2.1 to 3.0 cm

17274 lesion diameter 3.1 to 4.0 cm

17276 lesion diameter over 4.0 cm

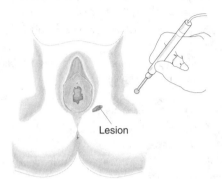

Lesion

The physician may use laser, fulguration, or cryosurgery, etc. to destroy the malignant lesion

Explanation

The physician destroys a malignant lesion of the genitalia. Destruction may be accomplished by using a laser or electrocautery to burn the lesion, cryotherapy to freeze the lesion, chemicals to destroy the lesion, or surgical curettement to remove the lesion. Report 17270 for a lesion diameter 0.5 cm or less; 17271 for 0.6 cm to 1 cm; 17272 for 1.1 cm to 2 cm; 17273 for 2.1 cm to 3 cm; 17274 for 3.1 cm to 4 cm; and 17276 if the lesion diameter is greater than 4 cm.

Coding Tips

Destruction is defined as the ablation of malignant tissue, by any method, with or without curettement. Local anesthesia is included in these services. Closure is not typically required. For destruction of benign lesions other than skin tags or cutaneous vascular lesions, see 17110–17111. For excision of a malignant lesion, see 11620–11626.

ICD-10-CM Diagnostic Codes

C51.0	Malignant neoplasm of labium majus ♀
C51.1	Malignant neoplasm of labium minus ♀
C51.2	Malignant neoplasm of clitoris ♀
C51.8	Malignant neoplasm of overlapping sites of vulva ♀
C52	Malignant neoplasm of vagina ♀
C57.7	Malignant neoplasm of other specified female genital organs ♀
C57.8	Malignant neoplasm of overlapping sites of female genital organs ♀
C60.0	Malignant neoplasm of prepuce ♂
C60.1	Malignant neoplasm of glans penis ♂
C60.2	Malignant neoplasm of body of penis ♂
C60.8	Malignant neoplasm of overlapping sites of penis ♂
C63.2	Malignant neoplasm of scrotum ♂
C63.7	Malignant neoplasm of other specified male genital organs ♂
C63.8	Malignant neoplasm of overlapping sites of male genital organs ♂

C7B.1	Secondary Merkel cell carcinoma

AMA: 17270 2018,Jan,8; 2017,Jan,8; 2017,Dec,14; 2016,Jan,13; 2015,Jan,16; 2014,Jan,11 **17271** 2018,Jan,8; 2017,Jan,8; 2017,Dec,14; 2016,Jan,13; 2015,Jan,16; 2014,Jan,11 **17272** 2018,Jan,8; 2017,Jan,8; 2017,Dec,14; 2016,Jan,13; 2015,Jan,16; 2014,Jan,11 **17273** 2018,Jan,8; 2017,Jan,8; 2017,Dec,14; 2016,Jan,13; 2015,Jan,16; 2014,Jan,11 **17274** 2018,Jan,8; 2017,Jan,8; 2017,Dec,14; 2016,Jan,13; 2015,Jan,16; 2014,Jan,11 **17276** 2018,Jan,8; 2017,Jan,8; 2017,Dec,14; 2016,Jan,13; 2015,Jan,16; 2014,Jan,11

Relative Value Units/Medicare Edits

Non-Facility RVU	Work	PE	MP	Total
17270	1.37	2.72	0.13	4.22
17271	1.54	2.98	0.13	4.65
17272	1.82	3.32	0.18	5.32
17273	2.1	3.61	0.21	5.92
17274	2.64	4.07	0.26	6.97
17276	3.25	4.51	0.31	8.07
Facility RVU	Work	PE	MP	Total
17270	1.37	1.24	0.13	2.74
17271	1.54	1.35	0.13	3.02
17272	1.82	1.52	0.18	3.52
17273	2.1	1.68	0.21	3.99
17274	2.64	1.98	0.26	4.88
17276	3.25	2.3	0.31	5.86

	FUD	Status	MUE	Modifiers				IOM Reference
17270	10	A	6(3)	51	N/A	N/A	N/A	None
17271	10	A	4(3)	51	N/A	N/A	N/A	
17272	10	A	5(3)	51	N/A	N/A	N/A	
17273	10	A	4(3)	51	N/A	N/A	N/A	
17274	10	A	2(3)	51	N/A	N/A	N/A	
17276	10	A	2(3)	51	N/A	N/A	N/A	

* with documentation

Terms To Know

chemosurgery. Application of chemical agents to destroy tissue, originally referring to the in situ chemical fixation of premalignant or malignant lesions to facilitate surgical excision.

cryosurgery. Application of intense cold, usually produced using liquid nitrogen, to locally freeze diseased or unwanted tissue and induce tissue necrosis without causing harm to adjacent tissue.

electrocautery. Division or cutting of tissue using high-frequency electrical current to produce heat, which destroys cells.

laser surgery. Use of concentrated, sharply defined light beams to cut, cauterize, coagulate, seal, or vaporize tissue. The color and wavelength of the laser light is produced by its active medium, such as argon, CO_2, potassium titanyl phosphate (KTP), Krypton, and Nd:YAG, which determines the type of tissues it can best treat.

CPT © 2020 American Medical Association. All Rights Reserved. ● New ▲ Revised + Add On ★ Telemedicine AMA: CPT Assist [Resequenced] ☑ Laterality © 2020 Optum360, LLC

35840

35840 Exploration for postoperative hemorrhage, thrombosis or infection; abdomen

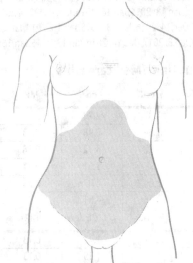

A surgical exploration is performed in the abdominal cavity for the purpose of finding and identifying postoperative hemorrhage, thrombosis (clotting), or infection

Explanation

The physician reopens the original incision site and inspects the operative area for active bleeding, hematoma, thrombus, and exudate. The physician removes or debrides any observed hematoma, thrombus, and infected tissues. The physician looks for and corrects any active bleeding sites using electrocautery or ligation of bleeding vessels. The physician may leave an infected wound open, but generally closes the incision, leaving drains in place.

Coding Tips

This code is used to report exploration for postoperative hemorrhage, thrombosis, or infection of veins and arteries of the abdomen only and is not used for exploration of vessels not followed by surgical repair.

ICD-10-CM Diagnostic Codes

G89.18	Other acute postprocedural pain
G89.28	Other chronic postprocedural pain
I77.2	Rupture of artery
K68.11	Postprocedural retroperitoneal abscess
N99.0	Postprocedural (acute) (chronic) kidney failure
N99.520	Hemorrhage of incontinent external stoma of urinary tract
N99.521	Infection of incontinent external stoma of urinary tract
N99.522	Malfunction of incontinent external stoma of urinary tract
N99.523	Herniation of incontinent stoma of urinary tract
N99.524	Stenosis of incontinent stoma of urinary tract
N99.528	Other complication of incontinent external stoma of urinary tract
N99.530	Hemorrhage of continent stoma of urinary tract
N99.531	Infection of continent stoma of urinary tract
N99.532	Malfunction of continent stoma of urinary tract
N99.533	Herniation of continent stoma of urinary tract
N99.534	Stenosis of continent stoma of urinary tract
N99.538	Other complication of continent stoma of urinary tract

N99.820	Postprocedural hemorrhage of a genitourinary system organ or structure following a genitourinary system procedure
N99.821	Postprocedural hemorrhage of a genitourinary system organ or structure following other procedure
N99.840	Postprocedural hematoma of a genitourinary system organ or structure following a genitourinary system procedure
N99.841	Postprocedural hematoma of a genitourinary system organ or structure following other procedure
N99.842	Postprocedural seroma of a genitourinary system organ or structure following a genitourinary system procedure
N99.843	Postprocedural seroma of a genitourinary system organ or structure following other procedure
N99.89	Other postprocedural complications and disorders of genitourinary system
T81.31XA	Disruption of external operation (surgical) wound, not elsewhere classified, initial encounter
T81.32XA	Disruption of internal operation (surgical) wound, not elsewhere classified, initial encounter
T81.41XA	Infection following a procedure, superficial incisional surgical site, initial encounter
T81.42XA	Infection following a procedure, deep incisional surgical site, initial encounter
T81.43XA	Infection following a procedure, organ and space surgical site, initial encounter
T81.710A	Complication of mesenteric artery following a procedure, not elsewhere classified, initial encounter
T81.711A	Complication of renal artery following a procedure, not elsewhere classified, initial encounter
T81.72XA	Complication of vein following a procedure, not elsewhere classified, initial encounter
T82.7XXA	Infection and inflammatory reaction due to other cardiac and vascular devices, implants and grafts, initial encounter
T82.818A	Embolism due to vascular prosthetic devices, implants and grafts, initial encounter
T82.828A	Fibrosis due to vascular prosthetic devices, implants and grafts, initial encounter
T82.838A	Hemorrhage due to vascular prosthetic devices, implants and grafts, initial encounter
T82.848A	Pain due to vascular prosthetic devices, implants and grafts, initial encounter
T82.858A	Stenosis of other vascular prosthetic devices, implants and grafts, initial encounter
T82.868A	Thrombosis due to vascular prosthetic devices, implants and grafts, initial encounter

AMA: 35840 1997,Nov,1; 1997,May,4

Relative Value Units/Medicare Edits

Non-Facility RVU	Work	PE	MP	Total
35840	20.75	9.38	4.73	34.86
Facility RVU	**Work**	**PE**	**MP**	**Total**
35840	20.75	9.38	4.73	34.86

	FUD	Status	MUE	Modifiers				IOM Reference
35840	90	A	2(3)	51	N/A	62*	80	None

* with documentation

36415-36416

36415 Collection of venous blood by venipuncture
36416 Collection of capillary blood specimen (eg, finger, heel, ear stick)

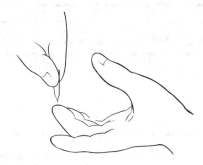

Capillary blood is collected.
The specimen is typically collected by finger stick

Explanation

A needle is inserted into the skin over a vein to puncture the blood vessel and withdraw blood for venous collection in 36415. In 36416, a prick is made into the finger, heel, or ear and capillary blood that pools at the puncture site is collected in a pipette. In either case, the blood is used for diagnostic study and no catheter is placed.

Coding Tips

These procedures do not include laboratory analysis. If a specimen is transported to an outside laboratory, report 99000 for handling or conveyance. For venipuncture, younger than 3 years of age, femoral or jugular vein, see 36400; scalp or other vein, see 36405–36406. For venipuncture, age 3 years or older, for non-routine diagnostic or therapeutic purposes, necessitating the skill of a physician or other qualified healthcare professional, see 36410. Do not append modifier 63 to 36415 as the description or nature of the procedure includes infants up to 4 kg. Medicare and some payers may require HCPCS Level II code G0471 to report this service when provided in an FQHC.

ICD-10-CM Diagnostic Codes

The application of this code is too broad to adequately present ICD-10-CM diagnostic code links here. Refer to your ICD-10-CM book.

Associated HCPCS Codes

G0471   Collection of venous blood by venipuncture or urine sample by catheterization from an individual in a skilled nursing facility (SNF) or by a laboratory on behalf of a home health agency (HHA)

AMA: 36415 2019,Aug,8; 2018,Jan,8; 2017,Jan,8; 2016,Jan,13; 2015,Jan,16; 2014,May,4; 2014,Jan,11

Relative Value Units/Medicare Edits

Non-Facility RVU	Work	PE	MP	Total
36415	0.0	0.0	0.0	0.0
36416	0.0	0.0	0.0	0.0
Facility RVU	**Work**	**PE**	**MP**	**Total**
36415	0.0	0.0	0.0	0.0
36416	0.0	0.0	0.0	0.0

	FUD	Status	MUE	Modifiers				IOM Reference
36415	N/A	X	2(3)	N/A	N/A	N/A	N/A	None
36416	N/A	B	0(3)	N/A	N/A	N/A	N/A	

* with documentation

Terms To Know

blood vessel. Tubular channel consisting of arteries, veins, and capillaries that transports blood throughout the body.

capillary. Tiny, minute blood vessel that connects the arterioles (smallest arteries) and the venules (smallest veins) and acts as a semipermeable membrane between the blood and the tissue fluid.

catheter. Flexible tube inserted into an area of the body for introducing or withdrawing fluid.

diagnostic. Examination or procedure to which the patient is subjected, or which is performed on materials derived from a hospital outpatient, to obtain information to aid in the assessment of a medical condition or the identification of a disease. Among these examinations and tests are diagnostic laboratory services such as hematology and chemistry, diagnostic x-rays, isotope studies, EKGs, pulmonary function studies, thyroid function tests, psychological tests, and other tests given to determine the nature and severity of an ailment or injury.

pipette. Small, narrow glass or plastic tube with both ends open used for measuring or transferring liquids.

specimen. Tissue cells or sample of fluid taken for analysis, pathologic examination, and diagnosis.

venipuncture. Piercing a vein through the skin by a needle and syringe or sharp-ended cannula or catheter to draw blood, start an intravenous infusion, instill medication, or inject another substance such as radiopaque dye.

venous. Relating to the veins.

Arteries and Veins

CPT © 2020 American Medical Association. All Rights Reserved.   ● New   ▲ Revised   + Add On   ★ Telemedicine   AMA: CPT Assist   [Resequenced]   ☑ Laterality   © 2020 Optum360, LLC

36593

36593 Declotting by thrombolytic agent of implanted vascular access device or catheter

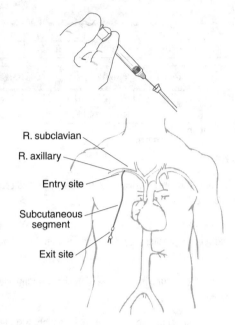

A thrombolytic agent is used to declot a catheter or implanted vascular access device

Explanation

To remove a clot from an implanted vascular access device or catheter, the physician injects a thrombolytic agent (e.g., Streptokinase) into the catheter to dissolve the clot. The patient is observed for any abnormal signs of bleeding.

Coding Tips

When 36593 is performed with another separately identifiable procedure, the highest dollar value code is listed as the primary procedure and subsequent procedures are appended with modifier 51. Supplies used when providing this procedure may be reported with the appropriate HCPCS Level II "J" code. Check with the specific payer to determine coverage.

ICD-10-CM Diagnostic Codes

T82.818A	Embolism due to vascular prosthetic devices, implants and grafts, initial encounter
T82.848A	Pain due to vascular prosthetic devices, implants and grafts, initial encounter
T82.856A	Stenosis of peripheral vascular stent, initial encounter
T82.858A	Stenosis of other vascular prosthetic devices, implants and grafts, initial encounter
T82.868A	Thrombosis due to vascular prosthetic devices, implants and grafts, initial encounter
T82.898A	Other specified complication of vascular prosthetic devices, implants and grafts, initial encounter

AMA: 36593 2018,Jan,8; 2017,Jan,8; 2016,Jan,13; 2015,Jan,16; 2014,Jan,11

Relative Value Units/Medicare Edits

Non-Facility RVU	Work	PE	MP	Total
36593	0.0	0.87	0.02	0.89
Facility RVU	**Work**	**PE**	**MP**	**Total**
36593	0.0	0.87	0.02	0.89

	FUD	Status	MUE	Modifiers				IOM Reference
36593	N/A	A	2(3)	N/A	N/A	N/A	80*	None

* with documentation

Terms To Know

arteriovenous fistula. Connecting passage between an artery and a vein.

blood clot. Semisolidified, coagulated mass of mainly platelets and fibrin in the bloodstream.

cannula. Tube inserted into a blood vessel, duct, or body cavity to facilitate passage.

catheter. Flexible tube inserted into an area of the body for introducing or withdrawing fluid.

embolism. Obstruction of a blood vessel resulting from a clot or foreign substance.

implantable venous access device. Catheter implanted for continuous access to the venous system for long-term parenteral feeding or for the administration of fluids or medications.

intravenous. Within a vein or veins.

stenosis. Narrowing or constriction of a passage.

thrombolytic agent. Drugs or other substances used to dissolve blood clots in blood vessels or in tubes that have been placed into the body.

thrombus. Stationary blood clot inside a blood vessel.

© 2020 Optum360, LLC   N Newborn: 0   P Pediatric: 0-17   M Maternity: 9-64   A Adult: 15-124   ♂ Male Only   ♀ Female Only   CPT © 2020 American Medical Association. All Rights Reserved.

Arteries and Veins

36598

36598 Contrast injection(s) for radiologic evaluation of existing central venous access device, including fluoroscopy, image documentation and report

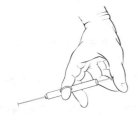

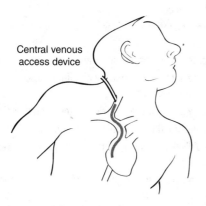

Contrast is injected into the central venous access device; this procedure includes image documentation, report, and fluoroscopy

Central venous access device

Explanation

A previously placed central venous access device is evaluated for complications that may be interfering with its proper functioning or the ability to draw blood from the catheter. Complications may include the presence of a fibrin sheath around the end of the catheter, migration of the catheter tip, patency of the tubing, kinking, fracture, or leaks. A small amount of contrast agent is injected into the catheter and the central venous access device is examined under fluoroscopy as the flow is evaluated. Images are documented and a radiological report is prepared.

Coding Tips

Fluoroscopic imaging (76000) is included in this code and not reported separately. Imaging is limited to the device and immediate areas of the vena cava or extremity vein. When a complete study of the vena cava or an extremity vein is performed, see 75820, 75825, and 75827. Do not report mechanical removal of pericatheter (36595) or intraluminal/intracatheter (36596) obstructive material separately.

ICD-10-CM Diagnostic Codes

T80.211A	Bloodstream infection due to central venous catheter, initial encounter
T80.212A	Local infection due to central venous catheter, initial encounter
T80.218A	Other infection due to central venous catheter, initial encounter
T82.41XA	Breakdown (mechanical) of vascular dialysis catheter, initial encounter
T82.42XA	Displacement of vascular dialysis catheter, initial encounter
T82.43XA	Leakage of vascular dialysis catheter, initial encounter
T82.49XA	Other complication of vascular dialysis catheter, initial encounter
T82.514A	Breakdown (mechanical) of infusion catheter, initial encounter
T82.524A	Displacement of infusion catheter, initial encounter
T82.534A	Leakage of infusion catheter, initial encounter
T82.594A	Other mechanical complication of infusion catheter, initial encounter
T82.598A	Other mechanical complication of other cardiac and vascular devices and implants, initial encounter
T82.7XXA	Infection and inflammatory reaction due to other cardiac and vascular devices, implants and grafts, initial encounter
T82.818A	Embolism due to vascular prosthetic devices, implants and grafts, initial encounter
T82.828A	Fibrosis due to vascular prosthetic devices, implants and grafts, initial encounter
T82.838A	Hemorrhage due to vascular prosthetic devices, implants and grafts, initial encounter
T82.848A	Pain due to vascular prosthetic devices, implants and grafts, initial encounter
T82.856A	Stenosis of peripheral vascular stent, initial encounter
T82.858A	Stenosis of other vascular prosthetic devices, implants and grafts, initial encounter
T82.868A	Thrombosis due to vascular prosthetic devices, implants and grafts, initial encounter
T82.898A	Other specified complication of vascular prosthetic devices, implants and grafts, initial encounter
Z45.2	Encounter for adjustment and management of vascular access device

AMA: 36598 2014,Jan,11

Relative Value Units/Medicare Edits

Non-Facility RVU	Work	PE	MP	Total
36598	0.74	2.62	0.08	3.44
Facility RVU	**Work**	**PE**	**MP**	**Total**
36598	0.74	0.25	0.08	1.07

	FUD	Status	MUE	Modifiers				IOM Reference
36598	0	T	2(3)	51	50	N/A	80*	None

* with documentation

Terms To Know

central venous catheter. Catheter positioned in the superior vena cava or right atrium and introduced through a large vein, such as the jugular or subclavian, and used to measure venous pressure or administer fluids or medication.

fibrin sheath. Obstructive material or thrombus that forms around or within the lumen of an indwelling catheter or central venous access device.

fluoroscopy. Radiology technique that allows visual examination of part of the body or a function of an organ using a device that projects an x-ray image on a fluorescent screen.

patency. State of a tube-like structure or conduit being open and unobstructed.

Arteries and Veins

36800-36815

36800   Insertion of cannula for hemodialysis, other purpose (separate procedure); vein to vein

36810   arteriovenous, external (Scribner type)

36815   arteriovenous, external revision, or closure

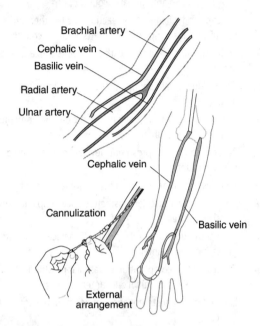

Brachial artery
Cephalic vein
Basilic vein
Radial artery
Ulnar artery

Cephalic vein

Cannulization

Basilic vein

External arrangement

Explanation

The physician isolates two veins, usually in the nondominant forearm, and inserts a needle through the skin and into each vessel. A guidance wire may be threaded through the needle into each vessel. The needle is removed. An end of a single cannula is inserted into each puncture, and any guidance wire removed. In 36810, an artery and a vein are isolated in the same procedure. A Scribner type cannula is inserted and any guide wire is removed. The cannulas remains external, and may be left in place for several days. (This hemodialysis cannula is used to remove blood from the vein, route it through the dialysis machine, then reinfuse it.) In 36815, an external cannula is repositioned or removed. Closure of the insertion site using sutures on the vessels or skin, as necessary, follows.

Coding Tips

This type of hemodialysis cannula is infrequently used; verify from the medical record that this is the type of procedure performed. This procedure includes venipuncture, when performed by the physician. Note that 36800, a separate procedure by definition, is usually a component of a more complex service and is not identified separately. When performed alone or with other unrelated procedures/services it may be reported. If performed alone, list the code; if performed with other procedures/services, list the code and append modifier 59 or an X{EPSU} modifier. For creation of an arteriovenous fistula, see 36825–36830. For open arteriovenous anastomosis, see 36818–36821.

ICD-10-CM Diagnostic Codes

D59.3	Hemolytic-uremic syndrome
E87.2	Acidosis
E87.5	Hyperkalemia
I12.0	Hypertensive chronic kidney disease with stage 5 chronic kidney disease or end stage renal disease
I13.11	Hypertensive heart and chronic kidney disease without heart failure, with stage 5 chronic kidney disease, or end stage renal disease
I13.2	Hypertensive heart and chronic kidney disease with heart failure and with stage 5 chronic kidney disease, or end stage renal disease
I16.0	Hypertensive urgency
I16.1	Hypertensive emergency
I82.3	Embolism and thrombosis of renal vein
N00.0	Acute nephritic syndrome with minor glomerular abnormality
N00.1	Acute nephritic syndrome with focal and segmental glomerular lesions
N00.2	Acute nephritic syndrome with diffuse membranous glomerulonephritis
N00.3	Acute nephritic syndrome with diffuse mesangial proliferative glomerulonephritis
N00.4	Acute nephritic syndrome with diffuse endocapillary proliferative glomerulonephritis
N00.5	Acute nephritic syndrome with diffuse mesangiocapillary glomerulonephritis
N00.6	Acute nephritic syndrome with dense deposit disease
N00.7	Acute nephritic syndrome with diffuse crescentic glomerulonephritis
N00.8	Acute nephritic syndrome with other morphologic changes
N00.A	Acute nephritic syndrome with C3 glomerulonephritis
N01.0	Rapidly progressive nephritic syndrome with minor glomerular abnormality
N01.1	Rapidly progressive nephritic syndrome with focal and segmental glomerular lesions
N01.2	Rapidly progressive nephritic syndrome with diffuse membranous glomerulonephritis
N01.3	Rapidly progressive nephritic syndrome with diffuse mesangial proliferative glomerulonephritis
N01.4	Rapidly progressive nephritic syndrome with diffuse endocapillary proliferative glomerulonephritis
N01.5	Rapidly progressive nephritic syndrome with diffuse mesangiocapillary glomerulonephritis
N01.6	Rapidly progressive nephritic syndrome with dense deposit disease
N01.7	Rapidly progressive nephritic syndrome with diffuse crescentic glomerulonephritis
N01.8	Rapidly progressive nephritic syndrome with other morphologic changes
N01.A	Rapidly progressive nephritic syndrome with C3 glomerulonephritis
N03.0	Chronic nephritic syndrome with minor glomerular abnormality
N03.1	Chronic nephritic syndrome with focal and segmental glomerular lesions
N03.2	Chronic nephritic syndrome with diffuse membranous glomerulonephritis
N03.3	Chronic nephritic syndrome with diffuse mesangial proliferative glomerulonephritis
N03.4	Chronic nephritic syndrome with diffuse endocapillary proliferative glomerulonephritis
N03.5	Chronic nephritic syndrome with diffuse mesangiocapillary glomerulonephritis

N03.6	Chronic nephritic syndrome with dense deposit disease	
N03.7	Chronic nephritic syndrome with diffuse crescentic glomerulonephritis	
N03.8	Chronic nephritic syndrome with other morphologic changes	
N03.A	Chronic nephritic syndrome with C3 glomerulonephritis	
N04.0	Nephrotic syndrome with minor glomerular abnormality	
N04.1	Nephrotic syndrome with focal and segmental glomerular lesions	
N04.2	Nephrotic syndrome with diffuse membranous glomerulonephritis	
N04.3	Nephrotic syndrome with diffuse mesangial proliferative glomerulonephritis	
N04.4	Nephrotic syndrome with diffuse endocapillary proliferative glomerulonephritis	
N04.5	Nephrotic syndrome with diffuse mesangiocapillary glomerulonephritis	
N04.6	Nephrotic syndrome with dense deposit disease	
N04.7	Nephrotic syndrome with diffuse crescentic glomerulonephritis	
N04.8	Nephrotic syndrome with other morphologic changes	
N04.A	Nephrotic syndrome with C3 glomerulonephritis	
N07.0	Hereditary nephropathy, not elsewhere classified with minor glomerular abnormality	
N07.1	Hereditary nephropathy, not elsewhere classified with focal and segmental glomerular lesions	
N07.2	Hereditary nephropathy, not elsewhere classified with diffuse membranous glomerulonephritis	
N07.3	Hereditary nephropathy, not elsewhere classified with diffuse mesangial proliferative glomerulonephritis	
N07.4	Hereditary nephropathy, not elsewhere classified with diffuse endocapillary proliferative glomerulonephritis	
N07.5	Hereditary nephropathy, not elsewhere classified with diffuse mesangiocapillary glomerulonephritis	
N07.6	Hereditary nephropathy, not elsewhere classified with dense deposit disease	
N07.7	Hereditary nephropathy, not elsewhere classified with diffuse crescentic glomerulonephritis	
N07.8	Hereditary nephropathy, not elsewhere classified with other morphologic lesions	
N07.A	Hereditary nephropathy, not elsewhere classified with C3 glomerulonephritis	
N10	Acute pyelonephritis	
N11.0	Nonobstructive reflux-associated chronic pyelonephritis	
N11.1	Chronic obstructive pyelonephritis	
N11.8	Other chronic tubulo-interstitial nephritis	
N12	Tubulo-interstitial nephritis, not specified as acute or chronic	
N15.8	Other specified renal tubulo-interstitial diseases	
N17.0	Acute kidney failure with tubular necrosis	
N17.1	Acute kidney failure with acute cortical necrosis	
N17.2	Acute kidney failure with medullary necrosis	
N17.8	Other acute kidney failure	
N18.5	Chronic kidney disease, stage 5	
N18.6	End stage renal disease	

AMA: 36800 2018,Jan,8; 2017,Jan,8; 2016,Jan,13; 2015,Jan,16; 2014,Jan,11
36810 2018,Jan,8; 2017,Jan,8; 2016,Jan,13; 2015,Jan,16; 2014,Jan,11 **36815**
2018,Jan,8; 2017,Jan,8; 2016,Jan,13; 2015,Jan,16; 2014,Jan,11

Relative Value Units/Medicare Edits

Non-Facility RVU	Work	PE	MP	Total
36800	2.43	0.81	0.31	3.55
36810	3.96	1.64	0.51	6.11
36815	2.62	0.68	0.62	3.92
Facility RVU	Work	PE	MP	Total
36800	2.43	0.81	0.31	3.55
36810	3.96	1.64	0.51	6.11
36815	2.62	0.68	0.62	3.92

	FUD	Status	MUE	Modifiers				IOM Reference
36800	0	A	1(3)	51	N/A	N/A	N/A	None
36810	0	A	1(3)	51	N/A	N/A	N/A	
36815	0	A	1(3)	51	N/A	N/A	N/A	

* with documentation

Terms To Know

artery. Vessel through which oxygenated blood passes away from the heart to any part of the body.

cannula. Tube inserted into a blood vessel, duct, or body cavity to facilitate passage.

guidewire. Flexible metal instrument designed to lead another instrument in its proper course.

hemodialysis. Cleansing of wastes and contaminating elements from the blood by virtue of different diffusion rates through a semipermeable membrane, which separates blood from a filtration solution that diffuses other elements out of the blood.

Scribner type arteriovenous access. External cannula or shunt with the ends inserted into both an artery and a vein, at a puncture site made into the vessels through the skin, usually in the forearm. The Scribner cannula remains external and may be left in place for several days and is generally placed to route blood outside the body for hemodialysis purposes.

vein. Vessel through which oxygen-depleted blood passes back to the heart.

Arteries and Veins

36818-36819

36818 Arteriovenous anastomosis, open; by upper arm cephalic vein transposition

36819 by upper arm basilic vein transposition

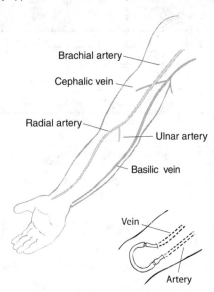

Explanation

A vascular surgeon creates a connection between an artery and a vein for a vascular access site in patients with end stage renal disease who require hemodialysis. In 36819, the surgeon dissects down to the basilic vein on the medial side of the upper arm and mobilizes the vein. A subcutaneous tunnel on the anterior side of the arm is created, and the mobilized basilic vein is transposed to this tunnel and anastomosed to the brachial artery. Report 36818 if a similar arteriovenous connection is made in the upper arm by anastomosing the cephalic vein to the brachial artery.

Coding Tips

This is a unilateral procedure. If performed bilaterally, some payers require that the service be reported twice with modifier 50 appended to the second code while others require identification of the service only once with modifier 50 appended. Check with individual payers. Modifier 50 identifies a procedure performed identically on the opposite side of the body (mirror image). Do not report these codes with each other or with 36820, 36821, or 36830 during a unilateral upper extremity procedure. For bilateral upper extremity open arteriovenous anastomosis performed at the same operative session, use modifier 50 or 59 as appropriate.

ICD-10-CM Diagnostic Codes

D59.3	Hemolytic-uremic syndrome
I12.0	Hypertensive chronic kidney disease with stage 5 chronic kidney disease or end stage renal disease
I13.11	Hypertensive heart and chronic kidney disease without heart failure, with stage 5 chronic kidney disease, or end stage renal disease
I13.2	Hypertensive heart and chronic kidney disease with heart failure and with stage 5 chronic kidney disease, or end stage renal disease
I16.0	Hypertensive urgency
I16.1	Hypertensive emergency
I82.3	Embolism and thrombosis of renal vein

N00.0	Acute nephritic syndrome with minor glomerular abnormality
N00.1	Acute nephritic syndrome with focal and segmental glomerular lesions
N00.2	Acute nephritic syndrome with diffuse membranous glomerulonephritis
N00.3	Acute nephritic syndrome with diffuse mesangial proliferative glomerulonephritis
N00.4	Acute nephritic syndrome with diffuse endocapillary proliferative glomerulonephritis
N00.5	Acute nephritic syndrome with diffuse mesangiocapillary glomerulonephritis
N00.6	Acute nephritic syndrome with dense deposit disease
N00.7	Acute nephritic syndrome with diffuse crescentic glomerulonephritis
N00.8	Acute nephritic syndrome with other morphologic changes
N00.A	Acute nephritic syndrome with C3 glomerulonephritis
N01.0	Rapidly progressive nephritic syndrome with minor glomerular abnormality
N01.1	Rapidly progressive nephritic syndrome with focal and segmental glomerular lesions
N01.2	Rapidly progressive nephritic syndrome with diffuse membranous glomerulonephritis
N01.3	Rapidly progressive nephritic syndrome with diffuse mesangial proliferative glomerulonephritis
N01.4	Rapidly progressive nephritic syndrome with diffuse endocapillary proliferative glomerulonephritis
N01.5	Rapidly progressive nephritic syndrome with diffuse mesangiocapillary glomerulonephritis
N01.6	Rapidly progressive nephritic syndrome with dense deposit disease
N01.7	Rapidly progressive nephritic syndrome with diffuse crescentic glomerulonephritis
N01.8	Rapidly progressive nephritic syndrome with other morphologic changes
N01.A	Rapidly progressive nephritic syndrome with C3 glomerulonephritis
N03.0	Chronic nephritic syndrome with minor glomerular abnormality
N03.1	Chronic nephritic syndrome with focal and segmental glomerular lesions
N03.2	Chronic nephritic syndrome with diffuse membranous glomerulonephritis
N03.3	Chronic nephritic syndrome with diffuse mesangial proliferative glomerulonephritis
N03.4	Chronic nephritic syndrome with diffuse endocapillary proliferative glomerulonephritis
N03.5	Chronic nephritic syndrome with diffuse mesangiocapillary glomerulonephritis
N03.6	Chronic nephritic syndrome with dense deposit disease
N03.7	Chronic nephritic syndrome with diffuse crescentic glomerulonephritis
N03.8	Chronic nephritic syndrome with other morphologic changes
N03.A	Chronic nephritic syndrome with C3 glomerulonephritis
N04.0	Nephrotic syndrome with minor glomerular abnormality
N04.1	Nephrotic syndrome with focal and segmental glomerular lesions
N04.2	Nephrotic syndrome with diffuse membranous glomerulonephritis

N04.3	Nephrotic syndrome with diffuse mesangial proliferative glomerulonephritis
N04.4	Nephrotic syndrome with diffuse endocapillary proliferative glomerulonephritis
N04.5	Nephrotic syndrome with diffuse mesangiocapillary glomerulonephritis
N04.6	Nephrotic syndrome with dense deposit disease
N04.7	Nephrotic syndrome with diffuse crescentic glomerulonephritis
N04.8	Nephrotic syndrome with other morphologic changes
N04.A	Nephrotic syndrome with C3 glomerulonephritis
N07.0	Hereditary nephropathy, not elsewhere classified with minor glomerular abnormality
N07.1	Hereditary nephropathy, not elsewhere classified with focal and segmental glomerular lesions
N07.2	Hereditary nephropathy, not elsewhere classified with diffuse membranous glomerulonephritis
N07.3	Hereditary nephropathy, not elsewhere classified with diffuse mesangial proliferative glomerulonephritis
N07.4	Hereditary nephropathy, not elsewhere classified with diffuse endocapillary proliferative glomerulonephritis
N07.5	Hereditary nephropathy, not elsewhere classified with diffuse mesangiocapillary glomerulonephritis
N07.6	Hereditary nephropathy, not elsewhere classified with dense deposit disease
N07.7	Hereditary nephropathy, not elsewhere classified with diffuse crescentic glomerulonephritis
N07.8	Hereditary nephropathy, not elsewhere classified with other morphologic lesions
N07.A	Hereditary nephropathy, not elsewhere classified with C3 glomerulonephritis
N10	Acute pyelonephritis
N11.0	Nonobstructive reflux-associated chronic pyelonephritis
N11.1	Chronic obstructive pyelonephritis
N11.8	Other chronic tubulo-interstitial nephritis
N12	Tubulo-interstitial nephritis, not specified as acute or chronic
N15.8	Other specified renal tubulo-interstitial diseases
N17.0	Acute kidney failure with tubular necrosis
N17.1	Acute kidney failure with acute cortical necrosis
N17.2	Acute kidney failure with medullary necrosis
N17.8	Other acute kidney failure
N18.5	Chronic kidney disease, stage 5
N18.6	End stage renal disease

AMA: 36818 2018,Jan,8; 2017,Mar,3; 2017,Jan,8; 2016,Mar,10; 2016,Jan,13; 2015,Jan,16; 2014,Jan,11 **36819** 2018,Jan,8; 2017,Mar,3; 2017,Jan,8; 2016,Jan,13; 2015,Jan,16; 2014,Jan,11

Relative Value Units/Medicare Edits

Non-Facility RVU	Work	PE	MP	Total
36818	12.39	4.78	2.94	20.11
36819	13.29	4.83	3.15	21.27
Facility RVU	**Work**	**PE**	**MP**	**Total**
36818	12.39	4.78	2.94	20.11
36819	13.29	4.83	3.15	21.27

	FUD	Status	MUE	Modifiers				IOM Reference
36818	90	A	1(3)	51	N/A	62*	80	None
36819	90	A	1(3)	51	N/A	62*	80	

* with documentation

Terms To Know

access. Ability or the means necessary to read, write, modify, or communicate data and other information.

anastomosis. Surgically created connection between ducts, blood vessels, or bowel segments to allow flow from one to the other.

anterior. Situated in the front area or toward the belly surface of the body.

dissection. Separating by cutting tissue or body structures apart.

hemodialysis. Cleansing of wastes and contaminating elements from the blood by virtue of different diffusion rates through a semipermeable membrane, which separates blood from a filtration solution that diffuses other elements out of the blood.

subcutaneous. Below the skin.

transposition. Removal or exchange from one side to another; change of position from one place to another.

vascular. Pertaining to blood vessels.

CPT © 2020 American Medical Association. All Rights Reserved. ● New ▲ Revised + Add On ★ Telemedicine AMA: CPT Assist [Resequenced] ☑ Laterality © 2020 Optum360, LLC

36820

36820   Arteriovenous anastomosis, open; by forearm vein transposition

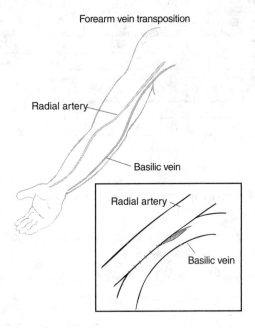

Forearm vein transposition

Radial artery

Basilic vein

Radial artery

Basilic vein

Explanation

The physician creates a connection between an artery or vein, using a forearm vein in the arm—inverted end to end. The physician dissects down to the vein and artery. The subfascial plane is identified and elevated laterally to the flexor carpi radialis (FCR) and medially to the brachioradialis (BR). The plane between the BR and FCR is dissected and the perforating vessels are identified and cauterized. The pedicle is followed to the antecubital fossa. The tourniquet is released, and the vessels are further cleaned of their adventitia under loupe visualization. Using microvascular techniques, a suture for the arterial anastomosis is performed and closure is completed. Suction drains are placed in the neck. If a Doppler is to be used for postoperative assessment, a suture is placed to mark the pedicle site. A splint is fabricated and secured to the arm with an elastic bandage.

Coding Tips

When this procedure is performed on the upper arm, basilic vein, see 36819; cephalic vein, see 36818. For insertion of a cannula for hemodialysis, other purpose (separate procedure), see 36800–36815.

ICD-10-CM Diagnostic Codes

D59.3	Hemolytic-uremic syndrome
I12.0	Hypertensive chronic kidney disease with stage 5 chronic kidney disease or end stage renal disease
I13.11	Hypertensive heart and chronic kidney disease without heart failure, with stage 5 chronic kidney disease, or end stage renal disease
I13.2	Hypertensive heart and chronic kidney disease with heart failure and with stage 5 chronic kidney disease, or end stage renal disease
I16.0	Hypertensive urgency
I16.1	Hypertensive emergency
I82.3	Embolism and thrombosis of renal vein
N00.0	Acute nephritic syndrome with minor glomerular abnormality

N00.1	Acute nephritic syndrome with focal and segmental glomerular lesions
N00.2	Acute nephritic syndrome with diffuse membranous glomerulonephritis
N00.3	Acute nephritic syndrome with diffuse mesangial proliferative glomerulonephritis
N00.4	Acute nephritic syndrome with diffuse endocapillary proliferative glomerulonephritis
N00.5	Acute nephritic syndrome with diffuse mesangiocapillary glomerulonephritis
N00.6	Acute nephritic syndrome with dense deposit disease
N00.7	Acute nephritic syndrome with diffuse crescentic glomerulonephritis
N00.8	Acute nephritic syndrome with other morphologic changes
N00.A	Acute nephritic syndrome with C3 glomerulonephritis
N01.0	Rapidly progressive nephritic syndrome with minor glomerular abnormality
N01.1	Rapidly progressive nephritic syndrome with focal and segmental glomerular lesions
N01.2	Rapidly progressive nephritic syndrome with diffuse membranous glomerulonephritis
N01.3	Rapidly progressive nephritic syndrome with diffuse mesangial proliferative glomerulonephritis
N01.4	Rapidly progressive nephritic syndrome with diffuse endocapillary proliferative glomerulonephritis
N01.5	Rapidly progressive nephritic syndrome with diffuse mesangiocapillary glomerulonephritis
N01.6	Rapidly progressive nephritic syndrome with dense deposit disease
N01.7	Rapidly progressive nephritic syndrome with diffuse crescentic glomerulonephritis
N01.8	Rapidly progressive nephritic syndrome with other morphologic changes
N01.A	Rapidly progressive nephritic syndrome with C3 glomerulonephritis
N03.0	Chronic nephritic syndrome with minor glomerular abnormality
N03.1	Chronic nephritic syndrome with focal and segmental glomerular lesions
N03.2	Chronic nephritic syndrome with diffuse membranous glomerulonephritis
N03.3	Chronic nephritic syndrome with diffuse mesangial proliferative glomerulonephritis
N03.4	Chronic nephritic syndrome with diffuse endocapillary proliferative glomerulonephritis
N03.5	Chronic nephritic syndrome with diffuse mesangiocapillary glomerulonephritis
N03.6	Chronic nephritic syndrome with dense deposit disease
N03.7	Chronic nephritic syndrome with diffuse crescentic glomerulonephritis
N03.8	Chronic nephritic syndrome with other morphologic changes
N03.A	Chronic nephritic syndrome with C3 glomerulonephritis
N04.0	Nephrotic syndrome with minor glomerular abnormality
N04.1	Nephrotic syndrome with focal and segmental glomerular lesions
N04.2	Nephrotic syndrome with diffuse membranous glomerulonephritis

© 2020 Optum360, LLC   N Newborn: 0   P Pediatric: 0-17   M Maternity: 9-64   A Adult: 15-124   ♂ Male Only   ♀ Female Only   CPT © 2020 American Medical Association. All Rights Reserved.

Arteries and Veins

N04.3	Nephrotic syndrome with diffuse mesangial proliferative glomerulonephritis
N04.4	Nephrotic syndrome with diffuse endocapillary proliferative glomerulonephritis
N04.5	Nephrotic syndrome with diffuse mesangiocapillary glomerulonephritis
N04.6	Nephrotic syndrome with dense deposit disease
N04.7	Nephrotic syndrome with diffuse crescentic glomerulonephritis
N04.8	Nephrotic syndrome with other morphologic changes
N04.A	Nephrotic syndrome with C3 glomerulonephritis
N07.0	Hereditary nephropathy, not elsewhere classified with minor glomerular abnormality
N07.1	Hereditary nephropathy, not elsewhere classified with focal and segmental glomerular lesions
N07.2	Hereditary nephropathy, not elsewhere classified with diffuse membranous glomerulonephritis
N07.3	Hereditary nephropathy, not elsewhere classified with diffuse mesangial proliferative glomerulonephritis
N07.4	Hereditary nephropathy, not elsewhere classified with diffuse endocapillary proliferative glomerulonephritis
N07.5	Hereditary nephropathy, not elsewhere classified with diffuse mesangiocapillary glomerulonephritis
N07.6	Hereditary nephropathy, not elsewhere classified with dense deposit disease
N07.7	Hereditary nephropathy, not elsewhere classified with diffuse crescentic glomerulonephritis
N07.8	Hereditary nephropathy, not elsewhere classified with other morphologic lesions
N07.A	Hereditary nephropathy, not elsewhere classified with C3 glomerulonephritis
N10	Acute pyelonephritis
N11.0	Nonobstructive reflux-associated chronic pyelonephritis
N11.1	Chronic obstructive pyelonephritis
N11.8	Other chronic tubulo-interstitial nephritis
N12	Tubulo-interstitial nephritis, not specified as acute or chronic
N15.8	Other specified renal tubulo-interstitial diseases
N17.0	Acute kidney failure with tubular necrosis
N17.1	Acute kidney failure with acute cortical necrosis
N17.2	Acute kidney failure with medullary necrosis
N17.8	Other acute kidney failure
N18.5	Chronic kidney disease, stage 5
N18.6	End stage renal disease

AMA: 36820 2018,Jan,8; 2017,Mar,3; 2017,Jan,8; 2016,Jan,13; 2015,Jan,16; 2014,Jan,11

Relative Value Units/Medicare Edits

Non-Facility RVU	Work	PE	MP	Total
36820	13.07	5.04	3.09	21.2
Facility RVU	Work	PE	MP	Total
36820	13.07	5.04	3.09	21.2

	FUD	Status	MUE	Modifiers				IOM Reference
36820	90	A	1(3)	51	50	62*	80	None

* with documentation

36821

36821 Arteriovenous anastomosis, open; direct, any site (eg, Cimino type) (separate procedure)

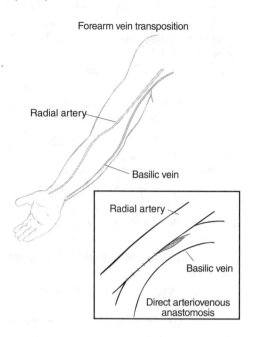

Forearm vein transposition

Radial artery

Basilic vein

Radial artery

Basilic vein

Direct arteriovenous anastomosis

Explanation

Through an incision, usually in the skin over an artery in the nondominant wrist or antecubital fossa, the physician isolates a desired section of artery and neighboring vein. Vessel clamps are placed on the vein and adjacent artery. The vein is dissected free, divided, and the downstream portion of the vein is sutured to an opening created in the adjacent artery, usually in an end-to-side fashion, allowing blood to flow both down the artery and into the vein. Large branches of the vein may be tied off to cause flow down a single vein. The skin incision is repaired with a layered closure. This arteriovenous anastomosis will allow an increased blood flow through the vein, usually for hemodialysis.

Coding Tips

This separate procedure by definition is usually a component of a more complex service and is not identified separately. When performed alone or with other unrelated procedures/services, it may be reported. If performed alone, list the code; if performed with other unrelated procedures/services, list the code and append modifier 59 or an X{EPSU} modifier. For insertion of a cannula for hemodialysis, other purpose, see 36800–36815. For creation of an arteriovenous fistula, by other than direct anastomosis, see 36825–36830.

ICD-10-CM Diagnostic Codes

D59.3	Hemolytic-uremic syndrome
E87.2	Acidosis
E87.5	Hyperkalemia
I12.0	Hypertensive chronic kidney disease with stage 5 chronic kidney disease or end stage renal disease
I13.11	Hypertensive heart and chronic kidney disease without heart failure, with stage 5 chronic kidney disease, or end stage renal disease
I13.2	Hypertensive heart and chronic kidney disease with heart failure and with stage 5 chronic kidney disease, or end stage renal disease

I16.0	Hypertensive urgency
I16.1	Hypertensive emergency
I82.3	Embolism and thrombosis of renal vein
N00.0	Acute nephritic syndrome with minor glomerular abnormality
N00.1	Acute nephritic syndrome with focal and segmental glomerular lesions
N00.2	Acute nephritic syndrome with diffuse membranous glomerulonephritis
N00.3	Acute nephritic syndrome with diffuse mesangial proliferative glomerulonephritis
N00.4	Acute nephritic syndrome with diffuse endocapillary proliferative glomerulonephritis
N00.5	Acute nephritic syndrome with diffuse mesangiocapillary glomerulonephritis
N00.6	Acute nephritic syndrome with dense deposit disease
N00.7	Acute nephritic syndrome with diffuse crescentic glomerulonephritis
N00.8	Acute nephritic syndrome with other morphologic changes
N00.A	Acute nephritic syndrome with C3 glomerulonephritis
N01.0	Rapidly progressive nephritic syndrome with minor glomerular abnormality
N01.1	Rapidly progressive nephritic syndrome with focal and segmental glomerular lesions
N01.2	Rapidly progressive nephritic syndrome with diffuse membranous glomerulonephritis
N01.3	Rapidly progressive nephritic syndrome with diffuse mesangial proliferative glomerulonephritis
N01.4	Rapidly progressive nephritic syndrome with diffuse endocapillary proliferative glomerulonephritis
N01.5	Rapidly progressive nephritic syndrome with diffuse mesangiocapillary glomerulonephritis
N01.6	Rapidly progressive nephritic syndrome with dense deposit disease
N01.7	Rapidly progressive nephritic syndrome with diffuse crescentic glomerulonephritis
N01.8	Rapidly progressive nephritic syndrome with other morphologic changes
N01.A	Rapidly progressive nephritic syndrome with C3 glomerulonephritis
N03.0	Chronic nephritic syndrome with minor glomerular abnormality
N03.1	Chronic nephritic syndrome with focal and segmental glomerular lesions
N03.2	Chronic nephritic syndrome with diffuse membranous glomerulonephritis
N03.3	Chronic nephritic syndrome with diffuse mesangial proliferative glomerulonephritis
N03.4	Chronic nephritic syndrome with diffuse endocapillary proliferative glomerulonephritis
N03.5	Chronic nephritic syndrome with diffuse mesangiocapillary glomerulonephritis
N03.6	Chronic nephritic syndrome with dense deposit disease
N03.7	Chronic nephritic syndrome with diffuse crescentic glomerulonephritis
N03.8	Chronic nephritic syndrome with other morphologic changes
N03.A	Chronic nephritic syndrome with C3 glomerulonephritis
N04.0	Nephrotic syndrome with minor glomerular abnormality
N04.1	Nephrotic syndrome with focal and segmental glomerular lesions
N04.2	Nephrotic syndrome with diffuse membranous glomerulonephritis
N04.3	Nephrotic syndrome with diffuse mesangial proliferative glomerulonephritis
N04.4	Nephrotic syndrome with diffuse endocapillary proliferative glomerulonephritis
N04.5	Nephrotic syndrome with diffuse mesangiocapillary glomerulonephritis
N04.6	Nephrotic syndrome with dense deposit disease
N04.7	Nephrotic syndrome with diffuse crescentic glomerulonephritis
N04.8	Nephrotic syndrome with other morphologic changes
N04.A	Nephrotic syndrome with C3 glomerulonephritis
N07.0	Hereditary nephropathy, not elsewhere classified with minor glomerular abnormality
N07.1	Hereditary nephropathy, not elsewhere classified with focal and segmental glomerular lesions
N07.2	Hereditary nephropathy, not elsewhere classified with diffuse membranous glomerulonephritis
N07.3	Hereditary nephropathy, not elsewhere classified with diffuse mesangial proliferative glomerulonephritis
N07.4	Hereditary nephropathy, not elsewhere classified with diffuse endocapillary proliferative glomerulonephritis
N07.5	Hereditary nephropathy, not elsewhere classified with diffuse mesangiocapillary glomerulonephritis
N07.6	Hereditary nephropathy, not elsewhere classified with dense deposit disease
N07.7	Hereditary nephropathy, not elsewhere classified with diffuse crescentic glomerulonephritis
N07.8	Hereditary nephropathy, not elsewhere classified with other morphologic lesions
N07.A	Hereditary nephropathy, not elsewhere classified with C3 glomerulonephritis
N10	Acute pyelonephritis
N11.0	Nonobstructive reflux-associated chronic pyelonephritis
N11.1	Chronic obstructive pyelonephritis
N11.8	Other chronic tubulo-interstitial nephritis
N12	Tubulo-interstitial nephritis, not specified as acute or chronic
N15.8	Other specified renal tubulo-interstitial diseases
N17.0	Acute kidney failure with tubular necrosis
N17.1	Acute kidney failure with acute cortical necrosis
N17.2	Acute kidney failure with medullary necrosis
N17.8	Other acute kidney failure
N18.5	Chronic kidney disease, stage 5
N18.6	End stage renal disease

AMA: **36821** 2018,Jan,8; 2017,Mar,3; 2017,Jan,8; 2016,Jan,13; 2015,Jan,16; 2015,Aug,8; 2014,Jan,11

Relative Value Units/Medicare Edits

Non-Facility RVU	Work	PE	MP	Total
36821	11.9	4.58	2.83	19.31
Facility RVU	**Work**	**PE**	**MP**	**Total**
36821	11.9	4.58	2.83	19.31

	FUD	Status	MUE	Modifiers				IOM Reference
36821	90	A	2(3)	51	N/A	62*	80	None

* with documentation

Terms To Know

artery. Vessel through which oxygenated blood passes away from the heart to any part of the body.

Cimino type arteriovenous anastomosis. Direct anastomosis of a vein to an artery, usually at the wrist of the nondominant hand. Using only a moderate amount of arterial and venous dissection, a portion of the vein is sutured in an end-to-side fashion to the adjacent artery, allowing blood to flow both down the artery and into the vein. The increased blood flow through the vein is used for hemodialysis.

clamp. Tool used to grip, compress, join, or fasten body parts.

dissect. Cut apart or separate tissue for surgical purposes or for visual or microscopic study.

fossa. Indentation or shallow depression.

hemodialysis. Cleansing of wastes and contaminating elements from the blood by virtue of different diffusion rates through a semipermeable membrane, which separates blood from a filtration solution that diffuses other elements out of the blood.

vein. Vessel through which oxygen-depleted blood passes back to the heart.

36825-36830

36825   Creation of arteriovenous fistula by other than direct arteriovenous anastomosis (separate procedure); autogenous graft

36830   nonautogenous graft (eg, biological collagen, thermoplastic graft)

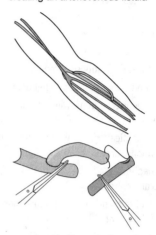

The artery and vein are connected by a vein graft in an end-to-side manner, creating an arteriovenous fistula

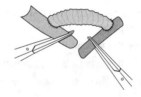

The artery and vein are corrected by a synthetic graft

Explanation

The physician creates an arteriovenous fistula by other than direct anastomosis. The physician makes an incision in the skin over an artery and vein, and the vein and artery are dissected free. A vessel clamp is affixed to each. A length of harvested vein from the patient is used for an autogenous graft in 36825 and is sutured to the incised artery and vein, usually in an end-to-side fashion. The graft is passed in a superficial subcutaneous tunnel that is created bluntly and connects the arterial and venous sites. The clamps are removed, allowing the blood to flow through the graft, creating an arteriovenous fistula. The skin incision is repaired with a layered closure. Report 36830 if a nonautogenous graft, such as biological collagen or a thermoplastic graft, is used.

Coding Tips

These separate procedures by definition are usually a component of a more complex service and are not identified separately. When performed alone or with other unrelated procedures/services, they may be reported. If performed alone, list the code; if performed with other unrelated procedures/services, list the code and append modifier 59 or an X{EPSU} modifier. Because the anastomosis created in this procedure must mature before use, an external cannulization or placement of central venous catheter for hemodialysis is often performed in the same operative session and is reported separately.

ICD-10-CM Diagnostic Codes

D59.3	Hemolytic-uremic syndrome
E87.2	Acidosis
E87.5	Hyperkalemia
I12.0	Hypertensive chronic kidney disease with stage 5 chronic kidney disease or end stage renal disease
I13.11	Hypertensive heart and chronic kidney disease without heart failure, with stage 5 chronic kidney disease, or end stage renal disease
I13.2	Hypertensive heart and chronic kidney disease with heart failure and with stage 5 chronic kidney disease, or end stage renal disease
I16.0	Hypertensive urgency
I16.1	Hypertensive emergency
I82.3	Embolism and thrombosis of renal vein
N00.0	Acute nephritic syndrome with minor glomerular abnormality
N00.1	Acute nephritic syndrome with focal and segmental glomerular lesions
N00.2	Acute nephritic syndrome with diffuse membranous glomerulonephritis
N00.3	Acute nephritic syndrome with diffuse mesangial proliferative glomerulonephritis
N00.4	Acute nephritic syndrome with diffuse endocapillary proliferative glomerulonephritis
N00.5	Acute nephritic syndrome with diffuse mesangiocapillary glomerulonephritis
N00.6	Acute nephritic syndrome with dense deposit disease
N00.7	Acute nephritic syndrome with diffuse crescentic glomerulonephritis
N00.8	Acute nephritic syndrome with other morphologic changes
N00.A	Acute nephritic syndrome with C3 glomerulonephritis
N01.0	Rapidly progressive nephritic syndrome with minor glomerular abnormality
N01.1	Rapidly progressive nephritic syndrome with focal and segmental glomerular lesions
N01.2	Rapidly progressive nephritic syndrome with diffuse membranous glomerulonephritis
N01.3	Rapidly progressive nephritic syndrome with diffuse mesangial proliferative glomerulonephritis
N01.4	Rapidly progressive nephritic syndrome with diffuse endocapillary proliferative glomerulonephritis
N01.5	Rapidly progressive nephritic syndrome with diffuse mesangiocapillary glomerulonephritis
N01.6	Rapidly progressive nephritic syndrome with dense deposit disease
N01.7	Rapidly progressive nephritic syndrome with diffuse crescentic glomerulonephritis
N01.8	Rapidly progressive nephritic syndrome with other morphologic changes
N01.A	Rapidly progressive nephritic syndrome with C3 glomerulonephritis
N03.0	Chronic nephritic syndrome with minor glomerular abnormality
N03.1	Chronic nephritic syndrome with focal and segmental glomerular lesions
N03.2	Chronic nephritic syndrome with diffuse membranous glomerulonephritis
N03.3	Chronic nephritic syndrome with diffuse mesangial proliferative glomerulonephritis
N03.4	Chronic nephritic syndrome with diffuse endocapillary proliferative glomerulonephritis
N03.5	Chronic nephritic syndrome with diffuse mesangiocapillary glomerulonephritis
N03.6	Chronic nephritic syndrome with dense deposit disease
N03.7	Chronic nephritic syndrome with diffuse crescentic glomerulonephritis
N03.8	Chronic nephritic syndrome with other morphologic changes
N03.A	Chronic nephritic syndrome with C3 glomerulonephritis
N04.0	Nephrotic syndrome with minor glomerular abnormality
N04.1	Nephrotic syndrome with focal and segmental glomerular lesions
N04.2	Nephrotic syndrome with diffuse membranous glomerulonephritis
N04.3	Nephrotic syndrome with diffuse mesangial proliferative glomerulonephritis
N04.4	Nephrotic syndrome with diffuse endocapillary proliferative glomerulonephritis
N04.5	Nephrotic syndrome with diffuse mesangiocapillary glomerulonephritis
N04.6	Nephrotic syndrome with dense deposit disease
N04.7	Nephrotic syndrome with diffuse crescentic glomerulonephritis
N04.8	Nephrotic syndrome with other morphologic changes
N04.A	Nephrotic syndrome with C3 glomerulonephritis
N07.0	Hereditary nephropathy, not elsewhere classified with minor glomerular abnormality
N07.1	Hereditary nephropathy, not elsewhere classified with focal and segmental glomerular lesions
N07.2	Hereditary nephropathy, not elsewhere classified with diffuse membranous glomerulonephritis
N07.3	Hereditary nephropathy, not elsewhere classified with diffuse mesangial proliferative glomerulonephritis
N07.4	Hereditary nephropathy, not elsewhere classified with diffuse endocapillary proliferative glomerulonephritis
N07.5	Hereditary nephropathy, not elsewhere classified with diffuse mesangiocapillary glomerulonephritis
N07.6	Hereditary nephropathy, not elsewhere classified with dense deposit disease
N07.7	Hereditary nephropathy, not elsewhere classified with diffuse crescentic glomerulonephritis
N07.8	Hereditary nephropathy, not elsewhere classified with other morphologic lesions
N07.A	Hereditary nephropathy, not elsewhere classified with C3 glomerulonephritis
N10	Acute pyelonephritis
N11.0	Nonobstructive reflux-associated chronic pyelonephritis
N11.1	Chronic obstructive pyelonephritis
N11.8	Other chronic tubulo-interstitial nephritis
N12	Tubulo-interstitial nephritis, not specified as acute or chronic
N15.8	Other specified renal tubulo-interstitial diseases
N17.0	Acute kidney failure with tubular necrosis
N17.1	Acute kidney failure with acute cortical necrosis
N17.2	Acute kidney failure with medullary necrosis
N17.8	Other acute kidney failure

N18.5   Chronic kidney disease, stage 5

N18.6   End stage renal disease

AMA: **36825** 2018,Jan,8; 2017,Mar,3; 2017,Jan,8; 2016,Jan,13; 2015,Jan,16; 2014,Jan,11 **36830** 2018,Jan,8; 2017,Mar,3; 2017,Jan,8; 2016,Jan,13; 2015,Jan,13; 2015,Jan,16; 2014,Jan,11

Relative Value Units/Medicare Edits

Non-Facility RVU	Work	PE	MP	Total
36825	14.17	5.57	3.37	23.11
36830	12.03	4.51	2.87	19.41
Facility RVU	**Work**	**PE**	**MP**	**Total**
36825	14.17	5.57	3.37	23.11
36830	12.03	4.51	2.87	19.41

	FUD	Status	MUE	Modifiers				IOM Reference
36825	90	A	1(3)	51	N/A	62*	80	None
36830	90	A	2(3)	51	N/A	62*	80	

* with documentation

Terms To Know

anastomosis. Surgically created connection between ducts, blood vessels, or bowel segments to allow flow from one to the other.

arteriovenous fistula. Connecting passage between an artery and a vein.

artery. Vessel through which oxygenated blood passes away from the heart to any part of the body.

clamp. Tool used to grip, compress, join, or fasten body parts.

collagen. Protein based substance of strength and flexibility that is the major component of connective tissue, found in cartilage, bone, tendons, and skin.

graft. Tissue implant from another part of the body or another person.

nonautogenous. Derived from a source other than the same individual or recipient (e.g., cells, tissue, blood vessels, and other organs donated from another human).

subcutaneous. Below the skin.

vein. Vessel through which oxygen-depleted blood passes back to the heart.

36831

36831   Thrombectomy, open, arteriovenous fistula without revision, autogenous or nonautogenous dialysis graft (separate procedure)

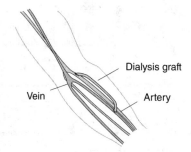

A previously placed dialysis graft, autogenous or nonautogenous, has developed a thrombus

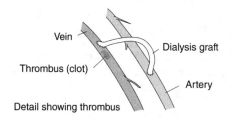

Detail showing thrombus

Explanation

The physician removes a blood clot from a surgically created connection between an artery and a vein (arteriovenous fistula). The procedure involves making an incision over the site of an existing fistula. The fistula is isolated and dissected free. Vessel clamps are affixed above and below the fistula. The blood clot is removed, the clamps are taken off, and the incision is repaired by layered sutures. The procedure may involve a vein acquired from the patient or the construction of a synthetic graft.

Coding Tips

This separate procedure by definition is usually a component of a more complex service and is not identified separately. When performed alone or with other unrelated procedures/services it may be reported. If performed alone, list the code; if performed with other procedures/services, list the code and append modifier 59 or an X{EPSU} modifier. Report this procedure for thrombectomy associated with reduced flow. This code reports open thrombectomy. For percutaneous transluminal mechanical thrombectomy and/or infusion for thrombolysis within the dialysis circuit, see 36904-36906. For external cannula declotting without balloon catheter, see 36860; with balloon catheter, see 36861. For thrombectomy with revision of an arteriovenous fistula, see 36833.

ICD-10-CM Diagnostic Codes

T82.818A   Embolism due to vascular prosthetic devices, implants and grafts, initial encounter

T82.828A   Fibrosis due to vascular prosthetic devices, implants and grafts, initial encounter

T82.848A   Pain due to vascular prosthetic devices, implants and grafts, initial encounter

T82.856A   Stenosis of peripheral vascular stent, initial encounter

T82.858A   Stenosis of other vascular prosthetic devices, implants and grafts, initial encounter

T82.868A   Thrombosis due to vascular prosthetic devices, implants and grafts, initial encounter

Arteries and Veins

T82.898A   Other specified complication of vascular prosthetic devices, implants and grafts, initial encounter

AMA: 36831 2018,Jan,8; 2017,Mar,3; 2017,Jan,8; 2016,Jan,13; 2015,Jan,16; 2014,Jan,11

Relative Value Units/Medicare Edits

Non-Facility RVU	Work	PE	MP	Total
36831	11.0	4.28	2.62	17.9
Facility RVU	Work	PE	MP	Total
36831	11.0	4.28	2.62	17.9

	FUD	Status	MUE	Modifiers				IOM Reference
36831	90	A	1(3)	51	N/A	62*	80	None

* with documentation

Terms To Know

arteriovenous fistula. Connecting passage between an artery and a vein.

autograft. Any tissue harvested from one anatomical site of a person and grafted to another anatomical site of the same person. Most commonly, blood vessels, skin, tendons, fascia, and bone are used as autografts.

blood clot. Semisolidified, coagulated mass of mainly platelets and fibrin in the bloodstream.

clamp. Tool used to grip, compress, join, or fasten body parts.

dissect. Cut apart or separate tissue for surgical purposes or for visual or microscopic study.

embolism. Obstruction of a blood vessel resulting from a clot or foreign substance.

fistula. Abnormal tube-like passage between two body cavities or organs or from an organ to the outside surface.

nonautogenous. Derived from a source other than the same individual or recipient (e.g., cells, tissue, blood vessels, and other organs donated from another human).

stenosis. Narrowing or constriction of a passage.

thrombectomy. Removal of a clot (thrombus) from a blood vessel utilizing various methods.

thrombosis. Condition arising from the presence or formation of blood clots within a blood vessel that may cause vascular obstruction and insufficient oxygenation.

36832-36833

36832   Revision, open, arteriovenous fistula; without thrombectomy, autogenous or nonautogenous dialysis graft (separate procedure)
36833   with thrombectomy, autogenous or nonautogenous dialysis graft (separate procedure)

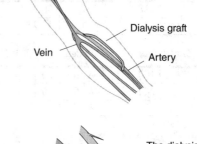

A previously placed dialysis graft, autogenous or nonautogenous, is revisited and the graft is revised

Dialysis graft

Vein

Artery

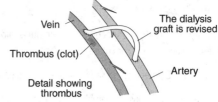

Vein

Thrombus (clot)

The dialysis graft is revised

Artery

Detail showing thrombus

Explanation

In 36832, the physician makes an incision at the site of an already existing artificial fistula between an artery and a vein. The fistula is dissected free. Vessel clamps are affixed above and below the fistula, which is incised. Revisions are made to the fistula at its juncture to the vein and/or artery and may require creating a new anastomosis with a graft obtained from a separate site or created with synthetic material. After the repair has been made, the fistula is sutured, the clamps removed, and the skin incision repaired with a layered closure. Report 36833 when the physician removes a blood clot at the fistula site in addition to revising the existing arteriovenous fistula.

Coding Tips

These separate procedures by definition are usually a component of a more complex service and are not identified separately. When performed alone or with other unrelated procedures/services they may be reported. If performed alone, list the code; if performed with other procedures, list the code and append modifier 59 or an X{EPSU} modifier. Report percutaneous thrombectomy within the dialysis circuit with codes 36904–36906. For central dialysis segment angioplasty performed with 36818–36833, see 36907; for stent placement, see 36908. These codes should not be reported with codes 36901–36906 for revision of the dialysis circuit.

ICD-10-CM Diagnostic Codes

T82.318A	Breakdown (mechanical) of other vascular grafts, initial encounter
T82.328A	Displacement of other vascular grafts, initial encounter
T82.338A	Leakage of other vascular grafts, initial encounter
T82.398A	Other mechanical complication of other vascular grafts, initial encounter
T82.510A	Breakdown (mechanical) of surgically created arteriovenous fistula, initial encounter

© 2020 Optum360, LLC   **N** Newborn: 0   **P** Pediatric: 0-17   **M** Maternity: 9-64   **A** Adult: 15-124   ♂ Male Only   ♀ Female Only   CPT © 2020 American Medical Association. All Rights Reserved.

Coding Companion for Urology/Nephrology

Arteries and Veins

T82.518A	Breakdown (mechanical) of other cardiac and vascular devices and implants, initial encounter
T82.520A	Displacement of surgically created arteriovenous fistula, initial encounter
T82.528A	Displacement of other cardiac and vascular devices and implants, initial encounter
T82.530A	Leakage of surgically created arteriovenous fistula, initial encounter
T82.538A	Leakage of other cardiac and vascular devices and implants, initial encounter
T82.590A	Other mechanical complication of surgically created arteriovenous fistula, initial encounter
T82.598A	Other mechanical complication of other cardiac and vascular devices and implants, initial encounter
T82.7XXA	Infection and inflammatory reaction due to other cardiac and vascular devices, implants and grafts, initial encounter
T82.818A	Embolism due to vascular prosthetic devices, implants and grafts, initial encounter
T82.828A	Fibrosis due to vascular prosthetic devices, implants and grafts, initial encounter
T82.848A	Pain due to vascular prosthetic devices, implants and grafts, initial encounter
T82.856A	Stenosis of peripheral vascular stent, initial encounter
T82.858A	Stenosis of other vascular prosthetic devices, implants and grafts, initial encounter
T82.868A	Thrombosis due to vascular prosthetic devices, implants and grafts, initial encounter
T82.898A	Other specified complication of vascular prosthetic devices, implants and grafts, initial encounter
Z45.89	Encounter for adjustment and management of other implanted devices
Z46.89	Encounter for fitting and adjustment of other specified devices

AMA: **36832** 2018,Jan,8; 2017,Mar,3; 2017,Jan,8; 2016,Jan,13; 2015,Jan,16; 2014,Jan,11 **36833** 2018,Jan,8; 2017,Mar,3; 2017,Jan,8; 2016,Jan,13; 2015,Jan,16; 2014,Jan,11

Relative Value Units/Medicare Edits

Non-Facility RVU	Work	PE	MP	Total
36832	13.5	5.28	3.19	21.97
36833	14.5	5.61	3.45	23.56
Facility RVU	Work	PE	MP	Total
36832	13.5	5.28	3.19	21.97
36833	14.5	5.61	3.45	23.56

	FUD	Status	MUE	Modifiers				IOM Reference
36832	90	A	2(3)	51	N/A	62*	80	None
36833	90	A	1(3)	51	N/A	62*	80	

* with documentation

36835

36835 Insertion of Thomas shunt (separate procedure)

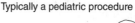

Typically a pediatric procedure

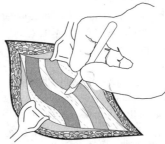

Major vein or artery is exposed and Thomas shunt established

Thomas shunt

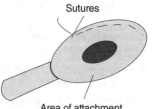

Sutures

Area of attachment to vessel (underside view)

Explanation

Through an incision in the skin overlying a large vein or artery of a child, the physician dissects the vessel that will receive a synthetic shunt. The vessel may be clamped. The vessel is nicked, and a needle threads a guidance wire into the vein or artery. The shunt follows, and the wire is removed. The physician sutures the synthetic shunt end-to-end, or end-to-side, to the vein or artery. The shunt is most often used for access in hemodialysis.

Coding Tips

This separate procedure by definition is usually a component of a more complex service and is not identified separately. When performed alone or with other unrelated procedures/services, it may be reported. If performed alone, list the code; if performed with other unrelated procedures/services, list the code and append modifier 59 or an X{EPSU} modifier. This type of shunt is infrequently used; verify in the medical record that this is the correct code. This code includes venipuncture when performed by the physician.

ICD-10-CM Diagnostic Codes

D59.3	Hemolytic-uremic syndrome
E87.2	Acidosis
E87.5	Hyperkalemia
I12.0	Hypertensive chronic kidney disease with stage 5 chronic kidney disease or end stage renal disease
I13.11	Hypertensive heart and chronic kidney disease without heart failure, with stage 5 chronic kidney disease, or end stage renal disease
I13.2	Hypertensive heart and chronic kidney disease with heart failure and with stage 5 chronic kidney disease, or end stage renal disease
I16.0	Hypertensive urgency
I16.1	Hypertensive emergency

Arteries and Veins

I82.3	Embolism and thrombosis of renal vein
N00.0	Acute nephritic syndrome with minor glomerular abnormality
N00.1	Acute nephritic syndrome with focal and segmental glomerular lesions
N00.2	Acute nephritic syndrome with diffuse membranous glomerulonephritis
N00.3	Acute nephritic syndrome with diffuse mesangial proliferative glomerulonephritis
N00.4	Acute nephritic syndrome with diffuse endocapillary proliferative glomerulonephritis
N00.5	Acute nephritic syndrome with diffuse mesangiocapillary glomerulonephritis
N00.6	Acute nephritic syndrome with dense deposit disease
N00.7	Acute nephritic syndrome with diffuse crescentic glomerulonephritis
N00.8	Acute nephritic syndrome with other morphologic changes
N00.A	Acute nephritic syndrome with C3 glomerulonephritis
N01.0	Rapidly progressive nephritic syndrome with minor glomerular abnormality
N01.1	Rapidly progressive nephritic syndrome with focal and segmental glomerular lesions
N01.2	Rapidly progressive nephritic syndrome with diffuse membranous glomerulonephritis
N01.3	Rapidly progressive nephritic syndrome with diffuse mesangial proliferative glomerulonephritis
N01.4	Rapidly progressive nephritic syndrome with diffuse endocapillary proliferative glomerulonephritis
N01.5	Rapidly progressive nephritic syndrome with diffuse mesangiocapillary glomerulonephritis
N01.6	Rapidly progressive nephritic syndrome with dense deposit disease
N01.7	Rapidly progressive nephritic syndrome with diffuse crescentic glomerulonephritis
N01.8	Rapidly progressive nephritic syndrome with other morphologic changes
N01.A	Rapidly progressive nephritic syndrome with C3 glomerulonephritis
N03.0	Chronic nephritic syndrome with minor glomerular abnormality
N03.1	Chronic nephritic syndrome with focal and segmental glomerular lesions
N03.2	Chronic nephritic syndrome with diffuse membranous glomerulonephritis
N03.3	Chronic nephritic syndrome with diffuse mesangial proliferative glomerulonephritis
N03.4	Chronic nephritic syndrome with diffuse endocapillary proliferative glomerulonephritis
N03.5	Chronic nephritic syndrome with diffuse mesangiocapillary glomerulonephritis
N03.6	Chronic nephritic syndrome with dense deposit disease
N03.7	Chronic nephritic syndrome with diffuse crescentic glomerulonephritis
N03.8	Chronic nephritic syndrome with other morphologic changes
N03.A	Chronic nephritic syndrome with C3 glomerulonephritis
N04.0	Nephrotic syndrome with minor glomerular abnormality
N04.1	Nephrotic syndrome with focal and segmental glomerular lesions
N04.2	Nephrotic syndrome with diffuse membranous glomerulonephritis
N04.3	Nephrotic syndrome with diffuse mesangial proliferative glomerulonephritis
N04.4	Nephrotic syndrome with diffuse endocapillary proliferative glomerulonephritis
N04.5	Nephrotic syndrome with diffuse mesangiocapillary glomerulonephritis
N04.6	Nephrotic syndrome with dense deposit disease
N04.7	Nephrotic syndrome with diffuse crescentic glomerulonephritis
N04.8	Nephrotic syndrome with other morphologic changes
N04.A	Nephrotic syndrome with C3 glomerulonephritis
N10	Acute pyelonephritis
N11.0	Nonobstructive reflux-associated chronic pyelonephritis
N11.1	Chronic obstructive pyelonephritis
N11.8	Other chronic tubulo-interstitial nephritis
N12	Tubulo-interstitial nephritis, not specified as acute or chronic
N15.8	Other specified renal tubulo-interstitial diseases
N17.0	Acute kidney failure with tubular necrosis
N17.1	Acute kidney failure with acute cortical necrosis
N17.2	Acute kidney failure with medullary necrosis
N17.8	Other acute kidney failure
N18.5	Chronic kidney disease, stage 5
N18.6	End stage renal disease
T80.211A	Bloodstream infection due to central venous catheter, initial encounter
T80.212A	Local infection due to central venous catheter, initial encounter
T80.218A	Other infection due to central venous catheter, initial encounter
T82.318A	Breakdown (mechanical) of other vascular grafts, initial encounter
T82.328A	Displacement of other vascular grafts, initial encounter
T82.338A	Leakage of other vascular grafts, initial encounter
T82.398A	Other mechanical complication of other vascular grafts, initial encounter
T82.41XA	Breakdown (mechanical) of vascular dialysis catheter, initial encounter
T82.42XA	Displacement of vascular dialysis catheter, initial encounter
T82.43XA	Leakage of vascular dialysis catheter, initial encounter
T82.49XA	Other complication of vascular dialysis catheter, initial encounter
T82.510A	Breakdown (mechanical) of surgically created arteriovenous fistula, initial encounter
T82.514A	Breakdown (mechanical) of infusion catheter, initial encounter
T82.518A	Breakdown (mechanical) of other cardiac and vascular devices and implants, initial encounter
T82.520A	Displacement of surgically created arteriovenous fistula, initial encounter
T82.524A	Displacement of infusion catheter, initial encounter
T82.528A	Displacement of other cardiac and vascular devices and implants, initial encounter
T82.530A	Leakage of surgically created arteriovenous fistula, initial encounter
T82.534A	Leakage of infusion catheter, initial encounter
T82.538A	Leakage of other cardiac and vascular devices and implants, initial encounter
T82.590A	Other mechanical complication of surgically created arteriovenous fistula, initial encounter

T82.594A	Other mechanical complication of infusion catheter, initial encounter
T82.598A	Other mechanical complication of other cardiac and vascular devices and implants, initial encounter
T82.7XXA	Infection and inflammatory reaction due to other cardiac and vascular devices, implants and grafts, initial encounter
T82.818A	Embolism due to vascular prosthetic devices, implants and grafts, initial encounter
T82.828A	Fibrosis due to vascular prosthetic devices, implants and grafts, initial encounter
T82.838A	Hemorrhage due to vascular prosthetic devices, implants and grafts, initial encounter
T82.848A	Pain due to vascular prosthetic devices, implants and grafts, initial encounter
T82.856A	Stenosis of peripheral vascular stent, initial encounter
T82.858A	Stenosis of other vascular prosthetic devices, implants and grafts, initial encounter
T82.868A	Thrombosis due to vascular prosthetic devices, implants and grafts, initial encounter
T82.898A	Other specified complication of vascular prosthetic devices, implants and grafts, initial encounter

AMA: 36835 2014,Jan,11

Relative Value Units/Medicare Edits

Non-Facility RVU	Work	PE	MP	Total
36835	7.51	4.66	1.69	13.86
Facility RVU	Work	PE	MP	Total
36835	7.51	4.66	1.69	13.86

	FUD	Status	MUE	Modifiers				IOM Reference
36835	90	A	1(3)	51	N/A	N/A	N/A	None

* with documentation

Terms To Know

artery. Vessel through which oxygenated blood passes away from the heart to any part of the body.

clamp. Tool used to grip, compress, join, or fasten body parts.

dissect. Cut apart or separate tissue for surgical purposes or for visual or microscopic study.

guidewire. Flexible metal instrument designed to lead another instrument in its proper course.

hemodialysis. Cleansing of wastes and contaminating elements from the blood by virtue of different diffusion rates through a semipermeable membrane, which separates blood from a filtration solution that diffuses other elements out of the blood.

shunt. Surgically created passage between blood vessels or other natural passages, such as an arteriovenous anastomosis, to divert or bypass blood flow from the normal channel.

vein. Vessel through which oxygen-depleted blood passes back to the heart.

36860-36861

| 36860 | External cannula declotting (separate procedure); without balloon catheter |
| 36861 | with balloon catheter |

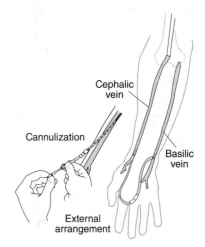

Cephalic vein

Cannulization

Basilic vein

External arrangement

Explanation

To remove a blood clot lodged in a previously placed cannula, the physician may inject a solution containing enzymes into the cannula to dissolve the clot (in 36860) or the physician may, after injecting a solution containing enzymes, insert a balloon catheter (in 36861) into the cannula to retrieve a clot there. The balloon is inserted and inflated beyond the clot. The catheter is slowly pulled out, capturing and retrieving the clot. Once the clot is dissolved or retrieved, the catheter is removed and the cannula is left in place.

Coding Tips

These separate procedures by definition are usually a component of a more complex service and are not identified separately. When performed alone or with other unrelated procedures/services, they may be reported. If performed alone, list the code; if performed with other unrelated procedures/services, list the code and append modifier 59 or an X{EPSU} modifier. For declotting of an implanted vascular access device or catheter by thrombolytic agent, see 36593. Imaging guidance is reported with 76000, when performed.

ICD-10-CM Diagnostic Codes

T82.49XA	Other complication of vascular dialysis catheter, initial encounter
T82.594A	Other mechanical complication of infusion catheter, initial encounter
T82.818A	Embolism due to vascular prosthetic devices, implants and grafts, initial encounter
T82.828A	Fibrosis due to vascular prosthetic devices, implants and grafts, initial encounter
T82.848A	Pain due to vascular prosthetic devices, implants and grafts, initial encounter
T82.856A	Stenosis of peripheral vascular stent, initial encounter
T82.858A	Stenosis of other vascular prosthetic devices, implants and grafts, initial encounter
T82.868A	Thrombosis due to vascular prosthetic devices, implants and grafts, initial encounter
T82.898A	Other specified complication of vascular prosthetic devices, implants and grafts, initial encounter

AMA: **36860** 2018,Jan,8; 2017,Jan,8; 2016,Jan,13; 2015,Jan,16; 2014,Jan,11
36861 2018,Jan,8; 2017,Jan,8; 2016,Jan,13; 2015,Jan,16; 2014,Jan,11

Relative Value Units/Medicare Edits

Non-Facility RVU	Work	PE	MP	Total
36860	2.01	4.55	0.49	7.05
36861	2.52	0.91	0.62	4.05
Facility RVU	Work	PE	MP	Total
36860	2.01	0.73	0.49	3.23
36861	2.52	0.91	0.62	4.05

	FUD	Status	MUE	Modifiers				IOM Reference
36860	0	A	2(3)	51	N/A	N/A	N/A	None
36861	0	A	2(3)	51	N/A	N/A	N/A	

* with documentation

Terms To Know

balloon catheter. Any catheter equipped with an inflatable balloon at the end to hold it in place in a body cavity or to be used for dilation of a vessel lumen.

blood clot. Semisolidified, coagulated mass of mainly platelets and fibrin in the bloodstream.

cannula. Tube inserted into a blood vessel, duct, or body cavity to facilitate passage.

embolism. Obstruction of a blood vessel resulting from a clot or foreign substance.

enzyme. Complex proteins produced by cells that provide specific chemical functions within the body.

fibrosis. Formation of fibrous tissue as part of the restorative process.

stenosis. Narrowing or constriction of a passage.

thrombolytic agent. Drugs or other substances used to dissolve blood clots in blood vessels or in tubes that have been placed into the body.

thrombosis. Condition arising from the presence or formation of blood clots within a blood vessel that may cause vascular obstruction and insufficient oxygenation.

37788-37790

37788 Penile revascularization, artery, with or without vein graft
37790 Penile venous occlusive procedure

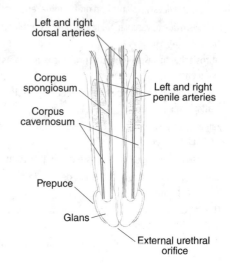

Explanation

Through an incision in the skin near the base of the penis, the physician isolates the penile artery and separates it from critical structures. In 37788, a neighboring artery in the groin or lower abdomen is also isolated and dissected and a vessel clamp applied. The end of the neighboring artery is sewn into the penile artery in an end-to-side fashion, or a piece of harvested vein may be used to connect the two arteries to establish an adequate blood flow to the penis. The clamps are removed and incision is repaired with a layered closure. In 37790, through an inguinoscrotal incision, lateral to the root of the penis, and along the spermatic cord, the physician exposes the suspensory ligaments and detaches them from the pubic bone, The physician incises the superficial layer of Buck's fascia, exposing and suture-ligating each leaking vein. A segment of deep dorsal vein is dissected, ligated at both ends, and resected. The physician reattaches the suspensory ligaments and when the procedure is complete, closes the skin incision with a layered closure.

Coding Tips

Vein graft harvest, when performed, is included in the service and not reported separately.

ICD-10-CM Diagnostic Codes

N50.1 Vascular disorders of male genital organs ♂
N50.89 Other specified disorders of the male genital organs ♂
N52.02 Corporo-venous occlusive erectile dysfunction 🅰 ♂
N52.03 Combined arterial insufficiency and corporo-venous occlusive erectile dysfunction 🅰 ♂

AMA: **37788** 2014,Jan,11 **37790** 2014,Jan,11

Relative Value Units/Medicare Edits

Non-Facility RVU	Work	PE	MP	Total
37788	23.33	10.5	2.69	36.52
37790	8.43	4.64	0.96	14.03
Facility RVU	**Work**	**PE**	**MP**	**Total**
37788	23.33	10.5	2.69	36.52
37790	8.43	4.64	0.96	14.03

	FUD	Status	MUE	Modifiers				IOM Reference
37788	90	A	1(2)	51	N/A	62*	80	None
37790	90	A	1(2)	51	N/A	N/A	80*	

* with documentation

Terms To Know

artery. Vessel through which oxygenated blood passes away from the heart to any part of the body.

clamp. Tool used to grip, compress, join, or fasten body parts.

dissect. Cut apart or separate tissue for surgical purposes or for visual or microscopic study.

dorsal. Pertaining to the back or posterior aspect.

dysfunction. Abnormal or impaired function of an organ, part, or system.

fascia. Fibrous sheet or band of tissue that envelops organs, muscles, and groupings of muscles.

graft. Tissue implant from another part of the body or another person.

incision. Act of cutting into tissue or an organ.

insufficiency. Inadequate closure of the valve that allows abnormal backward blood flow.

lateral. On/to the side.

ligate. To tie off a blood vessel or duct with a suture or a soft, thin wire (ligature wire).

occlusion. Constriction, closure, or blockage of a passage.

revascularization. Restoration of blood flow and oxygen supply to a body part. This may apply to an extremity, the heart, or penis.

vein. Vessel through which oxygen-depleted blood passes back to the heart.

venous. Relating to the veins.

38500-38505, 38531

38500 Biopsy or excision of lymph node(s); open, superficial
38505 by needle, superficial (eg, cervical, inguinal, axillary)
38531 open, inguinofemoral node(s)

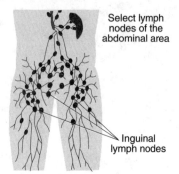

Select lymph nodes of the abdominal area

Inguinal lymph nodes

Explanation

The physician performs a biopsy on or removes one or more superficial lymph nodes. The physician makes a small incision through the skin overlying the lymph node. The tissue is dissected to the node. A small piece of the node and surrounding tissue are removed, or the node may be removed. The incision is repaired with a layered closure. Report 38505 if a needle is used. For biopsy or excision of the inguinofemoral nodes, report 38531.

Coding Tips

Code 38531 is a unilateral procedure. If performed bilaterally, some payers require that the service be reported twice with modifier 50 appended to the second code while others require identification of the service only once with modifier 50 appended. Check with individual payers. Modifier 50 identifies a procedure performed identically on the opposite side of the body (mirror image). Do not report 38500 with 38700–38780. When imaging guidance is performed, see 76942, 77002, 77012, or 77021. For fine needle aspiration, see 10004–10012 and 10021. For evaluation of fine needle aspirate, see 88172–88173. For injection of a sentinel node for identification, see 38792.

ICD-10-CM Diagnostic Codes

C60.0	Malignant neoplasm of prepuce ♂
C60.1	Malignant neoplasm of glans penis ♂
C60.2	Malignant neoplasm of body of penis ♂
C60.8	Malignant neoplasm of overlapping sites of penis ♂
C61	Malignant neoplasm of prostate ♂
C62.11	Malignant neoplasm of descended right testis ♂ ☑
C62.12	Malignant neoplasm of descended left testis ♂ ☑
C63.01	Malignant neoplasm of right epididymis ♂ ☑
C63.02	Malignant neoplasm of left epididymis ♂ ☑
C63.11	Malignant neoplasm of right spermatic cord ♂ ☑
C63.12	Malignant neoplasm of left spermatic cord ♂ ☑
C63.2	Malignant neoplasm of scrotum ♂
C77.4	Secondary and unspecified malignant neoplasm of inguinal and lower limb lymph nodes
C79.82	Secondary malignant neoplasm of genital organs
C81.05	Nodular lymphocyte predominant Hodgkin lymphoma, lymph nodes of inguinal region and lower limb
C81.15	Nodular sclerosis Hodgkin lymphoma, lymph nodes of inguinal region and lower limb
C81.25	Mixed cellularity Hodgkin lymphoma, lymph nodes of inguinal region and lower limb
C81.35	Lymphocyte depleted Hodgkin lymphoma, lymph nodes of inguinal region and lower limb
C81.45	Lymphocyte-rich Hodgkin lymphoma, lymph nodes of inguinal region and lower limb
C81.75	Other Hodgkin lymphoma, lymph nodes of inguinal region and lower limb
C82.05	Follicular lymphoma grade I, lymph nodes of inguinal region and lower limb
C82.15	Follicular lymphoma grade II, lymph nodes of inguinal region and lower limb
C82.35	Follicular lymphoma grade IIIa, lymph nodes of inguinal region and lower limb
C82.45	Follicular lymphoma grade IIIb, lymph nodes of inguinal region and lower limb
C82.55	Diffuse follicle center lymphoma, lymph nodes of inguinal region and lower limb
C82.65	Cutaneous follicle center lymphoma, lymph nodes of inguinal region and lower limb
C82.85	Other types of follicular lymphoma, lymph nodes of inguinal region and lower limb
C83.15	Mantle cell lymphoma, lymph nodes of inguinal region and lower limb
C83.35	Diffuse large B-cell lymphoma, lymph nodes of inguinal region and lower limb
C83.55	Lymphoblastic (diffuse) lymphoma, lymph nodes of inguinal region and lower limb
C83.75	Burkitt lymphoma, lymph nodes of inguinal region and lower limb
C83.85	Other non-follicular lymphoma, lymph nodes of inguinal region and lower limb
C84.05	Mycosis fungoides, lymph nodes of inguinal region and lower limb
C84.45	Peripheral T-cell lymphoma, not classified, lymph nodes of inguinal region and lower limb
C84.65	Anaplastic large cell lymphoma, ALK-positive, lymph nodes of inguinal region and lower limb
C84.75	Anaplastic large cell lymphoma, ALK-negative, lymph nodes of inguinal region and lower limb
C84.Z5	Other mature T/NK-cell lymphomas, lymph nodes of inguinal region and lower limb
C85.25	Mediastinal (thymic) large B-cell lymphoma, lymph nodes of inguinal region and lower limb
C85.85	Other specified types of non-Hodgkin lymphoma, lymph nodes of inguinal region and lower limb
D86.84	Sarcoid pyelonephritis
I88.1	Chronic lymphadenitis, except mesenteric
L04.8	Acute lymphadenitis of other sites
R59.0	Localized enlarged lymph nodes
R59.1	Generalized enlarged lymph nodes

AMA: 38500 2019,Feb,8; 2018,Jan,8; 2017,Jan,8; 2016,Jan,13; 2015,Jan,16; 2014,Jan,11 **38505** 2019,Feb,8; 2018,Jan,8; 2017,Jan,8; 2016,Jan,13; 2015,Jan,16; 2014,Jan,11 **38531** 2019,Feb,8

Lymph Nodes

Relative Value Units/Medicare Edits

Non-Facility RVU	Work	PE	MP	Total
38500	3.79	5.03	0.86	9.68
38505	1.14	2.3	0.11	3.55
38531	6.74	4.67	1.11	12.52
Facility RVU	**Work**	**PE**	**MP**	**Total**
38500	3.79	2.73	0.86	7.38
38505	1.14	0.77	0.11	2.02
38531	6.74	4.67	1.11	12.52

	FUD	Status	MUE	Modifiers				IOM Reference
38500	10	A	2(3)	51	50	N/A	N/A	None
38505	0	A	2(3)	51	50	N/A	N/A	
38531	90	A	1(2)	51	50	N/A	80*	

* with documentation

Terms To Know

axillary. Area under the arm.

biopsy. Tissue or fluid removed for diagnostic purposes through analysis of the cells in the biopsy material.

dissect. Cut apart or separate tissue for surgical purposes or for visual or microscopic study.

inguinal. Within the groin region.

lymph nodes. Bean-shaped structures along the lymphatic vessels that intercept and destroy foreign materials in the tissue and bloodstream.

superficial. On the skin surface or near the surface of any involved structure or field of interest.

38562-38564

38562   Limited lymphadenectomy for staging (separate procedure); pelvic and para-aortic

38564   retroperitoneal (aortic and/or splenic)

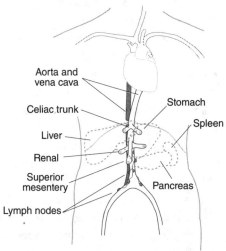

The aorta and other structures of the posterior abdominal cavity are lined with lymph nodes

Explanation

The physician makes a midline abdominal incision just below the navel. The surrounding tissue, nerves, and blood vessels are dissected away, and the pelvic and/or para-aortic lymph nodes are visualized. The nodes are removed. The wound is closed with sutures or staples. Report 38564 if retroperitoneal lymphadenectomy is performed.

Coding Tips

These separate procedures by definition are usually a component of a more complex service and are not identified separately. When performed alone or with other unrelated procedures/services they may be reported. If performed alone, list the code; if performed with other procedures/services, list the code and append modifier 59 or an X{EPSU} modifier. For limited pelvic lymphadenectomy combined with prostatectomy, see 55812 or 55842; combined with prostate exposure for insertion of radioactive substance, see 55862. For retroperitoneal transabdominal lymphadenectomy, see 38780.

ICD-10-CM Diagnostic Codes

C60.0	Malignant neoplasm of prepuce ♂
C60.1	Malignant neoplasm of glans penis ♂
C60.2	Malignant neoplasm of body of penis ♂
C60.8	Malignant neoplasm of overlapping sites of penis ♂
C61	Malignant neoplasm of prostate ♂
C62.11	Malignant neoplasm of descended right testis ♂ ☑
C62.12	Malignant neoplasm of descended left testis ♂ ☑
C63.01	Malignant neoplasm of right epididymis ♂ ☑
C63.02	Malignant neoplasm of left epididymis ♂ ☑
C63.11	Malignant neoplasm of right spermatic cord ♂ ☑
C63.12	Malignant neoplasm of left spermatic cord ♂ ☑
C63.2	Malignant neoplasm of scrotum ♂
C63.7	Malignant neoplasm of other specified male genital organs ♂

Lymph Nodes

Lymph Nodes

C63.8	Malignant neoplasm of overlapping sites of male genital organs ♂
C64.1	Malignant neoplasm of right kidney, except renal pelvis ☑
C64.2	Malignant neoplasm of left kidney, except renal pelvis ☑
C65.1	Malignant neoplasm of right renal pelvis ☑
C65.2	Malignant neoplasm of left renal pelvis ☑
C66.1	Malignant neoplasm of right ureter ☑
C66.2	Malignant neoplasm of left ureter ☑
C67.0	Malignant neoplasm of trigone of bladder
C67.1	Malignant neoplasm of dome of bladder
C67.2	Malignant neoplasm of lateral wall of bladder
C67.3	Malignant neoplasm of anterior wall of bladder
C67.4	Malignant neoplasm of posterior wall of bladder
C67.5	Malignant neoplasm of bladder neck
C67.6	Malignant neoplasm of ureteric orifice
C67.8	Malignant neoplasm of overlapping sites of bladder
C68.0	Malignant neoplasm of urethra
C68.1	Malignant neoplasm of paraurethral glands
C68.8	Malignant neoplasm of overlapping sites of urinary organs
C77.2	Secondary and unspecified malignant neoplasm of intra-abdominal lymph nodes
C77.5	Secondary and unspecified malignant neoplasm of intrapelvic lymph nodes
C78.6	Secondary malignant neoplasm of retroperitoneum and peritoneum
C7A.093	Malignant carcinoid tumor of the kidney
C7B.01	Secondary carcinoid tumors of distant lymph nodes
C7B.04	Secondary carcinoid tumors of peritoneum
C81.03	Nodular lymphocyte predominant Hodgkin lymphoma, intra-abdominal lymph nodes
C81.06	Nodular lymphocyte predominant Hodgkin lymphoma, intrapelvic lymph nodes
C81.13	Nodular sclerosis Hodgkin lymphoma, intra-abdominal lymph nodes
C81.16	Nodular sclerosis Hodgkin lymphoma, intrapelvic lymph nodes
C81.23	Mixed cellularity Hodgkin lymphoma, intra-abdominal lymph nodes
C81.26	Mixed cellularity Hodgkin lymphoma, intrapelvic lymph nodes
C81.32	Lymphocyte depleted Hodgkin lymphoma, intrathoracic lymph nodes
C81.33	Lymphocyte depleted Hodgkin lymphoma, intra-abdominal lymph nodes
C81.36	Lymphocyte depleted Hodgkin lymphoma, intrapelvic lymph nodes
C81.37	Lymphocyte depleted Hodgkin lymphoma, spleen
C81.38	Lymphocyte depleted Hodgkin lymphoma, lymph nodes of multiple sites
C81.42	Lymphocyte-rich Hodgkin lymphoma, intrathoracic lymph nodes
C81.43	Lymphocyte-rich Hodgkin lymphoma, intra-abdominal lymph nodes
C81.46	Lymphocyte-rich Hodgkin lymphoma, intrapelvic lymph nodes
C81.47	Lymphocyte-rich Hodgkin lymphoma, spleen
C81.48	Lymphocyte-rich Hodgkin lymphoma, lymph nodes of multiple sites
C82.03	Follicular lymphoma grade I, intra-abdominal lymph nodes
C82.06	Follicular lymphoma grade I, intrapelvic lymph nodes
C82.13	Follicular lymphoma grade II, intra-abdominal lymph nodes
C82.16	Follicular lymphoma grade II, intrapelvic lymph nodes
C82.33	Follicular lymphoma grade IIIa, intra-abdominal lymph nodes
C82.36	Follicular lymphoma grade IIIa, intrapelvic lymph nodes
C82.43	Follicular lymphoma grade IIIb, intra-abdominal lymph nodes
C82.46	Follicular lymphoma grade IIIb, intrapelvic lymph nodes
C82.53	Diffuse follicle center lymphoma, intra-abdominal lymph nodes
C82.56	Diffuse follicle center lymphoma, intrapelvic lymph nodes
C82.63	Cutaneous follicle center lymphoma, intra-abdominal lymph nodes
C82.66	Cutaneous follicle center lymphoma, intrapelvic lymph nodes
C83.03	Small cell B-cell lymphoma, intra-abdominal lymph nodes
C83.06	Small cell B-cell lymphoma, intrapelvic lymph nodes
C83.13	Mantle cell lymphoma, intra-abdominal lymph nodes
C83.16	Mantle cell lymphoma, intrapelvic lymph nodes
C83.33	Diffuse large B-cell lymphoma, intra-abdominal lymph nodes
C83.36	Diffuse large B-cell lymphoma, intrapelvic lymph nodes
C83.53	Lymphoblastic (diffuse) lymphoma, intra-abdominal lymph nodes
C83.56	Lymphoblastic (diffuse) lymphoma, intrapelvic lymph nodes
C83.73	Burkitt lymphoma, intra-abdominal lymph nodes
C83.76	Burkitt lymphoma, intrapelvic lymph nodes
C84.03	Mycosis fungoides, intra-abdominal lymph nodes
C84.06	Mycosis fungoides, intrapelvic lymph nodes
C84.13	Sezary disease, intra-abdominal lymph nodes
C84.16	Sezary disease, intrapelvic lymph nodes
C84.63	Anaplastic large cell lymphoma, ALK-positive, intra-abdominal lymph nodes
C84.66	Anaplastic large cell lymphoma, ALK-positive, intrapelvic lymph nodes
C84.67	Anaplastic large cell lymphoma, ALK-positive, spleen
C84.68	Anaplastic large cell lymphoma, ALK-positive, lymph nodes of multiple sites
C84.69	Anaplastic large cell lymphoma, ALK-positive, extranodal and solid organ sites
C84.72	Anaplastic large cell lymphoma, ALK-negative, intrathoracic lymph nodes
C84.73	Anaplastic large cell lymphoma, ALK-negative, intra-abdominal lymph nodes
C84.76	Anaplastic large cell lymphoma, ALK-negative, intrapelvic lymph nodes
C84.77	Anaplastic large cell lymphoma, ALK-negative, spleen
C84.78	Anaplastic large cell lymphoma, ALK-negative, lymph nodes of multiple sites
C84.79	Anaplastic large cell lymphoma, ALK-negative, extranodal and solid organ sites
C85.23	Mediastinal (thymic) large B-cell lymphoma, intra-abdominal lymph nodes
C85.26	Mediastinal (thymic) large B-cell lymphoma, intrapelvic lymph nodes

AMA: 38562 2019,Feb,8; 2018,Jan,8; 2017,Jan,8; 2016,Jan,13; 2015,Jan,16; 2014,Jan,11 **38564** 2019,Feb,8; 2014,Jan,11

Relative Value Units/Medicare Edits

Non-Facility RVU	Work	PE	MP	Total
38562	11.06	7.39	1.96	20.41
38564	11.38	6.7	2.35	20.43
Facility RVU	Work	PE	MP	Total
38562	11.06	7.39	1.96	20.41
38564	11.38	6.7	2.35	20.43

	FUD	Status	MUE	Modifiers				IOM Reference
38562	90	A	1(2)	51	N/A	62*	80	None
38564	90	A	1(2)	51	N/A	62*	80	

* with documentation

Terms To Know

dissect. Cut apart or separate tissue for surgical purposes or for visual or microscopic study.

lymph nodes. Bean-shaped structures along the lymphatic vessels that intercept and destroy foreign materials in the tissue and bloodstream.

lymphadenectomy. Dissection of lymph nodes free from the vessels and removal for examination by frozen section in a separate procedure to detect early-stage metastases.

lymphoma. Tumors occurring in the lymphoid tissues that are most commonly malignant.

malignant neoplasm. Any cancerous tumor or lesion exhibiting uncontrolled tissue growth that can progressively invade other parts of the body with its disease-generating cells.

para-. Indicates near, similar, beside, or past.

retroperitoneal. Located behind the peritoneum, the membrane that lines the abdominopelvic walls and forms a covering for the internal organs.

secondary. Second in order of occurrence or importance, or appearing during the course of another disease or condition.

wound. Injury to living tissue often involving a cut or break in the skin.

38570-38573

38570	Laparoscopy, surgical; with retroperitoneal lymph node sampling (biopsy), single or multiple
38571	with bilateral total pelvic lymphadenectomy
38572	with bilateral total pelvic lymphadenectomy and peri-aortic lymph node sampling (biopsy), single or multiple
38573	with bilateral total pelvic lymphadenectomy and peri-aortic lymph node sampling, peritoneal washings, peritoneal biopsy(ies), omentectomy, and diaphragmatic washings, including diaphragmatic and other serosal biopsy(ies), when performed

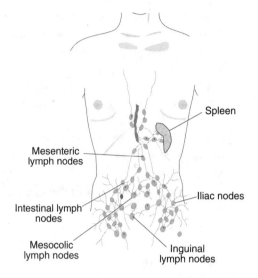

Spleen

Mesenteric lymph nodes

Iliac nodes

Intestinal lymph nodes

Mesocolic lymph nodes

Inguinal lymph nodes

Explanation

The physician performs a surgical laparoscopy. A trocar is placed at the umbilicus into the abdominal or retroperitoneal space to insufflate the abdominal, peritoneal, or retroperitoneal space. The laparoscope is placed through the umbilical trocar and additional trocars are placed into the peritoneal or retroperitoneal space. In 38570, retroperitoneal lymph node sampling is also performed. The lymph nodes are identified, dissected free of surrounding structures, and sampled for further separately reported analysis. In 38571, a bilateral pelvic lymphadenectomy is performed. The iliac vessels are identified and the lymph nodes are dissected from the surrounding structures and removed. When dissection is continued to the aorta for periaortic lymph node sampling, report 38572. In 38573, the services from 38571 and 38572 are performed, as well as peritoneal washing and biopsies, an omentectomy (removal of the membrane containing fat, lymph, and blood vessels that acts as a protective layer extending from the stomach to the transverse colon), and diaphragmatic washings. Diaphragmatic and other serosal biopsies are included in the procedure, when performed. When each procedure is complete, the trocars are removed and the incisions are closed.

Coding Tips

Surgical laparoscopy always includes diagnostic laparoscopy. Codes 38571–38573 are bilateral procedures and as such are reported once even if the procedure is performed on both sides. To report a diagnostic laparoscopy (peritoneoscopy), see 49320. For open biopsy or excision of superficial lymph nodes, see 38500–38505. For limited pelvic and retroperitoneal lymphadenectomy performed for staging (other than laparoscopic approach), see 38562-38564. Do not report 38573 with 38562, 38564, 38570-38572, 38589, 38770, 38780, 49255, 49320, 49326, 58541-58544, 58548, 58550, or 58552-58554.

Lymph Nodes

ICD-10-CM Diagnostic Codes

C61	Malignant neoplasm of prostate ♂
C77.2	Secondary and unspecified malignant neoplasm of intra-abdominal lymph nodes
C77.5	Secondary and unspecified malignant neoplasm of intrapelvic lymph nodes
C7B.01	Secondary carcinoid tumors of distant lymph nodes
C7B.04	Secondary carcinoid tumors of peritoneum
C7B.09	Secondary carcinoid tumors of other sites
C7B.1	Secondary Merkel cell carcinoma
C7B.8	Other secondary neuroendocrine tumors
C82.03	Follicular lymphoma grade I, intra-abdominal lymph nodes
C82.13	Follicular lymphoma grade II, intra-abdominal lymph nodes
C82.33	Follicular lymphoma grade IIIa, intra-abdominal lymph nodes
C82.43	Follicular lymphoma grade IIIb, intra-abdominal lymph nodes
C82.53	Diffuse follicle center lymphoma, intra-abdominal lymph nodes
C82.63	Cutaneous follicle center lymphoma, intra-abdominal lymph nodes
C82.83	Other types of follicular lymphoma, intra-abdominal lymph nodes
C83.13	Mantle cell lymphoma, intra-abdominal lymph nodes
C83.33	Diffuse large B-cell lymphoma, intra-abdominal lymph nodes
C83.53	Lymphoblastic (diffuse) lymphoma, intra-abdominal lymph nodes
C83.83	Other non-follicular lymphoma, intra-abdominal lymph nodes
C84.43	Peripheral T-cell lymphoma, not classified, intra-abdominal lymph nodes
C84.63	Anaplastic large cell lymphoma, ALK-positive, intra-abdominal lymph nodes
C84.73	Anaplastic large cell lymphoma, ALK-negative, intra-abdominal lymph nodes
C84.Z3	Other mature T/NK-cell lymphomas, intra-abdominal lymph nodes
C85.23	Mediastinal (thymic) large B-cell lymphoma, intra-abdominal lymph nodes
C85.83	Other specified types of non-Hodgkin lymphoma, intra-abdominal lymph nodes
C86.2	Enteropathy-type (intestinal) T-cell lymphoma
C86.3	Subcutaneous panniculitis-like T-cell lymphoma
C88.4	Extranodal marginal zone B-cell lymphoma of mucosa-associated lymphoid tissue [MALT-lymphoma]
D72.89	Other specified disorders of white blood cells
I88.1	Chronic lymphadenitis, except mesenteric
I89.8	Other specified noninfective disorders of lymphatic vessels and lymph nodes
L04.8	Acute lymphadenitis of other sites
R59.0	Localized enlarged lymph nodes
R59.1	Generalized enlarged lymph nodes

AMA: **38570** 2019,Feb,8; 2018,Jan,8; 2017,Jan,8; 2016,Jan,13; 2015,Jan,16; 2014,Jan,11 **38571** 2019,Feb,8; 2018,Jan,8; 2017,Jan,8; 2016,Jan,13; 2015,Jan,16; 2014,Jan,11 **38572** 2019,Feb,8; 2018,Jan,8; 2017,Jan,8; 2016,Jan,13; 2015,Jan,13; 2015,Jan,16; 2014,Jan,11 **38573** 2019,Mar,5; 2018,Apr,10

Relative Value Units/Medicare Edits

Non-Facility RVU	Work	PE	MP	Total
38570	8.49	4.88	1.42	14.79
38571	12.0	5.71	1.46	19.17
38572	15.6	8.36	2.36	26.32
38573	20.0	10.45	3.07	33.52
Facility RVU	Work	PE	MP	Total
38570	8.49	4.88	1.42	14.79
38571	12.0	5.71	1.46	19.17
38572	15.6	8.36	2.36	26.32
38573	20.0	10.45	3.07	33.52

	FUD	Status	MUE	Modifiers				IOM Reference
38570	10	A	1(2)	51	N/A	62	80	None
38571	10	A	1(2)	51	N/A	62	80	
38572	10	A	1(2)	51	N/A	62	80	
38573	10	A	1(2)	51	N/A	62	80	

* with documentation

Terms To Know

biopsy. Tissue or fluid removed for diagnostic purposes through analysis of the cells in the biopsy material.

dissection. (dis. apart; -section, act of cutting) Separating by cutting tissue or body structures apart.

insufflation. Blowing air or gas into a body cavity.

laparoscopy. Direct visualization utilizing a thin, flexible, fiberoptic tube.

lymph nodes. Bean-shaped structures along the lymphatic vessels that intercept and destroy foreign materials in the tissue and bloodstream.

lymphadenectomy. Dissection of lymph nodes free from the vessels and removal for examination by frozen section in a separate procedure to detect early-stage metastases.

lymphadenitis. Inflammation or enlargement of the lymph nodes.

lymphoma. Tumors occurring in the lymphoid tissues that are most commonly malignant.

membrane. Thin, flexible tissue layer that covers or functions to separate or connect anatomic areas, structures, or organs. May also be described as having the characteristic of allowing certain substances to permeate or pass through but not others (semipermeable).

omentum. Fold of peritoneal tissue suspended between the stomach and neighboring visceral organs of the abdominal cavity.

peritoneal. Space between the lining of the abdominal wall, or parietal peritoneum, and the surface layer of the abdominal organs, or visceral peritoneum. It contains a thin, watery fluid that keeps the peritoneal surfaces moist.

retroperitoneal. Located behind the peritoneum, the membrane that lines the abdominopelvic walls and forms a covering for the internal organs.

trocar. Cannula or a sharp pointed instrument used to puncture and aspirate fluid from cavities.

38747

+ **38747** Abdominal lymphadenectomy, regional, including celiac, gastric, portal, peripancreatic, with or without para-aortic and vena caval nodes (List separately in addition to code for primary procedure)

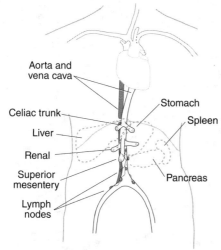

Abdominal lymph nodes are removed

Explanation

The physician makes a midline abdominal incision. The abdominal contents are exposed, allowing the physician to locate the lymph nodes. Each lymph node grouping, with or without para-aortic and vena caval nodes, is dissected away from the surrounding tissue, nerves, and blood vessels, and removed. The incision is closed with sutures or staples.

Coding Tips

Report 38747 in addition to the code for the primary procedure. For laparoscopic lymphadenectomy, see 38571–38572. For retroperitoneal transabdominal lymphadenectomy, see 38780.

ICD-10-CM Diagnostic Codes

This/these CPT code(s) are add-on codes. See the primary procedure code that this code is performed with for your ICD-10-CM code selections.

AMA: 38747 2020,Apr,10; 2019,Feb,8; 2014,Jan,11

Relative Value Units/Medicare Edits

Non-Facility RVU	Work	PE	MP	Total
38747	4.88	1.78	1.12	7.78
Facility RVU	Work	PE	MP	Total
38747	4.88	1.78	1.12	7.78

	FUD	Status	MUE	Modifiers				IOM Reference
38747	N/A	A	1(2)	N/A	N/A	62*	80	None

* with documentation

Terms To Know

lymph nodes. Bean-shaped structures along the lymphatic vessels that intercept and destroy foreign materials in the tissue and bloodstream.

38760-38765

38760 Inguinofemoral lymphadenectomy, superficial, including Cloquet's node (separate procedure)

38765 Inguinofemoral lymphadenectomy, superficial, in continuity with pelvic lymphadenectomy, including external iliac, hypogastric, and obturator nodes (separate procedure)

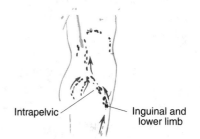

Superficial nodes of the inguinal region are removed along with certain pelvic nodes. Cloquet's node is of the deep inguinal group, but lies closest to the skin just under the inguinal ligament

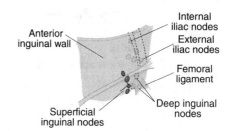

Explanation

The physician makes an incision across the groin area. The surrounding tissue, nerves, and blood vessels are dissected away, and the inguinal and femoral lymph nodes are visualized. The nodes are removed by group. The wound is closed with sutures or staples. Report 38765 if performing pelvic lymphadenectomy concurrently.

Coding Tips

These separate procedures by definition are usually a component of a more complex service and are not identified separately. When performed alone or with other unrelated procedures/services they may be reported. If performed alone, list the code; if performed with other procedures/services, list the code and append modifier 59 or an X{EPSU} modifier. These are unilateral procedures. If performed bilaterally, some payers require that the service be reported twice with modifier 50 appended to the second code while others require identification of the service only once with modifier 50 appended. Check with individual payers. Modifier 50 identifies a procedure performed identically on the opposite side of the body (mirror image).

ICD-10-CM Diagnostic Codes

C60.0	Malignant neoplasm of prepuce ♂
C60.1	Malignant neoplasm of glans penis ♂
C60.2	Malignant neoplasm of body of penis ♂
C60.8	Malignant neoplasm of overlapping sites of penis ♂
C61	Malignant neoplasm of prostate ♂
C62.11	Malignant neoplasm of descended right testis ♂ ☑
C62.12	Malignant neoplasm of descended left testis ♂ ☑
C63.01	Malignant neoplasm of right epididymis ♂ ☑

Lymph Nodes

C63.02	Malignant neoplasm of left epididymis ♂ ☑
C63.11	Malignant neoplasm of right spermatic cord ♂ ☑
C63.12	Malignant neoplasm of left spermatic cord ♂ ☑
C63.2	Malignant neoplasm of scrotum ♂
C63.7	Malignant neoplasm of other specified male genital organs ♂
C63.8	Malignant neoplasm of overlapping sites of male genital organs ♂
C66.1	Malignant neoplasm of right ureter ☑
C66.2	Malignant neoplasm of left ureter ☑
C67.0	Malignant neoplasm of trigone of bladder
C67.1	Malignant neoplasm of dome of bladder
C67.2	Malignant neoplasm of lateral wall of bladder
C67.3	Malignant neoplasm of anterior wall of bladder
C67.4	Malignant neoplasm of posterior wall of bladder
C67.5	Malignant neoplasm of bladder neck
C67.6	Malignant neoplasm of ureteric orifice
C67.7	Malignant neoplasm of urachus
C67.8	Malignant neoplasm of overlapping sites of bladder
C68.0	Malignant neoplasm of urethra
C68.1	Malignant neoplasm of paraurethral glands
C77.4	Secondary and unspecified malignant neoplasm of inguinal and lower limb lymph nodes
C7B.01	Secondary carcinoid tumors of distant lymph nodes
C7B.09	Secondary carcinoid tumors of other sites
C82.55	Diffuse follicle center lymphoma, lymph nodes of inguinal region and lower limb
C84.Z5	Other mature T/NK-cell lymphomas, lymph nodes of inguinal region and lower limb
C85.25	Mediastinal (thymic) large B-cell lymphoma, lymph nodes of inguinal region and lower limb
C85.85	Other specified types of non-Hodgkin lymphoma, lymph nodes of inguinal region and lower limb
D36.0	Benign neoplasm of lymph nodes
I88.8	Other nonspecific lymphadenitis
R59.0	Localized enlarged lymph nodes
R59.1	Generalized enlarged lymph nodes

AMA: 38760 2019,Feb,8; 2018,Jan,8; 2017,Jan,8; 2016,Jan,13; 2015,Jan,16; 2014,Jan,11 **38765** 2019,Feb,8; 2018,Jan,8; 2017,Jan,8; 2016,Jan,13; 2015,Jan,16; 2014,Jan,11

Relative Value Units/Medicare Edits

Non-Facility RVU	Work	PE	MP	Total
38760	13.62	7.85	2.82	24.29
38765	21.91	11.38	4.43	37.72
Facility RVU	Work	PE	MP	Total
38760	13.62	7.85	2.82	24.29
38765	21.91	11.38	4.43	37.72

	FUD	Status	MUE	Modifiers				IOM Reference
38760	90	A	1(2)	51	50	62*	80	None
38765	90	A	1(2)	51	50	62*	80	

* with documentation

38770

38770	Pelvic lymphadenectomy, including external iliac, hypogastric, and obturator nodes (separate procedure)

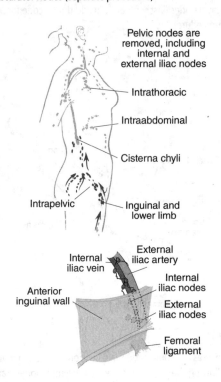

Explanation

The physician makes a low abdominal vertical incision. The surrounding tissue, nerves, and blood vessels are dissected away, and the pelvic lymph nodes are visualized. The nodes are removed by group. The wound is closed with sutures or staples.

Coding Tips

This separate procedure by definition is usually a component of a more complex service and is not identified separately. When performed alone or with other unrelated procedures/services it may be reported. If performed alone, list the code; if performed with other procedures/services, list the code and append modifier 59 or an X{EPSU} modifier. This is a unilateral procedure. If performed bilaterally, some payers require that the service be reported twice with modifier 50 appended to the second code while others require identification of the service only once with modifier 50 appended. Check with individual payers. Modifier 50 identifies a procedure performed identically on the opposite side of the body (mirror image). If significant additional time and effort is documented, append modifier 22 and submit a cover letter and operative report. For open limited pelvic and retroperitoneal lymphadenectomy staging procedures, see 38562 and 38564. For laparoscopic lymphadenectomy, see 38571–38572.

ICD-10-CM Diagnostic Codes

C60.0	Malignant neoplasm of prepuce ♂
C60.1	Malignant neoplasm of glans penis ♂
C60.2	Malignant neoplasm of body of penis ♂
C60.8	Malignant neoplasm of overlapping sites of penis ♂
C61	Malignant neoplasm of prostate ♂
C62.11	Malignant neoplasm of descended right testis ♂ ☑

© 2020 Optum360, LLC   **N** Newborn: 0   **P** Pediatric: 0-17   **M** Maternity: 9-64   **A** Adult: 15-124   ♂ Male Only   ♀ Female Only   CPT © 2020 American Medical Association. All Rights Reserved.

C62.12	Malignant neoplasm of descended left testis ♂ ☑
C63.01	Malignant neoplasm of right epididymis ♂ ☑
C63.02	Malignant neoplasm of left epididymis ♂ ☑
C63.11	Malignant neoplasm of right spermatic cord ♂ ☑
C63.12	Malignant neoplasm of left spermatic cord ♂ ☑
C63.2	Malignant neoplasm of scrotum ♂
C63.7	Malignant neoplasm of other specified male genital organs ♂
C63.8	Malignant neoplasm of overlapping sites of male genital organs ♂
C66.1	Malignant neoplasm of right ureter ☑
C66.2	Malignant neoplasm of left ureter ☑
C67.0	Malignant neoplasm of trigone of bladder
C67.1	Malignant neoplasm of dome of bladder
C67.2	Malignant neoplasm of lateral wall of bladder
C67.3	Malignant neoplasm of anterior wall of bladder
C67.4	Malignant neoplasm of posterior wall of bladder
C67.5	Malignant neoplasm of bladder neck
C67.6	Malignant neoplasm of ureteric orifice
C67.7	Malignant neoplasm of urachus
C67.8	Malignant neoplasm of overlapping sites of bladder
C68.0	Malignant neoplasm of urethra
C68.1	Malignant neoplasm of paraurethral glands
C77.5	Secondary and unspecified malignant neoplasm of intrapelvic lymph nodes
C79.89	Secondary malignant neoplasm of other specified sites
C7A.093	Malignant carcinoid tumor of the kidney
C7A.098	Malignant carcinoid tumors of other sites
C7B.01	Secondary carcinoid tumors of distant lymph nodes
C7B.09	Secondary carcinoid tumors of other sites
D48.7	Neoplasm of uncertain behavior of other specified sites

AMA: 38770 2019,Feb,8; 2014,Jan,11

Relative Value Units/Medicare Edits

Non-Facility RVU	Work	PE	MP	Total
38770	14.06	7.21	1.95	23.22
Facility RVU	**Work**	**PE**	**MP**	**Total**
38770	14.06	7.21	1.95	23.22

	FUD	Status	MUE	Modifiers				IOM Reference
38770	90	A	1(2)	51	50	62*	80	None

* with documentation

Terms To Know

dissection. Separating by cutting tissue or body structures apart.

lymph nodes. Bean-shaped structures along the lymphatic vessels that intercept and destroy foreign materials in the tissue and bloodstream.

lymphadenectomy. Dissection of lymph nodes free from the vessels and removal for examination by frozen section in a separate procedure to detect early-stage metastases.

tissue. Group of similar cells with a similar function that form definite structures and organs. Tissue types include epithelial tissue, muscle tissue, connective tissue, and nervous tissue.

38780

38780 Retroperitoneal transabdominal lymphadenectomy, extensive, including pelvic, aortic, and renal nodes (separate procedure)

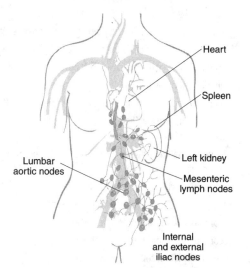

Extensive removal of lymph nodes of the retroperitoneal area is performed by a transabdominal approach

Explanation

The physician makes a large midline abdominal incision. The surrounding tissue, nerves, and blood vessels are dissected away, and the lymph nodes are visualized. The nodes are removed by group. Some surrounding tissues may also be removed. The wound is closed with sutures or staples.

Coding Tips

This separate procedure by definition is usually a component of a more complex service and is not identified separately. When performed alone or with other unrelated procedures/services it may be reported. If performed alone, list the code; if performed with other procedures/services, list the code and append modifier 59 or an X{EPSU} modifier. For open limited pelvic and retroperitoneal lymphadenectomy staging procedures, see 38562 and 38564. For laparoscopic lymphadenectomy, see 38571–38572.

ICD-10-CM Diagnostic Codes

C48.0	Malignant neoplasm of retroperitoneum
C48.1	Malignant neoplasm of specified parts of peritoneum
C48.8	Malignant neoplasm of overlapping sites of retroperitoneum and peritoneum
C61	Malignant neoplasm of prostate ♂
C62.11	Malignant neoplasm of descended right testis ♂ ☑
C62.12	Malignant neoplasm of descended left testis ♂ ☑
C64.1	Malignant neoplasm of right kidney, except renal pelvis ☑
C64.2	Malignant neoplasm of left kidney, except renal pelvis ☑
C65.1	Malignant neoplasm of right renal pelvis ☑
C65.2	Malignant neoplasm of left renal pelvis ☑
C66.1	Malignant neoplasm of right ureter ☑
C66.2	Malignant neoplasm of left ureter ☑
C67.0	Malignant neoplasm of trigone of bladder
C67.1	Malignant neoplasm of dome of bladder
C67.2	Malignant neoplasm of lateral wall of bladder
C67.3	Malignant neoplasm of anterior wall of bladder

C67.4	Malignant neoplasm of posterior wall of bladder	
C67.5	Malignant neoplasm of bladder neck	
C67.6	Malignant neoplasm of ureteric orifice	
C67.8	Malignant neoplasm of overlapping sites of bladder	
C68.0	Malignant neoplasm of urethra	
C68.1	Malignant neoplasm of paraurethral glands	
C68.8	Malignant neoplasm of overlapping sites of urinary organs	
C74.01	Malignant neoplasm of cortex of right adrenal gland	☑
C74.02	Malignant neoplasm of cortex of left adrenal gland	☑
C74.11	Malignant neoplasm of medulla of right adrenal gland	☑
C74.12	Malignant neoplasm of medulla of left adrenal gland	☑
C77.2	Secondary and unspecified malignant neoplasm of intra-abdominal lymph nodes	
C78.6	Secondary malignant neoplasm of retroperitoneum and peritoneum	
C7A.093	Malignant carcinoid tumor of the kidney	
C7B.01	Secondary carcinoid tumors of distant lymph nodes	
C7B.04	Secondary carcinoid tumors of peritoneum	
C7B.09	Secondary carcinoid tumors of other sites	
C7B.1	Secondary Merkel cell carcinoma	
C7B.8	Other secondary neuroendocrine tumors	
D48.3	Neoplasm of uncertain behavior of retroperitoneum	
D48.4	Neoplasm of uncertain behavior of peritoneum	

AMA: **38780** 2019,Feb,8; 2014,Jan,11

Relative Value Units/Medicare Edits

Non-Facility RVU	Work	PE	MP	Total
38780	17.7	9.33	2.89	29.92
Facility RVU	**Work**	**PE**	**MP**	**Total**
38780	17.7	9.33	2.89	29.92

	FUD	Status	MUE	Modifiers				IOM Reference
38780	90	A	1(2)	51	N/A	62*	80	None

* with documentation

Terms To Know

dissection. Separating by cutting tissue or body structures apart.

lymph nodes. Bean-shaped structures along the lymphatic vessels that intercept and destroy foreign materials in the tissue and bloodstream.

lymphadenectomy. Dissection of lymph nodes free from the vessels and removal for examination by frozen section in a separate procedure to detect early-stage metastases.

retroperitoneal. Located behind the peritoneum, the membrane that lines the abdominopelvic walls and forms a covering for the internal organs.

tissue. Group of similar cells with a similar function that form definite structures and organs. Tissue types include epithelial tissue, muscle tissue, connective tissue, and nervous tissue.

44660-44661

44660   Closure of enterovesical fistula; without intestinal or bladder resection
44661   with intestine and/or bladder resection

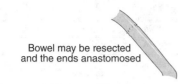

Bowel may be resected
and the ends anastomosed

Bladder may be resected and closed with sutures

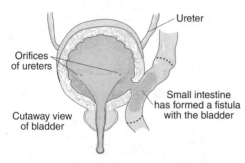

An enterovesical fistula (communication
between bowel and bladder) is repaired

Explanation

The physician closes a connection between the small bowel and bladder (enterovesical fistula). The physician makes an abdominal incision. Next, the enterovesical fistula is identified and divided. The ends of the fistula are closed with sutures. In 44661, the connection of the fistula to the bladder is resected and the bladder is closed with sutures; the segment of intestine containing the fistula is resected and the ends are reapproximated. The incision is closed.

Coding Tips

For closure of an intestinal cutaneous fistula, see 44640; enteroenteric or enterocolic, see 44650; renocolic, abdominal approach, see 50525; thoracic approach, see 50526; gastrocolic, see 43880; rectovesical, see 45800–45805.

ICD-10-CM Diagnostic Codes

N32.1   Vesicointestinal fistula
N32.2   Vesical fistula, not elsewhere classified
N49.8   Inflammatory disorders of other specified male genital organs ♂
Q64.73   Congenital urethrorectal fistula
Q64.79   Other congenital malformations of bladder and urethra
Q64.8   Other specified congenital malformations of urinary system
T81.83XA   Persistent postprocedural fistula, initial encounter

AMA: 44660 2014,Jan,11 **44661** 2014,Jan,11

Relative Value Units/Medicare Edits

Non-Facility RVU	Work	PE	MP	Total
44660	23.91	10.69	4.12	38.72
44661	27.35	12.18	5.54	45.07
Facility RVU	**Work**	**PE**	**MP**	**Total**
44660	23.91	10.69	4.12	38.72
44661	27.35	12.18	5.54	45.07

	FUD	Status	MUE	Modifiers				IOM Reference
44660	90	A	1(3)	51	N/A	62*	80	None
44661	90	A	1(3)	51	N/A	62*	80	

* with documentation

Terms To Know

anastomosis. Surgically created connection between ducts, blood vessels, or bowel segments to allow flow from one to the other.

enterovesical fistula. Abnormal communication between the small intestine and the bladder.

incision. Act of cutting into tissue or an organ.

peritonitis. Inflammation and infection within the peritoneal cavity, the space between the membrane lining the abdominopelvic walls and covering the internal organs.

regional enteritis. Chronic inflammation of unknown origin affecting the ileum and/or colon.

resection. Surgical removal of a part or all of an organ or body part.

suture. Numerous stitching techniques employed in wound closure.

Abdomen

46744-46746

46744 Repair of cloacal anomaly by anorectovaginoplasty and urethroplasty, sacroperineal approach

46746 Repair of cloacal anomaly by anorectovaginoplasty and urethroplasty, combined abdominal and sacroperineal approach;

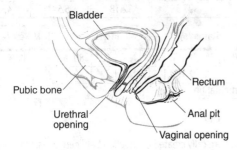

Persistent cloaca: common urinary, fecal, and reproductive passage

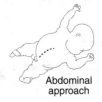 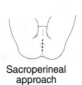

Abdominal approach   Sacroperineal approach

During early stages of fetal development, the rectal, urinary, and reproductive tracts drain through a common passage—the cloaca. In some anomalies, the cloaca persists or is abnormal

Explanation

The physician repairs a cloacal anomaly. The patient is placed in a lithotomy position. The physician makes a small incision in the perineum. The bladder, urethra, and vagina are dissected free of each other. A new rectum is formed by interposing muscle posterior to the rectum. The incision is closed with sutures. Report 46746 when a combined abdominal and sacroperineal approach is used.

Coding Tips

Coding surgical repair of cloacal anomaly is dependent on the approach (sacroperineal or combined abdominal/sacroperineal) and the need for intestinal grafting or pedicle flaps. Do not append modifier 63 to 46744 as the description or nature of the procedure includes infants up to 4 kg.

ICD-10-CM Diagnostic Codes

K63.89	Other specified diseases of intestine
N36.5	Urethral false passage
N36.8	Other specified disorders of urethra
Q43.3	Congenital malformations of intestinal fixation
Q43.6	Congenital fistula of rectum and anus
Q43.7	Persistent cloaca
Q43.8	Other specified congenital malformations of intestine
Q52.4	Other congenital malformations of vagina ♀
Q52.8	Other specified congenital malformations of female genitalia ♀
Q64.79	Other congenital malformations of bladder and urethra
Q64.8	Other specified congenital malformations of urinary system

AMA: **46744** 2014,Jan,11 **46746** 2014,Jan,11

Relative Value Units/Medicare Edits

Non-Facility RVU	Work	PE	MP	Total
46744	58.94	29.64	14.48	103.06
46746	65.44	32.09	16.18	113.71
Facility RVU	**Work**	**PE**	**MP**	**Total**
46744	58.94	29.64	14.48	103.06
46746	65.44	32.09	16.18	113.71

	FUD	Status	MUE	Modifiers				IOM Reference
46744	90	A	1(2)	51	N/A	62*	80	None
46746	90	A	1(2)	51	N/A	62*	80	

* with documentation

Terms To Know

anomaly. Irregularity in the structure or position of an organ or tissue.

approach. Method or anatomical location used to gain access to a body organ or specific area for procedures.

cloacal anomaly. Congenital anomaly resulting from the failure of one common urinary, anal, and reproductive vaginal passage of the early embryonic stage to develop into the properly divided rectal and urogenital sections.

congenital. Present at birth, occurring through heredity or an influence during gestation up to the moment of birth.

dissection. Separating by cutting tissue or body structures apart.

lithotomy position. Common position patients may be placed in for some surgical procedures and examinations involving the pelvis and/or lower abdomen. The patient is placed supine (on their back), hips and knees flexed, thighs apart, with feet supported in raised stirrups.

perineal. Pertaining to the pelvic floor area between the thighs; the diamond-shaped area bordered by the pubic symphysis in front, the ischial tuberosities on the sides, and the coccyx in back.

posterior. Located in the back part or caudal end of the body.

suture. Numerous stitching techniques employed in wound closure.

buried suture. Continuous or interrupted suture placed under the skin for a layered closure.

continuous suture. Running stitch with tension evenly distributed across a single strand to provide a leakproof closure line.

interrupted suture. Series of single stitches with tension isolated at each stitch, in which all stitches are not affected if one becomes loose, and the isolated sutures cannot act as a wick to transport an infection.

purse-string suture. Continuous suture placed around a tubular structure and tightened, to reduce or close the lumen.

retention suture. Secondary stitching that bridges the primary suture, providing support for the primary repair; a plastic or rubber bolster may be placed over the primary repair and under the retention sutures.

© 2020 Optum360, LLC   **N** Newborn: 0   **P** Pediatric: 0-17   **M** Maternity: 9-64   **A** Adult: 15-124   ♂ Male Only   ♀ Female Only   CPT © 2020 American Medical Association. All Rights Reserved.

Abdomen

49000

49000   Exploratory laparotomy, exploratory celiotomy with or without biopsy(s) (separate procedure)

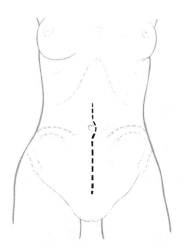

Typical incision for laparotomy

An access incision is made into the abdominal cavity for exploratory purposes

Explanation

To explore the intra-abdominal organs and structures, the physician makes a large incision extending from just above the pubic hairline to the rib cage. The abdominal cavity is opened for a systematic examination of all organs. The physician may take tissue samples of any or all intra-abdominal organs for diagnosis. The incision is closed with sutures.

Coding Tips

This separate procedure by definition is usually a component of a more complex service and is not identified separately. When performed alone or with other unrelated procedures/services it may be reported. If performed alone, list the code; if performed with other procedures/services, list the code and append modifier 59 or an X{EPSU} modifier. Steps in this procedure vary according to each case, depending on the condition of the patient, the nature of the suspected problem, and/or other circumstances. For reopening of a recent laparotomy, see 49002. For exploration, retroperitoneal area, see 49010. If a diagnostic laparoscopy is performed, see 49320. For wound exploration due to a penetrating trauma without laparotomy, see 20102.

ICD-10-CM Diagnostic Codes

The application of this code is too broad to adequately present ICD-10-CM diagnostic code links here. Refer to your ICD-10-CM book.

AMA: **49000** 2020,Jan,6; 2019,Dec,5; 2018,Jan,8; 2017,Jan,8; 2017,Dec,3; 2016,Jan,13; 2015,Jan,16; 2014,Jan,11

Relative Value Units/Medicare Edits

Non-Facility RVU	Work	PE	MP	Total
49000	12.54	7.01	2.83	22.38
Facility RVU	Work	PE	MP	Total
49000	12.54	7.01	2.83	22.38

	FUD	Status	MUE	Modifiers				IOM Reference
49000	90	A	1(2)	51	N/A	62*	80	None

* with documentation

Terms To Know

biopsy. Tissue or fluid removed for diagnostic purposes through analysis of the cells in the biopsy material.

celiotomy. Incision into the abdominal cavity.

diagnostic. Examination or procedure to which the patient is subjected, or which is performed on materials derived from a hospital outpatient, to obtain information to aid in the assessment of a medical condition or the identification of a disease. Among these examinations and tests are diagnostic laboratory services such as hematology and chemistry, diagnostic x-rays, isotope studies, EKGs, pulmonary function studies, thyroid function tests, psychological tests, and other tests given to determine the nature and severity of an ailment or injury.

exploration. Examination for diagnostic purposes.

incision. Act of cutting into tissue or an organ.

intra. Within.

laparotomy. Incision through the flank or abdomen for therapeutic or diagnostic purposes.

tissue. Group of similar cells with a similar function that form definite structures and organs. Tissue types include epithelial tissue, muscle tissue, connective tissue, and nervous tissue.

Abdomen

CPT © 2020 American Medical Association. All Rights Reserved.   ● New   ▲ Revised   + Add On   ★ Telemedicine   AMA: CPT Assist   [Resequenced]   ☑ Laterality   © 2020 Optum360, LLC

49002

49002 Reopening of recent laparotomy

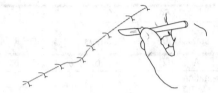

The site of a recent laparotomy incision is reopened

Explanation

The physician reopens the incision of a recent laparotomy before the incision has fully healed to control bleeding, remove packing, or drain a postoperative infection.

Coding Tips

Diagnosis codes should support the reason for reopening the laparotomy. For exploratory laparotomy, exploratory celiotomy, with or without biopsies, see 49000. For re-exploration of a pelvic wound to remove preperitoneal pelvic packing, see 49014.

ICD-10-CM Diagnostic Codes

D78.21	Postprocedural hemorrhage of the spleen following a procedure on the spleen
K56.51	Intestinal adhesions [bands], with partial obstruction
K56.52	Intestinal adhesions [bands] with complete obstruction
K56.600	Partial intestinal obstruction, unspecified as to cause
K56.601	Complete intestinal obstruction, unspecified as to cause
K56.690	Other partial intestinal obstruction
K56.691	Other complete intestinal obstruction
K65.0	Generalized (acute) peritonitis
K65.1	Peritoneal abscess
K65.2	Spontaneous bacterial peritonitis
K65.8	Other peritonitis
K66.1	Hemoperitoneum
K68.11	Postprocedural retroperitoneal abscess
K91.30	Postprocedural intestinal obstruction, unspecified as to partial versus complete
K91.31	Postprocedural partial intestinal obstruction
K91.32	Postprocedural complete intestinal obstruction
N73.6	Female pelvic peritoneal adhesions (postinfective) ♀
N99.0	Postprocedural (acute) (chronic) kidney failure
N99.520	Hemorrhage of incontinent external stoma of urinary tract
N99.521	Infection of incontinent external stoma of urinary tract
N99.522	Malfunction of incontinent external stoma of urinary tract
N99.523	Herniation of incontinent stoma of urinary tract
N99.524	Stenosis of incontinent stoma of urinary tract
N99.528	Other complication of incontinent external stoma of urinary tract
N99.530	Hemorrhage of continent stoma of urinary tract
N99.531	Infection of continent stoma of urinary tract
N99.532	Malfunction of continent stoma of urinary tract
N99.533	Herniation of continent stoma of urinary tract
N99.534	Stenosis of continent stoma of urinary tract
N99.538	Other complication of continent stoma of urinary tract
R10.0	Acute abdomen
R10.11	Right upper quadrant pain
R10.12	Left upper quadrant pain
R10.13	Epigastric pain
R10.2	Pelvic and perineal pain
R10.31	Right lower quadrant pain
R10.32	Left lower quadrant pain
R10.33	Periumbilical pain
R10.84	Generalized abdominal pain
R19.01	Right upper quadrant abdominal swelling, mass and lump
R19.02	Left upper quadrant abdominal swelling, mass and lump
R19.03	Right lower quadrant abdominal swelling, mass and lump
R19.04	Left lower quadrant abdominal swelling, mass and lump
R19.05	Periumbilic swelling, mass or lump
R19.06	Epigastric swelling, mass or lump
R19.07	Generalized intra-abdominal and pelvic swelling, mass and lump
R19.09	Other intra-abdominal and pelvic swelling, mass and lump
T81.510A	Adhesions due to foreign body accidentally left in body following surgical operation, initial encounter
T81.511A	Adhesions due to foreign body accidentally left in body following infusion or transfusion, initial encounter
T81.512A	Adhesions due to foreign body accidentally left in body following kidney dialysis, initial encounter
T81.513A	Adhesions due to foreign body accidentally left in body following injection or immunization, initial encounter
T81.514A	Adhesions due to foreign body accidentally left in body following endoscopic examination, initial encounter
T81.516A	Adhesions due to foreign body accidentally left in body following aspiration, puncture or other catheterization, initial encounter
T81.517A	Adhesions due to foreign body accidentally left in body following removal of catheter or packing, initial encounter
T81.518A	Adhesions due to foreign body accidentally left in body following other procedure, initial encounter
T81.520A	Obstruction due to foreign body accidentally left in body following surgical operation, initial encounter
T81.521A	Obstruction due to foreign body accidentally left in body following infusion or transfusion, initial encounter
T81.522A	Obstruction due to foreign body accidentally left in body following kidney dialysis, initial encounter
T81.523A	Obstruction due to foreign body accidentally left in body following injection or immunization, initial encounter
T81.524A	Obstruction due to foreign body accidentally left in body following endoscopic examination, initial encounter
T81.526A	Obstruction due to foreign body accidentally left in body following aspiration, puncture or other catheterization, initial encounter
T81.527A	Obstruction due to foreign body accidentally left in body following removal of catheter or packing, initial encounter
T81.528A	Obstruction due to foreign body accidentally left in body following other procedure, initial encounter
T81.530A	Perforation due to foreign body accidentally left in body following surgical operation, initial encounter

Abdomen

T81.531A	Perforation due to foreign body accidentally left in body following infusion or transfusion, initial encounter
T81.532A	Perforation due to foreign body accidentally left in body following kidney dialysis, initial encounter
T81.533A	Perforation due to foreign body accidentally left in body following injection or immunization, initial encounter
T81.534A	Perforation due to foreign body accidentally left in body following endoscopic examination, initial encounter
T81.536A	Perforation due to foreign body accidentally left in body following aspiration, puncture or other catheterization, initial encounter
T81.537A	Perforation due to foreign body accidentally left in body following removal of catheter or packing, initial encounter
T81.538A	Perforation due to foreign body accidentally left in body following other procedure, initial encounter
T81.590A	Other complications of foreign body accidentally left in body following surgical operation, initial encounter
T81.591A	Other complications of foreign body accidentally left in body following infusion or transfusion, initial encounter
T81.592A	Other complications of foreign body accidentally left in body following kidney dialysis, initial encounter
T81.593A	Other complications of foreign body accidentally left in body following injection or immunization, initial encounter
T81.594A	Other complications of foreign body accidentally left in body following endoscopic examination, initial encounter
T81.596A	Other complications of foreign body accidentally left in body following aspiration, puncture or other catheterization, initial encounter
T81.597A	Other complications of foreign body accidentally left in body following removal of catheter or packing, initial encounter
T81.598A	Other complications of foreign body accidentally left in body following other procedure, initial encounter

AMA: 49002 2020,Jan,6; 2018,Jan,8; 2017,Jan,8; 2016,Jan,13; 2015,Jan,16; 2014,Jan,11

Relative Value Units/Medicare Edits

Non-Facility RVU	Work	PE	MP	Total
49002	17.63	8.81	4.0	30.44
Facility RVU	Work	PE	MP	Total
49002	17.63	8.81	4.0	30.44

	FUD	Status	MUE	Modifiers				IOM Reference
49002	90	A	1(3)	51	N/A	62*	80	None

* with documentation

Terms To Know

adhesion. Abnormal fibrous connection between two structures, soft tissue or bony structures, that may occur as the result of surgery, infection, or trauma.

obstruction. Blockage that prevents normal function of the valve or structure.

peritonitis. Inflammation and infection within the peritoneal cavity, the space between the membrane lining the abdominopelvic walls and covering the internal organs.

49010

| 49010 | Exploration, retroperitoneal area with or without biopsy(s) (separate procedure) |

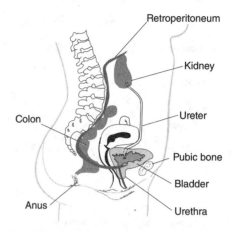

The retroperitoneal area can generally be defined as the posterior wall cavity

Explanation

The physician explores the retroperitoneum and may obtain sample tissue for separately reportable diagnostic testing. The physician may approach the retroperitoneum through a flank or an abdominal incision. The surface of the retroperitoneum is inspected and any area of interest of the retroperitoneum may be opened and the retroperitoneum explored. Tissues may be sampled. The incision is closed.

Coding Tips

This separate procedure by definition is usually a component of a more complex service and is not identified separately. When performed alone or with other unrelated procedures/services it may be reported. If performed alone, list the code; if performed with other procedures/services, list the code and append modifier 59 or an X{EPSU} modifier. To report wound exploration due to a penetrating trauma without laparotomy, see 20102.

ICD-10-CM Diagnostic Codes

The application of this code is too broad to adequately present ICD-10-CM diagnostic code links here. Refer to your ICD-10-CM book.

AMA: 49010 2020,Jan,6; 2019,Dec,5; 2014,Jan,11

Relative Value Units/Medicare Edits

Non-Facility RVU	Work	PE	MP	Total
49010	16.06	7.37	3.46	26.89
Facility RVU	Work	PE	MP	Total
49010	16.06	7.37	3.46	26.89

	FUD	Status	MUE	Modifiers				IOM Reference
49010	90	A	1(3)	51	N/A	62*	80	None

* with documentation

CPT © 2020 American Medical Association. All Rights Reserved. ● New ▲ Revised + Add On ★ Telemedicine AMA: CPT Assist [Resequenced] ☑ Laterality © 2020 Optum360, LLC

Abdomen

49020

49020 Drainage of peritoneal abscess or localized peritonitis, exclusive of appendiceal abscess, open

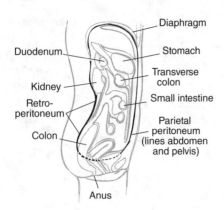

Peritonitis is an infectious irritation of the peritoneum, the viscous lining of internal organs and abdominal walls

Explanation

The physician makes an open abdominal or flank incision (laparotomy) to gain access to the peritoneal cavity. The peritoneum is explored and the abscess or isolated area of peritoneal inflammation is identified. The abscess is incised and drained and inflamed peritoneal tissue may be excised. The abscess and surrounding peritoneal cavity may be irrigated. A drain may be placed whereby a separate abdominal incision is made and the drain is drawn through it and sutured in place. The physician may completely reapproximate the abdominal incision or leave a portion of the incision open to allow for further drainage. Specimens taken during the procedure are typically sent to microbiology for identification and to determine antibiotic suitability. If a drain is placed, it is removed at a later date.

Coding Tips

For open drainage of a retroperitoneal abscess, see 49060. Report percutaneous, image-guided drainage of a peritoneal, retroperitoneal, subdiaphragmatic or subphrenic abscess or localized peritonitis, via catheter, with 49406.

ICD-10-CM Diagnostic Codes

K65.1	Peritoneal abscess
K65.2	Spontaneous bacterial peritonitis
K65.3	Choleperitonitis
K65.4	Sclerosing mesenteritis
K65.8	Other peritonitis
K66.1	Hemoperitoneum
K66.8	Other specified disorders of peritoneum
K68.11	Postprocedural retroperitoneal abscess
K68.12	Psoas muscle abscess
K68.19	Other retroperitoneal abscess
K68.9	Other disorders of retroperitoneum

AMA: **49020** 2014,Jan,11

Relative Value Units/Medicare Edits

Non-Facility RVU	Work	PE	MP	Total
49020	26.67	13.74	5.95	46.36
Facility RVU	**Work**	**PE**	**MP**	**Total**
49020	26.67	13.74	5.95	46.36

	FUD	Status	MUE	Modifiers				IOM Reference
49020	90	A	2(3)	51	N/A	N/A	80	None

* with documentation

Terms To Know

abscess. Circumscribed collection of pus resulting from bacteria, frequently associated with swelling and other signs of inflammation.

catheter. Flexible tube inserted into an area of the body for introducing or withdrawing fluid.

drainage. Releasing, taking, or letting out fluids and/or gases from a body part.

flank. Part of the body found between the posterior ribs and the uppermost crest of the ilium, or the lateral side of the hip, thigh, and buttock.

irrigate. Washing out, lavage.

peritoneal. Space between the lining of the abdominal wall, or parietal peritoneum, and the surface layer of the abdominal organs, or visceral peritoneum. It contains a thin, watery fluid that keeps the peritoneal surfaces moist.

peritoneal cavity. Space between the lining of the abdominal wall, or parietal peritoneum, and the surface layer of the abdominal organs, or visceral peritoneum. It contains a thin, watery fluid that keeps the peritoneal surfaces moist.

peritonitis. Inflammation and infection within the peritoneal cavity, the space between the membrane lining the abdominopelvic walls and covering the internal organs.

specimen. Tissue cells or sample of fluid taken for analysis, pathologic examination, and diagnosis.

tissue. Group of similar cells with a similar function that form definite structures and organs. Tissue types include epithelial tissue, muscle tissue, connective tissue, and nervous tissue.

ultrasound. Imaging using ultra-high sound frequency bounced off body structures.

© 2020 Optum360, LLC   **N Newborn: 0**   **P Pediatric: 0-17**   **M Maternity: 9-64**   **A Adult: 15-124**   ♂ Male Only   ♀ Female Only   CPT © 2020 American Medical Association. All Rights Reserved.

Abdomen

49060

49060   Drainage of retroperitoneal abscess, open

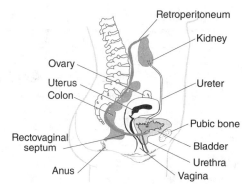

The retroperitoneal area can generally be defined as the posterior wall of the abdominal cavity

Explanation

The physician drains a retroperitoneal abscess. The physician makes an abdominal or flank incision. The abscess is identified and the retroperitoneal space is entered. The abscess cavity is opened and drained. Irrigation of the cavity is usually performed. A drain is usually placed in the abscess cavity and brought out through the abdominal wall. The incision is closed. The superficial portion of the incision may be packed open to allow drainage.

Coding Tips

For open drainage of a peritoneal abscess or localized peritonitis, see 49020. Report percutaneous, image-guided drainage of a peritoneal. retroperitoneal, subdiaphragmatic or subphrenic abscess or localized peritonitis, via catheter, with 49406.

ICD-10-CM Diagnostic Codes

K35.20	Acute appendicitis with generalized peritonitis, without abscess
K35.21	Acute appendicitis with generalized peritonitis, with abscess
K65.0	Generalized (acute) peritonitis
K65.2	Spontaneous bacterial peritonitis
K65.3	Choleperitonitis
K65.4	Sclerosing mesenteritis
K65.8	Other peritonitis
K66.1	Hemoperitoneum
K66.8	Other specified disorders of peritoneum
K67	Disorders of peritoneum in infectious diseases classified elsewhere
K68.11	Postprocedural retroperitoneal abscess
K68.12	Psoas muscle abscess
K68.19	Other retroperitoneal abscess
K68.9	Other disorders of retroperitoneum

AMA: **49060** 2018,Jan,8; 2017,Jan,8; 2016,Jan,13; 2015,Jan,16; 2014,Jan,11

Relative Value Units/Medicare Edits

Non-Facility RVU	Work	PE	MP	Total
49060	18.53	9.46	4.03	32.02
Facility RVU	**Work**	**PE**	**MP**	**Total**
49060	18.53	9.46	4.03	32.02

	FUD	Status	MUE	Modifiers				IOM Reference
49060	90	A	2(3)	51	N/A	62*	N/A	None

* with documentation

Terms To Know

abscess. Circumscribed collection of pus resulting from bacteria, frequently associated with swelling and other signs of inflammation.

cellulitis. Infection of the skin and subcutaneous tissues, most often caused by Staphylococcus or Streptococcus bacteria secondary to a cutaneous lesion. Progression of the inflammation may lead to abscess and tissue death, or even systemic infection-like bacteremia.

drainage. Releasing, taking, or letting out fluids and/or gases from a body part.

flank. Part of the body found between the posterior ribs and the uppermost crest of the ilium, or the lateral side of the hip, thigh, and buttock.

irrigation. To wash out or cleanse a body cavity, wound, or tissue with water or other fluid.

packing. Material placed into a cavity or wound, such as gels, gauze, pads, and sponges.

parametritis. Inflammation and infection of the tissue in the structures around the uterus.

percutaneous. Through the skin.

retroperitoneal. Located behind the peritoneum, the membrane that lines the abdominopelvic walls and forms a covering for the internal organs.

superficial. On the skin surface or near the surface of any involved structure or field of interest.

Abdomen

CPT © 2020 American Medical Association. All Rights Reserved.   ● New   ▲ Revised   + Add On   ★ Telemedicine   AMA: CPT Assist   [Resequenced]   ☑ Laterality   © 2020 Optum360, LLC

Coding Companion for Urology/Nephrology   **87**

49082-49083

49082 Abdominal paracentesis (diagnostic or therapeutic); without imaging guidance

49083 with imaging guidance

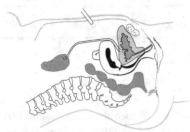

The peritoneum is accessed by a nick incision and a catheter is introduced into the cavity

Explanation

The physician inserts a needle or catheter into the abdominal cavity and withdraws and drains fluid for diagnostic or therapeutic purposes. The needle or catheter is removed at the completion of the procedure. Report 49082 if imaging guidance is not used and 49083 if imaging guidance is used.

Coding Tips

Do not report 49083 with 76942, 77002, 77012, or 77021. Peritoneal lavage with imaging guidance is reported with 49084, when performed. For percutaneous, image-guided drainage of a retroperitoneal abscess via catheter, see 49406.

ICD-10-CM Diagnostic Codes

A18.31	Tuberculous peritonitis
C78.6	Secondary malignant neoplasm of retroperitoneum and peritoneum
E87.2	Acidosis
E87.79	Other fluid overload
E87.8	Other disorders of electrolyte and fluid balance, not elsewhere classified
I81	Portal vein thrombosis
I89.8	Other specified noninfective disorders of lymphatic vessels and lymph nodes
K65.0	Generalized (acute) peritonitis
K65.1	Peritoneal abscess
K65.2	Spontaneous bacterial peritonitis
K65.8	Other peritonitis
K66.1	Hemoperitoneum
K66.8	Other specified disorders of peritoneum
N18.5	Chronic kidney disease, stage 5
N18.6	End stage renal disease
N25.89	Other disorders resulting from impaired renal tubular function
S36.81XA	Injury of peritoneum, initial encounter
S36.892A	Contusion of other intra-abdominal organs, initial encounter
S36.893A	Laceration of other intra-abdominal organs, initial encounter
S36.898A	Other injury of other intra-abdominal organs, initial encounter

AMA: 49082 2018,Jan,8; 2017,Jan,8; 2016,Jan,13; 2015,Jan,16; 2014,Jan,11
49083 2018,Jan,8; 2017,Jan,8; 2016,Jan,13; 2015,Jan,16; 2014,Mar,13; 2014,Jan,11

Relative Value Units/Medicare Edits

Non-Facility RVU	Work	PE	MP	Total
49082	1.24	4.4	0.18	5.82
49083	2.0	6.38	0.18	8.56
Facility RVU	**Work**	**PE**	**MP**	**Total**
49082	1.24	0.72	0.18	2.14
49083	2.0	0.93	0.18	3.11

	FUD	Status	MUE	Modifiers				IOM Reference
49082	0	A	1(3)	51	N/A	N/A	N/A	None
49083	0	A	2(3)	51	N/A	N/A	N/A	

* with documentation

Terms To Know

catheter. Flexible tube inserted into an area of the body for introducing or withdrawing fluid.

diagnostic. Examination or procedure to which the patient is subjected, or which is performed on materials derived from a hospital outpatient, to obtain information to aid in the assessment of a medical condition or the identification of a disease. Among these examinations and tests are diagnostic laboratory services such as hematology and chemistry, diagnostic x-rays, isotope studies, EKGs, pulmonary function studies, thyroid function tests, psychological tests, and other tests given to determine the nature and severity of an ailment or injury.

drain. Device that creates a channel to allow fluid from a cavity, wound, or infected area to exit the body.

imaging. Radiologic means of producing pictures for clinical study of the internal structures and functions of the body, such as x-ray, ultrasound, magnetic resonance, or positron emission tomography.

paracentesis. Surgical puncture of a body cavity with a specialized needle or hollow tubing to aspirate fluid for diagnostic or therapeutic reasons.

therapeutic. Act meant to alleviate a medical or mental condition.

Abdomen

49084

49084   Peritoneal lavage, including imaging guidance, when performed

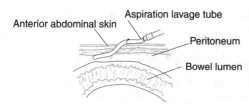

Anterior abdominal skin
Aspiration lavage tube
Peritoneum
Bowel lumen

The peritoneum is accessed by a nick incision
and a catheter is introduced into the cavity

Explanation

Peritoneal lavage is usually performed to determine the presence and/or extent of internal bleeding within the peritoneum. The physician makes a small incision to insert a catheter into the abdominal cavity. Fluids are infused into the cavity and subsequently aspirated for diagnostic testing. The catheter is removed at the completion of the procedure and the incision is closed.

Coding Tips

Imaging is included in this procedure and should not be reported separately. Do not report 49084 with 76942, 77002, 77012, or 77021. For percutaneous image-guided drainage of a retroperitoneal abscess by catheter, see 49406.

ICD-10-CM Diagnostic Codes

A18.31	Tuberculous peritonitis
C78.6	Secondary malignant neoplasm of retroperitoneum and peritoneum
I81	Portal vein thrombosis
I89.8	Other specified noninfective disorders of lymphatic vessels and lymph nodes
K56.600	Partial intestinal obstruction, unspecified as to cause
K56.601	Complete intestinal obstruction, unspecified as to cause
K56.690	Other partial intestinal obstruction
K56.691	Other complete intestinal obstruction
K65.0	Generalized (acute) peritonitis
K65.1	Peritoneal abscess
K65.2	Spontaneous bacterial peritonitis
K65.8	Other peritonitis
K66.1	Hemoperitoneum
K66.8	Other specified disorders of peritoneum
S36.81XA	Injury of peritoneum, initial encounter
S36.892A	Contusion of other intra-abdominal organs, initial encounter
S36.893A	Laceration of other intra-abdominal organs, initial encounter
S36.898A	Other injury of other intra-abdominal organs, initial encounter

AMA: 49084 2018,Jan,8; 2017,Jan,8; 2016,Jan,13; 2015,Jan,16; 2014,Jan,11

Relative Value Units/Medicare Edits

Non-Facility RVU	Work	PE	MP	Total
49084	2.0	0.73	0.43	3.16
Facility RVU	**Work**	**PE**	**MP**	**Total**
49084	2.0	0.73	0.43	3.16

	FUD	Status	MUE	Modifiers				IOM Reference
49084	0	A	1(3)	51	N/A	N/A	N/A	None

* with documentation

Terms To Know

catheter. Flexible tube inserted into an area of the body for introducing or withdrawing fluid.

diagnostic. Examination or procedure to which the patient is subjected, or which is performed on materials derived from a hospital outpatient, to obtain information to aid in the assessment of a medical condition or the identification of a disease. Among these examinations and tests are diagnostic laboratory services such as hematology and chemistry, diagnostic x-rays, isotope studies, EKGs, pulmonary function studies, thyroid function tests, psychological tests, and other tests given to determine the nature and severity of an ailment or injury.

imaging. Radiologic means of producing pictures for clinical study of the internal structures and functions of the body, such as x-ray, ultrasound, magnetic resonance, or positron emission tomography.

incision. Act of cutting into tissue or an organ.

infusion. Introduction of a therapeutic fluid, other than blood, into the bloodstream.

lavage. Washing.

peritoneal. Space between the lining of the abdominal wall, or parietal peritoneum, and the surface layer of the abdominal organs, or visceral peritoneum. It contains a thin, watery fluid that keeps the peritoneal surfaces moist.

Abdomen

49180

49180   Biopsy, abdominal or retroperitoneal mass, percutaneous needle

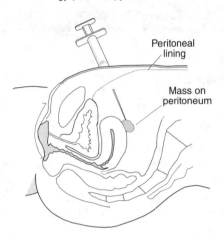

Biopsy needle guided to mass with aid of radiology (fluoroscopy, CT, ultrasound)

Peritoneal lining

Mass on peritoneum

Explanation

Using radiological supervision, the physician locates the mass within or immediately outside the peritoneal lining of the abdominal cavity. A biopsy needle is passed into the mass, a tissue sample is removed, and the needle is withdrawn. This may be repeated several times. No incision is necessary.

Coding Tips

If multiple areas are biopsied, report 49180 for each site taken and append modifier 51 to additional codes. Local anesthesia is included in this service. However, general anesthesia may be administered depending on the age or condition of the patient. Imaging guidance is reported with 76942, 77002, 77012, or 77021, when performed. For fine needle aspiration biopsy, see 10004–10012 and 10021. For evaluation of aspirate, see 88172–88173.

ICD-10-CM Diagnostic Codes

C48.0	Malignant neoplasm of retroperitoneum
C76.2	Malignant neoplasm of abdomen
C77.2	Secondary and unspecified malignant neoplasm of intra-abdominal lymph nodes
C78.6	Secondary malignant neoplasm of retroperitoneum and peritoneum
C7A.1	Malignant poorly differentiated neuroendocrine tumors
D20.0	Benign neoplasm of soft tissue of retroperitoneum
D48.3	Neoplasm of uncertain behavior of retroperitoneum
D48.4	Neoplasm of uncertain behavior of peritoneum
D48.7	Neoplasm of uncertain behavior of other specified sites
D49.89	Neoplasm of unspecified behavior of other specified sites
R16.0	Hepatomegaly, not elsewhere classified
R19.01	Right upper quadrant abdominal swelling, mass and lump
R19.02	Left upper quadrant abdominal swelling, mass and lump
R19.03	Right lower quadrant abdominal swelling, mass and lump
R19.04	Left lower quadrant abdominal swelling, mass and lump
R19.05	Periumbilic swelling, mass or lump
R19.06	Epigastric swelling, mass or lump
R19.07	Generalized intra-abdominal and pelvic swelling, mass and lump
R19.09	Other intra-abdominal and pelvic swelling, mass and lump
R59.0	Localized enlarged lymph nodes
R59.1	Generalized enlarged lymph nodes

AMA: **49180** 2019,Feb,8; 2019,Apr,4; 2018,Jan,8; 2017,Jan,8; 2016,Jan,13; 2015,Jan,16; 2014,Jan,11

Relative Value Units/Medicare Edits

Non-Facility RVU	Work	PE	MP	Total
49180	1.73	3.0	0.13	4.86
Facility RVU	**Work**	**PE**	**MP**	**Total**
49180	1.73	0.57	0.13	2.43

	FUD	Status	MUE	Modifiers				IOM Reference
49180	0	A	2(3)	51	N/A	N/A	N/A	None

* with documentation

Terms To Know

biopsy. Tissue or fluid removed for diagnostic purposes through analysis of the cells in the biopsy material.

percutaneous. Through the skin.

retroperitoneal. Located behind the peritoneum, the membrane that lines the abdominopelvic walls and forms a covering for the internal organs.

specimen. Tissue cells or sample of fluid taken for analysis, pathologic examination, and diagnosis.

tissue. Group of similar cells with a similar function that form definite structures and organs. Tissue types include epithelial tissue, muscle tissue, connective tissue, and nervous tissue.

© 2020 Optum360, LLC   N Newborn: 0   P Pediatric: 0-17   M Maternity: 9-64   A Adult: 15-124   ♂ Male Only   ♀ Female Only   CPT © 2020 American Medical Association. All Rights Reserved.

Abdomen

49185

49185 Sclerotherapy of a fluid collection (eg, lymphocele, cyst, or seroma), percutaneous, including contrast injection(s), sclerosant injection(s), diagnostic study, imaging guidance (eg, ultrasound, fluoroscopy) and radiological supervision and interpretation when performed

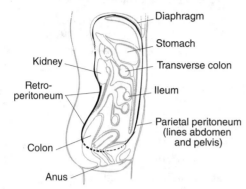

Fluid collection is treated with sclerotherapy

Explanation

Sclerotherapy is the therapeutic use of sclerosing agents (e.g., ethanol, povidone-iodine, tetracycline, doxycycline, bleomycin, talc, or fibrin glue) to systematically destroy undesired fluid collections such as cysts, lymphoceles, or seromas. This procedure is usually performed with the patient under moderate conscious sedation and involves a minimally invasive, percutaneous approach; depending on the size of the cyst or lymphocele, treatment may involve catheter drainage by gravity for approximately one day with subsequent administration of a sclerosing agent, such as ethanol, into the fluid collection under fluoroscopic guidance. For larger fluid collections, a catheter is placed using ultrasound or fluoroscopy and ethanol is administered via the catheter daily until the fluid collection has been reduced. The process involves percutaneous placement of a catheter over a guidewire into the area of fluid collection where the catheter is left in place and the sclerosing agent(s) is administered via the catheter as the patient remains in the supine position. The patient may be asked to change positions after the sclerosing agent has been injected in order to allow the entire area where the fluid collection is located to have contact with the sclerosing agent. Drainage of the sclerosing agent may take between 15 minutes and one hour depending on the agent used. Occasionally, depending on the size of the fluid collection, two catheters may be used. Aspirated fluid from the lymphocele, seroma, or cyst is sent for histopathology. The catheter is removed.

Coding Tips

For access or drainage using a needle, see 10160 or 50390; using a catheter, see 10030, 49405-49407, or 50390. Exchange of an existing catheter before or prior to sclerotherapy is reported with 49423 or 75984. Sclerotherapy treatment of a lymphatic or vascular malformation is reported with 37241. For sclerotherapy of veins or endovenous ablation of incompetent veins of an extremity, see 36468, 36470-36471, 36475-36476, and/or 36478-36479. Pleurodesis is reported with 32560. To report treatment of multiple lesions in a single session, via separate access, append modifier 59 or an X{EPSU} modifier to each additional, treated lesion. Do not report 49185 with 49424 or 76080.

ICD-10-CM Diagnostic Codes

B67.0	Echinococcus granulosus infection of liver
B67.5	Echinococcus multilocularis infection of liver
B67.99	Other echinococcosis
K76.89	Other specified diseases of liver
K86.2	Cyst of pancreas
N28.1	Cyst of kidney, acquired
N75.1	Abscess of Bartholin's gland ♀
Q44.6	Cystic disease of liver
Q45.2	Congenital pancreatic cyst
Q61.01	Congenital single renal cyst
Q61.02	Congenital multiple renal cysts
Q61.11	Cystic dilatation of collecting ducts
Q61.19	Other polycystic kidney, infantile type
Q61.2	Polycystic kidney, adult type
Q61.8	Other cystic kidney diseases
T79.2XXA	Traumatic secondary and recurrent hemorrhage and seroma, initial encounter
T88.8XXA	Other specified complications of surgical and medical care, not elsewhere classified, initial encounter

AMA: **49185** 2018,Jan,8; 2017,Jan,8; 2016,Mar,10

Relative Value Units/Medicare Edits

Non-Facility RVU	Work	PE	MP	Total
49185	2.35	30.85	0.22	33.42
Facility RVU	**Work**	**PE**	**MP**	**Total**
49185	2.35	0.9	0.22	3.47

	FUD	Status	MUE	Modifiers				IOM Reference
49185	0	A	2(3)	N/A	N/A	N/A	N/A	None

* with documentation

Terms To Know

catheter. Flexible tube inserted into an area of the body for introducing or withdrawing fluid.

contrast material. Any internally administered substance that has a different opacity from soft tissue on radiography or computed tomograph; includes barium, used to opacify parts of the gastrointestinal tract; water-soluble iodinated compounds, used to opacify blood vessels or the genitourinary tract; may refer to air occurring naturally or introduced into the body; also, paramagnetic substances used in magnetic resonance imaging. Substances may also be documented as contrast agent or contrast medium.

cyst. Elevated encapsulated mass containing fluid, semisolid, or solid material with a membranous lining.

drainage. Releasing, taking, or letting out fluids and/or gases from a body part.

guidewire. Flexible metal instrument designed to lead another instrument in its proper course.

sclerotherapy. Injection of a chemical agent that will irritate, inflame, and cause fibrosis in a vein, eventually obliterating hemorrhoids or varicose veins.

seroma. Swelling caused by the collection of serum, or clear fluid, in the tissues.

CPT © 2020 American Medical Association. All Rights Reserved.   ● New   ▲ Revised   + Add On   ★ Telemedicine   AMA: CPT Assist   [Resequenced]   ☑ Laterality   © 2020 Optum360, LLC

Abdomen

49320

49320 Laparoscopy, abdomen, peritoneum, and omentum, diagnostic, with or without collection of specimen(s) by brushing or washing (separate procedure)

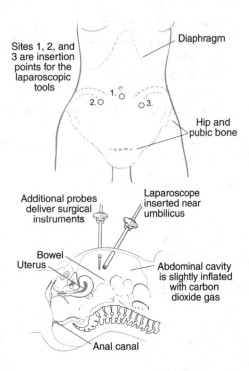

Sites 1, 2, and 3 are insertion points for the laparoscopic tools

Diaphragm

Hip and pubic bone

Additional probes deliver surgical instruments

Laparoscope inserted near umbilicus

Bowel
Uterus

Abdominal cavity is slightly inflated with carbon dioxide gas

Anal canal

Explanation

The physician makes a 1.0-centimeter incision in the umbilicus through which the abdomen is inflated and a fiberoptic laparoscope is inserted. Other incisions are also made through which trocars can be passed into the abdominal cavity to deliver instruments, a video camera, and when needed an additional light source. The physician manipulates the tools so that the pelvic organs, peritoneum, abdomen, and omentum can be viewed through the laparoscope and/or video monitor. Biopsy from any or all of the areas observed are obtained by brushing the surface and collecting the cells or by washing (bathing) the area with a saline solution, and suctioning out the cell rich solution. When the procedure is complete, the laparoscope, instruments, and light source are removed and the incisions are closed with sutures. If biopsy of pelvic organs is performed, the physician may also insert an instrument through the vagina to grasp the cervix and pass another instrument through the cervix, into the uterus to manipulate the uterus.

Coding Tips

For surgical laparoscopy with biopsy, see 49321. This separate procedure by definition is usually a component of a more complex service and is not identified separately. When performed alone or with other unrelated procedures/services it may be reported. If performed alone, list the code; if performed with other procedures/services, list the code and append modifier 59 or an X{EPSU} modifier. For exploratory laparotomy (open approach), exploratory celiotomy, with or without biopsies, see 49000.

ICD-10-CM Diagnostic Codes

C60.8	Malignant neoplasm of overlapping sites of penis ♂
C61	Malignant neoplasm of prostate ♂
C63.7	Malignant neoplasm of other specified male genital organs ♂
C63.8	Malignant neoplasm of overlapping sites of male genital organs ♂
C64.1	Malignant neoplasm of right kidney, except renal pelvis ☑
C64.2	Malignant neoplasm of left kidney, except renal pelvis ☑
C65.1	Malignant neoplasm of right renal pelvis ☑
C65.2	Malignant neoplasm of left renal pelvis ☑
C67.0	Malignant neoplasm of trigone of bladder
C67.1	Malignant neoplasm of dome of bladder
C67.2	Malignant neoplasm of lateral wall of bladder
C67.3	Malignant neoplasm of anterior wall of bladder
C67.4	Malignant neoplasm of posterior wall of bladder
C67.5	Malignant neoplasm of bladder neck
C74.01	Malignant neoplasm of cortex of right adrenal gland ☑
C74.02	Malignant neoplasm of cortex of left adrenal gland ☑
C74.11	Malignant neoplasm of medulla of right adrenal gland ☑
C74.12	Malignant neoplasm of medulla of left adrenal gland ☑
C79.01	Secondary malignant neoplasm of right kidney and renal pelvis ☑
C79.02	Secondary malignant neoplasm of left kidney and renal pelvis ☑
C79.11	Secondary malignant neoplasm of bladder
C79.19	Secondary malignant neoplasm of other urinary organs
D07.5	Carcinoma in situ of prostate ♂
D30.01	Benign neoplasm of right kidney ☑
D30.02	Benign neoplasm of left kidney ☑
D30.11	Benign neoplasm of right renal pelvis ☑
D30.12	Benign neoplasm of left renal pelvis ☑

AMA: **49320** 2018,Jan,8; 2017,Jan,8; 2017,Apr,7; 2016,Jan,13; 2015,Jan,16; 2015,Dec,16; 2014,Jan,11

Relative Value Units/Medicare Edits

Non-Facility RVU	Work	PE	MP	Total
49320	5.14	3.26	1.14	9.54
Facility RVU	**Work**	**PE**	**MP**	**Total**
49320	5.14	3.26	1.14	9.54

	FUD	Status	MUE	Modifiers				IOM Reference
49320	10	A	1(3)	51	N/A	N/A	80	None

* with documentation

Terms To Know

biopsy. Tissue or fluid removed for diagnostic purposes through analysis of the cells in the biopsy material.

brush. Tool used to gather cell samples or clean a body part.

peritoneum. Strong, continuous membrane that forms the lining of the abdominal and pelvic cavity. The parietal peritoneum, or outer layer, is attached to the abdominopelvic walls and the visceral peritoneum, or inner layer, surrounds the organs inside the abdominal cavity.

specimen. Tissue cells or sample of fluid taken for analysis, pathologic examination, and diagnosis.

trocar. Cannula or a sharp pointed instrument used to puncture and aspirate fluid from cavities.

© 2020 Optum360, LLC   N Newborn: 0   P Pediatric: 0-17   M Maternity: 9-64   A Adult: 15-124   ♂ Male Only   ♀ Female Only   CPT © 2020 American Medical Association. All Rights Reserved.

Abdomen

49321

49321 Laparoscopy, surgical; with biopsy (single or multiple)

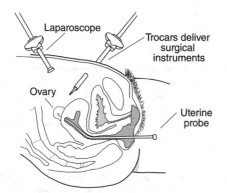

Laparoscope
Trocars deliver surgical instruments
Ovary
Uterine probe

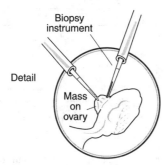

Biopsy instrument
Detail
Mass on ovary

Explanation

The physician makes a 1.0 centimeter incision in the umbilicus through which the abdomen is inflated and a fiberoptic laparoscope is inserted. Other incisions are also made through which trocars can be passed into the abdominal cavity to deliver instruments, a video camera, and, when needed, an additional light source. The physician manipulates the tools so that the pelvic organs, peritoneum, abdomen, and omentum can be viewed through the laparoscope and/or video monitor. Biopsy from any or all of the areas observed are obtained by grasping a sample with a biopsy forceps that is capable of "biting off" small pieces of tissue. When the procedure is complete, the laparoscope, instruments, and light source are removed and the incisions are closed with sutures. If a biopsy of female pelvic organs is performed, the physician may also insert an instrument through the vagina to grasp the cervix and pass another instrument through the cervix and into the uterus to manipulate the uterus.

Coding Tips

Surgical laparoscopy always includes diagnostic laparoscopy. To report a diagnostic laparoscopy (peritoneoscopy), see 49320. For laparoscopic aspiration (single or multiple), see 49322. For exploratory laparotomy, exploratory celiotomy, with or without biopsies, see 49000.

ICD-10-CM Diagnostic Codes

C45.1	Mesothelioma of peritoneum
C48.0	Malignant neoplasm of retroperitoneum
C48.1	Malignant neoplasm of specified parts of peritoneum
C48.8	Malignant neoplasm of overlapping sites of retroperitoneum and peritoneum
C64.1	Malignant neoplasm of right kidney, except renal pelvis ☑
C64.2	Malignant neoplasm of left kidney, except renal pelvis ☑
C65.1	Malignant neoplasm of right renal pelvis ☑
C65.2	Malignant neoplasm of left renal pelvis ☑
C66.1	Malignant neoplasm of right ureter ☑
C66.2	Malignant neoplasm of left ureter ☑
C67.8	Malignant neoplasm of overlapping sites of bladder
C79.01	Secondary malignant neoplasm of right kidney and renal pelvis ☑
C79.02	Secondary malignant neoplasm of left kidney and renal pelvis ☑
C79.11	Secondary malignant neoplasm of bladder
C79.19	Secondary malignant neoplasm of other urinary organs
D09.19	Carcinoma in situ of other urinary organs
D30.01	Benign neoplasm of right kidney ☑
D30.02	Benign neoplasm of left kidney ☑
D30.11	Benign neoplasm of right renal pelvis ☑
D30.12	Benign neoplasm of left renal pelvis ☑

AMA: **49321** 2018,Jan,8; 2018,Aug,10; 2017,Jan,8; 2016,Jan,13; 2015,Jan,16; 2014,Jan,11

Relative Value Units/Medicare Edits

Non-Facility RVU	Work	PE	MP	Total
49321	5.44	3.4	1.18	10.02
Facility RVU	**Work**	**PE**	**MP**	**Total**
49321	5.44	3.4	1.18	10.02

	FUD	Status	MUE	Modifiers				IOM Reference
49321	10	A	1(2)	51	N/A	62	80	None

* with documentation

Terms To Know

biopsy. Tissue or fluid removed for diagnostic purposes through analysis of the cells in the biopsy material.

carcinoma in situ. Malignancy that arises from the cells of the vessel, gland, or organ of origin that remains confined to that site or has not invaded neighboring tissue.

forceps. Tool used for grasping or compressing tissue.

incision. Act of cutting into tissue or an organ.

insufflation. Blowing air or gas into a body cavity.

laparoscopy. Direct visualization of the peritoneal cavity, outer fallopian tubes, uterus, and ovaries utilizing a laparoscope, a thin, flexible fiberoptic tube.

malignant neoplasm. Any cancerous tumor or lesion exhibiting uncontrolled tissue growth that can progressively invade other parts of the body with its disease-generating cells.

tissue. Group of similar cells with a similar function that form definite structures and organs. Tissue types include epithelial tissue, muscle tissue, connective tissue, and nervous tissue.

trocar. Cannula or a sharp pointed instrument used to puncture and aspirate fluid from cavities.

Abdomen

CPT © 2020 American Medical Association. All Rights Reserved.   ● New   ▲ Revised   + Add On   ★ Telemedicine   AMA: CPT Assist   [Resequenced]   ☑ Laterality   © 2020 Optum360, LLC

49324-49325

49324 Laparoscopy, surgical; with insertion of tunneled intraperitoneal catheter
49325 with revision of previously placed intraperitoneal cannula or catheter, with removal of intraluminal obstructive material if performed

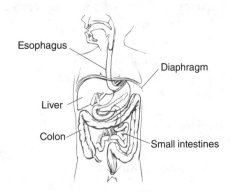

Esophagus
Diaphragm
Liver
Colon
Small intestines

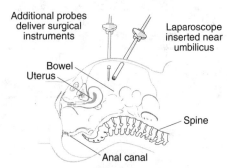

Additional probes deliver surgical instruments
Laparoscope inserted near umbilicus
Bowel
Uterus
Spine
Anal canal

Side view of laparoscopic surgical approach

Explanation

A permanent intraperitoneal catheter is inserted laparoscopically using a tunneling technique. The physician makes a 1 cm incision in the umbilicus through which the abdomen is inflated and a fiberoptic laparoscope is inserted. Other incisions are also made through which trocars can be passed into the abdominal cavity to deliver additional instruments. The physician manipulates the tools so that the pelvic organs, peritoneum, abdomen, and omentum can be viewed through the laparoscope and/or video monitor. Using various tunneling techniques, the physician inserts the intraperitoneal catheter, positioning the tip inside the peritoneal cavity. A separately reportable subcutaneous extension of the catheter with a remote chest exit site may also be performed. If the physician is revising an intraperitoneal catheter, the catheter is inspected and freed of occlusion or blockage. When either procedure is complete, the laparoscope and other instruments are removed and the incisions are closed with sutures. Report 49324 for the tunneled insertion of an intraperitoneal cannula or catheter and 49325 for its revision.

Coding Tips

Surgical laparoscopy always includes diagnostic laparoscopy. For diagnostic laparoscopy (peritoneoscopy), see 49320. Report subcutaneous extension of an intraperitoneal catheter with remote chest exit site (49435) with 49324, when performed. For open insertion of a tunneled intraperitoneal catheter, see 49421. When omentopexy is performed with these codes, report 49326.

ICD-10-CM Diagnostic Codes

R18.0   Malignant ascites
R18.8   Other ascites

Z49.02   Encounter for fitting and adjustment of peritoneal dialysis catheter
Z49.32   Encounter for adequacy testing for peritoneal dialysis

AMA: **49324** 2014,Jan,11 **49325** 2014,Jan,11

Relative Value Units/Medicare Edits

Non-Facility RVU	Work	PE	MP	Total
49324	6.32	3.52	1.5	11.34
49325	6.82	3.65	1.63	12.1
Facility RVU	Work	PE	MP	Total
49324	6.32	3.52	1.5	11.34
49325	6.82	3.65	1.63	12.1

	FUD	Status	MUE	Modifiers				IOM Reference
49324	10	A	1(2)	51	N/A	62	80	None
49325	10	A	1(2)	51	N/A	62	80	

* with documentation

Terms To Know

ascites. Abnormal accumulation of free fluid in the abdominal cavity, causing distention and tightness in addition to shortness of breath as the fluid accumulates. Ascites is usually an underlying disorder and can be a manifestation of any number of diseases.

intraperitoneal. Within the cavity or space created by the double-layered sac that lines the abdominopelvic walls and forms a covering for the internal organs.

laparoscopy. Direct visualization utilizing a thin, flexible, fiberoptic tube.

occlusion. Constriction, closure, or blockage of a passage.

omentum. Fold of peritoneal tissue suspended between the stomach and neighboring visceral organs of the abdominal cavity.

peritoneal dialysis. Dialysis that filters waste from blood inside the body using the peritoneum, the natural lining of the abdomen, as the semipermeable membrane across which ultrafiltration is accomplished. A special catheter is inserted into the abdomen and a dialysis solution is drained into the abdomen. This solution extracts fluids and wastes, which are then discarded when the fluid is drained. Various forms of peritoneal dialysis include CAPD, CCPD, and NIDP.

peritoneum. Strong, continuous membrane that forms the lining of the abdominal and pelvic cavity. The parietal peritoneum, or outer layer, is attached to the abdominopelvic walls and the visceral peritoneum, or inner layer, surrounds the organs inside the abdominal cavity.

tunneled catheter. Catheter inserted into a central vein via a chest incision and maneuvered under the skin to a distal outlet location enabling secure placement with decreased risk of infection and can stay in place for extended periods of time. This procedure is commonly performed in an operating room.

© 2020 Optum360, LLC **N** Newborn: 0 **P** Pediatric: 0-17 **M** Maternity: 9-64 **A** Adult: 15-124 ♂ Male Only ♀ Female Only CPT © 2020 American Medical Association. All Rights Reserved.

Coding Companion for Urology/Nephrology

Abdomen

49327

+ **49327** Laparoscopy, surgical; with placement of interstitial device(s) for radiation therapy guidance (eg, fiducial markers, dosimeter), intra-abdominal, intrapelvic, and/or retroperitoneum, including imaging guidance, if performed, single or multiple (List separately in addition to code for primary procedure)

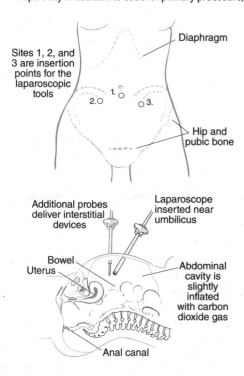

Sites 1, 2, and 3 are insertion points for the laparoscopic tools

Diaphragm

Hip and pubic bone

Additional probes deliver interstitial devices

Laparoscope inserted near umbilicus

Bowel

Uterus

Abdominal cavity is slightly inflated with carbon dioxide gas

Anal canal

Explanation

The physician makes a 1 cm incision in the umbilicus through which the abdomen is inflated and a fiberoptic laparoscope is inserted. Other incisions are also made through which trocars can be passed into the abdominal cavity to deliver instruments, a video camera, and, when needed, an additional light source. The physician manipulates the tools so that the pelvic organs, peritoneum, abdomen, and omentum can be viewed through the laparoscope and/or video monitor. In conjunction with other laparoscopic abdominal, pelvic, or retroperitoneal procedures that are performed concurrently, and using image guidance if necessary, the physician places one or more interstitial devices such as gold seeds (fiducial markers) for radiation therapy guidance or a dosimeter to gauge the amount of radiation received into the targeted soft tissue tumor. Allowing for precision in targeting radiation and/or for measuring the radiation doses received, a fiducial marker is visible by ultrasound and fluoroscopy and permits accurate triangulation of the tissue to be treated. A capsule dosimeter relays radiation dose information so that the clinical team can monitor for any deviation between the radiation plan and the actual radiation received. When the procedure is complete, the laparoscope, instruments, and light source are removed and the incisions are closed with sutures.

Coding Tips

Report 49327 with laparoscopic abdominal, pelvic, or retroperitoneal procedures, when performed at the same operative session. For placement of interstitial devices for intra-abdominal, intrapelvic, and/or retroperitoneal radiation therapy guidance at the same time as an open procedure, see 49412; percutaneous, see 49411.

ICD-10-CM Diagnostic Codes

This/these CPT code(s) are add-on code(s). See the primary procedure code that this code is performed with for your ICD-10-CM code selections.

AMA: **49327** 2014,Jan,11

Relative Value Units/Medicare Edits

Non-Facility RVU	Work	PE	MP	Total
49327	2.38	0.86	0.57	3.81
Facility RVU	**Work**	**PE**	**MP**	**Total**
49327	2.38	0.86	0.57	3.81

	FUD	Status	MUE	Modifiers				IOM Reference
49327	N/A	A	1(2)	N/A	N/A	62*	80	None

* with documentation

Terms To Know

dosimetry. Component in the administration of radiation oncology therapy in which a radiation dose is calculated to a specific site, including implant or beam orientation and exposure, isodose strengths, tissue inhomogeneities, and volume.

fiducial marker. Compact medical device or object placed in or near a tumor to serve as a landmark for the placement of radiation beams during treatment. Use of a fiducial marker allows the clinician to direct radiation to the tumor while preserving surrounding healthy tissue.

fluoroscopy. Radiology technique that allows visual examination of part of the body or a function of an organ using a device that projects an x-ray image on a fluorescent screen.

imaging. Radiologic means of producing pictures for clinical study of the internal structures and functions of the body, such as x-ray, ultrasound, magnetic resonance, or positron emission tomography.

interstitial. Within the small spaces or gaps occurring in tissue or organs.

intra. Within.

retroperitoneal. Located behind the peritoneum, the membrane that lines the abdominopelvic walls and forms a covering for the internal organs.

trocar. Cannula or a sharp pointed instrument used to puncture and aspirate fluid from cavities.

Abdomen

49400

49400   Injection of air or contrast into peritoneal cavity (separate procedure)

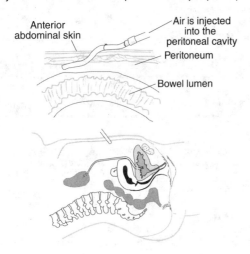

Air or contrast material is injected into the
peritoneal cavity. The procedure has broad
diagnostic and preparatory applications

Explanation

The physician injects air contrast into the peritoneal cavity. The physician inserts a needle or catheter into the peritoneal cavity and injects air as a diagnostic procedure. An x-ray is usually obtained to define the pattern of air in the abdomen. The needle or catheter is removed at the completion of the procedure.

Coding Tips

This separate procedure by definition is usually a component of a more complex service and is not identified separately. When performed alone or with other unrelated procedures/services it may be reported. If performed alone, list the code; if performed with other procedures/services, list the code and append modifier 59 or an X{EPSU} modifier. This code should be reported when injection of air or contrast into the peritoneal cavity is performed as an initial or subsequent procedure. For radiological supervision and interpretation, see 74190.

ICD-10-CM Diagnostic Codes

The application of this code is too broad to adequately present ICD-10-CM diagnostic code links here. Refer to your ICD-10-CM book.

AMA: 49400 2018,Jan,8; 2017,Jan,8; 2016,Jan,13; 2015,Jan,16; 2014,Jan,11

Relative Value Units/Medicare Edits

Non-Facility RVU	Work	PE	MP	Total
49400	1.88	2.06	0.21	4.15
Facility RVU	Work	PE	MP	Total
49400	1.88	0.59	0.21	2.68

	FUD	Status	MUE	Modifiers				IOM Reference
49400	0	A	1(3)	51	N/A	N/A	N/A	None

* with documentation

49402

49402   Removal of peritoneal foreign body from peritoneal cavity

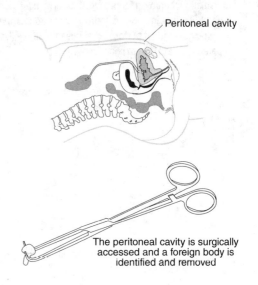

The peritoneal cavity is surgically
accessed and a foreign body is
identified and removed

Explanation

The physician removes a foreign body from the abdominal cavity. The physician makes an abdominal incision and explores the abdominal cavity. The foreign body is identified and removed. The incision is closed.

Coding Tips

For lysis of intestinal adhesions, see 44005. Report open or percutaneous abdominal or peritoneal drainage or lavage with 49020, 49040, 49082–49084 or 49406. For percutaneous insertion of a tunneled intraperitoneal catheter without a subcutaneous port, see 49418.

ICD-10-CM Diagnostic Codes

S31.620A	Laceration with foreign body of abdominal wall, right upper quadrant with penetration into peritoneal cavity, initial encounter ☑
S31.621A	Laceration with foreign body of abdominal wall, left upper quadrant with penetration into peritoneal cavity, initial encounter ☑
S31.622A	Laceration with foreign body of abdominal wall, epigastric region with penetration into peritoneal cavity, initial encounter
S31.623A	Laceration with foreign body of abdominal wall, right lower quadrant with penetration into peritoneal cavity, initial encounter ☑
S31.624A	Laceration with foreign body of abdominal wall, left lower quadrant with penetration into peritoneal cavity, initial encounter ☑
S31.625A	Laceration with foreign body of abdominal wall, periumbilic region with penetration into peritoneal cavity, initial encounter
S31.641A	Puncture wound with foreign body of abdominal wall, left upper quadrant with penetration into peritoneal cavity, initial encounter ☑
S31.642A	Puncture wound with foreign body of abdominal wall, epigastric region with penetration into peritoneal cavity, initial encounter
S31.643A	Puncture wound with foreign body of abdominal wall, right lower quadrant with penetration into peritoneal cavity, initial encounter ☑

© 2020 Optum360, LLC   **N** Newborn: 0   **P** Pediatric: 0-17   **M** Maternity: 9-64   **A** Adult: 15-124   ♂ Male Only   ♀ Female Only   CPT © 2020 American Medical Association. All Rights Reserved.

Abdomen

S31.644A	Puncture wound with foreign body of abdominal wall, left lower quadrant with penetration into peritoneal cavity, initial encounter ☑
S31.645A	Puncture wound with foreign body of abdominal wall, periumbilic region with penetration into peritoneal cavity, initial encounter
T81.516A	Adhesions due to foreign body accidentally left in body following aspiration, puncture or other catheterization, initial encounter
T81.517A	Adhesions due to foreign body accidentally left in body following removal of catheter or packing, initial encounter
T81.518A	Adhesions due to foreign body accidentally left in body following other procedure, initial encounter
T81.520A	Obstruction due to foreign body accidentally left in body following surgical operation, initial encounter
T81.526A	Obstruction due to foreign body accidentally left in body following aspiration, puncture or other catheterization, initial encounter
T81.527A	Obstruction due to foreign body accidentally left in body following removal of catheter or packing, initial encounter
T81.528A	Obstruction due to foreign body accidentally left in body following other procedure, initial encounter
T81.530A	Perforation due to foreign body accidentally left in body following surgical operation, initial encounter
T81.536A	Perforation due to foreign body accidentally left in body following aspiration, puncture or other catheterization, initial encounter
T81.537A	Perforation due to foreign body accidentally left in body following removal of catheter or packing, initial encounter
T81.538A	Perforation due to foreign body accidentally left in body following other procedure, initial encounter
T81.590A	Other complications of foreign body accidentally left in body following surgical operation, initial encounter
T81.596A	Other complications of foreign body accidentally left in body following aspiration, puncture or other catheterization, initial encounter
T81.597A	Other complications of foreign body accidentally left in body following removal of catheter or packing, initial encounter
T81.598A	Other complications of foreign body accidentally left in body following other procedure, initial encounter

AMA: 49402 2014,Jan,11

Relative Value Units/Medicare Edits

Non-Facility RVU	Work	PE	MP	Total
49402	14.09	7.62	3.22	24.93
Facility RVU	**Work**	**PE**	**MP**	**Total**
49402	14.09	7.62	3.22	24.93

	FUD	Status	MUE	Modifiers				IOM Reference
49402	90	A	1(3)	51	N/A	62*	N/A	None

* with documentation

Terms To Know

peritoneal cavity. Space between the lining of the abdominal wall, or parietal peritoneum, and the surface layer of the abdominal organs, or visceral peritoneum. It contains a thin, watery fluid that keeps the peritoneal surfaces moist.

49405

49405	Image-guided fluid collection drainage by catheter (eg, abscess, hematoma, seroma, lymphocele, cyst); visceral (eg, kidney, liver, spleen, lung/mediastinum), percutaneous

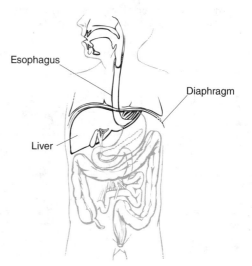

Percutaneous drainage of visceral organ abscess, hematoma, seroma, or lymphocele using image guidance

Explanation

A fluid collection in the visceral organs (kidney, liver, spleen, lung, mediastinum, etc.), such as a hematoma, seroma, abscess, lymphocele, or cyst, is drained using a catheter. The area over the affected organ is cleansed and local anesthesia is administered. Imaging is performed to assist in the insertion of a needle or guidewire into the fluid collection. Small tissue samples may be collected from the site for pathological examination. A catheter is inserted to drain and collect the fluid for analysis. The catheter is removed. More imaging may be performed to ensure hemostasis. A bandage is applied. In some cases, the catheter may be attached to a bag to allow for further drainage over the course of days.

Coding Tips

This code should be reported for each individual collection drained using a separate catheter. For image-guided drainage of fluid collection of the peritoneal/retroperitoneal (e.g., abscess, hematoma, seroma, cyst), via catheter, percutaneous, see 49406; transvaginal or transrectal, see 49407. For diagnostic or therapeutic abdominal/peritoneal paracentesis or lavage, see 49082–49084. For open drainage of an abscess, peritoneal, see 49020; retroperitoneal, see 49060; perirenal or renal, see 50020. To report percutaneous insertion of a tunneled intraperitoneal catheter without a subcutaneous port, see 49418. Do not report 49405 with 75989, 76942, 77002–77003, 77012, or 77021.

ICD-10-CM Diagnostic Codes

K68.12	Psoas muscle abscess
N15.1	Renal and perinephric abscess
N34.0	Urethral abscess
N41.2	Abscess of prostate ☒ ♂
N99.820	Postprocedural hemorrhage of a genitourinary system organ or structure following a genitourinary system procedure
N99.821	Postprocedural hemorrhage of a genitourinary system organ or structure following other procedure

CPT © 2020 American Medical Association. All Rights Reserved.   ● New   ▲ Revised   + Add On   ★ Telemedicine   AMA: CPT Assist   [Resequenced]   ☑ Laterality   © 2020 Optum360, LLC

Abdomen

N99.840	Postprocedural hematoma of a genitourinary system organ or structure following a genitourinary system procedure
N99.841	Postprocedural hematoma of a genitourinary system organ or structure following other procedure
N99.842	Postprocedural seroma of a genitourinary system organ or structure following a genitourinary system procedure
N99.843	Postprocedural seroma of a genitourinary system organ or structure following other procedure

AMA: 49405 2020,Feb,13; 2018,Jan,8; 2017,Jan,8; 2016,Jan,13; 2015,Jan,16; 2014,May,9; 2014,Jan,11

Relative Value Units/Medicare Edits

Non-Facility RVU	Work	PE	MP	Total
49405	4.0	20.79	0.35	25.14
Facility RVU	**Work**	**PE**	**MP**	**Total**
49405	4.0	1.36	0.35	5.71

	FUD	Status	MUE	Modifiers				IOM Reference
49405	0	A	2(3)	51	N/A	N/A	N/A	None

* with documentation

Terms To Know

catheter. Flexible tube inserted into an area of the body for introducing or withdrawing fluid.

drainage. Releasing, taking, or letting out fluids and/or gases from a body part.

guidewire. Flexible metal instrument designed to lead another instrument in its proper course.

hemostasis. Interruption of blood flow or the cessation or arrest of bleeding.

imaging. Radiologic means of producing pictures for clinical study of the internal structures and functions of the body, such as x-ray, ultrasound, magnetic resonance, or positron emission tomography.

percutaneous. Through the skin.

specimen. Tissue cells or sample of fluid taken for analysis, pathologic examination, and diagnosis.

tissue. Group of similar cells with a similar function that form definite structures and organs. Tissue types include epithelial tissue, muscle tissue, connective tissue, and nervous tissue.

viscera. Large interior organs enclosed within a cavity, generally referring to the abdominal organs.

49406

| 49406 | Image-guided fluid collection drainage by catheter (eg, abscess, hematoma, seroma, lymphocele, cyst); peritoneal or retroperitoneal, percutaneous |

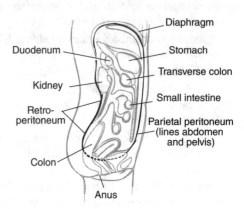

Percutaneous drainage of peritoneal or retroperitoneal abscess, hematoma, seroma, or lymphocele using image guidance

Explanation

A fluid collection in the peritoneum or retroperitoneum, such as a hematoma, a seroma, an abscess, a lymphocele, or a cyst, is drained using a catheter. The area over the affected site is cleansed and local anesthesia is administered. Imaging is performed to assist in the insertion of a needle or guidewire into the fluid collection. Small tissue samples may be collected from the site for pathological examination. A catheter is inserted to drain and collect the fluid for analysis and is then removed. More imaging may be performed to ensure hemostasis. A bandage is applied. In some cases, the catheter may be attached to a bag to allow for further drainage over the course of days.

Coding Tips

This code should be reported for each individual collection drained using a separate catheter. For percutaneous, image-guided drainage of fluid collection of the kidney (e.g., abscess, hematoma, seroma, cyst), via catheter, see 49405; transvaginal or transrectal, image-guided drainage of a peritoneal/retroperitoneal abscess, via catheter, see 49407. For open drainage of an abscess, peritoneal, see 49020; extraperitoneal to peritoneal cavity, see 49062; perirenal or renal, see 50020. For diagnostic or therapeutic abdominal/peritoneal paracentesis or lavage, see 49082–49084. For percutaneous insertion of a tunneled intraperitoneal catheter without a subcutaneous port, see 49418. Do not report 49406 with 75989, 76942, 77002–77003, 77012, or 77021.

ICD-10-CM Diagnostic Codes

K65.1	Peritoneal abscess
K68.11	Postprocedural retroperitoneal abscess
K68.19	Other retroperitoneal abscess
N15.1	Renal and perinephric abscess
N34.0	Urethral abscess
N41.2	Abscess of prostate 🄰 ♂
N99.820	Postprocedural hemorrhage of a genitourinary system organ or structure following a genitourinary system procedure
N99.821	Postprocedural hemorrhage of a genitourinary system organ or structure following other procedure

Abdomen

N99.840	Postprocedural hematoma of a genitourinary system organ or structure following a genitourinary system procedure
N99.841	Postprocedural hematoma of a genitourinary system organ or structure following other procedure
N99.842	Postprocedural seroma of a genitourinary system organ or structure following a genitourinary system procedure
N99.843	Postprocedural seroma of a genitourinary system organ or structure following other procedure

AMA: 49406 2020,Feb,13; 2018,Jan,8; 2017,Jan,8; 2016,Jan,13; 2015,Jan,16; 2014,May,9; 2014,Jan,11

Relative Value Units/Medicare Edits

Non-Facility RVU	Work	PE	MP	Total
49406	4.0	20.79	0.34	25.13
Facility RVU	**Work**	**PE**	**MP**	**Total**
49406	4.0	1.36	0.34	5.7

	FUD	Status	MUE	Modifiers				IOM Reference
49406	0	A	2(3)	51	N/A	N/A	N/A	None

* with documentation

Terms To Know

catheter. Flexible tube inserted into an area of the body for introducing or withdrawing fluid.

imaging. Radiologic means of producing pictures for clinical study of the internal structures and functions of the body, such as x-ray, ultrasound, magnetic resonance, or positron emission tomography.

percutaneous. Through the skin.

peritoneal. Space between the lining of the abdominal wall, or parietal peritoneum, and the surface layer of the abdominal organs, or visceral peritoneum. It contains a thin, watery fluid that keeps the peritoneal surfaces moist.

retroperitoneal. Located behind the peritoneum, the membrane that lines the abdominopelvic walls and forms a covering for the internal organs.

49407

| 49407 | Image-guided fluid collection drainage by catheter (eg, abscess, hematoma, seroma, lymphocele, cyst); peritoneal or retroperitoneal, transvaginal or transrectal |

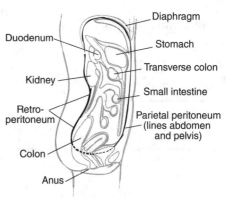

Transrectal or transvaginal approach is used to drain abscess, hematoma, seroma, or lymphocele using image guidance

Explanation

A fluid collection in the peritoneum or retroperitoneum, such as a hematoma, a seroma, an abscess, a lymphocele, or a cyst, is drained via a vaginal or rectal approach. An intracavitary probe is used to create access through the rectal or vaginal wall. Imaging is performed to assist in the insertion of a needle or guidewire into the fluid collection. Small tissue samples may be collected from the site for pathological examination. A catheter is inserted to drain and collect the fluid for analysis and is then removed. In some cases, the catheter may be attached to a bag to allow for further drainage over the course of days.

Coding Tips

This code should be reported for each individual collection drained using a separate catheter. For percutaneous, image-guided drainage of fluid collection of the kidney (e.g., abscess, hematoma, seroma, cyst), via catheter, see 49405; peritoneal/retroperitoneal, see 49406. For diagnostic or therapeutic abdominal/peritoneal paracentesis or lavage, see 49082–49084. For open drainage of an abscess, peritoneal, see 49020; retroperitoneal, see 49060; perirenal or renal, see 50020. For percutaneous insertion of a tunneled intraperitoneal catheter without a subcutaneous port, see 49418. Do not report 49407 with 75989, 76942, 77002–77003, 77012, or 77021. For percutaneous, image-guided fluid collection drainage, via catheter, for soft tissue, see 10030.

ICD-10-CM Diagnostic Codes

K65.1	Peritoneal abscess
K68.11	Postprocedural retroperitoneal abscess
K68.19	Other retroperitoneal abscess
N15.1	Renal and perinephric abscess
N34.0	Urethral abscess
N41.2	Abscess of prostate 🅰 ♂
N99.820	Postprocedural hemorrhage of a genitourinary system organ or structure following a genitourinary system procedure
N99.821	Postprocedural hemorrhage of a genitourinary system organ or structure following other procedure
N99.840	Postprocedural hematoma of a genitourinary system organ or structure following a genitourinary system procedure
N99.841	Postprocedural hematoma of a genitourinary system organ or structure following other procedure

CPT © 2020 American Medical Association. All Rights Reserved.   ● New   ▲ Revised   + Add On   ★ Telemedicine   AMA: CPT Assist   [Resequenced]   ☑ Laterality   © 2020 Optum360, LLC

Abdomen

| N99.842 | Postprocedural seroma of a genitourinary system organ or structure following a genitourinary system procedure |
| N99.843 | Postprocedural seroma of a genitourinary system organ or structure following other procedure |

AMA: **49407** 2018,Jan,8; 2017,Jan,8; 2016,Jan,13; 2015,Jan,16; 2014,May,9; 2014,Jan,11

Relative Value Units/Medicare Edits

Non-Facility RVU	Work	PE	MP	Total
49407	4.25	15.99	0.41	20.65
Facility RVU	**Work**	**PE**	**MP**	**Total**
49407	4.25	1.39	0.41	6.05

	FUD	Status	MUE	Modifiers				IOM Reference
49407	0	A	1(3)	51	N/A	N/A	N/A	None

* with documentation

Terms To Know

catheter. Flexible tube inserted into an area of the body for introducing or withdrawing fluid.

drainage. Releasing, taking, or letting out fluids and/or gases from a body part.

imaging. Radiologic means of producing pictures for clinical study of the internal structures and functions of the body, such as x-ray, ultrasound, magnetic resonance, or positron emission tomography.

intracavitary. Within a body cavity.

peritoneal. Space between the lining of the abdominal wall, or parietal peritoneum, and the surface layer of the abdominal organs, or visceral peritoneum. It contains a thin, watery fluid that keeps the peritoneal surfaces moist.

retroperitoneal. Located behind the peritoneum, the membrane that lines the abdominopelvic walls and forms a covering for the internal organs.

specimen. Tissue cells or sample of fluid taken for analysis, pathologic examination, and diagnosis.

tissue. Group of similar cells with a similar function that form definite structures and organs. Tissue types include epithelial tissue, muscle tissue, connective tissue, and nervous tissue.

49412

+ 49412 Placement of interstitial device(s) for radiation therapy guidance (eg, fiducial markers, dosimeter), open, intra-abdominal, intrapelvic, and/or retroperitoneum, including image guidance, if performed, single or multiple (List separately in addition to code for primary procedure)

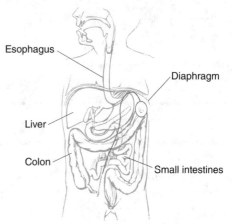

Interstitial devices are placed into the abdomen, pelvis, or retroperitoneum

Explanation

The physician places one or more interstitial devices such as gold seeds (fiducial markers) for radiation therapy guidance or a dosimeter to gauge the amount of radiation received into a targeted intra-abdominal, intrapelvic, or retroperitoneal soft tissue tumor. Implanted in conjunction with an open abdominal, pelvic, or retroperitoneal procedure performed concurrently, these act as radiographic landmarks to define the position of the target lesion. Using image guidance if necessary, the physician places a small capsule or seed into the targeted tissue. Allowing for precision in targeting radiation and/or for measuring the radiation doses received, a fiducial marker is visible by ultrasound and fluoroscopy and permits accurate triangulation of the tissue to be treated. A capsule dosimeter relays radiation dose information so that the clinical team can monitor for any deviation between the radiation plan and the actual radiation received. When the procedures are complete, the incisions are closed with sutures.

Coding Tips

Report 49412 with open abdominal, pelvic, or retroperitoneal procedures, when performed at the same operative session. For placement of interstitial devices for intra-abdominal, intrapelvic, and/or retroperitoneal radiation therapy guidance at the same time as a laparoscopic procedure, see 49327; percutaneous, see 49411.

ICD-10-CM Diagnostic Codes

This/these CPT code(s) are add-on code(s). See the primary procedure code that this code is performed with for your ICD-10-CM code selections.

AMA: **49412** 2014,Jan,11

Abdomen

Relative Value Units/Medicare Edits

Non-Facility RVU	Work	PE	MP	Total
49412	1.5	0.54	0.37	2.41
Facility RVU	Work	PE	MP	Total
49412	1.5	0.54	0.37	2.41

	FUD	Status	MUE	Modifiers				IOM Reference
49412	N/A	A	1(2)	N/A	N/A	62*	80*	None

* with documentation

Terms To Know

dosimetry. Component in the administration of radiation oncology therapy in which a radiation dose is calculated to a specific site, including implant or beam orientation and exposure, isodose strengths, tissue inhomogeneities, and volume.

fiducial marker. Compact medical device or object placed in or near a tumor to serve as a landmark for the placement of radiation beams during treatment. Use of a fiducial marker allows the clinician to direct radiation to the tumor while preserving surrounding healthy tissue.

fluoroscopy. Radiology technique that allows visual examination of part of the body or a function of an organ using a device that projects an x-ray image on a fluorescent screen.

interstitial. Within the small spaces or gaps occurring in tissue or organs.

retroperitoneal. Located behind the peritoneum, the membrane that lines the abdominopelvic walls and forms a covering for the internal organs.

soft tissue. Nonepithelial tissues outside of the skeleton.

tumor. Pathological swelling or enlargement; a neoplastic growth of uncontrolled, abnormal multiplication of cells.

ultrasound. Imaging using ultra-high sound frequency bounced off body structures.

49418

49418 Insertion of tunneled intraperitoneal catheter (eg, dialysis, intraperitoneal chemotherapy instillation, management of ascites), complete procedure, including imaging guidance, catheter placement, contrast injection when performed, and radiological supervision and interpretation, percutaneous

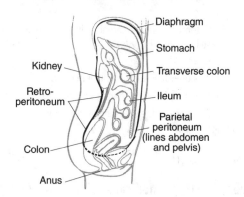

Explanation

The physician places a tunneled intraperitoneal catheter for drainage, dialysis, or chemotherapy instillation using a percutaneous approach. The physician makes a small abdominal incision, opens the peritoneum (the double-layered sac covering the internal organs and lining the abdominopelvic walls), and inserts the catheter into the cavity. The proximal end of the catheter is tunneled subcutaneously away from the initial incision and brought out through the skin. The incision is closed. Alternately, the physician may percutaneously insert the catheter over a wire placed through a needle inserted into the peritoneal cavity. This code reports the complete procedure and includes placement of the catheter under imaging guidance, contrast injection if performed, and radiological supervision and interpretation.

Coding Tips

For insertion of a tunneled intraperitoneal catheter, with subcutaneous port, see 49419; removal, see 49422. For open placement of a tunneled intraperitoneal catheter for dialysis, see 49421.

ICD-10-CM Diagnostic Codes

C45.1	Mesothelioma of peritoneum
C48.0	Malignant neoplasm of retroperitoneum
C48.1	Malignant neoplasm of specified parts of peritoneum
C48.8	Malignant neoplasm of overlapping sites of retroperitoneum and peritoneum
C78.6	Secondary malignant neoplasm of retroperitoneum and peritoneum
C7B.04	Secondary carcinoid tumors of peritoneum
C7B.09	Secondary carcinoid tumors of other sites
E10.21	Type 1 diabetes mellitus with diabetic nephropathy
E10.22	Type 1 diabetes mellitus with diabetic chronic kidney disease
E10.29	Type 1 diabetes mellitus with other diabetic kidney complication
E11.21	Type 2 diabetes mellitus with diabetic nephropathy
E11.22	Type 2 diabetes mellitus with diabetic chronic kidney disease
E11.29	Type 2 diabetes mellitus with other diabetic kidney complication
E13.10	Other specified diabetes mellitus with ketoacidosis without coma
E13.21	Other specified diabetes mellitus with diabetic nephropathy

Abdomen

E13.22	Other specified diabetes mellitus with diabetic chronic kidney disease
E13.29	Other specified diabetes mellitus with other diabetic kidney complication
I12.0	Hypertensive chronic kidney disease with stage 5 chronic kidney disease or end stage renal disease
I13.11	Hypertensive heart and chronic kidney disease without heart failure, with stage 5 chronic kidney disease, or end stage renal disease
I13.2	Hypertensive heart and chronic kidney disease with heart failure and with stage 5 chronic kidney disease, or end stage renal disease
N17.0	Acute kidney failure with tubular necrosis
N17.1	Acute kidney failure with acute cortical necrosis
N17.2	Acute kidney failure with medullary necrosis
N18.6	End stage renal disease

AMA: 49418 2014,Jan,11

Relative Value Units/Medicare Edits

Non-Facility RVU	Work	PE	MP	Total
49418	3.96	29.76	0.39	34.11
Facility RVU	**Work**	**PE**	**MP**	**Total**
49418	3.96	1.53	0.39	5.88

	FUD	Status	MUE	Modifiers				IOM Reference
49418	0	A	1(3)	51	N/A	N/A	80*	None

* with documentation

Terms To Know

approach. Method or anatomical location used to gain access to a body organ or specific area for procedures.

imaging. Radiologic means of producing pictures for clinical study of the internal structures and functions of the body, such as x-ray, ultrasound, magnetic resonance, or positron emission tomography.

intraperitoneal. Within the cavity or space created by the double-layered sac that lines the abdominopelvic walls and forms a covering for the internal organs.

percutaneous. Through the skin.

tunneled catheter. Catheter inserted into a central vein via a chest incision and maneuvered under the skin to a distal outlet location enabling secure placement with decreased risk of infection and can stay in place for extended periods of time. This procedure is commonly performed in an operating room.

49421

| 49421 | Insertion of tunneled intraperitoneal catheter for dialysis, open |

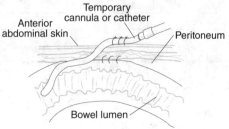

An intraperitoneal cannula or catheter
is placed for drainage or dialysis

Explanation

The physician places a tunneled intraperitoneal catheter for dialysis using an open technique. The physician makes a small abdominal incision, opens the peritoneum (the double-layered sac covering the internal organs and lining the abdominopelvic walls), and inserts the catheter into the cavity. The proximal end of the catheter is tunneled subcutaneously away from the initial incision and brought out through the skin. The incision is closed. A separately reportable subcutaneous extension of the intraperitoneal catheter with a remote chest exit site may also be performed at this time.

Coding Tips

For laparoscopic insertion of a tunneled intraperitoneal catheter, see 49324. For insertion of a tunneled intraperitoneal catheter, with a subcutaneous port, see 49419; removal, see 49422. Subcutaneous extension of an intraperitoneal catheter with remote chest exit site (49435) is reported with 49421, when performed. For removal of a non-tunneled catheter, report the appropriate E/M code.

ICD-10-CM Diagnostic Codes

B52.0	Plasmodium malariae malaria with nephropathy
E10.21	Type 1 diabetes mellitus with diabetic nephropathy
E10.22	Type 1 diabetes mellitus with diabetic chronic kidney disease
E10.29	Type 1 diabetes mellitus with other diabetic kidney complication
E11.21	Type 2 diabetes mellitus with diabetic nephropathy
E11.22	Type 2 diabetes mellitus with diabetic chronic kidney disease
E11.29	Type 2 diabetes mellitus with other diabetic kidney complication
E13.21	Other specified diabetes mellitus with diabetic nephropathy
E13.22	Other specified diabetes mellitus with diabetic chronic kidney disease
E13.29	Other specified diabetes mellitus with other diabetic kidney complication
I12.0	Hypertensive chronic kidney disease with stage 5 chronic kidney disease or end stage renal disease
I13.11	Hypertensive heart and chronic kidney disease without heart failure, with stage 5 chronic kidney disease, or end stage renal disease
I13.2	Hypertensive heart and chronic kidney disease with heart failure and with stage 5 chronic kidney disease, or end stage renal disease
I75.81	Atheroembolism of kidney
M32.14	Glomerular disease in systemic lupus erythematosus
M32.15	Tubulo-interstitial nephropathy in systemic lupus erythematosus

M35.04	Sicca syndrome with tubulo-interstitial nephropathy			
N17.0	Acute kidney failure with tubular necrosis			
N17.1	Acute kidney failure with acute cortical necrosis			
N17.2	Acute kidney failure with medullary necrosis			
N17.8	Other acute kidney failure			
N18.5	Chronic kidney disease, stage 5			
N18.6	End stage renal disease			
Z49.02	Encounter for fitting and adjustment of peritoneal dialysis catheter			
Z49.32	Encounter for adequacy testing for peritoneal dialysis			
Z76.89	Persons encountering health services in other specified circumstances			

AMA: **49421** 2018,Jan,8; 2017,Jan,8; 2016,Jan,13; 2015,Jan,16; 2014,Jan,11

Relative Value Units/Medicare Edits

Non-Facility RVU	Work	PE	MP	Total
49421	4.21	1.49	0.95	6.65
Facility RVU	**Work**	**PE**	**MP**	**Total**
49421	4.21	1.49	0.95	6.65

	FUD	Status	MUE	Modifiers				IOM Reference
49421	0	A	1(2)	51	N/A	N/A	N/A	None

* with documentation

Terms To Know

intra. Within.

peritoneal. Space between the lining of the abdominal wall, or parietal peritoneum, and the surface layer of the abdominal organs, or visceral peritoneum. It contains a thin, watery fluid that keeps the peritoneal surfaces moist.

tunneled catheter. Catheter inserted into a central vein via a chest incision and maneuvered under the skin to a distal outlet location enabling secure placement with decreased risk of infection and can stay in place for extended periods of time. This procedure is commonly performed in an operating room.

49422

49422	Removal of tunneled intraperitoneal catheter

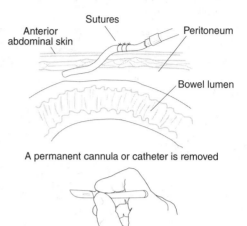

A permanent cannula or catheter is removed

Explanation

The physician removes a tunneled intraperitoneal catheter. The physician makes an incision over the insertion site of the catheter. The catheter is dissected free of surrounding scar tissue, transected, and removed from the peritoneal insertion site and skin exit site. The incision at the insertion site of the catheter is closed. The skin exit site is left open to allow drainage.

Coding Tips

When this procedure is performed with another separately identifiable procedure, the highest dollar value code is listed as the primary procedure and subsequent procedures are appended with modifier 51. For removal of a non-tunneled catheter, report the appropriate E/M code. Insertion of a tunneled intraperitoneal catheter, with subcutaneous port, is reported with 49419. For insertion of a tunneled intraperitoneal catheter for dialysis, open, see 49421; laparoscopic, see 49324; percutaneous, complete procedure, see 49418.

ICD-10-CM Diagnostic Codes

T82.818A	Embolism due to vascular prosthetic devices, implants and grafts, initial encounter
T82.828A	Fibrosis due to vascular prosthetic devices, implants and grafts, initial encounter
T82.838A	Hemorrhage due to vascular prosthetic devices, implants and grafts, initial encounter
T82.848A	Pain due to vascular prosthetic devices, implants and grafts, initial encounter
T82.856A	Stenosis of peripheral vascular stent, initial encounter
T82.858A	Stenosis of other vascular prosthetic devices, implants and grafts, initial encounter
T82.868A	Thrombosis due to vascular prosthetic devices, implants and grafts, initial encounter
T82.898A	Other specified complication of vascular prosthetic devices, implants and grafts, initial encounter
T85.611A	Breakdown (mechanical) of intraperitoneal dialysis catheter, initial encounter
T85.621A	Displacement of intraperitoneal dialysis catheter, initial encounter

Abdomen

T85.631A	Leakage of intraperitoneal dialysis catheter, initial encounter
T85.691A	Other mechanical complication of intraperitoneal dialysis catheter, initial encounter
T85.71XA	Infection and inflammatory reaction due to peritoneal dialysis catheter, initial encounter
Z49.02	Encounter for fitting and adjustment of peritoneal dialysis catheter
Z49.32	Encounter for adequacy testing for peritoneal dialysis

AMA: 49422 2014,Jan,11

Relative Value Units/Medicare Edits

Non-Facility RVU	Work	PE	MP	Total
49422	4.0	1.57	0.89	6.46
Facility RVU	**Work**	**PE**	**MP**	**Total**
49422	4.0	1.57	0.89	6.46

	FUD	Status	MUE	Modifiers				IOM Reference
49422	0	A	1(2)	51	N/A	N/A	N/A	None

* with documentation

Terms To Know

cannula. Tube inserted into a blood vessel, duct, or body cavity to facilitate passage.

dissect. Cut apart or separate tissue for surgical purposes or for visual or microscopic study.

drainage. Releasing, taking, or letting out fluids and/or gases from a body part.

intraperitoneal. Within the cavity or space created by the double-layered sac that lines the abdominopelvic walls and forms a covering for the internal organs.

scar tissue. Fibrous connective tissue that forms around a wounded area or injury, composed mainly of fibroblasts or collagenous fibers.

transection. Transverse dissection; to cut across a long axis; cross section.

tunneled catheter. Catheter inserted into a central vein via a chest incision and maneuvered under the skin to a distal outlet location enabling secure placement with decreased risk of infection and can stay in place for extended periods of time. This procedure is commonly performed in an operating room.

49435

+ **49435** Insertion of subcutaneous extension to intraperitoneal cannula or catheter with remote chest exit site (List separately in addition to code for primary procedure)

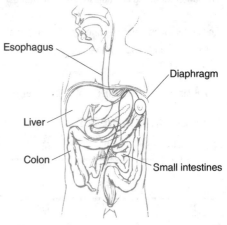

The catheter is extended to the intraperitoneal cannula/catheter and exits the chest

Explanation

A permanent, subcutaneous intraperitoneal catheter is lengthened with an extension and brought to the surface of the skin during the primary procedure in which a catheter/cannula is established. In the primary procedure, the physician makes a small abdominal incision, opens the peritoneum, and establishes the cannula. In 49435, the physician fits an extension to the cannula and tunnels subcutaneously to accommodate the extension. The physician makes a separate incision in the chest as an exit site for the extension. The extension is brought out through the skin and may be attached to the drug delivery system. The operative incision is closed.

Coding Tips

Report 49435 in addition to 49324 or 49421.

ICD-10-CM Diagnostic Codes

This/these CPT code(s) are add-on code(s). See the primary procedure code that this code is performed with for your ICD-10-CM code selections.

AMA: 49435 2014,Jan,11

Relative Value Units/Medicare Edits

Non-Facility RVU	Work	PE	MP	Total
49435	2.25	0.71	0.54	3.5
Facility RVU	**Work**	**PE**	**MP**	**Total**
49435	2.25	0.71	0.54	3.5

	FUD	Status	MUE	Modifiers				IOM Reference
49435	N/A	A	1(2)	N/A	N/A	62*	80	None

* with documentation

Abdomen

49436

49436   Delayed creation of exit site from embedded subcutaneous segment of intraperitoneal cannula or catheter

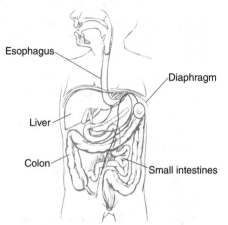

An exit site for the intraperitoneal catheter is created in a subsequent operative session

Explanation

A previously implanted, permanent subcutaneous intraperitoneal catheter is brought to the surface of the skin. The physician makes a small abdominal incision, opens the peritoneum, and locates the end of the existing intraperitoneal cannula. An extension may be fitted to the existing cannula. The physician makes a separate incision as an exit site for the cannula. The cannula is brought out through the skin and may be attached to the drug delivery system. The operative incision is closed.

Coding Tips

To indicate that this is a staged or related procedure performed during the postoperative period by the same physician, append modifier 58. For laparoscopic insertion of an intraperitoneal cannula or catheter, see 49324. For revision of a previously placed intraperitoneal cannula or catheter with removal of an intraluminal obstructive material if performed, see 49325; with omentopexy, see 49326. For insertion of a subcutaneous extension at the time of laparoscopic placement of an intraperitoneal catheter, see 49435.

ICD-10-CM Diagnostic Codes

K68.11	Postprocedural retroperitoneal abscess
T81.41XA	Infection following a procedure, superficial incisional surgical site, initial encounter
T81.42XA	Infection following a procedure, deep incisional surgical site, initial encounter
T81.43XA	Infection following a procedure, organ and space surgical site, initial encounter
T81.49XA	Infection following a procedure, other surgical site, initial encounter
T82.818A	Embolism due to vascular prosthetic devices, implants and grafts, initial encounter
T82.828A	Fibrosis due to vascular prosthetic devices, implants and grafts, initial encounter
T82.838A	Hemorrhage due to vascular prosthetic devices, implants and grafts, initial encounter
T82.848A	Pain due to vascular prosthetic devices, implants and grafts, initial encounter
T82.858A	Stenosis of other vascular prosthetic devices, implants and grafts, initial encounter
T82.868A	Thrombosis due to vascular prosthetic devices, implants and grafts, initial encounter
T82.898A	Other specified complication of vascular prosthetic devices, implants and grafts, initial encounter

AMA: 49436 2014,Jan,11

Relative Value Units/Medicare Edits

Non-Facility RVU	Work	PE	MP	Total
49436	2.72	2.06	0.64	5.42
Facility RVU	**Work**	**PE**	**MP**	**Total**
49436	2.72	2.06	0.64	5.42

	FUD	Status	MUE	Modifiers				IOM Reference
49436	10	A	1(2)	51	N/A	62*	80	None

* with documentation

Terms To Know

cannula. Tube inserted into a blood vessel, duct, or body cavity to facilitate passage.

catheter. Flexible tube inserted into an area of the body for introducing or withdrawing fluid.

embolism. Obstruction of a blood vessel resulting from a clot or foreign substance.

fibrosis. Formation of fibrous tissue as part of the restorative process.

hemorrhage. Internal or external bleeding with loss of significant amounts of blood.

intraperitoneal. Within the cavity or space created by the double-layered sac that lines the abdominopelvic walls and forms a covering for the internal organs.

peritoneum. Strong, continuous membrane that forms the lining of the abdominal and pelvic cavity. The parietal peritoneum, or outer layer, is attached to the abdominopelvic walls and the visceral peritoneum, or inner layer, surrounds the organs inside the abdominal cavity.

stenosis. Narrowing or constriction of a passage.

subcutaneous. Below the skin.

thrombosis. Condition arising from the presence or formation of blood clots within a blood vessel that may cause vascular obstruction and insufficient oxygenation.

Abdomen

CPT © 2020 American Medical Association. All Rights Reserved.   ● New   ▲ Revised   + Add On   ★ Telemedicine   AMA: CPT Assist   [Resequenced]   ☑ Laterality   © 2020 Optum360, LLC

50010

50010 Renal exploration, not necessitating other specific procedures

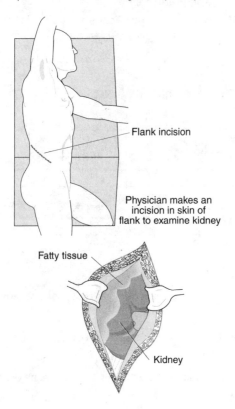

Flank incision

Physician makes an incision in skin of flank to examine kidney

Fatty tissue

Kidney

Explanation

The physician examines the kidney and renal pelvis. To access the kidney, the physician makes an incision in the skin of the flank, cuts the muscles, fat, and fibrous membranes (fascia) overlying the kidney, and sometimes removes a portion of the eleventh or twelfth rib. The physician clears away the fatty tissue surrounding the kidney, explores the area, and performs a layered closure.

Coding Tips

Nephrotomy with exploration is reported with 50045; pyelotomy, see 50120. For retroperitoneal exploration, see 49010.. If significant additional time and effort is documented, append modifier 22 and submit a cover letter and operative report.

ICD-10-CM Diagnostic Codes

C64.1	Malignant neoplasm of right kidney, except renal pelvis ☑
C64.2	Malignant neoplasm of left kidney, except renal pelvis ☑
C65.1	Malignant neoplasm of right renal pelvis ☑
C65.2	Malignant neoplasm of left renal pelvis ☑
C79.01	Secondary malignant neoplasm of right kidney and renal pelvis ☑
C79.02	Secondary malignant neoplasm of left kidney and renal pelvis ☑
C7A.093	Malignant carcinoid tumor of the kidney
C80.2	Malignant neoplasm associated with transplanted organ
D09.19	Carcinoma in situ of other urinary organs
D30.01	Benign neoplasm of right kidney ☑
D30.02	Benign neoplasm of left kidney ☑
D30.11	Benign neoplasm of right renal pelvis ☑
D30.12	Benign neoplasm of left renal pelvis ☑

D3A.093	Benign carcinoid tumor of the kidney
D41.01	Neoplasm of uncertain behavior of right kidney ☑
D41.02	Neoplasm of uncertain behavior of left kidney ☑
D41.11	Neoplasm of uncertain behavior of right renal pelvis ☑
D41.12	Neoplasm of uncertain behavior of left renal pelvis ☑
D49.511	Neoplasm of unspecified behavior of right kidney ☑
D49.512	Neoplasm of unspecified behavior of left kidney ☑
D49.59	Neoplasm of unspecified behavior of other genitourinary organ
K66.1	Hemoperitoneum
N13.0	Hydronephrosis with ureteropelvic junction obstruction
N13.1	Hydronephrosis with ureteral stricture, not elsewhere classified
N13.2	Hydronephrosis with renal and ureteral calculous obstruction
N13.39	Other hydronephrosis
N28.0	Ischemia and infarction of kidney
N28.1	Cyst of kidney, acquired
N28.81	Hypertrophy of kidney
N28.83	Nephroptosis
N28.89	Other specified disorders of kidney and ureter
Q61.01	Congenital single renal cyst
Q61.02	Congenital multiple renal cysts
Q61.19	Other polycystic kidney, infantile type
Q61.2	Polycystic kidney, adult type
Q61.4	Renal dysplasia
Q61.5	Medullary cystic kidney
Q61.8	Other cystic kidney diseases
Q62.0	Congenital hydronephrosis
Q62.39	Other obstructive defects of renal pelvis and ureter
S37.011A	Minor contusion of right kidney, initial encounter ☑
S37.012A	Minor contusion of left kidney, initial encounter ☑
S37.021A	Major contusion of right kidney, initial encounter ☑
S37.022A	Major contusion of left kidney, initial encounter ☑
S37.041A	Minor laceration of right kidney, initial encounter ☑
S37.042A	Minor laceration of left kidney, initial encounter ☑
S37.051A	Moderate laceration of right kidney, initial encounter ☑
S37.052A	Moderate laceration of left kidney, initial encounter ☑
S37.061A	Major laceration of right kidney, initial encounter ☑
S37.062A	Major laceration of left kidney, initial encounter ☑
S37.091A	Other injury of right kidney, initial encounter ☑
S37.092A	Other injury of left kidney, initial encounter ☑
T79.5XXA	Traumatic anuria, initial encounter

AMA: **50010** 2014,Jan,11

Relative Value Units/Medicare Edits

Non-Facility RVU	Work	PE	MP	Total
50010	12.28	6.98	1.98	21.24
Facility RVU	**Work**	**PE**	**MP**	**Total**
50010	12.28	6.98	1.98	21.24

	FUD	Status	MUE	Modifiers				IOM Reference
50010	90	A	1(2)	51	50	62*	80	None

* with documentation

Kidney

50020

50020   Drainage of perirenal or renal abscess, open

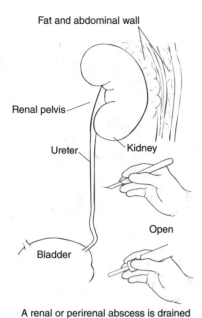

Fat and abdominal wall

Renal pelvis

Ureter

Kidney

Open

Bladder

A renal or perirenal abscess is drained

Explanation

The physician drains an infection (abscess) on the kidney or on the surrounding renal tissue in an open procedure. To access the renal or perirenal abscess, the physician makes a small incision in the skin of the flank, cuts the muscles, fat, and fibrous membranes (fascia) overlying the kidney, and sometimes removes a portion of the eleventh or twelfth rib. After exploring the abscess cavity, the physician irrigates the site, inserts multiple drain tubes through separate stab wounds, and sutures the drain tube ends to the skin. The physician packs the wound with gauze and sutures the fascia and muscles. The skin and subcutaneous tissue are usually left open to prevent formation of a secondary body wall abscess. The drainage catheters are later removed.

Coding Tips

For percutaneous, image-guided drainage of a perirenal/renal abscess, via catheter, see 49405; peritoneal. retroperitoneal, subdiaphragmatic or subphrenic abscess or localized peritonitis, see 49406. To report open drainage of a retroperitoneal abscess, see 49060.

ICD-10-CM Diagnostic Codes

N15.1   Renal and perinephric abscess

AMA: 50020 2018,Jan,8; 2017,Jan,8; 2016,Jan,13; 2015,Jan,16; 2014,May,9; 2014,Jan,11

Relative Value Units/Medicare Edits

Non-Facility RVU	Work	PE	MP	Total
50020	18.08	9.1	2.06	29.24
Facility RVU	**Work**	**PE**	**MP**	**Total**
50020	18.08	9.1	2.06	29.24

	FUD	Status	MUE	Modifiers				IOM Reference
50020	90	A	1(3)	51	N/A	62*	N/A	None

* with documentation

50040

50040   Nephrostomy, nephrotomy with drainage

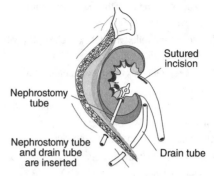

Sutured incision

Nephrostomy tube

Nephrostomy tube and drain tube are inserted

Drain tube

Physician passes curved clamp through renal pelvis, minor calyx, and kidney

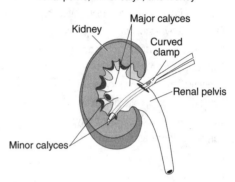

Kidney

Major calyces

Curved clamp

Renal pelvis

Minor calyces

Explanation

The physician creates an opening from the kidney to the exterior of the body by making an incision in the kidney. To access the kidney, the physician makes an incision in the skin of the flank, cuts the muscles, fat, and fibrous membranes (fascia) overlying the kidney, and sometimes removes a portion of the eleventh or twelfth rib. Using an incision to open the renal pelvis (pyelotomy), the physician passes a curved clamp into the renal pelvis, a middle or lower minor calyx, and the cortex of the kidney. The physician inserts a catheter tip through the same path as the clamp, and passes the tube through a stab incision in the skin of the flank. After suturing the incisions, the physician inserts a drain tube, bringing it out through a separate stab incision, and performs a layered closure.

Coding Tips

For dilation of an existing tract for an endourologic procedure, percutaneous, see 50436; including new access into the renal collecting system, see 50437. Cystourethroscopy with ureteral guidewire insertion for percutaneous nephrostomy, retrograde, is reported with 52334. For pyelotomy with drainage (pyelostomy), see 50125. For introduction of an intracatheter or a catheter into the renal pelvis for drainage/injection, percutaneous, see 50432. For change of a nephrostomy or pyelostomy tube, see 50435. For renal endoscopy through the nephrostomy or pyelostomy, with or without irrigation, instillation, or ureteropyelography, see 50551–50562.

ICD-10-CM Diagnostic Codes

N10   Acute pyelonephritis
N11.1   Chronic obstructive pyelonephritis
N12   Tubulo-interstitial nephritis, not specified as acute or chronic
N13.0   Hydronephrosis with ureteropelvic junction obstruction
N13.1   Hydronephrosis with ureteral stricture, not elsewhere classified

Kidney

CPT © 2020 American Medical Association. All Rights Reserved.   ● New   ▲ Revised   + Add On   ★ Telemedicine   AMA: CPT Assist   [Resequenced]   ☑ Laterality   © 2020 Optum360, LLC

N13.2	Hydronephrosis with renal and ureteral calculous obstruction
N13.39	Other hydronephrosis
N13.6	Pyonephrosis
N13.71	Vesicoureteral-reflux without reflux nephropathy
N13.721	Vesicoureteral-reflux with reflux nephropathy without hydroureter, unilateral
N13.722	Vesicoureteral-reflux with reflux nephropathy without hydroureter, bilateral
N13.731	Vesicoureteral-reflux with reflux nephropathy with hydroureter, unilateral
N13.732	Vesicoureteral-reflux with reflux nephropathy with hydroureter, bilateral
N13.8	Other obstructive and reflux uropathy
N15.1	Renal and perinephric abscess
N20.0	Calculus of kidney
N20.2	Calculus of kidney with calculus of ureter
N25.89	Other disorders resulting from impaired renal tubular function
N28.1	Cyst of kidney, acquired
N28.89	Other specified disorders of kidney and ureter
Q61.01	Congenital single renal cyst
Q61.02	Congenital multiple renal cysts
Q61.11	Cystic dilatation of collecting ducts
Q61.19	Other polycystic kidney, infantile type
Q61.2	Polycystic kidney, adult type
Q61.4	Renal dysplasia
Q61.5	Medullary cystic kidney
Q61.8	Other cystic kidney diseases
Q62.0	Congenital hydronephrosis
Q62.11	Congenital occlusion of ureteropelvic junction
Q62.12	Congenital occlusion of ureterovesical orifice
Q62.39	Other obstructive defects of renal pelvis and ureter
Q63.1	Lobulated, fused and horseshoe kidney
Q63.8	Other specified congenital malformations of kidney
S37.011A	Minor contusion of right kidney, initial encounter ☑
S37.012A	Minor contusion of left kidney, initial encounter ☑
S37.021A	Major contusion of right kidney, initial encounter ☑
S37.022A	Major contusion of left kidney, initial encounter ☑
T79.5XXA	Traumatic anuria, initial encounter

AMA: 50040 2018,Jan,8; 2017,Jan,8; 2016,Jan,13; 2015,Jan,16; 2014,Jan,11

Relative Value Units/Medicare Edits

Non-Facility RVU	Work	PE	MP	Total
50040	16.68	8.03	1.92	26.63
Facility RVU	Work	PE	MP	Total
50040	16.68	8.03	1.92	26.63

	FUD	Status	MUE	Modifiers				IOM Reference
50040	90	A	1(2)	51	50	62*	N/A	None

* with documentation

50045

50045   Nephrotomy, with exploration

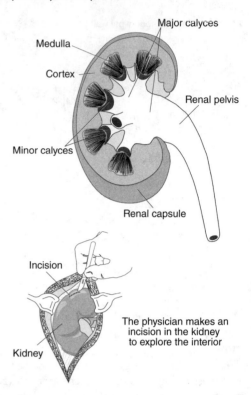

The physician makes an incision in the kidney to explore the interior

Explanation

The physician makes a small incision in the kidney to explore the interior of the kidney. To access the kidney, the physician makes an incision in the skin of the flank, cuts the muscles, fat, and fibrous membranes (fascia) overlying the kidney, and sometimes removes a portion of the eleventh or twelfth rib. The physician makes an incision in the kidney (nephrotomy) and sometimes places fine traction sutures at the edges of the incision. After exploration, the physician sutures the incision, inserts a drain tube, bringing it out through a separate stab incision, and performs a layered closure.

Coding Tips

For exploratory pyelotomy, see 50120. For renal exploration, see 50010. If the physician performs nephrotomy solely as an approach for renal endoscopy procedures, report the appropriate code from 50570–50580.

ICD-10-CM Diagnostic Codes

C64.1	Malignant neoplasm of right kidney, except renal pelvis ☑
C64.2	Malignant neoplasm of left kidney, except renal pelvis ☑
C65.1	Malignant neoplasm of right renal pelvis ☑
C65.2	Malignant neoplasm of left renal pelvis ☑
C79.01	Secondary malignant neoplasm of right kidney and renal pelvis ☑
C79.02	Secondary malignant neoplasm of left kidney and renal pelvis ☑
C7A.093	Malignant carcinoid tumor of the kidney
C80.2	Malignant neoplasm associated with transplanted organ
D09.19	Carcinoma in situ of other urinary organs
D30.01	Benign neoplasm of right kidney ☑
D30.02	Benign neoplasm of left kidney ☑
D30.11	Benign neoplasm of right renal pelvis ☑

D30.12	Benign neoplasm of left renal pelvis ☑
D3A.093	Benign carcinoid tumor of the kidney
D41.01	Neoplasm of uncertain behavior of right kidney ☑
D41.02	Neoplasm of uncertain behavior of left kidney ☑
D41.11	Neoplasm of uncertain behavior of right renal pelvis ☑
D41.12	Neoplasm of uncertain behavior of left renal pelvis ☑
D49.511	Neoplasm of unspecified behavior of right kidney ☑
D49.512	Neoplasm of unspecified behavior of left kidney ☑
D49.59	Neoplasm of unspecified behavior of other genitourinary organ
K66.1	Hemoperitoneum
N13.0	Hydronephrosis with ureteropelvic junction obstruction
N13.1	Hydronephrosis with ureteral stricture, not elsewhere classified
N13.2	Hydronephrosis with renal and ureteral calculous obstruction
N13.39	Other hydronephrosis
N28.0	Ischemia and infarction of kidney
N28.1	Cyst of kidney, acquired
N28.81	Hypertrophy of kidney
N28.83	Nephroptosis
N28.89	Other specified disorders of kidney and ureter
Q61.01	Congenital single renal cyst
Q61.02	Congenital multiple renal cysts
Q61.19	Other polycystic kidney, infantile type
Q61.2	Polycystic kidney, adult type
Q61.4	Renal dysplasia
Q61.5	Medullary cystic kidney
Q61.8	Other cystic kidney diseases
Q62.0	Congenital hydronephrosis
Q62.39	Other obstructive defects of renal pelvis and ureter
S37.011A	Minor contusion of right kidney, initial encounter ☑
S37.012A	Minor contusion of left kidney, initial encounter ☑
S37.021A	Major contusion of right kidney, initial encounter ☑
S37.022A	Major contusion of left kidney, initial encounter ☑
S37.041A	Minor laceration of right kidney, initial encounter ☑
S37.042A	Minor laceration of left kidney, initial encounter ☑
S37.051A	Moderate laceration of right kidney, initial encounter ☑
S37.052A	Moderate laceration of left kidney, initial encounter ☑
S37.061A	Major laceration of right kidney, initial encounter ☑
S37.062A	Major laceration of left kidney, initial encounter ☑
S37.091A	Other injury of right kidney, initial encounter ☑
S37.092A	Other injury of left kidney, initial encounter ☑
T79.5XXA	Traumatic anuria, initial encounter

AMA: 50045 2018,Jan,8; 2017,Jan,8; 2016,Jan,13; 2015,Jan,16; 2014,Jan,11

Relative Value Units/Medicare Edits

Non-Facility RVU	Work	PE	MP	Total
50045	16.82	8.17	1.92	26.91
Facility RVU	**Work**	**PE**	**MP**	**Total**
50045	16.82	8.17	1.92	26.91

	FUD	Status	MUE	Modifiers				IOM Reference
50045	90	A	1(2)	51	50	62*	80	None

* with documentation

50060-50075

50060	Nephrolithotomy; removal of calculus
50065	secondary surgical operation for calculus
50070	complicated by congenital kidney abnormality
50075	removal of large staghorn calculus filling renal pelvis and calyces (including anatrophic pyelolithotomy)

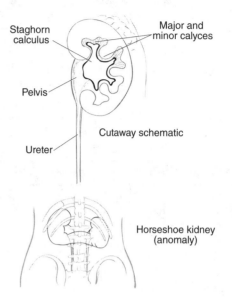

Staghorn calculus — Major and minor calyces — Pelvis — Cutaway schematic — Ureter — Horseshoe kidney (anomaly)

Explanation

The physician removes a kidney stone (calculus) by making an incision in the kidney. To access the calculus, the physician makes an incision in the skin of the flank, cuts the muscles, fat, and fibrous membranes (fascia) overlying the kidney, and sometimes removes a portion of the eleventh or twelfth rib. The physician isolates the calculus and removes it through an incision. After examining the kidney for other defects, the physician sutures the incision, inserts a drain tube, bringing it out through a separate stab incision, and performs a layered closure. Simple removal of the calculus by nephrotomy is reported with 50060. Report 50065 when a previous surgery on the kidney complicates the procedure. Report 50070 if the procedure is complicated because of a congenital kidney abnormality, wherein the physician usually repairs any calyces that are obstructed or abnormally narrowed. Report 50075 for removal of a staghorn calculus.

Coding Tips

For pyelotomy with removal of calculus, see 50130. Percutaneous nephrostolithotomy or pyelostolithotomy, with or without dilation, endoscopy, lithotripsy, stenting, or basket extraction, up to 2 cm, see 50080; over 2 cm, see 50081. For renal endoscopy procedures, with removal of foreign body or calculus, through established nephrostomy or pyelostomy, see 50561; through nephrotomy or pyelotomy, see 50580. For lithotripsy, extracorporeal shock wave, see 50590.

ICD-10-CM Diagnostic Codes

N20.0	Calculus of kidney
N20.2	Calculus of kidney with calculus of ureter
Q63.0	Accessory kidney
Q63.1	Lobulated, fused and horseshoe kidney
Q63.2	Ectopic kidney
Q63.3	Hyperplastic and giant kidney
Q63.8	Other specified congenital malformations of kidney

Kidney

AMA: 50060 2018,Jan,8; 2017,Jan,8; 2016,Jan,13; 2015,Jan,16; 2014,Jan,11 **50065** 2018,Jan,8; 2017,Jan,8; 2016,Jan,13; 2015,Jan,16; 2014,Jan,11 **50070** 2018,Jan,8; 2017,Jan,8; 2016,Jan,13; 2015,Jan,16; 2014,Jan,11 **50075** 2018,Jan,8; 2017,Jan,8; 2016,Jan,13; 2015,Jan,16; 2014,Jan,11

Relative Value Units/Medicare Edits

Non-Facility RVU	Work	PE	MP	Total
50060	20.95	9.57	2.4	32.92
50065	22.32	10.03	2.56	34.91
50070	21.85	9.87	2.5	34.22
50075	27.09	11.91	3.1	42.1
Facility RVU	Work	PE	MP	Total
50060	20.95	9.57	2.4	32.92
50065	22.32	10.03	2.56	34.91
50070	21.85	9.87	2.5	34.22
50075	27.09	11.91	3.1	42.1

	FUD	Status	MUE	Modifiers				IOM Reference
50060	90	A	1(2)	51	50	62*	80	None
50065	90	A	1(2)	51	50	N/A	80	
50070	90	A	1(2)	51	50	62*	80	
50075	90	A	1(2)	51	50	62*	80	

* with documentation

Terms To Know

anomaly. Irregularity in the structure or position of an organ or tissue.

calculus. Abnormal, stone-like concretion of calcium, cholesterol, mineral salts, or other substances that forms in any part of the body.

congenital. Present at birth, occurring through heredity or an influence during gestation up to the moment of birth.

defect. Imperfection, flaw, or absence.

fascia. Fibrous sheet or band of tissue that envelops organs, muscles, and groupings of muscles.

flank. Part of the body found between the posterior ribs and the uppermost crest of the ilium, or the lateral side of the hip, thigh, and buttock.

hematuria. Blood in urine, which may present as gross visible blood or as the presence of red blood cells visible only under a microscope.

horseshoe kidney. Congenital anomaly in which the kidneys are fused together at the lower end during fetal development, resulting in one large, horseshoe shaped kidney, often associated with cardiovascular, central nervous system, or genitourinary anomalies.

nephrolithotomy. Removal of a kidney stone or calculus through an incision made directly into the kidney.

nephrotomy. Incision into the body of the kidney.

staghorn calculus. Renal stone that develops in the pelvicaliceal system, and in advanced cases has a branching appearance that resembles the antlers of a stag.

ureterocele. Saccular formation of the lower part of the ureter, protruding into the bladder.

50080–50081

50080	Percutaneous nephrostolithotomy or pyelostolithotomy, with or without dilation, endoscopy, lithotripsy, stenting, or basket extraction; up to 2 cm
50081	over 2 cm

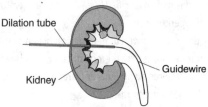

Physician creates nephrostomy tract by passing dilation tubes over guidewire

Dilation tube

Kidney

Guidewire

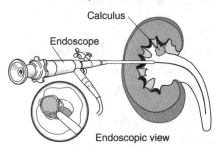

Physician passes instrument through endoscope to remove calculus

Calculus

Endoscope

Endoscopic view

Explanation

The physician creates a percutaneous passageway to remove kidney stones (calculi). The physician makes a small incision in the skin of the back, inserts a large needle, and radiologically guides it toward the kidney or renal pelvis. After passing a guidewire through the needle, the physician dilates the passageway by inserting and removing tubes with increasingly larger diameters. The physician inserts an endoscope over the guidewire and passes an instrument through the endoscope to crush or extract calculi. The physician may pass a ureteral stent from the pelvis into the bladder. The physician removes the guidewire and allows the passageway to seal on its own, or inserts a nephrostomy or pyelostomy tube before removing the guidewire. Report 50080 for removal of calculi measuring up to 2 cm; use 50081 for removal of calculi measuring more than 2 cm.

Coding Tips

For establishment of a nephrostomy without nephrostolithotomy, see 50040, 50432-50433, and 52334. For renal endoscopy with removal of foreign body or calculus, through established nephrostomy or pyelostomy, see 50561. For lithotripsy, extracorporeal shock wave, see 50590. For endoscopic removal of a renal calculus, see 50561 and 50580. Do not report 50080-50081 with 50436-50437 when performed by the same clinician. Fluoroscopic guidance is reported with 76000, when performed. Local or general anesthesia may be administered, depending on the age and/or condition of the patient.

ICD-10-CM Diagnostic Codes

N20.0	Calculus of kidney
N20.2	Calculus of kidney with calculus of ureter

AMA: 50080 2018,Jan,8; 2017,Jan,8; 2016,Jan,13; 2015,Jan,16; 2014,Jan,11 **50081** 2018,Jan,8; 2017,Jan,8; 2016,Jan,13; 2015,Jan,16; 2014,Jan,11

Relative Value Units/Medicare Edits

Non-Facility RVU	Work	PE	MP	Total
50080	15.74	7.55	1.8	25.09
50081	23.5	10.69	2.71	36.9
Facility RVU	**Work**	**PE**	**MP**	**Total**
50080	15.74	7.55	1.8	25.09
50081	23.5	10.69	2.71	36.9

	FUD	Status	MUE	Modifiers				IOM Reference
50080	90	A	1(2)	51	50	N/A	N/A	None
50081	90	A	1(2)	51	50	62*	80	

* with documentation

Terms To Know

calculus. Abnormal, stone-like concretion of calcium, cholesterol, mineral salts, or other substances that forms in any part of the body.

congenital. Present at birth, occurring through heredity or an influence during gestation up to the moment of birth.

dilation. Artificial increase in the diameter of an opening or lumen made by medication or by instrumentation.

guidewire. Flexible metal instrument designed to lead another instrument in its proper course.

hematuria. Blood in urine, which may present as gross visible blood or as the presence of red blood cells visible only under a microscope.

lithotripsy. Destruction of calcified substances in the gallbladder or urinary system by smashing the concretion into small particles to be washed out. This may be done by surgical or noninvasive methods, such as ultrasound.

nephrostolithotomy. Removal of a kidney stone through a percutaneous passageway created in the abdominal wall with a tube or stent inserted.

percutaneous approach. Method used to gain access to a body organ or specific area by puncture or minor incision through the skin or mucous membrane and/or any other body layers necessary to reach the procedure site.

pyelostolithotomy. Removal of a renal calculus via a tube placed through an opening in the abdominal wall into the pelvis of the kidney.

stent. Tube to provide support in a body cavity or lumen.

50100

50100   Transection or repositioning of aberrant renal vessels (separate procedure)

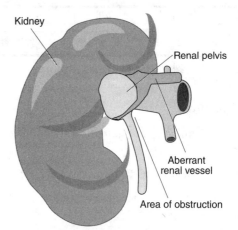

The physician corrects obstruction by cutting across or repositioning aberrant renal vessel

Explanation

The physician corrects an obstruction by cutting across or repositioning renal vessels that deviate from proper anatomical placement. To access the kidney, the physician makes an incision in the skin of the flank, cuts the muscles, fat, and fibrous membranes (fascia) overlying the kidney, and sometimes removes a portion of the twelfth rib. After repositioning the aberrant vessels to a more functional anatomic placement, the physician performs a layered closure.

Coding Tips

This separate procedure by definition is usually a component of a more complex service and is not identified separately. When performed alone, or with other unrelated procedures/services it may be reported. If performed alone, list the code; if performed with other procedures/services, list the code and append modifier 59 or an X{EPSU} modifier.

ICD-10-CM Diagnostic Codes

N11.1	Chronic obstructive pyelonephritis
N13.0	Hydronephrosis with ureteropelvic junction obstruction
N13.1	Hydronephrosis with ureteral stricture, not elsewhere classified
N13.2	Hydronephrosis with renal and ureteral calculus obstruction
N13.5	Crossing vessel and stricture of ureter without hydronephrosis
N28.0	Ischemia and infarction of kidney
Q27.1	Congenital renal artery stenosis
Q27.2	Other congenital malformations of renal artery
Q27.34	Arteriovenous malformation of renal vessel
Q62.0	Congenital hydronephrosis
Q62.11	Congenital occlusion of ureteropelvic junction
Q62.39	Other obstructive defects of renal pelvis and ureter
Q63.0	Accessory kidney
Q63.1	Lobulated, fused and horseshoe kidney
Q63.2	Ectopic kidney
Q63.3	Hyperplastic and giant kidney
Q63.8	Other specified congenital malformations of kidney

AMA: 50100 2018,Jan,8; 2017,Jan,8; 2016,Jan,13; 2015,Jan,16; 2014,Jan,11

Kidney

CPT © 2020 American Medical Association. All Rights Reserved.   ● New   ▲ Revised   + Add On   ★ Telemedicine   AMA: CPT Assist   [Resequenced]   ☑ Laterality   © 2020 Optum360, LLC

Relative Value Units/Medicare Edits

Non-Facility RVU	Work	PE	MP	Total
50100	17.45	9.78	4.24	31.47
Facility RVU	Work	PE	MP	Total
50100	17.45	9.78	4.24	31.47

	FUD	Status	MUE	Modifiers				IOM Reference
50100	90	A	1(2)	51	50	62*	80	None

* with documentation

Terms To Know

aberrant. Deviation or departure from the normal or usual course, condition, or pattern.

anomaly. Irregularity in the structure or position of an organ or tissue.

congenital. Present at birth, occurring through heredity or an influence during gestation up to the moment of birth.

fascia. Fibrous sheet or band of tissue that envelops organs, muscles, and groupings of muscles.

flank. Part of the body found between the posterior ribs and the uppermost crest of the ilium, or the lateral side of the hip, thigh, and buttock.

obstruction. Blockage that prevents normal function of the valve or structure.

renal. Referring to the kidney.

reposition. Placement of an organ or structure into another position or return of an organ or structure to its original position.

stricture. Narrowing of an anatomical structure.

transection. Transverse dissection; to cut across a long axis; cross section.

50120-50135

50120	Pyelotomy; with exploration
50125	with drainage, pyelostomy
50130	with removal of calculus (pyelolithotomy, pelviolithotomy, including coagulum pyelolithotomy)
50135	complicated (eg, secondary operation, congenital kidney abnormality)

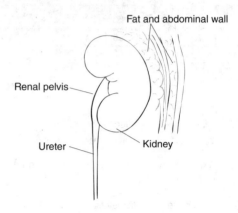

The renal pelvis is incised and explored

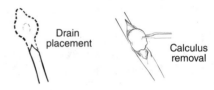

Drain placement

Calculus removal

Explanation

The physician makes an incision in the renal pelvis to explore the calyces and renal pelvis. To access the kidney, the physician makes an incision in the skin of the flank, cuts the muscles, fat, and fibrous membranes (fascia) overlying the kidney, and sometimes removes a portion of the eleventh or twelfth rib. An incision is made in the renal pelvis (pyelotomy). The physician may place fine traction sutures at the edges of the pyelotomy while exploring the calyces and renal pelvis. After closing the pyelotomy, the physician inserts a drain tube, bringing it out through a separate stab incision, and performs layered closure. In 50125, a pyelostomy tube for drainage is inserted; in 50130, calculi or coagulum are removed; in 50135, a complicated pyelotomy for a congenital kidney abnormality or secondary operation is performed.

Coding Tips

For nephrostomy, nephrotomy with drainage, see 50040; nephrotomy with exploration, see 50045. If the physician performs pyelotomy solely as an approach for renal endoscopy procedures, report the appropriate code from 50570–50580. For endoscopic procedures through an established pyelostomy, see 50551–50562.

ICD-10-CM Diagnostic Codes

C65.1	Malignant neoplasm of right renal pelvis ☑
C65.2	Malignant neoplasm of left renal pelvis ☑
C79.01	Secondary malignant neoplasm of right kidney and renal pelvis ☑
C79.02	Secondary malignant neoplasm of left kidney and renal pelvis ☑
D09.19	Carcinoma in situ of other urinary organs
D30.11	Benign neoplasm of right renal pelvis ☑
D30.12	Benign neoplasm of left renal pelvis ☑

© 2020 Optum360, LLC   N Newborn: 0   P Pediatric: 0-17   M Maternity: 9-64   A Adult: 15-124   ♂ Male Only   ♀ Female Only   CPT © 2020 American Medical Association. All Rights Reserved.

Kidney

D41.11	Neoplasm of uncertain behavior of right renal pelvis ☑
D41.12	Neoplasm of uncertain behavior of left renal pelvis ☑
D49.511	Neoplasm of unspecified behavior of right kidney ☑
D49.512	Neoplasm of unspecified behavior of left kidney ☑
D49.59	Neoplasm of unspecified behavior of other genitourinary organ
N10	Acute pyelonephritis
N11.0	Nonobstructive reflux-associated chronic pyelonephritis
N11.1	Chronic obstructive pyelonephritis
N11.8	Other chronic tubulo-interstitial nephritis
N12	Tubulo-interstitial nephritis, not specified as acute or chronic
N15.1	Renal and perinephric abscess
N20.0	Calculus of kidney
N20.2	Calculus of kidney with calculus of ureter
N25.89	Other disorders resulting from impaired renal tubular function
N28.84	Pyelitis cystica
N28.85	Pyeloureteritis cystica
N28.86	Ureteritis cystica
N28.89	Other specified disorders of kidney and ureter
Q62.39	Other obstructive defects of renal pelvis and ureter
Q63.0	Accessory kidney
Q63.1	Lobulated, fused and horseshoe kidney
Q63.2	Ectopic kidney
Q63.3	Hyperplastic and giant kidney
Q63.8	Other specified congenital malformations of kidney

AMA: 50120 2018,Jan,8; 2017,Jan,8; 2016,Jan,13; 2015,Jan,16; 2014,Jan,11 **50125** 2018,Jan,8; 2017,Jan,8; 2016,Jan,13; 2015,Jan,16; 2014,Jan,11 **50130** 2018,Jan,8; 2017,Jan,8; 2016,Jan,13; 2015,Jan,16; 2014,Jan,11 **50135** 2018,Jan,8; 2017,Jan,8; 2016,Jan,13; 2015,Jan,16; 2014,Jan,11

Relative Value Units/Medicare Edits

Non-Facility RVU	Work	PE	MP	Total
50120	17.21	8.23	1.97	27.41
50125	17.82	8.51	2.02	28.35
50130	18.82	8.85	2.16	29.83
50135	20.59	9.45	2.35	32.39
Facility RVU	**Work**	**PE**	**MP**	**Total**
50120	17.21	8.23	1.97	27.41
50125	17.82	8.51	2.02	28.35
50130	18.82	8.85	2.16	29.83
50135	20.59	9.45	2.35	32.39

	FUD	Status	MUE	Modifiers				IOM Reference
50120	90	A	1(2)	51	50	62*	80	None
50125	90	A	1(2)	51	50	62*	80	
50130	90	A	1(2)	51	50	62*	80	
50135	90	A	1(2)	51	50	62*	80	

* with documentation

50200-50205

50200 Renal biopsy; percutaneous, by trocar or needle
50205   by surgical exposure of kidney

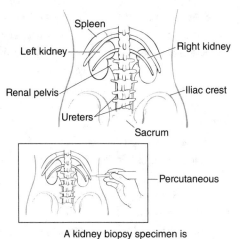

A kidney biopsy specimen is collected by trocar or needle

Explanation

The physician extracts a plug of biopsy tissue from the kidney by inserting a needle or trocar in the skin of the back. Using radiologic or ultrasonic guidance, the physician advances the instrument into the suspect tissue of the kidney. With the instrument's cutting sheath, the physician traps a specimen of renal tissue and removes the instrument. After repeating the process several times, the physician applies pressure to the puncture wound. In 50205, a specimen of biopsy tissue is excised from the kidney. An incision is made in the skin of the flank, through muscle, fat, and fibrous membranes (fascia), overlying the kidney. The incision is sutured with layered closure.

Coding Tips

Radiological supervision and interpretation is reported with 76942, 77002, 77012, and 77021. For fine needle aspiration biopsy services, see 10004–10012 and 10021. For pathological evaluation of fine needle aspirate, see 88172–88173. For laparoscopic ablation of renal mass lesions, see 50542.

ICD-10-CM Diagnostic Codes

B52.0	Plasmodium malariae malaria with nephropathy
C64.1	Malignant neoplasm of right kidney, except renal pelvis ☑
C64.2	Malignant neoplasm of left kidney, except renal pelvis ☑
C65.1	Malignant neoplasm of right renal pelvis ☑
C65.2	Malignant neoplasm of left renal pelvis ☑
C79.01	Secondary malignant neoplasm of right kidney and renal pelvis ☑
C79.02	Secondary malignant neoplasm of left kidney and renal pelvis ☑
C7A.093	Malignant carcinoid tumor of the kidney
C80.2	Malignant neoplasm associated with transplanted organ
D09.19	Carcinoma in situ of other urinary organs
D30.01	Benign neoplasm of right kidney ☑
D30.02	Benign neoplasm of left kidney ☑
D30.11	Benign neoplasm of right renal pelvis ☑
D30.12	Benign neoplasm of left renal pelvis ☑
D3A.093	Benign carcinoid tumor of the kidney
D41.01	Neoplasm of uncertain behavior of right kidney ☑

Kidney

D41.02	Neoplasm of uncertain behavior of left kidney ☑
D41.11	Neoplasm of uncertain behavior of right renal pelvis ☑
D41.12	Neoplasm of uncertain behavior of left renal pelvis ☑
D47.Z1	Post-transplant lymphoproliferative disorder (PTLD)
D47.Z2	Castleman disease
D49.511	Neoplasm of unspecified behavior of right kidney ☑
D49.512	Neoplasm of unspecified behavior of left kidney ☑
D49.59	Neoplasm of unspecified behavior of other genitourinary organ
D89.41	Monoclonal mast cell activation syndrome
D89.42	Idiopathic mast cell activation syndrome
D89.43	Secondary mast cell activation
D89.49	Other mast cell activation disorder
D89.810	Acute graft-versus-host disease
D89.811	Chronic graft-versus-host disease
D89.812	Acute on chronic graft-versus-host disease
I75.81	Atheroembolism of kidney
M04.1	Periodic fever syndromes
M04.2	Cryopyrin-associated periodic syndromes
M04.8	Other autoinflammatory syndromes
M32.14	Glomerular disease in systemic lupus erythematosus
M32.15	Tubulo-interstitial nephropathy in systemic lupus erythematosus
M35.04	Sicca syndrome with tubulo-interstitial nephropathy
M62.82	Rhabdomyolysis
N00.0	Acute nephritic syndrome with minor glomerular abnormality
N00.1	Acute nephritic syndrome with focal and segmental glomerular lesions
N00.2	Acute nephritic syndrome with diffuse membranous glomerulonephritis
N00.3	Acute nephritic syndrome with diffuse mesangial proliferative glomerulonephritis
N00.4	Acute nephritic syndrome with diffuse endocapillary proliferative glomerulonephritis
N00.5	Acute nephritic syndrome with diffuse mesangiocapillary glomerulonephritis
N00.6	Acute nephritic syndrome with dense deposit disease
N00.7	Acute nephritic syndrome with diffuse crescentic glomerulonephritis
N00.8	Acute nephritic syndrome with other morphologic changes
N00.A	Acute nephritic syndrome with C3 glomerulonephritis
N02.0	Recurrent and persistent hematuria with minor glomerular abnormality
N02.A	Recurrent and persistent hematuria with C3 glomerulonephritis
N03.2	Chronic nephritic syndrome with diffuse membranous glomerulonephritis
N03.4	Chronic nephritic syndrome with diffuse endocapillary proliferative glomerulonephritis
N03.5	Chronic nephritic syndrome with diffuse mesangiocapillary glomerulonephritis
N03.6	Chronic nephritic syndrome with dense deposit disease
N03.7	Chronic nephritic syndrome with diffuse crescentic glomerulonephritis
N03.8	Chronic nephritic syndrome with other morphologic changes
N03.A	Chronic nephritic syndrome with C3 glomerulonephritis
N04.0	Nephrotic syndrome with minor glomerular abnormality

N04.4	Nephrotic syndrome with diffuse endocapillary proliferative glomerulonephritis
N13.71	Vesicoureteral-reflux without reflux nephropathy
N17.0	Acute kidney failure with tubular necrosis
N17.1	Acute kidney failure with acute cortical necrosis
N17.2	Acute kidney failure with medullary necrosis
N17.8	Other acute kidney failure
N18.1	Chronic kidney disease, stage 1
N18.2	Chronic kidney disease, stage 2 (mild)
N18.31	Chronic kidney disease, stage 3a
N18.32	Chronic kidney disease, stage 3b
N18.4	Chronic kidney disease, stage 4 (severe)
N18.5	Chronic kidney disease, stage 5
N18.6	End stage renal disease
N25.0	Renal osteodystrophy
N28.1	Cyst of kidney, acquired
Q60.0	Renal agenesis, unilateral
Q60.1	Renal agenesis, bilateral
Q60.3	Renal hypoplasia, unilateral
Q60.4	Renal hypoplasia, bilateral
Q60.6	Potter's syndrome
T86.11	Kidney transplant rejection
T86.12	Kidney transplant failure
T86.13	Kidney transplant infection
T86.19	Other complication of kidney transplant
Z48.22	Encounter for aftercare following kidney transplant

AMA: **50200** 2019,Apr,4; 2018,Jan,8; 2017,Jan,8; 2016,Jan,13; 2015,Jan,16; 2014,Jan,11 **50205** 2018,Jan,8; 2017,Jan,8; 2016,Jan,13; 2015,Jan,16; 2014,Jan,11

Relative Value Units/Medicare Edits

Non-Facility RVU	Work	PE	MP	Total
50200	2.38	12.87	0.22	15.47
50205	12.29	6.9	2.75	21.94
Facility RVU	Work	PE	MP	Total
50200	2.38	1.1	0.22	3.7
50205	12.29	6.9	2.75	21.94

	FUD	Status	MUE	Modifiers				IOM Reference
50200	0	A	1(3)	51	50	N/A	N/A	None
50205	90	A	1(3)	51	50	62*	80	

* with documentation

50220-50230

50220 Nephrectomy, including partial ureterectomy, any open approach including rib resection;

50225 complicated because of previous surgery on same kidney

50230 radical, with regional lymphadenectomy and/or vena caval thrombectomy

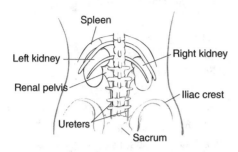

A kidney and part of a ureter is removed along with a portion of rib

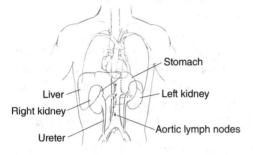

Explanation

The physician removes the kidney and upper portion of the ureter. To access the kidney and ureter, the physician usually makes an incision in the skin of the flank; cuts the muscles, fat, and fibrous membranes (fascia) overlying the kidney; and sometimes removes a portion of the eleventh or twelfth rib. After mobilizing the kidney and ureter, the physician clamps, ligates, and severs the upper ureter and major renal blood vessels (renal pedicle). The physician removes the kidney and upper ureter in 50220 and removes the kidney, upper ureter, neural and vascular structures at the apex of the renal pelvis, surrounding fat, Gerota's fascia, adrenal gland, and involved renal lymph nodes in 50230. The physician irrigates the site, places a drain tube, removes the clamps, and performs a layered closure. In a transthoracic approach, the lung is re-expanded and the chest tube left in. Report 50225 when a previous surgery on the kidney and/or ureter complicates the procedure.

Coding Tips

For a nephrectomy with total ureterectomy, see 50234–50236. For a partial nephrectomy, see 50240. For a laparoscopic radical nephrectomy, see 50545. For a laparoscopic nephrectomy with partial ureterectomy, see 50546. If significant additional time and effort is documented, append modifier 22 and submit a cover letter and operative report.

ICD-10-CM Diagnostic Codes

C64.1	Malignant neoplasm of right kidney, except renal pelvis ☑
C64.2	Malignant neoplasm of left kidney, except renal pelvis ☑
C65.1	Malignant neoplasm of right renal pelvis ☑
C65.2	Malignant neoplasm of left renal pelvis ☑
C66.1	Malignant neoplasm of right ureter ☑
C66.2	Malignant neoplasm of left ureter ☑
C68.8	Malignant neoplasm of overlapping sites of urinary organs
C79.01	Secondary malignant neoplasm of right kidney and renal pelvis ☑
C79.02	Secondary malignant neoplasm of left kidney and renal pelvis ☑
C7A.093	Malignant carcinoid tumor of the kidney
C80.2	Malignant neoplasm associated with transplanted organ
D09.19	Carcinoma in situ of other urinary organs
D30.01	Benign neoplasm of right kidney ☑
D30.02	Benign neoplasm of left kidney ☑
D30.11	Benign neoplasm of right renal pelvis ☑
D30.12	Benign neoplasm of left renal pelvis ☑
D30.21	Benign neoplasm of right ureter ☑
D30.22	Benign neoplasm of left ureter ☑
D3A.093	Benign carcinoid tumor of the kidney
D41.01	Neoplasm of uncertain behavior of right kidney ☑
D41.02	Neoplasm of uncertain behavior of left kidney ☑
D41.11	Neoplasm of uncertain behavior of right renal pelvis ☑
D41.12	Neoplasm of uncertain behavior of left renal pelvis ☑
D41.21	Neoplasm of uncertain behavior of right ureter ☑
D41.22	Neoplasm of uncertain behavior of left ureter ☑
D47.Z1	Post-transplant lymphoproliferative disorder (PTLD)
D47.Z2	Castleman disease
D49.511	Neoplasm of unspecified behavior of right kidney ☑
D49.512	Neoplasm of unspecified behavior of left kidney ☑
D49.59	Neoplasm of unspecified behavior of other genitourinary organ
I12.0	Hypertensive chronic kidney disease with stage 5 chronic kidney disease or end stage renal disease
I15.0	Renovascular hypertension
I16.0	Hypertensive urgency
I16.1	Hypertensive emergency
N00.0	Acute nephritic syndrome with minor glomerular abnormality
N00.1	Acute nephritic syndrome with focal and segmental glomerular lesions
N00.2	Acute nephritic syndrome with diffuse membranous glomerulonephritis
N00.3	Acute nephritic syndrome with diffuse mesangial proliferative glomerulonephritis
N00.4	Acute nephritic syndrome with diffuse endocapillary proliferative glomerulonephritis
N00.5	Acute nephritic syndrome with diffuse mesangiocapillary glomerulonephritis
N00.6	Acute nephritic syndrome with dense deposit disease
N00.7	Acute nephritic syndrome with diffuse crescentic glomerulonephritis
N00.A	Acute nephritic syndrome with C3 glomerulonephritis
N03.0	Chronic nephritic syndrome with minor glomerular abnormality
N03.1	Chronic nephritic syndrome with focal and segmental glomerular lesions
N03.2	Chronic nephritic syndrome with diffuse membranous glomerulonephritis
N03.3	Chronic nephritic syndrome with diffuse mesangial proliferative glomerulonephritis

Kidney

N03.4	Chronic nephritic syndrome with diffuse endocapillary proliferative glomerulonephritis
N03.5	Chronic nephritic syndrome with diffuse mesangiocapillary glomerulonephritis
N03.6	Chronic nephritic syndrome with dense deposit disease
N03.7	Chronic nephritic syndrome with diffuse crescentic glomerulonephritis
N03.8	Chronic nephritic syndrome with other morphologic changes
N03.A	Chronic nephritic syndrome with C3 glomerulonephritis
N04.0	Nephrotic syndrome with minor glomerular abnormality
N04.1	Nephrotic syndrome with focal and segmental glomerular lesions
N04.2	Nephrotic syndrome with diffuse membranous glomerulonephritis
N04.3	Nephrotic syndrome with diffuse mesangial proliferative glomerulonephritis
N04.4	Nephrotic syndrome with diffuse endocapillary proliferative glomerulonephritis
N04.5	Nephrotic syndrome with diffuse mesangiocapillary glomerulonephritis
N04.6	Nephrotic syndrome with dense deposit disease
N04.7	Nephrotic syndrome with diffuse crescentic glomerulonephritis
N04.8	Nephrotic syndrome with other morphologic changes
N04.A	Nephrotic syndrome with C3 glomerulonephritis
N11.0	Nonobstructive reflux-associated chronic pyelonephritis
N11.1	Chronic obstructive pyelonephritis
N11.8	Other chronic tubulo-interstitial nephritis
N13.0	Hydronephrosis with ureteropelvic junction obstruction
N13.1	Hydronephrosis with ureteral stricture, not elsewhere classified
N13.2	Hydronephrosis with renal and ureteral calculous obstruction
N13.39	Other hydronephrosis
N13.4	Hydroureter
N13.5	Crossing vessel and stricture of ureter without hydronephrosis
N13.6	Pyonephrosis
N13.71	Vesicoureteral-reflux without reflux nephropathy
N13.721	Vesicoureteral-reflux with reflux nephropathy without hydroureter, unilateral
N13.722	Vesicoureteral-reflux with reflux nephropathy without hydroureter, bilateral
N13.731	Vesicoureteral-reflux with reflux nephropathy with hydroureter, unilateral
N13.732	Vesicoureteral-reflux with reflux nephropathy with hydroureter, bilateral
N13.8	Other obstructive and reflux uropathy
N17.0	Acute kidney failure with tubular necrosis
N17.1	Acute kidney failure with acute cortical necrosis
N17.2	Acute kidney failure with medullary necrosis
N17.8	Other acute kidney failure
N18.4	Chronic kidney disease, stage 4 (severe)
N18.5	Chronic kidney disease, stage 5
N18.6	End stage renal disease
N20.0	Calculus of kidney
N20.2	Calculus of kidney with calculus of ureter
N26.1	Atrophy of kidney (terminal)
N26.2	Page kidney

N28.0	Ischemia and infarction of kidney
N28.1	Cyst of kidney, acquired
N28.81	Hypertrophy of kidney
N28.82	Megaloureter
N28.89	Other specified disorders of kidney and ureter
Q60.3	Renal hypoplasia, unilateral
Q60.4	Renal hypoplasia, bilateral
Q60.6	Potter's syndrome
Q61.01	Congenital single renal cyst
Q61.02	Congenital multiple renal cysts
Q61.11	Cystic dilatation of collecting ducts
Q61.19	Other polycystic kidney, infantile type
Q61.2	Polycystic kidney, adult type
Q61.4	Renal dysplasia
Q61.5	Medullary cystic kidney
Q61.8	Other cystic kidney diseases
Q62.0	Congenital hydronephrosis
Q62.11	Congenital occlusion of ureteropelvic junction
Q62.31	Congenital ureterocele, orthotopic
Q62.32	Cecoureterocele
Q62.39	Other obstructive defects of renal pelvis and ureter
S37.061A	Major laceration of right kidney, initial encounter ☑
S37.062A	Major laceration of left kidney, initial encounter ☑
S37.091A	Other injury of right kidney, initial encounter ☑
S37.092A	Other injury of left kidney, initial encounter ☑

AMA: **50220** 2018,Jan,8; 2017,Jan,8; 2016,Jan,13; 2015,Jan,16; 2014,Jan,11 **50225** 2018,Jan,8; 2017,Jan,8; 2016,Jan,13; 2015,Jan,16; 2014,Jan,11 **50230** 2018,Jan,8; 2017,Jan,8; 2016,Jan,13; 2015,Jan,16; 2014,Jan,11

Relative Value Units/Medicare Edits

Non-Facility RVU	Work	PE	MP	Total
50220	18.68	8.99	2.64	30.31
50225	21.88	9.98	2.87	34.73
50230	23.81	10.28	2.95	37.04
Facility RVU	Work	PE	MP	Total
50220	18.68	8.99	2.64	30.31
50225	21.88	9.98	2.87	34.73
50230	23.81	10.28	2.95	37.04

	FUD	Status	MUE	Modifiers				IOM Reference
50220	90	A	1(2)	51	50	62*	80	None
50225	90	A	1(2)	51	50	62*	80	
50230	90	A	1(2)	51	50	62	80	

* with documentation

50234-50236

50234 Nephrectomy with total ureterectomy and bladder cuff; through same incision

50236 through separate incision

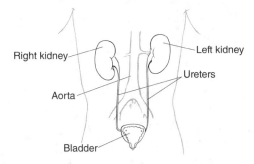

A kidney, ureter, and small bladder section are removed

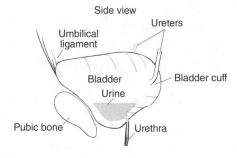

Explanation

The physician removes the kidney, ureter, and small cuff of the bladder through one excision in 50234 and through a separate incision in 50236. To access the kidney and ureter, the physician usually makes an incision in the skin of the flank, cuts the muscles, fat, and fibrous membranes (fascia) overlying the kidney, and sometimes removes a portion of the eleventh or twelfth rib. After mobilizing the kidney, ureter, and bladder, the physician clamps, ligates, and severs the ureter, major renal blood vessels (renal pedicle), and a small cuff of the bladder. The physician pulls the kidney, ureter, and bladder cuff upward through the flank incision. In both procedures, the physician does not remove the adrenal gland, surrounding fatty tissue, or Gerota's fascia. After controlling bleeding, the physician irrigates the site with normal saline and places a drain tube through a separate stab incision in the skin. In 50236, access to the lower ureter and bladder is made with an incision through the skin of the abdomen. Similarly to 50234, after mobilizing the bladder, the physician removes the lower ureter and a small cuff of the bladder. In both services, the physician sutures and catheterizes the bladder and after placing a drain tube behind the bladder, the clamps are removed and a layered closure is performed.

Coding Tips

For a partial nephrectomy, see 50240; via laparoscopic approach, see 50543. For laparoscopic nephrectomy with total ureterectomy, see 50548. For nephrectomy, including partial ureterectomy, see 50220–50230.

ICD-10-CM Diagnostic Codes

C64.1	Malignant neoplasm of right kidney, except renal pelvis ☑
C64.2	Malignant neoplasm of left kidney, except renal pelvis ☑
C65.1	Malignant neoplasm of right renal pelvis ☑
C65.2	Malignant neoplasm of left renal pelvis ☑
C66.1	Malignant neoplasm of right ureter ☑
C66.2	Malignant neoplasm of left ureter ☑
C68.8	Malignant neoplasm of overlapping sites of urinary organs
C79.01	Secondary malignant neoplasm of right kidney and renal pelvis ☑
C79.02	Secondary malignant neoplasm of left kidney and renal pelvis ☑
C79.11	Secondary malignant neoplasm of bladder
C79.19	Secondary malignant neoplasm of other urinary organs
C7A.093	Malignant carcinoid tumor of the kidney
C80.2	Malignant neoplasm associated with transplanted organ
D09.19	Carcinoma in situ of other urinary organs
D30.01	Benign neoplasm of right kidney ☑
D30.02	Benign neoplasm of left kidney ☑
D30.11	Benign neoplasm of right renal pelvis ☑
D30.12	Benign neoplasm of left renal pelvis ☑
D30.21	Benign neoplasm of right ureter ☑
D30.22	Benign neoplasm of left ureter ☑
D3A.093	Benign carcinoid tumor of the kidney
D41.01	Neoplasm of uncertain behavior of right kidney ☑
D41.02	Neoplasm of uncertain behavior of left kidney ☑
D41.11	Neoplasm of uncertain behavior of right renal pelvis ☑
D41.12	Neoplasm of uncertain behavior of left renal pelvis ☑
D41.21	Neoplasm of uncertain behavior of right ureter ☑
D41.22	Neoplasm of uncertain behavior of left ureter ☑
D47.Z1	Post-transplant lymphoproliferative disorder (PTLD)
D47.Z2	Castleman disease
D49.511	Neoplasm of unspecified behavior of right kidney ☑
D49.512	Neoplasm of unspecified behavior of left kidney ☑
D49.59	Neoplasm of unspecified behavior of other genitourinary organ
I12.0	Hypertensive chronic kidney disease with stage 5 chronic kidney disease or end stage renal disease
I13.11	Hypertensive heart and chronic kidney disease without heart failure, with stage 5 chronic kidney disease, or end stage renal disease
I15.0	Renovascular hypertension
I16.0	Hypertensive urgency
I16.1	Hypertensive emergency
I75.81	Atheroembolism of kidney
N00.0	Acute nephritic syndrome with minor glomerular abnormality
N00.1	Acute nephritic syndrome with focal and segmental glomerular lesions
N00.2	Acute nephritic syndrome with diffuse membranous glomerulonephritis
N00.3	Acute nephritic syndrome with diffuse mesangial proliferative glomerulonephritis
N00.4	Acute nephritic syndrome with diffuse endocapillary proliferative glomerulonephritis
N00.5	Acute nephritic syndrome with diffuse mesangiocapillary glomerulonephritis
N00.6	Acute nephritic syndrome with dense deposit disease
N00.7	Acute nephritic syndrome with diffuse crescentic glomerulonephritis
N03.0	Chronic nephritic syndrome with minor glomerular abnormality
N03.1	Chronic nephritic syndrome with focal and segmental glomerular lesions

Kidney

CPT © 2020 American Medical Association. All Rights Reserved.   ● New   ▲ Revised   + Add On   ★ Telemedicine   AMA: CPT Assist   [Resequenced]   ☑ Laterality   © 2020 Optum360, LLC

N03.2	Chronic nephritic syndrome with diffuse membranous glomerulonephritis
N03.3	Chronic nephritic syndrome with diffuse mesangial proliferative glomerulonephritis
N03.4	Chronic nephritic syndrome with diffuse endocapillary proliferative glomerulonephritis
N03.5	Chronic nephritic syndrome with diffuse mesangiocapillary glomerulonephritis
N03.6	Chronic nephritic syndrome with dense deposit disease
N03.7	Chronic nephritic syndrome with diffuse crescentic glomerulonephritis
N03.8	Chronic nephritic syndrome with other morphologic changes
N04.0	Nephrotic syndrome with minor glomerular abnormality
N04.1	Nephrotic syndrome with focal and segmental glomerular lesions
N04.2	Nephrotic syndrome with diffuse membranous glomerulonephritis
N04.3	Nephrotic syndrome with diffuse mesangial proliferative glomerulonephritis
N04.4	Nephrotic syndrome with diffuse endocapillary proliferative glomerulonephritis
N04.5	Nephrotic syndrome with diffuse mesangiocapillary glomerulonephritis
N04.6	Nephrotic syndrome with dense deposit disease
N04.7	Nephrotic syndrome with diffuse crescentic glomerulonephritis
N04.8	Nephrotic syndrome with other morphologic changes
N11.0	Nonobstructive reflux-associated chronic pyelonephritis
N11.1	Chronic obstructive pyelonephritis
N11.8	Other chronic tubulo-interstitial nephritis
N13.0	Hydronephrosis with ureteropelvic junction obstruction
N13.1	Hydronephrosis with ureteral stricture, not elsewhere classified
N13.2	Hydronephrosis with renal and ureteral calculous obstruction
N13.39	Other hydronephrosis
N13.4	Hydroureter
N13.5	Crossing vessel and stricture of ureter without hydronephrosis
N13.6	Pyonephrosis
N13.71	Vesicoureteral-reflux without reflux nephropathy
N13.721	Vesicoureteral-reflux with reflux nephropathy without hydroureter, unilateral
N13.722	Vesicoureteral-reflux with reflux nephropathy without hydroureter, bilateral
N13.731	Vesicoureteral-reflux with reflux nephropathy with hydroureter, unilateral
N13.732	Vesicoureteral-reflux with reflux nephropathy with hydroureter, bilateral
N13.8	Other obstructive and reflux uropathy
N17.0	Acute kidney failure with tubular necrosis
N17.1	Acute kidney failure with acute cortical necrosis
N17.2	Acute kidney failure with medullary necrosis
N18.4	Chronic kidney disease, stage 4 (severe)
N18.5	Chronic kidney disease, stage 5
N18.6	End stage renal disease
N20.0	Calculus of kidney
N20.2	Calculus of kidney with calculus of ureter
N26.1	Atrophy of kidney (terminal)
N26.2	Page kidney

N28.0	Ischemia and infarction of kidney
N28.1	Cyst of kidney, acquired
N28.81	Hypertrophy of kidney
N28.82	Megaloureter
Q60.3	Renal hypoplasia, unilateral
Q60.4	Renal hypoplasia, bilateral
Q60.6	Potter's syndrome
Q61.01	Congenital single renal cyst
Q61.02	Congenital multiple renal cysts
Q61.11	Cystic dilatation of collecting ducts
Q61.2	Polycystic kidney, adult type
Q61.4	Renal dysplasia
Q61.5	Medullary cystic kidney
Q62.0	Congenital hydronephrosis
Q62.11	Congenital occlusion of ureteropelvic junction
Q62.31	Congenital ureterocele, orthotopic
Q62.32	Cecoureterocele
Q62.39	Other obstructive defects of renal pelvis and ureter
S37.061A	Major laceration of right kidney, initial encounter ☑
S37.062A	Major laceration of left kidney, initial encounter ☑
S37.091A	Other injury of right kidney, initial encounter ☑
S37.092A	Other injury of left kidney, initial encounter ☑

AMA: 50234 2018,Jan,8; 2017,Jan,8; 2016,Jan,13; 2015,Jan,16; 2014,Jan,11
50236 2018,Jan,8; 2017,Jan,8; 2016,Jan,13; 2015,Jan,16; 2014,Jan,11

Relative Value Units/Medicare Edits

Non-Facility RVU	Work	PE	MP	Total
50234	24.05	10.64	2.93	37.62
50236	26.94	12.26	3.1	42.3
Facility RVU	Work	PE	MP	Total
50234	24.05	10.64	2.93	37.62
50236	26.94	12.26	3.1	42.3

	FUD	Status	MUE	Modifiers				IOM Reference
50234	90	A	1(2)	51	50	62*	80	None
50236	90	A	1(2)	51	50	62*	80	

* with documentation

Terms To Know

drain. Device that creates a channel to allow fluid from a cavity, wound, or infected area to exit the body.

flank. Part of the body found between the posterior ribs and the uppermost crest of the ilium, or the lateral side of the hip, thigh, and buttock.

nephrectomy. Partial or total removal of the kidney that may be performed for indications such as irreparable kidney damage, renal cell carcinoma, trauma, congenital abnormalities, or transplant purposes.

ureterectomy. Excision of all or part of a ureter. This procedure may be performed alone or as part of another procedure, such as urinary diversion or nephrectomy.

50240

50240 Nephrectomy, partial

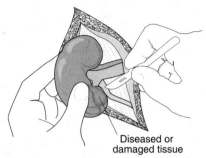

The physician excises a wedge of diseased or damaged kidney

Diseased or damaged tissue

Layered closure includes suturing of excision site

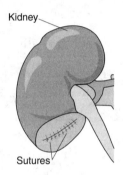

Kidney

Sutures

Explanation

The physician removes a portion of the kidney. To access the kidney and ureter, the physician usually makes an incision in the skin of the flank, cuts the muscles, fat, and fibrous membranes (fascia) overlying the kidney, and sometimes removes a portion of the eleventh or twelfth rib. After mobilizing the kidney and the major renal blood vessels (renal pedicle), the physician clamps the renal vessels, and sometimes induces hypothermia of the kidney with iced saline slush. The physician excises a wedge containing the diseased or damaged kidney tissue. After clamping and ligating the exposed arteries and veins, the physician inserts a drain tube, bringing it out through a separate stab incision in the skin, removes the clamps, and performs a layered closure.

Coding Tips

For nephrectomy, with partial ureterectomy, see 50220–50225; radical, with regional lymphadenectomy, see 50230. For nephrectomy, with total ureterectomy, see 50234–50236. For partial nephrectomy performed laparoscopically, see 50543.

ICD-10-CM Diagnostic Codes

C64.1	Malignant neoplasm of right kidney, except renal pelvis	☑
C64.2	Malignant neoplasm of left kidney, except renal pelvis	☑
C65.1	Malignant neoplasm of right renal pelvis	☑
C65.2	Malignant neoplasm of left renal pelvis	☑
C66.1	Malignant neoplasm of right ureter	☑
C66.2	Malignant neoplasm of left ureter	☑
C68.8	Malignant neoplasm of overlapping sites of urinary organs	
C79.01	Secondary malignant neoplasm of right kidney and renal pelvis	☑

C79.02	Secondary malignant neoplasm of left kidney and renal pelvis	☑
C7A.093	Malignant carcinoid tumor of the kidney	
C80.2	Malignant neoplasm associated with transplanted organ	
D09.19	Carcinoma in situ of other urinary organs	
D30.01	Benign neoplasm of right kidney	☑
D30.02	Benign neoplasm of left kidney	☑
D30.11	Benign neoplasm of right renal pelvis	☑
D30.12	Benign neoplasm of left renal pelvis	☑
D30.21	Benign neoplasm of right ureter	☑
D30.22	Benign neoplasm of left ureter	☑
D3A.093	Benign carcinoid tumor of the kidney	
D41.01	Neoplasm of uncertain behavior of right kidney	☑
D41.02	Neoplasm of uncertain behavior of left kidney	☑
D41.11	Neoplasm of uncertain behavior of right renal pelvis	☑
D41.12	Neoplasm of uncertain behavior of left renal pelvis	☑
D41.21	Neoplasm of uncertain behavior of right ureter	☑
D41.22	Neoplasm of uncertain behavior of left ureter	☑
D47.Z1	Post-transplant lymphoproliferative disorder (PTLD)	
D47.Z2	Castleman disease	
D49.511	Neoplasm of unspecified behavior of right kidney	☑
D49.512	Neoplasm of unspecified behavior of left kidney	☑
D49.59	Neoplasm of unspecified behavior of other genitourinary organ	
I12.0	Hypertensive chronic kidney disease with stage 5 chronic kidney disease or end stage renal disease	
I15.0	Renovascular hypertension	
I16.0	Hypertensive urgency	
I16.1	Hypertensive emergency	
N00.0	Acute nephritic syndrome with minor glomerular abnormality	
N00.1	Acute nephritic syndrome with focal and segmental glomerular lesions	
N00.2	Acute nephritic syndrome with diffuse membranous glomerulonephritis	
N00.3	Acute nephritic syndrome with diffuse mesangial proliferative glomerulonephritis	
N00.4	Acute nephritic syndrome with diffuse endocapillary proliferative glomerulonephritis	
N00.5	Acute nephritic syndrome with diffuse mesangiocapillary glomerulonephritis	
N00.6	Acute nephritic syndrome with dense deposit disease	
N00.7	Acute nephritic syndrome with diffuse crescentic glomerulonephritis	
N03.0	Chronic nephritic syndrome with minor glomerular abnormality	
N03.1	Chronic nephritic syndrome with focal and segmental glomerular lesions	
N03.2	Chronic nephritic syndrome with diffuse membranous glomerulonephritis	
N03.3	Chronic nephritic syndrome with diffuse mesangial proliferative glomerulonephritis	
N03.4	Chronic nephritic syndrome with diffuse endocapillary proliferative glomerulonephritis	
N03.5	Chronic nephritic syndrome with diffuse mesangiocapillary glomerulonephritis	
N03.6	Chronic nephritic syndrome with dense deposit disease	
N03.7	Chronic nephritic syndrome with diffuse crescentic glomerulonephritis	

Kidney

N03.8	Chronic nephritic syndrome with other morphologic changes
N04.0	Nephrotic syndrome with minor glomerular abnormality
N04.1	Nephrotic syndrome with focal and segmental glomerular lesions
N04.2	Nephrotic syndrome with diffuse membranous glomerulonephritis
N04.3	Nephrotic syndrome with diffuse mesangial proliferative glomerulonephritis
N04.4	Nephrotic syndrome with diffuse endocapillary proliferative glomerulonephritis
N04.5	Nephrotic syndrome with diffuse mesangiocapillary glomerulonephritis
N04.6	Nephrotic syndrome with dense deposit disease
N04.7	Nephrotic syndrome with diffuse crescentic glomerulonephritis
N04.8	Nephrotic syndrome with other morphologic changes
N11.0	Nonobstructive reflux-associated chronic pyelonephritis
N11.1	Chronic obstructive pyelonephritis
N11.8	Other chronic tubulo-interstitial nephritis
N13.0	Hydronephrosis with ureteropelvic junction obstruction
N13.1	Hydronephrosis with ureteral stricture, not elsewhere classified
N13.2	Hydronephrosis with renal and ureteral calculous obstruction
N13.39	Other hydronephrosis
N13.4	Hydroureter
N13.5	Crossing vessel and stricture of ureter without hydronephrosis
N13.6	Pyonephrosis
N13.71	Vesicoureteral-reflux without reflux nephropathy
N13.721	Vesicoureteral-reflux with reflux nephropathy without hydroureter, unilateral
N13.722	Vesicoureteral-reflux with reflux nephropathy without hydroureter, bilateral
N13.731	Vesicoureteral-reflux with reflux nephropathy with hydroureter, unilateral
N13.732	Vesicoureteral-reflux with reflux nephropathy with hydroureter, bilateral
N13.8	Other obstructive and reflux uropathy
N17.0	Acute kidney failure with tubular necrosis
N17.1	Acute kidney failure with acute cortical necrosis
N17.2	Acute kidney failure with medullary necrosis
N17.8	Other acute kidney failure
N18.4	Chronic kidney disease, stage 4 (severe)
N18.5	Chronic kidney disease, stage 5
N18.6	End stage renal disease
N20.0	Calculus of kidney
N20.2	Calculus of kidney with calculus of ureter
N26.1	Atrophy of kidney (terminal)
N26.2	Page kidney
N28.0	Ischemia and infarction of kidney
N28.1	Cyst of kidney, acquired
N28.81	Hypertrophy of kidney
N28.82	Megaloureter
N28.89	Other specified disorders of kidney and ureter
Q60.3	Renal hypoplasia, unilateral
Q60.4	Renal hypoplasia, bilateral
Q60.6	Potter's syndrome
Q61.01	Congenital single renal cyst

Q61.02	Congenital multiple renal cysts
Q61.11	Cystic dilatation of collecting ducts
Q61.2	Polycystic kidney, adult type
Q61.4	Renal dysplasia
Q61.5	Medullary cystic kidney
Q61.8	Other cystic kidney diseases
Q62.0	Congenital hydronephrosis
Q62.11	Congenital occlusion of ureteropelvic junction
Q62.31	Congenital ureterocele, orthotopic
Q62.32	Cecoureterocele
Q62.39	Other obstructive defects of renal pelvis and ureter
S37.061A	Major laceration of right kidney, initial encounter ☑
S37.062A	Major laceration of left kidney, initial encounter ☑
S37.091A	Other injury of right kidney, initial encounter ☑
S37.092A	Other injury of left kidney, initial encounter ☑

AMA: 50240 2018,Jan,8; 2017,Jan,8; 2016,Jan,13; 2015,Jan,16; 2014,Jan,11

Relative Value Units/Medicare Edits

Non-Facility RVU	Work	PE	MP	Total
50240	24.21	11.21	2.86	38.28
Facility RVU	**Work**	**PE**	**MP**	**Total**
50240	24.21	11.21	2.86	38.28

	FUD	Status	MUE	Modifiers				IOM Reference
50240	90	A	1(2)	51	50	62*	80	None

* with documentation

Terms To Know

acquired. Produced by outside influences and not by genetics or birth defect.

clamp. Tool used to grip, compress, join, or fasten body parts.

congenital. Present at birth, occurring through heredity or an influence during gestation up to the moment of birth.

drain. Device that creates a channel to allow fluid from a cavity, wound, or infected area to exit the body.

flank. Part of the body found between the posterior ribs and the uppermost crest of the ilium, or the lateral side of the hip, thigh, and buttock.

hydronephrosis. Distension of the kidney caused by an accumulation of urine that cannot flow out due to an obstruction that may be caused by conditions such as kidney stones or vesicoureteral reflux.

ligate. To tie off a blood vessel or duct with a suture or a soft, thin wire (ligature wire).

nephrectomy. Partial or total removal of the kidney that may be performed for indications such as irreparable kidney damage, renal cell carcinoma, trauma, congenital abnormalities, or transplant purposes.

tissue. Group of similar cells with a similar function that form definite structures and organs. Tissue types include epithelial tissue, muscle tissue, connective tissue, and nervous tissue.

50250

50250 Ablation, open, 1 or more renal mass lesion(s), cryosurgical, including intraoperative ultrasound guidance and monitoring, if performed

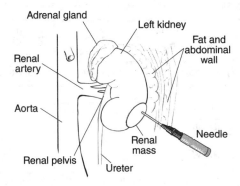

Explanation
The physician performs cryosurgical ablation of one or more renal mass lesions. The physician performs a laparotomy. Dissection is carried down to the kidney. Intraoperative ultrasound guidance and monitoring may be used to identify the lesion and monitor progress of the procedure. Cryosurgical probes are inserted into the kidney lesion. The cryosurgical probe delivers cryogen, a coolant, at subfreezing temperatures to freeze the lesion. The renal tissue is slowly thawed. A minimum of two cycles of freezing and thawing are performed. This is repeated for each lesion. When all lesions have been treated, the incision is closed with layered sutures.

Coding Tips
For laparoscopic ablation of a renal mass lesion, see 50542. Percutaneous ablation of renal tumors is reported with 50592–50593.

ICD-10-CM Diagnostic Codes
C64.1	Malignant neoplasm of right kidney, except renal pelvis ☑
C64.2	Malignant neoplasm of left kidney, except renal pelvis ☑
C65.1	Malignant neoplasm of right renal pelvis ☑
C65.2	Malignant neoplasm of left renal pelvis ☑
C79.01	Secondary malignant neoplasm of right kidney and renal pelvis ☑
C79.02	Secondary malignant neoplasm of left kidney and renal pelvis ☑
C7A.093	Malignant carcinoid tumor of the kidney
C80.2	Malignant neoplasm associated with transplanted organ
D09.19	Carcinoma in situ of other urinary organs
D30.01	Benign neoplasm of right kidney ☑
D30.02	Benign neoplasm of left kidney ☑
D30.11	Benign neoplasm of right renal pelvis ☑
D30.12	Benign neoplasm of left renal pelvis ☑
D3A.093	Benign carcinoid tumor of the kidney
D41.01	Neoplasm of uncertain behavior of right kidney ☑
D41.02	Neoplasm of uncertain behavior of left kidney ☑
D41.11	Neoplasm of uncertain behavior of right renal pelvis ☑
D41.12	Neoplasm of uncertain behavior of left renal pelvis ☑
D49.511	Neoplasm of unspecified behavior of right kidney ☑
D49.512	Neoplasm of unspecified behavior of left kidney ☑
D49.59	Neoplasm of unspecified behavior of other genitourinary organ
N28.1	Cyst of kidney, acquired
N28.89	Other specified disorders of kidney and ureter

Q61.01	Congenital single renal cyst
Q61.02	Congenital multiple renal cysts
Q61.11	Cystic dilatation of collecting ducts
Q61.19	Other polycystic kidney, infantile type
Q61.2	Polycystic kidney, adult type
Q61.4	Renal dysplasia
Q61.5	Medullary cystic kidney
Q61.8	Other cystic kidney diseases

AMA: 50250 2018,Jan,8; 2017,Jan,8; 2016,Jan,13; 2015,Jan,16; 2014,Jan,11

Relative Value Units/Medicare Edits

Non-Facility RVU	Work	PE	MP	Total
50250	22.22	10.36	2.56	35.14
Facility RVU	**Work**	**PE**	**MP**	**Total**
50250	22.22	10.36	2.56	35.14

	FUD	Status	MUE	Modifiers				IOM Reference
50250	90	A	1(3)	51	N/A	62*	80	None

* with documentation

Terms To Know

ablation. Removal or destruction of tissue by cutting, electrical energy, chemical substances, or excessive heat application.

cryosurgery. Application of intense cold, usually produced using liquid nitrogen, to locally freeze diseased or unwanted tissue and induce tissue necrosis without causing harm to adjacent tissue.

dissection. (dis. apart; -section, act of cutting) Separating by cutting tissue or body structures apart.

dysplasia. Abnormality or alteration in the size, shape, and organization of cells from their normal pattern of development.

laparotomy. Incision through the flank or abdomen for therapeutic or diagnostic purposes.

lesion. Area of damaged tissue that has lost continuity or function, due to disease or trauma.

malignant neoplasm. Any cancerous tumor or lesion exhibiting uncontrolled tissue growth that can progressively invade other parts of the body with its disease-generating cells.

renal. Referring to the kidney.

ultrasound. Imaging using ultra-high sound frequency bounced off body structures.

Kidney

CPT © 2020 American Medical Association. All Rights Reserved.   ● New   ▲ Revised   + Add On   ★ Telemedicine   AMA: CPT Assist   [Resequenced]   ☑ Laterality   © 2020 Optum360, LLC

50280-50290

50280   Excision or unroofing of cyst(s) of kidney
50290   Excision of perinephric cyst

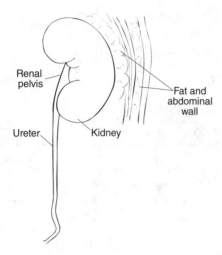

Renal pelvis

Fat and abdominal wall

Ureter

Kidney

Explanation

The physician excises a cyst on the kidney or in the surrounding renal tissue. To access the kidney, the physician makes an incision in the skin of the flank, cuts the muscles, fat, and fibrous membranes (fascia) overlying the kidney, and sometimes removes a portion of the twelfth rib. After clearing away the fatty tissue surrounding the kidney, the physician excises the cyst from the renal surface. The physician destroys tiny vessels bordering the cyst with high-frequency electric current (fulguration) to minimize the need for sutures. If the cyst requires a deep excision, the physician usually sutures the renal tissue. The physician inserts a drain tube, bringing it out through a separate stab incision in the skin, and performs a layered closure. 50280 reports excision of a cyst (or cysts) on the kidney; 50290 reports excision of a cyst (or cysts) in the tissue surrounding the kidney.

Coding Tips

For laparoscopic ablation of renal cysts, see 50541.

ICD-10-CM Diagnostic Codes

N28.1	Cyst of kidney, acquired
N28.89	Other specified disorders of kidney and ureter
Q61.01	Congenital single renal cyst
Q61.02	Congenital multiple renal cysts
Q61.11	Cystic dilatation of collecting ducts
Q61.19	Other polycystic kidney, infantile type
Q61.2	Polycystic kidney, adult type
Q61.8	Other cystic kidney diseases

AMA: 50280 2018,Jan,8; 2017,Jan,8; 2016,Jan,13; 2015,Jan,16; 2014,Jan,11
50290 2018,Jan,8; 2017,Jan,8; 2016,Jan,13; 2015,Jan,16; 2014,Jan,11

Relative Value Units/Medicare Edits

Non-Facility RVU	Work	PE	MP	Total
50280	17.09	8.37	2.23	27.69
50290	16.15	7.94	1.85	25.94
Facility RVU	**Work**	**PE**	**MP**	**Total**
50280	17.09	8.37	2.23	27.69
50290	16.15	7.94	1.85	25.94

	FUD	Status	MUE	Modifiers				IOM Reference
50280	90	A	1(2)	51	50	62*	80	None
50290	90	A	1(3)	51	N/A	62*	80	

* with documentation

Terms To Know

acquired. Produced by outside influences and not by genetics or birth defect.

congenital. Present at birth, occurring through heredity or an influence during gestation up to the moment of birth.

cyst. Elevated encapsulated mass containing fluid, semisolid, or solid material with a membranous lining.

excision. Surgical removal of an organ or tissue.

fascia. Fibrous sheet or band of tissue that envelops organs, muscles, and groupings of muscles.

flank. Part of the body found between the posterior ribs and the uppermost crest of the ilium, or the lateral side of the hip, thigh, and buttock.

fulguration. Destruction of living tissue by using sparks from a high-frequency electric current.

polycystic. Multiple cysts.

renal. Referring to the kidney.

suture. Numerous stitching techniques employed in wound closure.

buried suture. Continuous or interrupted suture placed under the skin for a layered closure.

continuous suture. Running stitch with tension evenly distributed across a single strand to provide a leakproof closure line.

interrupted suture. Series of single stitches with tension isolated at each stitch, in which all stitches are not affected if one becomes loose, and the isolated sutures cannot act as a wick to transport an infection.

purse-string suture. Continuous suture placed around a tubular structure and tightened, to reduce or close the lumen.

retention suture. Secondary stitching that bridges the primary suture, providing support for the primary repair; a plastic or rubber bolster may be placed over the primary repair and under the retention sutures.

tissue. Group of similar cells with a similar function that form definite structures and organs. Tissue types include epithelial tissue, muscle tissue, connective tissue, and nervous tissue.

Kidney

50300-50320

50300 Donor nephrectomy (including cold preservation); from cadaver donor, unilateral or bilateral
50320 open, from living donor

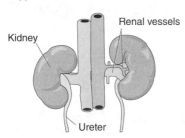

One or both kidneys, renal vessels, and upper ureter are removed from donor

Renal vessels
Kidney
Ureter

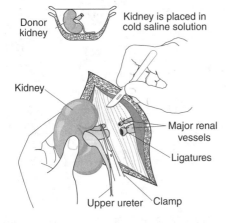

Donor kidney
Kidney is placed in cold saline solution

Kidney
Major renal vessels
Ligatures
Upper ureter
Clamp

Explanation

In 50300, the physician performs a donor nephrectomy by removing the kidney and upper ureter from a cadaver for transplantation. To access the kidney and upper ureter, the physician usually makes a midline incision in the skin from the xiphoid process to the symphysis pubis. After cutting the muscles, fat, and fibrous membranes (fascia) overlying the kidney, the physician uses clamps, ties, suture ligatures, and electrocoagulation to control bleeding. Before clamping the major renal blood vessels (renal pedicle), the physician administers heparin sodium to prevent intravascular clotting. The physician dissects and removes the kidney, renal vessels, and ureter, usually removing sections of the inferior vena cava and aorta with both kidneys. The donor kidney is preserved for transplantation into the recipient. The organ remains under refrigeration, packed in a sealable container with some preserving solution and kept on ice in a suitable carrier. In 50320, the physician performs an open donor nephrectomy from a living donor by removing one kidney and upper ureter for transplantation. To access the kidney, the physician usually makes an incision in the skin of the flank, cuts the muscles, fat, and fibrous membranes (fascia) overlying the kidney, and sometimes removes a portion of the eleventh or twelfth rib. After mobilizing the kidney and ureter, the physician administers an anticlogging agent. The physician clamps, ligates, and severs the upper ureter and major renal blood vessels (renal pedicle), and removes the kidney and upper ureter. The physician administers medication to reverse the effects of the anticlogging agent. After controlling bleeding, the physician irrigates the site, places a drain tube, and performs a layered closure. The donor kidney is preserved for transplantation into the recipient. The organ remains under refrigeration, packed in a sealable container with some preserving solution and kept on ice in a suitable carrier.

Coding Tips

For laparoscopic donor nephrectomy from living donor, see 50547. For backbench of cadaver donor renal allograft preparation prior to transplant, see 50323; living donor, see 50325. For backbench reconstruction of cadaver or living donor renal allograft procedures, see 50327–50329.

ICD-10-CM Diagnostic Codes

Z52.4 Kidney donor

AMA: 50300 2018,Jan,8; 2017,Jan,8; 2016,Jan,13; 2015,Jan,16; 2014,Jan,11
50320 2018,Jan,8; 2017,Jan,8; 2016,Jan,13; 2015,Jan,16; 2014,Jan,11

Relative Value Units/Medicare Edits

Non-Facility RVU	Work	PE	MP	Total
50300	0.0	0.0	0.0	0.0
50320	22.43	15.84	5.45	43.72
Facility RVU	**Work**	**PE**	**MP**	**Total**
50300	0.0	0.0	0.0	0.0
50320	22.43	15.84	5.45	43.72

	FUD	Status	MUE	Modifiers				IOM Reference
50300	N/A	X	1(2)	N/A	N/A	N/A	N/A	100-03,20.3;
50320	90	A	1(2)	51	50	62*	80	100-03,190.1; 100-04,3,90.1.1

* with documentation

Terms To Know

allograft. Graft from one individual to another of the same species.

cadaver. Dead body.

donor. Person from whom tissues or organs are removed for transplantation.

fascia. Fibrous sheet or band of tissue that envelops organs, muscles, and groupings of muscles.

homograft. Graft from one individual to another of the same species.

nephrectomy. Partial or total removal of the kidney that may be performed for indications such as irreparable kidney damage, renal cell carcinoma, trauma, congenital abnormalities, or transplant purposes.

transplantation. Grafting or movement of an organ or tissue from one site or person to another.

Kidney

50323

50323 Backbench standard preparation of cadaver donor renal allograft prior to transplantation, including dissection and removal of perinephric fat, diaphragmatic and retroperitoneal attachments, excision of adrenal gland, and preparation of ureter(s), renal vein(s), and renal artery(s), ligating branches, as necessary

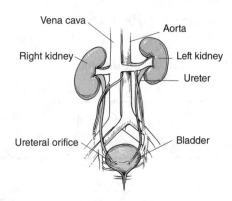

Explanation

The surgeon prepares a donor kidney from a cadaver prior to transplantation. Back table prep time is about an hour. The kidney and necessary vital structures removed en bloc usually contain some of the inferior vena cava, a cuff of aorta, perinephric tissue, the adrenal gland, and muscle, as well as some damaged blood vessels. The renal vein is dissected and the gonadal and adrenal veins are isolated and separated with ligatures. The renal artery is dissected from surrounding tissue along with the aortic patch. The adrenal gland, excess perinephric fat, and other tissue attachments are removed from the graft, taking care to leave fibrofatty tissue around the ureter to ensure its blood supply. The aortic patch, renal vein, and ureter are further repaired and/or modified to fit the recipient.

Coding Tips

Complete or partial adrenalectomy and excision of adjacent retroperitoneal tumor are included in this code and should not be reported separately. For donor nephrectomy from a cadaver, see 50300. Do not use 50323 in combination with 60540 or 60545.

ICD-10-CM Diagnostic Codes

This code is not identified as an add-on code by CPT® but is performed at the same time as another primary procedure. Refer to the corresponding primary procedure code for ICD-10-CM diagnosis code links.

AMA: 50323 2018,Jan,8; 2017,Jan,8; 2016,Jan,13; 2015,Jan,16; 2014,Jan,11

Relative Value Units/Medicare Edits

Non-Facility RVU	Work	PE	MP	Total
50323	0.0	0.0	0.0	0.0
Facility RVU	**Work**	**PE**	**MP**	**Total**
50323	0.0	0.0	0.0	0.0

	FUD	Status	MUE	Modifiers				IOM Reference
50323	N/A	C	1(2)	51	N/A	62*	80	None

* with documentation

50325

50325 Backbench standard preparation of living donor renal allograft (open or laparoscopic) prior to transplantation, including dissection and removal of perinephric fat and preparation of ureter(s), renal vein(s), and renal artery(s), ligating branches, as necessary

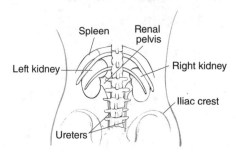

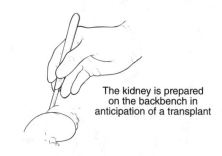

The kidney is prepared on the backbench in anticipation of a transplant

Explanation

The physician performs a standard backbench preparation of the kidney following procurement from a living donor. Backbench or back table preparation refers to procedures performed on the donor organ following procurement to prepare the donor organ for transplant. In a separately reportable procedure, the physician removes the kidney and upper ureter from a living donor. The kidney is flushed with a cold electrolyte solution to rinse any remaining donor blood from the kidney and lower its temperature. When the kidney is procured from a living donor, only minimal backbench preparation is required because most of the dissection is performed in situ during the nephrectomy. During the backbench preparation any excess perinephric fat and other tissue attachments are removed from the graft, taking care to leave fibrofatty tissue around the ureter to ensure its blood supply. Further separation of the renal artery or arteries from the renal veins is performed. The arterial and venous separation prevents the technical inconvenience of side-by-side anastomosis in the recipient. To reduce the risk of postoperative complications, the transplant ureter is shortened as needed leaving the vascularized periureteral fat intact. When all residual soft tissue has been removed and the blood vessels and ureters prepared, the kidney is ready for transplant.

Coding Tips

For donor nephrectomy from a living donor, see 50320. For laparoscopic donor nephrectomy, see 50547. For renal allotransplantation, see 50360–50365.

ICD-10-CM Diagnostic Codes

This code is not identified as an add-on code by CPT® but is performed at the same time as another primary procedure. Refer to the corresponding primary procedure code for ICD-10-CM diagnosis code links.

AMA: 50325 2014,Jan,11

Kidney

Relative Value Units/Medicare Edits

Non-Facility RVU	Work	PE	MP	Total
50325	0.0	0.0	0.0	0.0
Facility RVU	**Work**	**PE**	**MP**	**Total**
50325	0.0	0.0	0.0	0.0

	FUD	Status	MUE	Modifiers				IOM Reference
50325	N/A	C	1(2)	51	N/A	62*	80	None

* with documentation

Terms To Know

allograft. Graft from one individual to another of the same species.

anastomosis. Surgically created connection between ducts, blood vessels, or bowel segments to allow flow from one to the other.

backbench preparation. Procedures performed on a donor organ following procurement to prepare the organ for transplant into the recipient. Excess fat and other tissue may be removed, the organ may be perfused, and vital arteries may be sized, repaired, or modified to fit the patient. These procedures are done on a back table in the operating room before transplantation can begin.

dissection. (dis. apart; -section, act of cutting) Separating by cutting tissue or body structures apart.

donor. Person from whom tissues or organs are removed for transplantation.

in situ. Located in the natural position or contained within the origin site, not spread into neighboring tissue.

transplantation. Grafting or movement of an organ or tissue from one site or person to another.

ureter. Tube leading from the kidney to the urinary bladder made up of three layers of tissue: the mucous lining of the inner layer; the smooth, muscular middle layer that propels the urine from the kidney to the bladder by peristalsis; and the outer layer made of fibrous connective tissue. Each ureter leaves the kidney from the hilum, a concave notch on the middle surface, and enters the bladder through a narrow valve-like orifice that prevents the backflow of urine to the kidney.

50327

50327 Backbench reconstruction of cadaver or living donor renal allograft prior to transplantation; venous anastomosis, each

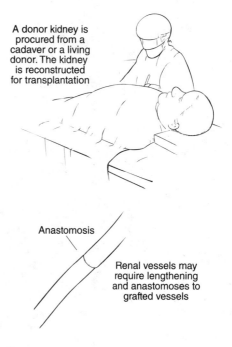

A donor kidney is procured from a cadaver or a living donor. The kidney is reconstructed for transplantation

Anastomosis

Renal vessels may require lengthening and anastomoses to grafted vessels

Explanation

The surgeon reconstructs a donor kidney from a cadaver or living donor prior to transplantation with a venous anastomosis. This procedure consists of performing venoplasties on the donor kidney to extend the renal vein before grafting. The inferior vena cava is used from a cadaver donor. When the donor organ comes from a living donor, a cuff of the inferior vena cava attached to the renal vein is used. When the donor organ comes from a cadaveric source, the external iliac vein is also routinely procured and prepared for venous grafting to extend the renal vein for the recipient. The vessels are tested for patency by flushing with a sterile preservation solution.

Coding Tips

For donor nephrectomy, see 50300–50320. For laparoscopic donor nephrectomy, see 50547. For renal allotransplantation, see 50360–50365.

ICD-10-CM Diagnostic Codes

This code is not identified as an add-on code by CPT® but is performed at the same time as another primary procedure. Refer to the corresponding primary procedure code for ICD-10-CM diagnosis code links.

AMA: 50327 2014,Jan,11

Relative Value Units/Medicare Edits

Non-Facility RVU	Work	PE	MP	Total
50327	4.0	1.41	0.9	6.31
Facility RVU	**Work**	**PE**	**MP**	**Total**
50327	4.0	1.41	0.9	6.31

	FUD	Status	MUE	Modifiers				IOM Reference
50327	N/A	A	2(3)	51	N/A	62*	80	None

* with documentation

Kidney

50328

50328   Backbench reconstruction of cadaver or living donor renal allograft prior to transplantation; arterial anastomosis, each

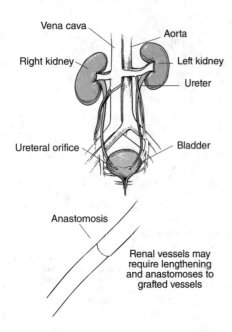

Vena cava

Aorta

Right kidney

Left kidney

Ureter

Ureteral orifice

Bladder

Anastomosis

Renal vessels may require lengthening and anastomoses to grafted vessels

Explanation

The surgeon performs arterial anastomosis reconstruction of a donor kidney from a cadaver or living donor prior to transplantation. The allograft is prepared with multiple renal arteries. When the donor organ comes from a cadaveric source, the aortic patch removed with the specimen is used for creating a viable renal artery graft for transplantation. Donor iliac arteries are routinely procured from cadaveric donors to be prepared and used as arterial grafting material. The segmental renal artery may also be anastomosed to the inferior epigastric artery when an aortic patch is not available, such as when the donor kidney is from a living donor. The vessels are tested for patency by flushing with a preservation solution.

Coding Tips

For donor nephrectomy, see 50300–50320. For laparoscopic donor nephrectomy, see 50547. For renal allotransplantation, see 50360–50365.

ICD-10-CM Diagnostic Codes

This code is not identified as an add-on code by CPT® but is performed at the same time as another primary procedure. Refer to the corresponding primary procedure code for ICD-10-CM diagnosis code links.

AMA: 50328 2014,Jan,11

Relative Value Units/Medicare Edits

Non-Facility RVU	Work	PE	MP	Total
50328	3.5	1.24	0.79	5.53
Facility RVU	**Work**	**PE**	**MP**	**Total**
50328	3.5	1.24	0.79	5.53

	FUD	Status	MUE	Modifiers				IOM Reference
50328	N/A	A	1(3)	51	N/A	62*	80	None

* with documentation

50329

50329   Backbench reconstruction of cadaver or living donor renal allograft prior to transplantation; ureteral anastomosis, each

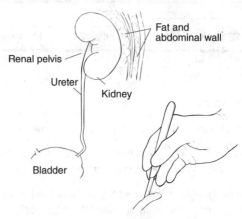

Fat and abdominal wall

Renal pelvis

Ureter

Kidney

Bladder

The ureter portion of a renal allograft is prepared on the backbonch in anticipation of transplantation. Ureteral anastomosis for anatomic variations on the donor/organ is done

Explanation

The physician performs a standard backbench reconstruction of the ureter following renal allograft procurement from a cadaver or living donor. Backbench or back table preparation refers to procedures performed on the donor organ following procurement to prepare the donor organ for transplant. In a separately reportable procedure, the physician removes the kidney en bloc from a cadaver donor or the kidney and upper ureter from a living donor. The kidney is flushed with a cold electrolyte solution to rinse any remaining donor blood from the kidney and lower its temperature. After preparing the kidney and blood vessels in a separately reportable procedure, the physician turns his attention to any required ureteral anastomosis. Ureteral anastomosis is generally required when anatomic variations are present in the donor organ. Anatomic variations for kidney donors include multiple ureters. When two or more ureters are present, the ureters may be separately implanted into the bladder or a side-to-side anastomosis of the ureters may be performed during the backbench preparation prior to implantation into the bladder. Code 50329 is reported when side-to-side anastomosis is performed and is reported for each anastomosis.

Coding Tips

For donor nephrectomy, see 50300–50320. For laparoscopic donor nephrectomy, see 50547. For renal allotransplantation, see 50360–50365.

ICD-10-CM Diagnostic Codes

This code is not identified as an add-on code by CPT® but is performed at the same time as another primary procedure. Refer to the corresponding primary procedure code for ICD-10-CM diagnosis code links.

AMA: 50329 2014,Jan,11

© 2020 Optum360, LLC   N Newborn: 0   P Pediatric: 0-17   M Maternity: 9-64   A Adult: 15-124   ♂ Male Only   ♀ Female Only   CPT © 2020 American Medical Association. All Rights Reserved.

Coding Companion for Urology/Nephrology

Kidney

Relative Value Units/Medicare Edits

Non-Facility RVU	Work	PE	MP	Total
50329	3.34	1.19	0.73	5.26
Facility RVU	Work	PE	MP	Total
50329	3.34	1.19	0.73	5.26

	FUD	Status	MUE	Modifiers				IOM Reference
50329	N/A	A	1(3)	51	N/A	62*	80	None

* with documentation

Terms To Know

allograft. Graft from one individual to another of the same species.

anastomosis. Surgically created connection between ducts, blood vessels, or bowel segments to allow flow from one to the other.

cadaver. Dead body.

donor. Person from whom tissues or organs are removed for transplantation.

en bloc. In total.

reconstruction. Recreating, restoring, or rebuilding a body part or organ.

transplantation. Grafting or movement of an organ or tissue from one site or person to another.

ureter. Tube leading from the kidney to the urinary bladder made up of three layers of tissue: the mucous lining of the inner layer; the smooth, muscular middle layer that propels the urine from the kidney to the bladder by peristalsis; and the outer layer made of fibrous connective tissue. Each ureter leaves the kidney from the hilum, a concave notch on the middle surface, and enters the bladder through a narrow valve-like orifice that prevents the backflow of urine to the kidney.

50340

50340   Recipient nephrectomy (separate procedure)

The physician removes the kidney and upper ureter of a transplant recipient

Explanation

The physician removes the kidney and the upper portion of the ureter in a patient who is to receive a kidney transplant. To access the kidney and ureter, the physician usually makes an incision in the skin of the flank, cuts the muscles, fat, and fibrous membranes (fascia) overlying the kidney, and sometimes removes a portion of the eleventh or twelfth rib. After mobilizing the kidney and ureter, the physician clamps, ligates, and severs the upper ureter and major renal blood vessels (renal pedicle). The physician removes the kidney and upper ureter, but does not remove the adrenal gland, surrounding fatty tissue, or Gerota's fascia. After controlling bleeding, the physician irrigates the site with normal saline and places a drain tube, bringing it out through a separate stab incision in the skin. The physician performs a layered closure.

Coding Tips

This separate procedure by definition is usually a component of a more complex service and is not identified separately. When performed alone or with other unrelated procedures/services it may be reported. If performed alone, list the code; if performed with other procedures/services, list the code and append modifier 59 or an X{EPSU} modifier. This is a unilateral procedure. If performed bilaterally, some payers require that the service be reported twice with modifier 50 appended to the second code while others require identification of the service only once with modifier 50 appended. Check with individual payers. Modifier 50 identifies a procedure performed identically on the opposite side of the body (mirror image). Nephrectomy with renal allotransplantation is reported with 50365. For donor nephrectomy, see 50300–50320 and 50547.

ICD-10-CM Diagnostic Codes

B52.0	Plasmodium malariae malaria with nephropathy
C64.1	Malignant neoplasm of right kidney, except renal pelvis ☑
C64.2	Malignant neoplasm of left kidney, except renal pelvis ☑
C65.1	Malignant neoplasm of right renal pelvis ☑
C65.2	Malignant neoplasm of left renal pelvis ☑
C66.1	Malignant neoplasm of right ureter ☑
C66.2	Malignant neoplasm of left ureter ☑
C68.8	Malignant neoplasm of overlapping sites of urinary organs
C79.01	Secondary malignant neoplasm of right kidney and renal pelvis ☑
C79.02	Secondary malignant neoplasm of left kidney and renal pelvis ☑

Kidney

C7A.093	Malignant carcinoid tumor of the kidney
C80.2	Malignant neoplasm associated with transplanted organ
D09.19	Carcinoma in situ of other urinary organs
D30.01	Benign neoplasm of right kidney ☑
D30.02	Benign neoplasm of left kidney ☑
D30.11	Benign neoplasm of right renal pelvis ☑
D30.12	Benign neoplasm of left renal pelvis ☑
D30.21	Benign neoplasm of right ureter ☑
D30.22	Benign neoplasm of left ureter ☑
D3A.093	Benign carcinoid tumor of the kidney
D41.01	Neoplasm of uncertain behavior of right kidney ☑
D41.02	Neoplasm of uncertain behavior of left kidney ☑
D41.11	Neoplasm of uncertain behavior of right renal pelvis ☑
D41.12	Neoplasm of uncertain behavior of left renal pelvis ☑
D41.21	Neoplasm of uncertain behavior of right ureter ☑
D41.22	Neoplasm of uncertain behavior of left ureter ☑
D47.Z1	Post-transplant lymphoproliferative disorder (PTLD)
D47.Z2	Castleman disease
I12.0	Hypertensive chronic kidney disease with stage 5 chronic kidney disease or end stage renal disease
I15.0	Renovascular hypertension
I16.0	Hypertensive urgency
I16.1	Hypertensive emergency
M31.31	Wegener's granulomatosis with renal involvement
N00.0	Acute nephritic syndrome with minor glomerular abnormality
N00.1	Acute nephritic syndrome with focal and segmental glomerular lesions
N00.2	Acute nephritic syndrome with diffuse membranous glomerulonephritis
N00.3	Acute nephritic syndrome with diffuse mesangial proliferative glomerulonephritis
N00.4	Acute nephritic syndrome with diffuse endocapillary proliferative glomerulonephritis
N00.5	Acute nephritic syndrome with diffuse mesangiocapillary glomerulonephritis
N00.6	Acute nephritic syndrome with dense deposit disease
N00.7	Acute nephritic syndrome with diffuse crescentic glomerulonephritis
N03.0	Chronic nephritic syndrome with minor glomerular abnormality
N03.1	Chronic nephritic syndrome with focal and segmental glomerular lesions
N03.2	Chronic nephritic syndrome with diffuse membranous glomerulonephritis
N03.3	Chronic nephritic syndrome with diffuse mesangial proliferative glomerulonephritis
N03.4	Chronic nephritic syndrome with diffuse endocapillary proliferative glomerulonephritis
N03.5	Chronic nephritic syndrome with diffuse mesangiocapillary glomerulonephritis
N03.6	Chronic nephritic syndrome with dense deposit disease
N03.7	Chronic nephritic syndrome with diffuse crescentic glomerulonephritis
N03.8	Chronic nephritic syndrome with other morphologic changes
N04.0	Nephrotic syndrome with minor glomerular abnormality
N04.1	Nephrotic syndrome with focal and segmental glomerular lesions

N04.2	Nephrotic syndrome with diffuse membranous glomerulonephritis
N04.3	Nephrotic syndrome with diffuse mesangial proliferative glomerulonephritis
N04.4	Nephrotic syndrome with diffuse endocapillary proliferative glomerulonephritis
N04.5	Nephrotic syndrome with diffuse mesangiocapillary glomerulonephritis
N04.6	Nephrotic syndrome with dense deposit disease
N04.7	Nephrotic syndrome with diffuse crescentic glomerulonephritis
N04.8	Nephrotic syndrome with other morphologic changes
N11.0	Nonobstructive reflux-associated chronic pyelonephritis
N11.1	Chronic obstructive pyelonephritis
N11.8	Other chronic tubulo-interstitial nephritis
N13.0	Hydronephrosis with ureteropelvic junction obstruction
N13.1	Hydronephrosis with ureteral stricture, not elsewhere classified
N13.2	Hydronephrosis with renal and ureteral calculous obstruction
N13.4	Hydroureter
N13.5	Crossing vessel and stricture of ureter without hydronephrosis
N13.6	Pyonephrosis
N13.71	Vesicoureteral-reflux without reflux nephropathy
N13.721	Vesicoureteral-reflux with reflux nephropathy without hydroureter, unilateral
N13.722	Vesicoureteral-reflux with reflux nephropathy without hydroureter, bilateral
N13.731	Vesicoureteral-reflux with reflux nephropathy with hydroureter, unilateral
N13.732	Vesicoureteral-reflux with reflux nephropathy with hydroureter, bilateral
N17.0	Acute kidney failure with tubular necrosis
N17.1	Acute kidney failure with acute cortical necrosis
N17.2	Acute kidney failure with medullary necrosis
N18.4	Chronic kidney disease, stage 4 (severe)
N18.5	Chronic kidney disease, stage 5
N18.6	End stage renal disease
N20.0	Calculus of kidney
N20.2	Calculus of kidney with calculus of ureter
N26.1	Atrophy of kidney (terminal)
N26.2	Page kidney
N28.0	Ischemia and infarction of kidney
N28.1	Cyst of kidney, acquired
N28.81	Hypertrophy of kidney
N28.82	Megaloureter
Q60.3	Renal hypoplasia, unilateral
Q60.4	Renal hypoplasia, bilateral
Q60.6	Potter's syndrome
Q61.01	Congenital single renal cyst
Q61.02	Congenital multiple renal cysts
Q61.11	Cystic dilatation of collecting ducts
Q61.2	Polycystic kidney, adult type
Q61.4	Renal dysplasia
Q61.5	Medullary cystic kidney
Q62.0	Congenital hydronephrosis
Q62.11	Congenital occlusion of ureteropelvic junction

Kidney

Q62.31	Congenital ureterocele, orthotopic
Q62.32	Cecoureterocele
S37.061A	Major laceration of right kidney, initial encounter ☑
S37.062A	Major laceration of left kidney, initial encounter ☑
S37.091A	Other injury of right kidney, initial encounter ☑
S37.092A	Other injury of left kidney, initial encounter ☑
T86.11	Kidney transplant rejection
T86.12	Kidney transplant failure
T86.13	Kidney transplant infection
T86.19	Other complication of kidney transplant

AMA: 50340 2014,Jan,11

Relative Value Units/Medicare Edits

Non-Facility RVU	Work	PE	MP	Total
50340	14.04	10.13	3.41	27.58
Facility RVU	Work	PE	MP	Total
50340	14.04	10.13	3.41	27.58

	FUD	Status	MUE	Modifiers				IOM Reference
50340	90	A	1(2)	51	50	62*	80	100-03,20.3

* with documentation

Terms To Know

clamp. Tool used to grip, compress, join, or fasten body parts.

drain. Device that creates a channel to allow fluid from a cavity, wound, or infected area to exit the body.

fascia. Fibrous sheet or band of tissue that envelops organs, muscles, and groupings of muscles.

flank. Part of the body found between the posterior ribs and the uppermost crest of the ilium, or the lateral side of the hip, thigh, and buttock.

irrigate. Washing out, lavage.

ligate. To tie off a blood vessel or duct with a suture or a soft, thin wire (ligature wire).

nephrectomy. Partial or total removal of the kidney that may be performed for indications such as irreparable kidney damage, renal cell carcinoma, trauma, congenital abnormalities, or transplant purposes.

renal. Referring to the kidney.

transplant. Insertion of an organ or tissue from one person or site into another.

ureter. Tube leading from the kidney to the urinary bladder made up of three layers of tissue: the mucous lining of the inner layer; the smooth, muscular middle layer that propels the urine from the kidney to the bladder by peristalsis; and the outer layer made of fibrous connective tissue. Each ureter leaves the kidney from the hilum, a concave notch on the middle surface, and enters the bladder through a narrow valve-like orifice that prevents the backflow of urine to the kidney.

50360-50365

| 50360 | Renal allotransplantation, implantation of graft; without recipient nephrectomy |
| 50365 | with recipient nephrectomy |

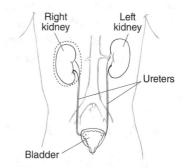

A kidney from a living donor or cadaver is implanted into a recipient

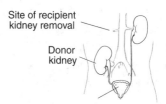

Explanation

In 50360, the physician surgically implants a human kidney and ureter from a living donor or cadaver into a transplant patient, without performing a concurrent nephrectomy on the recipient. To access the transplant site, the physician usually makes a curved, right or left lower quadrant incision in the skin. After cutting the muscles, fat, and fibrous membranes (fascia), the physician controls bleeding with clamps, ties, and electrocoagulation. The physician surgically connects the renal vein and artery of the donor kidney to the recipient's clamped and dissected internal iliac vein and hypogastric artery. After removing the clamps, the physician checks for leakage, bleeding, and insufficient blood supply. To implant the donor ureter, the physician makes an incision into the bladder and passes the ureter through the bladder. The physician sutures the ureter as well as the opening in the bladder (cystotomy). In 50365, the physician implants a donor kidney and upper ureter after removing the recipient's kidney and upper ureter. To access the recipient's kidney and ureter, the physician usually makes an incision in the skin of the flank, cuts the muscles, fat, and fibrous membranes (fascia) overlying the kidney, and sometimes removes a portion of the eleventh or twelfth rib. The physician clamps, ligates, and severs the upper ureter and major renal blood vessels (renal pedicle), and removes the kidney and upper ureter. To implant the donor kidney and upper ureter, the physician usually makes a curved lower quadrant incision in the skin. The physician surgically connects the renal vein and artery of the donor kidney to the recipient's clamped and dissected internal iliac vein and hypogastric artery. After incising the bladder, the physician passes the donor ureter through the bladder and sutures the ureter and opening in the bladder (cystotomy). In both cases, the physician performs a layered closure and a drain tube may be left in.

Coding Tips

Note that 50365 is a unilateral procedure. If performed bilaterally, some payers require that the service be reported twice with modifier 50 appended to the second code while others require identification of the service only once with modifier 50 appended. Check with individual payers. Modifier 50 identifies a

CPT © 2020 American Medical Association. All Rights Reserved.   ● New   ▲ Revised   + Add On   ★ Telemedicine   AMA: CPT Assist   [Resequenced]   ☑ Laterality   © 2020 Optum360, LLC

Kidney

procedure performed identically on the opposite side of the body (mirror image). For removal of the donor kidney, see 50300–50320; laparoscopic, see 50547.

ICD-10-CM Diagnostic Codes

B52.0	Plasmodium malariae malaria with nephropathy
C64.1	Malignant neoplasm of right kidney, except renal pelvis ☑
C64.2	Malignant neoplasm of left kidney, except renal pelvis ☑
C65.1	Malignant neoplasm of right renal pelvis ☑
C65.2	Malignant neoplasm of left renal pelvis ☑
C66.1	Malignant neoplasm of right ureter ☑
C66.2	Malignant neoplasm of left ureter ☑
C68.8	Malignant neoplasm of overlapping sites of urinary organs
C79.01	Secondary malignant neoplasm of right kidney and renal pelvis ☑
C79.02	Secondary malignant neoplasm of left kidney and renal pelvis ☑
C7A.093	Malignant carcinoid tumor of the kidney
C80.2	Malignant neoplasm associated with transplanted organ
D09.19	Carcinoma in situ of other urinary organs
D30.01	Benign neoplasm of right kidney ☑
D30.02	Benign neoplasm of left kidney ☑
D30.11	Benign neoplasm of right renal pelvis ☑
D30.12	Benign neoplasm of left renal pelvis ☑
D30.21	Benign neoplasm of right ureter ☑
D30.22	Benign neoplasm of left ureter ☑
D3A.093	Benign carcinoid tumor of the kidney
D41.01	Neoplasm of uncertain behavior of right kidney ☑
D41.02	Neoplasm of uncertain behavior of left kidney ☑
D41.11	Neoplasm of uncertain behavior of right renal pelvis ☑
D41.12	Neoplasm of uncertain behavior of left renal pelvis ☑
D41.21	Neoplasm of uncertain behavior of right ureter ☑
D41.22	Neoplasm of uncertain behavior of left ureter ☑
D47.Z1	Post-transplant lymphoproliferative disorder (PTLD)
D47.Z2	Castleman disease
D49.511	Neoplasm of unspecified behavior of right kidney ☑
D49.512	Neoplasm of unspecified behavior of left kidney ☑
D49.59	Neoplasm of unspecified behavior of other genitourinary organ
I12.0	Hypertensive chronic kidney disease with stage 5 chronic kidney disease or end stage renal disease
I15.0	Renovascular hypertension
I16.0	Hypertensive urgency
I16.1	Hypertensive emergency
M31.31	Wegener's granulomatosis with renal involvement
N00.0	Acute nephritic syndrome with minor glomerular abnormality
N00.1	Acute nephritic syndrome with focal and segmental glomerular lesions
N00.2	Acute nephritic syndrome with diffuse membranous glomerulonephritis
N00.3	Acute nephritic syndrome with diffuse mesangial proliferative glomerulonephritis
N00.4	Acute nephritic syndrome with diffuse endocapillary proliferative glomerulonephritis
N00.5	Acute nephritic syndrome with diffuse mesangiocapillary glomerulonephritis
N00.6	Acute nephritic syndrome with dense deposit disease
N00.7	Acute nephritic syndrome with diffuse crescentic glomerulonephritis
N03.0	Chronic nephritic syndrome with minor glomerular abnormality
N03.1	Chronic nephritic syndrome with focal and segmental glomerular lesions
N03.2	Chronic nephritic syndrome with diffuse membranous glomerulonephritis
N03.3	Chronic nephritic syndrome with diffuse mesangial proliferative glomerulonephritis
N03.4	Chronic nephritic syndrome with diffuse endocapillary proliferative glomerulonephritis
N03.5	Chronic nephritic syndrome with diffuse mesangiocapillary glomerulonephritis
N03.6	Chronic nephritic syndrome with dense deposit disease
N03.7	Chronic nephritic syndrome with diffuse crescentic glomerulonephritis
N03.8	Chronic nephritic syndrome with other morphologic changes
N04.0	Nephrotic syndrome with minor glomerular abnormality
N04.1	Nephrotic syndrome with focal and segmental glomerular lesions
N04.2	Nephrotic syndrome with diffuse membranous glomerulonephritis
N04.3	Nephrotic syndrome with diffuse mesangial proliferative glomerulonephritis
N04.4	Nephrotic syndrome with diffuse endocapillary proliferative glomerulonephritis
N04.5	Nephrotic syndrome with diffuse mesangiocapillary glomerulonephritis
N04.6	Nephrotic syndrome with dense deposit disease
N04.7	Nephrotic syndrome with diffuse crescentic glomerulonephritis
N04.8	Nephrotic syndrome with other morphologic changes
N11.0	Nonobstructive reflux-associated chronic pyelonephritis
N11.1	Chronic obstructive pyelonephritis
N11.8	Other chronic tubulo-interstitial nephritis
N13.0	Hydronephrosis with ureteropelvic junction obstruction
N13.1	Hydronephrosis with ureteral stricture, not elsewhere classified
N13.2	Hydronephrosis with renal and ureteral calculous obstruction
N13.39	Other hydronephrosis
N13.4	Hydroureter
N13.5	Crossing vessel and stricture of ureter without hydronephrosis
N13.6	Pyonephrosis
N13.71	Vesicoureteral-reflux without reflux nephropathy
N13.721	Vesicoureteral-reflux with reflux nephropathy without hydroureter, unilateral
N13.722	Vesicoureteral-reflux with reflux nephropathy without hydroureter, bilateral
N13.731	Vesicoureteral-reflux with reflux nephropathy with hydroureter, unilateral
N13.732	Vesicoureteral-reflux with reflux nephropathy with hydroureter, bilateral
N13.8	Other obstructive and reflux uropathy
N17.0	Acute kidney failure with tubular necrosis
N17.1	Acute kidney failure with acute cortical necrosis
N17.2	Acute kidney failure with medullary necrosis
N17.8	Other acute kidney failure

Kidney

N18.4	Chronic kidney disease, stage 4 (severe)
N18.5	Chronic kidney disease, stage 5
N18.6	End stage renal disease
N20.0	Calculus of kidney
N20.2	Calculus of kidney with calculus of ureter
N26.1	Atrophy of kidney (terminal)
N26.2	Page kidney
N28.0	Ischemia and infarction of kidney
N28.1	Cyst of kidney, acquired
N28.81	Hypertrophy of kidney
N28.82	Megaloureter
N28.89	Other specified disorders of kidney and ureter
Q60.3	Renal hypoplasia, unilateral
Q60.4	Renal hypoplasia, bilateral
Q60.6	Potter's syndrome
Q61.01	Congenital single renal cyst
Q61.02	Congenital multiple renal cysts
Q61.11	Cystic dilatation of collecting ducts
Q61.19	Other polycystic kidney, infantile type
Q61.2	Polycystic kidney, adult type
Q61.4	Renal dysplasia
Q61.5	Medullary cystic kidney
Q61.8	Other cystic kidney diseases
Q62.0	Congenital hydronephrosis
Q62.11	Congenital occlusion of ureteropelvic junction
Q62.31	Congenital ureterocele, orthotopic
Q62.32	Cecoureterocele
Q62.39	Other obstructive defects of renal pelvis and ureter
S37.061A	Major laceration of right kidney, initial encounter ☑
S37.062A	Major laceration of left kidney, initial encounter ☑
S37.091A	Other injury of right kidney, initial encounter ☑
S37.092A	Other injury of left kidney, initial encounter ☑
T86.11	Kidney transplant rejection
T86.12	Kidney transplant failure
T86.13	Kidney transplant infection
T86.19	Other complication of kidney transplant

AMA: **50360** 2014,Jan,11 **50365** 2018,Jan,8; 2017,Jan,8; 2016,Jan,13; 2015,Jan,16; 2014,Jan,11

Relative Value Units/Medicare Edits

Non-Facility RVU	Work	PE	MP	Total
50360	39.88	21.27	9.19	70.34
50365	46.13	26.77	10.66	83.56
Facility RVU	**Work**	**PE**	**MP**	**Total**
50360	39.88	21.27	9.19	70.34
50365	46.13	26.77	10.66	83.56

	FUD	Status	MUE	Modifiers				IOM Reference
50360	90	A	1(2)	51	N/A	62	80	100-03,190.1;
50365	90	A	1(2)	51	50	62	80	100-03,260.7
* with documentation								

50370

50370	Removal of transplanted renal allograft

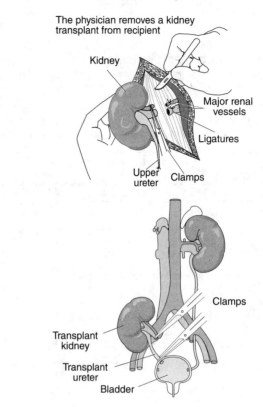

The physician removes a kidney transplant from recipient

Kidney · Major renal vessels · Ligatures · Upper ureter · Clamps

Transplant kidney · Transplant ureter · Clamps · Bladder

Explanation

The physician removes a transplanted donor kidney from the recipient. To access the rejected kidney, the physician usually reopens the original kidney transplant incision, and cuts the muscles, fat, and fibrous membranes (fascia) overlying the kidney. After mobilizing the kidney, the physician clamps, ligates, and severs the major renal blood vessels (renal pedicle). The physician removes the rejected kidney. After controlling bleeding, the physician irrigates the site with normal saline. The physician may place a drain tube, bringing it out through a separate stab incision in the skin. After removing the clamps, the physician performs a layered closure.

Coding Tips

For allotransplantation of the donor kidney, see 50360–50365. For removal of the donor kidney, see 50300–50320; laparoscopic, see 50547. For a nephrectomy that is not part of a renal transplant, see 50220–50240, 50545–50546, and 50548.

ICD-10-CM Diagnostic Codes

C80.2	Malignant neoplasm associated with transplanted organ
D47.Z1	Post-transplant lymphoproliferative disorder (PTLD)
D47.Z2	Castleman disease
D89.41	Monoclonal mast cell activation syndrome
D89.42	Idiopathic mast cell activation syndrome
D89.43	Secondary mast cell activation
D89.49	Other mast cell activation disorder
D89.810	Acute graft-versus-host disease
D89.811	Chronic graft-versus-host disease
D89.812	Acute on chronic graft-versus-host disease

Kidney

T86.11	Kidney transplant rejection
T86.12	Kidney transplant failure
T86.13	Kidney transplant infection
T86.19	Other complication of kidney transplant

AMA: 50370 2014,Jan,11

Relative Value Units/Medicare Edits

Non-Facility RVU	Work	PE	MP	Total
50370	18.88	11.9	4.28	35.06
Facility RVU	**Work**	**PE**	**MP**	**Total**
50370	18.88	11.9	4.28	35.06

	FUD	Status	MUE	Modifiers				IOM Reference
50370	90	A	1(2)	51	N/A	62*	80	100-03,190.1; 100-03,260.7

* with documentation

Terms To Know

allograft. Graft from one individual to another of the same species.

anastomosis. Surgically created connection between ducts, blood vessels, or bowel segments to allow flow from one to the other.

clamp. Tool used to grip, compress, join, or fasten body parts.

closure. Repairing an incision or wound by suture or other means.

donor. Person from whom tissues or organs are removed for transplantation.

drain. Device that creates a channel to allow fluid from a cavity, wound, or infected area to exit the body.

fascia. Fibrous sheet or band of tissue that envelops organs, muscles, and groupings of muscles.

irrigate. Washing out, lavage.

ligate. To tie off a blood vessel or duct with a suture or a soft, thin wire (ligature wire).

nephrectomy. Partial or total removal of the kidney that may be performed for indications such as irreparable kidney damage, renal cell carcinoma, trauma, congenital abnormalities, or transplant purposes.

transplant. Insertion of an organ or tissue from one person or site into another.

50380

50380   Renal autotransplantation, reimplantation of kidney

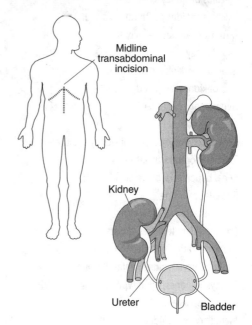

Physician revascularizes kidney by moving it to a new anatomical site

Explanation

The physician moves the kidney from its original anatomic site and revascularizes the kidney by connecting the renal and iliac vessels to a new site. To access the transplant site, the physician usually makes a midline transabdominal incision in the skin and cuts the muscles, fat, and fibrous membranes (fascia). After exposing the kidney, the physician clamps, ligates, and severs the renal vessels, keeping the ureter intact. The physician flushes the kidney with cold, anticoagulant electrolyte solution, and surgically connects the renal vessels to another appropriate arterial and venous site. The physician removes the clamps and checks for leakage, bleeding, and infarction. After placing a drain tube and bringing it out through a separate stab incision in the skin, the physician removes the clamps and performs a layered closure.

Coding Tips

When two surgeons are needed to perform the autotransplantation, each performing distinct parts of the procedure, both surgeons can report 50380 with modifier 62. When the kidney requires reimplantation for revascularization, other procedures such as partial nephrectomy or nephrolithotomy may be required. When autotransplantation is performed with another of these separately identifiable procedures, report 50380 as the primary procedure and indicate any secondary procedures with modifier 51. For implantation of a donor kidney, see 50360–50365.

ICD-10-CM Diagnostic Codes

C64.1	Malignant neoplasm of right kidney, except renal pelvis ☑
C64.2	Malignant neoplasm of left kidney, except renal pelvis ☑
C65.1	Malignant neoplasm of right renal pelvis ☑
C65.2	Malignant neoplasm of left renal pelvis ☑
C66.1	Malignant neoplasm of right ureter ☑
C66.2	Malignant neoplasm of left ureter ☑
C68.8	Malignant neoplasm of overlapping sites of urinary organs

© 2020 Optum360, LLC   **N** Newborn: 0   **P** Pediatric: 0-17   **M** Maternity: 9-64   **A** Adult: 15-124   ♂ Male Only   ♀ Female Only   CPT © 2020 American Medical Association. All Rights Reserved.

Kidney

Coding Companion for Urology/Nephrology

C79.01	Secondary malignant neoplasm of right kidney and renal pelvis ☑
C79.02	Secondary malignant neoplasm of left kidney and renal pelvis ☑
C7A.093	Malignant carcinoid tumor of the kidney
D30.01	Benign neoplasm of right kidney ☑
D30.02	Benign neoplasm of left kidney ☑
D30.11	Benign neoplasm of right renal pelvis ☑
D30.12	Benign neoplasm of left renal pelvis ☑
D30.21	Benign neoplasm of right ureter ☑
D30.22	Benign neoplasm of left ureter ☑
D3A.093	Benign carcinoid tumor of the kidney
D41.01	Neoplasm of uncertain behavior of right kidney ☑
D41.02	Neoplasm of uncertain behavior of left kidney ☑
D41.11	Neoplasm of uncertain behavior of right renal pelvis ☑
D41.12	Neoplasm of uncertain behavior of left renal pelvis ☑
D41.21	Neoplasm of uncertain behavior of right ureter ☑
D41.22	Neoplasm of uncertain behavior of left ureter ☑
I15.0	Renovascular hypertension
I16.0	Hypertensive urgency
I16.1	Hypertensive emergency
I70.1	Atherosclerosis of renal artery ▲
I72.2	Aneurysm of renal artery
I75.81	Atheroembolism of kidney
I82.3	Embolism and thrombosis of renal vein
N13.5	Crossing vessel and stricture of ureter without hydronephrosis
N20.0	Calculus of kidney
N28.0	Ischemia and infarction of kidney
Q27.1	Congenital renal artery stenosis
Q27.2	Other congenital malformations of renal artery
S35.411A	Laceration of right renal artery, initial encounter ☑
S35.412A	Laceration of left renal artery, initial encounter ☑
S35.414A	Laceration of right renal vein, initial encounter ☑
S35.415A	Laceration of left renal vein, initial encounter ☑
S35.491A	Other specified injury of right renal artery, initial encounter ☑
S35.492A	Other specified injury of left renal artery, initial encounter ☑
S35.494A	Other specified injury of right renal vein, initial encounter ☑
S35.495A	Other specified injury of left renal vein, initial encounter ☑
S37.12XA	Contusion of ureter, initial encounter
S37.13XA	Laceration of ureter, initial encounter
S37.19XA	Other injury of ureter, initial encounter
T86.19	Other complication of kidney transplant

AMA: 50380 2019,Sep,10; 2018,Jan,8; 2017,Jan,8; 2016,Jan,13; 2015,Jan,16; 2014,Jan,11

Relative Value Units/Medicare Edits

Non-Facility RVU	Work	PE	MP	Total
50380	30.11	21.04	7.32	58.47
Facility RVU	**Work**	**PE**	**MP**	**Total**
50380	30.11	21.04	7.32	58.47

	FUD	Status	MUE	Modifiers				IOM Reference
50380	90	A	1(2)	51	N/A	62*	80	100-03,20.3; 100-03,260.7

* with documentation

Terms To Know

autotransplantation. Excising tissue from the patient and transplanting it into another location in the same patient.

ligation. Tying off a blood vessel or duct with a suture or a soft, thin wire.

revascularize. Restoring blood flow or blood supply to a body part.

transabdominal. Across or through the belly or abdomen.

ureter. Tube leading from the kidney to the urinary bladder made up of three layers of tissue: the mucous lining of the inner layer; the smooth, muscular middle layer that propels the urine from the kidney to the bladder by peristalsis; and the outer layer made of fibrous connective tissue. Each ureter leaves the kidney from the hilum, a concave notch on the middle surface, and enters the bladder through a narrow valve-like orifice that prevents the backflow of urine to the kidney.

Kidney

50382-50384

50382 Removal (via snare/capture) and replacement of internally dwelling ureteral stent via percutaneous approach, including radiological supervision and interpretation

50384 Removal (via snare/capture) of internally dwelling ureteral stent via percutaneous approach, including radiological supervision and interpretation

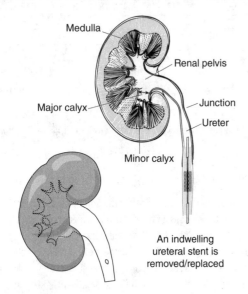

Medulla
Renal pelvis
Major calyx
Junction
Ureter
Minor calyx

An indwelling ureteral stent is removed/replaced

Explanation

The physician percutaneously removes an internally dwelling ureteral stent through the renal pelvis in 50384. With the patient under moderate sedation, a long, thin needle is advanced into the renal calyx under imaging guidance and the position is confirmed with contrast and fluoroscopy. A guidewire is threaded over the needle into the renal pelvis, the needle is removed, and a sheath placed over the guidewire. A snare device is threaded through the sheath into position, the indwelling stent is grasped, and pulled out partially through the sheath until the proximal end is outside the ureter. A guidewire is threaded through the stent, which is guided completely out. In 50382, the physician replaces the indwelling ureteral stent after removal of the old stent. The guidewire is left in place, the length of the old stent is noted, and the replacement stent is advanced into the ureter until the distal end is in the bladder and the distal loop is deployed. Stent position is confirmed with the proximal loop in the renal pelvis. The instruments are removed.

Coding Tips

Do not report 50382-50384 with 50436-50437. These are unilateral procedures. If performed bilaterally, some payers require that the service be reported twice with modifier 50 appended to the second code while others require identification of the service only once with modifier 50 appended. Check with individual payers. Modifier 50 identifies a procedure performed identically on the opposite side of the body (mirror image). Percutaneous introduction of a guidewire into the renal pelvis and ureter is included in these codes. For removal and replacement of an internally dwelling ureteral stent placed via a transurethral approach, see 50385.

ICD-10-CM Diagnostic Codes

T83.112A	Breakdown (mechanical) of indwelling ureteral stent, initial encounter
T83.113A	Breakdown (mechanical) of other urinary stents, initial encounter
T83.122A	Displacement of indwelling ureteral stent, initial encounter
T83.123A	Displacement of other urinary stents, initial encounter
T83.192A	Other mechanical complication of indwelling ureteral stent, initial encounter
T83.193A	Other mechanical complication of other urinary stent, initial encounter
T83.592A	Infection and inflammatory reaction due to indwelling ureteral stent, initial encounter
T83.593A	Infection and inflammatory reaction due to other urinary stents, initial encounter
T83.82XA	Fibrosis due to genitourinary prosthetic devices, implants and grafts, initial encounter
T83.83XA	Hemorrhage due to genitourinary prosthetic devices, implants and grafts, initial encounter
T83.84XA	Pain due to genitourinary prosthetic devices, implants and grafts, initial encounter
T83.85XA	Stenosis due to genitourinary prosthetic devices, implants and grafts, initial encounter
T83.86XA	Thrombosis due to genitourinary prosthetic devices, implants and grafts, initial encounter
T83.89XA	Other specified complication of genitourinary prosthetic devices, implants and grafts, initial encounter

AMA: 50382 2018,Jan,8; 2017,Jan,8; 2016,Jan,3; 2016,Jan,13; 2015,Jan,16; 2014,Jan,11 **50384** 2018,Jan,8; 2017,Jan,8; 2016,Jan,13; 2016,Jan,3; 2015,Jan,16; 2014,Jan,11

Relative Value Units/Medicare Edits

Non-Facility RVU	Work	PE	MP	Total
50382	5.25	25.6	0.48	31.33
50384	4.75	20.4	0.44	25.59
Facility RVU	**Work**	**PE**	**MP**	**Total**
50382	5.25	1.7	0.48	7.43
50384	4.75	1.46	0.44	6.65

	FUD	Status	MUE	Modifiers				IOM Reference
50382	0	A	1(3)	51	50	N/A	N/A	None
50384	0	A	1(3)	51	50	N/A	N/A	

* with documentation

Terms To Know

percutaneous approach. Method used to gain access to a body organ or specific area by puncture or minor incision through the skin or mucous membrane and/or any other body layers necessary to reach the procedure site.

renal calyces. Cuplike structures formed by the papilla, where urine is collected for transfer via the renal pelvis out of the kidney and into the ureter.

stent. Tube to provide support in a body cavity or lumen.

Kidney

50385-50386

50385 Removal (via snare/capture) and replacement of internally dwelling ureteral stent via transurethral approach, without use of cystoscopy, including radiological supervision and interpretation

50386 Removal (via snare/capture) of internally dwelling ureteral stent via transurethral approach, without use of cystoscopy, including radiological supervision and interpretation

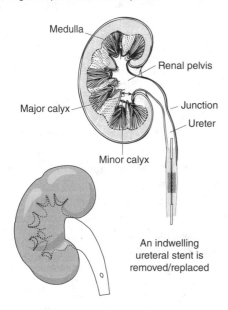

An indwelling ureteral stent is removed/replaced

Explanation

Using snare or capture, the physician removes (50386) or removes and replaces (50385) an internally dwelling ureteral stent (a thin, flexible tube that is inserted into the ureter to assist in the drainage of urine from the kidney). In one method, under appropriate sedation and sonographic guidance, a rigid biopsy forceps is introduced through the urethra, advanced to the urinary bladder, and the stent is grasped and removed. These codes are appropriate only when the procedure is performed via a transurethral approach, without the use of cystoscopy. Radiological supervision and interpretation is included and should not be reported separately.

Coding Tips

These are unilateral procedures. If performed bilaterally, some payers require that the service be reported twice with modifier 50 appended to the second code while others require identification of the service only once with modifier 50 appended. Check with individual payers. Modifier 50 identifies a procedure performed identically on the opposite side of the body (mirror image).

ICD-10-CM Diagnostic Codes

T83.112A	Breakdown (mechanical) of indwelling ureteral stent, initial encounter
T83.113A	Breakdown (mechanical) of other urinary stents, initial encounter
T83.122A	Displacement of indwelling ureteral stent, initial encounter
T83.123A	Displacement of other urinary stents, initial encounter
T83.192A	Other mechanical complication of indwelling ureteral stent, initial encounter
T83.193A	Other mechanical complication of other urinary stent, initial encounter
T83.592A	Infection and inflammatory reaction due to indwelling ureteral stent, initial encounter
T83.593A	Infection and inflammatory reaction due to other urinary stents, initial encounter
T83.82XA	Fibrosis due to genitourinary prosthetic devices, implants and grafts, initial encounter
T83.83XA	Hemorrhage due to genitourinary prosthetic devices, implants and grafts, initial encounter
T83.84XA	Pain due to genitourinary prosthetic devices, implants and grafts, initial encounter
T83.85XA	Stenosis due to genitourinary prosthetic devices, implants and grafts, initial encounter
T83.86XA	Thrombosis due to genitourinary prosthetic devices, implants and grafts, initial encounter
T83.89XA	Other specified complication of genitourinary prosthetic devices, implants and grafts, initial encounter

AMA: 50385 2018,Jan,8; 2017,Jan,8; 2016,Jan,3; 2016,Jan,13; 2015,Jan,16; 2014,Jan,11 **50386** 2018,Jan,8; 2017,Jan,8; 2016,Jan,3; 2016,Jan,13; 2015,Jan,16; 2014,Jan,11

Relative Value Units/Medicare Edits

Non-Facility RVU	Work	PE	MP	Total
50385	4.19	26.18	0.43	30.8
50386	3.05	17.72	0.34	21.11
Facility RVU	**Work**	**PE**	**MP**	**Total**
50385	4.19	1.7	0.43	6.32
50386	3.05	1.29	0.34	4.68

	FUD	Status	MUE	Modifiers				IOM Reference
50385	0	A	1(3)	51	50	N/A	80*	None
50386	0	A	1(3)	51	50	N/A	80*	

* with documentation

Terms To Know

approach. Method or anatomical location used to gain access to a body organ or specific area for procedures.

forceps. Tool used for grasping or compressing tissue.

imaging. Radiologic means of producing pictures for clinical study of the internal structures and functions of the body, such as x-ray, ultrasound, magnetic resonance, or positron emission tomography.

snare. Wire used as a loop to excise a polyp or lesion.

stent. Tube to provide support in a body cavity or lumen.

supervision and interpretation. Radiology services that usually contain an invasive component and are reported by the radiologist for supervision of the procedure and the personnel involved with performing the examination, reading the film, and preparing the written report.

ureter. Tube leading from the kidney to the urinary bladder made up of three layers of tissue: the mucous lining of the inner layer; the smooth, muscular middle layer that propels the urine from the kidney to the bladder by peristalsis; and the outer layer made of fibrous connective tissue. Each ureter leaves the kidney from the hilum, a concave notch on the middle surface, and enters the bladder through a narrow valve-like orifice that prevents the backflow of urine to the kidney.

Kidney

CPT © 2020 American Medical Association. All Rights Reserved.   ● New   ▲ Revised   + Add On   ★ Telemedicine   AMA: CPT Assist   [Resequenced]   ☑ Laterality   © 2020 Optum360, LLC

50387

50387 Removal and replacement of externally accessible nephroureteral catheter (eg, external/internal stent) requiring fluoroscopic guidance, including radiological supervision and interpretation

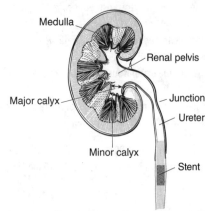

An external/internal ureteral stent is removed/replaced

Explanation

The physician removes and replaces an externally accessible nephroureteral catheter under fluoroscopic guidance. A nephroureteral catheter is placed within the renal collecting system, through the renal pelvis and into the bladder; the other end remains outside the body for drainage. Contrast may be injected at the entry site to assess anatomy and positioning. The suture holding the pigtail in place is cut and a guidewire is threaded through the stent lumen until it exits the distal end. The original stent is removed over the guidewire. Diameter and length are noted for a new stent, which is threaded over the guidewire until the distal end forms within the bladder. Fluoroscopy is used to assess the proximal position of formation within the renal pelvis. After position is verified, the guidewire is removed and the suture is put in position to hold the pigtail in place. Contrast may be injected to check position and function. Final adjustments are made for patient comfort, and the catheter may be sutured to the skin, capped, or a drainage bag may be attached.

Coding Tips

This is a unilateral procedure. If performed bilaterally, some payers require that the service be reported twice with modifier 50 appended to the second code while others require identification of the service only once with modifier 50 appended. Check with individual payers. Modifier 50 identifies a procedure performed identically on the opposite side of the body (mirror image). For removal of an externally accessible ureteral stent without fluoroscopy or replacement, see E/M service codes. For removal and replacement of an externally accessible ureteral stent through a ureterostomy or an ileal conduit, see 50688.

ICD-10-CM Diagnostic Codes

T83.112A	Breakdown (mechanical) of indwelling ureteral stent, initial encounter
T83.122A	Displacement of indwelling ureteral stent, initial encounter
T83.123A	Displacement of other urinary stents, initial encounter
T83.128A	Displacement of other urinary devices and implants, initial encounter
T83.192A	Other mechanical complication of indwelling ureteral stent, initial encounter
T83.193A	Other mechanical complication of other urinary stent, initial encounter
T83.510A	Infection and inflammatory reaction due to cystostomy catheter, initial encounter
T83.511A	Infection and inflammatory reaction due to indwelling urethral catheter, initial encounter
T83.512A	Infection and inflammatory reaction due to nephrostomy catheter, initial encounter
T83.518A	Infection and inflammatory reaction due to other urinary catheter, initial encounter
T83.592A	Infection and inflammatory reaction due to indwelling ureteral stent, initial encounter
T83.593A	Infection and inflammatory reaction due to other urinary stents, initial encounter
T83.81XA	Embolism due to genitourinary prosthetic devices, implants and grafts, initial encounter
T83.82XA	Fibrosis due to genitourinary prosthetic devices, implants and grafts, initial encounter
T83.83XA	Hemorrhage due to genitourinary prosthetic devices, implants and grafts, initial encounter
T83.84XA	Pain due to genitourinary prosthetic devices, implants and grafts, initial encounter
T83.85XA	Stenosis due to genitourinary prosthetic devices, implants and grafts, initial encounter
T83.86XA	Thrombosis due to genitourinary prosthetic devices, implants and grafts, initial encounter
T83.89XA	Other specified complication of genitourinary prosthetic devices, implants and grafts, initial encounter

AMA: **50387** 2018,Jan,8; 2017,Jan,8; 2016,Mar,10; 2016,Jan,13; 2016,Jan,3; 2015,Oct,5; 2015,Jan,16; 2014,Jan,11

Relative Value Units/Medicare Edits

Non-Facility RVU	Work	PE	MP	Total
50387	1.75	13.72	0.15	15.62
Facility RVU	**Work**	**PE**	**MP**	**Total**
50387	1.75	0.53	0.15	2.43

	FUD	Status	MUE	Modifiers				IOM Reference
50387	0	A	1(3)	51	50	N/A	80*	None

* with documentation

Terms To Know

catheter. Flexible tube inserted into an area of the body for introducing or withdrawing fluid.

contrast material. Any internally administered substance that has a different opacity from soft tissue on radiography or computed tomograph; includes barium, used to opacify parts of the gastrointestinal tract; water-soluble iodinated compounds, used to opacify blood vessels or the genitourinary tract; may refer to air occurring naturally or introduced into the body; also, paramagnetic substances used in magnetic resonance imaging. Substances may also be documented as contrast agent or contrast medium.

fluoroscopy. Radiology technique that allows visual examination of part of the body or a function of an organ using a device that projects an x-ray image on a fluorescent screen.

© 2020 Optum360, LLC   **N Newborn: 0   P Pediatric: 0-17   M Maternity: 9-64   A Adult: 15-124   ♂ Male Only   ♀ Female Only**   CPT © 2020 American Medical Association. All Rights Reserved.

Coding Companion for Urology/Nephrology

Kidney

50389

50389   Removal of nephrostomy tube, requiring fluoroscopic guidance (eg, with concurrent indwelling ureteral stent)

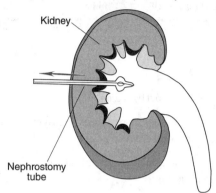

Under fluoroscopic guidance, the physician removes a nephrostomy tube

Kidney

Nephrostomy tube

Explanation

The physician removes an indwelling nephrostomy tube under fluoroscopic guidance that was previously placed concurrently with an indwelling ureteral stent. Nephrostomy tube removal may be done to avoid displacement of the stent. Contrast may first be injected through the indwelling catheter tube to verify placement and functioning of the stent. The suture holding the pigtail in place is cut and a guidewire is threaded through the nephrostomy tube under fluoroscopy, making certain that the pigtail or suture does not hook the stent and that the stent remains in proper position. The nephrostomy tube is pulled out over the guidewire, stent position is checked again, and the access site is dressed.

Coding Tips

If the indwelling nephrostomy tube is removed without fluoroscopic guidance, report with an appropriate E/M service code.

ICD-10-CM Diagnostic Codes

T83.118A   Breakdown (mechanical) of other urinary devices and implants, initial encounter

T83.128A   Displacement of other urinary devices and implants, initial encounter

T83.198A   Other mechanical complication of other urinary devices and implants, initial encounter

T83.512A   Infection and inflammatory reaction due to nephrostomy catheter, initial encounter

T83.518A   Infection and inflammatory reaction due to other urinary catheter, initial encounter

T83.592A   Infection and inflammatory reaction due to indwelling ureteral stent, initial encounter

T83.593A   Infection and inflammatory reaction due to other urinary stents, initial encounter

T83.81XA   Embolism due to genitourinary prosthetic devices, implants and grafts, initial encounter

T83.82XA   Fibrosis due to genitourinary prosthetic devices, implants and grafts, initial encounter

T83.83XA   Hemorrhage due to genitourinary prosthetic devices, implants and grafts, initial encounter

T83.84XA   Pain due to genitourinary prosthetic devices, implants and grafts, initial encounter

T83.85XA   Stenosis due to genitourinary prosthetic devices, implants and grafts, initial encounter

T83.86XA   Thrombosis due to genitourinary prosthetic devices, implants and grafts, initial encounter

T83.89XA   Other specified complication of genitourinary prosthetic devices, implants and grafts, initial encounter

T86.19   Other complication of kidney transplant

AMA: 50389 2018,Jan,8; 2017,Jan,8; 2016,Jan,13; 2016,Jan,3; 2015,Oct,5; 2015,Jan,16; 2014,Jan,11

Relative Value Units/Medicare Edits

Non-Facility RVU	Work	PE	MP	Total
50389	1.1	9.5	0.09	10.69
Facility RVU	Work	PE	MP	Total
50389	1.1	0.36	0.09	1.55

	FUD	Status	MUE	Modifiers				IOM Reference
50389	0	A	1(3)	51	50	N/A	N/A	None

* with documentation

Terms To Know

bone conduction. Transportation of sound through the bones of the skull to the inner ear.

contrast material. Any internally administered substance that has a different opacity from soft tissue on radiography or computed tomograph; includes barium, used to opacify parts of the gastrointestinal tract; water-soluble iodinated compounds, used to opacify blood vessels or the genitourinary tract; may refer to air occurring naturally or introduced into the body; also, paramagnetic substances used in magnetic resonance imaging. Substances may also be documented as contrast agent or contrast medium.

dressing. Material applied to a wound or surgical site for protection, absorption, or drainage of the area.

fluoroscopy. Radiology technique that allows visual examination of part of the body or a function of an organ using a device that projects an x-ray image on a fluorescent screen.

guidewire. Flexible metal instrument designed to lead another instrument in its proper course.

nephrostomy. Placement of a stent, tube, or catheter that forms a passage from the exterior of the body into the renal pelvis or calyx, often for drainage of urine or an abscess, for exploration, or calculus extraction.

stent. Tube to provide support in a body cavity or lumen.

tube. Long, hollow cylindrical instrument or body structure.

Kidney

50390

50390 Aspiration and/or injection of renal cyst or pelvis by needle, percutaneous

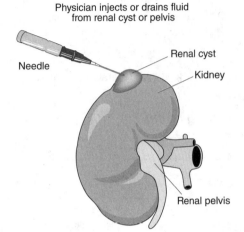

Physician injects or drains fluid from renal cyst or pelvis

Needle

Renal cyst

Kidney

Renal pelvis

Explanation

The physician inserts a needle through the skin to inject or drain fluid from the renal pelvis or a renal cyst. The physician usually inserts a long, thin needle in the skin of the back. Using radiologic guidance, the physician advances the needle toward the renal pelvis or renal cyst and injects or drains fluid.

Coding Tips

Local anesthesia is included in this service. However, general anesthesia may be administered depending on the age or condition of the patient. Radiological supervision and interpretation is reported with 74425, 74470, 76942, 77002, 77012, and 77021, when performed. For fine needle aspirate evaluation, see 88172–88173. For excision of cyst from a kidney, see 50280–50290. For antegrade nephrostogram and/or pyelogram, see 50430-50431.

ICD-10-CM Diagnostic Codes

N13.0	Hydronephrosis with ureteropelvic junction obstruction
N13.1	Hydronephrosis with ureteral stricture, not elsewhere classified
N13.2	Hydronephrosis with renal and ureteral calculous obstruction
N13.39	Other hydronephrosis
N13.6	Pyonephrosis
N15.1	Renal and perinephric abscess
N28.1	Cyst of kidney, acquired
N28.89	Other specified disorders of kidney and ureter
Q61.01	Congenital single renal cyst
Q61.02	Congenital multiple renal cysts
Q61.11	Cystic dilatation of collecting ducts
Q61.19	Other polycystic kidney, infantile type
Q61.2	Polycystic kidney, adult type
Q61.8	Other cystic kidney diseases
Q62.0	Congenital hydronephrosis

AMA: 50390 2018,Jan,8; 2017,Jan,8; 2016,Jan,13; 2015,Oct,5; 2015,Jan,16; 2014,Jan,11

Relative Value Units/Medicare Edits

Non-Facility RVU	Work	PE	MP	Total
50390	1.96	0.65	0.16	2.77
Facility RVU	**Work**	**PE**	**MP**	**Total**
50390	1.96	0.65	0.16	2.77

	FUD	Status	MUE	Modifiers				IOM Reference
50390	0	A	2(3)	51	50	N/A	N/A	None

* with documentation

Terms To Know

aspiration. Drawing fluid out by suction.

congenital. Present at birth, occurring through heredity or an influence during gestation up to the moment of birth.

cyst. Elevated encapsulated mass containing fluid, semisolid, or solid material with a membranous lining.

drainage. Releasing, taking, or letting out fluids and/or gases from a body part.

hydronephrosis. Distension of the kidney caused by an accumulation of urine that cannot flow out due to an obstruction that may be caused by conditions such as kidney stones or vesicoureteral reflux.

percutaneous. Through the skin.

polycystic. Multiple cysts.

pyonephrosis. Destruction of the kidney parenchyma wherein pus is produced and there is partial or total loss of kidney function.

renal. Referring to the kidney.

ureterocele. Saccular formation of the lower part of the ureter, protruding into the bladder.

Kidney

© 2020 Optum360, LLC   **N** Newborn: 0   **P** Pediatric: 0-17   **M** Maternity: 9-64   **A** Adult: 15-124   ♂ Male Only   ♀ Female Only   CPT © 2020 American Medical Association. All Rights Reserved.

Coding Companion for Urology/Nephrology

50391

50391   Instillation(s) of therapeutic agent into renal pelvis and/or ureter through established nephrostomy, pyelostomy or ureterostomy tube (eg, anticarcinogenic or antifungal agent)

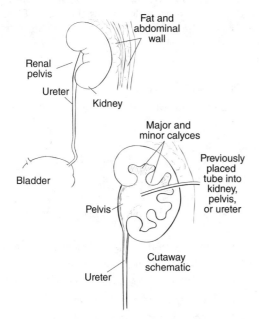

A therapeutic agent is instilled through an established opening into the kidney, renal pelvis, and/or ureter via established nephrostomy, pyelostomy, or ureterostomy tube

Explanation

The physician instills a therapeutic agent, such as an anticarcinogenic or an antifungal, through the tube of an established opening between the skin and kidney (nephrostomy), renal pelvis (pyelostomy), or ureter (ureterostomy). This type of intracavitary topical therapy is reliably done through a tube left in place following a previous surgery. After inserting a guidewire, an endoscope or flexible delivery catheter is passed through the tube into the kidney, renal pelvis, or ureter. To better view renal and ureteric structures, the physician may flush (irrigate) or introduce by drops (instillate) a saline solution. The physician introduces the therapeutic agent to the target area. After examination, the physician removes the instruments and reinserts the nephrostomy, pyelostomy, or ureterostomy tube or allows the surgical passageway to seal on its own.

Coding Tips

For renal endoscopy through established nephrostomy or pyelostomy, with or without irrigation or instillation, see 50551.

ICD-10-CM Diagnostic Codes

B37.89	Other sites of candidiasis
B48.8	Other specified mycoses
C64.1	Malignant neoplasm of right kidney, except renal pelvis ☑
C64.2	Malignant neoplasm of left kidney, except renal pelvis ☑
C65.1	Malignant neoplasm of right renal pelvis ☑
C65.2	Malignant neoplasm of left renal pelvis ☑
C66.1	Malignant neoplasm of right ureter ☑
C66.2	Malignant neoplasm of left ureter ☑
C67.6	Malignant neoplasm of ureteric orifice

C79.01	Secondary malignant neoplasm of right kidney and renal pelvis ☑
C79.02	Secondary malignant neoplasm of left kidney and renal pelvis ☑
C79.11	Secondary malignant neoplasm of bladder
C79.19	Secondary malignant neoplasm of other urinary organs
C7A.093	Malignant carcinoid tumor of the kidney
C80.2	Malignant neoplasm associated with transplanted organ
D09.0	Carcinoma in situ of bladder
D09.19	Carcinoma in situ of other urinary organs
D41.01	Neoplasm of uncertain behavior of right kidney ☑
D41.02	Neoplasm of uncertain behavior of left kidney ☑
D41.11	Neoplasm of uncertain behavior of right renal pelvis ☑
D41.12	Neoplasm of uncertain behavior of left renal pelvis ☑
D41.21	Neoplasm of uncertain behavior of right ureter ☑
D41.22	Neoplasm of uncertain behavior of left ureter ☑
D41.4	Neoplasm of uncertain behavior of bladder
D49.511	Neoplasm of unspecified behavior of right kidney ☑
D49.512	Neoplasm of unspecified behavior of left kidney ☑
D49.59	Neoplasm of unspecified behavior of other genitourinary organ
N10	Acute pyelonephritis
N11.0	Nonobstructive reflux-associated chronic pyelonephritis
N11.1	Chronic obstructive pyelonephritis
N11.8	Other chronic tubulo-interstitial nephritis
N12	Tubulo-interstitial nephritis, not specified as acute or chronic
N13.6	Pyonephrosis

AMA: **50391** 2018,Jan,8; 2017,Jan,8; 2016,Jan,13; 2015,Oct,5; 2015,Jan,16; 2014,Jan,11

Relative Value Units/Medicare Edits

Non-Facility RVU	Work	PE	MP	Total
50391	1.96	1.36	0.23	3.55
Facility RVU	Work	PE	MP	Total
50391	1.96	0.66	0.23	2.85

	FUD	Status	MUE	Modifiers				IOM Reference
50391	0	A	1(3)	51	50	N/A	N/A	None

* with documentation

Terms To Know

catheter. Flexible tube inserted into an area of the body for introducing or withdrawing fluid.

instillation. Administering a liquid slowly over time, drop by drop.

nephrostomy. Placement of a stent, tube, or catheter that forms a passage from the exterior of the body into the renal pelvis or calyx, often for drainage of urine or an abscess, for exploration, or calculus extraction.

pyelostomy. Surgical creation of an opening through the abdominal wall into the renal pelvis.

ureterostomy. Placement of a stent, tube, or catheter into the ureter, forming a passageway from the exterior of the body to the ureter.

CPT © 2020 American Medical Association. All Rights Reserved.   ● New   ▲ Revised   + Add On   ★ Telemedicine   AMA: CPT Assist   [Resequenced]   ☑ Laterality   © 2020 Optum360, LLC

[50436, 50437]

50436   Dilation of existing tract, percutaneous, for an endourologic procedure including imaging guidance (eg, ultrasound and/or fluoroscopy) and all associated radiological supervision and interpretation, with postprocedure tube placement, when performed

50437   Dilation of existing tract, percutaneous, for an endourologic procedure including imaging guidance (eg, ultrasound and/or fluoroscopy) and all associated radiological supervision and interpretation, with postprocedure tube placement, when performed; including new access into the renal collecting system

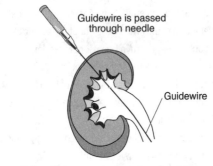

Guidewire is passed through needle

Guidewire

Tubes dilate passageway and nephrostomy tube is inserted; guidewire is withdrawn

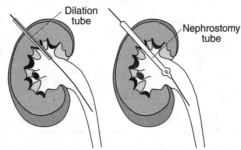

Dilation tube

Nephrostomy tube

Explanation

A guide is inserted into the renal pelvis and/or ureter to enlarge the passageway between the skin and kidney. The physician makes a small incision in the skin of the back, inserts a large needle, and ultrasonographically guides it toward the kidney. After passing a guidewire through the needle and through the kidney into the renal pelvis, the physician removes the needle by passing it backward over the guidewire. The physician enlarges (dilates) the guidewire passageway by inserting and removing tubes with increasingly larger diameters. When the passageway is sufficiently dilated, the physician passes a nephrostomy tube over the guidewire, removes the guidewire, and sutures the tube to the skin. All imaging, including radiologic supervision and interpretation, is included and should not be reported separately. Report 50436 when the physician enlarges an existing percutaneous nephrostomy tract and inserts a needle into the renal collecting system in order to allow for the introduction of large instruments to be utilized in an endoscopic urologic procedure. Report 50437 when the physician creates new access into the renal collecting system in the same operative session where an existing tract is not present.

Coding Tips

Diagnostic nephrostogram and/or ureterogram are often included with these services and should not be reported separately. Do not report 50436–50437 with the following services: 50080–50081, 50382, 50384, 50430–50434, or 74485. Imaging, including radiological supervision and interpretation, is included in these services. For creation of nephrostomy or pyelostomy, see 50040 and 50125. Report nephrostolithotomy with 50080-50081. For cystourethroscopy, with insertion of a ureteral guidewire through the kidney to establish a percutaneous nephrostomy, see 52334. For renal endoscopic procedures, see 50551–50561.

ICD-10-CM Diagnostic Codes

C64.1	Malignant neoplasm of right kidney, except renal pelvis ☑
C64.2	Malignant neoplasm of left kidney, except renal pelvis ☑
C65.1	Malignant neoplasm of right renal pelvis ☑
C65.2	Malignant neoplasm of left renal pelvis ☑
C66.1	Malignant neoplasm of right ureter ☑
C66.2	Malignant neoplasm of left ureter ☑
C79.01	Secondary malignant neoplasm of right kidney and renal pelvis ☑
C79.02	Secondary malignant neoplasm of left kidney and renal pelvis ☑
C79.11	Secondary malignant neoplasm of bladder
C79.19	Secondary malignant neoplasm of other urinary organs
C7A.093	Malignant carcinoid tumor of the kidney
C80.2	Malignant neoplasm associated with transplanted organ
D09.19	Carcinoma in situ of other urinary organs
D30.11	Benign neoplasm of right renal pelvis ☑
D30.12	Benign neoplasm of left renal pelvis ☑
D30.21	Benign neoplasm of right ureter ☑
D30.22	Benign neoplasm of left ureter ☑
D3A.093	Benign carcinoid tumor of the kidney
D41.01	Neoplasm of uncertain behavior of right kidney ☑
D41.02	Neoplasm of uncertain behavior of left kidney ☑
D41.11	Neoplasm of uncertain behavior of right renal pelvis ☑
D41.12	Neoplasm of uncertain behavior of left renal pelvis ☑
D41.21	Neoplasm of uncertain behavior of right ureter ☑
D41.22	Neoplasm of uncertain behavior of left ureter ☑
D47.Z1	Post-transplant lymphoproliferative disorder (PTLD)
D47.Z2	Castleman disease
D49.511	Neoplasm of unspecified behavior of right kidney ☑
D49.512	Neoplasm of unspecified behavior of left kidney ☑
D49.59	Neoplasm of unspecified behavior of other genitourinary organ
N10	Acute pyelonephritis
N11.0	Nonobstructive reflux-associated chronic pyelonephritis
N11.1	Chronic obstructive pyelonephritis
N11.8	Other chronic tubulo-interstitial nephritis
N12	Tubulo-interstitial nephritis, not specified as acute or chronic
N13.0	Hydronephrosis with ureteropelvic junction obstruction
N13.1	Hydronephrosis with ureteral stricture, not elsewhere classified
N13.2	Hydronephrosis with renal and ureteral calculous obstruction
N13.39	Other hydronephrosis
N13.4	Hydroureter
N13.5	Crossing vessel and stricture of ureter without hydronephrosis
N13.6	Pyonephrosis

Kidney

N13.721	Vesicoureteral-reflux with reflux nephropathy without hydroureter, unilateral
N13.722	Vesicoureteral-reflux with reflux nephropathy without hydroureter, bilateral
N13.731	Vesicoureteral-reflux with reflux nephropathy with hydroureter, unilateral
N13.732	Vesicoureteral-reflux with reflux nephropathy with hydroureter, bilateral
N13.8	Other obstructive and reflux uropathy
N15.1	Renal and perinephric abscess
N20.0	Calculus of kidney
N20.1	Calculus of ureter
N20.2	Calculus of kidney with calculus of ureter
N22	Calculus of urinary tract in diseases classified elsewhere
N25.81	Secondary hyperparathyroidism of renal origin
N25.89	Other disorders resulting from impaired renal tubular function
N28.82	Megaloureter
N28.84	Pyelitis cystica
N28.85	Pyeloureteritis cystica
N28.86	Ureteritis cystica
N28.89	Other specified disorders of kidney and ureter
N29	Other disorders of kidney and ureter in diseases classified elsewhere
N39.3	Stress incontinence (female) (male)
N39.41	Urge incontinence
N39.42	Incontinence without sensory awareness
N39.43	Post-void dribbling
N39.44	Nocturnal enuresis
N39.45	Continuous leakage
N39.46	Mixed incontinence
N39.490	Overflow incontinence
N39.491	Coital incontinence
N39.492	Postural (urinary) incontinence
N39.498	Other specified urinary incontinence
N39.8	Other specified disorders of urinary system
N82.1	Other female urinary-genital tract fistulae ♀
Q62.0	Congenital hydronephrosis
Q62.11	Congenital occlusion of ureteropelvic junction
Q62.12	Congenital occlusion of ureterovesical orifice
Q62.2	Congenital megaureter
Q62.31	Congenital ureterocele, orthotopic
Q62.32	Cecoureterocele
Q62.39	Other obstructive defects of renal pelvis and ureter
Q62.5	Duplication of ureter
Q62.61	Deviation of ureter
Q62.62	Displacement of ureter
Q62.63	Anomalous implantation of ureter
Q62.69	Other malposition of ureter
Q62.8	Other congenital malformations of ureter
R82.71	Bacteriuria
R82.79	Other abnormal findings on microbiological examination of urine
T86.11	Kidney transplant rejection
T86.12	Kidney transplant failure
T86.13	Kidney transplant infection
T86.19	Other complication of kidney transplant

Relative Value Units/Medicare Edits

Non-Facility RVU	Work	PE	MP	Total
50436	2.78	1.3	0.27	4.35
50437	4.85	1.97	0.47	7.29
Facility RVU	Work	PE	MP	Total
50436	2.78	1.3	0.27	4.35
50437	4.85	1.97	0.47	7.29

	FUD	Status	MUE	Modifiers				IOM Reference
50436	0	A	1(3)	51	50	N/A	N/A	None
50437	0	A	1(3)	51	50	N/A	N/A	

* with documentation

Terms To Know

dilation. Artificial increase in the diameter of an opening or lumen made by medication or by instrumentation.

guidewire. Flexible metal instrument designed to lead another instrument in its proper course.

imaging. Radiologic means of producing pictures for clinical study of the internal structures and functions of the body, such as x-ray, ultrasound, magnetic resonance, or positron emission tomography.

nephrostomy. Placement of a stent, tube, or catheter that forms a passage from the exterior of the body into the renal pelvis or calyx, often for drainage of urine or an abscess, for exploration, or calculus extraction.

percutaneous approach. Method used to gain access to a body organ or specific area by puncture or minor incision through the skin or mucous membrane and/or any other body layers necessary to reach the procedure site.

supervision and interpretation. Radiology services that usually contain an invasive component and are reported by the radiologist for supervision of the procedure and the personnel involved with performing the examination, reading the film, and preparing the written report.

Kidney

CPT © 2020 American Medical Association. All Rights Reserved.   ● New   ▲ Revised   + Add On   ★ Telemedicine   AMA: CPT Assist   [Resequenced]   ☑ Laterality   © 2020 Optum360, LLC

50396

50396 Manometric studies through nephrostomy or pyelostomy tube, or indwelling ureteral catheter

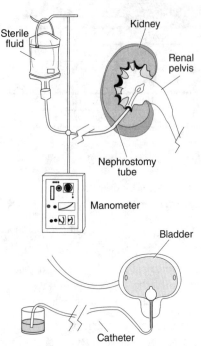

Manometer measures pressure flow in kidney and ureter

Sterile fluid

Kidney

Renal pelvis

Nephrostomy tube

Manometer

Bladder

Catheter

Explanation

The physician connects an indwelling ureteral catheter or existing pyelostomy or nephrostomy tube to a manometer line to measure pressure and flow in the kidneys and ureters. The physician connects a ureteral catheter or pyelostomy or nephrostomy tube to a manometer line filled with fluid. The physician inserts a bladder catheter that may be irrigated. The physician measures intrarenal and/or extrarenal pressure. After discontinuing perfusion of fluid, the physician aspirates residual fluid from the kidney and disconnects the manometer line. The physician may remove the ureteral catheter or pyelostomy or nephrostomy tube and dress the wound.

Coding Tips

Anesthesia is not administered with this procedure. For creation of a nephrostomy or pyelostomy, see 50040 and 50125. For dilation of an existing tract for an endourologic procedure, percutaneous, see 50436; including new access into the renal collecting system, see 50437. Report exchange of a percutaneous nephrostomy catheter with 50435. For radiological supervision and interpretation, see 74425.

ICD-10-CM Diagnostic Codes

N13.0	Hydronephrosis with ureteropelvic junction obstruction
N13.1	Hydronephrosis with ureteral stricture, not elsewhere classified
N13.2	Hydronephrosis with renal and ureteral calculous obstruction
N13.39	Other hydronephrosis
N39.3	Stress incontinence (female) (male)
N39.41	Urge incontinence
N39.42	Incontinence without sensory awareness
N39.43	Post-void dribbling
N39.44	Nocturnal enuresis
N39.45	Continuous leakage
N39.46	Mixed incontinence
N39.490	Overflow incontinence
N39.491	Coital incontinence
N39.492	Postural (urinary) incontinence
N39.498	Other specified urinary incontinence
Q62.0	Congenital hydronephrosis
Q62.11	Congenital occlusion of ureteropelvic junction
Q62.12	Congenital occlusion of ureterovesical orifice
Q62.2	Congenital megaureter
Q62.31	Congenital ureterocele, orthotopic
Q62.32	Cecoureterocele
Q62.39	Other obstructive defects of renal pelvis and ureter

AMA: **50396** 2018,Jan,8; 2017,Jan,8; 2016,Jan,13; 2015,Jan,16; 2014,Jan,11

Relative Value Units/Medicare Edits

Non-Facility RVU	Work	PE	MP	Total
50396	2.09	1.11	0.16	3.36
Facility RVU	**Work**	**PE**	**MP**	**Total**
50396	2.09	1.11	0.16	3.36

	FUD	Status	MUE	Modifiers				IOM Reference
50396	0	A	1(3)	51	50	N/A	80*	None

* with documentation

Terms To Know

aspirate. To withdraw fluid or air from a body cavity by suction.

catheter. Flexible tube inserted into an area of the body for introducing or withdrawing fluid.

dressing. Material applied to a wound or surgical site for protection, absorption, or drainage of the area.

intra. Within.

manometric. Pertaining to pressure, as measured in a meter.

nephrostomy. Placement of a stent, tube, or catheter that forms a passage from the exterior of the body into the renal pelvis or calyx, often for drainage of urine or an abscess, for exploration, or calculus extraction.

perfusion. Act of pouring over or through, especially the passage of a fluid through the vessels of a specific organ.

pyelostomy. Surgical creation of an opening through the abdominal wall into the renal pelvis.

renal. Referring to the kidney.

tube. Long, hollow cylindrical instrument or body structure.

Kidney

© 2020 Optum360, LLC

N Newborn: 0   **P** Pediatric: 0-17   **M** Maternity: 9-64   **A** Adult: 15-124   ♂ Male Only   ♀ Female Only   CPT © 2020 American Medical Association. All Rights Reserved.

[50430, 50431]

50430 Injection procedure for antegrade nephrostogram and/or ureterogram, complete diagnostic procedure including imaging guidance (eg, ultrasound and fluoroscopy) and all associated radiological supervision and interpretation; new access

50431 Injection procedure for antegrade nephrostogram and/or ureterogram, complete diagnostic procedure including imaging guidance (eg, ultrasound and fluoroscopy) and all associated radiological supervision and interpretation; existing access

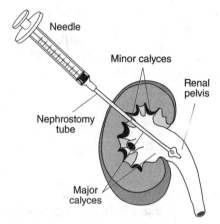

Physician injects contrast agent through tube or catheter to study kidney and renal collecting system

Needle

Minor calyces

Renal pelvis

Nephrostomy tube

Major calyces

Explanation

The physician injects a contrast agent through a tube or indwelling catheter into the renal pelvis to study the kidney and renal collecting system. The physician determines immediate allergic response to the contrast agent by injecting a small initial dose of contrast material through an existing nephrostomy tube or indwelling ureteral catheter. If no allergic response occurs, a large quantity of contrast material is injected into the renal pelvis. The contrast is visualized as it passes from the kidneys into the ureters and the urinary bladder. Imaging guidance via fluoroscopy or ultrasound is used to observe the contrast path. When an obstruction is present, it can be readily identified on imaging because the contrast is unable to progress properly through the urinary tract. The radiologist produces a representation of the kidney, renal pelvis, and/or ureter with an x-ray. Report 50431 when this test is performed through an existing access.

Coding Tips

Do not report 50430-50431 with 50432–50435, 50693–50695, or 74425 for the same renal collection system and/or associated ureter. These codes are diagnostic services that include injection of contrast material, all associated radiological supervision and interpretation, and procedural imaging guidance (i.e., fluoroscopy, ultrasound, etc.). Code 50430 includes accessing the collecting system and/or associated ureter with a needle or catheter.

ICD-10-CM Diagnostic Codes

C64.1	Malignant neoplasm of right kidney, except renal pelvis ☑
C64.2	Malignant neoplasm of left kidney, except renal pelvis ☑
C65.1	Malignant neoplasm of right renal pelvis ☑
C65.2	Malignant neoplasm of left renal pelvis ☑
C66.1	Malignant neoplasm of right ureter ☑
C66.2	Malignant neoplasm of left ureter ☑
C68.8	Malignant neoplasm of overlapping sites of urinary organs
C79.01	Secondary malignant neoplasm of right kidney and renal pelvis ☑
C79.02	Secondary malignant neoplasm of left kidney and renal pelvis ☑
C79.19	Secondary malignant neoplasm of other urinary organs
C7A.093	Malignant carcinoid tumor of the kidney
D09.19	Carcinoma in situ of other urinary organs
D30.01	Benign neoplasm of right kidney ☑
D30.02	Benign neoplasm of left kidney ☑
D30.11	Benign neoplasm of right renal pelvis ☑
D30.12	Benign neoplasm of left renal pelvis ☑
D30.21	Benign neoplasm of right ureter ☑
D30.22	Benign neoplasm of left ureter ☑
D3A.093	Benign carcinoid tumor of the kidney
D41.01	Neoplasm of uncertain behavior of right kidney ☑
D41.02	Neoplasm of uncertain behavior of left kidney ☑
D41.11	Neoplasm of uncertain behavior of right renal pelvis ☑
D41.12	Neoplasm of uncertain behavior of left renal pelvis ☑
D41.21	Neoplasm of uncertain behavior of right ureter ☑
D41.22	Neoplasm of uncertain behavior of left ureter ☑
D47.Z1	Post-transplant lymphoproliferative disorder (PTLD)
D47.Z2	Castleman disease
D49.511	Neoplasm of unspecified behavior of right kidney ☑
D49.512	Neoplasm of unspecified behavior of left kidney ☑
D49.59	Neoplasm of unspecified behavior of other genitourinary organ
N11.0	Nonobstructive reflux-associated chronic pyelonephritis
N11.1	Chronic obstructive pyelonephritis
N11.8	Other chronic tubulo-interstitial nephritis
N13.0	Hydronephrosis with ureteropelvic junction obstruction
N13.1	Hydronephrosis with ureteral stricture, not elsewhere classified
N13.2	Hydronephrosis with renal and ureteral calculous obstruction
N13.39	Other hydronephrosis
N13.5	Crossing vessel and stricture of ureter without hydronephrosis
N13.71	Vesicoureteral-reflux without reflux nephropathy
N13.721	Vesicoureteral-reflux with reflux nephropathy without hydroureter, unilateral
N13.722	Vesicoureteral-reflux with reflux nephropathy without hydroureter, bilateral
N13.731	Vesicoureteral-reflux with reflux nephropathy with hydroureter, unilateral
N13.732	Vesicoureteral-reflux with reflux nephropathy with hydroureter, bilateral
N13.8	Other obstructive and reflux uropathy
N20.0	Calculus of kidney
N20.1	Calculus of ureter
N20.2	Calculus of kidney with calculus of ureter
N25.81	Secondary hyperparathyroidism of renal origin
N25.89	Other disorders resulting from impaired renal tubular function
N26.1	Atrophy of kidney (terminal)
N28.1	Cyst of kidney, acquired
N28.82	Megaloureter
N28.84	Pyelitis cystica
N28.85	Pyeloureteritis cystica

N28.86	Ureteritis cystica
N28.89	Other specified disorders of kidney and ureter
N41.1	Chronic prostatitis 🅐 ♂
N99.0	Postprocedural (acute) (chronic) kidney failure
N99.81	Other intraoperative complications of genitourinary system
N99.89	Other postprocedural complications and disorders of genitourinary system
Q60.3	Renal hypoplasia, unilateral
Q60.4	Renal hypoplasia, bilateral
Q60.6	Potter's syndrome
Q61.01	Congenital single renal cyst
Q61.02	Congenital multiple renal cysts
Q61.11	Cystic dilatation of collecting ducts
Q61.19	Other polycystic kidney, infantile type
Q61.2	Polycystic kidney, adult type
Q61.4	Renal dysplasia
Q61.5	Medullary cystic kidney
Q61.8	Other cystic kidney diseases
Q62.0	Congenital hydronephrosis
Q62.11	Congenital occlusion of ureteropelvic junction
Q62.12	Congenital occlusion of ureterovesical orifice
Q62.2	Congenital megaureter
Q62.31	Congenital ureterocele, orthotopic
Q62.32	Cecoureterocele
Q62.39	Other obstructive defects of renal pelvis and ureter
Q64.8	Other specified congenital malformations of urinary system
T86.19	Other complication of kidney transplant

AMA: **50430** 2018,Jan,8; 2017,Jan,8; 2016,Jan,3; 2016,Jan,13; 2015,Oct,5
50431 2018,Jan,8; 2017,Jan,8; 2016,Jan,3; 2016,Jan,13; 2015,Oct,5

Relative Value Units/Medicare Edits

Non-Facility RVU	Work	PE	MP	Total
50430	2.9	13.0	0.27	16.17
50431	1.1	6.17	0.09	7.36
Facility RVU	**Work**	**PE**	**MP**	**Total**
50430	2.9	1.29	0.27	4.46
50431	1.1	0.69	0.09	1.88

	FUD	Status	MUE	Modifiers				IOM Reference
50430	0	A	2(3)	51	50	N/A	80*	None
50431	0	A	2(3)	51	50	N/A	N/A	

* with documentation

Terms To Know

catheter. Flexible tube inserted into an area of the body for introducing or withdrawing fluid.

contrast material. Any internally administered substance that has a different opacity from soft tissue on radiography or computed tomograph; includes barium, used to opacify parts of the gastrointestinal tract; water-soluble iodinated compounds, used to opacify blood vessels or the genitourinary tract; may refer to air occurring naturally or introduced into the body; also, paramagnetic substances used in magnetic resonance imaging. Substances may also be documented as contrast agent or contrast medium.

[50432, 50433]

50432 Placement of nephrostomy catheter, percutaneous, including diagnostic nephrostogram and/or ureterogram when performed, imaging guidance (eg, ultrasound and/or fluoroscopy) and all associated radiological supervision and interpretation

50433 Placement of nephroureteral catheter, percutaneous, including diagnostic nephrostogram and/or ureterogram when performed, imaging guidance (eg, ultrasound and/or fluoroscopy) and all associated radiological supervision and interpretation, new access

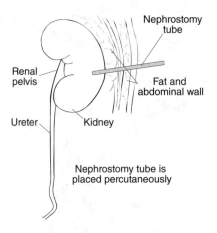

Explanation

The physician inserts a catheter through the skin and into the kidney for drainage of urine and/or for an injection. With the patient lying face down and the puncture site having been identified, a local anesthetic is injected. A needle with a guidewire is slowly advanced into the kidney under fluoroscopic guidance. The needle is removed when urine flows back through and, if necessary, the tract may be dilated to accommodate the catheter or nephrostomy tube, which is advanced over the needle, and the needle is removed. The catheter or nephrostomy tube is fixed in place and secured on the skin with a drainage bag attached. These codes include diagnostic nephrostogram and ureterogram, imaging guidance, and all radiological supervision and interpretation. Report 50433 for placement of a nephroureteral catheter via a new access.

Coding Tips

Do not report 50432–50433 with 50430–50431 (injection procedure for antegrade nephrostogram and/or ureterogram), 50436–50437 (dilation of the nephrostomy tube tract), 50694–50695 (percutaneous ureteral stent placement with/without separate nephrostomy catheter), 74425, or each other; additionally, 50433 should not be reported with 50693. Report 50435 when the nephrostomy tube remains in place and in the kidney. For removal and replacement of a nephroureteral catheter, see 50387.

ICD-10-CM Diagnostic Codes

C64.1	Malignant neoplasm of right kidney, except renal pelvis ☑
C64.2	Malignant neoplasm of left kidney, except renal pelvis ☑
C65.1	Malignant neoplasm of right renal pelvis ☑
C65.2	Malignant neoplasm of left renal pelvis ☑
C66.1	Malignant neoplasm of right ureter ☑
C66.2	Malignant neoplasm of left ureter ☑
C79.01	Secondary malignant neoplasm of right kidney and renal pelvis ☑
C79.02	Secondary malignant neoplasm of left kidney and renal pelvis ☑

Kidney

C79.19	Secondary malignant neoplasm of other urinary organs
C7A.093	Malignant carcinoid tumor of the kidney
C80.2	Malignant neoplasm associated with transplanted organ
D09.19	Carcinoma in situ of other urinary organs
D30.11	Benign neoplasm of right renal pelvis ☑
D30.12	Benign neoplasm of left renal pelvis ☑
D30.21	Benign neoplasm of right ureter ☑
D30.22	Benign neoplasm of left ureter ☑
D3A.093	Benign carcinoid tumor of the kidney
D41.01	Neoplasm of uncertain behavior of right kidney ☑
D41.02	Neoplasm of uncertain behavior of left kidney ☑
D41.11	Neoplasm of uncertain behavior of right renal pelvis ☑
D41.12	Neoplasm of uncertain behavior of left renal pelvis ☑
D41.21	Neoplasm of uncertain behavior of right ureter ☑
D41.22	Neoplasm of uncertain behavior of left ureter ☑
D47.Z1	Post-transplant lymphoproliferative disorder (PTLD)
D47.Z2	Castleman disease
D49.511	Neoplasm of unspecified behavior of right kidney ☑
D49.512	Neoplasm of unspecified behavior of left kidney ☑
D49.59	Neoplasm of unspecified behavior of other genitourinary organ
N10	Acute pyelonephritis
N11.0	Nonobstructive reflux-associated chronic pyelonephritis
N11.1	Chronic obstructive pyelonephritis
N11.8	Other chronic tubulo-interstitial nephritis
N12	Tubulo-interstitial nephritis, not specified as acute or chronic
N13.0	Hydronephrosis with ureteropelvic junction obstruction
N13.1	Hydronephrosis with ureteral stricture, not elsewhere classified
N13.2	Hydronephrosis with renal and ureteral calculous obstruction
N13.39	Other hydronephrosis
N13.4	Hydroureter
N13.5	Crossing vessel and stricture of ureter without hydronephrosis
N13.6	Pyonephrosis
N13.721	Vesicoureteral-reflux with reflux nephropathy without hydroureter, unilateral
N13.722	Vesicoureteral-reflux with reflux nephropathy without hydroureter, bilateral
N13.731	Vesicoureteral-reflux with reflux nephropathy with hydroureter, unilateral
N13.732	Vesicoureteral-reflux with reflux nephropathy with hydroureter, bilateral
N13.8	Other obstructive and reflux uropathy
N15.1	Renal and perinephric abscess
N20.0	Calculus of kidney
N20.1	Calculus of ureter
N20.2	Calculus of kidney with calculus of ureter
N25.81	Secondary hyperparathyroidism of renal origin
N25.89	Other disorders resulting from impaired renal tubular function
N28.82	Megaloureter
N28.84	Pyelitis cystica
N28.85	Pyeloureteritis cystica
N28.86	Ureteritis cystica
N28.89	Other specified disorders of kidney and ureter
N39.3	Stress incontinence (female) (male)

N39.41	Urge incontinence
N39.42	Incontinence without sensory awareness
N39.43	Post-void dribbling
N39.44	Nocturnal enuresis
N39.45	Continuous leakage
N39.46	Mixed incontinence
N39.490	Overflow incontinence
N39.491	Coital incontinence
N39.492	Postural (urinary) incontinence
N39.498	Other specified urinary incontinence
N39.8	Other specified disorders of urinary system
N82.1	Other female urinary-genital tract fistulae ♀
Q62.0	Congenital hydronephrosis
Q62.11	Congenital occlusion of ureteropelvic junction
Q62.12	Congenital occlusion of ureterovesical orifice
Q62.2	Congenital megaureter
Q62.31	Congenital ureterocele, orthotopic
Q62.32	Cecoureterocele
Q62.39	Other obstructive defects of renal pelvis and ureter
Q62.5	Duplication of ureter
Q62.61	Deviation of ureter
Q62.62	Displacement of ureter
Q62.63	Anomalous implantation of ureter
Q62.69	Other malposition of ureter
Q62.8	Other congenital malformations of ureter
R82.71	Bacteriuria
R82.79	Other abnormal findings on microbiological examination of urine
T86.11	Kidney transplant rejection
T86.12	Kidney transplant failure
T86.13	Kidney transplant infection
T86.19	Other complication of kidney transplant

AMA: **50432** 2018,Mar,11; 2018,Jan,8; 2017,Jan,8; 2016,Jan,3; 2016,Jan,13; 2015,Oct,5 **50433** 2018,Mar,11; 2018,Jan,8; 2017,Jan,8; 2016,Jan,3; 2016,Jan,13; 2015,Oct,5

Relative Value Units/Medicare Edits

Non-Facility RVU	Work	PE	MP	Total
50432	4.0	20.95	0.35	25.3
50433	5.05	27.24	0.44	32.73
Facility RVU	**Work**	**PE**	**MP**	**Total**
50432	4.0	1.61	0.35	5.96
50433	5.05	1.91	0.44	7.4

	FUD	Status	MUE	Modifiers				IOM Reference
50432	0	A	2(3)	51	50	N/A	N/A	None
50433	0	A	2(3)	51	50	N/A	N/A	

* with documentation

Terms To Know

calculus. Abnormal, stone-like concretion of calcium, cholesterol, mineral salts, or other substances that forms in any part of the body.

Kidney

[50434]

50434 Convert nephrostomy catheter to nephroureteral catheter, percutaneous, including diagnostic nephrostogram and/or ureterogram when performed, imaging guidance (eg, ultrasound and/or fluoroscopy) and all associated radiological supervision and interpretation, via pre-existing nephrostomy tract

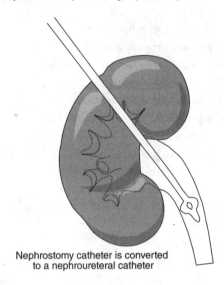

Nephrostomy catheter is converted to a nephroureteral catheter

Explanation

A previously placed nephrostomy catheter is converted to a nephroureteral catheter via percutaneous approach along the current nephrostomy tract. The patient is placed face down and the conversion is performed over a stiff wire. Contrast is injected through the catheter to better visualize the kidneys and ureter. The wire is advanced and the catheter is replaced over the wire and the wire removed. Imaging guidance assures proper placement and the new catheter is secured to the skin with sutures. This procedure includes diagnostic nephrostogram and/or ureterogram, imaging guidance, and all radiological supervision and interpretation.

Coding Tips

Do not report 50434 with 50430–50431, 50435, 50684, 50693, or 74425 for the same renal collecting system and/or associated ureter.

ICD-10-CM Diagnostic Codes

C64.1	Malignant neoplasm of right kidney, except renal pelvis ☑
C64.2	Malignant neoplasm of left kidney, except renal pelvis ☑
C65.1	Malignant neoplasm of right renal pelvis ☑
C65.2	Malignant neoplasm of left renal pelvis ☑
C66.1	Malignant neoplasm of right ureter ☑
C66.2	Malignant neoplasm of left ureter ☑
C79.01	Secondary malignant neoplasm of right kidney and renal pelvis ☑
C79.02	Secondary malignant neoplasm of left kidney and renal pelvis ☑
C79.19	Secondary malignant neoplasm of other urinary organs
C7A.093	Malignant carcinoid tumor of the kidney
C80.2	Malignant neoplasm associated with transplanted organ
D09.19	Carcinoma in situ of other urinary organs
D30.11	Benign neoplasm of right renal pelvis ☑
D30.12	Benign neoplasm of left renal pelvis ☑
D30.21	Benign neoplasm of right ureter ☑

D30.22	Benign neoplasm of left ureter ☑
D3A.093	Benign carcinoid tumor of the kidney
D41.01	Neoplasm of uncertain behavior of right kidney ☑
D41.02	Neoplasm of uncertain behavior of left kidney ☑
D41.11	Neoplasm of uncertain behavior of right renal pelvis ☑
D41.12	Neoplasm of uncertain behavior of left renal pelvis ☑
D41.21	Neoplasm of uncertain behavior of right ureter ☑
D41.22	Neoplasm of uncertain behavior of left ureter ☑
D47.Z1	Post-transplant lymphoproliferative disorder (PTLD)
N10	Acute pyelonephritis
N11.0	Nonobstructive reflux-associated chronic pyelonephritis
N11.1	Chronic obstructive pyelonephritis
N11.8	Other chronic tubulo-interstitial nephritis
N13.0	Hydronephrosis with ureteropelvic junction obstruction
N13.1	Hydronephrosis with ureteral stricture, not elsewhere classified
N13.2	Hydronephrosis with renal and ureteral calculous obstruction
N13.39	Other hydronephrosis
N13.4	Hydroureter
N13.5	Crossing vessel and stricture of ureter without hydronephrosis
N13.6	Pyonephrosis
N13.721	Vesicoureteral-reflux with reflux nephropathy without hydroureter, unilateral
N13.722	Vesicoureteral-reflux with reflux nephropathy without hydroureter, bilateral
N13.731	Vesicoureteral-reflux with reflux nephropathy with hydroureter, unilateral
N13.732	Vesicoureteral-reflux with reflux nephropathy with hydroureter, bilateral
N13.8	Other obstructive and reflux uropathy
N15.1	Renal and perinephric abscess
N20.0	Calculus of kidney
N20.1	Calculus of ureter
N20.2	Calculus of kidney with calculus of ureter
N25.81	Secondary hyperparathyroidism of renal origin
N25.89	Other disorders resulting from impaired renal tubular function
N28.82	Megaloureter
N28.84	Pyelitis cystica
N28.85	Pyeloureteritis cystica
N28.86	Ureteritis cystica
N28.89	Other specified disorders of kidney and ureter
N39.3	Stress incontinence (female) (male)
N39.41	Urge incontinence
N39.42	Incontinence without sensory awareness
N39.43	Post-void dribbling
N39.44	Nocturnal enuresis
N39.45	Continuous leakage
N39.46	Mixed incontinence
N39.490	Overflow incontinence
N39.498	Other specified urinary incontinence
N39.8	Other specified disorders of urinary system
N82.1	Other female urinary-genital tract fistulae ♀
Q62.0	Congenital hydronephrosis
Q62.11	Congenital occlusion of ureteropelvic junction

Kidney

Q62.12	Congenital occlusion of ureterovesical orifice
Q62.2	Congenital megaureter
Q62.31	Congenital ureterocele, orthotopic
Q62.32	Cecoureterocele
Q62.39	Other obstructive defects of renal pelvis and ureter
Q62.5	Duplication of ureter
Q62.61	Deviation of ureter
Q62.62	Displacement of ureter
Q62.63	Anomalous implantation of ureter
Q62.69	Other malposition of ureter
Q62.8	Other congenital malformations of ureter
R82.71	Bacteriuria
R82.79	Other abnormal findings on microbiological examination of urine
T83.118A	Breakdown (mechanical) of other urinary devices and implants, initial encounter
T83.128A	Displacement of other urinary devices and implants, initial encounter
T83.198A	Other mechanical complication of other urinary devices and implants, initial encounter
T83.81XA	Embolism due to genitourinary prosthetic devices, implants and grafts, initial encounter
T83.82XA	Fibrosis due to genitourinary prosthetic devices, implants and grafts, initial encounter
T83.83XA	Hemorrhage due to genitourinary prosthetic devices, implants and grafts, initial encounter
T83.84XA	Pain due to genitourinary prosthetic devices, implants and grafts, initial encounter
T83.85XA	Stenosis due to genitourinary prosthetic devices, implants and grafts, initial encounter
T83.86XA	Thrombosis due to genitourinary prosthetic devices, implants and grafts, initial encounter
T83.89XA	Other specified complication of genitourinary prosthetic devices, implants and grafts, initial encounter
Z46.6	Encounter for fitting and adjustment of urinary device

AMA: 50434 2018,Jan,8; 2017,Jan,8; 2016,Jan,3; 2016,Jan,13; 2015,Oct,5

Relative Value Units/Medicare Edits

Non-Facility RVU	Work	PE	MP	Total
50434	3.75	21.99	0.32	26.06
Facility RVU	**Work**	**PE**	**MP**	**Total**
50434	3.75	1.49	0.32	5.56

	FUD	Status	MUE	Modifiers				IOM Reference
50434	0	A	2(3)	51	50	N/A	N/A	None

* with documentation

[50435]

50435 Exchange nephrostomy catheter, percutaneous, including diagnostic nephrostogram and/or ureterogram when performed, imaging guidance (eg, ultrasound and/or fluoroscopy) and all associated radiological supervision and interpretation

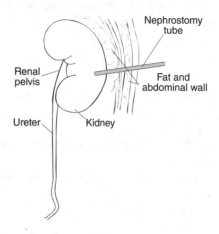

Explanation

The provider changes a nephrostomy catheter by replacing the existing tube. Sutures holding an existing tube in place are removed. A guidewire is inserted through the tube and pulls the tube back out over the wire. A new tube is threaded over the wire until proper placement is achieved. The wire is removed and the new catheter is sutured to the skin. This procedure includes diagnostic nephrostogram and/or ureterogram, imaging guidance, and all radiological supervision and interpretation.

Coding Tips

This code should only be reported if the nephrostomy tube remains in place and in the kidney. For replacement of a nephrostomy catheter via a prior skin incision, see 50432; for new access, see 50433. Do not report 50435 with 50430–50431, 50434, 50693, or 74425 for the same renal collecting system and/or associated ureter. For removal of a nephrostomy catheter under fluoroscopic guidance, see 50389.

ICD-10-CM Diagnostic Codes

C64.1	Malignant neoplasm of right kidney, except renal pelvis ☑
C64.2	Malignant neoplasm of left kidney, except renal pelvis ☑
C65.1	Malignant neoplasm of right renal pelvis ☑
C65.2	Malignant neoplasm of left renal pelvis ☑
C66.1	Malignant neoplasm of right ureter ☑
C66.2	Malignant neoplasm of left ureter ☑
C79.01	Secondary malignant neoplasm of right kidney and renal pelvis ☑
C79.02	Secondary malignant neoplasm of left kidney and renal pelvis ☑
C7A.093	Malignant carcinoid tumor of the kidney
D09.19	Carcinoma in situ of other urinary organs
D30.11	Benign neoplasm of right renal pelvis ☑
D30.12	Benign neoplasm of left renal pelvis ☑
D30.21	Benign neoplasm of right ureter ☑
D30.22	Benign neoplasm of left ureter ☑
D41.01	Neoplasm of uncertain behavior of right kidney ☑
D41.02	Neoplasm of uncertain behavior of left kidney ☑
D41.11	Neoplasm of uncertain behavior of right renal pelvis ☑

Kidney

D41.12	Neoplasm of uncertain behavior of left renal pelvis ☑	
D41.21	Neoplasm of uncertain behavior of right ureter ☑	
D41.22	Neoplasm of uncertain behavior of left ureter ☑	
N11.0	Nonobstructive reflux-associated chronic pyelonephritis	
N11.1	Chronic obstructive pyelonephritis	
N11.8	Other chronic tubulo-interstitial nephritis	
N13.0	Hydronephrosis with ureteropelvic junction obstruction	
N13.1	Hydronephrosis with ureteral stricture, not elsewhere classified	
N13.2	Hydronephrosis with renal and ureteral calculus obstruction	
N13.39	Other hydronephrosis	
N13.4	Hydroureter	
N13.5	Crossing vessel and stricture of ureter without hydronephrosis	
N13.721	Vesicoureteral-reflux with reflux nephropathy without hydroureter, unilateral	
N13.722	Vesicoureteral-reflux with reflux nephropathy without hydroureter, bilateral	
N13.731	Vesicoureteral-reflux with reflux nephropathy with hydroureter, unilateral	
N13.732	Vesicoureteral-reflux with reflux nephropathy with hydroureter, bilateral	
N13.8	Other obstructive and reflux uropathy	
N20.0	Calculus of kidney	
N20.1	Calculus of ureter	
N20.2	Calculus of kidney with calculus of ureter	
N25.81	Secondary hyperparathyroidism of renal origin	
N25.89	Other disorders resulting from impaired renal tubular function	
N28.82	Megaloureter	
N28.84	Pyelitis cystica	
N28.85	Pyeloureteritis cystica	
N28.86	Ureteritis cystica	
N28.89	Other specified disorders of kidney and ureter	
N39.3	Stress incontinence (female) (male)	
N39.41	Urge incontinence	
N39.42	Incontinence without sensory awareness	
N39.43	Post-void dribbling	
N39.44	Nocturnal enuresis	
N39.45	Continuous leakage	
N39.46	Mixed incontinence	
N39.490	Overflow incontinence	
N39.498	Other specified urinary incontinence	
N39.8	Other specified disorders of urinary system	
N82.1	Other female urinary-genital tract fistulae ♀	
Q62.0	Congenital hydronephrosis	
Q62.11	Congenital occlusion of ureteropelvic junction	
Q62.12	Congenital occlusion of ureterovesical orifice	
Q62.2	Congenital megaureter	
Q62.31	Congenital ureterocele, orthotopic	
Q62.32	Cecoureterocele	
Q62.39	Other obstructive defects of renal pelvis and ureter	
Q62.5	Duplication of ureter	
Q62.61	Deviation of ureter	
Q62.62	Displacement of ureter	
Q62.63	Anomalous implantation of ureter	

Q62.69	Other malposition of ureter
Q62.8	Other congenital malformations of ureter
R82.71	Bacteriuria
R82.79	Other abnormal findings on microbiological examination of urine
T83.118A	Breakdown (mechanical) of other urinary devices and implants, initial encounter
T83.128A	Displacement of other urinary devices and implants, initial encounter
T83.198A	Other mechanical complication of other urinary devices and implants, initial encounter
T83.512A	Infection and inflammatory reaction due to nephrostomy catheter, initial encounter
T83.518A	Infection and inflammatory reaction due to other urinary catheter, initial encounter
T83.81XA	Embolism due to genitourinary prosthetic devices, implants and grafts, initial encounter
T83.82XA	Fibrosis due to genitourinary prosthetic devices, implants and grafts, initial encounter
T83.83XA	Hemorrhage due to genitourinary prosthetic devices, implants and grafts, initial encounter
T83.84XA	Pain due to genitourinary prosthetic devices, implants and grafts, initial encounter
T83.85XA	Stenosis due to genitourinary prosthetic devices, implants and grafts, initial encounter
T83.86XA	Thrombosis due to genitourinary prosthetic devices, implants and grafts, initial encounter
T83.89XA	Other specified complication of genitourinary prosthetic devices, implants and grafts, initial encounter
Z46.6	Encounter for fitting and adjustment of urinary device

AMA: **50435** 2018,Mar,11; 2018,Jan,8; 2017,Jan,8; 2016,Jan,3; 2016,Jan,13; 2015,Oct,5

Relative Value Units/Medicare Edits

Non-Facility RVU	Work	PE	MP	Total
50435	1.82	14.06	0.15	16.03
Facility RVU	Work	PE	MP	Total
50435	1.82	0.91	0.15	2.88

	FUD	Status	MUE	Modifiers				IOM Reference
50435	0	A	2(3)	51	50	N/A	N/A	None

* with documentation

Terms To Know

catheter. Flexible tube inserted into an area of the body for introducing or withdrawing fluid.

imaging. Radiologic means of producing pictures for clinical study of the internal structures and functions of the body, such as x-ray, ultrasound, magnetic resonance, or positron emission tomography.

supervision and interpretation. Radiology services that usually contain an invasive component and are reported by the radiologist for supervision of the procedure and the personnel involved with performing the examination, reading the film, and preparing the written report.

50400-50405

50400 Pyeloplasty (Foley Y-pyeloplasty), plastic operation on renal pelvis, with or without plastic operation on ureter, nephropexy, nephrostomy, pyelostomy, or ureteral splinting; simple

50405 complicated (congenital kidney abnormality, secondary pyeloplasty, solitary kidney, calycoplasty)

For Foley Y-pyeloplasty, physician advances Y-shaped flap of renal pelvis into ureter

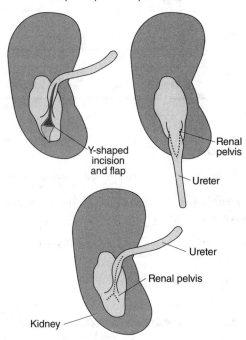

Y-shaped incision and flap

Renal pelvis

Ureter

Ureter

Renal pelvis

Kidney

Explanation

The physician uses plastic surgery to correct an obstruction or defect in the renal pelvis or ureteropelvic junction. To access the renal pelvis and ureter, the physician usually makes an incision in the skin of the flank. The physician incises, trims, and shapes the renal pelvis and ureter, using absorbable sutures or soft rubber drains for traction. The physician usually inserts a slender tube into the renal pelvis to provide support during healing. In Foley Y-pyeloplasty, the physician advances a Y-shaped flap of the renal pelvis into a vertical incision in the upper ureter. The physician may surgically fixate (nephropexy) a floating or mobile kidney, and/or establish an opening between the kidney (nephrostomy) or renal pelvis (pyelostomy) and the exterior of the body. The physician places a drain tube, bringing it out through a separate stab incision in the skin, and performs a layered closure. Report 50405 if a congenital abnormality, secondary pyeloplasty, solitary kidney, or calycoplasty complicates the procedure.

Coding Tips

For laparoscopic approach, see 50544. Symphysiotomy for a horseshoe kidney, with or without pyeloplasty, is reported with 50540.

ICD-10-CM Diagnostic Codes

N11.1	Chronic obstructive pyelonephritis
N12	Tubulo-interstitial nephritis, not specified as acute or chronic
N13.0	Hydronephrosis with ureteropelvic junction obstruction
N13.1	Hydronephrosis with ureteral stricture, not elsewhere classified
N13.2	Hydronephrosis with renal and ureteral calculous obstruction
N13.39	Other hydronephrosis
N20.0	Calculus of kidney
N20.1	Calculus of ureter
N20.2	Calculus of kidney with calculus of ureter
Q62.11	Congenital occlusion of ureteropelvic junction
Q62.12	Congenital occlusion of ureterovesical orifice
Q62.31	Congenital ureterocele, orthotopic
Q62.32	Cecoureterocele
Q62.39	Other obstructive defects of renal pelvis and ureter

AMA: 50400 2018,Jan,8; 2017,Jan,8; 2016,Jan,13; 2015,Jan,16; 2014,Jan,11
50405 2018,Jan,8; 2017,Jan,8; 2016,Jan,13; 2015,Jan,16; 2014,Jan,11

Relative Value Units/Medicare Edits

Non-Facility RVU	Work	PE	MP	Total
50400	21.27	9.73	2.61	33.61
50405	25.86	11.49	2.96	40.31
Facility RVU	**Work**	**PE**	**MP**	**Total**
50400	21.27	9.73	2.61	33.61
50405	25.86	11.49	2.96	40.31

	FUD	Status	MUE	Modifiers				IOM Reference
50400	90	A	1(2)	51	50	62*	80	None
50405	90	A	1(2)	51	50	62*	80	

* with documentation

Terms To Know

agenesis. Absence of an organ due to developmental failure in the prenatal period.

congenital. Present at birth, occurring through heredity or an influence during gestation up to the moment of birth.

defect. Imperfection, flaw, or absence.

dysgenesis. Defective development of an organ.

flank. Part of the body found between the posterior ribs and the uppermost crest of the ilium, or the lateral side of the hip, thigh, and buttock.

Foley Y-pyeloplasty. Y-shaped flap prepared from the renal pelvis of the kidney and advanced into the ureter to correct a defect.

horseshoe kidney. Congenital anomaly in which the kidneys are fused together at the lower end during fetal development, resulting in one large, horseshoe shaped kidney, often associated with cardiovascular, central nervous system, or genitourinary anomalies.

hydronephrosis. Distension of the kidney caused by an accumulation of urine that cannot flow out due to an obstruction that may be caused by conditions such as kidney stones or vesicoureteral reflux.

nephropexy. Surgical fixation or suspension of a floating or mobile kidney.

obstruction. Blockage that prevents normal function of the valve or structure.

Kidney

CPT © 2020 American Medical Association. All Rights Reserved. ● New ▲ Revised + Add On ★ Telemedicine AMA: CPT Assist [Resequenced] ☑ Laterality © 2020 Optum360, LLC

50500

50500 Nephrorrhaphy, suture of kidney wound or injury

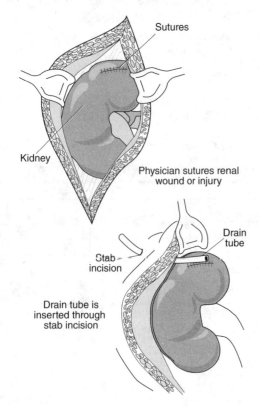

Sutures

Kidney

Physician sutures renal
wound or injury

Drain
tube

Stab
incision

Drain tube is
inserted through
stab incision

Explanation

The physician uses sutures to surgically fixate a wound or injury of the kidney. To access the kidney, the physician makes an incision in the skin of the flank, cuts the muscles, fat, and fibrous membranes (fascia) overlying the kidney, and sometimes removes a portion of the eleventh or twelfth rib. After using sutures to close or surgically fixate a kidney wound or injury, the physician places a drain tube, bringing it out through a separate stab incision in the skin, and performs a layered closure.

Coding Tips

Closure of a nephrocutaneous or pyelocutaneous fistula is reported with 50520. For closure of a nephrovisceral fistula, including visceral repair, abdominal approach, see 50525; thoracic approach, see 50526.

ICD-10-CM Diagnostic Codes

N99.71	Accidental puncture and laceration of a genitourinary system organ or structure during a genitourinary system procedure
N99.72	Accidental puncture and laceration of a genitourinary system organ or structure during other procedure
S37.011A	Minor contusion of right kidney, initial encounter ☑
S37.012A	Minor contusion of left kidney, initial encounter ☑
S37.021A	Major contusion of right kidney, initial encounter ☑
S37.022A	Major contusion of left kidney, initial encounter ☑
S37.041A	Minor laceration of right kidney, initial encounter ☑
S37.042A	Minor laceration of left kidney, initial encounter ☑
S37.051A	Moderate laceration of right kidney, initial encounter ☑
S37.052A	Moderate laceration of left kidney, initial encounter ☑
S37.061A	Major laceration of right kidney, initial encounter ☑
S37.062A	Major laceration of left kidney, initial encounter ☑
S37.091A	Other injury of right kidney, initial encounter ☑
S37.092A	Other injury of left kidney, initial encounter ☑
T88.8XXA	Other specified complications of surgical and medical care, not elsewhere classified, initial encounter

AMA: 50500 2014,Jan,11

Relative Value Units/Medicare Edits

Non-Facility RVU	Work	PE	MP	Total
50500	21.22	10.54	4.15	35.91
Facility RVU	**Work**	**PE**	**MP**	**Total**
50500	21.22	10.54	4.15	35.91

	FUD	Status	MUE	Modifiers				IOM Reference
50500	90	A	1(3)	51	N/A	62*	80	None

* with documentation

Terms To Know

closure. Repairing an incision or wound by suture or other means.

drain. Device that creates a channel to allow fluid from a cavity, wound, or infected area to exit the body.

fascia. Fibrous sheet or band of tissue that envelops organs, muscles, and groupings of muscles.

fixate. Hold, secure, or fasten in position.

flank. Part of the body found between the posterior ribs and the uppermost crest of the ilium, or the lateral side of the hip, thigh, and buttock.

laceration. Tearing injury; a torn, ragged-edged wound.

nephrorrhaphy. Open surgical repair or suture of a wound or injury of the kidney.

puncture. Creating a hole.

suture. Numerous stitching techniques employed in wound closure.

wound. Injury to living tissue often involving a cut or break in the skin.

Kidney

50520

50520   Closure of nephrocutaneous or pyelocutaneous fistula

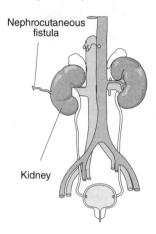

Physician closes fistula between
kidney or renal pelvis and skin

Nephrocutaneous
fistula

Kidney

Explanation

The physician closes a fistula that is an abnormal opening between the skin and the kidney (nephrocutaneous) or the renal pelvis (pyelocutaneous). After excising the fistula, the physician sutures the clean percutaneous tissues together to create a smooth surface.

Coding Tips

Local anesthesia is included in the service. However, general anesthesia may be administered depending on the age or condition of the patient. For closure of a nephrovisceral fistula, including visceral repair, abdominal approach, see 50525; thoracic approach, see 50526.

ICD-10-CM Diagnostic Codes

N28.89   Other specified disorders of kidney and ureter

AMA: **50520** 2014,Jan,11

Relative Value Units/Medicare Edits

Non-Facility RVU	Work	PE	MP	Total
50520	18.88	10.29	4.58	33.75
Facility RVU	**Work**	**PE**	**MP**	**Total**
50520	18.88	10.29	4.58	33.75

	FUD	Status	MUE	Modifiers				IOM Reference
50520	90	A	1(3)	51	N/A	62*	80	None

* with documentation

Terms To Know

fistula. Abnormal tube-like passage between two body cavities or organs or from an organ to the outside surface.

tissue. Group of similar cells with a similar function that form definite structures and organs. Tissue types include epithelial tissue, muscle tissue, connective tissue, and nervous tissue.

50525-50526

50525   Closure of nephrovisceral fistula (eg, renocolic), including visceral repair; abdominal approach
50526   thoracic approach

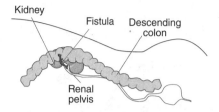

Kidney   Fistula   Descending
colon

Renal
pelvis

The physician closes a fistula between the kidney
or renal pelvis and an organ of the digestive,
respiratory, urogenital, or endocrine system

Explanation

The physician closes a fistula that is an abnormal opening between the kidney and an organ of the digestive, respiratory, urogenital, or endocrine system. In 50525, the physician usually makes an incision in the abdomen, cuts the muscles, fat, and fibrous membranes (fascia) overlying the kidney to access the fistula. In 50526, the physician makes an incision in the skin of the chest, opens the chest cavity, collapses the lung, and separates the leaves of the diaphragm to expose the kidney. After excising the fistula, the physician sutures the clean tissues together to create a smooth surface. The physician places a drain tube, bringing it out through a separate stab incision in the skin, and performs a layered closure. In 50526, the physician inserts a chest tube to re-expand the lung.

Coding Tips

Closure of a nephrocutaneous or pyelocutaneous fistula is reported with 50520.

ICD-10-CM Diagnostic Codes

N28.89   Other specified disorders of kidney and ureter

AMA: **50525** 2014,Jan,11 **50526** 2014,Jan,11

Relative Value Units/Medicare Edits

Non-Facility RVU	Work	PE	MP	Total
50525	24.39	12.53	5.92	42.84
50526	26.31	13.23	6.39	45.93
Facility RVU	**Work**	**PE**	**MP**	**Total**
50525	24.39	12.53	5.92	42.84
50526	26.31	13.23	6.39	45.93

	FUD	Status	MUE	Modifiers				IOM Reference
50525	90	A	1(3)	51	N/A	62*	80	None
50526	90	A	1(3)	51	N/A	N/A	80	

* with documentation

Terms To Know

approach. Method or anatomical location used to gain access to a body organ or specific area for procedures.

fistula. Abnormal tube-like passage between two body cavities or organs or from an organ to the outside surface.

CPT © 2020 American Medical Association. All Rights Reserved.   ● New   ▲ Revised   + Add On   ★ Telemedicine   AMA: CPT Assist   [Resequenced]   ☑ Laterality   © 2020 Optum360, LLC

50540

50540 Symphysiotomy for horseshoe kidney with or without pyeloplasty and/or other plastic procedure, unilateral or bilateral (1 operation)

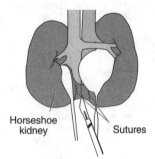

Horseshoe kidney   Sutures

Physician incises and sutures horseshoe kidney union

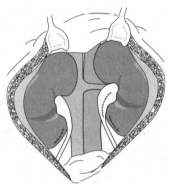

Physician may perform pyeloplasty

Explanation

The physician divides an abnormal union of the kidneys to correct a horseshoe kidney. To access the horseshoe kidney, the physician usually makes an incision in the skin of the lower abdomen and cuts the muscles, fat, and fibrous membranes (fascia) overlying the kidney. After incising the union and placing two rows of sutures to control bleeding, the physician usually performs pyeloplasty or another plastic procedure on one or both sides of the divided kidney. After completion of repair, the physician may rotate the kidney to effect drainage. The physician irrigates the site with normal saline, places a drain tube, bringing it out through a separate stab incision in the skin, and performs a layered closure.

Coding Tips

Code 50540 includes pyeloplasty or any other plastic procedure performed on the kidney during the same surgical session as the symphysiotomy. The plastic procedure may be performed on one or both sides of the sutured division. For pyeloplasty, simple, see 50400; complicated, see 50405; laparoscopic approach, 50544.

ICD-10-CM Diagnostic Codes

Q63.1   Lobulated, fused and horseshoe kidney

AMA: **50540** 2014,Jan,11

Relative Value Units/Medicare Edits

Non-Facility RVU	Work	PE	MP	Total
50540	21.1	9.62	2.41	33.13
Facility RVU	**Work**	**PE**	**MP**	**Total**
50540	21.1	9.62	2.41	33.13

	FUD	Status	MUE	Modifiers				IOM Reference
50540	90	A	1(2)	51	N/A	62*	80	None

* with documentation

Terms To Know

anomaly. Irregularity in the structure or position of an organ or tissue.

closure. Repairing an incision or wound by suture or other means.

congenital. Present at birth, occurring through heredity or an influence during gestation up to the moment of birth.

drainage. Releasing, taking, or letting out fluids and/or gases from a body part.

fascia. Fibrous sheet or band of tissue that envelops organs, muscles, and groupings of muscles.

horseshoe kidney. Congenital anomaly in which the kidneys are fused together at the lower end during fetal development, resulting in one large, horseshoe shaped kidney, often associated with cardiovascular, central nervous system, or genitourinary anomalies.

incision. Act of cutting into tissue or an organ.

irrigate. Washing out, lavage.

pyeloplasty. Surgical correction of an obstruction or defect in the renal pelvis of the kidney or its junction with the ureter.

suture. Numerous stitching techniques employed in wound closure.

buried suture. Continuous or interrupted suture placed under the skin for a layered closure.

continuous suture. Running stitch with tension evenly distributed across a single strand to provide a leakproof closure line.

interrupted suture. Series of single stitches with tension isolated at each stitch, in which all stitches are not affected if one becomes loose, and the isolated sutures cannot act as a wick to transport an infection.

purse-string suture. Continuous suture placed around a tubular structure and tightened, to reduce or close the lumen.

retention suture. Secondary stitching that bridges the primary suture, providing support for the primary repair; a plastic or rubber bolster may be placed over the primary repair and under the retention sutures.

Kidney

50541-50542

50541 Laparoscopy, surgical; ablation of renal cysts
50542 ablation of renal mass lesion(s), including intraoperative ultrasound guidance and monitoring, when performed

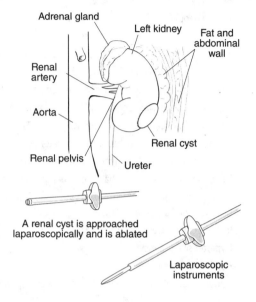

Adrenal gland
Left kidney
Fat and abdominal wall
Renal artery
Aorta
Renal cyst
Renal pelvis
Ureter

A renal cyst is approached laparoscopically and is ablated

Laparoscopic instruments

Explanation

The physician performs a laparoscopic surgical ablation of renal cysts in 50541 or a renal mass lesion in 50542 through the abdomen or back. With the abdominal approach, an umbilical port is created by placing a trocar at the level of the umbilicus. The abdominal wall is insufflated. The laparoscope is placed through the umbilical port and additional trocars are placed into the abdominal cavity. In the back approach, the trocar is placed at the back proximate to the retroperitoneal space near to the kidney with additional ports placed nearby for appropriate access to the operative site. The physician uses the laparoscope fitted with a fiberoptic camera and/or an operating instrument. The renal cysts or lesions are visualized through the scope and are ablated by fulguration or another method that can be utilized endoscopically, such as cryotherapy or radiofrequency thermal coagulation. The instruments are removed and the abdominal or back incisions are closed by staples or sutures. Code 50542 includes intraoperative ultrasound guidance and monitoring, if performed.

Coding Tips

Surgical laparoscopy always includes diagnostic laparoscopy; the diagnostic laparoscopy should not be reported separately. To report open ablation of renal mass lesion(s), including intraoperative ultrasound guidance and monitoring, when performed, see 50250; percutaneous ablation of renal tumors, see 50592–50593. For percutaneous aspiration and/or injection of a renal cyst, see 50390. For excision or unroofing of renal cyst(s), open, see 50280; perinephric cyst, see 50290.

ICD-10-CM Diagnostic Codes

C64.1	Malignant neoplasm of right kidney, except renal pelvis ☑
C64.2	Malignant neoplasm of left kidney, except renal pelvis ☑
C65.1	Malignant neoplasm of right renal pelvis ☑
C65.2	Malignant neoplasm of left renal pelvis ☑
C79.01	Secondary malignant neoplasm of right kidney and renal pelvis ☑
C79.02	Secondary malignant neoplasm of left kidney and renal pelvis ☑
C7A.093	Malignant carcinoid tumor of the kidney
C80.2	Malignant neoplasm associated with transplanted organ
D09.19	Carcinoma in situ of other urinary organs
D30.01	Benign neoplasm of right kidney ☑
D30.02	Benign neoplasm of left kidney ☑
D30.11	Benign neoplasm of right renal pelvis ☑
D30.12	Benign neoplasm of left renal pelvis ☑
D3A.093	Benign carcinoid tumor of the kidney
D41.01	Neoplasm of uncertain behavior of right kidney ☑
D41.02	Neoplasm of uncertain behavior of left kidney ☑
D41.11	Neoplasm of uncertain behavior of right renal pelvis ☑
D41.12	Neoplasm of uncertain behavior of left renal pelvis ☑
D49.511	Neoplasm of unspecified behavior of right kidney ☑
D49.512	Neoplasm of unspecified behavior of left kidney ☑
D49.59	Neoplasm of unspecified behavior of other genitourinary organ
N28.1	Cyst of kidney, acquired
N28.89	Other specified disorders of kidney and ureter
Q61.01	Congenital single renal cyst
Q61.02	Congenital multiple renal cysts
Q61.11	Cystic dilatation of collecting ducts
Q61.19	Other polycystic kidney, infantile type
Q61.2	Polycystic kidney, adult type
Q61.4	Renal dysplasia
Q61.5	Medullary cystic kidney
Q61.8	Other cystic kidney diseases

AMA: 50541 2018,Jan,8; 2017,Jan,8; 2016,Jan,13; 2015,Jan,16; 2014,Jan,11
50542 2018,Jan,8; 2017,Jan,8; 2016,Jan,13; 2015,Jan,16; 2014,Jan,11

Relative Value Units/Medicare Edits

Non-Facility RVU	Work	PE	MP	Total
50541	16.86	7.68	1.96	26.5
50542	21.36	9.85	2.45	33.66
Facility RVU	Work	PE	MP	Total
50541	16.86	7.68	1.96	26.5
50542	21.36	9.85	2.45	33.66

	FUD	Status	MUE	Modifiers				IOM Reference
50541	90	A	1(2)	51	50	62*	80	None
50542	90	A	1(2)	51	50	62*	80	

* with documentation

Terms To Know

ablation. Removal or destruction of a body part or tissue or its function. Ablation may be performed by surgical means, hormones, drugs, radiofrequency, heat, chemical application, or other methods.

cyst. Elevated encapsulated mass containing fluid, semisolid, or solid material with a membranous lining.

fulguration. Destruction of living tissue by using sparks from a high-frequency electric current.

Kidney

50543

50543 Laparoscopy, surgical; partial nephrectomy

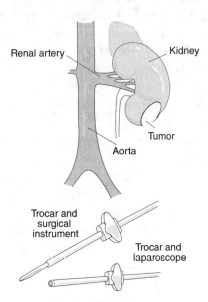

Renal artery

Kidney

Tumor

Aorta

Trocar and surgical instrument

Trocar and laparoscope

A partial nephrectomy is performed to treat renal lesions or tumors

Explanation

The physician performs a laparoscopic partial nephrectomy to treat small renal lesions or tumors. With an abdominal approach, an umbilical port is created by placing a trocar at the level of the umbilicus. The abdominal wall is insufflated. The laparoscope is placed through the umbilical port and additional trocars are placed into the abdominal cavity. In a back approach, the trocar is placed at the back proximate to the retroperitoneal space near to the kidney with additional ports placed nearby for appropriate access to the operative site. The physician uses the laparoscope fitted with a fiberoptic camera for direct vision and/or an operating instrument. Direct vision and the use of laparoscopic ultrasonography allow the physician to identify the tumors and assess the appropriate surgical margin that should be allowed. The diseased kidney tissue is removed with emphasis on hemostasis. Methods such as electrocautery, argon beam coagulator, topical agents, and microwave thermotherapy may be employed to help reduce bleeding during resection. Retrieval pouches used in endoscopic surgery allow removal of the tumor specimen without spilling. The instruments are removed and the abdominal or back incisions are closed by staples or sutures.

Coding Tips

Surgical laparoscopy always includes diagnostic laparoscopy; the diagnostic laparoscopy should not be reported separately. For open partial nephrectomy, use 50240.

ICD-10-CM Diagnostic Codes

C64.1	Malignant neoplasm of right kidney, except renal pelvis ☑
C64.2	Malignant neoplasm of left kidney, except renal pelvis ☑
C65.1	Malignant neoplasm of right renal pelvis ☑
C65.2	Malignant neoplasm of left renal pelvis ☑
C66.1	Malignant neoplasm of right ureter ☑
C66.2	Malignant neoplasm of left ureter ☑
C68.8	Malignant neoplasm of overlapping sites of urinary organs
C79.01	Secondary malignant neoplasm of right kidney and renal pelvis ☑
C79.02	Secondary malignant neoplasm of left kidney and renal pelvis ☑
C7A.093	Malignant carcinoid tumor of the kidney
C80.2	Malignant neoplasm associated with transplanted organ
D09.19	Carcinoma in situ of other urinary organs
D30.01	Benign neoplasm of right kidney ☑
D30.02	Benign neoplasm of left kidney ☑
D30.11	Benign neoplasm of right renal pelvis ☑
D30.12	Benign neoplasm of left renal pelvis ☑
D41.01	Neoplasm of uncertain behavior of right kidney ☑
D41.02	Neoplasm of uncertain behavior of left kidney ☑
D41.11	Neoplasm of uncertain behavior of right renal pelvis ☑
D41.12	Neoplasm of uncertain behavior of left renal pelvis ☑
D41.21	Neoplasm of uncertain behavior of right ureter ☑
D41.22	Neoplasm of uncertain behavior of left ureter ☑
D47.Z1	Post-transplant lymphoproliferative disorder (PTLD)
D49.59	Neoplasm of unspecified behavior of other genitourinary organ
I12.0	Hypertensive chronic kidney disease with stage 5 chronic kidney disease or end stage renal disease
I15.0	Renovascular hypertension
I16.0	Hypertensive urgency
I16.1	Hypertensive emergency
N11.0	Nonobstructive reflux-associated chronic pyelonephritis
N11.1	Chronic obstructive pyelonephritis
N11.8	Other chronic tubulo-interstitial nephritis
N13.0	Hydronephrosis with ureteropelvic junction obstruction
N13.1	Hydronephrosis with ureteral stricture, not elsewhere classified
N13.2	Hydronephrosis with renal and ureteral calculous obstruction
N13.39	Other hydronephrosis
N13.4	Hydroureter
N13.5	Crossing vessel and stricture of ureter without hydronephrosis
N13.6	Pyonephrosis
N13.71	Vesicoureteral-reflux without reflux nephropathy
N13.721	Vesicoureteral-reflux with reflux nephropathy without hydroureter, unilateral
N13.722	Vesicoureteral-reflux with reflux nephropathy without hydroureter, bilateral
N13.731	Vesicoureteral-reflux with reflux nephropathy with hydroureter, unilateral
N13.732	Vesicoureteral-reflux with reflux nephropathy with hydroureter, bilateral
N13.8	Other obstructive and reflux uropathy
N20.0	Calculus of kidney
N20.2	Calculus of kidney with calculus of ureter
N26.1	Atrophy of kidney (terminal)
N26.2	Page kidney
N28.0	Ischemia and infarction of kidney
N28.1	Cyst of kidney, acquired
N28.81	Hypertrophy of kidney
N28.82	Megaloureter
N28.89	Other specified disorders of kidney and ureter
Q60.3	Renal hypoplasia, unilateral
Q60.4	Renal hypoplasia, bilateral

Kidney

Q60.6	Potter's syndrome
Q61.01	Congenital single renal cyst
Q61.02	Congenital multiple renal cysts
Q61.11	Cystic dilatation of collecting ducts
Q61.19	Other polycystic kidney, infantile type
Q61.2	Polycystic kidney, adult type
Q61.4	Renal dysplasia
Q61.5	Medullary cystic kidney
Q62.0	Congenital hydronephrosis
Q62.11	Congenital occlusion of ureteropelvic junction
Q62.31	Congenital ureterocele, orthotopic
Q62.32	Cecoureterocele
S37.061A	Major laceration of right kidney, initial encounter ☑
S37.062A	Major laceration of left kidney, initial encounter ☑
S37.091A	Other injury of right kidney, initial encounter ☑
S37.092A	Other injury of left kidney, initial encounter ☑

AMA: 50543 2018,Jan,8; 2017,Jan,8; 2016,Jan,13; 2015,Jan,16; 2014,Jan,11

Relative Value Units/Medicare Edits

Non-Facility RVU	Work	PE	MP	Total
50543	27.41	12.43	3.16	43.0
Facility RVU	**Work**	**PE**	**MP**	**Total**
50543	27.41	12.43	3.16	43.0

	FUD	Status	MUE	Modifiers				IOM Reference
50543	90	A	1(2)	51	50	62*	80	None

* with documentation

Terms To Know

approach. Method or anatomical location used to gain access to a body organ or specific area for procedures.

hemostasis. Interruption of blood flow or the cessation or arrest of bleeding.

laparoscopy. Direct visualization of the peritoneal cavity, outer fallopian tubes, uterus, and ovaries utilizing a laparoscope, a thin, flexible fiberoptic tube.

lesion. Area of damaged tissue that has lost continuity or function, due to disease or trauma.

margin. Boundary, edge, or border, as of a surface or structure.

nephrectomy. Partial or total removal of the kidney that may be performed for indications such as irreparable kidney damage, renal cell carcinoma, trauma, congenital abnormalities, or transplant purposes.

renal. Referring to the kidney.

retroperitoneal. Located behind the peritoneum, the membrane that lines the abdominopelvic walls and forms a covering for the internal organs.

specimen. Tissue cells or sample of fluid taken for analysis, pathologic examination, and diagnosis.

tissue. Group of similar cells with a similar function that form definite structures and organs. Tissue types include epithelial tissue, muscle tissue, connective tissue, and nervous tissue.

50544

50544   Laparoscopy, surgical; pyeloplasty

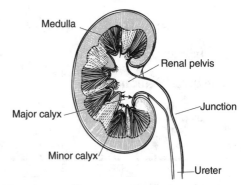

Cutaway detail of normal right kidney and ureter

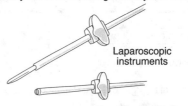

The kidney is approached laparoscopically and the renal pelvis and/or ureteropelvic junction is surgically altered

Explanation

The physician performs a laparoscopic pyeloplasty to correct an obstruction or defect in the renal pelvis or ureteropelvic junction through the abdomen or back. With the abdominal approach, an umbilical port is created by placing a trocar at the level of the umbilicus. The abdominal wall is insufflated. The laparoscope is placed through the umbilical port and additional trocars are placed into the abdominal cavity. In the back approach, the trocar is placed at the back proximate to the retroperitoneal space near to the kidney with additional ports placed nearby for appropriate access to the operative site. The physician uses the laparoscope fitted with a fiberoptic camera and/or an operating instrument. The physician incises, trims, and/or shapes the renal pelvis and ureter using absorbable sutures or soft rubber drains for traction. A tube is usually inserted to promote healing. The instruments are removed and abdominal or back incisions are closed by staples or sutures.

Coding Tips

Surgical laparoscopy always includes diagnostic laparoscopy; the diagnostic laparoscopy should not be reported separately. For an open pyeloplasty, see 50400–50405. For pyeloplasty with symphysiotomy for horseshoe kidney, see 50540.

ICD-10-CM Diagnostic Codes

N10	Acute pyelonephritis
N11.1	Chronic obstructive pyelonephritis
N12	Tubulo-interstitial nephritis, not specified as acute or chronic
N13.0	Hydronephrosis with ureteropelvic junction obstruction
N13.1	Hydronephrosis with ureteral stricture, not elsewhere classified
N13.2	Hydronephrosis with renal and ureteral calculous obstruction
N13.39	Other hydronephrosis
N20.0	Calculus of kidney
N20.1	Calculus of ureter

Kidney

CPT © 2020 American Medical Association. All Rights Reserved.   ● New   ▲ Revised   + Add On   ★ Telemedicine   AMA: CPT Assist   [Resequenced]   ☑ Laterality   © 2020 Optum360, LLC

N20.2	Calculus of kidney with calculus of ureter			
Q62.11	Congenital occlusion of ureteropelvic junction			
Q62.12	Congenital occlusion of ureterovesical orifice			
Q62.31	Congenital ureterocele, orthotopic			
Q62.32	Cecoureterocele			
Q62.39	Other obstructive defects of renal pelvis and ureter			

AMA: **50544** 2018,Jan,8; 2017,Jan,8; 2016,Jan,13; 2015,Jan,16; 2014,Jan,11

Relative Value Units/Medicare Edits

Non-Facility RVU	Work	PE	MP	Total
50544	23.37	9.88	2.71	35.96
Facility RVU	**Work**	**PE**	**MP**	**Total**
50544	23.37	9.88	2.71	35.96

	FUD	Status	MUE	Modifiers				IOM Reference
50544	90	A	1(2)	51	50	62*	80	None

* with documentation

Terms To Know

agenesis. Absence of an organ due to developmental failure in the prenatal period.

approach. Method or anatomical location used to gain access to a body organ or specific area for procedures.

calculus. Abnormal, stone-like concretion of calcium, cholesterol, mineral salts, or other substances that forms in any part of the body.

congenital. Present at birth, occurring through heredity or an influence during gestation up to the moment of birth.

defect. Imperfection, flaw, or absence.

dysgenesis. Defective development of an organ.

hydronephrosis. Distension of the kidney caused by an accumulation of urine that cannot flow out due to an obstruction that may be caused by conditions such as kidney stones or vesicoureteral reflux.

laparoscopy. Direct visualization of the peritoneal cavity, outer fallopian tubes, uterus, and ovaries utilizing a laparoscope, a thin, flexible fiberoptic tube.

obstruction. Blockage that prevents normal function of the valve or structure.

pyeloplasty. Surgical correction of an obstruction or defect in the renal pelvis of the kidney or its junction with the ureter.

stricture. Narrowing of an anatomical structure.

ureterocele. Saccular formation of the lower part of the ureter, protruding into the bladder.

vesicoureteral reflux. Urine passage from the bladder flows backward up into the ureter and kidneys that can lead to bacterial infection and an increase in hydrostatic pressure, causing kidney damage.

50545

50545 Laparoscopy, surgical; radical nephrectomy (includes removal of Gerota's fascia and surrounding fatty tissue, removal of regional lymph nodes, and adrenalectomy)

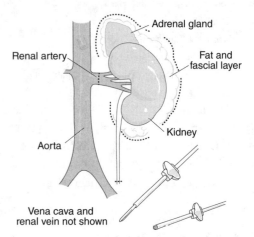

A radical nephrectomy is performed laparoscopically

Explanation

The physician performs a radical nephrectomy, including removal of Gerota's fascia and surrounding fatty tissue, regional lymph nodes, and the adrenal gland through a laparoscope. The physician makes a 1 centimeter periumbilical incision and inserts a trocar. The abdominal cavity is insufflated with carbon dioxide. A fiberoptic laparoscope fitted with a camera and light source is inserted through the trocar. Other incisions (ports) are made in the abdomen or flank to allow other instruments or an additional light source to be passed into the abdomen or retroperitoneum. The colon is mobilized, and the laparoscope is advanced to the operative site. The ureter is transected at the ureterovesical junction. The physician clamps, ligates, and severs the renal vein and renal artery. The Gerota's fascia is dissected to expose the upper pole of the kidney. The adrenal gland is visualized. Clips are placed on the suprarenal vein and adrenal arteries (diaphragmatic [inferior phrenic], aortic, and renal) which are cut. Any lymph nodes in the surrounding area are excised and removed. The kidney, adrenal gland, renal (Gerota's) fascia, and surrounding fat are dissected free; they are bagged and removed through an enlarged port site. The instruments are removed. The incisions are closed with staples or suture.

Coding Tips

Surgical laparoscopy always includes diagnostic laparoscopy; the diagnostic laparoscopy should not be reported separately. For laparoscopic nephrectomy with ureterectomy, partial, see 50546; complete, see 50548. For laparoscopic donor nephrectomy, see 50547. Radical nephrectomy, open, see 50230.

ICD-10-CM Diagnostic Codes

C64.1	Malignant neoplasm of right kidney, except renal pelvis	☑
C64.2	Malignant neoplasm of left kidney, except renal pelvis	☑
C65.1	Malignant neoplasm of right renal pelvis	☑
C65.2	Malignant neoplasm of left renal pelvis	☑
C66.1	Malignant neoplasm of right ureter	☑
C66.2	Malignant neoplasm of left ureter	☑
C68.8	Malignant neoplasm of overlapping sites of urinary organs	
C79.01	Secondary malignant neoplasm of right kidney and renal pelvis	☑

© 2020 Optum360, LLC   **N** Newborn: 0   **P** Pediatric: 0-17   **M** Maternity: 9-64   **A** Adult: 15-124   ♂ Male Only   ♀ Female Only   CPT © 2020 American Medical Association. All Rights Reserved.

Kidney

C79.02	Secondary malignant neoplasm of left kidney and renal pelvis ☑
C7A.093	Malignant carcinoid tumor of the kidney
C80.2	Malignant neoplasm associated with transplanted organ
D09.19	Carcinoma in situ of other urinary organs
D30.01	Benign neoplasm of right kidney ☑
D30.02	Benign neoplasm of left kidney ☑
D30.11	Benign neoplasm of right renal pelvis ☑
D30.12	Benign neoplasm of left renal pelvis ☑
D30.21	Benign neoplasm of right ureter ☑
D30.22	Benign neoplasm of left ureter ☑
D3A.093	Benign carcinoid tumor of the kidney
D41.01	Neoplasm of uncertain behavior of right kidney ☑
D41.02	Neoplasm of uncertain behavior of left kidney ☑
D41.11	Neoplasm of uncertain behavior of right renal pelvis ☑
D41.12	Neoplasm of uncertain behavior of left renal pelvis ☑
D41.21	Neoplasm of uncertain behavior of right ureter ☑
D41.22	Neoplasm of uncertain behavior of left ureter ☑
D47.Z1	Post-transplant lymphoproliferative disorder (PTLD)
D47.Z2	Castleman disease
D49.511	Neoplasm of unspecified behavior of right kidney ☑
D49.512	Neoplasm of unspecified behavior of left kidney ☑
D49.59	Neoplasm of unspecified behavior of other genitourinary organ
I12.0	Hypertensive chronic kidney disease with stage 5 chronic kidney disease or end stage renal disease
I15.0	Renovascular hypertension
I16.0	Hypertensive urgency
I16.1	Hypertensive emergency
I75.81	Atheroembolism of kidney
I82.220	Acute embolism and thrombosis of inferior vena cava
I82.221	Chronic embolism and thrombosis of inferior vena cava
N11.0	Nonobstructive reflux-associated chronic pyelonephritis
N11.1	Chronic obstructive pyelonephritis
N11.8	Other chronic tubulo-interstitial nephritis
N13.0	Hydronephrosis with ureteropelvic junction obstruction
N13.1	Hydronephrosis with ureteral stricture, not elsewhere classified
N13.2	Hydronephrosis with renal and ureteral calculous obstruction
N13.39	Other hydronephrosis
N13.4	Hydroureter
N13.5	Crossing vessel and stricture of ureter without hydronephrosis
N13.6	Pyonephrosis
N13.71	Vesicoureteral-reflux without reflux nephropathy
N13.721	Vesicoureteral-reflux with reflux nephropathy without hydroureter, unilateral
N13.722	Vesicoureteral-reflux with reflux nephropathy without hydroureter, bilateral
N13.731	Vesicoureteral-reflux with reflux nephropathy with hydroureter, unilateral
N13.732	Vesicoureteral-reflux with reflux nephropathy with hydroureter, bilateral
N13.8	Other obstructive and reflux uropathy
N20.0	Calculus of kidney
N20.2	Calculus of kidney with calculus of ureter
N26.1	Atrophy of kidney (terminal)

N26.2	Page kidney
N28.0	Ischemia and infarction of kidney
N28.1	Cyst of kidney, acquired
N28.81	Hypertrophy of kidney
N28.82	Megaloureter
N28.89	Other specified disorders of kidney and ureter
Q60.3	Renal hypoplasia, unilateral
Q60.4	Renal hypoplasia, bilateral
Q60.6	Potter's syndrome
Q61.01	Congenital single renal cyst
Q61.02	Congenital multiple renal cysts
Q61.11	Cystic dilatation of collecting ducts
Q61.19	Other polycystic kidney, infantile type
Q61.2	Polycystic kidney, adult type
Q61.4	Renal dysplasia
Q61.5	Medullary cystic kidney
Q61.8	Other cystic kidney diseases
Q62.0	Congenital hydronephrosis
Q62.11	Congenital occlusion of ureteropelvic junction
Q62.31	Congenital ureterocele, orthotopic
Q62.32	Cecoureterocele
Q62.39	Other obstructive defects of renal pelvis and ureter
S37.061A	Major laceration of right kidney, initial encounter ☑
S37.062A	Major laceration of left kidney, initial encounter ☑
S37.091A	Other injury of right kidney, initial encounter ☑
S37.092A	Other injury of left kidney, initial encounter ☑

AMA: 50545 2018,Jan,8; 2017,Jan,8; 2016,Jan,13; 2015,Jan,16; 2014,Jan,11

Relative Value Units/Medicare Edits

Non-Facility RVU	Work	PE	MP	Total
50545	25.06	10.67	2.93	38.66
Facility RVU	**Work**	**PE**	**MP**	**Total**
50545	25.06	10.67	2.93	38.66

	FUD	Status	MUE	Modifiers				IOM Reference
50545	90	A	1(2)	51	50	62*	80	None

* with documentation

Terms To Know

dissect. Cut apart or separate tissue for surgical purposes or for visual or microscopic study.

fascia. Fibrous sheet or band of tissue that envelops organs, muscles, and groupings of muscles.

ligate. To tie off a blood vessel or duct with a suture or a soft, thin wire (ligature wire).

lymph nodes. Bean-shaped structures along the lymphatic vessels that intercept and destroy foreign materials in the tissue and bloodstream.

nephrectomy. Partial or total removal of the kidney that may be performed for indications such as irreparable kidney damage, renal cell carcinoma, trauma, congenital abnormalities, or transplant purposes.

radical. Extensive surgery.

Kidney

50546

50546   Laparoscopy, surgical; nephrectomy, including partial ureterectomy

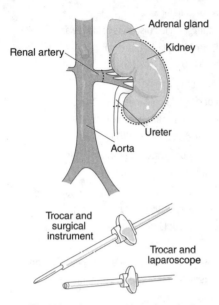

The kidney is removed laparoscopically

Explanation

The physician removes the kidney and a portion of the ureter through a laparoscope. The physician makes a 1 cm periumbilical incision and inserts a trocar. The abdominal cavity is insufflated with carbon dioxide. A fiberoptic laparoscope fitted with a camera and light source is inserted through the trocar. Other incisions (ports) are made in the abdomen or flank to allow other instruments or an additional light source to be passed into the abdomen or retroperitoneum. The colon is mobilized and the laparoscope is advanced to the operative site. The physician mobilizes the kidney and clamps, ligates, and severs part of the ureter and major renal blood vessels (renal pedicle). The kidney and upper ureter are bagged and brought through one of the port sites (e.g., periumbilical) that has been slightly enlarged. The instruments are removed, and the small abdominal or flank incisions are closed with staples or suture.

Coding Tips

For laparoscopic nephrectomy with complete ureterectomy, see 50548. For laparoscopic donor nephrectomy, see 50547. For open nephrectomy procedures, see 50220–50240.

ICD-10-CM Diagnostic Codes

C64.1	Malignant neoplasm of right kidney, except renal pelvis ☑
C64.2	Malignant neoplasm of left kidney, except renal pelvis ☑
C65.1	Malignant neoplasm of right renal pelvis ☑
C65.2	Malignant neoplasm of left renal pelvis ☑
C66.1	Malignant neoplasm of right ureter ☑
C66.2	Malignant neoplasm of left ureter ☑
C68.8	Malignant neoplasm of overlapping sites of urinary organs
C79.01	Secondary malignant neoplasm of right kidney and renal pelvis ☑
C79.02	Secondary malignant neoplasm of left kidney and renal pelvis ☑
C7A.093	Malignant carcinoid tumor of the kidney
C80.2	Malignant neoplasm associated with transplanted organ

D09.19	Carcinoma in situ of other urinary organs
D30.01	Benign neoplasm of right kidney ☑
D30.02	Benign neoplasm of left kidney ☑
D30.11	Benign neoplasm of right renal pelvis ☑
D30.12	Benign neoplasm of left renal pelvis ☑
D30.21	Benign neoplasm of right ureter ☑
D30.22	Benign neoplasm of left ureter ☑
D3A.093	Benign carcinoid tumor of the kidney
D41.01	Neoplasm of uncertain behavior of right kidney ☑
D41.02	Neoplasm of uncertain behavior of left kidney ☑
D41.11	Neoplasm of uncertain behavior of right renal pelvis ☑
D41.12	Neoplasm of uncertain behavior of left renal pelvis ☑
D41.21	Neoplasm of uncertain behavior of right ureter ☑
D41.22	Neoplasm of uncertain behavior of left ureter ☑
D47.Z1	Post-transplant lymphoproliferative disorder (PTLD)
D47.Z2	Castleman disease
I12.0	Hypertensive chronic kidney disease with stage 5 chronic kidney disease or end stage renal disease
I15.0	Renovascular hypertension
I16.0	Hypertensive urgency
I16.1	Hypertensive emergency
N11.0	Nonobstructive reflux-associated chronic pyelonephritis
N11.1	Chronic obstructive pyelonephritis
N11.8	Other chronic tubulo-interstitial nephritis
N13.0	Hydronephrosis with ureteropelvic junction obstruction
N13.1	Hydronephrosis with ureteral stricture, not elsewhere classified
N13.2	Hydronephrosis with renal and ureteral calculous obstruction
N13.4	Hydroureter
N13.5	Crossing vessel and stricture of ureter without hydronephrosis
N13.6	Pyonephrosis
N13.71	Vesicoureteral-reflux without reflux nephropathy
N13.721	Vesicoureteral-reflux with reflux nephropathy without hydroureter, unilateral
N13.722	Vesicoureteral-reflux with reflux nephropathy without hydroureter, bilateral
N13.731	Vesicoureteral-reflux with reflux nephropathy with hydroureter, unilateral
N13.732	Vesicoureteral-reflux with reflux nephropathy with hydroureter, bilateral
N20.0	Calculus of kidney
N20.2	Calculus of kidney with calculus of ureter
N26.1	Atrophy of kidney (terminal)
N26.2	Page kidney
N28.0	Ischemia and infarction of kidney
N28.1	Cyst of kidney, acquired
N28.81	Hypertrophy of kidney
N28.82	Megaloureter
Q60.3	Renal hypoplasia, unilateral
Q60.4	Renal hypoplasia, bilateral
Q60.6	Potter's syndrome
Q61.01	Congenital single renal cyst
Q61.02	Congenital multiple renal cysts
Q61.11	Cystic dilatation of collecting ducts

© 2020 Optum360, LLC   N Newborn: 0   P Pediatric: 0-17   M Maternity: 9-64   A Adult: 15-124   ♂ Male Only   ♀ Female Only   CPT © 2020 American Medical Association. All Rights Reserved.

Kidney

Q61.2	Polycystic kidney, adult type
Q61.4	Renal dysplasia
Q61.5	Medullary cystic kidney
Q62.0	Congenital hydronephrosis
Q62.11	Congenital occlusion of ureteropelvic junction
Q62.31	Congenital ureterocele, orthotopic
Q62.32	Cecoureterocele
S37.061A	Major laceration of right kidney, initial encounter ☑
S37.062A	Major laceration of left kidney, initial encounter ☑
S37.091A	Other injury of right kidney, initial encounter ☑
S37.092A	Other injury of left kidney, initial encounter ☑

AMA: 50546 2018,Jan,8; 2017,Jan,8; 2016,Jan,13; 2015,Jan,16; 2014,Jan,11

Relative Value Units/Medicare Edits

Non-Facility RVU	Work	PE	MP	Total
50546	21.87	10.17	2.74	34.78
Facility RVU	**Work**	**PE**	**MP**	**Total**
50546	21.87	10.17	2.74	34.78

	FUD	Status	MUE	Modifiers				IOM Reference
50546	90	A	1(2)	51	50	62*	80	None

* with documentation

Terms To Know

clamp. Tool used to grip, compress, join, or fasten body parts.

flank. Part of the body found between the posterior ribs and the uppermost crest of the ilium, or the lateral side of the hip, thigh, and buttock.

insufflation. Blowing air or gas into a body cavity.

laparoscopy. Direct visualization of the peritoneal cavity, outer fallopian tubes, uterus, and ovaries utilizing a laparoscope, a thin, flexible fiberoptic tube.

ligate. To tie off a blood vessel or duct with a suture or a soft, thin wire (ligature wire).

nephrectomy. Partial or total removal of the kidney that may be performed for indications such as irreparable kidney damage, renal cell carcinoma, trauma, congenital abnormalities, or transplant purposes.

retroperitoneal. Located behind the peritoneum, the membrane that lines the abdominopelvic walls and forms a covering for the internal organs.

trocar. Cannula or a sharp pointed instrument used to puncture and aspirate fluid from cavities.

ureterectomy. Excision of all or part of a ureter. This procedure may be performed alone or as part of another procedure, such as urinary diversion or nephrectomy.

50547

50547   Laparoscopy, surgical; donor nephrectomy (including cold preservation), from living donor

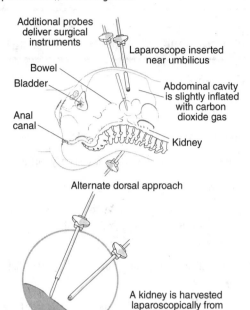

A kidney is harvested laparoscopically from a living donor

Explanation

The physician performs a donor nephrectomy from a living donor by removing the kidney and upper portion of the ureter laparoscopically through the abdomen or back. With the abdominal approach, an umbilical port is created by placing a trocar at the level of the umbilicus. The abdominal wall is insufflated. The laparoscope is placed through the umbilical port and additional trocars are placed into the abdominal cavity. In the back approach, the trocar is placed at the back proximate to the retroperitoneal space near the kidney with additional ports placed nearby for appropriate access to the operative site. The physician uses the laparoscope fitted with a fiberoptic camera and/or operating instruments to explore the area. After mobilization of the kidney and ureter, an anti-clotting agent is administered. The physician clamps, ligates, and severs the upper ureter and major renal blood vessels (renal pedicle), and removes the kidney and upper ureter. The physician administers medication to reverse the effects of the anti-clotting agent. The small abdominal or back incisions are closed by staple or suture in the usual fashion. The donor kidney is preserved for transplantation into the recipient. The organ remains under refrigeration, packed in a sealable container with some preserving solution and kept on ice in a suitable carrier.

Coding Tips

This code reports removal of one kidney from a living donor. For open donor nephrectomy from a living donor, see 50320. For donor nephrectomy from a cadaver, see 50300. For laparoscopic nephrectomy procedures that are not part of a renal transplant, see 50545–50546 and 50548. Backbench renal allograft standard preparation prior to transplantation is reported with 50325; reconstruction, see 50327-50329.

ICD-10-CM Diagnostic Codes

Z52.4   Kidney donor

AMA: 50547 2018,Jan,8; 2017,Jan,8; 2016,Jan,13; 2015,Jan,16; 2014,Jan,11

CPT © 2020 American Medical Association. All Rights Reserved.   ● New   ▲ Revised   + Add On   ★ Telemedicine   AMA: CPT Assist   [Resequenced]   ☑ Laterality   © 2020 Optum360, LLC

Relative Value Units/Medicare Edits

Non-Facility RVU	Work	PE	MP	Total
50547	26.34	14.72	5.57	46.63
Facility RVU	Work	PE	MP	Total
50547	26.34	14.72	5.57	46.63

	FUD	Status	MUE	Modifiers				IOM Reference
50547	90	A	1(2)	51	50	62*	80	100-04,3,90.1.1

* with documentation

Terms To Know

allograft. Graft from one individual to another of the same species.

clamp. Tool used to grip, compress, join, or fasten body parts.

donor. Person from whom tissues or organs are removed for transplantation.

laparoscopy. Direct visualization of the peritoneal cavity, outer fallopian tubes, uterus, and ovaries utilizing a laparoscope, a thin, flexible fiberoptic tube.

ligate. To tie off a blood vessel or duct with a suture or a soft, thin wire (ligature wire).

nephrectomy. Partial or total removal of the kidney that may be performed for indications such as irreparable kidney damage, renal cell carcinoma, trauma, congenital abnormalities, or transplant purposes.

pedicle. Stem-like, narrow base or stalk attached to a new growth.

renal. Referring to the kidney.

retroperitoneal. Located behind the peritoneum, the membrane that lines the abdominopelvic walls and forms a covering for the internal organs.

transplantation. Grafting or movement of an organ or tissue from one site or person to another.

50548

50548   Laparoscopy, surgical; nephrectomy with total ureterectomy

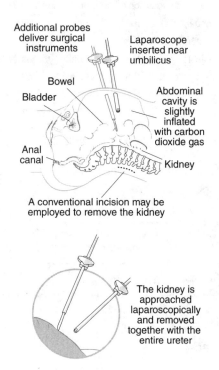

Additional probes deliver surgical instruments

Laparoscope inserted near umbilicus

Bowel

Bladder

Abdominal cavity is slightly inflated with carbon dioxide gas

Anal canal

Kidney

A conventional incision may be employed to remove the kidney

The kidney is approached laparoscopically and removed together with the entire ureter

Explanation

The physician removes the kidney and all of the ureter through a laparoscope. The physician makes a 1.0-centimeter periumbilical incision and inserts a trocar. The abdominal cavity is insufflated with carbon dioxide. A fiberoptic laparoscope fitted with a camera and light source is inserted through the trocar. Other incisions (ports) are made in the abdomen or flank to allow other instruments or an additional light source to be passed into the abdomen or retroperitoneum. The colon is mobilized and the laparoscope is advanced to the operative site. The physician mobilizes the kidney and clamps, ligates, and severs the all of the ureter at the ureterovesical junction and major renal blood vessels (renal pedicle). The kidney and ureter are bagged and brought through one of the port sites (e.g., periumbilical) that has been slightly enlarged. The instruments are removed, and the small abdominal or flank incisions are closed with staple or suture.

Coding Tips

Surgical laparoscopy always includes diagnostic laparoscopy; the diagnostic laparoscopy should not be reported separately. For open nephrectomy with total ureterectomy, see 50234–50236. For open nephrectomy with partial ureterectomy, see 50220–50230.

ICD-10-CM Diagnostic Codes

C64.1	Malignant neoplasm of right kidney, except renal pelvis ☑
C64.2	Malignant neoplasm of left kidney, except renal pelvis ☑
C65.1	Malignant neoplasm of right renal pelvis ☑
C65.2	Malignant neoplasm of left renal pelvis ☑
C66.1	Malignant neoplasm of right ureter ☑
C66.2	Malignant neoplasm of left ureter ☑
C68.8	Malignant neoplasm of overlapping sites of urinary organs

Kidney

C79.01	Secondary malignant neoplasm of right kidney and renal pelvis ☑
C79.02	Secondary malignant neoplasm of left kidney and renal pelvis ☑
C79.11	Secondary malignant neoplasm of bladder
C79.19	Secondary malignant neoplasm of other urinary organs
C7A.093	Malignant carcinoid tumor of the kidney
C80.2	Malignant neoplasm associated with transplanted organ
D09.19	Carcinoma in situ of other urinary organs
D30.01	Benign neoplasm of right kidney ☑
D30.02	Benign neoplasm of left kidney ☑
D30.11	Benign neoplasm of right renal pelvis ☑
D30.12	Benign neoplasm of left renal pelvis ☑
D30.21	Benign neoplasm of right ureter ☑
D30.22	Benign neoplasm of left ureter ☑
D3A.093	Benign carcinoid tumor of the kidney
D41.01	Neoplasm of uncertain behavior of right kidney ☑
D41.02	Neoplasm of uncertain behavior of left kidney ☑
D41.11	Neoplasm of uncertain behavior of right renal pelvis ☑
D41.12	Neoplasm of uncertain behavior of left renal pelvis ☑
D41.21	Neoplasm of uncertain behavior of right ureter ☑
D41.22	Neoplasm of uncertain behavior of left ureter ☑
D47.Z1	Post-transplant lymphoproliferative disorder (PTLD)
D47.Z2	Castleman disease
D49.511	Neoplasm of unspecified behavior of right kidney ☑
D49.512	Neoplasm of unspecified behavior of left kidney ☑
D49.59	Neoplasm of unspecified behavior of other genitourinary organ
I12.0	Hypertensive chronic kidney disease with stage 5 chronic kidney disease or end stage renal disease
I13.11	Hypertensive heart and chronic kidney disease without heart failure, with stage 5 chronic kidney disease, or end stage renal disease
I15.0	Renovascular hypertension
I16.0	Hypertensive urgency
I16.1	Hypertensive emergency
I75.81	Atheroembolism of kidney
N11.0	Nonobstructive reflux-associated chronic pyelonephritis
N11.1	Chronic obstructive pyelonephritis
N11.8	Other chronic tubulo-interstitial nephritis
N13.0	Hydronephrosis with ureteropelvic junction obstruction
N13.1	Hydronephrosis with ureteral stricture, not elsewhere classified
N13.2	Hydronephrosis with renal and ureteral calculous obstruction
N13.39	Other hydronephrosis
N13.4	Hydroureter
N13.5	Crossing vessel and stricture of ureter without hydronephrosis
N13.6	Pyonephrosis
N13.71	Vesicoureteral-reflux without reflux nephropathy
N13.721	Vesicoureteral-reflux with reflux nephropathy without hydroureter, unilateral
N13.722	Vesicoureteral-reflux with reflux nephropathy without hydroureter, bilateral
N13.731	Vesicoureteral-reflux with reflux nephropathy with hydroureter, unilateral
N13.732	Vesicoureteral-reflux with reflux nephropathy with hydroureter, bilateral

N20.0	Calculus of kidney
N20.2	Calculus of kidney with calculus of ureter
N26.1	Atrophy of kidney (terminal)
N26.2	Page kidney
N28.0	Ischemia and infarction of kidney
N28.1	Cyst of kidney, acquired
N28.81	Hypertrophy of kidney
N28.82	Megaloureter
N28.89	Other specified disorders of kidney and ureter
Q60.3	Renal hypoplasia, unilateral
Q60.4	Renal hypoplasia, bilateral
Q60.6	Potter's syndrome
Q61.01	Congenital single renal cyst
Q61.02	Congenital multiple renal cysts
Q61.11	Cystic dilatation of collecting ducts
Q61.2	Polycystic kidney, adult type
Q61.4	Renal dysplasia
Q61.5	Medullary cystic kidney
Q61.8	Other cystic kidney diseases
Q62.0	Congenital hydronephrosis
Q62.11	Congenital occlusion of ureteropelvic junction
Q62.31	Congenital ureterocele, orthotopic
Q62.32	Cecoureterocele
Q62.39	Other obstructive defects of renal pelvis and ureter
S37.061A	Major laceration of right kidney, initial encounter ☑
S37.062A	Major laceration of left kidney, initial encounter ☑
S37.091A	Other injury of right kidney, initial encounter ☑
S37.092A	Other injury of left kidney, initial encounter ☑

AMA: **50548** 2018,Jan,8; 2017,Jan,8; 2016,Jan,13; 2015,Jan,16; 2014,Jan,11

Relative Value Units/Medicare Edits

Non-Facility RVU	Work	PE	MP	Total
50548	25.36	10.57	2.95	38.88
Facility RVU	**Work**	**PE**	**MP**	**Total**
50548	25.36	10.57	2.95	38.88

	FUD	Status	MUE	Modifiers				IOM Reference
50548	90	A	1(2)	51	50	62*	80	None

* with documentation

Terms To Know

flank. Part of the body found between the posterior ribs and the uppermost crest of the ilium, or the lateral side of the hip, thigh, and buttock.

insufflation. Blowing air or gas into a body cavity.

laparoscopy. Direct visualization of the peritoneal cavity, outer fallopian tubes, uterus, and ovaries utilizing a laparoscope, a thin, flexible fiberoptic tube.

nephrectomy. Partial or total removal of the kidney that may be performed for indications such as irreparable kidney damage, renal cell carcinoma, trauma, congenital abnormalities, or transplant purposes.

Kidney

50551-50555

50551 Renal endoscopy through established nephrostomy or pyelostomy, with or without irrigation, instillation, or ureteropyelography, exclusive of radiologic service;
50553 with ureteral catheterization, with or without dilation of ureter
50555 with biopsy

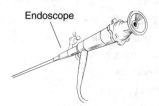

Endoscope

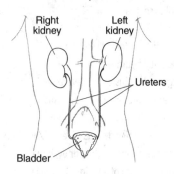

A variety of procedures are performed endoscopically through an already established incision to the kidney or renal pelvis

Right kidney
Left kidney
Ureters
Bladder

Explanation

The physician examines the kidney and ureter with an endoscope passed through an established opening between the skin and kidney (nephrostomy) or renal pelvis (pyelostomy). After inserting a guidewire, the physician removes the nephrostomy or pyelostomy tube and passes the endoscope through the opening into the kidney or renal pelvis. To better view renal and ureteric structures, the physician may flush (irrigate) or introduce by drops (instillate) a saline solution. The physician may introduce contrast medium for radiologic study of the renal pelvis and ureter (ureteropyelogram). In 50551, the physician removes the endoscope and guidewire and reinserts the nephrostomy tube or allows the surgical passageway to seal on its own. In 50553, the physician passes a thin tube through the endoscope into the ureter. The physician may insert a balloon catheter to dilate a ureteral constriction. In 50555, the physician passes a cutting instrument through the endoscope into the suspect renal tissue and takes a biopsy specimen. The physician removes the endoscope and reinserts the nephrostomy or pyelostomy tube or allows the passageway to seal on its own.

Coding Tips

For percutaneous renal endoscopy (through established nephrostomy/pyelostomy) with fulguration and/or incision, with or without biopsy, see 50557; removal of foreign body or calculus, see 50561; with resection of tumor, see 50562. For open renal endoscopic procedures (through nephrotomy or pyelotomy), see 50570–50580. Report image-guided dilation of a ureter, without endoscopic guidance, with 50706; imaged-guided biopsy, ureter and/or renal pelvis, see 50606. Local anesthesia is included in these services. However, general anesthesia may be administered depending on the age or condition of the patient. Supplies used when providing these procedures may be reported with the appropriate HCPCS Level II code. Check with the specific payer to determine coverage.

ICD-10-CM Diagnostic Codes

C64.1	Malignant neoplasm of right kidney, except renal pelvis ☑
C64.2	Malignant neoplasm of left kidney, except renal pelvis ☑
C65.1	Malignant neoplasm of right renal pelvis ☑
C65.2	Malignant neoplasm of left renal pelvis ☑
C66.1	Malignant neoplasm of right ureter ☑
C66.2	Malignant neoplasm of left ureter ☑
C67.6	Malignant neoplasm of ureteric orifice
C79.01	Secondary malignant neoplasm of right kidney and renal pelvis ☑
C79.02	Secondary malignant neoplasm of left kidney and renal pelvis ☑
C7A.093	Malignant carcinoid tumor of the kidney
C80.2	Malignant neoplasm associated with transplanted organ
D09.19	Carcinoma in situ of other urinary organs
D30.01	Benign neoplasm of right kidney ☑
D30.02	Benign neoplasm of left kidney ☑
D30.11	Benign neoplasm of right renal pelvis ☑
D30.12	Benign neoplasm of left renal pelvis ☑
D30.21	Benign neoplasm of right ureter ☑
D30.22	Benign neoplasm of left ureter ☑
D3A.093	Benign carcinoid tumor of the kidney
D41.01	Neoplasm of uncertain behavior of right kidney ☑
D41.02	Neoplasm of uncertain behavior of left kidney ☑
D41.11	Neoplasm of uncertain behavior of right renal pelvis ☑
D41.12	Neoplasm of uncertain behavior of left renal pelvis ☑
D41.21	Neoplasm of uncertain behavior of right ureter ☑
D41.22	Neoplasm of uncertain behavior of left ureter ☑
D49.511	Neoplasm of unspecified behavior of right kidney ☑
D49.512	Neoplasm of unspecified behavior of left kidney ☑
D49.59	Neoplasm of unspecified behavior of other genitourinary organ
N11.1	Chronic obstructive pyelonephritis
N13.0	Hydronephrosis with ureteropelvic junction obstruction
N13.1	Hydronephrosis with ureteral stricture, not elsewhere classified
N13.2	Hydronephrosis with renal and ureteral calculous obstruction
N13.39	Other hydronephrosis
N13.4	Hydroureter
N13.5	Crossing vessel and stricture of ureter without hydronephrosis
N13.8	Other obstructive and reflux uropathy
N15.1	Renal and perinephric abscess
N20.0	Calculus of kidney
N20.1	Calculus of ureter
N20.2	Calculus of kidney with calculus of ureter
N25.81	Secondary hyperparathyroidism of renal origin
N28.0	Ischemia and infarction of kidney
N28.1	Cyst of kidney, acquired
N28.81	Hypertrophy of kidney
N28.82	Megaloureter
N28.83	Nephroptosis
N28.89	Other specified disorders of kidney and ureter
Q61.01	Congenital single renal cyst
Q61.02	Congenital multiple renal cysts
Q61.19	Other polycystic kidney, infantile type
Q61.2	Polycystic kidney, adult type

© 2020 Optum360, LLC   **N** Newborn: 0   **P** Pediatric: 0-17   **M** Maternity: 9-64   **A** Adult: 15-124   ♂ Male Only   ♀ Female Only   CPT © 2020 American Medical Association. All Rights Reserved.

Kidney

Q61.4	Renal dysplasia
Q61.5	Medullary cystic kidney
Q61.8	Other cystic kidney diseases
Q62.0	Congenital hydronephrosis
Q62.11	Congenital occlusion of ureteropelvic junction
Q62.12	Congenital occlusion of ureterovesical orifice
Q62.2	Congenital megaureter
Q62.31	Congenital ureterocele, orthotopic
Q62.32	Cecoureterocele
Q62.39	Other obstructive defects of renal pelvis and ureter

AMA: **50551** 2018,Jan,8; 2017,Jan,8; 2016,Jan,13; 2015,Jan,16; 2014,Jan,11
50553 2018,Jan,8; 2017,Jan,8; 2016,Jan,3; 2016,Jan,13; 2015,Jan,16; 2014,Jan,11
50555 2018,Jan,8; 2017,Jan,8; 2016,Jan,3; 2016,Jan,13; 2015,Jan,16; 2014,Jan,11

Relative Value Units/Medicare Edits

Non-Facility RVU	Work	PE	MP	Total
50551	5.59	4.14	0.63	10.36
50553	5.98	4.43	0.66	11.07
50555	6.52	4.6	0.76	11.88
Facility RVU	Work	PE	MP	Total
50551	5.59	2.26	0.63	8.48
50553	5.98	2.4	0.66	9.04
50555	6.52	2.58	0.76	9.86

	FUD	Status	MUE	Modifiers				IOM Reference
50551	0	A	1(3)	51	50	N/A	80*	None
50553	0	A	1(3)	51	50	N/A	N/A	
50555	0	A	1(2)	51	50	N/A	80*	

* with documentation

Terms To Know

biopsy. Tissue or fluid removed for diagnostic purposes through analysis of the cells in the biopsy material.

endoscopy. Visual inspection of the body using a fiberoptic scope.

guidewire. Flexible metal instrument designed to lead another instrument in its proper course.

irrigate. Washing out, lavage.

nephrostomy. Placement of a stent, tube, or catheter that forms a passage from the exterior of the body into the renal pelvis or calyx, often for drainage of urine or an abscess, for exploration, or calculus extraction.

pyelostomy. Surgical creation of an opening through the abdominal wall into the renal pelvis.

renal. Referring to the kidney.

specimen. Tissue cells or sample of fluid taken for analysis, pathologic examination, and diagnosis.

50557-50561

| 50557 | Renal endoscopy through established nephrostomy or pyelostomy, with or without irrigation, instillation, or ureteropyelography, exclusive of radiologic service; with fulguration and/or incision, with or without biopsy |
| 50561 | with removal of foreign body or calculus |

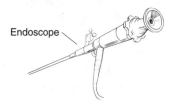

Endoscope

A variety of procedures are performed endoscopically through an already established incision to the kidney or pelvis

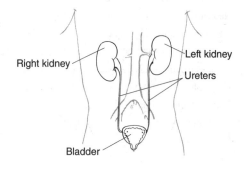

Right kidney
Left kidney
Ureters
Bladder

Explanation

The physician examines the kidney and ureter with an endoscope passed through an established opening between the skin and kidney (nephrostomy) or renal pelvis (pyelostomy) and removes renal lesions by electric current (fulguration) or incision in 50557, and removes a foreign body or calculus in 50561. After inserting a guidewire, the physician removes the nephrostomy or pyelostomy tube and passes the endoscope through the opening into the kidney or renal pelvis. To better view renal and ureteric structures, the physician may flush (irrigate) or introduce by drops (instillate) a saline solution. The physician may introduce contrast medium for radiologic study of the renal pelvis and ureter (ureteropyelogram). After examination, the physician passes through the endoscope an instrument that destroys lesions with electric current or incises lesions. The physician may insert a cutting instrument to biopsy renal tissue. The physician removes the endoscope and reinserts the nephrostomy/pyelostomy tube or allows the passageway to seal on its own.

Coding Tips

For percutaneous renal endoscopy (through established nephrostomy or pyelostomy), with ureteral catheterization, with or without dilation, see 50553; with biopsy, see 50555. For open renal endoscopic procedures (through nephrotomy or pyelotomy), see 50570–50580. Local anesthesia is included in the service. However, general anesthesia may be administered depending on the age or condition of the patient. Supplies used when providing these procedures may be reported with the appropriate HCPCS Level II code. Check with the specific payer to determine coverage.

ICD-10-CM Diagnostic Codes

C64.1	Malignant neoplasm of right kidney, except renal pelvis ☑
C64.2	Malignant neoplasm of left kidney, except renal pelvis ☑
C65.1	Malignant neoplasm of right renal pelvis ☑
C65.2	Malignant neoplasm of left renal pelvis ☑

Kidney

C66.1	Malignant neoplasm of right ureter ☑
C66.2	Malignant neoplasm of left ureter ☑
C67.6	Malignant neoplasm of ureteric orifice
C79.01	Secondary malignant neoplasm of right kidney and renal pelvis ☑
C79.02	Secondary malignant neoplasm of left kidney and renal pelvis ☑
C7A.093	Malignant carcinoid tumor of the kidney
C80.2	Malignant neoplasm associated with transplanted organ
D09.19	Carcinoma in situ of other urinary organs
D30.01	Benign neoplasm of right kidney ☑
D30.02	Benign neoplasm of left kidney ☑
D30.11	Benign neoplasm of right renal pelvis ☑
D30.12	Benign neoplasm of left renal pelvis ☑
D30.21	Benign neoplasm of right ureter ☑
D30.22	Benign neoplasm of left ureter ☑
D3A.093	Benign carcinoid tumor of the kidney
D41.01	Neoplasm of uncertain behavior of right kidney ☑
D41.02	Neoplasm of uncertain behavior of left kidney ☑
D41.11	Neoplasm of uncertain behavior of right renal pelvis ☑
D41.12	Neoplasm of uncertain behavior of left renal pelvis ☑
D41.21	Neoplasm of uncertain behavior of right ureter ☑
D41.22	Neoplasm of uncertain behavior of left ureter ☑
N13.4	Hydroureter
N13.8	Other obstructive and reflux uropathy
N15.1	Renal and perinephric abscess
N20.0	Calculus of kidney
N20.1	Calculus of ureter
N20.2	Calculus of kidney with calculus of ureter
N25.81	Secondary hyperparathyroidism of renal origin
N28.0	Ischemia and infarction of kidney
N28.1	Cyst of kidney, acquired
N28.81	Hypertrophy of kidney
N28.82	Megaloureter
N28.83	Nephroptosis
N28.89	Other specified disorders of kidney and ureter
T19.8XXA	Foreign body in other parts of genitourinary tract, initial encounter
T81.510A	Adhesions due to foreign body accidentally left in body following surgical operation, initial encounter
T81.512A	Adhesions due to foreign body accidentally left in body following kidney dialysis, initial encounter
T81.514A	Adhesions due to foreign body accidentally left in body following endoscopic examination, initial encounter
T81.516A	Adhesions due to foreign body accidentally left in body following aspiration, puncture or other catheterization, initial encounter
T81.517A	Adhesions due to foreign body accidentally left in body following removal of catheter or packing, initial encounter
T81.518A	Adhesions due to foreign body accidentally left in body following other procedure, initial encounter
T81.520A	Obstruction due to foreign body accidentally left in body following surgical operation, initial encounter
T81.522A	Obstruction due to foreign body accidentally left in body following kidney dialysis, initial encounter
T81.524A	Obstruction due to foreign body accidentally left in body following endoscopic examination, initial encounter
T81.526A	Obstruction due to foreign body accidentally left in body following aspiration, puncture or other catheterization, initial encounter
T81.527A	Obstruction due to foreign body accidentally left in body following removal of catheter or packing, initial encounter
T81.528A	Obstruction due to foreign body accidentally left in body following other procedure, initial encounter
T81.530A	Perforation due to foreign body accidentally left in body following surgical operation, initial encounter
T81.532A	Perforation due to foreign body accidentally left in body following kidney dialysis, initial encounter
T81.534A	Perforation due to foreign body accidentally left in body following endoscopic examination, initial encounter
T81.536A	Perforation due to foreign body accidentally left in body following aspiration, puncture or other catheterization, initial encounter
T81.537A	Perforation due to foreign body accidentally left in body following removal of catheter or packing, initial encounter
T81.538A	Perforation due to foreign body accidentally left in body following other procedure, initial encounter
T81.590A	Other complications of foreign body accidentally left in body following surgical operation, initial encounter
T81.592A	Other complications of foreign body accidentally left in body following kidney dialysis, initial encounter
T81.594A	Other complications of foreign body accidentally left in body following endoscopic examination, initial encounter
T81.596A	Other complications of foreign body accidentally left in body following aspiration, puncture or other catheterization, initial encounter
T81.597A	Other complications of foreign body accidentally left in body following removal of catheter or packing, initial encounter
T81.598A	Other complications of foreign body accidentally left in body following other procedure, initial encounter

AMA: **50557** 2018,Jan,8; 2017,Jan,8; 2016,Jan,13; 2015,Jan,16; 2014,Jan,11
50561 2018,Jan,8; 2017,Jan,8; 2016,Jan,13; 2015,Jan,16; 2014,Jan,11

Relative Value Units/Medicare Edits

Non-Facility RVU	Work	PE	MP	Total
50557	6.61	4.7	0.77	12.08
50561	7.58	5.22	0.86	13.66
Facility RVU	Work	PE	MP	Total
50557	6.61	2.61	0.77	9.99
50561	7.58	2.92	0.86	11.36

	FUD	Status	MUE	Modifiers				IOM Reference
50557	0	A	1(2)	51	50	N/A	80*	None
50561	0	A	1(2)	51	50	N/A	80*	

* with documentation

Kidney

50562

50562 Renal endoscopy through established nephrostomy or pyelostomy, with or without irrigation, instillation, or ureteropyelography, exclusive of radiologic service; with resection of tumor

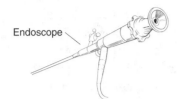

Endoscope

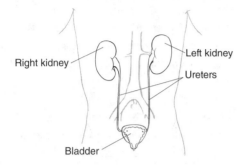

A tumor is removed through established nephrostomy or pyelostomy

Right kidney

Left kidney

Ureters

Bladder

Explanation

The physician examines the kidney and ureter with an endoscope passed through an established opening between the skin and kidney (nephrostomy) or renal pelvis (pyelostomy). After inserting a guidewire, the physician removes the nephrostomy or pyelostomy tube and passes the endoscope through the opening into the kidney or renal pelvis. To better view renal and ureteric structures, the physician may flush (irrigate) or introduce by drops (instillate) a saline solution. The physician may introduce contrast medium for radiologic study of the renal pelvis and ureter (ureteropyelogram). After examination, the physician passes an instrument through the endoscope to resect a tumor. The tumor may be removed by cold-cup biopsy forceps with the bulk of the tumor being grasped and removed in piecemeal fashion until the base is reached. Alternately, a cutting loop may be used to remove the tumor to the base, or the tumor may be ablated with YAG laser. After the tumor resection, the physician removes the endoscope and other instruments and reinserts the nephrostomy tube or allows the surgical passageway to seal on its own.

Coding Tips

This procedure is performed through an already established stoma. Previously, there was no code to capture the difficult technical work and skill involved in resecting a renal pelvic tumor through a nephrostomy site. This procedure is usually reported in high-tech research facilities and hospitals.

ICD-10-CM Diagnostic Codes

C64.1	Malignant neoplasm of right kidney, except renal pelvis ☑
C64.2	Malignant neoplasm of left kidney, except renal pelvis ☑
C65.1	Malignant neoplasm of right renal pelvis ☑
C65.2	Malignant neoplasm of left renal pelvis ☑
C79.01	Secondary malignant neoplasm of right kidney and renal pelvis ☑
C79.02	Secondary malignant neoplasm of left kidney and renal pelvis ☑
C7A.093	Malignant carcinoid tumor of the kidney
C80.2	Malignant neoplasm associated with transplanted organ

D09.19	Carcinoma in situ of other urinary organs
D30.01	Benign neoplasm of right kidney ☑
D30.02	Benign neoplasm of left kidney ☑
D30.11	Benign neoplasm of right renal pelvis ☑
D30.12	Benign neoplasm of left renal pelvis ☑
D3A.093	Benign carcinoid tumor of the kidney
D41.01	Neoplasm of uncertain behavior of right kidney ☑
D41.02	Neoplasm of uncertain behavior of left kidney ☑
D41.11	Neoplasm of uncertain behavior of right renal pelvis ☑
D41.12	Neoplasm of uncertain behavior of left renal pelvis ☑
D41.21	Neoplasm of uncertain behavior of right ureter ☑
D41.22	Neoplasm of uncertain behavior of left ureter ☑
D49.511	Neoplasm of unspecified behavior of right kidney ☑
D49.512	Neoplasm of unspecified behavior of left kidney ☑
D49.59	Neoplasm of unspecified behavior of other genitourinary organ

AMA: **50562** 2018,Jan,8; 2017,Jan,8; 2016,Jan,13; 2015,Jan,16; 2014,Jan,11

Relative Value Units/Medicare Edits

Non-Facility RVU	Work	PE	MP	Total
50562	10.9	4.58	1.25	16.73
Facility RVU	**Work**	**PE**	**MP**	**Total**
50562	10.9	4.58	1.25	16.73

	FUD	Status	MUE	Modifiers				IOM Reference
50562	90	A	1(3)	51	N/A	62*	80	None

* with documentation

Terms To Know

benign lesion. Neoplasm or change in tissue that is not cancerous (nonmalignant).

carcinoma in situ. Malignancy that arises from the cells of the vessel, gland, or organ of origin that remains confined to that site or has not invaded neighboring tissue.

malignant neoplasm. Any cancerous tumor or lesion exhibiting uncontrolled tissue growth that can progressively invade other parts of the body with its disease-generating cells.

nephrostomy. Placement of a stent, tube, or catheter that forms a passage from the exterior of the body into the renal pelvis or calyx, often for drainage of urine or an abscess, for exploration, or calculus extraction.

resection. Surgical removal of a part or all of an organ or body part.

tumor. Pathological swelling or enlargement; a neoplastic growth of uncontrolled, abnormal multiplication of cells.

ureteropyelogram. Radiologic study of the renal pelvis and the ureter.

Kidney

50570-50574

50570 Renal endoscopy through nephrotomy or pyelotomy, with or without irrigation, instillation, or ureteropyelography, exclusive of radiologic service;

50572 with ureteral catheterization, with or without dilation of ureter

50574 with biopsy

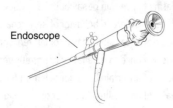

A variety of procedures are performed endoscopically through an incision into the kidney or renal pelvis

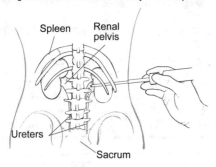

Explanation

The physician examines the kidney and ureter with an endoscope passed through an incision in the kidney (nephrotomy) or renal pelvis (pyelotomy). After accessing the renal and ureteric structures with an incision in the skin of the flank, the physician incises the kidney or renal pelvis and guides the endoscope through the incision. To better view renal and ureteric structures, the physician may flush (irrigate) or introduce by drops (instillate) a saline solution. The physician may also introduce contrast medium for radiologic study of the renal pelvis and ureter (ureteropyelogram). In 50572, the physician passes a thin tube through the endoscope into the ureter, and may insert a balloon catheter to dilate a ureteral constriction. In 50574, the physician passes a cutting instrument through the endoscope into the suspect renal tissue and takes a biopsy specimen. The physician removes the endoscope, sutures the incision, inserts a drain tube, and performs a layered closure.

Coding Tips

If the nephrotomy or pyelotomy is done for an additional, significantly identifiable endoscopic service, report both the appropriate endoscopic procedure code (50570–50580) and 50045 or 50120. For open renal endoscopy (through nephrotomy or pyelotomy), with fulguration and/or incision with or without biopsy, see 50576; removal of a foreign body or calculus, see 50580. For percutaneous renal endoscopic procedures (through established nephrostomy/pyelostomy), see 50551–50562.

ICD-10-CM Diagnostic Codes

C64.1	Malignant neoplasm of right kidney, except renal pelvis ☑
C64.2	Malignant neoplasm of left kidney, except renal pelvis ☑
C65.1	Malignant neoplasm of right renal pelvis ☑
C65.2	Malignant neoplasm of left renal pelvis ☑
C66.1	Malignant neoplasm of right ureter ☑
C66.2	Malignant neoplasm of left ureter ☑
C67.6	Malignant neoplasm of ureteric orifice
C79.01	Secondary malignant neoplasm of right kidney and renal pelvis ☑
C79.02	Secondary malignant neoplasm of left kidney and renal pelvis ☑
C7A.093	Malignant carcinoid tumor of the kidney
C80.2	Malignant neoplasm associated with transplanted organ
D09.19	Carcinoma in situ of other urinary organs
D30.01	Benign neoplasm of right kidney ☑
D30.02	Benign neoplasm of left kidney ☑
D30.11	Benign neoplasm of right renal pelvis ☑
D30.12	Benign neoplasm of left renal pelvis ☑
D30.21	Benign neoplasm of right ureter ☑
D30.22	Benign neoplasm of left ureter ☑
D3A.093	Benign carcinoid tumor of the kidney
D41.01	Neoplasm of uncertain behavior of right kidney ☑
D41.02	Neoplasm of uncertain behavior of left kidney ☑
D41.11	Neoplasm of uncertain behavior of right renal pelvis ☑
D41.12	Neoplasm of uncertain behavior of left renal pelvis ☑
D41.21	Neoplasm of uncertain behavior of right ureter ☑
D41.22	Neoplasm of uncertain behavior of left ureter ☑
D49.511	Neoplasm of unspecified behavior of right kidney ☑
D49.512	Neoplasm of unspecified behavior of left kidney ☑
D49.59	Neoplasm of unspecified behavior of other genitourinary organ
N11.1	Chronic obstructive pyelonephritis
N13.0	Hydronephrosis with ureteropelvic junction obstruction
N13.1	Hydronephrosis with ureteral stricture, not elsewhere classified
N13.2	Hydronephrosis with renal and ureteral calculous obstruction
N13.39	Other hydronephrosis
N13.4	Hydroureter
N13.5	Crossing vessel and stricture of ureter without hydronephrosis
N13.8	Other obstructive and reflux uropathy
N15.1	Renal and perinephric abscess
N20.0	Calculus of kidney
N20.1	Calculus of ureter
N20.2	Calculus of kidney with calculus of ureter
N25.81	Secondary hyperparathyroidism of renal origin
N28.0	Ischemia and infarction of kidney
N28.1	Cyst of kidney, acquired
N28.81	Hypertrophy of kidney
N28.82	Megaloureter
N28.83	Nephroptosis
N28.89	Other specified disorders of kidney and ureter
Q61.01	Congenital single renal cyst
Q61.02	Congenital multiple renal cysts
Q61.19	Other polycystic kidney, infantile type
Q61.2	Polycystic kidney, adult type
Q61.4	Renal dysplasia
Q61.5	Medullary cystic kidney
Q61.8	Other cystic kidney diseases
Q62.0	Congenital hydronephrosis
Q62.11	Congenital occlusion of ureteropelvic junction
Q62.12	Congenital occlusion of ureterovesical orifice
Q62.2	Congenital megaureter
Q62.31	Congenital ureterocele, orthotopic

Q62.32   Cecoureterocele

Q62.39   Other obstructive defects of renal pelvis and ureter

AMA: **50570** 2018,Jan,8; 2017,Jan,8; 2016,Jan,13; 2015,Jan,16; 2014,Jan,11
50572 2018,Jan,8; 2017,Jan,8; 2016,Jan,3; 2016,Jan,13; 2015,Jan,16; 2014,Jan,11
50574 2018,Jan,8; 2017,Jan,8; 2016,Jan,3; 2016,Jan,13; 2015,Jan,16; 2014,Jan,11

Relative Value Units/Medicare Edits

Non-Facility RVU	Work	PE	MP	Total
50570	9.53	3.56	1.09	14.18
50572	10.33	3.83	1.18	15.34
50574	11.0	4.06	1.25	16.31
Facility RVU	Work	PE	MP	Total
50570	9.53	3.56	1.09	14.18
50572	10.33	3.83	1.18	15.34
50574	11.0	4.06	1.25	16.31

	FUD	Status	MUE	Modifiers				IOM Reference
50570	0	A	1(3)	51	50	N/A	80*	None
50572	0	A	1(3)	51	50	N/A	80*	
50574	0	A	1(2)	51	50	N/A	80*	

* with documentation

Terms To Know

balloon catheter. Any catheter equipped with an inflatable balloon at the end to hold it in place in a body cavity or to be used for dilation of a vessel lumen.

biopsy. Tissue or fluid removed for diagnostic purposes through analysis of the cells in the biopsy material.

catheterization. Use or insertion of a tubular device into a duct, blood vessel, hollow organ, or body cavity for injecting or withdrawing fluids for diagnostic or therapeutic purposes.

dilation. Artificial increase in the diameter of an opening or lumen made by medication or by instrumentation.

endoscopy. Visual inspection of the body using a fiberoptic scope.

flank. Part of the body found between the posterior ribs and the uppermost crest of the ilium, or the lateral side of the hip, thigh, and buttock.

irrigation. To wash out or cleanse a body cavity, wound, or tissue with water or other fluid.

nephrotomy. Incision into the body of the kidney.

pyelotomy. Incision or opening made into the renal pelvis.

50575

50575   Renal endoscopy through nephrotomy or pyelotomy, with or without irrigation, instillation, or ureteropyelography, exclusive of radiologic service; with endopyelotomy (includes cystoscopy, ureteroscopy, dilation of ureter and ureteral pelvic junction, incision of ureteral pelvic junction and insertion of endopyelotomy stent)

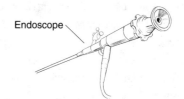

Endoscope

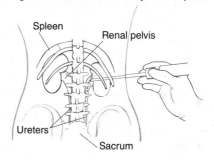

A variety of procedures are performed endoscopically through an incision into the kidney or renal pelvis

Spleen   Renal pelvis

Ureters

Sacrum

Explanation

The physician examines the kidney and ureter with an endoscope passed through an incision in the kidney (nephrotomy) or renal pelvis (pyelotomy), and dilates ureter and ureteropelvic junction. After accessing the renal and ureteric structures with an incision in the skin of the flank, the physician incises the kidney or renal pelvis and guides the endoscope through the incision. To better view renal and ureteric structures, the physician may flush (irrigate) or introduce by drops (instillate) a saline solution. The physician may introduce contrast medium for radiologic study of the renal pelvis and ureter (ureteropyelogram). For endopyelotomy, the physician places endoscope through the ureter and/or the pelvis, incises the pelvis, enlarges the ureteropelvic junction, and sutures the junction as in a Y-V pyeloplasty. The physician inserts the stent through the renal pelvis into the junction, sutures the incisions, inserts a drain tube, and performs a layered closure.

Coding Tips

Other open renal endoscopy procedures include examination (50570), ureteral catheterization (50572), biopsy (50574), fulguration/incision (50576), and removal of a foreign body or calculus (50580). If the nephrotomy or pyelotomy is done for an additional, significantly identifiable endoscopic service, report both the appropriate endoscopic procedure code (50570–50580) and 50045 or 50120. For percutaneous renal endoscopic procedures (through established nephrostomy/pyelostomy), see 50551–50562.

ICD-10-CM Diagnostic Codes

C64.1	Malignant neoplasm of right kidney, except renal pelvis	☑
C64.2	Malignant neoplasm of left kidney, except renal pelvis	☑
C65.1	Malignant neoplasm of right renal pelvis	☑
C65.2	Malignant neoplasm of left renal pelvis	☑
C79.01	Secondary malignant neoplasm of right kidney and renal pelvis	☑
C79.02	Secondary malignant neoplasm of left kidney and renal pelvis	☑
C7A.093	Malignant carcinoid tumor of the kidney	

Kidney

C80.2	Malignant neoplasm associated with transplanted organ	
D09.19	Carcinoma in situ of other urinary organs	
D30.01	Benign neoplasm of right kidney ☑	
D30.02	Benign neoplasm of left kidney ☑	
D30.11	Benign neoplasm of right renal pelvis ☑	
D30.12	Benign neoplasm of left renal pelvis ☑	
D3A.093	Benign carcinoid tumor of the kidney	
D41.01	Neoplasm of uncertain behavior of right kidney ☑	
D41.02	Neoplasm of uncertain behavior of left kidney ☑	
D41.11	Neoplasm of uncertain behavior of right renal pelvis ☑	
D41.12	Neoplasm of uncertain behavior of left renal pelvis ☑	
D41.21	Neoplasm of uncertain behavior of right ureter ☑	
D41.22	Neoplasm of uncertain behavior of left ureter ☑	
D49.511	Neoplasm of unspecified behavior of right kidney ☑	
D49.512	Neoplasm of unspecified behavior of left kidney ☑	
D49.59	Neoplasm of unspecified behavior of other genitourinary organ	
N10	Acute pyelonephritis	
N11.1	Chronic obstructive pyelonephritis	
N12	Tubulo-interstitial nephritis, not specified as acute or chronic	
N13.0	Hydronephrosis with ureteropelvic junction obstruction	
N13.1	Hydronephrosis with ureteral stricture, not elsewhere classified	
N13.2	Hydronephrosis with renal and ureteral calculous obstruction	
N13.39	Other hydronephrosis	
N13.8	Other obstructive and reflux uropathy	
Q62.0	Congenital hydronephrosis	
Q62.11	Congenital occlusion of ureteropelvic junction	
Q62.12	Congenital occlusion of ureterovesical orifice	
Q62.2	Congenital megaureter	
Q62.31	Congenital ureterocele, orthotopic	
Q62.32	Cecoureterocele	
Q62.39	Other obstructive defects of renal pelvis and ureter	

AMA: **50575** 2018,Jan,8; 2017,Jan,8; 2016,Jan,13; 2015,Jan,16; 2014,Jan,11

Relative Value Units/Medicare Edits

Non-Facility RVU	Work	PE	MP	Total
50575	13.96	5.07	1.61	20.64
Facility RVU	Work	PE	MP	Total
50575	13.96	5.07	1.61	20.64

	FUD	Status	MUE	Modifiers				IOM Reference
50575	0	A	1(2)	51	50	N/A	N/A	None

* with documentation

Terms To Know

flank. Part of the body found between the posterior ribs and the uppermost crest of the ilium, or the lateral side of the hip, thigh, and buttock.

stent. Tube to provide support in a body cavity or lumen.

50576-50580

50576	Renal endoscopy through nephrotomy or pyelotomy, with or without irrigation, instillation, or ureteropyelography, exclusive of radiologic service; with fulguration and/or incision, with or without biopsy
50580	with removal of foreign body or calculus

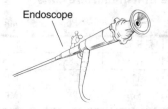

Endoscope

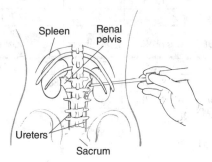

A variety of procedures are performed endoscopically through an incision into the kidney or renal pelvis

Spleen Renal pelvis

Ureters

Sacrum

Explanation

The physician examines the kidney and ureter with an endoscope passed through an incision in the kidney (nephrotomy) or renal pelvis (pyelotomy). After accessing the renal and ureteric structures with an incision in the skin of the flank, the physician incises the kidney or renal pelvis and guides the endoscope through the incision. To better view renal and ureteric structures, the physician may flush (irrigate) or introduce by drops (instillate) a saline solution. The physician may introduce contrast medium for radiologic study of the renal pelvis and ureter (ureteropyelogram). In 50576, the physician passes through the endoscope an instrument that destroys lesions by electric current or incision The physician may insert an instrument to biopsy renal tissue. In 50580, the physician passes instruments through the endoscope to remove a foreign body or calculus, and may pass a stent through the ureter into the bladder. The physician sutures the incision, inserts a drain tube, and performs a layered closure.

Coding Tips

If the nephrotomy or pyelotomy is done for an additional, significantly identifiable endoscopic service, report the appropriate endoscopic procedure code (50570–50580) and 50045 or 50120. For open renal endoscopy (through nephrotomy or pyelotomy), with examination only, see 50570; ureteral catheterization, with or without dilation of the ureter, see 50572; biopsy, see 50574. For percutaneous renal endoscopic procedures (through established nephrostomy/pyelostomy), see 50551–50562.

ICD-10-CM Diagnostic Codes

C64.1	Malignant neoplasm of right kidney, except renal pelvis ☑	
C64.2	Malignant neoplasm of left kidney, except renal pelvis ☑	
C65.1	Malignant neoplasm of right renal pelvis ☑	
C65.2	Malignant neoplasm of left renal pelvis ☑	
C79.01	Secondary malignant neoplasm of right kidney and renal pelvis ☑	

© 2020 Optum360, LLC

Kidney

C79.02	Secondary malignant neoplasm of left kidney and renal pelvis ☑
C7A.093	Malignant carcinoid tumor of the kidney
C80.2	Malignant neoplasm associated with transplanted organ
D09.19	Carcinoma in situ of other urinary organs
D30.01	Benign neoplasm of right kidney ☑
D30.02	Benign neoplasm of left kidney ☑
D30.11	Benign neoplasm of right renal pelvis ☑
D30.12	Benign neoplasm of left renal pelvis ☑
D3A.093	Benign carcinoid tumor of the kidney
D41.01	Neoplasm of uncertain behavior of right kidney ☑
D41.02	Neoplasm of uncertain behavior of left kidney ☑
D41.11	Neoplasm of uncertain behavior of right renal pelvis ☑
D41.12	Neoplasm of uncertain behavior of left renal pelvis ☑
D41.21	Neoplasm of uncertain behavior of right ureter ☑
D41.22	Neoplasm of uncertain behavior of left ureter ☑
D49.511	Neoplasm of unspecified behavior of right kidney ☑
D49.512	Neoplasm of unspecified behavior of left kidney ☑
D49.59	Neoplasm of unspecified behavior of other genitourinary organ
N13.8	Other obstructive and reflux uropathy
N15.1	Renal and perinephric abscess
N20.0	Calculus of kidney
N20.1	Calculus of ureter
N20.2	Calculus of kidney with calculus of ureter
N25.81	Secondary hyperparathyroidism of renal origin
N28.0	Ischemia and infarction of kidney
N28.82	Megaloureter
N28.83	Nephroptosis
N28.89	Other specified disorders of kidney and ureter
T19.8XXA	Foreign body in other parts of genitourinary tract, initial encounter
T81.510A	Adhesions due to foreign body accidentally left in body following surgical operation, initial encounter
T81.512A	Adhesions due to foreign body accidentally left in body following kidney dialysis, initial encounter
T81.514A	Adhesions due to foreign body accidentally left in body following endoscopic examination, initial encounter
T81.516A	Adhesions due to foreign body accidentally left in body following aspiration, puncture or other catheterization, initial encounter
T81.517A	Adhesions due to foreign body accidentally left in body following removal of catheter or packing, initial encounter
T81.518A	Adhesions due to foreign body accidentally left in body following other procedure, initial encounter
T81.520A	Obstruction due to foreign body accidentally left in body following surgical operation, initial encounter
T81.522A	Obstruction due to foreign body accidentally left in body following kidney dialysis, initial encounter
T81.524A	Obstruction due to foreign body accidentally left in body following endoscopic examination, initial encounter
T81.526A	Obstruction due to foreign body accidentally left in body following aspiration, puncture or other catheterization, initial encounter
T81.527A	Obstruction due to foreign body accidentally left in body following removal of catheter or packing, initial encounter
T81.528A	Obstruction due to foreign body accidentally left in body following other procedure, initial encounter

T81.530A	Perforation due to foreign body accidentally left in body following surgical operation, initial encounter
T81.532A	Perforation due to foreign body accidentally left in body following kidney dialysis, initial encounter
T81.534A	Perforation due to foreign body accidentally left in body following endoscopic examination, initial encounter
T81.536A	Perforation due to foreign body accidentally left in body following aspiration, puncture or other catheterization, initial encounter
T81.537A	Perforation due to foreign body accidentally left in body following removal of catheter or packing, initial encounter
T81.538A	Perforation due to foreign body accidentally left in body following other procedure, initial encounter
T81.590A	Other complications of foreign body accidentally left in body following surgical operation, initial encounter
T81.592A	Other complications of foreign body accidentally left in body following kidney dialysis, initial encounter
T81.594A	Other complications of foreign body accidentally left in body following endoscopic examination, initial encounter
T81.596A	Other complications of foreign body accidentally left in body following aspiration, puncture or other catheterization, initial encounter
T81.597A	Other complications of foreign body accidentally left in body following removal of catheter or packing, initial encounter
T81.598A	Other complications of foreign body accidentally left in body following other procedure, initial encounter

AMA: **50576** 2018,Jan,8; 2017,Jan,8; 2016,Jan,13; 2015,Jan,16; 2014,Jan,11 **50580** 2018,Jan,8; 2017,Jan,8; 2016,Jan,13; 2015,Jan,16; 2014,Jan,11

Relative Value Units/Medicare Edits

Non-Facility RVU	Work	PE	MP	Total
50576	10.97	4.05	1.25	16.27
50580	11.84	4.35	1.34	17.53
Facility RVU	**Work**	**PE**	**MP**	**Total**
50576	10.97	4.05	1.25	16.27
50580	11.84	4.35	1.34	17.53

	FUD	Status	MUE	Modifiers				IOM Reference
50576	0	A	1(2)	51	50	N/A	80*	None
50580	0	A	1(2)	51	50	N/A	80*	

* with documentation

Terms To Know

biopsy. Tissue or fluid removed for diagnostic purposes through analysis of the cells in the biopsy material.

calculus. Abnormal, stone-like concretion of calcium, cholesterol, mineral salts, or other substances that forms in any part of the body.

endoscopy. Visual inspection of the body using a fiberoptic scope.

foreign body. Any object or substance found in an organ and tissue that does not belong under normal circumstances.

fulguration. Destruction of living tissue by using sparks from a high-frequency electric current.

50590

50590   Lithotripsy, extracorporeal shock wave

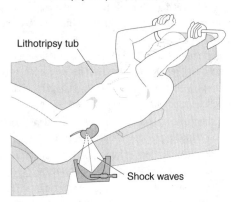

Shock waves delivered through a
lithotripsy tub pulverize calculus

Lithotripsy tub

Shock waves

Explanation

The physician pulverizes a kidney stone (renal calculus) by directing shock waves through a liquid medium. Two different methods are currently available to accomplish this procedure. The physician first uses radiological guidance to determine the location and size of the renal calculus. In the first method, the patient is immersed in a liquid medium (degassed, deionized water) with shock waves directed through the liquid to the kidney stone. In the second method, the one most often used, the patient is placed on a treatment table. A series of shock waves are directed through a water-cushion, or bellow that is placed against the patient's body at the location of the kidney stone. Each shock wave is directed to the stone for only a fraction of a second, and the procedure generally takes from 30 to 50 minutes. The treatment table is equipped with video x-ray so the physician can view the pulverization process. Over several days or weeks, the tiny stone fragments pass harmlessly though the patient's urinary system and are discharged during urination.

Coding Tips

For removal of a calculus, open, see 50060–50075; percutaneous, see 50080–50081; via pyelotomy, see 50130; via renal endoscopy, through a previously established nephrostomy or pyelostomy, see 50561; through a nephrotomy or pyelotomy, see 50580.

ICD-10-CM Diagnostic Codes

N20.0   Calculus of kidney
N20.1   Calculus of ureter
N20.2   Calculus of kidney with calculus of ureter

AMA: 50590 2018,Jan,8; 2017,Jan,8; 2016,Jan,13; 2015,Jan,16; 2014,Jan,11

Relative Value Units/Medicare Edits

Non-Facility RVU	Work	PE	MP	Total
50590	9.77	10.27	1.13	21.17
Facility RVU	**Work**	**PE**	**MP**	**Total**
50590	9.77	5.52	1.13	16.42

	FUD	Status	MUE	Modifiers				IOM Reference
50590	90	A	1(2)	51	50	N/A	N/A	None

* with documentation

50592-50593

50592   Ablation, 1 or more renal tumor(s), percutaneous, unilateral, radiofrequency
50593   Ablation, renal tumor(s), unilateral, percutaneous, cryotherapy

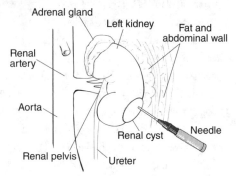

Through a small incision, a radiofrequency needle
electrode is introduced and directed at a renal tumor

Adrenal gland
Left kidney
Fat and abdominal wall
Renal artery
Aorta
Renal cyst
Needle
Renal pelvis
Ureter

Explanation

They physician performs percutaneous ablation of one or more renal tumors. Using appropriate anesthesia, a small incision is made and a probe or electrode is positioned in the lesion/tumor. In 50592, using an internally cooled radiofrequency needle electrode the tumor tissue is heated to a specified temperature with monitoring done before and after each treatment, depending on the ablation device used, until sufficient time results in permanent cell damage and tumor necrosis. Overlapping tumor tissue is ablated in the same manner until all margins are satisfactory. In 50593, a cryoprobe is used to provide cycles of freezing and thawing to ensure encapsulation of the tumor tissue and a sufficient margin within the ice ball created by the cryotherapy. After the second active thaw cycle, the cryoprobes are removed if the ice ball is judged to cover the tumor tissue. If freezing was insufficient, the probes may be removed and repositioned or additional probes may be added and freezing is continued until the tumor and margin receive two complete cycles. Hemostasis is ensured when the electrode or cryoprobe is removed. The ablated tissue remains in place and is absorbed over time and replaced with scar tissue. The incision site is closed and dressings are applied.

Coding Tips

These are unilateral procedures. If performed bilaterally, some payers require that the service be reported twice with modifier 50 appended to the second code while others require identification of the service only once with modifier 50 appended. Check with individual payers. Modifier 50 identifies a procedure performed identically on the opposite side of the body (mirror image). Imaging guidance and monitoring is reported with 76940, 77013, and 77022, when performed.

ICD-10-CM Diagnostic Codes

C64.1   Malignant neoplasm of right kidney, except renal pelvis ☑
C64.2   Malignant neoplasm of left kidney, except renal pelvis ☑
C65.1   Malignant neoplasm of right renal pelvis ☑
C65.2   Malignant neoplasm of left renal pelvis ☑
C79.01   Secondary malignant neoplasm of right kidney and renal pelvis ☑
C79.02   Secondary malignant neoplasm of left kidney and renal pelvis ☑
C7A.093   Malignant carcinoid tumor of the kidney
C80.2   Malignant neoplasm associated with transplanted organ
D09.19   Carcinoma in situ of other urinary organs

© 2020 Optum360, LLC   N Newborn: 0   P Pediatric: 0-17   M Maternity: 9-64   A Adult: 15-124   ♂ Male Only   ♀ Female Only   CPT © 2020 American Medical Association. All Rights Reserved.

Coding Companion for Urology/Nephrology

Kidney

D30.01	Benign neoplasm of right kidney ☑		
D30.02	Benign neoplasm of left kidney ☑		
D30.11	Benign neoplasm of right renal pelvis ☑		
D30.12	Benign neoplasm of left renal pelvis ☑		
D3A.093	Benign carcinoid tumor of the kidney		
D41.01	Neoplasm of uncertain behavior of right kidney ☑		
D41.02	Neoplasm of uncertain behavior of left kidney ☑		
D41.11	Neoplasm of uncertain behavior of right renal pelvis ☑		
D41.12	Neoplasm of uncertain behavior of left renal pelvis ☑		
D41.21	Neoplasm of uncertain behavior of right ureter ☑		
D41.22	Neoplasm of uncertain behavior of left ureter ☑		
D49.511	Neoplasm of unspecified behavior of right kidney ☑		
D49.512	Neoplasm of unspecified behavior of left kidney ☑		
D49.59	Neoplasm of unspecified behavior of other genitourinary organ		

AMA: 50592 2014,Jan,11 **50593** 2018,Jan,8; 2014,Jan,11

Relative Value Units/Medicare Edits

Non-Facility RVU	Work	PE	MP	Total
50592	6.55	84.08	0.56	91.19
50593	8.88	113.64	0.79	123.31
Facility RVU	**Work**	**PE**	**MP**	**Total**
50592	6.55	2.81	0.56	9.92
50593	8.88	3.64	0.79	13.31

	FUD	Status	MUE	Modifiers				IOM Reference
50592	10	A	1(2)	51	50	N/A	N/A	None
50593	10	A	1(2)	51	50	N/A	80	

* with documentation

Terms To Know

ablation. Removal or destruction of tissue by cutting, electrical energy, chemical substances, or excessive heat application.

cryotherapy. Any surgical procedure that uses intense cold for treatment.

imaging. Radiologic means of producing pictures for clinical study of the internal structures and functions of the body, such as x-ray, ultrasound, magnetic resonance, or positron emission tomography.

lesion. Area of damaged tissue that has lost continuity or function, due to disease or trauma.

necrosis. Death of cells or tissue within a living organ or structure.

percutaneous. Through the skin.

radiofrequency ablation. To destroy by electromagnetic wave frequencies.

renal. Referring to the kidney.

tissue. Group of similar cells with a similar function that form definite structures and organs. Tissue types include epithelial tissue, muscle tissue, connective tissue, and nervous tissue.

tumor. Pathological swelling or enlargement; a neoplastic growth of uncontrolled, abnormal multiplication of cells.

Kidney

50600

50600 Ureterotomy with exploration or drainage (separate procedure)

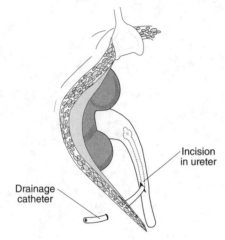

The physician incises the ureter for
examination or insertion of drainage catheter

Explanation

The physician makes an incision in the ureter (ureterotomy) for examination of the ureter or insertion of a drainage catheter (ureterostomy tube) between the ureter and skin. To access the ureter, the physician makes an incision in the skin of the flank, and cuts the muscles, fat, and fibrous membranes (fascia) overlying the ureter. The physician makes an incision in the ureter and sometimes places fine traction sutures at the edges of the incision. The physician examines the interior of the ureter or, if the incision is for drainage, the physician inserts a catheter tip into the ureter and passes the tube through a stab incision in the skin of the flank. The physician sutures the incision and performs a layered closure.

Coding Tips

This separate procedure by definition is usually a component of a more complex service and is not identified separately. When performed alone or with other unrelated procedures/services it may be reported. If performed alone, list the code; if performed with other procedures/services, list the code and append modifier 59 or an X{EPSU} modifier. If the ureterotomy is done for an additional, significantly identifiable endoscopic service, report both the appropriate endoscopic procedure code (50970–50980) and 50600. Report 50605 if the ureterotomy is for insertion of a stent.

ICD-10-CM Diagnostic Codes

C66.1	Malignant neoplasm of right ureter ☑
C66.2	Malignant neoplasm of left ureter ☑
C79.19	Secondary malignant neoplasm of other urinary organs
D09.19	Carcinoma in situ of other urinary organs
D30.21	Benign neoplasm of right ureter ☑
D30.22	Benign neoplasm of left ureter ☑
D41.21	Neoplasm of uncertain behavior of right ureter ☑
D41.22	Neoplasm of uncertain behavior of left ureter ☑
D49.511	Neoplasm of unspecified behavior of right kidney ☑
D49.512	Neoplasm of unspecified behavior of left kidney ☑
D49.59	Neoplasm of unspecified behavior of other genitourinary organ
N11.1	Chronic obstructive pyelonephritis
N13.0	Hydronephrosis with ureteropelvic junction obstruction
N13.1	Hydronephrosis with ureteral stricture, not elsewhere classified
N13.2	Hydronephrosis with renal and ureteral calculous obstruction
N13.5	Crossing vessel and stricture of ureter without hydronephrosis
N13.8	Other obstructive and reflux uropathy
N28.89	Other specified disorders of kidney and ureter
N99.71	Accidental puncture and laceration of a genitourinary system organ or structure during a genitourinary system procedure
N99.72	Accidental puncture and laceration of a genitourinary system organ or structure during other procedure
S37.12XA	Contusion of ureter, initial encounter
S37.13XA	Laceration of ureter, initial encounter
S37.19XA	Other injury of ureter, initial encounter

AMA: **50600** 2014,Jan,11

Relative Value Units/Medicare Edits

Non-Facility RVU	Work	PE	MP	Total
50600	17.17	7.96	1.97	27.1
Facility RVU	**Work**	**PE**	**MP**	**Total**
50600	17.17	7.96	1.97	27.1

	FUD	Status	MUE	Modifiers				IOM Reference
50600	90	A	1(3)	51	50	62*	80	None

* with documentation

Terms To Know

carcinoma in situ. Malignancy that arises from the cells of the vessel, gland, or organ of origin that remains confined to that site or has not invaded neighboring tissue.

catheter. Flexible tube inserted into an area of the body for introducing or withdrawing fluid.

drainage. Releasing, taking, or letting out fluids and/or gases from a body part.

exploration. Examination for diagnostic purposes.

fascia. Fibrous sheet or band of tissue that envelops organs, muscles, and groupings of muscles.

flank. Part of the body found between the posterior ribs and the uppermost crest of the ilium, or the lateral side of the hip, thigh, and buttock.

hydronephrosis. Distension of the kidney caused by an accumulation of urine that cannot flow out due to an obstruction that may be caused by conditions such as kidney stones or vesicoureteral reflux.

malignant neoplasm. Any cancerous tumor or lesion exhibiting uncontrolled tissue growth that can progressively invade other parts of the body with its disease-generating cells.

stricture. Narrowing of an anatomical structure.

ureter. Tube leading from the kidney to the urinary bladder made up of three layers of tissue: the mucous lining of the inner layer; the smooth, muscular middle layer that propels the urine from the kidney to the bladder by peristalsis; and the outer layer made of fibrous connective tissue. Each ureter leaves the kidney from the hilum, a concave notch on the middle surface, and enters the bladder through a narrow valve-like orifice that prevents the backflow of urine to the kidney.

Ureter

50605

50605 Ureterotomy for insertion of indwelling stent, all types

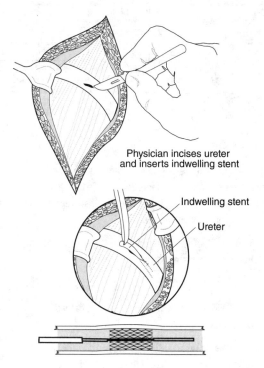

Physician incises ureter and inserts indwelling stent

Indwelling stent

Ureter

Stent expands to support the canal

Explanation

The physician makes an incision in the ureter (ureterotomy) to insert a catheter (stent) in the ureter. To access the ureter, the physician makes an incision in the skin of the flank, and cuts the muscles, fat, and fibrous membranes (fascia) overlying the ureter. The physician makes an incision in the ureter and sometimes places fine traction sutures at the edges of the incision. The physician inserts a slender rod or catheter into the ureter, sutures the incision, and performs a layered closure.

Coding Tips

For ureterotomy with exploration or drainage, see 50600. If the incision is for removal of a calculus, see 50610–50630.

ICD-10-CM Diagnostic Codes

C66.1	Malignant neoplasm of right ureter ☑
C66.2	Malignant neoplasm of left ureter ☑
C79.19	Secondary malignant neoplasm of other urinary organs
D09.19	Carcinoma in situ of other urinary organs
D30.21	Benign neoplasm of right ureter ☑
D30.22	Benign neoplasm of left ureter ☑
D41.21	Neoplasm of uncertain behavior of right ureter ☑
D41.22	Neoplasm of uncertain behavior of left ureter ☑
D49.511	Neoplasm of unspecified behavior of right kidney ☑
D49.512	Neoplasm of unspecified behavior of left kidney ☑
D49.59	Neoplasm of unspecified behavior of other genitourinary organ
N11.1	Chronic obstructive pyelonephritis
N13.0	Hydronephrosis with ureteropelvic junction obstruction
N13.1	Hydronephrosis with ureteral stricture, not elsewhere classified
N13.2	Hydronephrosis with renal and ureteral calculous obstruction
N13.5	Crossing vessel and stricture of ureter without hydronephrosis
N13.8	Other obstructive and reflux uropathy
N20.0	Calculus of kidney
N20.1	Calculus of ureter
N20.2	Calculus of kidney with calculus of ureter

AMA: **50605** 2018,Jan,8; 2017,Jan,8; 2016,Jan,13; 2015,Jan,16; 2014,Jan,11

Relative Value Units/Medicare Edits

Non-Facility RVU	Work	PE	MP	Total
50605	16.79	8.67	3.41	28.87
Facility RVU	**Work**	**PE**	**MP**	**Total**
50605	16.79	8.67	3.41	28.87

	FUD	Status	MUE	Modifiers				IOM Reference
50605	90	A	1(3)	51	50	62*	80	None

* with documentation

Terms To Know

calculus. Abnormal, stone-like concretion of calcium, cholesterol, mineral salts, or other substances that forms in any part of the body.

carcinoma in situ. Malignancy that arises from the cells of the vessel, gland, or organ of origin that remains confined to that site or has not invaded neighboring tissue.

catheter. Flexible tube inserted into an area of the body for introducing or withdrawing fluid.

fascia. Fibrous sheet or band of tissue that envelops organs, muscles, and groupings of muscles.

hydronephrosis. Distension of the kidney caused by an accumulation of urine that cannot flow out due to an obstruction that may be caused by conditions such as kidney stones or vesicoureteral reflux.

incision. Act of cutting into tissue or an organ.

malignant. Any condition tending to progress toward death, specifically an invasive tumor with a loss of cellular differentiation that has the ability to spread or metastasize to other body areas.

neoplasm. New abnormal growth, tumor.

stent. Tube to provide support in a body cavity or lumen.

stricture. Narrowing of an anatomical structure.

ureter. Tube leading from the kidney to the urinary bladder made up of three layers of tissue: the mucous lining of the inner layer; the smooth, muscular middle layer that propels the urine from the kidney to the bladder by peristalsis; and the outer layer made of fibrous connective tissue. Each ureter leaves the kidney from the hilum, a concave notch on the middle surface, and enters the bladder through a narrow valve-like orifice that prevents the backflow of urine to the kidney.

Ureter

CPT © 2020 American Medical Association. All Rights Reserved.   ● New   ▲ Revised   + Add On   ★ Telemedicine   AMA: CPT Assist   [Resequenced]   ☑ Laterality   © 2020 Optum360, LLC

50606

+ **50606** Endoluminal biopsy of ureter and/or renal pelvis, non-endoscopic, including imaging guidance (eg, ultrasound and/or fluoroscopy) and all associated radiological supervision and interpretation (List separately in addition to code for primary procedure)

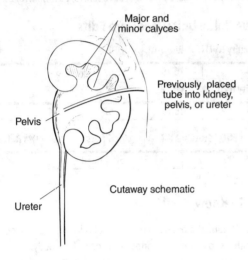

Major and minor calyces

Previously placed tube into kidney, pelvis, or ureter

Pelvis

Ureter

Cutaway schematic

Explanation

A nonendoscopic endoluminal biopsy of the ureter and/or renal pelvis is accomplished by incision into the skin overlying the target area. The patient is anesthetized and the incision is made. The target area is visualized by imaging guidance. A guidewire is inserted into the biopsy site followed by a sheath over the wire. A forceps device is inserted along the wire until it reaches the biopsy site and the sheath is withdrawn exposing the forceps. With the wings of the forceps open, the device is inserted into the target area where the wings are closed trapping the tissue sample. The device is pulled back with the biopsy sample intact. Another method uses a brush biopsy to retrieve the sample. The brush may be inserted through a scope until it reaches the target area. Biopsy is obtained with rubbing of the brush within the lumen. Upon removal, the sample is retrieved from the brush for examination. The guidewire is removed and any other instruments used in the primary procedure are also removed. The incision site is closed with sutures. This code includes procurement of biopsy sample, imaging guidance, and radiological supervision and interpretation. The biopsy may be performed via transrenal access, existing renal/ureteral access, transurethral access, an ileal conduit, or ureterostomy. This code reports the biopsy only; the procedure performed for access to the biopsy site is reported separately.

Coding Tips

Report 50606 with 50382, 50384–50387, 50389, 50430–50435, 50684, 50688, 50690, 50693–50695, and 51610. Do not report 50606 with 50555, 50574, 50955, 50974, 52007, or 74425 for the same renal collecting system and/or associated ureter. This code describes endoluminal biopsy using nonendoscopic imaging guidance and may be reported once per ureter per day. The biopsy work, imaging guidance, and radiological supervision and interpretation required to accomplish the biopsy are included. Diagnostic pyelography/ureterography is not included in this code and may be reported separately. This code is reported once for each renal collecting system/ureter accessed.

ICD-10-CM Diagnostic Codes

This/these CPT code(s) are add-on code(s). See the primary procedure code that this code is performed with for your ICD-10-CM code selections.

AMA: 50606 2018,Jan,8; 2017,Jan,8; 2016,Jan,3

Relative Value Units/Medicare Edits

Non-Facility RVU	Work	PE	MP	Total
50606	3.16	14.36	0.28	17.8
Facility RVU	**Work**	**PE**	**MP**	**Total**
50606	3.16	0.97	0.28	4.41

	FUD	Status	MUE	Modifiers				IOM Reference
50606	N/A	A	1(3)	N/A	50	N/A	N/A	None

* with documentation

Terms To Know

add-on code. Code representing a procedure performed in addition to the primary procedure and is represented with a + in the CPT book. Add-on codes are never reported for stand-alone services but are reported secondarily in addition to the primary procedure.

biopsy. Tissue or fluid removed for diagnostic purposes through analysis of the cells in the biopsy material.

forceps. Tool used for grasping or compressing tissue.

guidewire. Flexible metal instrument designed to lead another instrument in its proper course.

imaging. Radiologic means of producing pictures for clinical study of the internal structures and functions of the body, such as x-ray, ultrasound, magnetic resonance, or positron emission tomography.

lumen. Space inside an intestine, artery, vein, duct, or tube.

specimen. Tissue cells or sample of fluid taken for analysis, pathologic examination, and diagnosis.

supervision and interpretation. Radiology services that usually contain an invasive component and are reported by the radiologist for supervision of the procedure and the personnel involved with performing the examination, reading the film, and preparing the written report.

tissue. Group of similar cells with a similar function that form definite structures and organs. Tissue types include epithelial tissue, muscle tissue, connective tissue, and nervous tissue.

ureter. Tube leading from the kidney to the urinary bladder made up of three layers of tissue: the mucous lining of the inner layer; the smooth, muscular middle layer that propels the urine from the kidney to the bladder by peristalsis; and the outer layer made of fibrous connective tissue. Each ureter leaves the kidney from the hilum, a concave notch on the middle surface, and enters the bladder through a narrow valve-like orifice that prevents the backflow of urine to the kidney.

Ureter

© 2020 Optum360, LLC   **N** Newborn: 0   **P** Pediatric: 0-17   **M** Maternity: 9-64   **A** Adult: 15-124   ♂ Male Only   ♀ Female Only   CPT © 2020 American Medical Association. All Rights Reserved.

50610-50630

50610 Ureterolithotomy; upper one-third of ureter
50620 middle one-third of ureter
50630 lower one-third of ureter

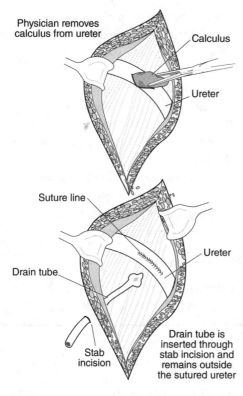

Physician removes calculus from ureter

Calculus

Ureter

Suture line

Ureter

Drain tube

Stab incision

Drain tube is inserted through stab incision and remains outside the sutured ureter

Explanation

The physician makes an incision in the ureter (ureterotomy) to remove a stone (calculus) from the ureter. To access the ureter, the physician makes an incision in the skin and cuts the muscles, fat, and fibrous membranes (fascia) overlying the ureter. For the upper or middle third of the ureter, the physician usually makes an incision in the skin of the flank; to access the lower third of the ureter, the physician usually makes a curved lower quadrant incision. The physician isolates the calculus and removes it through an incision in the ureter. After examining the ureter for other defects, the physician sutures the incision and performs a layered closure, inserting a drain tube through a stab incision in the skin. Report 50610 for calculus removal from the upper third of the ureter; 50620 for calculus removal from the middle third; and 50630 for calculus removal from the lower third.

Coding Tips

Report 50610–50630 for removal of one or more calculi. For laparoscopic approach, see 50945. Endoscopic removal or manipulation of ureteral calculus is reported with 50080–50081, 50561, 50961, 50980. 52320–52330, 52352–52353, or 52356. For removal of ureteral calculi through an incision in the bladder, see 51060–51065. For removal of calculi located in the kidney and/or renal pelvis, see 50060–50075 and 50130. For endoscopic removal of a calculus, see 50561, 50580, 50961, 50980, 52320–52325, 52352, and 52353. For extracorporeal shock wave lithotripsy (ESWL) to remove calculi, see 50590.

ICD-10-CM Diagnostic Codes

N20.1   Calculus of ureter
N20.2   Calculus of kidney with calculus of ureter

AMA: **50610** 2018,Jan,8; 2017,Jan,8; 2016,Jan,13; 2015,Jan,16; 2014,Jan,11 **50620** 2018,Jan,8; 2017,Jan,8; 2016,Jan,13; 2015,Jan,16; 2014,Jan,11 **50630** 2018,Jan,8; 2017,Jan,8; 2016,Jan,13; 2015,Jan,16; 2014,May,3; 2014,Jan,11

Relative Value Units/Medicare Edits

Non-Facility RVU	Work	PE	MP	Total
50610	17.25	8.06	1.98	27.29
50620	16.43	7.78	1.89	26.1
50630	16.21	7.7	1.86	25.77
Facility RVU	Work	PE	MP	Total
50610	17.25	8.06	1.98	27.29
50620	16.43	7.78	1.89	26.1
50630	16.21	7.7	1.86	25.77

	FUD	Status	MUE	Modifiers				IOM Reference
50610	90	A	1(2)	51	50	62*	80	None
50620	90	A	1(2)	51	50	62*	80	
50630	90	A	1(2)	51	50	62*	80	

* with documentation

Terms To Know

calculus. Abnormal, stone-like concretion of calcium, cholesterol, mineral salts, or other substances that forms in any part of the body.

closure. Repairing an incision or wound by suture or other means.

defect. Imperfection, flaw, or absence.

drain. Device that creates a channel to allow fluid from a cavity, wound, or infected area to exit the body.

fascia. Fibrous sheet or band of tissue that envelops organs, muscles, and groupings of muscles.

flank. Part of the body found between the posterior ribs and the uppermost crest of the ilium, or the lateral side of the hip, thigh, and buttock.

incision. Act of cutting into tissue or an organ.

ureter. Tube leading from the kidney to the urinary bladder made up of three layers of tissue: the mucous lining of the inner layer; the smooth, muscular middle layer that propels the urine from the kidney to the bladder by peristalsis; and the outer layer made of fibrous connective tissue. Each ureter leaves the kidney from the hilum, a concave notch on the middle surface, and enters the bladder through a narrow valve-like orifice that prevents the backflow of urine to the kidney.

ureterolithotomy. Surgical removal of a calculus or stone from the ureter.

ureterotomy. Incision made into the ureter for accomplishing a variety of procedures such as exploration, drainage, instillation, ureteropyelography, catheterization, dilation, biopsy, or foreign body removal.

Ureter

50650

50650 Ureterectomy, with bladder cuff (separate procedure)

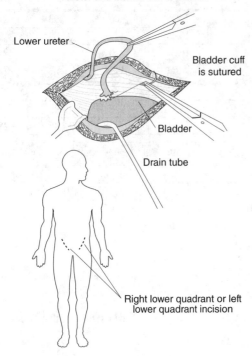

The physician removes the ureter and a small cuff of bladder

- Lower ureter
- Bladder cuff is sutured
- Bladder
- Drain tube
- Right lower quadrant or left lower quadrant incision

Explanation

The physician removes the ureter and a small cuff of the bladder. To access the ureter, the physician usually makes a curved lower quadrant incision in the skin of the abdomen, and cuts the muscles, fat, and fibrous membranes (fascia) overlying the ureter. The physician mobilizes the bladder, dissects a small cuff of the bladder, and ligates and dissects the ureter. After removing the bladder cuff and lower ureter, the physician sutures and catheterizes the bladder. The physician places a drain tube behind the bladder and performs a layered closure.

Coding Tips

This separate procedure by definition is usually a component of a more complex service and is not identified separately. When performed alone or with other unrelated procedures/services it may be reported. If performed alone, list the code; if performed with other procedures/services, list the code and append modifier 59 or an X{EPSU} modifier. When 50650 is performed with another separately identifiable procedure, the highest dollar value code is listed as the primary procedure and subsequent procedures are appended with modifier 51. If significant additional time and effort is documented, append modifier 22 and submit a cover letter and operative report. For ureterectomy and bladder cuff removal as part of a kidney removal (nephrectomy), see 50234–50236. Report 50660 for removal of a ureter that deviates from proper anatomic placement. Report ureterocele with 51535 and/or 52300.

ICD-10-CM Diagnostic Codes

C66.1	Malignant neoplasm of right ureter ☑
C66.2	Malignant neoplasm of left ureter ☑
C67.0	Malignant neoplasm of trigone of bladder
C67.1	Malignant neoplasm of dome of bladder
C67.2	Malignant neoplasm of lateral wall of bladder
C67.3	Malignant neoplasm of anterior wall of bladder
C67.4	Malignant neoplasm of posterior wall of bladder
C67.5	Malignant neoplasm of bladder neck
C67.6	Malignant neoplasm of ureteric orifice
C67.7	Malignant neoplasm of urachus
C79.11	Secondary malignant neoplasm of bladder
C79.19	Secondary malignant neoplasm of other urinary organs
D09.19	Carcinoma in situ of other urinary organs
D30.21	Benign neoplasm of right ureter ☑
D30.22	Benign neoplasm of left ureter ☑
D41.21	Neoplasm of uncertain behavior of right ureter ☑
D41.22	Neoplasm of uncertain behavior of left ureter ☑
D49.59	Neoplasm of unspecified behavior of other genitourinary organ
N28.82	Megaloureter
N28.89	Other specified disorders of kidney and ureter
S37.12XA	Contusion of ureter, initial encounter
S37.13XA	Laceration of ureter, initial encounter
S37.19XA	Other injury of ureter, initial encounter

AMA: **50650** 2014,Jan,11

Relative Value Units/Medicare Edits

Non-Facility RVU	Work	PE	MP	Total
50650	18.82	8.9	2.28	30.0
Facility RVU	**Work**	**PE**	**MP**	**Total**
50650	18.82	8.9	2.28	30.0

	FUD	Status	MUE	Modifiers				IOM Reference
50650	90	A	1(2)	51	50	62*	80	None

* with documentation

Terms To Know

carcinoma in situ. Malignancy that arises from the cells of the vessel, gland, or organ of origin that remains confined to that site or has not invaded neighboring tissue.

catheterization. Use or insertion of a tubular device into a duct, blood vessel, hollow organ, or body cavity for injecting or withdrawing fluids for diagnostic or therapeutic purposes.

dissection. Separating by cutting tissue or body structures apart.

drain. Device that creates a channel to allow fluid from a cavity, wound, or infected area to exit the body.

ligation. Tying off a blood vessel or duct with a suture or a soft, thin wire.

malignant. Any condition tending to progress toward death, specifically an invasive tumor with a loss of cellular differentiation that has the ability to spread or metastasize to other body areas.

urachus. Embryonic tube connecting the urinary bladder to the umbilicus during development of the fetus that normally closes before birth, generally in the fourth or fifth month of gestation.

ureterectomy. Excision of all or part of a ureter. This procedure may be performed alone or as part of another procedure, such as urinary diversion or nephrectomy.

Ureter

50660

50660 Ureterectomy, total, ectopic ureter, combination abdominal, vaginal and/or perineal approach

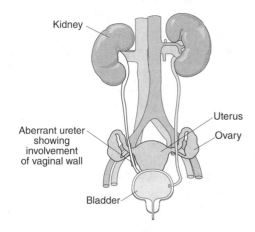

Kidney

Uterus

Ovary

Aberrant ureter showing involvement of vaginal wall

Bladder

Explanation

The physician removes a ureter that deviates from proper anatomical placement. To access the ureter, the physician makes an incision in the skin of the abdomen, perineum, and/or vagina. The physician cuts the muscles, fat, and fibrous membranes (fascia) overlying the ureter. After mobilizing the bladder and ureter, the physician ligates, dissects, and removes the ureter. The physician places a drain tube at the site of the incision and performs a layered closure.

Coding Tips

For removal of a non-deviant ureter, see 50650. For ureterectomy and bladder cuff removal as part of a kidney removal (nephrectomy), see 50234–50236. For partial ureterectomy as part of a kidney removal (nephrectomy), see 50220–50230. If the kidney and ureter removal is part of a renal transplant, see 50300–50340 or 50365. Report 50660 for removal of a ureter that deviates from proper anatomic placement. Report ureterocele with 51535 and/or 52300.

ICD-10-CM Diagnostic Codes

Q62.63   Anomalous implantation of ureter

AMA: 50660 2014,Jan,11

Relative Value Units/Medicare Edits

Non-Facility RVU	Work	PE	MP	Total
50660	21.02	9.6	2.4	33.02
Facility RVU	Work	PE	MP	Total
50660	21.02	9.6	2.4	33.02

	FUD	Status	MUE	Modifiers				IOM Reference
50660	90	A	1(3)	51	N/A	62*	80	None

* with documentation

Terms To Know

ectopic. Organ or other structure that is aberrant or out of place.

50684

50684 Injection procedure for ureterography or ureteropyelography through ureterostomy or indwelling ureteral catheter

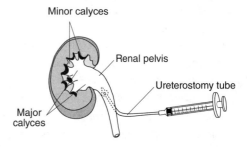

Physician injects contrast material through ureterostomy or ureteral catheter to study ureter and renal collecting system

Minor calyces

Renal pelvis

Ureterostomy tube

Major calyces

Explanation

The physician injects a contrast agent through an opening between the skin and the ureter (ureterostomy) or via an indwelling catheter into the ureter and renal pelvis to study the renal collecting system. To determine immediate allergic response to the contrast agent, the physician injects a dose of contrast material through the ureterostomy or indwelling catheter into the ureter and renal pelvis, and takes an x-ray.

Coding Tips

Injection procedure for antegrade nephrostogram and/or ureterogram is reported with 50430–50431. Report 50690 if the physician uses the injection procedure to visualize the ileal conduit and/or study the upper urinary system. For radiological supervision and interpretation, see 74425. Do not report 50684 with 50433–50434 or 50693–50695. Supplies used when providing this procedure may be reported with the appropriate HCPCS Level II code. Check with the specific payer to determine coverage.

ICD-10-CM Diagnostic Codes

C64.1	Malignant neoplasm of right kidney, except renal pelvis ☑
C64.2	Malignant neoplasm of left kidney, except renal pelvis ☑
C65.1	Malignant neoplasm of right renal pelvis ☑
C65.2	Malignant neoplasm of left renal pelvis ☑
C66.1	Malignant neoplasm of right ureter ☑
C66.2	Malignant neoplasm of left ureter ☑
C68.8	Malignant neoplasm of overlapping sites of urinary organs
C79.01	Secondary malignant neoplasm of right kidney and renal pelvis ☑
C79.02	Secondary malignant neoplasm of left kidney and renal pelvis ☑
C79.11	Secondary malignant neoplasm of bladder
C79.19	Secondary malignant neoplasm of other urinary organs
C7A.093	Malignant carcinoid tumor of the kidney
C80.2	Malignant neoplasm associated with transplanted organ
D09.19	Carcinoma in situ of other urinary organs
D30.01	Benign neoplasm of right kidney ☑
D30.02	Benign neoplasm of left kidney ☑
D30.11	Benign neoplasm of right renal pelvis ☑
D30.12	Benign neoplasm of left renal pelvis ☑
D30.21	Benign neoplasm of right ureter ☑

Ureter

D30.22	Benign neoplasm of left ureter ☑
D3A.093	Benign carcinoid tumor of the kidney
D41.01	Neoplasm of uncertain behavior of right kidney ☑
D41.02	Neoplasm of uncertain behavior of left kidney ☑
D41.11	Neoplasm of uncertain behavior of right renal pelvis ☑
D41.12	Neoplasm of uncertain behavior of left renal pelvis ☑
D41.21	Neoplasm of uncertain behavior of right ureter ☑
D41.22	Neoplasm of uncertain behavior of left ureter ☑
D47.Z1	Post-transplant lymphoproliferative disorder (PTLD)
D47.Z2	Castleman disease
D49.59	Neoplasm of unspecified behavior of other genitourinary organ
N11.0	Nonobstructive reflux-associated chronic pyelonephritis
N11.1	Chronic obstructive pyelonephritis
N11.8	Other chronic tubulo-interstitial nephritis
N13.0	Hydronephrosis with ureteropelvic junction obstruction
N13.1	Hydronephrosis with ureteral stricture, not elsewhere classified
N13.2	Hydronephrosis with renal and ureteral calculous obstruction
N13.39	Other hydronephrosis
N13.5	Crossing vessel and stricture of ureter without hydronephrosis
N13.71	Vesicoureteral-reflux without reflux nephropathy
N13.721	Vesicoureteral-reflux with reflux nephropathy without hydroureter, unilateral
N13.722	Vesicoureteral-reflux with reflux nephropathy without hydroureter, bilateral
N13.731	Vesicoureteral-reflux with reflux nephropathy with hydroureter, unilateral
N13.732	Vesicoureteral-reflux with reflux nephropathy with hydroureter, bilateral
N13.8	Other obstructive and reflux uropathy
N20.0	Calculus of kidney
N20.2	Calculus of kidney with calculus of ureter
N25.81	Secondary hyperparathyroidism of renal origin
N25.89	Other disorders resulting from impaired renal tubular function
N26.1	Atrophy of kidney (terminal)
N28.1	Cyst of kidney, acquired
N28.82	Megaloureter
N28.84	Pyelitis cystica
N28.85	Pyeloureteritis cystica
N28.86	Ureteritis cystica
N28.89	Other specified disorders of kidney and ureter
N39.3	Stress incontinence (female) (male)
N39.41	Urge incontinence
N39.42	Incontinence without sensory awareness
N39.43	Post-void dribbling
N39.44	Nocturnal enuresis
N39.45	Continuous leakage
N39.46	Mixed incontinence
N39.490	Overflow incontinence
N39.491	Coital incontinence
N39.492	Postural (urinary) incontinence
N39.498	Other specified urinary incontinence
N41.1	Chronic prostatitis ▲ ♂
N99.0	Postprocedural (acute) (chronic) kidney failure
N99.81	Other intraoperative complications of genitourinary system
N99.89	Other postprocedural complications and disorders of genitourinary system
Q60.3	Renal hypoplasia, unilateral
Q60.4	Renal hypoplasia, bilateral
Q60.6	Potter's syndrome
Q61.01	Congenital single renal cyst
Q61.02	Congenital multiple renal cysts
Q61.11	Cystic dilatation of collecting ducts
Q61.19	Other polycystic kidney, infantile type
Q61.2	Polycystic kidney, adult type
Q61.4	Renal dysplasia
Q61.5	Medullary cystic kidney
Q61.8	Other cystic kidney diseases
Q62.0	Congenital hydronephrosis
Q62.11	Congenital occlusion of ureteropelvic junction
Q62.12	Congenital occlusion of ureterovesical orifice
Q62.2	Congenital megaureter
Q62.31	Congenital ureterocele, orthotopic
Q62.32	Cecoureterocele
Q62.39	Other obstructive defects of renal pelvis and ureter
Q64.8	Other specified congenital malformations of urinary system
R82.71	Bacteriuria
R82.79	Other abnormal findings on microbiological examination of urine

AMA: 50684 2018,Jan,8; 2017,Jan,8; 2016,Jan,3; 2015,Oct,5; 2014,Jan,11

Relative Value Units/Medicare Edits

Non-Facility RVU	Work	PE	MP	Total
50684	0.76	2.49	0.09	3.34
Facility RVU	**Work**	**PE**	**MP**	**Total**
50684	0.76	0.6	0.09	1.45

	FUD	Status	MUE	Modifiers				IOM Reference
50684	0	A	1(3)	51	50	N/A	N/A	None

* with documentation

Terms To Know

contrast material. Any internally administered substance that has a different opacity from soft tissue on radiography or computed tomograph; includes barium, used to opacify parts of the gastrointestinal tract; water-soluble iodinated compounds, used to opacify blood vessels or the genitourinary tract; may refer to air occurring naturally or introduced into the body; also, paramagnetic substances used in magnetic resonance imaging. Substances may also be documented as contrast agent or contrast medium.

ureter. Tube leading from the kidney to the urinary bladder made up of three layers of tissue: the mucous lining of the inner layer; the smooth, muscular middle layer that propels the urine from the kidney to the bladder by peristalsis; and the outer layer made of fibrous connective tissue. Each ureter leaves the kidney from the hilum, a concave notch on the middle surface, and enters the bladder through a narrow valve-like orifice that prevents the backflow of urine to the kidney.

ureterostomy. Placement of a stent, tube, or catheter into the ureter, forming a passageway from the exterior of the body to the ureter.

50686

50686 Manometric studies through ureterostomy or indwelling ureteral catheter

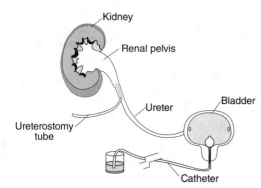

Manometer measures pressure flow in kidney and ureter

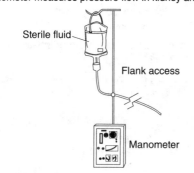

Explanation

The physician connects an indwelling ureteral catheter or existing ureterostomy to a manometer line to measure pressure and flow in the kidneys and ureters. The physician connects a ureteral catheter or ureterostomy to a manometer line filled with fluid. The physician inserts a bladder catheter that may be irrigated. The physician measures intrarenal and/or extra renal pressure. After discontinuing perfusion of fluid, the physician aspirates residual fluid from the kidney and disconnects the manometer line. The physician may remove the ureteral catheter or ureterostomy tube (if applicable) and dress the wound.

Coding Tips

No anesthesia is administered with this procedure. For manometric studies through a nephrostomy/pyelostomy tube or an indwelling ureteral catheter, see 50396. For urodynamics studies, see 51725–51797.

ICD-10-CM Diagnostic Codes

N11.1	Chronic obstructive pyelonephritis
N13.0	Hydronephrosis with ureteropelvic junction obstruction
N13.1	Hydronephrosis with ureteral stricture, not elsewhere classified
N13.2	Hydronephrosis with renal and ureteral calculous obstruction
N13.39	Other hydronephrosis
N13.5	Crossing vessel and stricture of ureter without hydronephrosis
Q62.0	Congenital hydronephrosis
Q62.11	Congenital occlusion of ureteropelvic junction
Q62.12	Congenital occlusion of ureterovesical orifice
Q62.2	Congenital megaureter
Q62.31	Congenital ureterocele, orthotopic
Q62.32	Cecoureterocele

Q62.39	Other obstructive defects of renal pelvis and ureter

AMA: 50686 2014,Jan,11

Relative Value Units/Medicare Edits

Non-Facility RVU	Work	PE	MP	Total
50686	1.51	2.34	0.18	4.03
Facility RVU	**Work**	**PE**	**MP**	**Total**
50686	1.51	0.85	0.18	2.54

	FUD	Status	MUE	Modifiers				IOM Reference
50686	0	A	2(3)	51	N/A	N/A	80*	None

* with documentation

Terms To Know

aspiration. Drawing fluid out by suction.

congenital. Present at birth, occurring through heredity or an influence during gestation up to the moment of birth.

defect. Imperfection, flaw, or absence.

dressing. Material applied to a wound or surgical site for protection, absorption, or drainage of the area.

Foley catheter. Temporary indwelling urethral catheter held in place in the bladder by an inflated balloon containing fluid or air.

hydronephrosis. Distension of the kidney caused by an accumulation of urine that cannot flow out due to an obstruction that may be caused by conditions such as kidney stones or vesicoureteral reflux.

irrigate. Washing out, lavage.

manometric. Pertaining to pressure, as measured in a meter.

obstruction. Blockage that prevents normal function of the valve or structure.

occlusion. Constriction, closure, or blockage of a passage.

perfusion. Act of pouring over or through, especially the passage of a fluid through the vessels of a specific organ.

stricture. Narrowing of an anatomical structure.

ureterocele. Saccular formation of the lower part of the ureter, protruding into the bladder.

ureterostomy. Placement of a stent, tube, or catheter into the ureter, forming a passageway from the exterior of the body to the ureter.

Ureter

50688

50688 Change of ureterostomy tube or externally accessible ureteral stent via ileal conduit

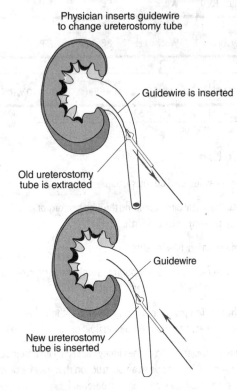

Physician inserts guidewire to change ureterostomy tube

Guidewire is inserted

Old ureterostomy tube is extracted

Guidewire

New ureterostomy tube is inserted

Explanation

The physician changes an ureterostomy tube or an externally accessible ureteral stent via an ileal conduit. To remove the existing tube, the physician takes out the sutures securing the tube to the skin. The physician inserts a guidewire through the tube and passes the tube back over the guidewire. The physician passes a new tube over the guidewire, removes the guidewire, and sutures the tube to the skin. To change an externally accessible ureteral stent via an ileal conduit, a guidewire is inserted through the ileal conduit. An ileal conduit is an isolated loop of ileum to which the ureter has been anastomosed at one end with the opposite end exiting through the skin and attached to an ostomy bag. The existing stent is retrieved and a new stent is placed. The guidewire is removed.

Coding Tips

Local anesthesia is included in the service. However, general anesthesia may be administered depending on the age or condition of the patient. For imaging guidance, see 75984.

ICD-10-CM Diagnostic Codes

T83.112A	Breakdown (mechanical) of indwelling ureteral stent, initial encounter
T83.113A	Breakdown (mechanical) of other urinary stents, initial encounter
T83.118A	Breakdown (mechanical) of other urinary devices and implants, initial encounter
T83.122A	Displacement of indwelling ureteral stent, initial encounter
T83.123A	Displacement of other urinary stents, initial encounter
T83.128A	Displacement of other urinary devices and implants, initial encounter

T83.192A	Other mechanical complication of indwelling ureteral stent, initial encounter
T83.193A	Other mechanical complication of other urinary stent, initial encounter
T83.198A	Other mechanical complication of other urinary devices and implants, initial encounter
T83.518A	Infection and inflammatory reaction due to other urinary catheter, initial encounter
T83.598A	Infection and inflammatory reaction due to other prosthetic device, implant and graft in urinary system, initial encounter
T83.81XA	Embolism due to genitourinary prosthetic devices, implants and grafts, initial encounter
T83.82XA	Fibrosis due to genitourinary prosthetic devices, implants and grafts, initial encounter
T83.83XA	Hemorrhage due to genitourinary prosthetic devices, implants and grafts, initial encounter
T83.84XA	Pain due to genitourinary prosthetic devices, implants and grafts, initial encounter
T83.85XA	Stenosis due to genitourinary prosthetic devices, implants and grafts, initial encounter
T83.86XA	Thrombosis due to genitourinary prosthetic devices, implants and grafts, initial encounter
T83.89XA	Other specified complication of genitourinary prosthetic devices, implants and grafts, initial encounter

AMA: 50688 2018,Jan,8; 2017,Jan,8; 2016,Jan,3; 2014,Jan,11

Relative Value Units/Medicare Edits

Non-Facility RVU	Work	PE	MP	Total
50688	1.2	0.93	0.11	2.24
Facility RVU	**Work**	**PE**	**MP**	**Total**
50688	1.2	0.93	0.11	2.24

	FUD	Status	MUE	Modifiers				IOM Reference
50688	10	A	2(3)	51	N/A	N/A	N/A	None

* with documentation

Terms To Know

fluoroscopy. Radiology technique that allows visual examination of part of the body or a function of an organ using a device that projects an x-ray image on a fluorescent screen.

guidewire. Flexible metal instrument designed to lead another instrument in its proper course.

hydronephrosis. Distension of the kidney caused by an accumulation of urine that cannot flow out due to an obstruction that may be caused by conditions such as kidney stones or vesicoureteral reflux.

stent. Tube to provide support in a body cavity or lumen.

ureter. Tube leading from the kidney to the urinary bladder made up of three layers of tissue: the mucous lining of the inner layer; the smooth, muscular middle layer that propels the urine from the kidney to the bladder by peristalsis; and the outer layer made of fibrous connective tissue. Each ureter leaves the kidney from the hilum, a concave notch on the middle surface, and enters the bladder through a narrow valve-like orifice that prevents the backflow of urine to the kidney.

Ureter

50690

50690 Injection procedure for visualization of ileal conduit and/or ureteropyelography, exclusive of radiologic service

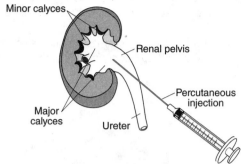

The physician injects contrast material into an ileal stoma or percutaneously or intravenously through a catheter to study the ureter and renal collecting system

Explanation

The physician injects a contrast agent through an existing ileal stoma into the renal pelvis or ureters to study the ileal conduit (where the ureters have been diverted into the ilium) or percutaneously or intravenously via a catheter to study the renal collecting system. To determine immediate allergic response to the contrast agent, the physician injects a small, initial dose of contrast material. If an allergic response is not evident, a larger amount of radiopaque dye is injected into the ureter and renal pelvis, and radiographic pictures are obtained for a ureteropyelogram or study of the ileal conduit diversion.

Coding Tips

Injection procedure for antegrade nephrostogram and/or ureterogram is reported with 50430–50431; for ureterography through ureterostomy or indwelling ureteral catheter, see 50684. For radiological supervision and interpretation, see 74420 for retrograde and 74425 for antegrade. Supplies used when providing this procedure may be reported with the appropriate HCPCS Level II code. Check with the specific payer to determine coverage.

ICD-10-CM Diagnostic Codes

C64.1	Malignant neoplasm of right kidney, except renal pelvis ☑
C64.2	Malignant neoplasm of left kidney, except renal pelvis ☑
C65.1	Malignant neoplasm of right renal pelvis ☑
C65.2	Malignant neoplasm of left renal pelvis ☑
C66.1	Malignant neoplasm of right ureter ☑
C66.2	Malignant neoplasm of left ureter ☑
C68.8	Malignant neoplasm of overlapping sites of urinary organs
C79.01	Secondary malignant neoplasm of right kidney and renal pelvis ☑
C79.02	Secondary malignant neoplasm of left kidney and renal pelvis ☑
C79.11	Secondary malignant neoplasm of bladder
C79.19	Secondary malignant neoplasm of other urinary organs
C7A.093	Malignant carcinoid tumor of the kidney
C80.2	Malignant neoplasm associated with transplanted organ
D30.01	Benign neoplasm of right kidney ☑
D30.02	Benign neoplasm of left kidney ☑
D30.11	Benign neoplasm of right renal pelvis ☑
D30.12	Benign neoplasm of left renal pelvis ☑
D30.21	Benign neoplasm of right ureter ☑

D30.22	Benign neoplasm of left ureter ☑
D3A.093	Benign carcinoid tumor of the kidney
D41.01	Neoplasm of uncertain behavior of right kidney ☑
D41.02	Neoplasm of uncertain behavior of left kidney ☑
D41.11	Neoplasm of uncertain behavior of right renal pelvis ☑
D41.12	Neoplasm of uncertain behavior of left renal pelvis ☑
D41.21	Neoplasm of uncertain behavior of right ureter ☑
D41.22	Neoplasm of uncertain behavior of left ureter ☑
D47.Z1	Post-transplant lymphoproliferative disorder (PTLD)
D47.Z2	Castleman disease
D49.511	Neoplasm of unspecified behavior of right kidney ☑
D49.512	Neoplasm of unspecified behavior of left kidney ☑
D49.59	Neoplasm of unspecified behavior of other genitourinary organ
N11.1	Chronic obstructive pyelonephritis
N13.0	Hydronephrosis with ureteropelvic junction obstruction
N13.1	Hydronephrosis with ureteral stricture, not elsewhere classified
N13.2	Hydronephrosis with renal and ureteral calculous obstruction
N13.39	Other hydronephrosis
N13.8	Other obstructive and reflux uropathy
N20.0	Calculus of kidney
N20.2	Calculus of kidney with calculus of ureter
N30.10	Interstitial cystitis (chronic) without hematuria
N30.11	Interstitial cystitis (chronic) with hematuria
N30.20	Other chronic cystitis without hematuria
N30.21	Other chronic cystitis with hematuria
N99.0	Postprocedural (acute) (chronic) kidney failure
N99.520	Hemorrhage of incontinent external stoma of urinary tract
N99.521	Infection of incontinent external stoma of urinary tract
N99.522	Malfunction of incontinent external stoma of urinary tract
N99.523	Herniation of incontinent stoma of urinary tract
N99.524	Stenosis of incontinent stoma of urinary tract
N99.528	Other complication of incontinent external stoma of urinary tract
N99.530	Hemorrhage of continent stoma of urinary tract
N99.531	Infection of continent stoma of urinary tract
N99.532	Malfunction of continent stoma of urinary tract
N99.533	Herniation of continent stoma of urinary tract
N99.534	Stenosis of continent stoma of urinary tract
N99.538	Other complication of continent stoma of urinary tract
N99.81	Other intraoperative complications of genitourinary system
N99.89	Other postprocedural complications and disorders of genitourinary system
Q64.11	Supravesical fissure of urinary bladder
Q64.5	Congenital absence of bladder and urethra
Q64.6	Congenital diverticulum of bladder
Q64.79	Other congenital malformations of bladder and urethra
Q64.8	Other specified congenital malformations of urinary system
R82.71	Bacteriuria
R82.79	Other abnormal findings on microbiological examination of urine
Z93.6	Other artificial openings of urinary tract status

AMA: 50690 2018,Jan,8; 2017,Jan,8; 2016,Jan,3; 2014,Jan,11

CPT © 2020 American Medical Association. All Rights Reserved.   ● New   ▲ Revised   + Add On   ★ Telemedicine   AMA: CPT Assist   [Resequenced]   ☑ Laterality   © 2020 Optum360, LLC

Relative Value Units/Medicare Edits

Non-Facility RVU	Work	PE	MP	Total
50690	1.16	1.82	0.11	3.09
Facility RVU	**Work**	**PE**	**MP**	**Total**
50690	1.16	0.75	0.11	2.02

	FUD	Status	MUE	Modifiers				IOM Reference
50690	0	A	2(3)	51	N/A	N/A	N/A	None

* with documentation

Terms To Know

calculus. Abnormal, stone-like concretion of calcium, cholesterol, mineral salts, or other substances that forms in any part of the body.

catheter. Flexible tube inserted into an area of the body for introducing or withdrawing fluid.

conduit. Surgically created channel for the passage of fluids.

contrast material. Any internally administered substance that has a different opacity from soft tissue on radiography or computed tomograph; includes barium, used to opacify parts of the gastrointestinal tract; water-soluble iodinated compounds, used to opacify blood vessels or the genitourinary tract; may refer to air occurring naturally or introduced into the body; also, paramagnetic substances used in magnetic resonance imaging. Substances may also be documented as contrast agent or contrast medium.

cystitis. Inflammation of the urinary bladder. Symptoms include dysuria, frequency of urination, urgency, and hematuria.

fissure. Deep furrow, groove, or cleft in tissue structures.

hydronephrosis. Distension of the kidney caused by an accumulation of urine that cannot flow out due to an obstruction that may be caused by conditions such as kidney stones or vesicoureteral reflux.

intravenous. Within a vein or veins.

malignant neoplasm. Any cancerous tumor or lesion exhibiting uncontrolled tissue growth that can progressively invade other parts of the body with its disease-generating cells.

percutaneous. Through the skin.

stoma. Opening created in the abdominal wall from an internal organ or structure for diversion of waste elimination, drainage, and access.

ureteropyelogram. Radiologic study of the renal pelvis and the ureter.

Ureter

50693-50695

50693 Placement of ureteral stent, percutaneous, including diagnostic nephrostogram and/or ureterogram when performed, imaging guidance (eg, ultrasound and/or fluoroscopy), and all associated radiological supervision and interpretation; pre-existing nephrostomy tract

50694 new access, without separate nephrostomy catheter

50695 new access, with separate nephrostomy catheter

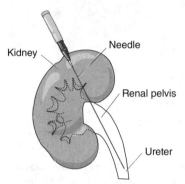

Physician advances needle toward renal pelvis into ureter

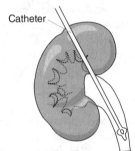

Catheter is passed over needle, which is withdrawn

Explanation

The physician inserts a catheter or stent percutaneously through the renal pelvis into the ureter for drainage of urine and/or an injection. With the patient face down, and the puncture site having been identified, a local anesthetic is injected. The physician inserts a long, thin needle with a removable probe in the skin of the back. The physician advances the needle toward the renal pelvis and into the ureter. When urine flows back through the needle, the physician advances a catheter over the needle and the needle is removed. An internal stent resides in the ureter and an external stent has one end that remains outside of the body. These codes report diagnostic nephrostogram and/or ureterogram, imaging guidance, and radiological supervision and interpretation. Report 50693 when this procedure is performed through an existing nephrostomy tract; 50694 when performed via a new access without a separate nephrostomy catheter; and 50695 when performed via a new access with a separate nephrostomy catheter.

Coding Tips

Do not report 50693–50695 with 50430–50435, 50684, or 74425 for the same renal collection system and/or associated ureter. These codes should be reported once for each renal collecting system/ureter accessed.

ICD-10-CM Diagnostic Codes

C64.1	Malignant neoplasm of right kidney, except renal pelvis ☑
C64.2	Malignant neoplasm of left kidney, except renal pelvis ☑
C65.1	Malignant neoplasm of right renal pelvis ☑

C65.2	Malignant neoplasm of left renal pelvis ☑
C66.1	Malignant neoplasm of right ureter ☑
C66.2	Malignant neoplasm of left ureter ☑
C79.01	Secondary malignant neoplasm of right kidney and renal pelvis ☑
C79.02	Secondary malignant neoplasm of left kidney and renal pelvis ☑
C79.19	Secondary malignant neoplasm of other urinary organs
C7A.093	Malignant carcinoid tumor of the kidney
D09.19	Carcinoma in situ of other urinary organs
D30.11	Benign neoplasm of right renal pelvis ☑
D30.12	Benign neoplasm of left renal pelvis ☑
D30.21	Benign neoplasm of right ureter ☑
D30.22	Benign neoplasm of left ureter ☑
D41.01	Neoplasm of uncertain behavior of right kidney ☑
D41.02	Neoplasm of uncertain behavior of left kidney ☑
D41.11	Neoplasm of uncertain behavior of right renal pelvis ☑
D41.12	Neoplasm of uncertain behavior of left renal pelvis ☑
D41.21	Neoplasm of uncertain behavior of right ureter ☑
D41.22	Neoplasm of uncertain behavior of left ureter ☑
D49.511	Neoplasm of unspecified behavior of right kidney ☑
D49.512	Neoplasm of unspecified behavior of left kidney ☑
D49.59	Neoplasm of unspecified behavior of other genitourinary organ
N10	Acute pyelonephritis
N11.0	Nonobstructive reflux-associated chronic pyelonephritis
N11.1	Chronic obstructive pyelonephritis
N11.8	Other chronic tubulo-interstitial nephritis
N12	Tubulo-interstitial nephritis, not specified as acute or chronic
N13.0	Hydronephrosis with ureteropelvic junction obstruction
N13.1	Hydronephrosis with ureteral stricture, not elsewhere classified
N13.2	Hydronephrosis with renal and ureteral calculous obstruction
N13.39	Other hydronephrosis
N13.4	Hydroureter
N13.5	Crossing vessel and stricture of ureter without hydronephrosis
N13.721	Vesicoureteral-reflux with reflux nephropathy without hydroureter, unilateral
N13.722	Vesicoureteral-reflux with reflux nephropathy without hydroureter, bilateral
N13.731	Vesicoureteral-reflux with reflux nephropathy with hydroureter, unilateral
N13.732	Vesicoureteral-reflux with reflux nephropathy with hydroureter, bilateral
N13.8	Other obstructive and reflux uropathy
N20.0	Calculus of kidney
N20.1	Calculus of ureter
N20.2	Calculus of kidney with calculus of ureter
N25.81	Secondary hyperparathyroidism of renal origin
N25.89	Other disorders resulting from impaired renal tubular function
N28.82	Megaloureter
N28.84	Pyelitis cystica
N28.85	Pyeloureteritis cystica
N28.86	Ureteritis cystica
N28.89	Other specified disorders of kidney and ureter
N39.3	Stress incontinence (female) (male)

N39.41	Urge incontinence
N39.42	Incontinence without sensory awareness
N39.43	Post-void dribbling
N39.44	Nocturnal enuresis
N39.45	Continuous leakage
N39.46	Mixed incontinence
N39.490	Overflow incontinence
N39.491	Coital incontinence
N39.492	Postural (urinary) incontinence
N39.498	Other specified urinary incontinence
N39.8	Other specified disorders of urinary system
N82.1	Other female urinary-genital tract fistulae ♀
Q62.0	Congenital hydronephrosis
Q62.11	Congenital occlusion of ureteropelvic junction
Q62.12	Congenital occlusion of ureterovesical orifice
Q62.2	Congenital megaureter
Q62.31	Congenital ureterocele, orthotopic
Q62.32	Cecoureterocele
Q62.39	Other obstructive defects of renal pelvis and ureter
Q62.5	Duplication of ureter
Q62.61	Deviation of ureter
Q62.62	Displacement of ureter
Q62.63	Anomalous implantation of ureter
Q62.69	Other malposition of ureter
Q62.8	Other congenital malformations of ureter
R82.71	Bacteriuria
R82.79	Other abnormal findings on microbiological examination of urine

AMA: **50693** 2018,Jan,8; 2017,Jan,8; 2016,Jan,3; 2016,Jan,13; 2015,Oct,5 **50694** 2018,Jan,8; 2017,Jan,8; 2016,Jan,3; 2016,Jan,13; 2015,Oct,5 **50695** 2018,Jan,8; 2017,Jan,8; 2016,Jan,3; 2016,Jan,13; 2015,Oct,5

Relative Value Units/Medicare Edits

Non-Facility RVU	Work	PE	MP	Total
50693	3.96	25.37	0.34	29.67
50694	5.25	27.24	0.46	32.95
50695	6.8	32.54	0.58	39.92
Facility RVU	**Work**	**PE**	**MP**	**Total**
50693	3.96	1.62	0.34	5.92
50694	5.25	2.07	0.46	7.78
50695	6.8	2.59	0.58	9.97

	FUD	Status	MUE	Modifiers				IOM Reference
50693	0	A	2(3)	51	50	N/A	N/A	None
50694	0	A	2(3)	51	50	N/A	N/A	
50695	0	A	2(3)	51	50	N/A	N/A	

* with documentation

50700

50700 Ureteroplasty, plastic operation on ureter (eg, stricture)

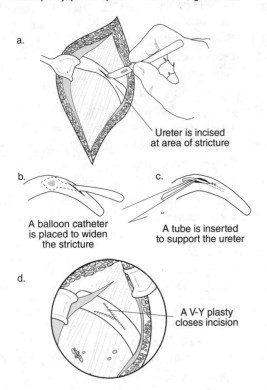

a. Ureter is incised at area of stricture

b. A balloon catheter is placed to widen the stricture

c. A tube is inserted to support the ureter

d. A V-Y plasty closes incision

Explanation

The physician uses plastic surgery to correct an obstruction or defect in the ureter. To access the ureter, the physician makes an incision in the skin and cuts the muscles, fat, and fibrous membranes (fascia) overlying the ureter. For the upper or middle third of the ureter, the physician usually makes an incision in the skin of the flank; to access the lower third of the ureter, the physician usually makes a curved lower quadrant incision. The physician inserts a catheter into the ureter to the point of obstruction. The balloon is inflated, sometimes using repeated inflation with increasing diameter of the catheter. The physician incises, trims, and shapes the ureter, using absorbable sutures or soft rubber drains for traction. The physician may insert a slender tube into the ureter to provide support during healing. The physician places a drain tube, bringing it out through a separate stab incision in the skin, and performs a layered closure.

Coding Tips

For plastic surgery on the renal pelvis and/or ureteropelvic junction, see 50400–50405. For plastic repair of the bladder and/or ureters, see 51800–51820.

ICD-10-CM Diagnostic Codes

N11.1	Chronic obstructive pyelonephritis
N13.5	Crossing vessel and stricture of ureter without hydronephrosis
N13.8	Other obstructive and reflux uropathy
N20.1	Calculus of ureter
N28.82	Megaloureter
N28.89	Other specified disorders of kidney and ureter
Q62.11	Congenital occlusion of ureteropelvic junction
Q62.12	Congenital occlusion of ureterovesical orifice
Q62.2	Congenital megaureter
Q62.31	Congenital ureterocele, orthotopic
Q62.32	Cecoureterocele
Q62.39	Other obstructive defects of renal pelvis and ureter

AMA: **50700** 2014,Jan,11

Relative Value Units/Medicare Edits

Non-Facility RVU	Work	PE	MP	Total
50700	16.69	8.12	1.91	26.72
Facility RVU	**Work**	**PE**	**MP**	**Total**
50700	16.69	8.12	1.91	26.72

	FUD	Status	MUE	Modifiers				IOM Reference
50700	90	A	1(2)	51	50	62*	80	None

* with documentation

Terms To Know

absorbable sutures. Strands used for suture or repair of tissue prepared from collagen or a synthetic polymer and capable of being absorbed by tissue over time.

balloon catheter. Any catheter equipped with an inflatable balloon at the end to hold it in place in a body cavity or to be used for dilation of a vessel lumen.

calculus. Abnormal, stone-like concretion of calcium, cholesterol, mineral salts, or other substances that forms in any part of the body.

congenital. Present at birth, occurring through heredity or an influence during gestation up to the moment of birth.

defect. Imperfection, flaw, or absence.

endometriosis. Aberrant uterine mucosal tissue appearing in areas of the pelvic cavity outside of its normal location, lining the uterus, and inflaming surrounding tissues often resulting in infertility or spontaneous abortion.

fascia. Fibrous sheet or band of tissue that envelops organs, muscles, and groupings of muscles.

flank. Part of the body found between the posterior ribs and the uppermost crest of the ilium, or the lateral side of the hip, thigh, and buttock.

obstruction. Blockage that prevents normal function of the valve or structure.

stricture. Narrowing of an anatomical structure.

ureter. Tube leading from the kidney to the urinary bladder made up of three layers of tissue: the mucous lining of the inner layer; the smooth, muscular middle layer that propels the urine from the kidney to the bladder by peristalsis; and the outer layer made of fibrous connective tissue. Each ureter leaves the kidney from the hilum, a concave notch on the middle surface, and enters the bladder through a narrow valve-like orifice that prevents the backflow of urine to the kidney.

ureterocele. Saccular formation of the lower part of the ureter, protruding into the bladder.

ureteroplasty. Plastic surgery to reconstruct a ureter when a congenital malformation or acquired narrowing blocks the normal flow of urine.

Ureter

50705

+ **50705** Ureteral embolization or occlusion, including imaging guidance (eg, ultrasound and/or fluoroscopy) and all associated radiological supervision and interpretation (List separately in addition to code for primary procedure)

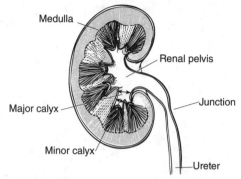

Cutaway detail of normal right kidney and ureter

Explanation

Ureteral embolization or occlusion performed non-endoscopically requires the patient to be under anesthesia. Typically a nephrostomy tube is introduced into both kidneys prior to embolization, being replaced with a sheath during the procedure. A nephrostogram may be performed. A catheter is positioned into the distal ureter with groups of coils in various sizes. These coils are used for the occlusion and it may take four to 12 coils to accomplish the end result. Gelatin sponges may also be placed within the coil groups to speed up the lumen occlusion. A nephrostogram may be performed again to verify success of the procedure at the coil positions. The sheath is replaced with a catheter allowing for drainage and may be replaced every eight weeks. This procedure may be performed via transrenal access, existing renal/ureteral access, transurethral access, an ileal conduit, or ureterostomy. It includes the embolization or dilation, imaging guidance, and radiological supervision and interpretation. The service performed for gaining access may be reported separately.

Coding Tips

This code is reported once per ureter per day. Diagnostic pyelography or ureterography is not a component of this service and may be reported separately in addition to other interventions or catheter placements performed at the same time. Report 50705 in addition to 50382, 50384–50387, 50389, 50430–50435, 50684, 50688, 50690, 50693–50695, and 51610.

ICD-10-CM Diagnostic Codes

This/these CPT code(s) are add-on code(s). See the primary procedure code that this code is performed with for your ICD-10-CM code selections.

AMA: **50705** 2018,Jan,8; 2017,Jan,8; 2016,Jan,3

Relative Value Units/Medicare Edits

Non-Facility RVU	Work	PE	MP	Total
50705	4.03	49.62	0.4	54.05
Facility RVU	Work	PE	MP	Total
50705	4.03	0.68	0.4	5.11

	FUD	Status	MUE	Modifiers				IOM Reference
50705	N/A	A	2(3)	N/A	50	N/A	N/A	None

* with documentation

50706

+ **50706** Balloon dilation, ureteral stricture, including imaging guidance (eg, ultrasound and/or fluoroscopy) and all associated radiological supervision and interpretation (List separately in addition to code for primary procedure)

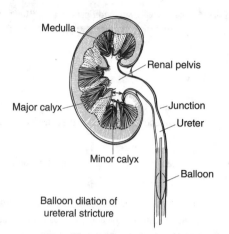

Balloon dilation of
ureteral stricture

Explanation

The physician treats a ureteral stricture by balloon dilation by making an incision into the skin overlying the target area. The patient is anesthetized and the incision is made. The target area is visualized by imaging guidance. A guidewire is inserted through the strictured area. A catheter containing the balloon is threaded over the wire to the stricture and the wire is removed. Balloon catheter sizes are determined based on normal ureter diameter as measured by radiological images. The balloon is inflated until stricture is minimalized; the process may be repeated until the desired result is achieved. Contrast may be injected to determine adequate flow through the ureter. The instruments are removed and the incision site is sutured closed. This procedure may be performed via transrenal access, existing renal/ureteral access, transurethral access, an ileal conduit, or ureterostomy. It includes the embolization or dilation, imaging guidance, and radiological supervision and interpretation. The service performed for gaining access may be reported separately.

Coding Tips

This code is reported once per ureter per day. Diagnostic pyelography or ureterography is not a component of this service and may be reported separately in addition to other interventions or catheter placements performed at the same time. For percutaneous nephrostomy, nephroureteral catheter, and/or ureteral catheter placement, see 50385, 50387, 50432–50435, and 50693–50695. Report 50706 in addition to 50382, 50384–50387, 50389, 50430–50435, 50684, 50688, 50690, 50693–50695, and 51610. Do not report 50706 with 50553, 50572, 50953, 50972, 52341, 52344, 52345, or 74485.

ICD-10-CM Diagnostic Codes

This/these CPT code(s) are add-on code(s). See the primary procedure code that this code is performed with for your ICD-10-CM code selections.

AMA: **50706** 2018,Jan,8; 2017,Jan,8; 2016,Jan,3

CPT © 2020 American Medical Association. All Rights Reserved.   ● New   ▲ Revised   + Add On   ★ Telemedicine   AMA: CPT Assist   [Resequenced]   ☑ Laterality   © 2020 Optum360, LLC

Relative Value Units/Medicare Edits

Non-Facility RVU	Work	PE	MP	Total
50706	3.8	22.82	0.34	26.96
Facility RVU	Work	PE	MP	Total
50706	3.8	1.16	0.34	5.3

	FUD	Status	MUE	Modifiers				IOM Reference
50706	N/A	A	2(3)	N/A	50	N/A	N/A	None

* with documentation

Terms To Know

balloon catheter. Any catheter equipped with an inflatable balloon at the end to hold it in place in a body cavity or to be used for dilation of a vessel lumen.

dilation. Artificial increase in the diameter of an opening or lumen made by medication or by instrumentation.

imaging. Radiologic means of producing pictures for clinical study of the internal structures and functions of the body, such as x-ray, ultrasound, magnetic resonance, or positron emission tomography.

stricture. Narrowing of an anatomical structure.

supervision and interpretation. Radiology services that usually contain an invasive component and are reported by the radiologist for supervision of the procedure and the personnel involved with performing the examination, reading the film, and preparing the written report.

ureter. Tube leading from the kidney to the urinary bladder made up of three layers of tissue: the mucous lining of the inner layer; the smooth, muscular middle layer that propels the urine from the kidney to the bladder by peristalsis; and the outer layer made of fibrous connective tissue. Each ureter leaves the kidney from the hilum, a concave notch on the middle surface, and enters the bladder through a narrow valve-like orifice that prevents the backflow of urine to the kidney.

50715

50715   Ureterolysis, with or without repositioning of ureter for retroperitoneal fibrosis

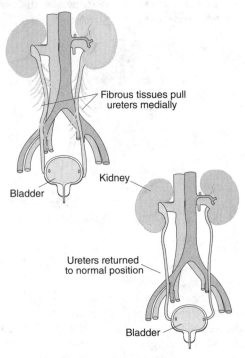

Fibrous tissues pull ureters medially

Kidney

Bladder

Ureters returned to normal position

Bladder

The physician surgically frees the ureter from the surrounding fibrotic tissue

Explanation

The physician surgically frees the ureter from localized inflammatory disease of retroperitoneal fibrous tissue. To access the ureter, the physician makes a midline incision in the skin of the abdomen and cuts the muscles, fat, and fibrous membranes (fascia) overlying the ureter. The physician incises surrounding fibrotic tissue to free the ureter, and may use sutures to reposition the ureter away from obstructive fibrous tissue. The physician places a drain tube, bringing it out through a separate stab incision in the skin, and performs a layered closure.

Coding Tips

This is a unilateral procedure. If performed bilaterally, some payers require that the service be reported twice with modifier 50 appended to the second code while others require identification of the service only once with modifier 50 appended. Check with individual payers. Modifier 50 identifies a procedure performed identically on the opposite side of the body (mirror image). If the physician performs ureterolysis for ovarian vein syndrome, see 50722. For ureterolysis to divide and reconnect a ureter that is positioned behind the vena cava, see 50725.

ICD-10-CM Diagnostic Codes

N11.1	Chronic obstructive pyelonephritis
N13.5	Crossing vessel and stricture of ureter without hydronephrosis
N13.8	Other obstructive and reflux uropathy
N28.89	Other specified disorders of kidney and ureter

AMA: 50715 2014,Jan,11

Ureter

Relative Value Units/Medicare Edits

Non-Facility RVU	Work	PE	MP	Total
50715	20.64	10.78	3.34	34.76
Facility RVU	**Work**	**PE**	**MP**	**Total**
50715	20.64	10.78	3.34	34.76

	FUD	Status	MUE	Modifiers				IOM Reference
50715	90	A	1(2)	51	50	62*	80	None

* with documentation

Terms To Know

adhesion. Abnormal fibrous connection between two structures, soft tissue or bony structures, that may occur as the result of surgery, infection, or trauma.

drain. Device that creates a channel to allow fluid from a cavity, wound, or infected area to exit the body.

fascia. Fibrous sheet or band of tissue that envelops organs, muscles, and groupings of muscles.

fibrosis. Formation of fibrous tissue as part of the restorative process.

fibrous tissue. Connective tissues.

obstruction. Blockage that prevents normal function of the valve or structure.

peritoneum. Strong, continuous membrane that forms the lining of the abdominal and pelvic cavity. The parietal peritoneum, or outer layer, is attached to the abdominopelvic walls and the visceral peritoneum, or inner layer, surrounds the organs inside the abdominal cavity.

retroperitoneal. Located behind the peritoneum, the membrane that lines the abdominopelvic walls and forms a covering for the internal organs.

ureter. Tube leading from the kidney to the urinary bladder made up of three layers of tissue: the mucous lining of the inner layer; the smooth, muscular middle layer that propels the urine from the kidney to the bladder by peristalsis; and the outer layer made of fibrous connective tissue. Each ureter leaves the kidney from the hilum, a concave notch on the middle surface, and enters the bladder through a narrow valve-like orifice that prevents the backflow of urine to the kidney.

ureterolysis. Surgical procedure to release or free the ureter from surrounding obstructive retroperitoneal fibrotic tissue, free the ureter from adhesions caused by obstructive ovarian veins, or divide and reconnect to free the ureter from an obstructive aberrant position behind the vena cava.

50722

50722   Ureterolysis for ovarian vein syndrome

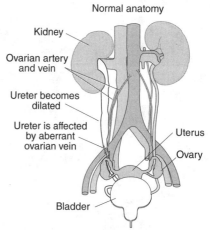

The physician surgically frees the ureter from obstruction caused by ovarian vein syndrome

Explanation

The physician surgically frees the ureter from ureteral obstruction caused by aberrant ovarian veins (ovarian vein syndrome). To access the ureter, the physician makes an incision in the skin above the pubic hairline, and cuts the muscles, fat, and fibrous membranes (fascia) overlying the ureter. The physician incises surrounding adhesions to free the ureter from the obstructing ovarian veins. The physician places a drain tube, bringing it out through a separate stab incision in the skin, and performs a layered closure.

Coding Tips

If the physician performs ureterolysis for retroperitoneal fibrosis, see 50715. For ureterolysis to divide and reconnect a ureter that is positioned behind the vena cava, see 50725.

ICD-10-CM Diagnostic Codes

N13.5   Crossing vessel and stricture of ureter without hydronephrosis

AMA: 50722 2014,Jan,11

Relative Value Units/Medicare Edits

Non-Facility RVU	Work	PE	MP	Total
50722	17.95	9.04	2.83	29.82
Facility RVU	**Work**	**PE**	**MP**	**Total**
50722	17.95	9.04	2.83	29.82

	FUD	Status	MUE	Modifiers				IOM Reference
50722	90	A	1(2)	51	N/A	62*	80	None

* with documentation

Terms To Know

ovarian vein syndrome. Retroperitoneal structures involving and often obstructing the ureters following certain types of chemical treatment; there is no identified cause.

Ureter

50725

50725 Ureterolysis for retrocaval ureter, with reanastomosis of upper urinary tract or vena cava

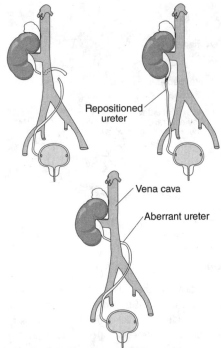

Physician divides and reconnects aberrantly placed ureter into normal anatomic position

Explanation

The physician divides and reconnects a ureter aberrantly positioned behind the vena cava. To access the ureter, the physician makes a midline incision in the skin of the abdomen, and cuts the muscles, fat, and fibrous membranes (fascia) overlying the ureter. The physician dissects the ureter on both sides of the vena cava, leaving the ureteric segment behind the vena cava in place. The physician connects (anastomosis) the distal end of the ureter to the upper ureter by fashioning a long, elliptical flap from the renal pelvis. The physician may alternatively dissect and connect the two ends of the vena cava, positioning the ureter in front. To provide support during healing, the physician may insert a slender tube into the renal pelvis. After wrapping the anastomosis with perinephric fat, the physician inserts a drain tube and performs a layered closure.

Coding Tips

If the physician performs ureterolysis for retroperitoneal fibrosis, see 50715. If the physician performs ureterolysis for ovarian vein syndrome, see 50722. Other ureteral repair codes include anastomosis of the ureter to the renal pelvis (50740), renal calyx (50750), ureter (50760–50770), bladder (50780–50785), or intestine (50800–50825). Supplies used when providing this procedure may be reported with the appropriate HCPCS Level II code. Check with the specific payer to determine coverage.

ICD-10-CM Diagnostic Codes

Q62.4	Agenesis of ureter
Q62.5	Duplication of ureter
Q62.61	Deviation of ureter
Q62.62	Displacement of ureter
Q62.63	Anomalous implantation of ureter
Q62.69	Other malposition of ureter
Q62.7	Congenital vesico-uretero-renal reflux
Q62.8	Other congenital malformations of ureter

AMA: **50725** 2014,Jan,11

Relative Value Units/Medicare Edits

Non-Facility RVU	Work	PE	MP	Total
50725	20.2	9.32	2.33	31.85
Facility RVU	**Work**	**PE**	**MP**	**Total**
50725	20.2	9.32	2.33	31.85

	FUD	Status	MUE	Modifiers				IOM Reference
50725	90	A	1(3)	51	N/A	62*	80	None

* with documentation

Terms To Know

aberrant. Deviation or departure from the normal or usual course, condition, or pattern.

adhesion. Abnormal fibrous connection between two structures, soft tissue or bony structures, that may occur as the result of surgery, infection, or trauma.

agenesis. Absence of an organ due to developmental failure in the prenatal period.

anastomosis. Surgically created connection between ducts, blood vessels, or bowel segments to allow flow from one to the other.

anomaly. Irregularity in the structure or position of an organ or tissue.

congenital. Present at birth, occurring through heredity or an influence during gestation up to the moment of birth.

dissect. Cut apart or separate tissue for surgical purposes or for visual or microscopic study.

distal. Located farther away from a specified reference point or the trunk.

drain. Device that creates a channel to allow fluid from a cavity, wound, or infected area to exit the body.

fascia. Fibrous sheet or band of tissue that envelops organs, muscles, and groupings of muscles.

malposition. Congenital or acquired condition in which an organ or body part is in an abnormal or uncharacteristic position.

ureterolysis. Surgical procedure to release or free the ureter from surrounding obstructive retroperitoneal fibrotic tissue, free the ureter from adhesions caused by obstructive ovarian veins, or divide and reconnect to free the ureter from an obstructive aberrant position behind the vena cava.

vena cava. Main venous trunk that empties into the right atrium from both the lower and upper regions, beginning at the junction of the common iliac veins inferiorly and the two brachiocephalic veins superiorly.

50727-50728

50727 Revision of urinary-cutaneous anastomosis (any type urostomy);
50728 with repair of fascial defect and hernia

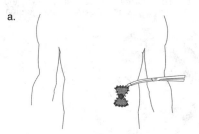

Physician removes sutures securing opening to skin

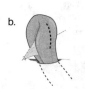

Physician revises surgical opening between skin and ureter

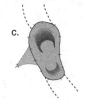

A tube may be inserted during healing to support the ureter

Explanation

The physician revises any surgical opening (anastomosis) between the skin and ureter, bladder, or colon segment. The physician removes the sutures securing the anastomosis to the skin and revises the anastomosis. The physician may make a midline incision in the skin of the abdomen to access the urinary tract. In 50728, the physician repairs a defect in surrounding fibrous membranes (fascia), and/or a rupture (hernia) in ureteral tissues.

Coding Tips

Other ureteral repair codes include anastomosis of the ureter to the renal pelvis (50740), renal calyx (50750), ureter (50760–50770), bladder (50780–50785), or intestine (50800–50825). For repair of the kidney pelvis, see 50400–50405. Supplies used when providing these procedures may be reported with the appropriate HCPCS Level II code. Check with the specific payer to determine coverage.

ICD-10-CM Diagnostic Codes

C66.1	Malignant neoplasm of right ureter ☑
C66.2	Malignant neoplasm of left ureter ☑
C67.0	Malignant neoplasm of trigone of bladder
C67.1	Malignant neoplasm of dome of bladder
C67.2	Malignant neoplasm of lateral wall of bladder
C67.3	Malignant neoplasm of anterior wall of bladder
C67.4	Malignant neoplasm of posterior wall of bladder
C67.5	Malignant neoplasm of bladder neck
C67.6	Malignant neoplasm of ureteric orifice
C67.8	Malignant neoplasm of overlapping sites of bladder
C68.0	Malignant neoplasm of urethra
C78.6	Secondary malignant neoplasm of retroperitoneum and peritoneum
K50.014	Crohn's disease of small intestine with abscess
K50.114	Crohn's disease of large intestine with abscess
K50.814	Crohn's disease of both small and large intestine with abscess

K51.014	Ulcerative (chronic) pancolitis with abscess
K51.214	Ulcerative (chronic) proctitis with abscess
K51.314	Ulcerative (chronic) rectosigmoiditis with abscess
K51.414	Inflammatory polyps of colon with abscess
K51.514	Left sided colitis with abscess
K51.814	Other ulcerative colitis with abscess
K56.51	Intestinal adhesions [bands], with partial obstruction
K56.52	Intestinal adhesions [bands] with complete obstruction
K57.00	Diverticulitis of small intestine with perforation and abscess without bleeding
K57.01	Diverticulitis of small intestine with perforation and abscess with bleeding
K57.20	Diverticulitis of large intestine with perforation and abscess without bleeding
K57.21	Diverticulitis of large intestine with perforation and abscess with bleeding
K57.40	Diverticulitis of both small and large intestine with perforation and abscess without bleeding
K57.41	Diverticulitis of both small and large intestine with perforation and abscess with bleeding
K63.0	Abscess of intestine
K63.1	Perforation of intestine (nontraumatic)
K63.3	Ulcer of intestine
K63.4	Enteroptosis
K63.89	Other specified diseases of intestine
K92.89	Other specified diseases of the digestive system
K94.01	Colostomy hemorrhage
K94.02	Colostomy infection
K94.03	Colostomy malfunction
K94.09	Other complications of colostomy
K94.11	Enterostomy hemorrhage
K94.12	Enterostomy infection
K94.13	Enterostomy malfunction
K94.19	Other complications of enterostomy
L02.211	Cutaneous abscess of abdominal wall
L02.214	Cutaneous abscess of groin
L03.311	Cellulitis of abdominal wall
L03.314	Cellulitis of groin
L03.321	Acute lymphangitis of abdominal wall
L03.324	Acute lymphangitis of groin
N11.1	Chronic obstructive pyelonephritis
N13.5	Crossing vessel and stricture of ureter without hydronephrosis
N13.8	Other obstructive and reflux uropathy
N28.82	Megaloureter
N28.89	Other specified disorders of kidney and ureter
N73.6	Female pelvic peritoneal adhesions (postinfective) ♀
N99.0	Postprocedural (acute) (chronic) kidney failure
N99.520	Hemorrhage of incontinent external stoma of urinary tract
N99.521	Infection of incontinent external stoma of urinary tract
N99.522	Malfunction of incontinent external stoma of urinary tract
N99.523	Herniation of incontinent stoma of urinary tract
N99.524	Stenosis of incontinent stoma of urinary tract
N99.528	Other complication of incontinent external stoma of urinary tract
N99.530	Hemorrhage of continent stoma of urinary tract

Ureter

N99.531	Infection of continent stoma of urinary tract
N99.532	Malfunction of continent stoma of urinary tract
N99.533	Herniation of continent stoma of urinary tract
N99.534	Stenosis of continent stoma of urinary tract
N99.538	Other complication of continent stoma of urinary tract
N99.81	Other intraoperative complications of genitourinary system
N99.89	Other postprocedural complications and disorders of genitourinary system
Z43.6	Encounter for attention to other artificial openings of urinary tract

AMA: **50727** 2014,Jan,11 **50728** 2014,Jan,11

Relative Value Units/Medicare Edits

Non-Facility RVU	Work	PE	MP	Total
50727	8.28	5.37	1.04	14.69
50728	12.18	7.14	1.95	21.27
Facility RVU	Work	PE	MP	Total
50727	8.28	5.37	1.04	14.69
50728	12.18	7.14	1.95	21.27

	FUD	Status	MUE	Modifiers				IOM Reference
50727	90	A	1(3)	51	N/A	62	80	None
50728	90	A	1(3)	51	N/A	62	80	

* with documentation

Terms To Know

anastomosis. Surgically created connection between ducts, blood vessels, or bowel segments to allow flow from one to the other.

cutaneous. Relating to the skin.

defect. Imperfection, flaw, or absence.

enteroptosis. Condition in which the intestines are abnormally positioned downward in the abdominal cavity and often associated with displacement of other internal organs.

fascia. Fibrous sheet or band of tissue that envelops organs, muscles, and groupings of muscles.

hernia. Protrusion of a body structure through tissue.

tissue. Group of similar cells with a similar function that form definite structures and organs. Tissue types include epithelial tissue, muscle tissue, connective tissue, and nervous tissue.

urostomy. Creation of an opening from the ureter to the abdominal surface to divert urine flow.

50740

50740   Ureteropyelostomy, anastomosis of ureter and renal pelvis

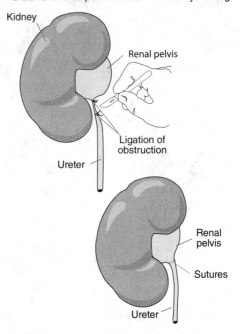

The physician divides and surgically rejoins the ureter and renal pelvis to allow for urinary drainage

Explanation

The physician surgically connects the upper ureter and renal pelvis to allow for urinary drainage. To access the renal pelvis and ureter, the physician makes an incision in the skin of the flank, cuts the muscles, fat, and fibrous membranes (fascia) overlying the kidney, and sometimes removes a portion of the eleventh or twelfth rib. The physician ligates the renal pelvis and ureter at the point of blockage. After excising the obstructing part of the ureter or pelvis, the physician surgically connects (anastomosis) the two structures, bypassing the obstructing point. To provide support during healing, the physician may insert a slender tube into the renal pelvis. After wrapping the anastomosis with perinephric fat, the physician inserts a drain tube and performs a layered closure.

Coding Tips

For anastomosis of the ureter to the renal calyx, see 50750; to the ureter, see 50760–50770; to the bladder, see 50780–50785; and to the intestine, see 50800–50825.

ICD-10-CM Diagnostic Codes

C65.1	Malignant neoplasm of right renal pelvis ☑
C65.2	Malignant neoplasm of left renal pelvis ☑
C79.01	Secondary malignant neoplasm of right kidney and renal pelvis ☑
C79.02	Secondary malignant neoplasm of left kidney and renal pelvis ☑
C79.19	Secondary malignant neoplasm of other urinary organs
C80.2	Malignant neoplasm associated with transplanted organ
D30.11	Benign neoplasm of right renal pelvis ☑
D30.12	Benign neoplasm of left renal pelvis ☑
D3A.093	Benign carcinoid tumor of the kidney
N11.1	Chronic obstructive pyelonephritis

Ureter

N13.5	Crossing vessel and stricture of ureter without hydronephrosis
N13.8	Other obstructive and reflux uropathy
N28.89	Other specified disorders of kidney and ureter
Q62.0	Congenital hydronephrosis
Q62.11	Congenital occlusion of ureteropelvic junction
Q62.31	Congenital ureterocele, orthotopic
Q62.32	Cecoureterocele
Q62.39	Other obstructive defects of renal pelvis and ureter

AMA: 50740 2018,Jan,8; 2017,Jan,8; 2016,Jan,13; 2015,Jan,16; 2014,Jan,11

Relative Value Units/Medicare Edits

Non-Facility RVU	Work	PE	MP	Total
50740	20.07	10.72	4.86	35.65
Facility RVU	**Work**	**PE**	**MP**	**Total**
50740	20.07	10.72	4.86	35.65

	FUD	Status	MUE	Modifiers				IOM Reference
50740	90	A	1(2)	51	50	62*	80	None

* with documentation

Terms To Know

anastomosis. Surgically created connection between ducts, blood vessels, or bowel segments to allow flow from one to the other.

benign. Mild or nonmalignant in nature.

congenital. Present at birth, occurring through heredity or an influence during gestation up to the moment of birth.

cyst. Elevated encapsulated mass containing fluid, semisolid, or solid material with a membranous lining.

drain. Device that creates a channel to allow fluid from a cavity, wound, or infected area to exit the body.

flank. Part of the body found between the posterior ribs and the uppermost crest of the ilium, or the lateral side of the hip, thigh, and buttock.

ligate. To tie off a blood vessel or duct with a suture or a soft, thin wire (ligature wire).

malignant neoplasm. Any cancerous tumor or lesion exhibiting uncontrolled tissue growth that can progressively invade other parts of the body with its disease-generating cells.

obstruction. Blockage that prevents normal function of the valve or structure.

stent. Tube to provide support in a body cavity or lumen.

stricture. Narrowing of an anatomical structure.

ureterocele. Saccular formation of the lower part of the ureter, protruding into the bladder.

50750

| 50750 | Ureterocalycostomy, anastomosis of ureter to renal calyx |

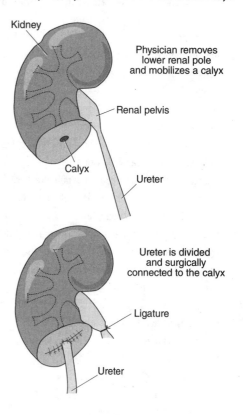

Explanation

The physician connects the upper ureter and a renal calyx to allow for urinary drainage. To access the renal calyces and ureter, the physician makes an incision in the skin of the flank, cuts the muscles, fat, and fibrous membranes (fascia) overlying the kidney, and sometimes removes a portion of the eleventh or twelfth rib. The physician ligates the appropriate renal arteries and performs a partial nephrectomy by removing a part of the kidney. The physician partially mobilizes the calyx and ureter, and places a nephrostomy tube and stent. After surgically joining (anastomosing) the calyx and ureter, the physician closes the renal pelvis and wraps the anastomosis with perinephric fat. The physician inserts a drain tube and performs a layered closure.

Coding Tips

The partial nephrectomy is part of this procedure and should not be reported separately. For anastomosis of the ureter to the renal pelvis, see 50740; to the ureter, see 50760–50770; to the bladder, see 50780–50785; and to the intestine, see 50800–50825.

ICD-10-CM Diagnostic Codes

C64.1	Malignant neoplasm of right kidney, except renal pelvis ☑
C64.2	Malignant neoplasm of left kidney, except renal pelvis ☑
C65.1	Malignant neoplasm of right renal pelvis ☑
C65.2	Malignant neoplasm of left renal pelvis ☑
C66.1	Malignant neoplasm of right ureter ☑
C66.2	Malignant neoplasm of left ureter ☑
C68.8	Malignant neoplasm of overlapping sites of urinary organs
C79.01	Secondary malignant neoplasm of right kidney and renal pelvis ☑

Ureter

C79.02	Secondary malignant neoplasm of left kidney and renal pelvis ☑
C79.19	Secondary malignant neoplasm of other urinary organs
C7A.093	Malignant carcinoid tumor of the kidney
C80.2	Malignant neoplasm associated with transplanted organ
D30.01	Benign neoplasm of right kidney ☑
D30.02	Benign neoplasm of left kidney ☑
D30.11	Benign neoplasm of right renal pelvis ☑
D30.12	Benign neoplasm of left renal pelvis ☑
D3A.093	Benign carcinoid tumor of the kidney
D41.01	Neoplasm of uncertain behavior of right kidney ☑
D41.02	Neoplasm of uncertain behavior of left kidney ☑
D41.11	Neoplasm of uncertain behavior of right renal pelvis ☑
D41.12	Neoplasm of uncertain behavior of left renal pelvis ☑
D41.21	Neoplasm of uncertain behavior of right ureter ☑
D41.22	Neoplasm of uncertain behavior of left ureter ☑
N11.1	Chronic obstructive pyelonephritis
N13.0	Hydronephrosis with ureteropelvic junction obstruction
N13.1	Hydronephrosis with ureteral stricture, not elsewhere classified
N13.2	Hydronephrosis with renal and ureteral calculous obstruction
N13.39	Other hydronephrosis
N13.5	Crossing vessel and stricture of ureter without hydronephrosis
N13.8	Other obstructive and reflux uropathy
N20.0	Calculus of kidney
N20.1	Calculus of ureter
N20.2	Calculus of kidney with calculus of ureter
N28.89	Other specified disorders of kidney and ureter
Q61.02	Congenital multiple renal cysts
Q61.8	Other cystic kidney diseases
Q62.0	Congenital hydronephrosis
Q62.11	Congenital occlusion of ureteropelvic junction
Q62.31	Congenital ureterocele, orthotopic
Q62.32	Cecoureterocele
Q62.39	Other obstructive defects of renal pelvis and ureter

AMA: **50750** 2018,Jan,8; 2017,Jan,8; 2016,Jan,13; 2015,Jan,16; 2014,Jan,11

Relative Value Units/Medicare Edits

Non-Facility RVU	Work	PE	MP	Total
50750	21.22	9.66	2.43	33.31
Facility RVU	Work	PE	MP	Total
50750	21.22	9.66	2.43	33.31

	FUD	Status	MUE	Modifiers				IOM Reference
50750	90	A	1(2)	51	50	N/A	80	None

* with documentation

Terms To Know

anastomosis. Surgically created connection between ducts, blood vessels, or bowel segments to allow flow from one to the other.

congenital. Present at birth, occurring through heredity or an influence during gestation up to the moment of birth.

50760

50760   Ureteroureterostomy

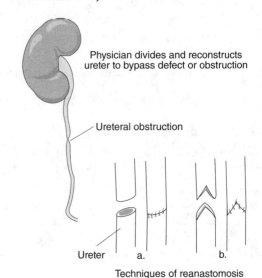

Physician divides and reconstructs ureter to bypass defect or obstruction

Ureteral obstruction

Ureter

a.   b.

Techniques of reanastomosis

Explanation

The physician divides and reconnects the ureter to bypass a defect or obstruction. To access the ureter, the physician makes an incision in the skin of the abdomen and cuts the muscles, fat, and fibrous membranes (fascia) overlying the ureter. For the upper or middle third of the ureter, the physician usually makes an incision in the skin of the flank; to access the lower third of the ureter, the physician usually makes a curved lower quadrant incision. The physician ligates and dissects the ureter at the point of blockage, and surgically rejoins (anastomosis) the two ends, bypassing the obstructing point. To provide support during healing, the physician may insert a slender tube into the ureter. The physician inserts a drain tube and performs a layered closure.

Coding Tips

For connection of one ureter to the ureter on the opposite side, see 50770. If the ureteroureterostomy is performed on a ureter that previously diverted urine flow through a colon segment or to the skin, see 50830. If the ureter is anastomosed to the bladder, see 50780–50785.

ICD-10-CM Diagnostic Codes

C66.1	Malignant neoplasm of right ureter ☑
C66.2	Malignant neoplasm of left ureter ☑
N11.1	Chronic obstructive pyelonephritis
N13.5	Crossing vessel and stricture of ureter without hydronephrosis
N13.8	Other obstructive and reflux uropathy
Q62.0	Congenital hydronephrosis
Q62.11	Congenital occlusion of ureteropelvic junction
Q62.12	Congenital occlusion of ureterovesical orifice
Q62.2	Congenital megaureter
Q62.31	Congenital ureterocele, orthotopic
Q62.32	Cecoureterocele
Q62.39	Other obstructive defects of renal pelvis and ureter
Q62.61	Deviation of ureter
Q62.62	Displacement of ureter
Q62.63	Anomalous implantation of ureter
Q62.69	Other malposition of ureter

Ureter

Q62.8	Other congenital malformations of ureter
S37.12XA	Contusion of ureter, initial encounter
S37.13XA	Laceration of ureter, initial encounter
S37.19XA	Other injury of ureter, initial encounter

AMA: **50760** 2018,Jan,8; 2017,Jan,8; 2016,Jan,13; 2015,Jan,16; 2014,Jan,11

Relative Value Units/Medicare Edits

Non-Facility RVU	Work	PE	MP	Total
50760	20.07	9.6	3.01	32.68
Facility RVU	**Work**	**PE**	**MP**	**Total**
50760	20.07	9.6	3.01	32.68

	FUD	Status	MUE	Modifiers				IOM Reference
50760	90	A	1(2)	51	50	62*	80	None

* with documentation

Terms To Know

anastomosis. Surgically created connection between ducts, blood vessels, or bowel segments to allow flow from one to the other.

benign. Mild or nonmalignant in nature.

bypass. Auxiliary or diverted route to maintain continuous flow.

congenital. Present at birth, occurring through heredity or an influence during gestation up to the moment of birth.

defect. Imperfection, flaw, or absence.

dissection. Separating by cutting tissue or body structures apart.

flank. Part of the body found between the posterior ribs and the uppermost crest of the ilium, or the lateral side of the hip, thigh, and buttock.

ligation. Tying off a blood vessel or duct with a suture or a soft, thin wire.

malignant. Any condition tending to progress toward death, specifically an invasive tumor with a loss of cellular differentiation that has the ability to spread or metastasize to other body areas.

obstruction. Blockage that prevents normal function of the valve or structure.

stent. Tube to provide support in a body cavity or lumen.

stricture. Narrowing of an anatomical structure.

ureterocele. Saccular formation of the lower part of the ureter, protruding into the bladder.

50770

50770	Transureteroureterostomy, anastomosis of ureter to contralateral ureter

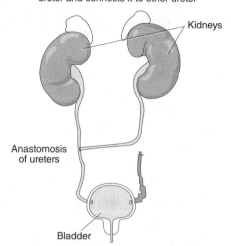

Physician divides diseased or obstructed ureter and connects it to other ureter

Kidneys

Anastomosis of ureters

Bladder

Diseased or obstructed ureter

Explanation

The physician divides and connects a diseased or obstructed ureter to the other ureter. To access the ureters, the physician usually makes a midline incision in the skin of the abdomen, and cuts the muscles, fat, and fibrous membranes (fascia) overlying the ureters. The physician ligates and dissects the ureter at the point of disease or blockage, and surgically attaches (anastomosis) the end of the usable ureteric portion to the other ureter. To provide support during healing, the physician may insert a slender tube into the ureter. The physician inserts a drain tube and performs a layered closure.

Coding Tips

If the physician divides and reconnects the same ureter to bypass the point of disease or obstruction, see 50760. Ureteroureterostomy performed on a ureter that previously diverted urine flow through a colon segment or to the skin is reported with 50830. If the ureter is implanted into the bladder, see 50780–50785.

ICD-10-CM Diagnostic Codes

C66.1	Malignant neoplasm of right ureter ☑
C66.2	Malignant neoplasm of left ureter ☑
N11.1	Chronic obstructive pyelonephritis
N13.5	Crossing vessel and stricture of ureter without hydronephrosis
N13.71	Vesicoureteral-reflux without reflux nephropathy
N13.721	Vesicoureteral-reflux with reflux nephropathy without hydroureter, unilateral
N13.722	Vesicoureteral-reflux with reflux nephropathy without hydroureter, bilateral
N13.731	Vesicoureteral-reflux with reflux nephropathy with hydroureter, unilateral
N13.732	Vesicoureteral-reflux with reflux nephropathy with hydroureter, bilateral
N13.8	Other obstructive and reflux uropathy
Q62.0	Congenital hydronephrosis

Ureter

Q62.11	Congenital occlusion of ureteropelvic junction
Q62.12	Congenital occlusion of ureterovesical orifice
Q62.2	Congenital megaureter
Q62.31	Congenital ureterocele, orthotopic
Q62.32	Cecoureterocele
Q62.39	Other obstructive defects of renal pelvis and ureter
Q62.61	Deviation of ureter
Q62.62	Displacement of ureter
Q62.63	Anomalous implantation of ureter
Q62.69	Other malposition of ureter
Q62.7	Congenital vesico-uretero-renal reflux
Q62.8	Other congenital malformations of ureter
S37.12XA	Contusion of ureter, initial encounter
S37.13XA	Laceration of ureter, initial encounter
S37.19XA	Other injury of ureter, initial encounter

AMA: 50770 2014,Jan,11

Relative Value Units/Medicare Edits

Non-Facility RVU	Work	PE	MP	Total
50770	21.22	9.66	2.43	33.31
Facility RVU	Work	PE	MP	Total
50770	21.22	9.66	2.43	33.31

	FUD	Status	MUE	Modifiers				IOM Reference
50770	90	A	1(2)	51	N/A	62*	80	None

* with documentation

Terms To Know

anastomosis. Surgically created connection between ducts, blood vessels, or bowel segments to allow flow from one to the other.

anomaly. Irregularity in the structure or position of an organ or tissue.

benign. Mild or nonmalignant in nature.

congenital. Present at birth, occurring through heredity or an influence during gestation up to the moment of birth.

dissect. Cut apart or separate tissue for surgical purposes or for visual or microscopic study.

ligate. To tie off a blood vessel or duct with a suture or a soft, thin wire (ligature wire).

malignant neoplasm. Any cancerous tumor or lesion exhibiting uncontrolled tissue growth that can progressively invade other parts of the body with its disease-generating cells.

peritoneum. Strong, continuous membrane that forms the lining of the abdominal and pelvic cavity. The parietal peritoneum, or outer layer, is attached to the abdominopelvic walls and the visceral peritoneum, or inner layer, surrounds the organs inside the abdominal cavity.

retroperitoneal. Located behind the peritoneum, the membrane that lines the abdominopelvic walls and forms a covering for the internal organs.

50780-50785

50780	Ureteroneocystostomy; anastomosis of single ureter to bladder
50782	anastomosis of duplicated ureter to bladder
50783	with extensive ureteral tailoring
50785	with vesico-psoas hitch or bladder flap

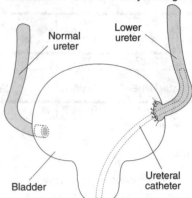

The physician connects the lower ureter and bladder to allow for urinary drainage

Normal ureter

Lower ureter

Bladder

Ureteral catheter

Explanation

The physician connects the lower ureter and bladder to allow for urinary drainage. The physician usually makes an incision in the skin of the abdomen. After dissecting the ureter at the point of disease or obstruction, the physician brings the ureter through a stab incision in the bladder and sutures the ureter to the bladder. To provide support during healing, the physician may insert a catheter into the ureter. The physician inserts a drain tube and performs a layered single ureter to the bladder (50780). Report 50782 if the physician attaches a duplicated ureter to the bladder. Report 50783 if the anastomosis requires extensive ureter reconstruction. Report 50785 if the anastomosis requires suturing the bladder and psoas, or by fashioning a long, elliptical flap from the bladder.

Coding Tips

Note that 50780 and 50785 are unilateral procedures. If performed bilaterally, some payers require that the service be reported twice with modifier 50 appended to the second code while others require identification of the service only once with modifier 50 appended. Check with individual payers. Modifier 50 identifies a procedure performed identically on the opposite side of the body (mirror image). For ureteroneocystostomy combined with plastic reconstruction on the bladder and urethra (cystourethroplasty), see 51820. If the physician performs a ureteroneocystostomy to restore urethral continuity after surgical diversion, see 50830. For ureteroneocystostomy combined with partial removal of the bladder, see 51565.

ICD-10-CM Diagnostic Codes

C66.1	Malignant neoplasm of right ureter ☑
C66.2	Malignant neoplasm of left ureter ☑
C79.19	Secondary malignant neoplasm of other urinary organs
D30.21	Benign neoplasm of right ureter ☑
D30.22	Benign neoplasm of left ureter ☑
D41.11	Neoplasm of uncertain behavior of right renal pelvis ☑
D41.12	Neoplasm of uncertain behavior of left renal pelvis ☑
D41.21	Neoplasm of uncertain behavior of right ureter ☑
D41.22	Neoplasm of uncertain behavior of left ureter ☑

Ureter

D41.8	Neoplasm of uncertain behavior of other specified urinary organs			
D47.Z1	Post-transplant lymphoproliferative disorder (PTLD)			
D47.Z2	Castleman disease			
D49.511	Neoplasm of unspecified behavior of right kidney ☑			
D49.512	Neoplasm of unspecified behavior of left kidney ☑			
D49.59	Neoplasm of unspecified behavior of other genitourinary organ			
N11.1	Chronic obstructive pyelonephritis			
N13.5	Crossing vessel and stricture of ureter without hydronephrosis			
N13.71	Vesicoureteral-reflux without reflux nephropathy			
N13.721	Vesicoureteral-reflux with reflux nephropathy without hydroureter, unilateral			
N13.722	Vesicoureteral-reflux with reflux nephropathy without hydroureter, bilateral			
N13.731	Vesicoureteral-reflux with reflux nephropathy with hydroureter, unilateral			
N13.732	Vesicoureteral-reflux with reflux nephropathy with hydroureter, bilateral			
N13.8	Other obstructive and reflux uropathy			
Q62.0	Congenital hydronephrosis			
Q62.11	Congenital occlusion of ureteropelvic junction			
Q62.12	Congenital occlusion of ureterovesical orifice			
Q62.2	Congenital megaureter			
Q62.31	Congenital ureterocele, orthotopic			
Q62.32	Cecoureterocele			
Q62.39	Other obstructive defects of renal pelvis and ureter			
Q62.5	Duplication of ureter			
Q62.61	Deviation of ureter			
Q62.62	Displacement of ureter			
Q62.63	Anomalous implantation of ureter			
Q62.69	Other malposition of ureter			
Q62.7	Congenital vesico-uretero-renal reflux			
Q62.8	Other congenital malformations of ureter			
Q64.8	Other specified congenital malformations of urinary system			
S37.12XA	Contusion of ureter, initial encounter			
S37.13XA	Laceration of ureter, initial encounter			
S37.19XA	Other injury of ureter, initial encounter			
T86.11	Kidney transplant rejection			
T86.12	Kidney transplant failure			
T86.13	Kidney transplant infection			
T86.19	Other complication of kidney transplant			

AMA: **50780** 2018,Jan,8; 2018,Feb,11; 2017,Jan,8; 2016,Jan,13; 2015,Jan,16; 2014,Jan,11 **50782** 2018,Jan,8; 2017,Jan,8; 2016,Jan,13; 2015,Jan,16; 2014,Jan,11 **50783** 2018,Jan,8; 2017,Jan,8; 2016,Jan,13; 2015,Jan,16; 2014,Jan,11 **50785** 2018,Jan,8; 2017,Jan,8; 2016,Jan,13; 2015,Jan,16; 2014,Jan,11

Relative Value Units/Medicare Edits

Non-Facility RVU	Work	PE	MP	Total
50780	19.95	9.41	2.64	32.0
50782	19.66	9.13	2.25	31.04
50783	20.7	9.49	2.36	32.55
50785	22.23	10.11	2.71	35.05
Facility RVU	**Work**	**PE**	**MP**	**Total**
50780	19.95	9.41	2.64	32.0
50782	19.66	9.13	2.25	31.04
50783	20.7	9.49	2.36	32.55
50785	22.23	10.11	2.71	35.05

	FUD	Status	MUE	Modifiers				IOM Reference
50780	90	A	1(2)	51	50	62*	80	None
50782	90	A	1(2)	51	50	62	80	
50783	90	A	1(2)	51	50	62	80	
50785	90	A	1(2)	51	50	62*	80	

* with documentation

Terms To Know

anastomosis. Surgically created connection between ducts, blood vessels, or bowel segments to allow flow from one to the other.

anomaly. Irregularity in the structure or position of an organ or tissue.

catheter. Flexible tube inserted into an area of the body for introducing or withdrawing fluid.

congenital. Present at birth, occurring through heredity or an influence during gestation up to the moment of birth.

dissect. Cut apart or separate tissue for surgical purposes or for visual or microscopic study.

drain. Device that creates a channel to allow fluid from a cavity, wound, or infected area to exit the body.

malposition. Congenital or acquired condition in which an organ or body part is in an abnormal or uncharacteristic position.

obstruction. Blockage that prevents normal function of the valve or structure.

psoas. Muscles of the loins, the part of the side and back between the ribs and the pelvis.

reconstruction. Recreating, restoring, or rebuilding a body part or organ.

ureteroneocystostomy. Surgical procedure that divides the ureter at a point of disease or obstruction and reconnects it to the bladder to form a new junction with the bladder and allow for urinary drainage and prevent vesicoureteral reflux.

Ureter

CPT © 2020 American Medical Association. All Rights Reserved. ● New ▲ Revised + Add On ★ Telemedicine AMA: CPT Assist [Resequenced] ☑ Laterality © 2020 Optum360, LLC

50800

50800 Ureteroenterostomy, direct anastomosis of ureter to intestine

The physician connects the ureter to a segment of intestine to divert urine flow

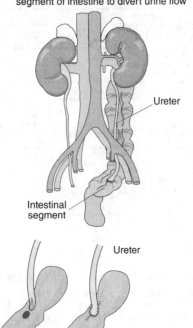

Ureter

Intestinal segment

Ureter

Intestinal segment

Explanation

The physician connects the ureter to a segment of intestine to divert urine flow. To access the ureter and intestine, the physician makes an incision in the skin of the abdomen and cuts the corresponding muscles, fat, and fibrous membranes (fascia). The physician dissects the ureter, makes small incisions in the intestine segment, and surgically connects (anastomosis) the ureter to the intestine. To provide support during healing, the physician may insert a slender tube into the ureter. The physician inserts a drain tube and performs a layered closure.

Coding Tips

This is a unilateral procedure. If performed bilaterally, some payers require that the service be reported twice with modifier 50 appended to the second code while others require identification of the service only once with modifier 50 appended. Check with individual payers. Modifier 50 identifies a procedure performed identically on the opposite side of the body (mirror image). If the physician connects the ureter to a segment of sigmoid colon fashioned into a bladder with an opening in the skin, see 50810. For connection of one ureter to the ureter on the opposite side, see 50770. For anastomosis of the ureter to the bladder, see 50780–50785.

ICD-10-CM Diagnostic Codes

C67.0	Malignant neoplasm of trigone of bladder
C67.1	Malignant neoplasm of dome of bladder
C67.2	Malignant neoplasm of lateral wall of bladder
C67.3	Malignant neoplasm of anterior wall of bladder
C67.4	Malignant neoplasm of posterior wall of bladder
C67.5	Malignant neoplasm of bladder neck
C67.6	Malignant neoplasm of ureteric orifice
C67.8	Malignant neoplasm of overlapping sites of bladder

C79.11	Secondary malignant neoplasm of bladder
C79.19	Secondary malignant neoplasm of other urinary organs
D09.0	Carcinoma in situ of bladder
D41.4	Neoplasm of uncertain behavior of bladder
D49.4	Neoplasm of unspecified behavior of bladder
N21.0	Calculus in bladder
N99.520	Hemorrhage of incontinent external stoma of urinary tract
N99.521	Infection of incontinent external stoma of urinary tract
N99.522	Malfunction of incontinent external stoma of urinary tract
N99.523	Herniation of incontinent stoma of urinary tract
N99.524	Stenosis of incontinent stoma of urinary tract
N99.528	Other complication of incontinent external stoma of urinary tract
N99.530	Hemorrhage of continent stoma of urinary tract
N99.531	Infection of continent stoma of urinary tract
N99.532	Malfunction of continent stoma of urinary tract
N99.533	Herniation of continent stoma of urinary tract
N99.534	Stenosis of continent stoma of urinary tract
N99.538	Other complication of continent stoma of urinary tract
N99.81	Other intraoperative complications of genitourinary system
N99.89	Other postprocedural complications and disorders of genitourinary system
S37.22XA	Contusion of bladder, initial encounter
S37.23XA	Laceration of bladder, initial encounter
S37.29XA	Other injury of bladder, initial encounter

AMA: 50800 2018,Jan,8; 2017,Jan,8; 2016,Jan,13; 2015,Jan,16; 2014,Jan,11

Relative Value Units/Medicare Edits

Non-Facility RVU	Work	PE	MP	Total
50800	16.41	8.34	2.0	26.75
Facility RVU	**Work**	**PE**	**MP**	**Total**
50800	16.41	8.34	2.0	26.75

	FUD	Status	MUE	Modifiers				IOM Reference
50800	90	A	1(2)	51	50	62*	80	None

* with documentation

Terms To Know

anastomosis. Surgically created connection between ducts, blood vessels, or bowel segments to allow flow from one to the other.

calculus. Abnormal, stone-like concretion of calcium, cholesterol, mineral salts, or other substances that forms in any part of the body.

drain. Device that creates a channel to allow fluid from a cavity, wound, or infected area to exit the body.

fascia. Fibrous sheet or band of tissue that envelops organs, muscles, and groupings of muscles.

malignant neoplasm. Any cancerous tumor or lesion exhibiting uncontrolled tissue growth that can progressively invade other parts of the body with its disease-generating cells.

stent. Tube to provide support in a body cavity or lumen.

stricture. Narrowing of an anatomical structure.

Ureter

50810

50810 Ureterosigmoidostomy, with creation of sigmoid bladder and establishment of abdominal or perineal colostomy, including intestine anastomosis

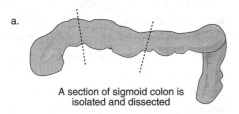

a.

A section of sigmoid colon is isolated and dissected

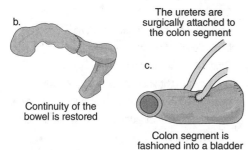

b.

Continuity of the bowel is restored

The ureters are surgically attached to the colon segment

c.

Colon segment is fashioned into a bladder

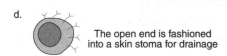

d.

The open end is fashioned into a skin stoma for drainage

Explanation

The physician connects the ureters to a segment of sigmoid colon to create a bladder with an opening to the skin. To access the ureters and sigmoid colon, the physician makes a midline incision in the skin of the abdomen and cuts the corresponding muscles, fat, and fibrous membranes (fascia). After dissecting an isolated segment of sigmoid colon, the physician reconnects (anastomosis) the divided colon to restore bowel continuity. The sigmoid section is closed by sutures on one end. The physician dissects each ureter, makes small incisions in the sigmoid segment, and surgically connects each ureter to the sigmoid segment. To provide support during healing, the physician may insert a slender tube into each ureter. The physician fashions a bladder by closing the proximal end of the sigmoid segment, and brings the distal end through an incision in the skin of the abdomen to establish an opening (colostomy) for intermittent emptying of urine. The physician inserts a drain tube and performs a layered closure.

Coding Tips

If the physician connects the ureter to an intestine segment without creation of a bladder or opening in the skin, see 50800. For anastomosis of ureters to an intestine segment that diverts urine directly through an opening in the skin, see 50815–50820. If the physician reverses the diversion and restores ureter continuity, see 50830. For ureterosigmoidostomy in combination with cystectomy, see 51580–51585.

ICD-10-CM Diagnostic Codes

C67.0	Malignant neoplasm of trigone of bladder
C67.1	Malignant neoplasm of dome of bladder
C67.2	Malignant neoplasm of lateral wall of bladder
C67.3	Malignant neoplasm of anterior wall of bladder
C67.4	Malignant neoplasm of posterior wall of bladder
C67.5	Malignant neoplasm of bladder neck
C67.6	Malignant neoplasm of ureteric orifice
C67.7	Malignant neoplasm of urachus
C67.8	Malignant neoplasm of overlapping sites of bladder
C79.11	Secondary malignant neoplasm of bladder
D09.0	Carcinoma in situ of bladder
D41.4	Neoplasm of uncertain behavior of bladder
N21.0	Calculus in bladder
N30.40	Irradiation cystitis without hematuria
N30.41	Irradiation cystitis with hematuria
N30.80	Other cystitis without hematuria
N30.81	Other cystitis with hematuria
N31.0	Uninhibited neuropathic bladder, not elsewhere classified
N31.1	Reflex neuropathic bladder, not elsewhere classified
N32.0	Bladder-neck obstruction
N32.3	Diverticulum of bladder
N99.520	Hemorrhage of incontinent external stoma of urinary tract
N99.521	Infection of incontinent external stoma of urinary tract
N99.522	Malfunction of incontinent external stoma of urinary tract
N99.528	Other complication of incontinent external stoma of urinary tract
N99.530	Hemorrhage of continent stoma of urinary tract
N99.531	Infection of continent stoma of urinary tract
N99.532	Malfunction of continent stoma of urinary tract
N99.538	Other complication of continent stoma of urinary tract
N99.81	Other intraoperative complications of genitourinary system
N99.89	Other postprocedural complications and disorders of genitourinary system
Q64.11	Supravesical fissure of urinary bladder
Q64.12	Cloacal exstrophy of urinary bladder
Q64.19	Other exstrophy of urinary bladder
Q64.5	Congenital absence of bladder and urethra
Q64.6	Congenital diverticulum of bladder
Q64.79	Other congenital malformations of bladder and urethra
S37.22XA	Contusion of bladder, initial encounter
S37.23XA	Laceration of bladder, initial encounter

AMA: **50810** 2018,Jan,8; 2017,Jan,8; 2016,Jan,13; 2015,Jan,16; 2014,Jan,11

Relative Value Units/Medicare Edits

Non-Facility RVU	Work	PE	MP	Total
50810	22.61	12.7	5.49	40.8
Facility RVU	**Work**	**PE**	**MP**	**Total**
50810	22.61	12.7	5.49	40.8

	FUD	Status	MUE	Modifiers				IOM Reference
50810	90	A	1(3)	51	N/A	62*	80	None

* with documentation

Terms To Know

anastomosis. Surgically created connection between ducts, blood vessels, or bowel segments to allow flow from one to the other.

drain. Device that creates a channel to allow fluid from a cavity, wound, or infected area to exit the body.

CPT © 2020 American Medical Association. All Rights Reserved.   ● New   ▲ Revised   + Add On   ★ Telemedicine   AMA: CPT Assist   [Resequenced]   ☑ Laterality   © 2020 Optum360, LLC

50815-50820

50815 Ureterocolon conduit, including intestine anastomosis
50820 Ureteroileal conduit (ileal bladder), including intestine anastomosis (Bricker operation)

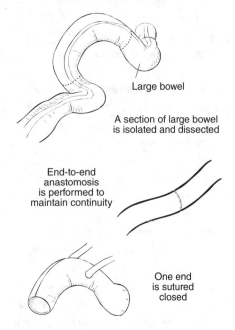

Large bowel

A section of large bowel is isolated and dissected

End-to-end anastomosis is performed to maintain continuity

One end is sutured closed

Ureters are surgically attached to the segment of bowel, which serves as a conduit to divert urine. The open end is fashioned into a skin stoma for drainage

Explanation

The physician connects the ureters to a segment of intestine to divert urine flow through an opening in the skin. To access the ureters and intestine, the physician makes a midline incision in the skin of the abdomen and cuts the corresponding muscles, fat, and fibrous membranes (fascia). After dissecting an isolated segment of intestine, the physician reconnects (anastomosis) the divided intestine to restore bowel continuity. The colon segment is closed by sutures on one end. The physician dissects each ureter, makes small incisions in the intestine segment, and surgically connects each ureter to the colon segment. To provide support during healing, the physician may insert a slender tube into each ureter. The physician closes the proximal end of the intestine segment and brings the distal end through an incision in the skin of the abdomen to establish an opening (stoma) for direct emptying of urine. The physician inserts a drain tube and performs a layered closure. Report 50820 if the physician dissects a segment of ileal colon to divert urine flow.

Coding Tips

Note that 50815 and 50820 are unilateral procedures. If performed bilaterally, some payers require that the service be reported twice with modifier 50 appended to the second code while others require identification of the service only once with modifier 50 appended. Check with individual payers. Modifier 50 identifies a procedure performed identically on the opposite side of the body (mirror image). For ureteroileal conduit in combination with cystectomy, see 51590–51595. If the physician connects the ureter to a segment of sigmoid colon fashioned into a bladder with an opening in the skin, see 50810. For reversal of the diversion and restoration of ureter continuity, see 50830.

ICD-10-CM Diagnostic Codes

C67.0	Malignant neoplasm of trigone of bladder
C67.1	Malignant neoplasm of dome of bladder
C67.2	Malignant neoplasm of lateral wall of bladder
C67.3	Malignant neoplasm of anterior wall of bladder
C67.4	Malignant neoplasm of posterior wall of bladder
C67.5	Malignant neoplasm of bladder neck
C67.6	Malignant neoplasm of ureteric orifice
C67.7	Malignant neoplasm of urachus
C67.8	Malignant neoplasm of overlapping sites of bladder
C79.11	Secondary malignant neoplasm of bladder
D09.0	Carcinoma in situ of bladder
D41.4	Neoplasm of uncertain behavior of bladder
D49.4	Neoplasm of unspecified behavior of bladder
N21.0	Calculus in bladder
N30.40	Irradiation cystitis without hematuria
N30.41	Irradiation cystitis with hematuria
N30.80	Other cystitis without hematuria
N30.81	Other cystitis with hematuria
N31.0	Uninhibited neuropathic bladder, not elsewhere classified
N31.1	Reflex neuropathic bladder, not elsewhere classified
N32.0	Bladder-neck obstruction
N32.3	Diverticulum of bladder
N32.89	Other specified disorders of bladder
Q64.11	Supravesical fissure of urinary bladder
Q64.12	Cloacal exstrophy of urinary bladder
Q64.19	Other exstrophy of urinary bladder
Q64.5	Congenital absence of bladder and urethra
Q64.6	Congenital diverticulum of bladder
Q64.79	Other congenital malformations of bladder and urethra
S37.22XA	Contusion of bladder, initial encounter
S37.23XA	Laceration of bladder, initial encounter
S37.29XA	Other injury of bladder, initial encounter

AMA: **50815** 2018,Jan,8; 2017,Jan,8; 2016,Jan,13; 2015,Jan,16; 2014,Jan,11 **50820** 2018,Jan,8; 2017,Jan,8; 2016,Jan,13; 2015,Jan,16; 2014,Jan,11

Relative Value Units/Medicare Edits

Non-Facility RVU	Work	PE	MP	Total
50815	22.26	10.52	2.56	35.34
50820	24.07	10.96	2.92	37.95
Facility RVU	Work	PE	MP	Total
50815	22.26	10.52	2.56	35.34
50820	24.07	10.96	2.92	37.95

	FUD	Status	MUE	Modifiers				IOM Reference
50815	90	A	1(2)	51	50	62*	80	None
50820	90	A	1(2)	51	50	62*	80	

* with documentation

Terms To Know

Bricker operation. Surgical procedure to connect the ureters to a segment of the ileal colon to divert urine flow through the bowel.

Ureter

50825

50825 Continent diversion, including intestine anastomosis using any segment of small and/or large intestine (Kock pouch or Camey enterocystoplasty)

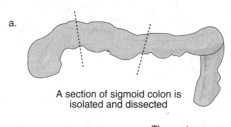

a.

A section of sigmoid colon is isolated and dissected

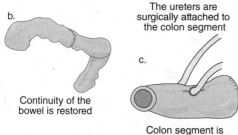

b.

The ureters are surgically attached to the colon segment

Continuity of the bowel is restored

c.

Colon segment is fashioned into a bladder

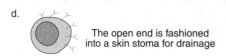

d.

The open end is fashioned into a skin stoma for drainage

Explanation

The physician connects the ureter(s) to loops of intestine fashioned into a reservoir with a valve opening. To access the intestine and ureters, the physician makes a midline incision in the skin of the abdomen and cuts the corresponding muscles, fat, and fibrous membranes (fascia). After dissecting an isolated segment of intestine, the physician reconnects (anastomosis) the divided intestine to restore bowel continuity. After shaping the intestine segment into a pouch, the physician dissects each ureter, makes small incisions in the intestine segment, and surgically connects each ureter to the intestine segment. To provide support during healing, the physician inserts a slender tube into each ureter, and closes the pouch. The physician brings part of the pouch out through an abdominal wall opening, or anastomosis the pouch to the male urethra. The physician inserts a drain tube and performs a layered closure.

Coding Tips

If the physician reconstructs or enlarges the bladder with an intestine segment, without reimplantation of the ureters, see 51960. For creation of an opening between the bladder and skin using the vermiform appendix, see 50845. For connection of the ureters to an intestine segment without creating a bladder or opening to the skin, see 50800. If the physician connects the ureter to a segment of sigmoid colon fashioned into a bladder with an opening in the skin, see 50810. For continent diversion in combination with bladder removal (cystectomy), see 51596.

ICD-10-CM Diagnostic Codes

C67.0	Malignant neoplasm of trigone of bladder
C67.1	Malignant neoplasm of dome of bladder
C67.2	Malignant neoplasm of lateral wall of bladder
C67.3	Malignant neoplasm of anterior wall of bladder
C67.4	Malignant neoplasm of posterior wall of bladder
C67.5	Malignant neoplasm of bladder neck
C67.6	Malignant neoplasm of ureteric orifice
C67.7	Malignant neoplasm of urachus
C67.8	Malignant neoplasm of overlapping sites of bladder
C68.0	Malignant neoplasm of urethra
C79.11	Secondary malignant neoplasm of bladder
D09.0	Carcinoma in situ of bladder
D41.4	Neoplasm of uncertain behavior of bladder
D49.4	Neoplasm of unspecified behavior of bladder
N21.0	Calculus in bladder
N30.40	Irradiation cystitis without hematuria
N30.41	Irradiation cystitis with hematuria
N30.80	Other cystitis without hematuria
N30.81	Other cystitis with hematuria
N31.0	Uninhibited neuropathic bladder, not elsewhere classified
N31.1	Reflex neuropathic bladder, not elsewhere classified
N32.0	Bladder-neck obstruction
N32.3	Diverticulum of bladder
N32.89	Other specified disorders of bladder
Q64.11	Supravesical fissure of urinary bladder
Q64.12	Cloacal exstrophy of urinary bladder
Q64.19	Other exstrophy of urinary bladder
Q64.31	Congenital bladder neck obstruction
Q64.39	Other atresia and stenosis of urethra and bladder neck
Q64.5	Congenital absence of bladder and urethra
Q64.6	Congenital diverticulum of bladder
Q64.79	Other congenital malformations of bladder and urethra
S37.22XA	Contusion of bladder, initial encounter
S37.23XA	Laceration of bladder, initial encounter
S37.29XA	Other injury of bladder, initial encounter

AMA: **50825** 2018,Jan,8; 2017,Jan,8; 2016,Jan,13; 2015,Jan,16; 2014,Jan,11

Relative Value Units/Medicare Edits

Non-Facility RVU	Work	PE	MP	Total
50825	30.68	13.47	3.71	47.86
Facility RVU	**Work**	**PE**	**MP**	**Total**
50825	30.68	13.47	3.71	47.86

	FUD	Status	MUE	Modifiers				IOM Reference
50825	90	A	1(3)	51	N/A	62*	80	None

* with documentation

Terms To Know

anastomosis. Surgically created connection between ducts, blood vessels, or bowel segments to allow flow from one to the other.

congenital. Present at birth, occurring through heredity or an influence during gestation up to the moment of birth.

cystitis. Inflammation of the urinary bladder. Symptoms include dysuria, frequency of urination, urgency, and hematuria.

Ureter

CPT © 2020 American Medical Association. All Rights Reserved. ● New ▲ Revised + Add On ★ Telemedicine AMA: CPT Assist [Resequenced] ☑ Laterality © 2020 Optum360, LLC

50830

50830 Urinary undiversion (eg, taking down of ureteroileal conduit, ureterosigmoidostomy or ureteroenterostomy with ureteroureterostomy or ureteroneocystostomy)

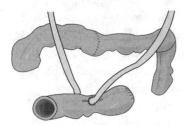

Old diversion and ureter attachments

A previous diversion is surgically addressed to restore urinary continence

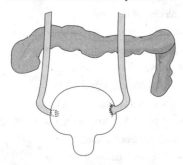

Ureters are reattached to bladder; support tubes and drains are used during healing

Explanation

The physician restores continuity of a ureter through which urine flow was previously diverted. To access the ureter, the physician usually reopens the original ureteral diversion incision and cuts the corresponding muscles, fat, and fibrous membranes (fascia). The physician reverses the diversion by removing sutures connecting the ureter and colon, colon segment, and/or skin. The physician closes the opening in the skin used for the diversionary anastomosis. To restore ureteral continuity, the physician either reconnects the upper and lower ureter segments or connects the ureter to the other ureter (ureteroureterostomy), or reimplants the ureter into the bladder (ureteroneocystostomy). To provide support during healing, the physician inserts a slender tube into the ureter. The physician inserts a drain tube and performs a layered closure.

Coding Tips

For initial connection of the ureter to a segment of sigmoid colon fashioned into a bladder with an opening in the skin (ureterosigmoidostomy), see 50810. For initial ureterocolon or ureteroileal conduit, see 50815–50820.

ICD-10-CM Diagnostic Codes

N31.0	Uninhibited neuropathic bladder, not elsewhere classified
N31.1	Reflex neuropathic bladder, not elsewhere classified
N31.2	Flaccid neuropathic bladder, not elsewhere classified
N31.8	Other neuromuscular dysfunction of bladder
Z43.6	Encounter for attention to other artificial openings of urinary tract

AMA: **50830** 2018,Jan,8; 2017,Jan,8; 2016,Jan,13; 2015,Jan,16; 2014,Jan,11

Relative Value Units/Medicare Edits

Non-Facility RVU	Work	PE	MP	Total
50830	33.77	14.42	3.86	52.05
Facility RVU	**Work**	**PE**	**MP**	**Total**
50830	33.77	14.42	3.86	52.05

	FUD	Status	MUE	Modifiers				IOM Reference
50830	90	A	1(3)	51	N/A	62*	80	None

* with documentation

Terms To Know

anastomosis. Surgically created connection between ducts, blood vessels, or bowel segments to allow flow from one to the other.

colostomy. Artificial surgical opening anywhere along the length of the colon to the skin surface for the diversion of feces.

conduit. Surgically created channel for the passage of fluids.

cystostomy. Formation of an opening through the abdominal wall into the bladder.

drain. Device that creates a channel to allow fluid from a cavity, wound, or infected area to exit the body.

enterostomy. Surgically created opening into the intestine through the abdominal wall.

fascia. Fibrous sheet or band of tissue that envelops organs, muscles, and groupings of muscles.

malignant neoplasm. Any cancerous tumor or lesion exhibiting uncontrolled tissue growth that can progressively invade other parts of the body with its disease-generating cells.

undiversion. Restoration of continuity, flow, or passage through the normal channel.

ureteroneocystostomy. Surgical procedure that divides the ureter at a point of disease or obstruction and reconnects it to the bladder to form a new junction with the bladder and allow for urinary drainage and prevent vesicoureteral reflux.

ureteroureterostomy. Surgical procedure to divide and reconnect a damaged or diseased ureter to bypass a defect or obstruction. The ureter may be anastomosed after excision of the defect or it may be connected to the other ureter in a contralateral ureteroureterostomy.

50840

50840 Replacement of all or part of ureter by intestine segment, including intestine anastomosis

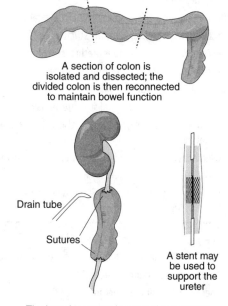

A section of colon is isolated and dissected; the divided colon is then reconnected to maintain bowel function

Drain tube

Sutures

A stent may be used to support the ureter

The bowel segment is sutured to a ureter; stents and drains are employed to enhance healing

Explanation

The physician replaces part or all of the ureter with a segment of intestine. To access the ureters and intestine, the physician makes a midline incision in the skin of the abdomen and cuts the corresponding muscles, fat, and fibrous membranes (fascia). After dissecting an isolated segment of intestine, the physician reconnects (anastomosis) the divided intestine to restore bowel continuity. The physician dissects and removes the diseased or defective ureteral segment, replacing it with the intestine segment. To provide support during healing, the physician may insert a slender tube into the ureter. The physician inserts a drain tube and performs a layered closure.

Coding Tips

This is a unilateral procedure. If performed bilaterally, some payers require that the service be reported twice with modifier 50 appended to the second code while others require identification of the service only once with modifier 50 appended. Check with individual payers. Modifier 50 identifies a procedure performed identically on the opposite side of the body (mirror image). For connection of ureters to an intestine segment without creation of a bladder or percutaneous opening, see 50800. For connection of ureters to a segment of sigmoid colon fashioned into a bladder, see 50810.

ICD-10-CM Diagnostic Codes

C66.1	Malignant neoplasm of right ureter ☑
C66.2	Malignant neoplasm of left ureter ☑
D41.21	Neoplasm of uncertain behavior of right ureter ☑
D41.22	Neoplasm of uncertain behavior of left ureter ☑
G83.4	Cauda equina syndrome
N20.1	Calculus of ureter
N20.2	Calculus of kidney with calculus of ureter
N99.520	Hemorrhage of incontinent external stoma of urinary tract
N99.521	Infection of incontinent external stoma of urinary tract
N99.522	Malfunction of incontinent external stoma of urinary tract
N99.523	Herniation of incontinent stoma of urinary tract
N99.524	Stenosis of incontinent stoma of urinary tract
N99.528	Other complication of incontinent external stoma of urinary tract
N99.530	Hemorrhage of continent stoma of urinary tract
N99.531	Infection of continent stoma of urinary tract
N99.532	Malfunction of continent stoma of urinary tract
N99.533	Herniation of continent stoma of urinary tract
N99.534	Stenosis of continent stoma of urinary tract
N99.538	Other complication of continent stoma of urinary tract
N99.81	Other intraoperative complications of genitourinary system
N99.89	Other postprocedural complications and disorders of genitourinary system
S37.12XA	Contusion of ureter, initial encounter
S37.13XA	Laceration of ureter, initial encounter
S37.19XA	Other injury of ureter, initial encounter

AMA: 50840 2018,Jan,8; 2017,Jan,8; 2016,Jan,13; 2015,Jan,16; 2014,Jan,11

Relative Value Units/Medicare Edits

Non-Facility RVU	Work	PE	MP	Total
50840	22.39	10.56	2.56	35.51
Facility RVU	**Work**	**PE**	**MP**	**Total**
50840	22.39	10.56	2.56	35.51

	FUD	Status	MUE	Modifiers				IOM Reference
50840	90	A	1(2)	51	50	62*	80	None

* with documentation

Terms To Know

anastomosis. Surgically created connection between ducts, blood vessels, or bowel segments to allow flow from one to the other.

calculus. Abnormal, stone-like concretion of calcium, cholesterol, mineral salts, or other substances that forms in any part of the body.

dissection. Separating by cutting tissue or body structures apart.

endometriosis. Aberrant uterine mucosal tissue appearing in areas of the pelvic cavity outside of its normal location, lining the uterus, and inflaming surrounding tissues often resulting in infertility or spontaneous abortion.

fascia. Fibrous sheet or band of tissue that envelops organs, muscles, and groupings of muscles.

malignant neoplasm. Any cancerous tumor or lesion exhibiting uncontrolled tissue growth that can progressively invade other parts of the body with its disease-generating cells.

neurogenic bladder. Dysfunctional bladder due to a central or peripheral nervous system lesion that may result in incontinence, residual urine retention, infection, stones, and renal failure.

stenosis. Narrowing or constriction of a passage.

stent. Tube to provide support in a body cavity or lumen.

stoma. Opening created in the abdominal wall from an internal organ or structure for diversion of waste elimination, drainage, and access.

Ureter

50845

50845 Cutaneous appendico-vesicostomy

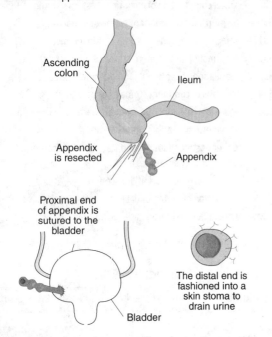

Ascending colon

Ileum

Appendix is resected

Appendix

Proximal end of appendix is sutured to the bladder

The distal end is fashioned into a skin stoma to drain urine

Bladder

Explanation

The physician connects a segment of cecum colon (vermiform appendix) to the bladder to directly divert urine flow through an opening in the skin (cutaneous appendico-vesicostomy). To access the bladder and cecum colon, the physician makes a midline incision in the skin of the abdomen and cuts the corresponding muscles, fat, and fibrous membranes (fascia). After dissecting vermiform appendix, the physician sutures the colon to restore bowel continuity. The physician makes an incision in the bladder and surgically connects the proximal end of the vermiform appendix to the bladder. The physician brings the distal end of vermiform appendix through an incision in the skin of the abdomen to establish an opening (stoma) for direct emptying of urine. The physician inserts a drain tube and performs a layered closure.

Coding Tips

For connection of the bladder alone to the skin (cutaneous vesicostomy), see 51980. For urinary diversion performed with bladder removal, see 51580–51596.

ICD-10-CM Diagnostic Codes

C67.5	Malignant neoplasm of bladder neck
C68.0	Malignant neoplasm of urethra
C68.8	Malignant neoplasm of overlapping sites of urinary organs
D30.3	Benign neoplasm of bladder
D30.4	Benign neoplasm of urethra
D41.3	Neoplasm of uncertain behavior of urethra
D49.511	Neoplasm of unspecified behavior of right kidney ☑
D49.512	Neoplasm of unspecified behavior of left kidney ☑
G83.4	Cauda equina syndrome
N21.1	Calculus in urethra
N31.0	Uninhibited neuropathic bladder, not elsewhere classified
N31.1	Reflex neuropathic bladder, not elsewhere classified
N31.2	Flaccid neuropathic bladder, not elsewhere classified

N31.8	Other neuromuscular dysfunction of bladder
N32.0	Bladder-neck obstruction
N32.81	Overactive bladder
N34.0	Urethral abscess
N34.1	Nonspecific urethritis
N34.2	Other urethritis
N35.010	Post-traumatic urethral stricture, male, meatal ♂
N35.011	Post-traumatic bulbous urethral stricture ♂
N35.012	Post-traumatic membranous urethral stricture ♂
N35.013	Post-traumatic anterior urethral stricture ♂
N35.021	Urethral stricture due to childbirth ♀
N35.028	Other post-traumatic urethral stricture, female ♀
N35.111	Postinfective urethral stricture, not elsewhere classified, male, meatal ♂
N35.112	Postinfective bulbous urethral stricture, not elsewhere classified, male ♂
N35.113	Postinfective membranous urethral stricture, not elsewhere classified, male ♂
N35.114	Postinfective anterior urethral stricture, not elsewhere classified, male ♂
N35.12	Postinfective urethral stricture, not elsewhere classified, female ♀
N35.811	Other urethral stricture, male, meatal ♂
N35.812	Other urethral bulbous stricture, male ♂
N35.813	Other membranous urethral stricture, male ♂
N35.814	Other anterior urethral stricture, male ♂
N36.0	Urethral fistula
N36.1	Urethral diverticulum
N36.8	Other specified disorders of urethra
N99.110	Postprocedural urethral stricture, male, meatal ♂
N99.111	Postprocedural bulbous urethral stricture, male ♂
N99.112	Postprocedural membranous urethral stricture, male ♂
N99.113	Postprocedural anterior bulbous urethral stricture, male ♂
N99.115	Postprocedural fossa navicularis urethral stricture ♂
N99.12	Postprocedural urethral stricture, female ♀
Q64.0	Epispadias ♂
Q64.12	Cloacal exstrophy of urinary bladder
Q64.19	Other exstrophy of urinary bladder
Q64.2	Congenital posterior urethral valves
Q64.31	Congenital bladder neck obstruction
Q64.32	Congenital stricture of urethra
Q64.33	Congenital stricture of urinary meatus

AMA: **50845** 2014,Jan,11

Relative Value Units/Medicare Edits

Non-Facility RVU	Work	PE	MP	Total
50845	22.46	11.09	2.58	36.13
Facility RVU	**Work**	**PE**	**MP**	**Total**
50845	22.46	11.09	2.58	36.13

	FUD	Status	MUE	Modifiers				IOM Reference
50845	90	A	1(2)	51	N/A	62*	80	None

* with documentation

50860

50860 Ureterostomy, transplantation of ureter to skin

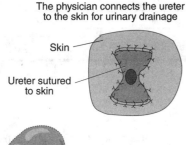

The physician connects the ureter to the skin for urinary drainage

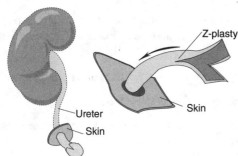

Explanation

The physician connects the ureter to the skin for urinary drainage. To access the ureter, the physician makes a midline incision in the skin of the abdomen and cuts the corresponding muscles, fat, and fibrous membranes (fascia). The physician ligates the distal ureter and brings the proximal end to the skin. The physician splits the end of the ureter and sutures it to the skin with a double Z-plasty to prevent the ureter from narrowing. To provide support during healing, the physician may insert a slender tube into the ureter. The physician inserts a drain tube and performs a layered closure.

Coding Tips

This is a unilateral procedure. If performed bilaterally, some payers require that the service be reported twice with modifier 50 appended to the second code while others require identification of the service only once with modifier 50 appended. Check with individual payers. Modifier 50 identifies a procedure performed identically on the opposite side of the body (mirror image). Ureteroureterostomy is reported with 50760. For transureteroureterostomy (connection of one ureter to the ureter on the opposite side), see 50770. If a urinary diversion is performed with bladder removal (cystectomy), see 51580–51596.

ICD-10-CM Diagnostic Codes

C67.0	Malignant neoplasm of trigone of bladder
C67.1	Malignant neoplasm of dome of bladder
C67.2	Malignant neoplasm of lateral wall of bladder
C67.3	Malignant neoplasm of anterior wall of bladder
C67.4	Malignant neoplasm of posterior wall of bladder
C67.5	Malignant neoplasm of bladder neck
C67.6	Malignant neoplasm of ureteric orifice
C67.7	Malignant neoplasm of urachus
C67.8	Malignant neoplasm of overlapping sites of bladder
C68.0	Malignant neoplasm of urethra
C79.11	Secondary malignant neoplasm of bladder
D09.0	Carcinoma in situ of bladder
D41.4	Neoplasm of uncertain behavior of bladder
D49.4	Neoplasm of unspecified behavior of bladder
G83.4	Cauda equina syndrome
N11.1	Chronic obstructive pyelonephritis
N13.8	Other obstructive and reflux uropathy
N20.1	Calculus of ureter
N21.0	Calculus in bladder
N30.40	Irradiation cystitis without hematuria
N30.41	Irradiation cystitis with hematuria
N30.80	Other cystitis without hematuria
N30.81	Other cystitis with hematuria
N31.0	Uninhibited neuropathic bladder, not elsewhere classified
N31.1	Reflex neuropathic bladder, not elsewhere classified
N31.2	Flaccid neuropathic bladder, not elsewhere classified
N31.8	Other neuromuscular dysfunction of bladder
N32.0	Bladder-neck obstruction
N32.3	Diverticulum of bladder
N32.89	Other specified disorders of bladder
Q62.0	Congenital hydronephrosis
Q62.11	Congenital occlusion of ureteropelvic junction
Q62.12	Congenital occlusion of ureterovesical orifice
Q62.2	Congenital megaureter
Q62.39	Other obstructive defects of renal pelvis and ureter
Q64.2	Congenital posterior urethral valves
Q64.31	Congenital bladder neck obstruction
Q64.32	Congenital stricture of urethra
Q64.33	Congenital stricture of urinary meatus
Q64.39	Other atresia and stenosis of urethra and bladder neck
Q64.5	Congenital absence of bladder and urethra
Q64.6	Congenital diverticulum of bladder
Q64.79	Other congenital malformations of bladder and urethra
S37.22XA	Contusion of bladder, initial encounter
S37.23XA	Laceration of bladder, initial encounter
S37.29XA	Other injury of bladder, initial encounter
S37.32XA	Contusion of urethra, initial encounter
S37.33XA	Laceration of urethra, initial encounter
S37.39XA	Other injury of urethra, initial encounter

AMA: **50860** 2014,Jan,11

Relative Value Units/Medicare Edits

Non-Facility RVU	Work	PE	MP	Total
50860	17.08	8.26	1.96	27.3
Facility RVU	**Work**	**PE**	**MP**	**Total**
50860	17.08	8.26	1.96	27.3

	FUD	Status	MUE	Modifiers				IOM Reference
50860	90	A	1(2)	51	50	62*	80	None

* with documentation

CPT © 2020 American Medical Association. All Rights Reserved.   ● New   ▲ Revised   + Add On   ★ Telemedicine   AMA: CPT Assist   [Resequenced]   ☑ Laterality   © 2020 Optum360, LLC

50900

50900   Ureterorrhaphy, suture of ureter (separate procedure)

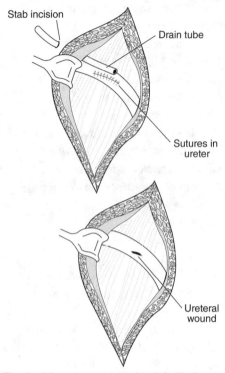

The physician sutures a wound or defect in the ureter

Explanation

The physician sutures a wound or defect in the ureter. To access the ureter, the physician makes an incision in the skin and cuts the muscles, fat, and fibrous membranes (fascia) overlying the ureter. For the upper or middle third of the ureter, the physician usually makes an incision in the skin of the flank; to access the lower third of the ureter, the physician usually makes a curved lower quadrant incision. The physician uses sutures to close or surgically fixate a ureteral wound or defect. To provide support during healing, the physician may insert a slender tube into the ureter. The physician inserts a drain tube and performs a layered closure.

Coding Tips

This separate procedure by definition is usually a component of a more complex service and is not identified separately. When performed alone or with other unrelated procedures/ services it may be reported. If performed alone, list the code; if performed with other procedures/services, list the code and append modifier 59 or an X{EPSU} modifier. If the physician uses sutures to close an opening (fistula) between the ureter and skin or the ureter and an organ of the urogenital, digestive, respiratory, or endocrine system, see 50920–50930. Report ureteroplasty and ureterolysis with 50700–50860.

ICD-10-CM Diagnostic Codes

S37.12XA   Contusion of ureter, initial encounter
S37.13XA   Laceration of ureter, initial encounter
S37.19XA   Other injury of ureter, initial encounter

AMA: 50900 2014,Jan,11

Relative Value Units/Medicare Edits

Non-Facility RVU	Work	PE	MP	Total
50900	15.04	7.57	1.7	24.31
Facility RVU	**Work**	**PE**	**MP**	**Total**
50900	15.04	7.57	1.7	24.31

	FUD	Status	MUE	Modifiers				IOM Reference
50900	90	A	1(3)	51	50	62*	80	None

* with documentation

Terms To Know

absorbable sutures. Strands used for suture or repair of tissue prepared from collagen or a synthetic polymer and capable of being absorbed by tissue over time.

closure. Repairing an incision or wound by suture or other means.

defect. Imperfection, flaw, or absence.

drain. Device that creates a channel to allow fluid from a cavity, wound, or infected area to exit the body.

fascia. Fibrous sheet or band of tissue that envelops organs, muscles, and groupings of muscles.

fixate. Hold, secure, or fasten in position.

flank. Part of the body found between the posterior ribs and the uppermost crest of the ilium, or the lateral side of the hip, thigh, and buttock.

laceration. Tearing injury; a torn, ragged-edged wound.

nonabsorbable sutures. Strands of natural or synthetic material that resist absorption into living tissue and are removed once healing is under way. Nonabsorbable sutures are commonly used to close skin wounds and repair tendons or collagenous tissue. Examples include surgical silk, surgical cotton, linen, stainless steel, surgical nylon, polyester fiber, polybutester (Novofil), polyethylene (Dermalene), and polypropylene (Prolene, Surilene).

perforation. Hole in an object, organ, or tissue, or the act of punching or boring holes through a part.

puncture. Creating a hole.

stent. Tube to provide support in a body cavity or lumen.

tube. Long, hollow cylindrical instrument or body structure.

ureterorrhaphy. Surgical repair using sutures to close an open wound or injury of the ureter.

wound. Injury to living tissue often involving a cut or break in the skin.

Ureter

50920

50920   Closure of ureterocutaneous fistula

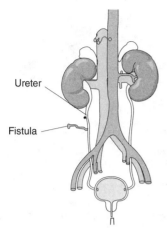

The physician closes a fistula
between the ureter and the skin

Explanation

The physician closes an abnormal opening (fistula) between the skin and the ureter (ureterocutaneous). After excising the fistula, the physician sutures the clean percutaneous tissues together to create a smooth surface.

Coding Tips

For take down of a ureteroileal conduit (50820) or ureterosigmoidostomy with colostomy (50810), see 50830. For closure of an abnormal opening between the ureter and an organ of the digestive, respiratory, urogenital, or endocrine system, see 50930.

ICD-10-CM Diagnostic Codes

N28.89   Other specified disorders of kidney and ureter

AMA: **50920** 2014,Jan,11

Relative Value Units/Medicare Edits

Non-Facility RVU	Work	PE	MP	Total
50920	15.81	7.82	1.8	25.43
Facility RVU	Work	PE	MP	Total
50920	15.81	7.82	1.8	25.43

	FUD	Status	MUE	Modifiers				IOM Reference
50920	90	A	2(3)	51	N/A	62*	80	None

* with documentation

Terms To Know

cutaneous. Relating to the skin.

fistula. Abnormal tube-like passage between two body cavities or organs or from an organ to the outside surface.

percutaneous. Through the skin.

tissue. Group of similar cells with a similar function that form definite structures and organs. Tissue types include epithelial tissue, muscle tissue, connective tissue, and nervous tissue.

50930

50930   Closure of ureterovisceral fistula (including visceral repair)

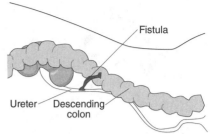

The physician closes a fistula between the ureter
and an organ of the digestive, respiratory,
urogenital, or endocrine system

Explanation

The physician closes an abnormal opening (fistula) between the ureter and an organ of the digestive, respiratory, urogenital, or endocrine system. To access the ureter, the physician makes a midline incision in the skin of the abdomen and cuts the corresponding muscles, fat, and fibrous membranes (fascia). After excising the fistula, the physician sutures the clean tissues together to create a smooth surface. The physician places a drain tube, bringing it out through a separate stab incision in the skin, and performs a layered closure.

Coding Tips

For closure of an abnormal opening between the ureter and the skin, see 50920.

ICD-10-CM Diagnostic Codes

N28.89   Other specified disorders of kidney and ureter

AMA: **50930** 2014,Jan,11

Relative Value Units/Medicare Edits

Non-Facility RVU	Work	PE	MP	Total
50930	20.19	9.31	2.33	31.83
Facility RVU	Work	PE	MP	Total
50930	20.19	9.31	2.33	31.83

	FUD	Status	MUE	Modifiers				IOM Reference
50930	90	A	2(3)	51	N/A	62*	80	None

* with documentation

Terms To Know

drain. Device that creates a channel to allow fluid from a cavity, wound, or infected area to exit the body.

fascia. Fibrous sheet or band of tissue that envelops organs, muscles, and groupings of muscles.

fistula. Abnormal tube-like passage between two body cavities or organs or from an organ to the outside surface.

viscera. Large interior organs enclosed within a cavity, generally referring to the abdominal organs.

Ureter

50940

50940   Deligation of ureter

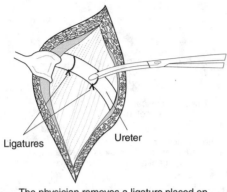

The physician removes a ligature placed on the ureter during a previous operative session

Explanation

The physician removes a thread, wire, or constricting band (ligature) placed on the ureter during a previous operative session. To access the ureter, the physician usually reopens the incision used for the previous operative session. After removing the ligature(s) from the ureter, the physician places a drain tube, bringing it out through a separate stab incision in the skin, and performs a layered closure.

Coding Tips

For plastic repair on the ureter (ureteroplasty), see 50700. For removal of the ureter from surrounding adhesions (ureterolysis), see 50715–50725.

ICD-10-CM Diagnostic Codes

Z48.02   Encounter for removal of sutures
Z48.89   Encounter for other specified surgical aftercare

AMA: 50940 2014,Jan,11

Relative Value Units/Medicare Edits

Non-Facility RVU	Work	PE	MP	Total
50940	15.93	7.86	1.82	25.61
Facility RVU	Work	PE	MP	Total
50940	15.93	7.86	1.82	25.61

	FUD	Status	MUE	Modifiers				IOM Reference
50940	90	A	1(2)	51	50	62*	80	None

* with documentation

Terms To Know

closure. Repairing an incision or wound by suture or other means.

deligation. Closure by tying up; sutures, ligatures.

drain. Device that creates a channel to allow fluid from a cavity, wound, or infected area to exit the body.

50945

50945   Laparoscopy, surgical; ureterolithotomy

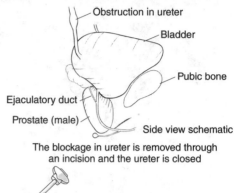

The blockage in ureter is removed through an incision and the ureter is closed

The procedures are performed laparoscopically

Explanation

The physician performs a laparoscopic surgical removal of a stone (calculus) lodged in the ureter (ureterolithotomy). In an abdominal approach, the physician creates an umbilical port by placing a trocar at the level of the umbilicus. The abdominal wall is insufflated. The laparoscope is placed through the umbilical port and additional trocars are placed into the abdominal cavity. In the back (flank) approach, the trocar is placed at the back proximate to the retroperitoneal space near the kidney with additional ports placed nearby for appropriate access to the operative site. The physician uses the laparoscope fitted with a fiberoptic camera and/or an operating instrument to isolate the calculus and remove it through an incision in the ureter. The ureter is surgically closed. The small abdominal or back (flank) incisions are closed with staples or sutures.

Coding Tips

Surgical laparoscopy always includes diagnostic laparoscopy; the diagnostic laparoscopy should not be reported separately. For open ureterolithotomy, see 50610–50630. For open transvesical ureterolithotomy, see 51060. For cystotomy with stone calculus basket extraction of a ureteral calculus, see 51065. For endoscopic extraction or manipulation of a ureteral calculus, see 50961, 50980, 52320–52330, 52352, and 52353.

ICD-10-CM Diagnostic Codes

N20.1   Calculus of ureter
N20.2   Calculus of kidney with calculus of ureter

AMA: 50945 2018,Jan,8; 2017,Jan,8; 2016,Jan,13; 2015,Jan,16; 2014,Jan,11

Relative Value Units/Medicare Edits

Non-Facility RVU	Work	PE	MP	Total
50945	17.97	8.05	2.05	28.07
Facility RVU	Work	PE	MP	Total
50945	17.97	8.05	2.05	28.07

	FUD	Status	MUE	Modifiers				IOM Reference
50945	90	A	1(2)	51	50	62*	80	None

* with documentation

Ureter

50947-50948

50947 Laparoscopy, surgical; ureteroneocystostomy with cystoscopy and ureteral stent placement
50948 ureteroneocystostomy without cystoscopy and ureteral stent placement

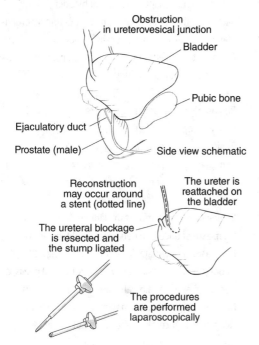

Obstruction in ureterovesical junction

Bladder

Pubic bone

Ejaculatory duct

Prostate (male)

Side view schematic

Reconstruction may occur around a stent (dotted line)

The ureter is reattached on the bladder

The ureteral blockage is resected and the stump ligated

The procedures are performed laparoscopically

Explanation

The physician repositions the ureter on the bladder (due to an obstruction of the ureterovesical junction), using a laparoscopic approach. A stent may be placed with a cystoscope. In both procedures the physician makes a 1 centimeter periumbilical incision and inserts a trocar. The abdominal cavity is insufflated with carbon dioxide. A fiberoptic laparoscope fitted with a camera and light source is inserted through the trocar. Other incisions (ports) are made in the abdomen to allow other instruments or an additional light source to be passed into the abdomen. The physician manipulates the tools so the ureter and bladder can be observed through the laparoscope. The physician transects the ureter above the point of obstruction, brings the ureter through a stab incision in the bladder, and sutures the ureter to the new site on the bladder. In 50947, the physician inserts a cystoscope and places a stent in the repositioned ureter to provide support of the ureter. In 50948, the ureter is repositioned without cystoscopy or stent placement. The instruments are removed. The incisions are closed with staples or suture.

Coding Tips

Surgical laparoscopy always includes diagnostic laparoscopy; the diagnostic laparoscopy should not be reported separately. For ureteroneocystostomy, via an open approach, see 50780–50785.

ICD-10-CM Diagnostic Codes

C66.1	Malignant neoplasm of right ureter ☑
C66.2	Malignant neoplasm of left ureter ☑
D30.21	Benign neoplasm of right ureter ☑
D30.22	Benign neoplasm of left ureter ☑
D41.11	Neoplasm of uncertain behavior of right renal pelvis ☑
D41.12	Neoplasm of uncertain behavior of left renal pelvis ☑
D41.21	Neoplasm of uncertain behavior of right ureter ☑
D41.22	Neoplasm of uncertain behavior of left ureter ☑
D41.8	Neoplasm of uncertain behavior of other specified urinary organs
D47.Z1	Post-transplant lymphoproliferative disorder (PTLD)
N11.1	Chronic obstructive pyelonephritis
N13.5	Crossing vessel and stricture of ureter without hydronephrosis
N13.71	Vesicoureteral-reflux without reflux nephropathy
N13.721	Vesicoureteral-reflux with reflux nephropathy without hydroureter, unilateral
N13.722	Vesicoureteral-reflux with reflux nephropathy without hydroureter, bilateral
N13.731	Vesicoureteral-reflux with reflux nephropathy with hydroureter, unilateral
N13.732	Vesicoureteral-reflux with reflux nephropathy with hydroureter, bilateral
N13.8	Other obstructive and reflux uropathy
Q62.0	Congenital hydronephrosis
Q62.11	Congenital occlusion of ureteropelvic junction
Q62.12	Congenital occlusion of ureterovesical orifice
Q62.2	Congenital megaureter
Q62.31	Congenital ureterocele, orthotopic
Q62.32	Cecoureterocele
Q62.5	Duplication of ureter
Q62.61	Deviation of ureter
Q62.62	Displacement of ureter
Q62.63	Anomalous implantation of ureter
Q62.69	Other malposition of ureter
Q62.7	Congenital vesico-uretero-renal reflux
Q62.8	Other congenital malformations of ureter
Q64.8	Other specified congenital malformations of urinary system
S37.12XA	Contusion of ureter, initial encounter
S37.13XA	Laceration of ureter, initial encounter
T86.11	Kidney transplant rejection
T86.12	Kidney transplant failure
T86.13	Kidney transplant infection
T86.19	Other complication of kidney transplant

AMA: **50947** 2018,Jan,8; 2017,Jan,8; 2016,Jan,13; 2015,Jan,16; 2014,Jan,11
50948 2018,Jan,8; 2017,Jan,8; 2016,Jan,13; 2015,Jan,16; 2014,Jan,11

Relative Value Units/Medicare Edits

Non-Facility RVU	Work	PE	MP	Total
50947	25.78	11.27	3.0	40.05
50948	23.82	10.23	2.74	36.79
Facility RVU	**Work**	**PE**	**MP**	**Total**
50947	25.78	11.27	3.0	40.05
50948	23.82	10.23	2.74	36.79

	FUD	Status	MUE	Modifiers				IOM Reference
50947	90	A	1(2)	51	50	62*	80	None
50948	90	A	1(2)	51	50	62*	80	

* with documentation

Ureter

50951-50955

50951 Ureteral endoscopy through established ureterostomy, with or without irrigation, instillation, or ureteropyelography, exclusive of radiologic service;

50953 with ureteral catheterization, with or without dilation of ureter

50955 with biopsy

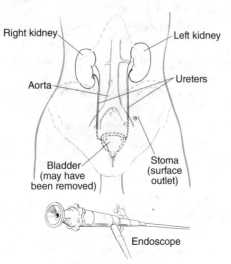

Right kidney

Left kidney

Aorta

Ureters

Bladder (may have been removed)

Stoma (surface outlet)

Endoscope

An endoscope is inserted through an existing ureterostomy. A variety of procedures may be performed

Explanation

The physician examines renal and ureteral structures with an endoscope passed through an established opening between the skin and ureter (ureterostomy). In 50951, the physician inserts a guidewire, removes the ureterostomy tube, and passes the endoscope into the kidney or renal pelvis. The physician may flush (irrigate) or introduce by drops (instillate) a saline solution to better view the renal and ureteral structures, and/or may introduce contrast medium for radiologic study of the renal pelvis and ureter (ureteropyelogram). In 50953, the physician passes a thin tube through the endoscope into the ureter, and may insert a balloon catheter to dilate a ureteral constriction. In, 50955, the physician passes a cutting instrument through the endoscope into the suspect tissue and takes a biopsy specimen. The physician removes the endoscope and guidewire and reinserts the ureterostomy tube or allows the passageway to seal on its own.

Coding Tips

Local anesthesia is included in these services. However, these procedures may be performed under general anesthesia, depending on the age and/or condition of the patient. Report image-guided dilation of ureter, without endoscopic guidance, with 50706. For percutaneous ureteral endoscopy (through an established ureterostomy), with fulguration and/or incision with or without biopsy, see 50957; removal of a foreign body or calculus, see 50961. For open ureteral endoscopic procedures (through ureterotomy), see 50970–50980. Supplies used when providing these procedures may be reported with the appropriate HCPCS Level II code. Check with the specific payer to determine coverage.

ICD-10-CM Diagnostic Codes

C64.1	Malignant neoplasm of right kidney, except renal pelvis ☑
C64.2	Malignant neoplasm of left kidney, except renal pelvis ☑
C65.1	Malignant neoplasm of right renal pelvis ☑
C65.2	Malignant neoplasm of left renal pelvis ☑
C66.1	Malignant neoplasm of right ureter ☑
C66.2	Malignant neoplasm of left ureter ☑
C67.6	Malignant neoplasm of ureteric orifice
C79.01	Secondary malignant neoplasm of right kidney and renal pelvis ☑
C79.02	Secondary malignant neoplasm of left kidney and renal pelvis ☑
C79.11	Secondary malignant neoplasm of bladder
C79.19	Secondary malignant neoplasm of other urinary organs
C7A.093	Malignant carcinoid tumor of the kidney
C80.2	Malignant neoplasm associated with transplanted organ
D09.0	Carcinoma in situ of bladder
D09.19	Carcinoma in situ of other urinary organs
D30.01	Benign neoplasm of right kidney ☑
D30.02	Benign neoplasm of left kidney ☑
D30.11	Benign neoplasm of right renal pelvis ☑
D30.12	Benign neoplasm of left renal pelvis ☑
D30.21	Benign neoplasm of right ureter ☑
D30.22	Benign neoplasm of left ureter ☑
D3A.093	Benign carcinoid tumor of the kidney
D41.01	Neoplasm of uncertain behavior of right kidney ☑
D41.02	Neoplasm of uncertain behavior of left kidney ☑
D41.11	Neoplasm of uncertain behavior of right renal pelvis ☑
D41.12	Neoplasm of uncertain behavior of left renal pelvis ☑
D41.21	Neoplasm of uncertain behavior of right ureter ☑
D41.22	Neoplasm of uncertain behavior of left ureter ☑
D41.4	Neoplasm of uncertain behavior of bladder
D49.511	Neoplasm of unspecified behavior of right kidney ☑
D49.512	Neoplasm of unspecified behavior of left kidney ☑
D49.59	Neoplasm of unspecified behavior of other genitourinary organ
N11.1	Chronic obstructive pyelonephritis
N13.0	Hydronephrosis with ureteropelvic junction obstruction
N13.1	Hydronephrosis with ureteral stricture, not elsewhere classified
N13.2	Hydronephrosis with renal and ureteral calculous obstruction
N13.39	Other hydronephrosis
N13.4	Hydroureter
N13.5	Crossing vessel and stricture of ureter without hydronephrosis
N13.8	Other obstructive and reflux uropathy
N15.1	Renal and perinephric abscess
N20.0	Calculus of kidney
N20.1	Calculus of ureter
N20.2	Calculus of kidney with calculus of ureter
N25.81	Secondary hyperparathyroidism of renal origin
N28.0	Ischemia and infarction of kidney
N28.1	Cyst of kidney, acquired
N28.81	Hypertrophy of kidney
N28.82	Megaloureter
N28.83	Nephroptosis
N28.89	Other specified disorders of kidney and ureter
Q61.01	Congenital single renal cyst
Q61.02	Congenital multiple renal cysts
Q61.19	Other polycystic kidney, infantile type
Q61.2	Polycystic kidney, adult type
Q61.4	Renal dysplasia

Ureter

Q61.5	Medullary cystic kidney
Q61.8	Other cystic kidney diseases
Q62.0	Congenital hydronephrosis
Q62.11	Congenital occlusion of ureteropelvic junction
Q62.12	Congenital occlusion of ureterovesical orifice
Q62.2	Congenital megaureter
Q62.31	Congenital ureterocele, orthotopic
Q62.32	Cecoureterocele
Q62.39	Other obstructive defects of renal pelvis and ureter

AMA: 50951 2018,Jan,8; 2017,Jan,8; 2016,Jan,13; 2015,Jan,16; 2014,Jan,11
50953 2018,Jan,8; 2017,Jan,8; 2016,Jan,13; 2016,Jan,3; 2015,Jan,16; 2014,Jan,11
50955 2018,Jan,8; 2017,Jan,8; 2016,Jan,13; 2016,Jan,3; 2015,Jan,16; 2014,Jan,11

Relative Value Units/Medicare Edits

Non-Facility RVU	Work	PE	MP	Total
50951	5.83	4.36	0.65	10.84
50953	6.23	4.56	0.7	11.49
50955	6.74	4.76	0.78	12.28
Facility RVU	Work	PE	MP	Total
50951	5.83	2.35	0.65	8.83
50953	6.23	2.48	0.7	9.41
50955	6.74	2.66	0.78	10.18

	FUD	Status	MUE	Modifiers				IOM Reference
50951	0	A	1(3)	51	50	N/A	80*	None
50953	0	A	1(3)	51	50	N/A	80*	
50955	0	A	1(2)	51	50	N/A	80*	

* with documentation

Terms To Know

balloon catheter. Any catheter equipped with an inflatable balloon at the end to hold it in place in a body cavity or to be used for dilation of a vessel lumen.

biopsy. Tissue or fluid removed for diagnostic purposes through analysis of the cells in the biopsy material.

catheterization. Use or insertion of a tubular device into a duct, blood vessel, hollow organ, or body cavity for injecting or withdrawing fluids for diagnostic or therapeutic purposes.

dilation. Artificial increase in the diameter of an opening or lumen made by medication or by instrumentation.

guidewire. Flexible metal instrument designed to lead another instrument in its proper course.

hydroureter. Abnormal enlargement or distension of the ureter with water or urine caused by an obstruction.

irrigation. To wash out or cleanse a body cavity, wound, or tissue with water or other fluid.

specimen. Tissue cells or sample of fluid taken for analysis, pathologic examination, and diagnosis.

50957-50961

50957 Ureteral endoscopy through established ureterostomy, with or without irrigation, instillation, or ureteropyelography, exclusive of radiologic service; with fulguration and/or incision, with or without biopsy

50961 with removal of foreign body or calculus

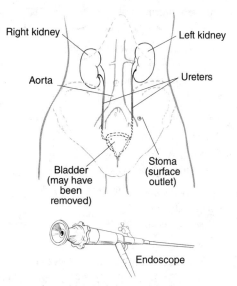

An endoscope is inserted through an existing ureterostomy. A variety of procedures may be performed

Explanation

The physician examines renal and ureteral structures with an endoscope passed through an established opening between the skin and ureter (ureterostomy). The physician inserts a guidewire, removes the ureterostomy tube, and passes the endoscope into the kidney or renal pelvis. The physician may flush (irrigate) or introduce by drops (instillate) a saline solution to better view the renal and ureteral structures, and/or may introduce contrast medium for radiologic study of the renal pelvis and ureter (ureteropyelogram). In 50957, the physician passes through the endoscope an instrument that destroys lesions by electric current or incision. The physician may insert an instrument to biopsy renal tissue. In 50961, the physician passes an instrument through the endoscope to remove a foreign body or calculus. The physician removes the endoscope and guidewire and reinserts the ureterostomy tube or allows the passageway to seal on its own.

Coding Tips

For percutaneous ureteral endoscopy (through an established ureterostomy), with examination alone, see 50951; with ureteral catheterization, with or without dilation of the ureter, see 50953; with biopsy, see 50955. For open ureteral endoscopic procedures (through ureterotomy), see 50970–50980. Supplies used when providing these procedures may be reported with the appropriate HCPCS Level II code. Check with the specific payer to determine coverage.

ICD-10-CM Diagnostic Codes

C66.1	Malignant neoplasm of right ureter ☑
C66.2	Malignant neoplasm of left ureter ☑
C67.6	Malignant neoplasm of ureteric orifice
C79.11	Secondary malignant neoplasm of bladder
C79.19	Secondary malignant neoplasm of other urinary organs

Ureter

D09.0	Carcinoma in situ of bladder
D09.19	Carcinoma in situ of other urinary organs
D30.21	Benign neoplasm of right ureter ☑
D30.22	Benign neoplasm of left ureter ☑
D41.21	Neoplasm of uncertain behavior of right ureter ☑
D41.22	Neoplasm of uncertain behavior of left ureter ☑
D41.4	Neoplasm of uncertain behavior of bladder
N11.1	Chronic obstructive pyelonephritis
N13.5	Crossing vessel and stricture of ureter without hydronephrosis
N13.8	Other obstructive and reflux uropathy
N20.1	Calculus of ureter
N20.2	Calculus of kidney with calculus of ureter
N25.81	Secondary hyperparathyroidism of renal origin
N28.82	Megaloureter
N28.89	Other specified disorders of kidney and ureter
Q62.0	Congenital hydronephrosis
Q62.11	Congenital occlusion of ureteropelvic junction
Q62.12	Congenital occlusion of ureterovesical orifice
Q62.2	Congenital megaureter
Q62.31	Congenital ureterocele, orthotopic
Q62.32	Cecoureterocele
Q62.39	Other obstructive defects of renal pelvis and ureter
T19.8XXA	Foreign body in other parts of genitourinary tract, initial encounter
T81.510A	Adhesions due to foreign body accidentally left in body following surgical operation, initial encounter
T81.512A	Adhesions due to foreign body accidentally left in body following kidney dialysis, initial encounter
T81.514A	Adhesions due to foreign body accidentally left in body following endoscopic examination, initial encounter
T81.516A	Adhesions due to foreign body accidentally left in body following aspiration, puncture or other catheterization, initial encounter
T81.517A	Adhesions due to foreign body accidentally left in body following removal of catheter or packing, initial encounter
T81.518A	Adhesions due to foreign body accidentally left in body following other procedure, initial encounter
T81.520A	Obstruction due to foreign body accidentally left in body following surgical operation, initial encounter
T81.522A	Obstruction due to foreign body accidentally left in body following kidney dialysis, initial encounter
T81.524A	Obstruction due to foreign body accidentally left in body following endoscopic examination, initial encounter
T81.526A	Obstruction due to foreign body accidentally left in body following aspiration, puncture or other catheterization, initial encounter
T81.527A	Obstruction due to foreign body accidentally left in body following removal of catheter or packing, initial encounter
T81.528A	Obstruction due to foreign body accidentally left in body following other procedure, initial encounter
T81.530A	Perforation due to foreign body accidentally left in body following surgical operation, initial encounter
T81.532A	Perforation due to foreign body accidentally left in body following kidney dialysis, initial encounter
T81.534A	Perforation due to foreign body accidentally left in body following endoscopic examination, initial encounter

T81.536A	Perforation due to foreign body accidentally left in body following aspiration, puncture or other catheterization, initial encounter
T81.537A	Perforation due to foreign body accidentally left in body following removal of catheter or packing, initial encounter
T81.538A	Perforation due to foreign body accidentally left in body following other procedure, initial encounter
T81.590A	Other complications of foreign body accidentally left in body following surgical operation, initial encounter
T81.592A	Other complications of foreign body accidentally left in body following kidney dialysis, initial encounter
T81.594A	Other complications of foreign body accidentally left in body following endoscopic examination, initial encounter
T81.596A	Other complications of foreign body accidentally left in body following aspiration, puncture or other catheterization, initial encounter
T81.597A	Other complications of foreign body accidentally left in body following removal of catheter or packing, initial encounter
T81.598A	Other complications of foreign body accidentally left in body following other procedure, initial encounter

AMA: **50957** 2018,Jan,8; 2017,Jan,8; 2016,Jan,13; 2015,Jan,16; 2014,Jan,11
50961 2018,Jan,8; 2017,Jan,8; 2016,Jan,13; 2015,Jan,16; 2014,Jan,11

Relative Value Units/Medicare Edits

Non-Facility RVU	Work	PE	MP	Total
50957	6.78	4.83	0.79	12.4
50961	6.04	4.44	0.68	11.16
Facility RVU	**Work**	**PE**	**MP**	**Total**
50957	6.78	2.67	0.79	10.24
50961	6.04	2.42	0.68	9.14

	FUD	Status	MUE	Modifiers				IOM Reference
50957	0	A	1(2)	51	50	N/A	80*	None
50961	0	A	1(2)	51	50	N/A	80*	

* with documentation

Terms To Know

biopsy. Tissue or fluid removed for diagnostic purposes through analysis of the cells in the biopsy material.

calculus. Abnormal, stone-like concretion of calcium, cholesterol, mineral salts, or other substances that forms in any part of the body.

foreign body. Any object or substance found in an organ and tissue that does not belong under normal circumstances.

fulguration. Destruction of living tissue by using sparks from a high-frequency electric current.

guidewire. Flexible metal instrument designed to lead another instrument in its proper course.

irrigate. Washing out, lavage.

© 2020 Optum360, LLC   **N Newborn: 0**   **P Pediatric: 0-17**   **M Maternity: 9-64**   **A Adult: 15-124**   ♂ Male Only   ♀ Female Only   CPT © 2020 American Medical Association. All Rights Reserved.

Ureter

50970-50974

50970 Ureteral endoscopy through ureterotomy, with or without irrigation, instillation, or ureteropyelography, exclusive of radiologic service;

50972 with ureteral catheterization, with or without dilation of ureter

50974 with biopsy

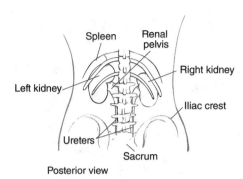

Posterior view

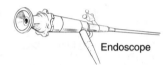

Endoscope

An endoscope is inserted through an incision in the ureter. A variety of procedures may be performed

Explanation

The physician examines renal and ureteral structures with an endoscope passed through an incision in the ureter (ureterotomy). After accessing the ureter with an incision in the skin of the flank, the physician incises the ureter and guides the endoscope through the incision. The physician may flush (irrigate) or introduce by drops (instillate) a solution to better view the renal and ureteral structures, and/or may introduce contrast medium for radiologic study of the renal pelvis and ureter (ureteropyelogram). After examination, the physician sutures the incision, inserts a drain tube, and performs a layered closure. In 50972, to catheterize the ureter, the physician passes a thin tube through the endoscope into the ureter and may insert a balloon catheter to dilate a ureteral constriction. In 50974, the physician passes a cutting instrument through the endoscope into the suspect tissue and takes a biopsy specimen. The physician removes the endoscope, sutures the incision, inserts a drain tube, and performs a layered closure.

Coding Tips

If the ureterotomy is done for an additional, significantly identifiable endoscopic service, report the appropriate endoscopic procedure code (50970–50980) and 50600. For open ureteral endoscopic procedures (through ureterotomy), with fulguration and/or incision with or without biopsy, see 50976; with removal of a foreign body or calculus, see 50980. For percutaneous ureteral endoscopic procedures (through established ureterostomy), see 50951–50961. Report image-guided dilation or ureter, without endoscopic guidance, with 50706; biopsy of ureter and/or renal pelvis, see 50606.

ICD-10-CM Diagnostic Codes

C64.1	Malignant neoplasm of right kidney, except renal pelvis ☑
C64.2	Malignant neoplasm of left kidney, except renal pelvis ☑
C65.1	Malignant neoplasm of right renal pelvis ☑
C65.2	Malignant neoplasm of left renal pelvis ☑
C66.1	Malignant neoplasm of right ureter ☑
C66.2	Malignant neoplasm of left ureter ☑
C67.6	Malignant neoplasm of ureteric orifice
C79.01	Secondary malignant neoplasm of right kidney and renal pelvis ☑
C79.02	Secondary malignant neoplasm of left kidney and renal pelvis ☑
C79.11	Secondary malignant neoplasm of bladder
C79.19	Secondary malignant neoplasm of other urinary organs
C7A.093	Malignant carcinoid tumor of the kidney
C80.2	Malignant neoplasm associated with transplanted organ
D09.0	Carcinoma in situ of bladder
D09.19	Carcinoma in situ of other urinary organs
D30.01	Benign neoplasm of right kidney ☑
D30.02	Benign neoplasm of left kidney ☑
D30.11	Benign neoplasm of right renal pelvis ☑
D30.12	Benign neoplasm of left renal pelvis ☑
D30.21	Benign neoplasm of right ureter ☑
D30.22	Benign neoplasm of left ureter ☑
D3A.093	Benign carcinoid tumor of the kidney
D41.01	Neoplasm of uncertain behavior of right kidney ☑
D41.02	Neoplasm of uncertain behavior of left kidney ☑
D41.11	Neoplasm of uncertain behavior of right renal pelvis ☑
D41.12	Neoplasm of uncertain behavior of left renal pelvis ☑
D41.21	Neoplasm of uncertain behavior of right ureter ☑
D41.22	Neoplasm of uncertain behavior of left ureter ☑
D41.4	Neoplasm of uncertain behavior of bladder
D49.511	Neoplasm of unspecified behavior of right kidney ☑
D49.512	Neoplasm of unspecified behavior of left kidney ☑
D49.59	Neoplasm of unspecified behavior of other genitourinary organ
N11.1	Chronic obstructive pyelonephritis
N13.0	Hydronephrosis with ureteropelvic junction obstruction
N13.1	Hydronephrosis with ureteral stricture, not elsewhere classified
N13.2	Hydronephrosis with renal and ureteral calculous obstruction
N13.39	Other hydronephrosis
N13.4	Hydroureter
N13.5	Crossing vessel and stricture of ureter without hydronephrosis
N13.8	Other obstructive and reflux uropathy
N15.1	Renal and perinephric abscess
N20.0	Calculus of kidney
N20.1	Calculus of ureter
N20.2	Calculus of kidney with calculus of ureter
N25.81	Secondary hyperparathyroidism of renal origin
N28.0	Ischemia and infarction of kidney
N28.1	Cyst of kidney, acquired
N28.81	Hypertrophy of kidney
N28.82	Megaloureter
N28.83	Nephroptosis
N28.89	Other specified disorders of kidney and ureter
Q61.01	Congenital single renal cyst
Q61.02	Congenital multiple renal cysts
Q61.19	Other polycystic kidney, infantile type
Q61.2	Polycystic kidney, adult type
Q61.4	Renal dysplasia
Q61.5	Medullary cystic kidney
Q61.8	Other cystic kidney diseases

CPT © 2020 American Medical Association. All Rights Reserved.   ● New   ▲ Revised   + Add On   ★ Telemedicine   **AMA: CPT Assist**   [Resequenced]   ☑ Laterality   © 2020 Optum360, LLC

Ureter

Q62.0	Congenital hydronephrosis		
Q62.11	Congenital occlusion of ureteropelvic junction		
Q62.12	Congenital occlusion of ureterovesical orifice		
Q62.2	Congenital megaureter		
Q62.31	Congenital ureterocele, orthotopic		
Q62.32	Cecoureterocele		
Q62.39	Other obstructive defects of renal pelvis and ureter		

AMA: 50970 2018,Jan,8; 2017,Jan,8; 2016,Jan,13; 2015,Jan,16; 2014,Jan,11
50972 2018,Jan,8; 2017,Jan,8; 2016,Jan,3; 2016,Jan,13; 2015,Jan,16; 2014,Jan,11
50974 2018,Jan,8; 2017,Jan,8; 2016,Jan,3; 2016,Jan,13; 2015,Jan,16; 2014,Jan,11

Relative Value Units/Medicare Edits

Non-Facility RVU	Work	PE	MP	Total
50970	7.13	2.75	0.81	10.69
50972	6.88	2.67	0.79	10.34
50974	9.16	3.44	1.04	13.64
Facility RVU	Work	PE	MP	Total
50970	7.13	2.75	0.81	10.69
50972	6.88	2.67	0.79	10.34
50974	9.16	3.44	1.04	13.64

	FUD	Status	MUE	Modifiers				IOM Reference
50970	0	A	1(3)	51	50	N/A	80*	None
50972	0	A	1(3)	51	50	N/A	80*	
50974	0	A	1(2)	51	50	N/A	80*	

* with documentation

Terms To Know

biopsy. Tissue or fluid removed for diagnostic purposes through analysis of the cells in the biopsy material.

catheterization. Use or insertion of a tubular device into a duct, blood vessel, hollow organ, or body cavity for injecting or withdrawing fluids for diagnostic or therapeutic purposes.

flank. Part of the body found between the posterior ribs and the uppermost crest of the ilium, or the lateral side of the hip, thigh, and buttock.

hematuria. Blood in urine, which may present as gross visible blood or as the presence of red blood cells visible only under a microscope.

hydroureter. Abnormal enlargement or distension of the ureter with water or urine caused by an obstruction.

irrigation. To wash out or cleanse a body cavity, wound, or tissue with water or other fluid.

neoplasm. New abnormal growth, tumor.

specimen. Tissue cells or sample of fluid taken for analysis, pathologic examination, and diagnosis.

stricture. Narrowing of an anatomical structure.

tissue. Group of similar cells with a similar function that form definite structures and organs. Tissue types include epithelial tissue, muscle tissue, connective tissue, and nervous tissue.

50976-50980

50976	Ureteral endoscopy through ureterotomy, with or without irrigation, instillation, or ureteropyelography, exclusive of radiologic service; with fulguration and/or incision, with or without biopsy
50980	with removal of foreign body or calculus

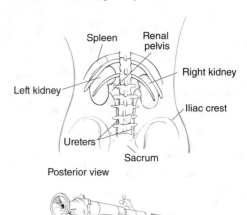

An endoscope is inserted through an incision in the ureter. A variety of procedures may be performed

Explanation

The physician examines renal and ureteral structures with an endoscope passed through an incision in the ureter (ureterotomy), and removes renal or ureteral lesions by electric current (fulguration) or incision. After accessing the ureter with an incision in the skin of the flank, the physician incises the ureter and guides the endoscope through the incision. The physician may flush (irrigate) or introduce by drops (instillate) a solution to better view the renal and ureteral structures, and/or may introduce contrast medium for radiologic study of the renal pelvis and ureter (ureteropyelogram). In 50976, the physician passes through the endoscope an instrument that destroys lesions with electric sparks or incises lesions. The physician may insert an instrument to biopsy renal tissue. In 50980, the physician passes an instrument through the endoscope to remove a foreign body or calculus, and may pass a stent through the ureter into the bladder. The physician removes the endoscope, sutures the incision, inserts a drain tube, and performs a layered closure.

Coding Tips

For open ureteral endoscopy (through ureterotomy) with examination alone, see 50970; with ureteral catheterization, with or without dilation of the ureter, see 50972; with biopsy, see 50974. For percutaneous ureteral endoscopy procedures (through established ureterostomy), see 50951–50961.

ICD-10-CM Diagnostic Codes

C66.1	Malignant neoplasm of right ureter ☑	
C66.2	Malignant neoplasm of left ureter ☑	
C67.6	Malignant neoplasm of ureteric orifice	
C79.11	Secondary malignant neoplasm of bladder	
C79.19	Secondary malignant neoplasm of other urinary organs	
D09.0	Carcinoma in situ of bladder	
D09.19	Carcinoma in situ of other urinary organs	
D30.21	Benign neoplasm of right ureter ☑	
D30.22	Benign neoplasm of left ureter ☑	

Ureter

D41.21	Neoplasm of uncertain behavior of right ureter ☑	
D41.22	Neoplasm of uncertain behavior of left ureter ☑	
D41.4	Neoplasm of uncertain behavior of bladder	
N11.1	Chronic obstructive pyelonephritis	
N13.5	Crossing vessel and stricture of ureter without hydronephrosis	
N13.8	Other obstructive and reflux uropathy	
N20.1	Calculus of ureter	
N20.2	Calculus of kidney with calculus of ureter	
N25.81	Secondary hyperparathyroidism of renal origin	
N28.82	Megaloureter	
N28.89	Other specified disorders of kidney and ureter	
Q62.0	Congenital hydronephrosis	
Q62.11	Congenital occlusion of ureteropelvic junction	
Q62.12	Congenital occlusion of ureterovesical orifice	
Q62.2	Congenital megaureter	
Q62.31	Congenital ureterocele, orthotopic	
Q62.32	Cecoureterocele	
Q62.39	Other obstructive defects of renal pelvis and ureter	
T19.8XXA	Foreign body in other parts of genitourinary tract, initial encounter	
T81.510A	Adhesions due to foreign body accidentally left in body following surgical operation, initial encounter	
T81.512A	Adhesions due to foreign body accidentally left in body following kidney dialysis, initial encounter	
T81.514A	Adhesions due to foreign body accidentally left in body following endoscopic examination, initial encounter	
T81.516A	Adhesions due to foreign body accidentally left in body following aspiration, puncture or other catheterization, initial encounter	
T81.517A	Adhesions due to foreign body accidentally left in body following removal of catheter or packing, initial encounter	
T81.518A	Adhesions due to foreign body accidentally left in body following other procedure, initial encounter	
T81.520A	Obstruction due to foreign body accidentally left in body following surgical operation, initial encounter	
T81.522A	Obstruction due to foreign body accidentally left in body following kidney dialysis, initial encounter	
T81.524A	Obstruction due to foreign body accidentally left in body following endoscopic examination, initial encounter	
T81.526A	Obstruction due to foreign body accidentally left in body following aspiration, puncture or other catheterization, initial encounter	
T81.527A	Obstruction due to foreign body accidentally left in body following removal of catheter or packing, initial encounter	
T81.528A	Obstruction due to foreign body accidentally left in body following other procedure, initial encounter	
T81.530A	Perforation due to foreign body accidentally left in body following surgical operation, initial encounter	
T81.532A	Perforation due to foreign body accidentally left in body following kidney dialysis, initial encounter	
T81.534A	Perforation due to foreign body accidentally left in body following endoscopic examination, initial encounter	
T81.536A	Perforation due to foreign body accidentally left in body following aspiration, puncture or other catheterization, initial encounter	
T81.537A	Perforation due to foreign body accidentally left in body following removal of catheter or packing, initial encounter	

T81.538A	Perforation due to foreign body accidentally left in body following other procedure, initial encounter
T81.590A	Other complications of foreign body accidentally left in body following surgical operation, initial encounter
T81.592A	Other complications of foreign body accidentally left in body following kidney dialysis, initial encounter
T81.594A	Other complications of foreign body accidentally left in body following endoscopic examination, initial encounter
T81.596A	Other complications of foreign body accidentally left in body following aspiration, puncture or other catheterization, initial encounter
T81.597A	Other complications of foreign body accidentally left in body following removal of catheter or packing, initial encounter
T81.598A	Other complications of foreign body accidentally left in body following other procedure, initial encounter

AMA: **50976** 2018,Jan,8; 2017,Jan,8; 2016,Jan,13; 2015,Jan,16; 2014,Jan,11
50980 2018,Jan,8; 2017,Jan,8; 2016,Jan,13; 2015,Jan,16; 2014,Jan,11

Relative Value Units/Medicare Edits

Non-Facility RVU	Work	PE	MP	Total
50976	9.03	3.39	1.04	13.46
50980	6.84	2.66	0.79	10.29
Facility RVU	Work	PE	MP	Total
50976	9.03	3.39	1.04	13.46
50980	6.84	2.66	0.79	10.29

	FUD	Status	MUE	Modifiers				IOM Reference
50976	0	A	1(2)	51	50	N/A	80*	None
50980	0	A	1(2)	51	50	N/A	80*	

* with documentation

Terms To Know

biopsy. Tissue or fluid removed for diagnostic purposes through analysis of the cells in the biopsy material.

calculus. Abnormal, stone-like concretion of calcium, cholesterol, mineral salts, or other substances that forms in any part of the body.

fistula. Abnormal tube-like passage between two body cavities or organs or from an organ to the outside surface.

foreign body. Any object or substance found in an organ and tissue that does not belong under normal circumstances.

fulguration. Destruction of living tissue by using sparks from a high-frequency electric current.

irrigation. To wash out or cleanse a body cavity, wound, or tissue with water or other fluid.

ureteropyelogram. Radiologic study of the renal pelvis and the ureter.

ureterotomy. Incision made into the ureter for accomplishing a variety of procedures such as exploration, drainage, instillation, ureteropyelography, catheterization, dilation, biopsy, or foreign body removal.

Ureter

51020-51030

51020 Cystotomy or cystostomy; with fulguration and/or insertion of radioactive material
51030 with cryosurgical destruction of intravesical lesion

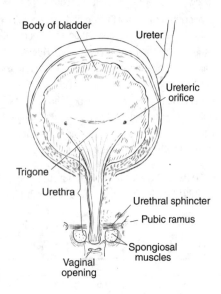

Body of bladder
Ureter
Ureteric orifice
Trigone
Urethra
Urethral sphincter
Pubic ramus
Spongiosal muscles
Vaginal opening

Frontal section of the female bladder, urethra, and select bone and musculature

Explanation

The physician makes an incision (cystotomy) or creates an opening (cystostomy) into the bladder to destroy abnormal tissue. To access the bladder, the physician makes an incision in the skin of the lower abdomen and cuts the corresponding muscles, fat, fibrous membranes (fascia), and bladder wall. Report 51020 if the physician uses electric current (fulguration) or inserts radioactive material to destroy a lesion on the bladder (usually with the aid of a radiation oncologist). Report 51030 if the physician uses cryosurgery to destroy the lesion. The bladder wall and lower abdomen is sutured closed. If a cystostomy is made, the cystostomy tube is sutured in place and the bladder and abdominal wall is closed.

Coding Tips

For fulguration and cryosurgery of lesions and/or tumors of the bladder through a cystourethroscope, see 52214–52240. For insertion of a radioactive substance into the bladder, with or without biopsy or fulguration of lesions, through a cystourethroscope, see 52250. Report 51880 for closure of the cystostomy in a separate operative session. For a cystotomy for excision of a bladder tumor, see 51530.

ICD-10-CM Diagnostic Codes

C67.0	Malignant neoplasm of trigone of bladder
C67.1	Malignant neoplasm of dome of bladder
C67.2	Malignant neoplasm of lateral wall of bladder
C67.3	Malignant neoplasm of anterior wall of bladder
C67.4	Malignant neoplasm of posterior wall of bladder
C67.5	Malignant neoplasm of bladder neck
C67.6	Malignant neoplasm of ureteric orifice
C67.7	Malignant neoplasm of urachus
C67.8	Malignant neoplasm of overlapping sites of bladder
C79.11	Secondary malignant neoplasm of bladder
D09.0	Carcinoma in situ of bladder
D30.3	Benign neoplasm of bladder
D41.4	Neoplasm of uncertain behavior of bladder
D49.4	Neoplasm of unspecified behavior of bladder
N21.0	Calculus in bladder
N30.10	Interstitial cystitis (chronic) without hematuria
N30.11	Interstitial cystitis (chronic) with hematuria
N32.89	Other specified disorders of bladder

AMA: 51020 2014,Jan,11 **51030** 2014,Jan,11

Relative Value Units/Medicare Edits

Non-Facility RVU	Work	PE	MP	Total
51020	7.69	4.94	0.88	13.51
51030	7.81	4.91	0.89	13.61
Facility RVU	Work	PE	MP	Total
51020	7.69	4.94	0.88	13.51
51030	7.81	4.91	0.89	13.61

	FUD	Status	MUE	Modifiers				IOM Reference
51020	90	A	1(2)	51	N/A	62*	80	None
51030	90	A	1(2)	51	N/A	N/A	80*	

* with documentation

Terms To Know

benign. Mild or nonmalignant in nature.

carcinoma in situ. Malignancy that arises from the cells of the vessel, gland, or organ of origin that remains confined to that site or has not invaded neighboring tissue.

cryosurgery. Application of intense cold, usually produced using liquid nitrogen, to locally freeze diseased or unwanted tissue and induce tissue necrosis without causing harm to adjacent tissue.

cystostomy. Formation of an opening through the abdominal wall into the bladder.

fulguration. Destruction of living tissue by using sparks from a high-frequency electric current.

malignant. Any condition tending to progress toward death, specifically an invasive tumor with a loss of cellular differentiation that has the ability to spread or metastasize to other body areas.

trigone. Triangular, smooth area of mucous membrane at the base of the bladder, located between the ureteric openings in back and the urethral opening in front.

urachus. Embryonic tube connecting the urinary bladder to the umbilicus during development of the fetus that normally closes before birth, generally in the fourth or fifth month of gestation.

© 2020 Optum360, LLC
N Newborn: 0   **P** Pediatric: 0-17   **M** Maternity: 9-64   **A** Adult: 15-124   ♂ Male Only   ♀ Female Only   CPT © 2020 American Medical Association. All Rights Reserved.

Coding Companion for Urology/Nephrology

Bladder

51040

51040   Cystostomy, cystotomy with drainage

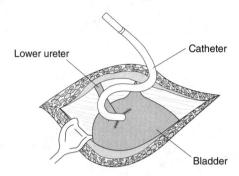

Lower ureter

Catheter

Bladder

The physician incises the bladder
and places a catheter for drainage

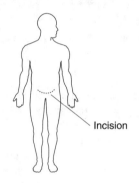

Incision

Explanation

The physician creates an opening into the bladder (cystostomy) through an incision in the bladder (cystotomy). To access the bladder, the physician makes an incision in the skin of the lower abdomen and cuts the corresponding muscles, fat, and fibrous membranes (fascia). The physician makes a small incision and inserts a catheter (cystostomy tube) into the bladder, passing the tube through a stab incision in the skin of the abdomen. The physician may insert a drain tube for the cystostomy. If only a cystotomy is performed the wound can be repaired with a layered closure using absorbable sutures.

Coding Tips

For cystotomy or cystostomy for the destruction of lesions, see 51020–51030. For cystotomy with the insertion of a ureteral catheter or stent, see 51045. For cystotomy for the removal of a calculus, see 51050 and 51065. For cystotomy for excision of the vesical neck, see 51520; excision of the bladder diverticulum, see 51525; and excision of a bladder tumor, see 51530. For cystotomy for repair of a ureterocele, see 52300–52301.

ICD-10-CM Diagnostic Codes

A56.01	Chlamydial cystitis and urethritis
C61	Malignant neoplasm of prostate ♂
C67.0	Malignant neoplasm of trigone of bladder
C67.2	Malignant neoplasm of lateral wall of bladder
C67.3	Malignant neoplasm of anterior wall of bladder

C67.4	Malignant neoplasm of posterior wall of bladder
C67.5	Malignant neoplasm of bladder neck
C67.6	Malignant neoplasm of ureteric orifice
D07.5	Carcinoma in situ of prostate ♂
D29.1	Benign neoplasm of prostate ♂
D40.0	Neoplasm of uncertain behavior of prostate ♂
G83.4	Cauda equina syndrome
N11.0	Nonobstructive reflux-associated chronic pyelonephritis
N13.71	Vesicoureteral-reflux without reflux nephropathy
N21.1	Calculus in urethra
N28.84	Pyelitis cystica
N28.85	Pyeloureteritis cystica
N28.86	Ureteritis cystica
N30.00	Acute cystitis without hematuria
N30.01	Acute cystitis with hematuria
N30.10	Interstitial cystitis (chronic) without hematuria
N30.11	Interstitial cystitis (chronic) with hematuria
N30.30	Trigonitis without hematuria
N30.31	Trigonitis with hematuria
N30.80	Other cystitis without hematuria
N30.81	Other cystitis with hematuria
N32.0	Bladder-neck obstruction
N32.1	Vesicointestinal fistula
N32.3	Diverticulum of bladder
N32.81	Overactive bladder
N36.0	Urethral fistula
N39.3	Stress incontinence (female) (male)
N40.1	Benign prostatic hyperplasia with lower urinary tract symptoms 🄰 ♂
N40.3	Nodular prostate with lower urinary tract symptoms 🄰 ♂
N81.11	Cystocele, midline ♀
N81.12	Cystocele, lateral ♀
N82.0	Vesicovaginal fistula ♀
Q64.2	Congenital posterior urethral valves
Q64.31	Congenital bladder neck obstruction
Q64.32	Congenital stricture of urethra
Q64.33	Congenital stricture of urinary meatus
R82.71	Bacteriuria
S37.22XA	Contusion of bladder, initial encounter
S37.23XA	Laceration of bladder, initial encounter
S37.32XA	Contusion of urethra, initial encounter
S37.33XA	Laceration of urethra, initial encounter

AMA: **51040** 2014,Jan,11

Bladder

Relative Value Units/Medicare Edits

Non-Facility RVU	Work	PE	MP	Total
51040	4.49	3.33	0.52	8.34
Facility RVU	**Work**	**PE**	**MP**	**Total**
51040	4.49	3.33	0.52	8.34

	FUD	Status	MUE	Modifiers				IOM Reference
51040	90	A	1(3)	51	N/A	62*	80	None

* with documentation

Terms To Know

benign prostatic hyperplasia. Enlargement of the prostate gland due to an abnormal proliferation of fibrostromal tissue in the paraurethral glands. This condition causes impingement of the urethra resulting in obstructed urinary flow.

catheter. Flexible tube inserted into an area of the body for introducing or withdrawing fluid.

closure. Repairing an incision or wound by suture or other means.

cystostomy. Formation of an opening through the abdominal wall into the bladder.

diversion. Rechanneling of body fluid through another conduit.

drainage. Releasing, taking, or letting out fluids and/or gases from a body part.

urinary stasis. Urinary retention.

51045

51045   Cystotomy, with insertion of ureteral catheter or stent (separate procedure)

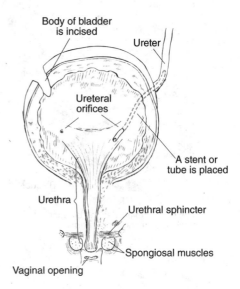

Explanation

The physician makes an incision in the bladder to insert a catheter or slender tube (stent) into the ureter. To access the bladder and ureters, the physician makes a midline incision in the skin of the abdomen and cuts the corresponding muscles, fat, and fibrous membranes (fascia). The physician incises the bladder (cystotomy) and inserts a stent or catheter in the ureter. Insertion of a ureteral catheter requires that the physician bring the tube end out through the urethra or bladder incision. The physician inserts a drain tube and performs a layered closure.

Coding Tips

This separate procedure by definition is usually a component of a more complex service and is not identified separately. When performed alone or with other unrelated procedures/services it may be reported. If performed alone, list the code; if performed with other procedures/services, list the code and append modifier 59 or an X{EPSU} modifier. For cystotomy or cystostomy for the destruction of lesions, see 51020–51030. For cystotomy, cystostomy with drainage, see 51040. For cystotomy for the removal of a calculus, see 51050 and 51065. For cystotomy for excision of the vesical neck, see 51520; excision of the bladder diverticulum, see 51525; or excision of a bladder tumor, see 51530. For cystotomy for repair of a ureterocele, see 52300–52301.

ICD-10-CM Diagnostic Codes

C66.1	Malignant neoplasm of right ureter ☑
C66.2	Malignant neoplasm of left ureter ☑
D30.21	Benign neoplasm of right ureter ☑
D30.22	Benign neoplasm of left ureter ☑
D41.21	Neoplasm of uncertain behavior of right ureter ☑
D41.22	Neoplasm of uncertain behavior of left ureter ☑
N11.1	Chronic obstructive pyelonephritis
N13.4	Hydroureter
N13.5	Crossing vessel and stricture of ureter without hydronephrosis
N13.8	Other obstructive and reflux uropathy
N20.1	Calculus of ureter

Bladder

© 2020 Optum360, LLC   **N** Newborn: 0   **P** Pediatric: 0-17   **M** Maternity: 9-64   **A** Adult: 15-124   ♂ Male Only   ♀ Female Only   CPT © 2020 American Medical Association. All Rights Reserved.

216   *Coding Companion for Urology/Nephrology*

N28.89	Other specified disorders of kidney and ureter	
Q62.0	Congenital hydronephrosis	
Q62.11	Congenital occlusion of ureteropelvic junction	
Q62.12	Congenital occlusion of ureterovesical orifice	
Q62.2	Congenital megaureter	
Q62.31	Congenital ureterocele, orthotopic	
Q62.32	Cecoureterocele	
Q62.39	Other obstructive defects of renal pelvis and ureter	
S37.12XA	Contusion of ureter, initial encounter	
S37.13XA	Laceration of ureter, initial encounter	
S37.19XA	Other injury of ureter, initial encounter	

AMA: 51045 2014,Jan,11

Relative Value Units/Medicare Edits

Non-Facility RVU	Work	PE	MP	Total
51045	7.81	5.33	1.29	14.43
Facility RVU	Work	PE	MP	Total
51045	7.81	5.33	1.29	14.43

	FUD	Status	MUE	Modifiers				IOM Reference
51045	90	A	2(3)	51	N/A	N/A	80	None

* with documentation

Terms To Know

calculus. Abnormal, stone-like concretion of calcium, cholesterol, mineral salts, or other substances that forms in any part of the body.

catheter. Flexible tube inserted into an area of the body for introducing or withdrawing fluid.

cystotomy. Surgical incision into the gallbladder or urinary bladder.

fistula. Abnormal tube-like passage between two body cavities or organs or from an organ to the outside surface.

hydroureter. Abnormal enlargement or distension of the ureter with water or urine caused by an obstruction.

neoplasm. New abnormal growth, tumor.

occlusion. Constriction, closure, or blockage of a passage.

stent. Tube to provide support in a body cavity or lumen.

stricture. Narrowing of an anatomical structure.

tube. Long, hollow cylindrical instrument or body structure.

ureter. Tube leading from the kidney to the urinary bladder made up of three layers of tissue: the mucous lining of the inner layer; the smooth, muscular middle layer that propels the urine from the kidney to the bladder by peristalsis; and the outer layer made of fibrous connective tissue. Each ureter leaves the kidney from the hilum, a concave notch on the middle surface, and enters the bladder through a narrow valve-like orifice that prevents the backflow of urine to the kidney.

51050

51050 Cystolithotomy, cystotomy with removal of calculus, without vesical neck resection

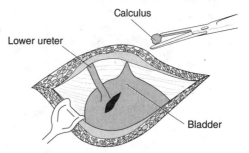

The physician incises the bladder to remove a calculus

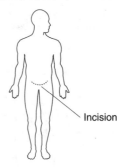

Explanation

The physician makes an incision in the bladder to remove a calculus. To access the bladder, the physician makes an incision in the skin of the lower abdomen and cuts the corresponding muscles, fat, and fibrous membranes (fascia). The physician performs a cystotomy, isolates the calculus, and removes it. The bladder neck is not excised. After examining the bladder for other defects, the physician sutures the incision and performs a layered closure using absorbable sutures, inserting a drain tube through a stab incision in the skin.

Coding Tips

If a cystourethroscope is used to remove a calculus, see 52310–52315 and 52352–52353. For litholapaxy, see 52317–52318. For cystotomy with removal of a calculus with a stone basket or ultrasonic/electrohydraulic fragmentation, see 51065.

ICD-10-CM Diagnostic Codes

N21.0	Calculus in bladder
N21.1	Calculus in urethra

AMA: 51050 2014,Jan,11

Relative Value Units/Medicare Edits

Non-Facility RVU	Work	PE	MP	Total
51050	7.97	4.72	0.91	13.6
Facility RVU	Work	PE	MP	Total
51050	7.97	4.72	0.91	13.6

	FUD	Status	MUE	Modifiers				IOM Reference
51050	90	A	1(3)	51	N/A	62*	80	None

* with documentation

CPT © 2020 American Medical Association. All Rights Reserved.   ● New   ▲ Revised   + Add On   ★ Telemedicine   AMA: CPT Assist   [Resequenced]   ☑ Laterality   © 2020 Optum360, LLC

Bladder

51060-51065

51060 Transvesical ureterolithotomy
51065 Cystotomy, with calculus basket extraction and/or ultrasonic or electrohydraulic fragmentation of ureteral calculus

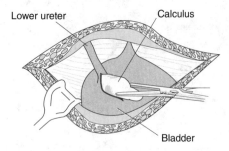

The physician incises the bladder to remove a calculus in the ureter

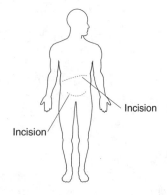

Explanation

The physician makes an incision in the bladder to remove a calculus in the ureter. To access the bladder and ureters, the physician makes a midline incision in the skin of the abdomen and cuts the corresponding muscles, fat, and fibrous membranes (fascia). In 51060, the physician isolates the calculus and removes it through incisions in the bladder (cystotomy) and ureter (ureterotomy). In 51065, the physician inserts an instrument (e.g., a stone basket) through the bladder incision into the ureter to remove or destroy a ureteral calculus. After examining the ureter for other defects, the physician inserts a ureteral catheter and sutures the incision. The physician inserts a drain tube and performs a layered closure.

Coding Tips

If significant additional time and effort is documented, append modifier 22 and submit a cover letter and operative report. When 51060 or 51065 is performed with another separately identifiable procedure, the highest dollar value code is listed as the primary procedure and subsequent procedures are appended with modifier 51. For removal of a calculus through an incision in the ureter, see 50610–50630. For removal of a calculus through a bladder incision only, see 51050.

ICD-10-CM Diagnostic Codes

N20.1   Calculus of ureter
N20.2   Calculus of kidney with calculus of ureter

AMA: 51060 2014,Jan,11 **51065** 2014,Jan,11

Relative Value Units/Medicare Edits

Non-Facility RVU	Work	PE	MP	Total
51060	9.95	5.7	1.15	16.8
51065	9.95	5.63	1.14	16.72
Facility RVU	**Work**	**PE**	**MP**	**Total**
51060	9.95	5.7	1.15	16.8
51065	9.95	5.63	1.14	16.72

	FUD	Status	MUE	Modifiers				IOM Reference
51060	90	A	1(3)	51	N/A	62*	80	None
51065	90	A	1(3)	51	N/A	N/A	80*	

* with documentation

Terms To Know

calculus. Abnormal, stone-like concretion of calcium, cholesterol, mineral salts, or other substances that forms in any part of the body.

catheter. Flexible tube inserted into an area of the body for introducing or withdrawing fluid.

cystotomy. Surgical incision into the gallbladder or urinary bladder.

defect. Imperfection, flaw, or absence.

destruction. Ablation or eradication of a structure or tissue.

drain. Device that creates a channel to allow fluid from a cavity, wound, or infected area to exit the body.

fascia. Fibrous sheet or band of tissue that envelops organs, muscles, and groupings of muscles.

fragment. Small piece broken off a larger whole; to divide into pieces.

tube. Long, hollow cylindrical instrument or body structure.

ureter. Tube leading from the kidney to the urinary bladder made up of three layers of tissue: the mucous lining of the inner layer; the smooth, muscular middle layer that propels the urine from the kidney to the bladder by peristalsis; and the outer layer made of fibrous connective tissue. Each ureter leaves the kidney from the hilum, a concave notch on the middle surface, and enters the bladder through a narrow valve-like orifice that prevents the backflow of urine to the kidney.

ureterotomy. Incision made into the ureter for accomplishing a variety of procedures such as exploration, drainage, instillation, ureteropyelography, catheterization, dilation, biopsy, or foreign body removal.

© 2020 Optum360, LLC   **N** Newborn: 0   **P** Pediatric: 0-17   **M** Maternity: 9-64   **A** Adult: 15-124   ♂ Male Only   ♀ Female Only   CPT © 2020 American Medical Association. All Rights Reserved.

Bladder

51080

51080   Drainage of perivesical or prevesical space abscess

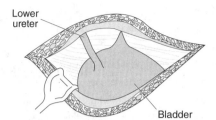

Lower ureter

Bladder

The physician drains an abscess
from the space around the bladder

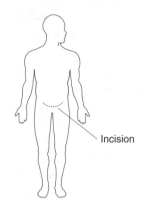

Incision

Explanation

The physician drains an infection (abscess) near the bladder. To access the bladder, the physician makes an incision in the skin of the lower abdomen and cuts the corresponding muscles, fat, and fibrous membranes (fascia). After exploring the abscess cavity, the physician irrigates the site, inserts multiple drain tubes through separate stab wounds, and sutures the drain tube ends to the skin. The physician inserts a urethral catheter and performs a layered closure.

Coding Tips

This procedure includes incision, exploration, biopsy, irrigation, and debridement. When 51080 is performed with another separately identifiable procedure, the highest dollar value code is listed as the primary procedure and subsequent procedures are appended with modifier 51. If significant additional time and effort is documented, append modifier 22 and submit a cover letter and operative report. If the physician makes an incision into the bladder and inserts a catheter for drainage, see 51040. For aspiration of the bladder, see 51100–51102. For drainage of an abscess in or surrounding the urethra, see 53040. To report percutaneous, image-guided fluid collection drainage of a perivesicular or prevesicular space abscess, via catheter, see 49406.

ICD-10-CM Diagnostic Codes

K65.1	Peritoneal abscess
K68.11	Postprocedural retroperitoneal abscess
K68.19	Other retroperitoneal abscess
N30.80	Other cystitis without hematuria
N30.81	Other cystitis with hematuria

AMA: **51080** 2014,Jan,11

Relative Value Units/Medicare Edits

Non-Facility RVU	Work	PE	MP	Total
51080	6.71	4.3	0.78	11.79
Facility RVU	Work	PE	MP	Total
51080	6.71	4.3	0.78	11.79

	FUD	Status	MUE	Modifiers				IOM Reference
51080	90	A	1(3)	51	N/A	62*	80	None

* with documentation

Terms To Know

abscess. Circumscribed collection of pus resulting from bacteria, frequently associated with swelling and other signs of inflammation.

catheter. Flexible tube inserted into an area of the body for introducing or withdrawing fluid.

cellulitis. Infection of the skin and subcutaneous tissues, most often caused by Staphylococcus or Streptococcus bacteria secondary to a cutaneous lesion. Progression of the inflammation may lead to abscess and tissue death, or even systemic infection-like bacteremia.

cystitis. Inflammation of the urinary bladder. Symptoms include dysuria, frequency of urination, urgency, and hematuria.

drainage. Releasing, taking, or letting out fluids and/or gases from a body part.

fascia. Fibrous sheet or band of tissue that envelops organs, muscles, and groupings of muscles.

hematuria. Blood in urine, which may present as gross visible blood or as the presence of red blood cells visible only under a microscope.

infected postoperative seroma. Infection within a pocket of serum following surgery.

irrigation. To wash out or cleanse a body cavity, wound, or tissue with water or other fluid.

parametritis. Inflammation and infection of the tissue in the structures around the uterus.

peritoneal. Space between the lining of the abdominal wall, or parietal peritoneum, and the surface layer of the abdominal organs, or visceral peritoneum. It contains a thin, watery fluid that keeps the peritoneal surfaces moist.

retroperitoneal. Located behind the peritoneum, the membrane that lines the abdominopelvic walls and forms a covering for the internal organs.

Bladder

CPT © 2020 American Medical Association. All Rights Reserved.   ● New   ▲ Revised   + Add On   ★ Telemedicine   AMA: CPT Assist   [Resequenced]   ☑ Laterality   © 2020 Optum360, LLC

51100-51102

51100 Aspiration of bladder; by needle
51101   by trocar or intracatheter
51102   with insertion of suprapubic catheter

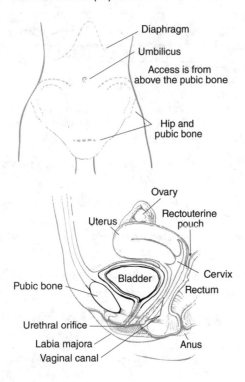

Diaphragm
Umbilicus
Access is from above the pubic bone
Hip and pubic bone

Ovary
Uterus
Rectouterine pouch
Cervix
Pubic bone
Bladder
Rectum
Urethral orifice
Labia majora
Anus
Vaginal canal

Explanation

In 51100, the physician inserts a needle through the skin into the bladder to withdraw urine. In 51101, the physician inserts a trocar or intracatheter through the skin into the bladder. In 51102, a suprapubic catheter is placed into the bladder. This procedure may also be performed after the abdomen has been surgically incised.

Coding Tips

Local anesthesia is included in these services. However, these procedures may be performed under general anesthesia, depending on the age and/or condition of the patient. If a specimen is transported to an outside laboratory, report 99000 for handling or conveyance. For radiology services, see 76942, 77002, and 77012.

ICD-10-CM Diagnostic Codes

A56.01	Chlamydial cystitis and urethritis
C61	Malignant neoplasm of prostate ♂
C67.0	Malignant neoplasm of trigone of bladder
C67.2	Malignant neoplasm of lateral wall of bladder
C67.3	Malignant neoplasm of anterior wall of bladder
C67.4	Malignant neoplasm of posterior wall of bladder
C67.5	Malignant neoplasm of bladder neck
C67.6	Malignant neoplasm of ureteric orifice
D07.5	Carcinoma in situ of prostate ♂
D29.1	Benign neoplasm of prostate ♂
D40.0	Neoplasm of uncertain behavior of prostate ♂
G83.4	Cauda equina syndrome
N11.0	Nonobstructive reflux-associated chronic pyelonephritis
N11.8	Other chronic tubulo-interstitial nephritis
N13.71	Vesicoureteral-reflux without reflux nephropathy
N16	Renal tubulo-interstitial disorders in diseases classified elsewhere
N21.1	Calculus in urethra
N28.84	Pyelitis cystica
N28.85	Pyeloureteritis cystica
N28.86	Ureteritis cystica
N30.00	Acute cystitis without hematuria
N30.01	Acute cystitis with hematuria
N30.10	Interstitial cystitis (chronic) without hematuria
N30.11	Interstitial cystitis (chronic) with hematuria
N30.30	Trigonitis without hematuria
N30.31	Trigonitis with hematuria
N30.80	Other cystitis without hematuria
N30.81	Other cystitis with hematuria
N32.0	Bladder-neck obstruction
N32.1	Vesicointestinal fistula
N32.3	Diverticulum of bladder
N32.81	Overactive bladder
N32.89	Other specified disorders of bladder
N36.0	Urethral fistula
N37	Urethral disorders in diseases classified elsewhere
N39.3	Stress incontinence (female) (male)
N40.1	Benign prostatic hyperplasia with lower urinary tract symptoms 🅰 ♂
N40.3	Nodular prostate with lower urinary tract symptoms 🅰 ♂
N47.1	Phimosis ♂
N99.81	Other intraoperative complications of genitourinary system
N99.89	Other postprocedural complications and disorders of genitourinary system
Q54.0	Hypospadias, balanic ♂
Q54.1	Hypospadias, penile ♂
Q54.2	Hypospadias, penoscrotal ♂
Q54.3	Hypospadias, perineal ♂
Q54.4	Congenital chordee ♂
Q54.8	Other hypospadias ♂
Q55.5	Congenital absence and aplasia of penis ♂
Q55.61	Curvature of penis (lateral) ♂
Q55.62	Hypoplasia of penis ♂
Q55.63	Congenital torsion of penis ♂
Q55.64	Hidden penis ♂
Q55.69	Other congenital malformation of penis ♂
Q64.0	Epispadias ♂
Q64.2	Congenital posterior urethral valves
Q64.31	Congenital bladder neck obstruction
Q64.32	Congenital stricture of urethra
Q64.33	Congenital stricture of urinary meatus
Q64.39	Other atresia and stenosis of urethra and bladder neck
R82.71	Bacteriuria
R82.79	Other abnormal findings on microbiological examination of urine
S37.22XA	Contusion of bladder, initial encounter
S37.23XA	Laceration of bladder, initial encounter
S37.29XA	Other injury of bladder, initial encounter

Bladder

S37.32XA	Contusion of urethra, initial encounter
S37.33XA	Laceration of urethra, initial encounter
S37.39XA	Other injury of urethra, initial encounter

AMA: 51100 2018,Jan,8; 2017,Jan,8; 2016,Jan,13; 2015,Jan,16; 2014,Jan,11
51101 2018,Jan,8; 2017,Jan,8; 2016,Jan,13; 2015,Jan,16; 2014,Jan,11 **51102** 2018,Jan,8; 2017,Jan,8; 2016,Jan,13; 2015,Jan,16; 2014,Jan,11

Relative Value Units/Medicare Edits

Non-Facility RVU	Work	PE	MP	Total
51100	0.78	1.08	0.09	1.95
51101	1.02	2.92	0.12	4.06
51102	2.7	3.78	0.3	6.78
Facility RVU	**Work**	**PE**	**MP**	**Total**
51100	0.78	0.25	0.09	1.12
51101	1.02	0.35	0.12	1.49
51102	2.7	1.2	0.3	4.2

	FUD	Status	MUE	Modifiers				IOM Reference
51100	0	A	1(3)	51	N/A	N/A	N/A	None
51101	0	A	1(3)	51	N/A	N/A	N/A	
51102	0	A	1(3)	51	N/A	N/A	N/A	

* with documentation

Terms To Know

aspiration. Drawing fluid out by suction.

bacteriuria. Bacteria in the urine. The presence of large amounts may be a sign of infection in the urinary tract.

catheter. Flexible tube inserted into an area of the body for introducing or withdrawing fluid.

congenital. Present at birth, occurring through heredity or an influence during gestation up to the moment of birth.

cystitis. Inflammation of the urinary bladder. Symptoms include dysuria, frequency of urination, urgency, and hematuria.

hypoplasia. Condition in which there is underdevelopment of an organ or tissue.

insertion. Placement or implantation into a body part.

intra. Within.

nocturia. Frequent urination during the night that affects sleep patterns.

polyuria. Excessive urination.

supra. Above.

trocar. Cannula or a sharp pointed instrument used to puncture and aspirate fluid from cavities.

51500

| 51500 | Excision of urachal cyst or sinus, with or without umbilical hernia repair |

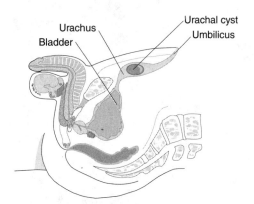

The physician excises the urachal cyst from the fibrous cord

Explanation

The physician removes a cyst or dilated urachus (the remnant of bladder development that attaches from bladder to umbilicus). To access the urachus, the physician makes an incision in the skin of the lower abdomen through the umbilicus, and cuts the corresponding muscles, fat, and fibrous membranes (fascia). After isolating the urachus with a clamp, the physician excises the urachal cyst or sinus and a small cuff of the bladder. The physician sutures the bladder and removes the urachal tissue, leaving the navel intact. The physician may also repair a rupture (hernia) of tissue in the umbilicus. After inserting a drain tube and urethral catheter, the physician performs a layered closure.

Coding Tips

For excision of the vesical neck, see 51520. For excision of the bladder diverticulum, see 51525. For excision of a bladder tumor, see 51530. For excision or repair of a ureterocele, see 51535.

ICD-10-CM Diagnostic Codes

K42.0	Umbilical hernia with obstruction, without gangrene
K42.1	Umbilical hernia with gangrene
K42.9	Umbilical hernia without obstruction or gangrene
Q64.4	Malformation of urachus

AMA: 51500 2014,Jan,11

Relative Value Units/Medicare Edits

Non-Facility RVU	Work	PE	MP	Total
51500	11.05	6.06	1.26	18.37
Facility RVU	**Work**	**PE**	**MP**	**Total**
51500	11.05	6.06	1.26	18.37

	FUD	Status	MUE	Modifiers				IOM Reference
51500	90	A	1(2)	51	N/A	62*	80	None

* with documentation

Terms To Know

anomaly. Irregularity in the structure or position of an organ or tissue.

Bladder

51520

51520 Cystotomy; for simple excision of vesical neck (separate procedure)

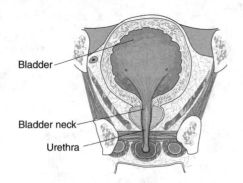

Bladder
Bladder neck
Urethra

The physician uses a bladder cuff
to help excise the bladder neck

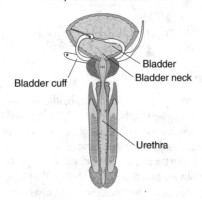

Bladder cuff
Bladder
Bladder neck
Urethra

Explanation

The physician removes part or all of the bladder neck. The physician makes an incision in the skin of the lower abdomen and cuts the corresponding muscles, fat, and fibrous membranes (fascia). Through this incision, the physician accesses the bladder neck and removes diseased or enlarged bladder neck tissue. The bladder is sutured and the abdominal wall is closed.

Coding Tips

This separate procedure by definition is usually a component of a more complex service and is not identified separately. When performed alone or with other unrelated procedures/services it may be reported. If performed alone, list the code; if performed with other procedures/services, list the code and append modifier 59 or an X{EPSU} modifier. For resection of vesical neck congenital defects through a cystourethroscope, see 52400. For endoscopic excision of the bladder neck through the urethra, see 52500. For fulguration of the bladder neck through a cystourethroscope, see 52214.

ICD-10-CM Diagnostic Codes

C67.5	Malignant neoplasm of bladder neck
C79.11	Secondary malignant neoplasm of bladder
D09.0	Carcinoma in situ of bladder
D30.3	Benign neoplasm of bladder
D41.4	Neoplasm of uncertain behavior of bladder
D49.4	Neoplasm of unspecified behavior of bladder
N32.0	Bladder-neck obstruction
N32.89	Other specified disorders of bladder
Q64.31	Congenital bladder neck obstruction
Q64.39	Other atresia and stenosis of urethra and bladder neck

AMA: 51520 2014,Jan,11

Relative Value Units/Medicare Edits

Non-Facility RVU	Work	PE	MP	Total
51520	10.21	5.79	1.17	17.17
Facility RVU	**Work**	**PE**	**MP**	**Total**
51520	10.21	5.79	1.17	17.17

	FUD	Status	MUE	Modifiers				IOM Reference
51520	90	A	1(2)	51	N/A	62*	80	None

* with documentation

Terms To Know

carcinoma in situ. Malignancy that arises from the cells of the vessel, gland, or organ of origin that remains confined to that site or has not invaded neighboring tissue.

cystitis. Inflammation of the urinary bladder. Symptoms include dysuria, frequency of urination, urgency, and hematuria.

cystotomy. Surgical incision into the gallbladder or urinary bladder.

nocturnal enuresis. Bed-wetting.

stress incontinence. Involuntary escape of urine at times of minor stress against the bladder, such as coughing, sneezing, or laughing.

Bladder

51525

51525   Cystotomy; for excision of bladder diverticulum, single or multiple (separate procedure)

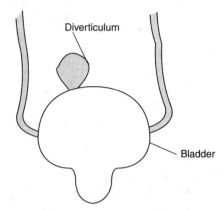

The physician enters through the abdomen and excises the diverticulum, suturing the remaining musculature and mucosa

Diverticulum

Bladder

Saccular defect, or diverticulum, is excised

Explanation

The physician removes a diverticulum, a herniated defect of the bladder. To access the diverticulum, the physician makes an incision in the skin of the lower abdomen and cuts the corresponding muscles, fat, and fibrous membranes (fascia). The physician makes an incision in the bladder and may insert a ureteral stent if the diverticulum is close to the ureter. After dissecting the diverticulum from surrounding tissues and arteries, the physician excises the defective tissue and closes the remaining musculature and mucosa with absorbable sutures. This process may be repeated in other diverticula. The incision is repaired with a layered closure.

Coding Tips

This separate procedure by definition is usually a component of a more complex service and is not identified separately. When performed alone or with other unrelated procedures/services it may be reported. If performed alone, list the code; if performed with other procedures/services, list the code and append modifier 59 or an X{EPSU} modifier. For incision or removal of the opening of a bladder diverticulum through a cystourethroscope, see 52305. For fulguration of the bladder neck through a cystourethroscope, see 52214.

ICD-10-CM Diagnostic Codes

N32.3   Diverticulum of bladder

AMA: 51525 2014,Jan,11

Relative Value Units/Medicare Edits

Non-Facility RVU	Work	PE	MP	Total
51525	15.42	7.58	1.81	24.81
Facility RVU	Work	PE	MP	Total
51525	15.42	7.58	1.81	24.81

	FUD	Status	MUE	Modifiers				IOM Reference
51525	90	A	1(2)	51	N/A	62*	80	None

* with documentation

51530

51530   Cystotomy; for excision of bladder tumor

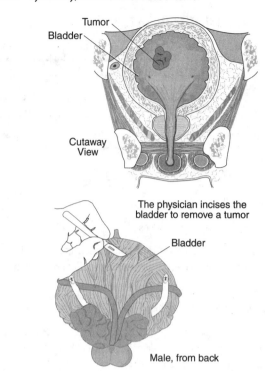

Tumor

Bladder

Cutaway View

The physician incises the bladder to remove a tumor

Bladder

Male, from back

Explanation

The physician makes an incision in the bladder to remove a tumor of the bladder. To access the bladder, the physician makes an incision in the skin of the lower abdomen and cuts the corresponding muscles, fat, and fibrous membranes (fascia). The bladder is incised (cystotomy). After removing the tumor and surrounding diseased vesical tissue, the physician inserts a drain tube and performs a layered closure.

Coding Tips

If significant additional time and effort is documented, append modifier 22 and submit a cover letter and operative report. For removal of bladder tumors through a cystourethroscope, see 52234–52240. For removal of minor lesions of the bladder through a cystourethroscope, see 52224. For resection of a ureteral or renal pelvic tumor through a cystourethroscope, see 52355. For cystourethroscopy with incision or resection of orifice of bladder diverticulum, single or multiple, see 52305.

ICD-10-CM Diagnostic Codes

C67.0	Malignant neoplasm of trigone of bladder
C67.1	Malignant neoplasm of dome of bladder
C67.2	Malignant neoplasm of lateral wall of bladder
C67.3	Malignant neoplasm of anterior wall of bladder
C67.4	Malignant neoplasm of posterior wall of bladder
C67.5	Malignant neoplasm of bladder neck
C67.6	Malignant neoplasm of ureteric orifice
C67.7	Malignant neoplasm of urachus
C79.11	Secondary malignant neoplasm of bladder
C79.19	Secondary malignant neoplasm of other urinary organs
D09.0	Carcinoma in situ of bladder
D30.3	Benign neoplasm of bladder

Bladder

D41.4	Neoplasm of uncertain behavior of bladder	
D49.4	Neoplasm of unspecified behavior of bladder	

AMA: 51530 2014,Jan,11

Relative Value Units/Medicare Edits

Non-Facility RVU	Work	PE	MP	Total
51530	13.71	6.96	1.57	22.24
Facility RVU	Work	PE	MP	Total
51530	13.71	6.96	1.57	22.24

	FUD	Status	MUE	Modifiers				IOM Reference
51530	90	A	1(2)	51	N/A	62*	80	None

* with documentation

Terms To Know

benign. Mild or nonmalignant in nature.

carcinoma in situ. Malignancy that arises from the cells of the vessel, gland, or organ of origin that remains confined to that site or has not invaded neighboring tissue.

cystotomy. Surgical incision into the gallbladder or urinary bladder.

malignant. Any condition tending to progress toward death, specifically an invasive tumor with a loss of cellular differentiation that has the ability to spread or metastasize to other body areas.

neoplasm. New abnormal growth, tumor.

trigone. Triangular, smooth area of mucous membrane at the base of the bladder, located between the ureteric openings in back and the urethral opening in front.

urachus. Embryonic tube connecting the urinary bladder to the umbilicus during development of the fetus that normally closes before birth, generally in the fourth or fifth month of gestation.

51535

51535   Cystotomy for excision, incision, or repair of ureterocele

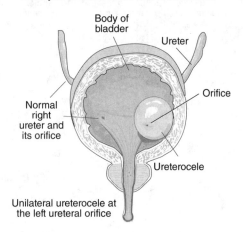

A ureterocele is a saccular dilation of the ureter, usually at its orifice in the wall of the bladder

The physician surgically excises, incises, or otherwise repairs the ureterocele defect

Explanation

The physician makes an incision in the bladder to remove or repair a saccular dilation of the ureteral end (ureterocele) that protrudes into the bladder. To access the bladder and ureters, the physician makes a midline incision in the skin of the abdomen and cuts the corresponding muscles, fat, and fibrous membranes (fascia). The physician incises the bladder (cystotomy) and excises or fulgurates the ureterocele. After examining the ureter for other defects, the physician sutures the bladder incision and inserts a ureteral catheter. The physician inserts a drain tube and performs a layered closure.

Coding Tips

This is a unilateral procedure. If performed bilaterally, some payers require that the service be reported twice with modifier 50 appended to the second code while others require identification of the service only once with modifier 50 appended. Check with individual payers. Modifier 50 identifies a procedure performed identically on the opposite side of the body (mirror image). For repair of a ureterocele through a cystourethroscope, see 52300–52301. For cystotomy for excision of a bladder tumor, see 51530. For cystotomy for excision of a bladder diverticulum, see 51525. For cystourethroscopy with incision or resection of orifice of bladder diverticulum, single or multiple, see 52305.

ICD-10-CM Diagnostic Codes

N28.89	Other specified disorders of kidney and ureter
Q62.31	Congenital ureterocele, orthotopic
Q62.32	Cecoureterocele

AMA: 51535 2014,Jan,11

Relative Value Units/Medicare Edits

Non-Facility RVU	Work	PE	MP	Total
51535	13.9	7.03	1.61	22.54
Facility RVU	**Work**	**PE**	**MP**	**Total**
51535	13.9	7.03	1.61	22.54

	FUD	Status	MUE	Modifiers				IOM Reference
51535	90	A	1(2)	51	50	62*	80	None

* with documentation

Terms To Know

catheter. Flexible tube inserted into an area of the body for introducing or withdrawing fluid.

congenital. Present at birth, occurring through heredity or an influence during gestation up to the moment of birth.

suture. Numerous stitching techniques employed in wound closure.

buried suture. Continuous or interrupted suture placed under the skin for a layered closure.

continuous suture. Running stitch with tension evenly distributed across a single strand to provide a leakproof closure line.

interrupted suture. Series of single stitches with tension isolated at each stitch, in which all stitches are not affected if one becomes loose, and the isolated sutures cannot act as a wick to transport an infection.

purse-string suture. Continuous suture placed around a tubular structure and tightened, to reduce or close the lumen.

retention suture. Secondary stitching that bridges the primary suture, providing support for the primary repair; a plastic or rubber bolster may be placed over the primary repair and under the retention sutures.

ureterocele. Saccular formation of the lower part of the ureter, protruding into the bladder.

vesicoureteral reflux. Urine passage from the bladder flows backward up into the ureter and kidneys that can lead to bacterial infection and an increase in hydrostatic pressure, causing kidney damage.

51550-51555

51550   Cystectomy, partial; simple
51555   complicated (eg, postradiation, previous surgery, difficult location)

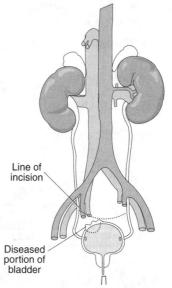

Line of incision

Diseased portion of bladder

The physician removes the diseased portion of the bladder only

Explanation

The physician removes a portion of diseased or damaged bladder tissue. To access the bladder, the physician makes an incision in the skin above the pubic bone and cuts the corresponding muscles, fat, and fibrous membranes (fascia). The physician mobilizes the bladder and the major vesical blood vessels, and incises the bladder wall to access the diseased or damaged bladder tissue. After removing the tissue, the physician inserts catheters into the bladder and urethra and sutures the bladder tissues. The physician performs a layered closure and inserts a drain tube, bringing it out through a separate stab incision in the skin. Report 51550 if the cystectomy presents few complications; report 51555 if the procedure is complicated because of prior administration of radiation, a previous surgery, or difficult access to the diseased or damaged bladder tissue.

Coding Tips

For removal of diseased or damaged bladder tissue with reimplantation of the ureter into the bladder (ureteroneocystostomy), see 51565. For excision of the bladder cuff as part of the removal of a ureter, see 50650. For complete removal of the bladder, see 51570–51596.

ICD-10-CM Diagnostic Codes

C67.0	Malignant neoplasm of trigone of bladder
C67.1	Malignant neoplasm of dome of bladder
C67.2	Malignant neoplasm of lateral wall of bladder
C67.3	Malignant neoplasm of anterior wall of bladder
C67.4	Malignant neoplasm of posterior wall of bladder
C67.5	Malignant neoplasm of bladder neck
C67.6	Malignant neoplasm of ureteric orifice
C67.8	Malignant neoplasm of overlapping sites of bladder
C79.11	Secondary malignant neoplasm of bladder
D09.0	Carcinoma in situ of bladder

Bladder

D30.3	Benign neoplasm of bladder	
D41.4	Neoplasm of uncertain behavior of bladder	
D48.7	Neoplasm of uncertain behavior of other specified sites	
D49.4	Neoplasm of unspecified behavior of bladder	
N30.10	Interstitial cystitis (chronic) without hematuria	
N30.11	Interstitial cystitis (chronic) with hematuria	
N32.1	Vesicointestinal fistula	
N32.3	Diverticulum of bladder	
N80.8	Other endometriosis ♀	
N82.0	Vesicovaginal fistula ♀	

AMA: 51550 2014,Jan,11 **51555** 2014,Jan,11

Relative Value Units/Medicare Edits

Non-Facility RVU	Work	PE	MP	Total
51550	17.23	8.36	2.23	27.82
51555	23.18	10.52	2.88	36.58
Facility RVU	**Work**	**PE**	**MP**	**Total**
51550	17.23	8.36	2.23	27.82
51555	23.18	10.52	2.88	36.58

	FUD	Status	MUE	Modifiers				IOM Reference
51550	90	A	1(2)	51	N/A	62*	80	None
51555	90	A	1(2)	51	N/A	62*	80	

* with documentation

Terms To Know

carcinoma in situ. Malignancy that arises from the cells of the vessel, gland, or organ of origin that remains confined to that site or has not invaded neighboring tissue.

catheter. Flexible tube inserted into an area of the body for introducing or withdrawing fluid.

chronic. Persistent, continuing, or recurring.

cystitis. Inflammation of the urinary bladder. Symptoms include dysuria, frequency of urination, urgency, and hematuria.

diverticulum. Pouch or sac in the walls of an organ or canal.

fistula. Abnormal tube-like passage between two body cavities or organs or from an organ to the outside surface.

neurogenic bladder. Dysfunctional bladder due to a central or peripheral nervous system lesion that may result in incontinence, residual urine retention, infection, stones, and renal failure.

Bladder

51565

51565   Cystectomy, partial, with reimplantation of ureter(s) into bladder (ureteroneocystostomy)

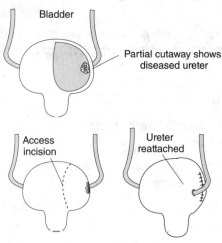

The physician removes diseased or damaged bladder tissue close to the ureteral orifice

Explanation

The physician removes diseased or damaged bladder tissue close to the ureteral orifice, and reimplants ureter(s) into the bladder (ureteroneocystostomy). To access the bladder and ureters, the physician makes a midline incision in the skin of the abdomen and cuts the corresponding muscles, fat, and fibrous membranes (fascia). The physician mobilizes the bladder, ureter(s), and the major vesical blood vessels, and may incise the bladder wall to access the diseased or damaged bladder tissue. The physician removes the diseased or damaged bladder tissue, requiring removal of the ureteral orifice and/or ureteral division. The physician brings the cut end of the ureter through a stab wound in the bladder and sutures the ureter to the bladder. To provide support during healing, the physician inserts a ureteral catheter, bringing the tube end out through the urethra or bladder incision. The physician inserts a drain tube and performs a layered closure.

Coding Tips

Report 51550–51555 for removal of diseased or damaged bladder tissue not requiring reimplantation of the ureter. For implantation of the ureter into the bladder without removal of diseased or damaged bladder tissue, see 50780–50785. Report 50830 if the physician performs a ureteroneocystostomy to restore urethral continuity after surgical diversion. For ureteroneocystostomy following plastic reconstruction on the bladder and urethra (cystourethroplasty), see 51820.

ICD-10-CM Diagnostic Codes

C67.0	Malignant neoplasm of trigone of bladder
C67.1	Malignant neoplasm of dome of bladder
C67.2	Malignant neoplasm of lateral wall of bladder
C67.3	Malignant neoplasm of anterior wall of bladder
C67.4	Malignant neoplasm of posterior wall of bladder
C67.5	Malignant neoplasm of bladder neck
C67.6	Malignant neoplasm of ureteric orifice
C67.8	Malignant neoplasm of overlapping sites of bladder
C79.11	Secondary malignant neoplasm of bladder
D09.0	Carcinoma in situ of bladder

D30.3	Benign neoplasm of bladder
D41.4	Neoplasm of uncertain behavior of bladder
D48.7	Neoplasm of uncertain behavior of other specified sites
D49.4	Neoplasm of unspecified behavior of bladder
N30.10	Interstitial cystitis (chronic) without hematuria
N30.11	Interstitial cystitis (chronic) with hematuria
N32.1	Vesicointestinal fistula
N32.3	Diverticulum of bladder
N80.8	Other endometriosis ♀
N82.0	Vesicovaginal fistula ♀

AMA: 51565 2014,Jan,11

Relative Value Units/Medicare Edits

Non-Facility RVU	Work	PE	MP	Total
51565	23.68	10.95	2.96	37.59
Facility RVU	**Work**	**PE**	**MP**	**Total**
51565	23.68	10.95	2.96	37.59

	FUD	Status	MUE	Modifiers				IOM Reference
51565	90	A	1(2)	51	N/A	62*	80	None

* with documentation

Terms To Know

carcinoma in situ. Malignancy that arises from the cells of the vessel, gland, or organ of origin that remains confined to that site or has not invaded neighboring tissue.

cystitis. Inflammation of the urinary bladder. Symptoms include dysuria, frequency of urination, urgency, and hematuria.

diverticulum. Pouch or sac in the walls of an organ or canal.

fistula. Abnormal tube-like passage between two body cavities or organs or from an organ to the outside surface.

malignant. Any condition tending to progress toward death, specifically an invasive tumor with a loss of cellular differentiation that has the ability to spread or metastasize to other body areas.

neurogenic bladder. Dysfunctional bladder due to a central or peripheral nervous system lesion that may result in incontinence, residual urine retention, infection, stones, and renal failure.

51570-51575

51570 Cystectomy, complete; (separate procedure)
51575   with bilateral pelvic lymphadenectomy, including external iliac, hypogastric, and obturator nodes

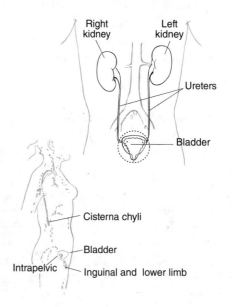

Explanation

The physician removes the bladder (cystectomy). To access the bladder, the physician makes an incision in the skin of the lower abdomen and cuts the corresponding muscles, fat, and fibrous membranes (fascia). Report 51570 if the physician dissects and ties (ligates) the hypogastric and vesical vessels, and severs the bladder from the urethra, rectum, surrounding peritoneum, vas deferens, and prostate (if applicable). After removing the bladder and controlling bleeding, the physician inserts drain tubes and performs a layered closure. If the physician bilaterally removes the pelvic lymph nodes, report 51575.

Coding Tips

Note that 51570, a separate procedure by definition, is usually a component of a more complex service and is not identified separately. When performed alone or with other unrelated procedures/services it may be reported. If performed alone, list the code; if performed with other procedures/services, list the code and append modifier 59 or an X{EPSU} modifier. For removal of the bladder with urinary diversion, see 51580–51585. For complete removal of the bladder in combination with a continent diversion, see 51596. If the bladder removal is part of pelvic exenteration, see 51597.

ICD-10-CM Diagnostic Codes

C67.0	Malignant neoplasm of trigone of bladder
C67.1	Malignant neoplasm of dome of bladder
C67.2	Malignant neoplasm of lateral wall of bladder
C67.3	Malignant neoplasm of anterior wall of bladder
C67.4	Malignant neoplasm of posterior wall of bladder
C67.5	Malignant neoplasm of bladder neck
C67.6	Malignant neoplasm of ureteric orifice
C67.8	Malignant neoplasm of overlapping sites of bladder
C77.5	Secondary and unspecified malignant neoplasm of intrapelvic lymph nodes
C79.11	Secondary malignant neoplasm of bladder

Bladder

D09.0	Carcinoma in situ of bladder
D30.3	Benign neoplasm of bladder
D41.4	Neoplasm of uncertain behavior of bladder
D49.4	Neoplasm of unspecified behavior of bladder
D49.511	Neoplasm of unspecified behavior of right kidney ☑
D49.512	Neoplasm of unspecified behavior of left kidney ☑
D49.59	Neoplasm of unspecified behavior of other genitourinary organ
N30.10	Interstitial cystitis (chronic) without hematuria
N30.11	Interstitial cystitis (chronic) with hematuria

AMA: **51570** 2014,Jan,11 **51575** 2014,Jan,11

Relative Value Units/Medicare Edits

Non-Facility RVU	Work	PE	MP	Total
51570	27.46	11.89	3.26	42.61
51575	34.18	14.51	3.97	52.66
Facility RVU	**Work**	**PE**	**MP**	**Total**
51570	27.46	11.89	3.26	42.61
51575	34.18	14.51	3.97	52.66

	FUD	Status	MUE	Modifiers				IOM Reference
51570	90	A	1(2)	51	N/A	62*	80	None
51575	90	A	1(2)	51	N/A	62*	80	

* with documentation

Terms To Know

bilateral. Consisting of or affecting two sides.

carcinoma in situ. Malignancy that arises from the cells of the vessel, gland, or organ of origin that remains confined to that site or has not invaded neighboring tissue.

chronic. Persistent, continuing, or recurring.

cystitis. Inflammation of the urinary bladder. Symptoms include dysuria, frequency of urination, urgency, and hematuria.

lymphadenectomy. Dissection of lymph nodes free from the vessels and removal for examination by frozen section in a separate procedure to detect early-stage metastases.

malignant. Any condition tending to progress toward death, specifically an invasive tumor with a loss of cellular differentiation that has the ability to spread or metastasize to other body areas.

neoplasm. New abnormal growth, tumor.

51580-51585

51580 Cystectomy, complete, with ureterosigmoidostomy or ureterocutaneous transplantations;
51585 with bilateral pelvic lymphadenectomy, including external iliac, hypogastric, and obturator nodes

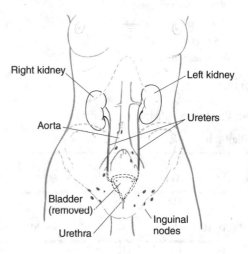

Explanation

In 51580, the physician removes the bladder (cystectomy) and connects the ureters to the skin or sigmoid colon. To access the bladder and ureters, the physician makes a midline incision in the skin of the abdomen and cuts the corresponding muscles, fat, and fibrous membranes (fascia). The physician dissects and ligates the hypogastric and vesical vessels, and severs the bladder from the ureters and urethra. Blunt dissection from adherent rectum, surrounding peritoneum, and vas deferens and prostate may be needed. After controlling bleeding, the physician diverts urine by implanting the ureters to the skin (ureterocutaneous transplant), or connecting (anastomosing) the ureters to the sigmoid colon (ureterosigmoidostomy). To provide support during healing, the physician inserts a slender tube into each ureter. After completing the urinary diversion procedure, the physician inserts drain tubes and performs a layered closure. In 51585, the physician removes the bladder (cystectomy) and pelvic lymph nodes, and connects the ureters to the skin or sigmoid colon. The physician also removes external iliac, hypogastric, and obturator lymph nodes. After controlling bleeding, the physician diverts urine by implanting the ureters to the skin (ureterocutaneous transplant), or connecting the ureters to the sigmoid colon (ureterosigmoidostomy). The physician also inserts a slender tube into each ureter for support. After completing the urinary diversion procedure, the physician inserts drain tubes and performs a layered closure.

Coding Tips

For cystectomy, complete, with ureteroileal conduit or sigmoid bladder, including bowel anastomosis, see 51590; with bilateral pelvic lymphadenectomy, including external iliac, hypogastric, and obturator nodes, see 51595. If the bladder removal is part of pelvic exenteration, see 51597.

ICD-10-CM Diagnostic Codes

C67.0	Malignant neoplasm of trigone of bladder
C67.1	Malignant neoplasm of dome of bladder
C67.2	Malignant neoplasm of lateral wall of bladder
C67.3	Malignant neoplasm of anterior wall of bladder
C67.4	Malignant neoplasm of posterior wall of bladder
C67.5	Malignant neoplasm of bladder neck

Bladder

C67.6	Malignant neoplasm of ureteric orifice
C67.8	Malignant neoplasm of overlapping sites of bladder
C77.5	Secondary and unspecified malignant neoplasm of intrapelvic lymph nodes
C79.11	Secondary malignant neoplasm of bladder
D09.0	Carcinoma in situ of bladder
D30.3	Benign neoplasm of bladder
D41.4	Neoplasm of uncertain behavior of bladder
D49.4	Neoplasm of unspecified behavior of bladder
N30.10	Interstitial cystitis (chronic) without hematuria
N30.11	Interstitial cystitis (chronic) with hematuria

AMA: **51580** 2014,Jan,11 **51585** 2014,Jan,11

Relative Value Units/Medicare Edits

Non-Facility RVU	Work	PE	MP	Total
51580	35.37	15.35	4.04	54.76
51585	39.64	16.79	4.53	60.96
Facility RVU	Work	PE	MP	Total
51580	35.37	15.35	4.04	54.76
51585	39.64	16.79	4.53	60.96

	FUD	Status	MUE	Modifiers				IOM Reference
51580	90	A	1(2)	51	N/A	62*	80	None
51585	90	A	1(2)	51	N/A	62*	80	

* with documentation

Terms To Know

chronic. Persistent, continuing, or recurring.

cystitis. Inflammation of the urinary bladder. Symptoms include dysuria, frequency of urination, urgency, and hematuria.

malignant. Any condition tending to progress toward death, specifically an invasive tumor with a loss of cellular differentiation that has the ability to spread or metastasize to other body areas.

secondary. Second in order of occurrence or importance, or appearing during the course of another disease or condition.

51590-51595

51590 Cystectomy, complete, with ureteroileal conduit or sigmoid bladder, including intestine anastomosis;
51595 with bilateral pelvic lymphadenectomy, including external iliac, hypogastric, and obturator nodes

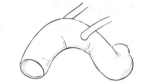

Ureteral remnants attached to bowel

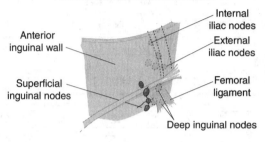

Explanation

In 51590, the physician removes the bladder (cystectomy) and diverts urine by connecting the ureters to a ureteroileal conduit or sigmoid bladder with an opening into the skin. To access the bladder and ureters, the physician makes a midline incision in the skin of the abdomen and cuts the corresponding muscles, fat, and fibrous membranes (fascia). The physician dissects and ligates the hypogastric and vesical vessels, and severs the bladder from the ureters and urethra. Blunt dissection from adherent rectum, surrounding peritoneum, and vas deferens and prostate may be needed. After controlling bleeding, the physician diverts urine by connecting the ureters to a segment of ileal or sigmoid colon fashioned into a conduit or bladder, respectively, with an opening into the skin. To provide support during healing, the physician inserts a slender tube into each ureter. After completing the urinary diversion procedure, the physician inserts drain tubes and performs a layered closure. In 51595, the physician removes the bladder (cystectomy) and pelvic lymph nodes, and diverts urine by connecting the ureters to a ureteroileal conduit or sigmoid bladder with an opening into the skin and anastomoses the bowel as described above. The physician also removes external iliac, hypogastric, and obturator lymph nodes. After completing the urinary diversion procedure, the physician inserts drain tubes and performs a layered closure.

Coding Tips

For cystectomy, complete, with ureterosigmoidostomy or ureterocutaneous transplantations, see 51580; with bilateral pelvic lymphadenectomy, including external iliac, hypogastric, and obturator nodes, see 51585. For ureteroileal or ureterocolon conduit alone (without cystectomy), see 50815 and 50820.

ICD-10-CM Diagnostic Codes

C67.0	Malignant neoplasm of trigone of bladder
C67.1	Malignant neoplasm of dome of bladder
C67.2	Malignant neoplasm of lateral wall of bladder
C67.3	Malignant neoplasm of anterior wall of bladder
C67.4	Malignant neoplasm of posterior wall of bladder
C67.5	Malignant neoplasm of bladder neck
C67.6	Malignant neoplasm of ureteric orifice

Bladder

CPT © 2020 American Medical Association. All Rights Reserved.   ● New   ▲ Revised   + Add On   ★ Telemedicine   AMA: CPT Assist   [Resequenced]   ☑ Laterality   © 2020 Optum360, LLC

C67.8	Malignant neoplasm of overlapping sites of bladder
C77.5	Secondary and unspecified malignant neoplasm of intrapelvic lymph nodes
C79.11	Secondary malignant neoplasm of bladder
D09.0	Carcinoma in situ of bladder
D30.3	Benign neoplasm of bladder
D41.4	Neoplasm of uncertain behavior of bladder
D49.4	Neoplasm of unspecified behavior of bladder
N30.10	Interstitial cystitis (chronic) without hematuria
N30.11	Interstitial cystitis (chronic) with hematuria

AMA: **51590** 2014,Jan,11 **51595** 2014,Jan,11

Relative Value Units/Medicare Edits

Non-Facility RVU	Work	PE	MP	Total
51590	36.33	15.23	4.33	55.89
51595	41.32	17.09	4.8	63.21
Facility RVU	Work	PE	MP	Total
51590	36.33	15.23	4.33	55.89
51595	41.32	17.09	4.8	63.21

	FUD	Status	MUE	Modifiers				IOM Reference
51590	90	A	1(2)	51	N/A	62*	80	None
51595	90	A	1(2)	51	N/A	62*	80	

* with documentation

Terms To Know

conduit. Surgically created channel for the passage of fluids.

lymphadenectomy. Dissection of lymph nodes free from the vessels and removal for examination by frozen section in a separate procedure to detect early-stage metastases.

prostate. Male gland surrounding the bladder neck and urethra that secretes a substance into the seminal fluid.

trigone. Triangular, smooth area of mucous membrane at the base of the bladder, located between the ureteric openings in back and the urethral opening in front.

51596

51596 Cystectomy, complete, with continent diversion, any open technique, using any segment of small and/or large intestine to construct neobladder

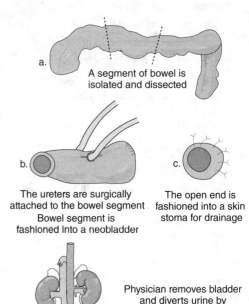

a. A segment of bowel is isolated and dissected

b. The ureters are surgically attached to the bowel segment Bowel segment is fashioned into a neobladder

c. The open end is fashioned into a skin stoma for drainage

Physician removes bladder and diverts urine by connecting ureters to any segment of bowel

Bladder removed

Explanation

The physician removes the bladder (cystectomy) and diverts urine by any method, using any bowel segment to create a new bladder. To access the bladder and ureters, the physician makes a midline incision in the skin of the abdomen and cuts the corresponding muscles, fat, and fibrous membranes (fascia). The physician dissects and ligates the hypogastric and vesical vessels, and severs the bladder from the urethra. Blunt dissection from adherent rectum, surrounding peritoneum, and vas deferens and prostate may be needed. After controlling bleeding, the physician diverts urine by connecting the ureters to a segment of large or small bowel fashioned into a bladder with an opening into the skin. To provide support during healing, the physician inserts a slender tube into each ureter. After completing the urinary diversion procedure, the physician inserts drain tubes and performs a layered closure.

Coding Tips

For cystectomy, complete, with ureterosigmoidostomy or ureterocutaneous transplantations, see 51580; with bilateral pelvic lymphadenectomy, including external iliac, hypogastric, and obturator nodes, see 51585. For cystectomy, complete, with ureteroileal conduit or sigmoid bladder, including bowel anastomosis, see 51590; with bilateral pelvic lymphadenectomy, including external iliac, hypogastric, and obturator nodes, see 51595. For continent diversion performed without bladder removal, see 50825.

ICD-10-CM Diagnostic Codes

C67.0	Malignant neoplasm of trigone of bladder
C67.1	Malignant neoplasm of dome of bladder
C67.2	Malignant neoplasm of lateral wall of bladder

C67.3	Malignant neoplasm of anterior wall of bladder
C67.4	Malignant neoplasm of posterior wall of bladder
C67.5	Malignant neoplasm of bladder neck
C67.6	Malignant neoplasm of ureteric orifice
C67.8	Malignant neoplasm of overlapping sites of bladder
C79.11	Secondary malignant neoplasm of bladder
D09.0	Carcinoma in situ of bladder
D30.3	Benign neoplasm of bladder
D41.4	Neoplasm of uncertain behavior of bladder
D49.4	Neoplasm of unspecified behavior of bladder
N30.10	Interstitial cystitis (chronic) without hematuria
N30.11	Interstitial cystitis (chronic) with hematuria

AMA: **51596** 2014,Jan,11

Relative Value Units/Medicare Edits

Non-Facility RVU	Work	PE	MP	Total
51596	44.26	18.58	5.14	67.98
Facility RVU	**Work**	**PE**	**MP**	**Total**
51596	44.26	18.58	5.14	67.98

	FUD	Status	MUE	Modifiers				IOM Reference
51596	90	A	1(2)	51	N/A	62*	80	None

* with documentation

Terms To Know

blunt dissection. Surgical technique used to expose an underlying area by separating along natural cleavage lines of tissue, without cutting.

chronic interstitial cystitis. Persistently inflamed lesion of the bladder wall, usually accompanied by urinary frequency, pain, nocturia, and a distended bladder.

ligation. Tying off a blood vessel or duct with a suture or a soft, thin wire.

malignant. Any condition tending to progress toward death, specifically an invasive tumor with a loss of cellular differentiation that has the ability to spread or metastasize to other body areas.

neoplasm. New abnormal growth, tumor.

prostate. Male gland surrounding the bladder neck and urethra that secretes a substance into the seminal fluid.

secondary. Second in order of occurrence or importance, or appearing during the course of another disease or condition.

trigone. Triangular, smooth area of mucous membrane at the base of the bladder, located between the ureteric openings in back and the urethral opening in front.

51597

51597 Pelvic exenteration, complete, for vesical, prostatic or urethral malignancy, with removal of bladder and ureteral transplantations, with or without hysterectomy and/or abdominoperineal resection of rectum and colon and colostomy, or any combination thereof

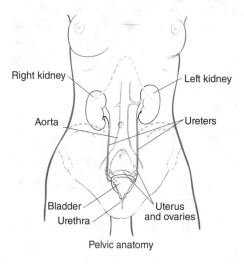

Pelvic anatomy

Explanation

The physician removes the bladder, lower ureters, lymph nodes, urethra, prostate (if applicable), colon, and rectum, due to a vesical, prostatic, or urethral malignancy. To access the bladder and ureters, the physician makes a midline incision in the skin of the abdomen and cuts the corresponding muscles, fat, and fibrous membranes (fascia). The physician dissects and ligates the hypogastric and vesical vessels, and severs the bladder, urethra, lower ureters, lymph nodes, and prostate (if applicable) from surrounding structures. The physician removes the bladder and diverts urine flow by transplanting the ureters to the skin or colon. The vagina and uterus (if applicable) and/or rectum and part of the colon may be removed and an artificial abdominal opening in the skin surface created for waste (colostomy). After completing the urinary diversion procedure, the physician inserts drain tubes and performs a layered closure.

Coding Tips

Note that this pelvic exenteration procedure is for a lower urinary tract or male genital malignancy (bladder, urethra, or prostate) and not for a gynecological malignancy. Pelvic exenteration for a gynecological malignancy is reported with 58240.

ICD-10-CM Diagnostic Codes

C61	Malignant neoplasm of prostate ♂
C67.0	Malignant neoplasm of trigone of bladder
C67.1	Malignant neoplasm of dome of bladder
C67.2	Malignant neoplasm of lateral wall of bladder
C67.3	Malignant neoplasm of anterior wall of bladder
C67.4	Malignant neoplasm of posterior wall of bladder
C67.5	Malignant neoplasm of bladder neck
C67.6	Malignant neoplasm of ureteric orifice
C67.8	Malignant neoplasm of overlapping sites of bladder
C68.0	Malignant neoplasm of urethra
C79.11	Secondary malignant neoplasm of bladder
C79.19	Secondary malignant neoplasm of other urinary organs

Bladder

AMA: **51597** 2014,Jan,11

Relative Value Units/Medicare Edits

Non-Facility RVU	Work	PE	MP	Total
51597	42.86	18.26	5.16	66.28
Facility RVU	**Work**	**PE**	**MP**	**Total**
51597	42.86	18.26	5.16	66.28

	FUD	Status	MUE	Modifiers				IOM Reference
51597	90	A	1(2)	51	N/A	62*	80	None

* with documentation

Terms To Know

dissection. Separating by cutting tissue or body structures apart.

diversion. Rechanneling of body fluid through another conduit.

drain. Device that creates a channel to allow fluid from a cavity, wound, or infected area to exit the body.

exenteration. Surgical removal of the entire contents of a body cavity, such as the pelvis or orbit.

fascia. Fibrous sheet or band of tissue that envelops organs, muscles, and groupings of muscles.

ligate. To tie off a blood vessel or duct with a suture or a soft, thin wire (ligature wire).

lymph nodes. Bean-shaped structures along the lymphatic vessels that intercept and destroy foreign materials in the tissue and bloodstream.

malignant neoplasm. Any cancerous tumor or lesion exhibiting uncontrolled tissue growth that can progressively invade other parts of the body with its disease-generating cells.

resection. Surgical removal of a part or all of an organ or body part.

secondary. Second in order of occurrence or importance, or appearing during the course of another disease or condition.

transplant. Insertion of an organ or tissue from one person or site into another.

tube. Long, hollow cylindrical instrument or body structure.

51600-51610

51600 Injection procedure for cystography or voiding urethrocystography
51605 Injection procedure and placement of chain for contrast and/or chain urethrocystography
51610 Injection procedure for retrograde urethrocystography

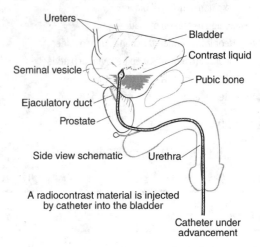

A radiocontrast material is injected by catheter into the bladder

Explanation

The physician injects a radiocontrast agent through a catheter inserted in the bladder to study the lower urinary tract. Using radiologic instruments, the physician produces an image of the bladder with x-rays (cystogram). Filling, voiding, and post-voiding x-rays are obtained. The catheter is partially or completely withdrawn and the urethra is studied by x-ray. Report 51605 if the physician inserts a chain in the bladder or through the urethra as part of the injection procedure for contrast x-rays of the bladder and urethra (chain urethrocystogram). Report 51610 if contrast material is injected through a urethral catheter or catheter-tipped syringe for x-rays of the urethra and bladder (retrograde urethrocystogram).

Coding Tips

For insertion of a drainage catheter (cystostomy tube) through an incision in the bladder, see 51040. For radiological supervision and interpretation, see 74430, 74450, and 74455. Supplies used when providing these procedures may be reported with the appropriate HCPCS Level II code. Check with the specific payer to determine coverage.

ICD-10-CM Diagnostic Codes

A54.09	Other gonococcal infection of lower genitourinary tract
A54.1	Gonococcal infection of lower genitourinary tract with periurethral and accessory gland abscess
A56.01	Chlamydial cystitis and urethritis
C61	Malignant neoplasm of prostate ♂
C67.0	Malignant neoplasm of trigone of bladder
C67.1	Malignant neoplasm of dome of bladder
C67.2	Malignant neoplasm of lateral wall of bladder
C67.3	Malignant neoplasm of anterior wall of bladder
C67.4	Malignant neoplasm of posterior wall of bladder
C67.5	Malignant neoplasm of bladder neck
C67.6	Malignant neoplasm of ureteric orifice
C67.7	Malignant neoplasm of urachus
C67.8	Malignant neoplasm of overlapping sites of bladder
D30.3	Benign neoplasm of bladder

Bladder

D30.4	Benign neoplasm of urethra
D30.8	Benign neoplasm of other specified urinary organs
D49.4	Neoplasm of unspecified behavior of bladder
N10	Acute pyelonephritis
N11.1	Chronic obstructive pyelonephritis
N13.0	Hydronephrosis with ureteropelvic junction obstruction
N13.1	Hydronephrosis with ureteral stricture, not elsewhere classified
N13.2	Hydronephrosis with renal and ureteral calculous obstruction
N13.39	Other hydronephrosis
N13.71	Vesicoureteral-reflux without reflux nephropathy
N13.721	Vesicoureteral-reflux with reflux nephropathy without hydroureter, unilateral
N13.722	Vesicoureteral-reflux with reflux nephropathy without hydroureter, bilateral
N13.731	Vesicoureteral-reflux with reflux nephropathy with hydroureter, unilateral
N13.732	Vesicoureteral-reflux with reflux nephropathy with hydroureter, bilateral
N13.8	Other obstructive and reflux uropathy
N20.0	Calculus of kidney
N20.1	Calculus of ureter
N20.2	Calculus of kidney with calculus of ureter
N21.0	Calculus in bladder
N21.1	Calculus in urethra
N21.8	Other lower urinary tract calculus
N30.00	Acute cystitis without hematuria
N30.01	Acute cystitis with hematuria
N30.20	Other chronic cystitis without hematuria
N30.21	Other chronic cystitis with hematuria
N30.30	Trigonitis without hematuria
N30.31	Trigonitis with hematuria
N30.40	Irradiation cystitis without hematuria
N30.41	Irradiation cystitis with hematuria
N30.80	Other cystitis without hematuria
N30.81	Other cystitis with hematuria
N31.0	Uninhibited neuropathic bladder, not elsewhere classified
N31.1	Reflex neuropathic bladder, not elsewhere classified
N31.2	Flaccid neuropathic bladder, not elsewhere classified
N31.8	Other neuromuscular dysfunction of bladder
N32.1	Vesicointestinal fistula
N32.2	Vesical fistula, not elsewhere classified
N32.3	Diverticulum of bladder
N32.81	Overactive bladder
N34.2	Other urethritis
N35.010	Post-traumatic urethral stricture, male, meatal ♂
N35.011	Post-traumatic bulbous urethral stricture ♂
N35.012	Post-traumatic membranous urethral stricture ♂
N35.013	Post-traumatic anterior urethral stricture ♂
N35.021	Urethral stricture due to childbirth ♀
N35.028	Other post-traumatic urethral stricture, female ♀
N35.111	Postinfective urethral stricture, not elsewhere classified, male, meatal ♂
N35.112	Postinfective bulbous urethral stricture, not elsewhere classified, male ♂

N35.113	Postinfective membranous urethral stricture, not elsewhere classified, male ♂
N35.114	Postinfective anterior urethral stricture, not elsewhere classified, male ♂
N35.12	Postinfective urethral stricture, not elsewhere classified, female ♀
N35.811	Other urethral stricture, male, meatal ♂
N35.812	Other urethral bulbous stricture, male ♂
N35.813	Other membranous urethral stricture, male ♂
N35.814	Other anterior urethral stricture, male ♂
N35.816	Other urethral stricture, male, overlapping sites ♂
N35.82	Other urethral stricture, female ♀
N36.0	Urethral fistula
N36.41	Hypermobility of urethra
N36.42	Intrinsic sphincter deficiency (ISD)
N36.43	Combined hypermobility of urethra and intrinsic sphincter deficiency
N36.44	Muscular disorders of urethra
N36.8	Other specified disorders of urethra
N39.3	Stress incontinence (female) (male)
N39.41	Urge incontinence
N39.42	Incontinence without sensory awareness
N39.43	Post-void dribbling
N39.44	Nocturnal enuresis
N39.45	Continuous leakage
N39.46	Mixed incontinence
N39.490	Overflow incontinence
N39.491	Coital incontinence
N39.492	Postural (urinary) incontinence
N39.498	Other specified urinary incontinence
N39.8	Other specified disorders of urinary system
N40.0	Benign prostatic hyperplasia without lower urinary tract symptoms 🄰 ♂
N40.1	Benign prostatic hyperplasia with lower urinary tract symptoms 🄰 ♂
N40.2	Nodular prostate without lower urinary tract symptoms 🄰 ♂
N40.3	Nodular prostate with lower urinary tract symptoms 🄰 ♂
N41.1	Chronic prostatitis 🄰 ♂
N42.83	Cyst of prostate 🄰 ♂
N42.89	Other specified disorders of prostate 🄰 ♂
N81.0	Urethrocele ♀
N81.11	Cystocele, midline ♀
N81.12	Cystocele, lateral ♀
N82.0	Vesicovaginal fistula ♀
N82.1	Other female urinary-genital tract fistulae ♀
N99.0	Postprocedural (acute) (chronic) kidney failure
N99.110	Postprocedural urethral stricture, male, meatal ♂
N99.111	Postprocedural bulbous urethral stricture, male ♂
N99.112	Postprocedural membranous urethral stricture, male ♂
N99.113	Postprocedural anterior bulbous urethral stricture, male ♂
N99.115	Postprocedural fossa navicularis urethral stricture ♂
N99.12	Postprocedural urethral stricture, female ♀
N99.520	Hemorrhage of incontinent external stoma of urinary tract
N99.521	Infection of incontinent external stoma of urinary tract

N99.522	Malfunction of incontinent external stoma of urinary tract
N99.528	Other complication of incontinent external stoma of urinary tract
N99.530	Hemorrhage of continent stoma of urinary tract
N99.531	Infection of continent stoma of urinary tract
N99.532	Malfunction of continent stoma of urinary tract
N99.538	Other complication of continent stoma of urinary tract
N99.81	Other intraoperative complications of genitourinary system
N99.89	Other postprocedural complications and disorders of genitourinary system
Q64.11	Supravesical fissure of urinary bladder
Q64.12	Cloacal exstrophy of urinary bladder
Q64.19	Other exstrophy of urinary bladder
Q64.2	Congenital posterior urethral valves
Q64.31	Congenital bladder neck obstruction
Q64.32	Congenital stricture of urethra
Q64.33	Congenital stricture of urinary meatus
Q64.39	Other atresia and stenosis of urethra and bladder neck
O64.5	Congenital absence of bladder and urethra
Q64.6	Congenital diverticulum of bladder
Q64.71	Congenital prolapse of urethra
Q64.72	Congenital prolapse of urinary meatus
Q64.73	Congenital urethrorectal fistula
Q64.74	Double urethra
Q64.75	Double urinary meatus
Q64.79	Other congenital malformations of bladder and urethra
Q64.8	Other specified congenital malformations of urinary system
R82.71	Bacteriuria
R82.79	Other abnormal findings on microbiological examination of urine
S37.22XA	Contusion of bladder, initial encounter
S37.23XA	Laceration of bladder, initial encounter
S37.29XA	Other injury of bladder, initial encounter
S37.32XA	Contusion of urethra, initial encounter
S37.33XA	Laceration of urethra, initial encounter
S37.39XA	Other injury of urethra, initial encounter

AMA: 51600 2019,Oct,10; 2014,Jan,11 51605 2014,Jan,11 51610 2019,Oct,10; 2018,Jan,8; 2017,Jan,8; 2016,Jan,3; 2014,Jan,11

Relative Value Units/Medicare Edits

Non-Facility RVU	Work	PE	MP	Total
51600	0.88	4.91	0.09	5.88
51605	0.64	0.39	0.09	1.12
51610	1.05	2.27	0.11	3.43
Facility RVU	Work	PE	MP	Total
51600	0.88	0.31	0.09	1.28
51605	0.64	0.39	0.09	1.12
51610	1.05	0.69	0.11	1.85

	FUD	Status	MUE	Modifiers				IOM Reference
51600	0	A	1(3)	51	N/A	N/A	N/A	None
51605	0	A	1(3)	51	N/A	N/A	N/A	
51610	0	A	1(3)	51	N/A	N/A	N/A	

* with documentation

51700

51700 Bladder irrigation, simple, lavage and/or instillation

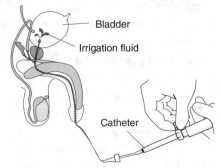

Bladder
Irrigation fluid
Catheter

The physician flushes the bladder and/or instills a saline solution

Explanation

The physician irrigates the bladder with saline solution that is flushed, injected, or introduced by drops (instillation) through a catheter. The physician initially places the catheter into the bladder and irrigates by hand until the bladder is free of clots or debris. A three-way Foley catheter may be inserted for continuous bladder irrigation.

Coding Tips

For insertion of a drainage catheter (cystostomy tube) through an incision in the bladder, see 51040. For instillation of an anticarcinogenic agent into the bladder, see 51720. Supplies used when providing this procedure may be reported with the appropriate HCPCS Level II code. Check with the specific payer to determine coverage.

ICD-10-CM Diagnostic Codes

A56.01	Chlamydial cystitis and urethritis
C67.0	Malignant neoplasm of trigone of bladder
C67.1	Malignant neoplasm of dome of bladder
C67.2	Malignant neoplasm of lateral wall of bladder
C67.3	Malignant neoplasm of anterior wall of bladder
C67.4	Malignant neoplasm of posterior wall of bladder
C67.5	Malignant neoplasm of bladder neck
C67.8	Malignant neoplasm of overlapping sites of bladder
D09.0	Carcinoma in situ of bladder
G83.4	Cauda equina syndrome
N30.00	Acute cystitis without hematuria
N30.01	Acute cystitis with hematuria
N30.10	Interstitial cystitis (chronic) without hematuria
N30.11	Interstitial cystitis (chronic) with hematuria
N30.20	Other chronic cystitis without hematuria
N30.21	Other chronic cystitis with hematuria
N30.30	Trigonitis without hematuria
N30.31	Trigonitis with hematuria
N30.40	Irradiation cystitis without hematuria
N30.41	Irradiation cystitis with hematuria
N30.80	Other cystitis without hematuria
N30.81	Other cystitis with hematuria
N31.2	Flaccid neuropathic bladder, not elsewhere classified

Bladder

© 2020 Optum360, LLC **N** Newborn: 0 **P** Pediatric: 0-17 **M** Maternity: 9-64 **A** Adult: 15-124 ♂ Male Only ♀ Female Only CPT © 2020 American Medical Association. All Rights Reserved.

N32.0	Bladder-neck obstruction
N32.89	Other specified disorders of bladder
N33	Bladder disorders in diseases classified elsewhere
N99.510	Cystostomy hemorrhage
N99.511	Cystostomy infection
R31.0	Gross hematuria
R31.1	Benign essential microscopic hematuria
R31.21	Asymptomatic microscopic hematuria
R31.29	Other microscopic hematuria
R33.0	Drug induced retention of urine
R33.8	Other retention of urine
R34	Anuria and oliguria
R39.191	Need to immediately re-void
R39.82	Chronic bladder pain

AMA: 51700 2014,Jan,11

Relative Value Units/Medicare Edits

Non-Facility RVU	Work	PE	MP	Total
51700	0.6	1.45	0.09	2.14
Facility RVU	**Work**	**PE**	**MP**	**Total**
51700	0.6	0.21	0.09	0.9

	FUD	Status	MUE	Modifiers				IOM Reference
51700	0	A	1(3)	51	N/A	N/A	N/A	None

* with documentation

Terms To Know

Foley catheter. Temporary indwelling urethral catheter held in place in the bladder by an inflated balloon containing fluid or air.

hematuria. Blood in urine, which may present as gross visible blood or as the presence of red blood cells visible only under a microscope.

instillation. Administering a liquid slowly over time, drop by drop.

irrigation. To wash out or cleanse a body cavity, wound, or tissue with water or other fluid.

lavage. Washing.

prostatitis. Inflammation of the prostate that may be acute or chronic.

trigonitis. Inflammation of the triangular area of mucous membrane at the base of the bladder, called the trigonum vesicae.

51701-51703

51701 Insertion of non-indwelling bladder catheter (eg, straight catheterization for residual urine)
51702 Insertion of temporary indwelling bladder catheter; simple (eg, Foley)
51703 complicated (eg, altered anatomy, fractured catheter/balloon)

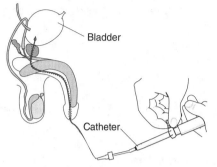

Insertion of bladder catheter

Explanation

The patient is catheterized with a non-indwelling bladder catheter (e.g., for residual urine) in 51701; simple catheterization with a temporary indwelling bladder catheter (Foley) is performed in 51702. The area is properly cleaned and sterilized. A water-soluble lubricant may be injected into the urethra before catheterization begins. The distal part of the catheter is coated with lubricant. In males, the penis is held perpendicular to the body and pulled up gently and the catheter is steadily inserted about 8 inches until urine is noted. In females, the catheter is gently inserted until urine is noted. With an indwelling catheter, insertion continues into the bladder until the retention balloon can be inflated. The catheter is gently pulled until the retention balloon is snuggled against the neck of the bladder. The catheter is secured to the abdomen or thigh and the drainage bag is secured below bladder level. Report 51703 if a change in anatomy, such as enlarging of the prostate or a fractured catheter or balloon, complicate the catheterization process.

Coding Tips

Codes 51701 and 51702 should not be reported in addition to any other procedure that includes catheter insertion as a component. Report 51701 and 51702 only when performed independently. Supplies used when providing these procedures may be reported with the appropriate HCPCS Level II code. Check with the specific payer to determine coverage. Do not report code 51702 with CPT category III codes 0071T or 0072T

ICD-10-CM Diagnostic Codes

C61	Malignant neoplasm of prostate ♂
C67.5	Malignant neoplasm of bladder neck
C68.0	Malignant neoplasm of urethra
C68.1	Malignant neoplasm of paraurethral glands
C68.8	Malignant neoplasm of overlapping sites of urinary organs
N21.1	Calculus in urethra
N21.8	Other lower urinary tract calculus
N31.2	Flaccid neuropathic bladder, not elsewhere classified
N31.8	Other neuromuscular dysfunction of bladder
N32.89	Other specified disorders of bladder
N33	Bladder disorders in diseases classified elsewhere
N35.010	Post-traumatic urethral stricture, male, meatal ♂
N35.011	Post-traumatic bulbous urethral stricture ♂

Bladder

N35.012	Post-traumatic membranous urethral stricture ♂
N35.013	Post-traumatic anterior urethral stricture ♂
N35.016	Post-traumatic urethral stricture, male, overlapping sites ♂
N35.021	Urethral stricture due to childbirth ♀
N35.028	Other post-traumatic urethral stricture, female ♀
N35.111	Postinfective urethral stricture, not elsewhere classified, male, meatal ♂
N35.112	Postinfective bulbous urethral stricture, not elsewhere classified, male ♂
N35.113	Postinfective membranous urethral stricture, not elsewhere classified, male ♂
N35.114	Postinfective anterior urethral stricture, not elsewhere classified, male ♂
N35.116	Postinfective urethral stricture, not elsewhere classified, male, overlapping sites ♂
N35.12	Postinfective urethral stricture, not elsewhere classified, female ♀
N35.811	Other urethral stricture, male, meatal ♂
N35.812	Other urethral bulbous stricture, male ♂
N35.813	Other membranous urethral stricture, male ♂
N35.814	Other anterior urethral stricture, male ♂
N35.816	Other urethral stricture, male, overlapping sites ♂
N35.82	Other urethral stricture, female ♀
N36.2	Urethral caruncle
N36.5	Urethral false passage
N36.8	Other specified disorders of urethra
N37	Urethral disorders in diseases classified elsewhere
N39.3	Stress incontinence (female) (male)
N39.45	Continuous leakage
N39.490	Overflow incontinence
N40.0	Benign prostatic hyperplasia without lower urinary tract symptoms 🅰 ♂
N40.1	Benign prostatic hyperplasia with lower urinary tract symptoms 🅰 ♂
N40.2	Nodular prostate without lower urinary tract symptoms 🅰 ♂
N99.110	Postprocedural urethral stricture, male, meatal ♂
N99.111	Postprocedural bulbous urethral stricture, male ♂
N99.112	Postprocedural membranous urethral stricture, male ♂
N99.113	Postprocedural anterior bulbous urethral stricture, male ♂
N99.115	Postprocedural fossa navicularis urethral stricture ♂
N99.116	Postprocedural urethral stricture, male, overlapping sites ♂
N99.12	Postprocedural urethral stricture, female ♀
N99.81	Other intraoperative complications of genitourinary system
N99.89	Other postprocedural complications and disorders of genitourinary system
R30.0	Dysuria
R30.1	Vesical tenesmus
R31.0	Gross hematuria
R31.1	Benign essential microscopic hematuria
R31.21	Asymptomatic microscopic hematuria
R31.29	Other microscopic hematuria
R33.0	Drug induced retention of urine
R33.8	Other retention of urine
R35.0	Frequency of micturition
R35.8	Other polyuria

R39.14	Feeling of incomplete bladder emptying
R39.81	Functional urinary incontinence
R39.89	Other symptoms and signs involving the genitourinary system
S34.3XXA	Injury of cauda equina, initial encounter
S37.32XA	Contusion of urethra, initial encounter
S37.33XA	Laceration of urethra, initial encounter
S37.39XA	Other injury of urethra, initial encounter
T83.010A	Breakdown (mechanical) of cystostomy catheter, initial encounter
T83.020A	Displacement of cystostomy catheter, initial encounter
T83.030A	Leakage of cystostomy catheter, initial encounter
T83.090A	Other mechanical complication of cystostomy catheter, initial encounter

AMA: **51701** 2018,Jan,8; 2017,Jan,8; 2016,Jan,13; 2015,Jan,16; 2014,Jan,11 **51702** 2018,Jan,8; 2017,Jan,8; 2016,Jan,13; 2015,Jan,16; 2014,May,3; 2014,Jan,11 **51703** 2018,Jan,8; 2017,Jan,8; 2016,Jan,13; 2015,Jan,16; 2014,Jan,11

Relative Value Units/Medicare Edits

Non-Facility RVU	Work	PE	MP	Total
51701	0.5	0.7	0.08	1.28
51702	0.5	1.18	0.06	1.74
51703	1.47	2.33	0.18	3.98
Facility RVU	Work	PE	MP	Total
51701	0.5	0.18	0.08	0.76
51702	0.5	0.18	0.06	0.74
51703	1.47	0.58	0.18	2.23

	FUD	Status	MUE	Modifiers				IOM Reference
51701	0	A	2(3)	51	N/A	N/A	N/A	None
51702	0	A	2(3)	51	N/A	N/A	N/A	
51703	0	A	2(3)	51	N/A	N/A	N/A	

* with documentation

Terms To Know

catheterization. Use or insertion of a tubular device into a duct, blood vessel, hollow organ, or body cavity for injecting or withdrawing fluids for diagnostic or therapeutic purposes.

distal. Located farther away from a specified reference point or the trunk.

Foley catheter. Temporary indwelling urethral catheter held in place in the bladder by an inflated balloon containing fluid or air.

Bladder

51705-51710

51705 Change of cystostomy tube; simple
51710   complicated

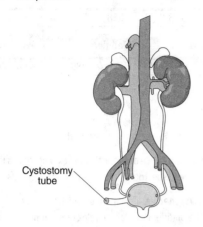

Cystostomy
tube

The physician changes the tube

Explanation

A cystostomy tube, also referred to as a suprapubic catheter, is inserted into the bladder through a small hole in the abdomen for patients with urinary incontinence or retention. The catheter must be changed every four to six weeks by a health care provider or the patient. The old catheter is slowly extracted after the area is cleansed and a balloon is deflated within the syringe. The new catheter is inserted and positioned in the same location. Once urine flows through the catheter, the balloon is inflated with saline or sterile water and the new catheter is attached to the collection bag. Report 51710 if complications such as infection, inflammation, hemorrhage, constriction, or dilation occur.

Coding Tips

These procedures may be performed under general anesthesia, depending on the age and/or condition of the patient. For creation of the cystostomy, see 51040. For closure of the cystostomy, see 51880. For imaging guidance, see 75984.

ICD-10-CM Diagnostic Codes

T83.010A	Breakdown (mechanical) of cystostomy catheter, initial encounter
T83.020A	Displacement of cystostomy catheter, initial encounter
T83.030A	Leakage of cystostomy catheter, initial encounter
T83.090A	Other mechanical complication of cystostomy catheter, initial encounter
T83.510A	Infection and inflammatory reaction due to cystostomy catheter, initial encounter
T83.518A	Infection and inflammatory reaction due to other urinary catheter, initial encounter
T83.598A	Infection and inflammatory reaction due to other prosthetic device, implant and graft in urinary system, initial encounter
T83.81XA	Embolism due to genitourinary prosthetic devices, implants and grafts, initial encounter
T83.82XA	Fibrosis due to genitourinary prosthetic devices, implants and grafts, initial encounter
T83.83XA	Hemorrhage due to genitourinary prosthetic devices, implants and grafts, initial encounter
T83.84XA	Pain due to genitourinary prosthetic devices, implants and grafts, initial encounter
T83.85XA	Stenosis due to genitourinary prosthetic devices, implants and grafts, initial encounter
T83.86XA	Thrombosis due to genitourinary prosthetic devices, implants and grafts, initial encounter
T83.89XA	Other specified complication of genitourinary prosthetic devices, implants and grafts, initial encounter
Z43.5	Encounter for attention to cystostomy

AMA: **51705** 2018,Jan,8; 2017,Jan,8; 2016,Jan,13; 2015,Jan,16; 2014,Jan,11
51710 2018,Jan,8; 2017,Jan,8; 2016,Jan,13; 2015,Jan,16; 2014,Jan,11

Relative Value Units/Medicare Edits

Non-Facility RVU	Work	PE	MP	Total
51705	0.9	1.7	0.11	2.71
51710	1.35	2.27	0.15	3.77
Facility RVU	**Work**	**PE**	**MP**	**Total**
51705	0.9	0.49	0.11	1.5
51710	1.35	0.78	0.15	2.28

	FUD	Status	MUE	Modifiers				IOM Reference
51705	0	A	1(3)	51	N/A	N/A	N/A	None
51710	0	A	1(3)	51	N/A	N/A	N/A	

* with documentation

Terms To Know

catheter. Flexible tube inserted into an area of the body for introducing or withdrawing fluid.

constriction. Narrowed or squeezed portion of a tubular or luminal structure, such as a duct, vessel, or tube (e.g., esophagus). The narrowing can be a defect that is occurring naturally, or one that is surgically induced for therapeutic reasons.

cystostomy. Formation of an opening through the abdominal wall into the bladder.

guidewire. Flexible metal instrument designed to lead another instrument in its proper course.

hemorrhage. Internal or external bleeding with loss of significant amounts of blood.

incontinence. Inability to control urination or defecation.

infection. Presence of microorganisms in body tissues that may result in cellular damage.

inflammation. Cytologic and chemical reactions that occur in affected blood vessels and adjacent tissues in response to injury or abnormal stimulation from a physical, chemical, or biologic agent.

supra. Above.

Bladder

51715

51715   Endoscopic injection of implant material into the submucosal tissues of the urethra and/or bladder neck

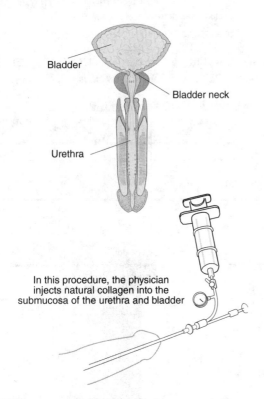

Bladder

Bladder neck

Urethra

In this procedure, the physician injects natural collagen into the submucosa of the urethra and bladder

Explanation

The physician injects natural proteins or synthetic material into the urethra and bladder neck, helping to prevent urinary incontinence. Before the injection, an endoscope is placed through the urethra into the bladder. Using local anesthesia, the physician makes one to three injections into the transurethra submucous. The injections are made through the endoscope into the affected area. The procedure can also be performed through the lower abdomen.

Coding Tips

Local or general anesthesia may be administered depending on the age or condition of the patient. For steroid injection for urethral stricture, see 52283. Supplies used when providing this procedure may be reported with the appropriate HCPCS Level II code. Check with the specific payer to determine coverage.

ICD-10-CM Diagnostic Codes

N36.41	Hypermobility of urethra
N36.42	Intrinsic sphincter deficiency (ISD)
N36.43	Combined hypermobility of urethra and intrinsic sphincter deficiency
N36.44	Muscular disorders of urethra
N39.3	Stress incontinence (female) (male)

AMA: **51715** 2014,Jan,11

Relative Value Units/Medicare Edits

Non-Facility RVU	Work	PE	MP	Total
51715	3.73	5.57	0.48	9.78
Facility RVU	**Work**	**PE**	**MP**	**Total**
51715	3.73	1.58	0.48	5.79

	FUD	Status	MUE	Modifiers				IOM Reference
51715	0	A	1(2)	51	N/A	N/A	80*	100-03,230.10

* with documentation

Terms To Know

atony. Absence of normal muscle tone and strength.

collagen. Protein based substance of strength and flexibility that is the major component of connective tissue, found in cartilage, bone, tendons, and skin.

detrusor sphincter dyssynergia. Condition in which urinary outflow is obstructed because the bladder neck fails to relax or tightens when the detrusor muscle contracts during urination.

endoscopy. Visual inspection of the body using a fiberoptic scope.

hypertonicity. Excessive muscle tone and augmented resistance to normal muscle stretching.

implant. Material or device inserted or placed within the body for therapeutic, reconstructive, or diagnostic purposes.

neurogenic bladder. Dysfunctional bladder due to a central or peripheral nervous system lesion that may result in incontinence, residual urine retention, infection, stones, and renal failure.

tissue. Group of similar cells with a similar function that form definite structures and organs. Tissue types include epithelial tissue, muscle tissue, connective tissue, and nervous tissue.

urethra. Small tube lined with mucous membrane that leads from the bladder to the exterior of the body.

© 2020 Optum360, LLC   N Newborn: 0   P Pediatric: 0-17   M Maternity: 9-64   A Adult: 15-124   ♂ Male Only   ♀ Female Only   CPT © 2020 American Medical Association. All Rights Reserved.

Bladder

51720

51720   Bladder instillation of anticarcinogenic agent (including retention time)

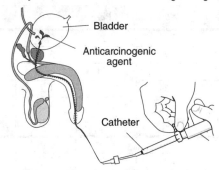

Physician introduces an anticarcinogenic agent

- Bladder
- Anticarcinogenic agent
- Catheter

Explanation

The physician introduces by drops (instillation) an anticarcinogenic agent into the bladder to treat a cancer. Prior to the instillation of the agent, a standard lavage is usually performed. The anticarcinogenic agent is introduced through a catheter and held in the bladder for a specified amount of time. This procedure may be used in conjunction with a cystostomy (51020) or with procedures such as cystectomy for the removal of a tumor.

Coding Tips

For resection of a bladder tumor, see 51530. Supplies used when providing this procedure may be reported with the appropriate HCPCS Level II code. Check with the specific payer to determine coverage.

ICD-10-CM Diagnostic Codes

C67.0	Malignant neoplasm of trigone of bladder
C67.1	Malignant neoplasm of dome of bladder
C67.2	Malignant neoplasm of lateral wall of bladder
C67.3	Malignant neoplasm of anterior wall of bladder
C67.4	Malignant neoplasm of posterior wall of bladder
C67.5	Malignant neoplasm of bladder neck
C67.6	Malignant neoplasm of ureteric orifice
C67.7	Malignant neoplasm of urachus
C67.8	Malignant neoplasm of overlapping sites of bladder
C79.11	Secondary malignant neoplasm of bladder
D09.0	Carcinoma in situ of bladder
Z51.11	Encounter for antineoplastic chemotherapy

AMA: **51720** 2020,Nov,1; 2020,Jan,11; 2018,Jan,8; 2017,Jan,8; 2016,Jan,13; 2015,Jan,16; 2014,Jan,11

Relative Value Units/Medicare Edits

Non-Facility RVU	Work	PE	MP	Total
51720	0.87	1.42	0.09	2.38
Facility RVU	**Work**	**PE**	**MP**	**Total**
51720	0.87	0.3	0.09	1.26

	FUD	Status	MUE	Modifiers				IOM Reference
51720	0	A	1(3)	51	N/A	N/A	N/A	None

* with documentation

51725-51729

51725	Simple cystometrogram (CMG) (eg, spinal manometer)
51726	Complex cystometrogram (ie, calibrated electronic equipment);
51727	with urethral pressure profile studies (ie, urethral closure pressure profile), any technique
51728	with voiding pressure studies (ie, bladder voiding pressure), any technique
51729	with voiding pressure studies (ie, bladder voiding pressure) and urethral pressure profile studies (ie, urethral closure pressure profile), any technique

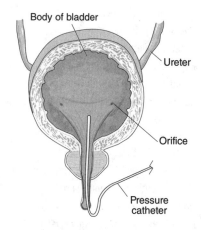

- Body of bladder
- Ureter
- Orifice
- Pressure catheter

A pressure catheter is introduced into the bladder and connected to a manometer to measure pressure

Explanation

A cystometrogram (a graphic record of urinary bladder pressure at different volumes) is used to distinguish bladder outlet obstruction from other voiding dysfunctions. For a simple cystometrogram (51725), the physician inserts a pressure catheter into the bladder and connects it to a manometer line filled with fluid to measure pressure and flow in the lower urinary tract. For a complex cystometrogram (51726), the physician typically uses a transurethral catheter to fill the bladder with water or gas while simultaneously obtaining rectal pressure. As the bladder is being filled, intravesical pressure is measured by a microtip transducer or fluid-filled catheter attached to the transducer. Code 51727 reports a complex cystometrogram performed in conjunction with a study for measuring urethral pressure. In one technique, the bladder is filled with fluid and the catheter withdrawn into the urethra while bladder sensations and volume are recorded. Urethral pressure changes are recorded as the patient follows specific instructions (Valsalva maneuver, cough). For voiding pressure studies performed in conjunction with a complex cystometrogram (51728), a transducer is placed into the bladder and the bladder is filled with fluid. The patient is instructed to attempt to void upon the feeling of bladder fullness, and recordings are taken of bladder sensation and volume at specific times. Report 51729 if complex cystometrogram is combined with both voiding pressure studies and urethral pressure profile studies.

Coding Tips

These codes imply that the service is performed by, or under the direct supervision of, a physician or other qualified health care professional. All instruments, equipment, fluids, gases, probes, catheters, technician fees, medications, gloves, trays, tubing, and other sterile supplies are presumed to be provided by the provider.

Bladder

ICD-10-CM Diagnostic Codes

N13.722	Vesicoureteral-reflux with reflux nephropathy without hydroureter, bilateral
N13.732	Vesicoureteral-reflux with reflux nephropathy with hydroureter, bilateral
N30.10	Interstitial cystitis (chronic) without hematuria
N30.11	Interstitial cystitis (chronic) with hematuria
N31.0	Uninhibited neuropathic bladder, not elsewhere classified
N31.1	Reflex neuropathic bladder, not elsewhere classified
N31.2	Flaccid neuropathic bladder, not elsewhere classified
N31.8	Other neuromuscular dysfunction of bladder
N32.0	Bladder-neck obstruction
N32.81	Overactive bladder
N32.89	Other specified disorders of bladder
N36.41	Hypermobility of urethra
N36.42	Intrinsic sphincter deficiency (ISD)
N36.43	Combined hypermobility of urethra and intrinsic sphincter deficiency
N36.44	Muscular disorders of urethra
N36.8	Other specified disorders of urethra
N37	Urethral disorders in diseases classified elsewhere
N39.3	Stress incontinence (female) (male)
N39.41	Urge incontinence
N39.42	Incontinence without sensory awareness
N39.43	Post-void dribbling
N39.44	Nocturnal enuresis
N39.45	Continuous leakage
N39.46	Mixed incontinence
N39.490	Overflow incontinence
N39.491	Coital incontinence
N39.492	Postural (urinary) incontinence
N39.498	Other specified urinary incontinence
Q64.74	Double urethra
Q64.79	Other congenital malformations of bladder and urethra
R30.0	Dysuria
R33.0	Drug induced retention of urine
R33.8	Other retention of urine
R35.0	Frequency of micturition
R35.1	Nocturia
R35.8	Other polyuria
R39.11	Hesitancy of micturition
R39.12	Poor urinary stream
R39.13	Splitting of urinary stream
R39.14	Feeling of incomplete bladder emptying
R39.15	Urgency of urination
R39.16	Straining to void
R39.191	Need to immediately re-void
R39.192	Position dependent micturition
R39.198	Other difficulties with micturition
R39.81	Functional urinary incontinence
R39.89	Other symptoms and signs involving the genitourinary system

Bladder

AMA: **51725** 2018,Jan,8; 2017,Jan,8; 2016,Jan,13; 2015,Jan,16; 2014,Jan,11 **51726** 2018,Jan,8; 2017,Jan,8; 2016,Jan,13; 2015,Jan,16; 2014,Jan,11 **51727** 2018,Jan,8; 2017,Jan,8; 2016,Jan,13; 2015,Jan,16; 2014,Jan,11 **51728** 2018,Jan,8; 2017,Jan,8; 2016,Jan,13; 2015,Jan,16; 2014,Jan,11 **51729** 2018,Jan,8; 2017,Jan,8; 2016,Jan,13; 2015,Jan,16; 2014,Jan,11

Relative Value Units/Medicare Edits

Non-Facility RVU	Work	PE	MP	Total
51725	1.51	4.38	0.15	6.04
51726	1.71	6.37	0.15	8.23
51727	2.11	7.54	0.23	9.88
51728	2.11	7.69	0.2	10.0
51729	2.51	7.89	0.27	10.67
Facility RVU	**Work**	**PE**	**MP**	**Total**
51725	1.51	4.38	0.15	6.04
51726	1.71	6.37	0.15	8.23
51727	2.11	7.54	0.23	9.88
51728	2.11	7.69	0.2	10.0
51729	2.51	7.89	0.27	10.67

	FUD	Status	MUE	Modifiers				IOM Reference
51725	0	A	1(3)	51	N/A	N/A	80*	None
51726	0	A	1(3)	51	N/A	N/A	N/A	
51727	0	A	1(3)	51	N/A	N/A	80*	
51728	0	A	1(3)	51	N/A	N/A	80*	
51729	0	A	1(3)	51	N/A	N/A	80*	

* with documentation

Terms To Know

catheter. Flexible tube inserted into an area of the body for introducing or withdrawing fluid.

complex cystometrogram. Medical test used to determine the size and functionality of the bladder, specifically the capacity, filling sensation, and intravesical pressure of the bladder. A rectal probe is used to further distinguish between abdominal pressure and bladder pressure.

simple cystometrogram. Test that measures the capacity of the bladder, sensation of filling, and intravesical pressure.

transducer. Apparatus that transfers or translates one type of energy into another, such as converting pressure to an electrical signal.

urethral pressure profile. Measures urethral pressure by pulling a transducer through the urethra and noting the pressure change.

voiding pressure study. Voiding pressure produced by the bladder and the resultant flow of urine is determined.

[51797]

+ **51797** Voiding pressure studies, intra-abdominal (ie, rectal, gastric, intraperitoneal) (List separately in addition to code for primary procedure)

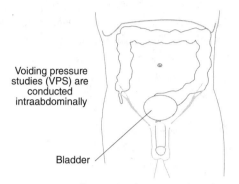

Voiding pressure studies (VPS) are conducted intraabdominally

Bladder

Explanation

The physician conducts an intraabdominal voiding pressure study. In one method, the physician places a rectal catheter simultaneously with a urethral catheter in order to determine how much the patient strains while attempting to void. This measures both the amount of pressure generated and the subsequent urine flow.

Coding Tips

Report 51797 in addition to 51728-51729. This code has both a technical and professional component. To claim only the professional component, append modifier 26. To claim only the technical component, append modifier TC. To claim the complete procedure (i.e., both the professional and technical components), submit without a modifier.

ICD-10-CM Diagnostic Codes

This/these CPT code(s) are add-on code(s). See the primary procedure code that this code is performed with for your ICD-10-CM code selections.

AMA: **51797** 2018,Jan,8; 2017,Jan,8; 2016,Jan,13; 2015,Jan,16; 2014,Jan,11

Relative Value Units/Medicare Edits

Non-Facility RVU	Work	PE	MP	Total
51797	0.8	3.73	0.08	4.61
Facility RVU	**Work**	**PE**	**MP**	**Total**
51797	0.8	3.73	0.08	4.61

	FUD	Status	MUE	Modifiers				IOM Reference
51797	N/A	A	1(3)	N/A	N/A	N/A	80*	None

* with documentation

Terms To Know

catheter. Flexible tube inserted into an area of the body for introducing or withdrawing fluid.

cystometrogram. Recorded measurement of bladder pressure from multiple volume amounts.

voiding pressure study. Voiding pressure produced by the bladder and the resultant flow of urine is determined.

51736-51741

51736 Simple uroflowmetry (UFR) (eg, stop-watch flow rate, mechanical uroflowmeter)
51741 Complex uroflowmetry (eg, calibrated electronic equipment)

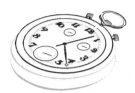

A simple flowmetry is performed typically with a stopwatch to measure the amount of time a patient needs to urinate into a calibrated vessel. The physician assesses the ratio

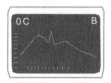

A complex flowmetry is performed typically with electronic equipment to record the volume of urine and elapsed time. The physician assesses the ratio

Explanation

For simple uroflowmetry (51736), the physician assesses the rate of emptying the bladder by stopwatch, recording the volume of urine per time. For complex uroflowmetry, (51741), the physician assesses the rate of emptying of the bladder by electronic equipment, recording the volume of urine per time.

Coding Tips

These codes imply that the service is performed by, or under the direct supervision of, a physician or other qualified health care professional, and that all instruments, equipment, fluids, gases, probes, catheters, technician's fee, medications, gloves, trays, tubing, and other sterile supplies be provided by the provider. These codes have both a technical and professional component. To claim only the professional component, append modifier 26. To claim only the technical component, append modifier TC. To claim the complete procedure (i.e., both the technical and professional components), submit without a modifier.

ICD-10-CM Diagnostic Codes

A56.01	Chlamydial cystitis and urethritis
C61	Malignant neoplasm of prostate ♂
D29.1	Benign neoplasm of prostate ♂
D40.0	Neoplasm of uncertain behavior of prostate ♂
D49.4	Neoplasm of unspecified behavior of bladder
N30.10	Interstitial cystitis (chronic) without hematuria
N30.11	Interstitial cystitis (chronic) with hematuria
N30.20	Other chronic cystitis without hematuria
N30.21	Other chronic cystitis with hematuria
N30.30	Trigonitis without hematuria
N30.31	Trigonitis with hematuria
N30.40	Irradiation cystitis without hematuria
N30.41	Irradiation cystitis with hematuria
N30.80	Other cystitis without hematuria
N30.81	Other cystitis with hematuria

Bladder

N31.0	Uninhibited neuropathic bladder, not elsewhere classified
N31.1	Reflex neuropathic bladder, not elsewhere classified
N31.2	Flaccid neuropathic bladder, not elsewhere classified
N31.8	Other neuromuscular dysfunction of bladder
N32.0	Bladder-neck obstruction
N32.81	Overactive bladder
N32.89	Other specified disorders of bladder
N33	Bladder disorders in diseases classified elsewhere
N35.010	Post-traumatic urethral stricture, male, meatal ♂
N35.011	Post-traumatic bulbous urethral stricture ♂
N35.012	Post-traumatic membranous urethral stricture ♂
N35.013	Post-traumatic anterior urethral stricture ♂
N35.016	Post-traumatic urethral stricture, male, overlapping sites ♂
N35.021	Urethral stricture due to childbirth ♀
N35.028	Other post-traumatic urethral stricture, female ♀
N35.111	Postinfective urethral stricture, not elsewhere classified, male, meatal ♂
N35.112	Postinfective bulbous urethral stricture, not elsewhere classified, male ♂
N35.113	Postinfective membranous urethral stricture, not elsewhere classified, male ♂
N35.114	Postinfective anterior urethral stricture, not elsewhere classified, male ♂
N35.12	Postinfective urethral stricture, not elsewhere classified, female ♀
N35.811	Other urethral stricture, male, meatal ♂
N35.812	Other urethral bulbous stricture, male ♂
N35.813	Other membranous urethral stricture, male ♂
N35.814	Other anterior urethral stricture, male ♂
N35.816	Other urethral stricture, male, overlapping sites ♂
N35.82	Other urethral stricture, female ♀
N36.41	Hypermobility of urethra
N36.42	Intrinsic sphincter deficiency (ISD)
N36.43	Combined hypermobility of urethra and intrinsic sphincter deficiency
N36.44	Muscular disorders of urethra
N36.8	Other specified disorders of urethra
N37	Urethral disorders in diseases classified elsewhere
N39.3	Stress incontinence (female) (male)
N39.41	Urge incontinence
N39.42	Incontinence without sensory awareness
N39.43	Post-void dribbling
N39.46	Mixed incontinence
N39.490	Overflow incontinence
N39.491	Coital incontinence
N39.492	Postural (urinary) incontinence
N39.498	Other specified urinary incontinence
N39.8	Other specified disorders of urinary system
N40.0	Benign prostatic hyperplasia without lower urinary tract symptoms 🅰 ♂
N40.1	Benign prostatic hyperplasia with lower urinary tract symptoms 🅰 ♂
N40.2	Nodular prostate without lower urinary tract symptoms 🅰 ♂
N40.3	Nodular prostate with lower urinary tract symptoms 🅰 ♂
N41.1	Chronic prostatitis 🅰 ♂

N81.84	Pelvic muscle wasting ♀
N99.110	Postprocedural urethral stricture, male, meatal ♂
N99.111	Postprocedural bulbous urethral stricture, male ♂
N99.112	Postprocedural membranous urethral stricture, male ♂
N99.113	Postprocedural anterior bulbous urethral stricture, male ♂
N99.115	Postprocedural fossa navicularis urethral stricture ♂
N99.116	Postprocedural urethral stricture, male, overlapping sites ♂
N99.12	Postprocedural urethral stricture, female ♀
Q62.11	Congenital occlusion of ureteropelvic junction
Q62.12	Congenital occlusion of ureterovesical orifice
Q62.2	Congenital megaureter
Q62.39	Other obstructive defects of renal pelvis and ureter
Q64.2	Congenital posterior urethral valves
Q64.31	Congenital bladder neck obstruction
Q64.32	Congenital stricture of urethra
Q64.33	Congenital stricture of urinary meatus
Q64.39	Other atresia and stenosis of urethra and bladder neck
R30.0	Dysuria
R33.0	Drug induced retention of urine
R33.8	Other retention of urine
R35.0	Frequency of micturition
R39.11	Hesitancy of micturition
R39.12	Poor urinary stream
R39.13	Splitting of urinary stream
R39.14	Feeling of incomplete bladder emptying
R39.15	Urgency of urination
R39.16	Straining to void

AMA: **51736** 2018,Jan,8; 2017,Jan,8; 2016,Jan,13; 2015,Jan,16; 2014,Jan,11 **51741** 2018,Jan,8; 2017,Jan,8; 2016,Jan,13; 2015,Jan,16; 2014,Sep,13; 2014,Jan,11

Relative Value Units/Medicare Edits

Non-Facility RVU	Work	PE	MP	Total
51736	0.17	0.2	0.02	0.39
51741	0.17	0.21	0.03	0.41
Facility RVU	Work	PE	MP	Total
51736	0.17	0.2	0.02	0.39
51741	0.17	0.21	0.03	0.41

	FUD	Status	MUE	Modifiers				IOM Reference
51736	N/A	A	1(3)	51	N/A	N/A	80*	None
51741	N/A	A	1(3)	51	N/A	N/A	N/A	

* with documentation

51784-51785

51784 Electromyography studies (EMG) of anal or urethral sphincter, other than needle, any technique
51785 Needle electromyography studies (EMG) of anal or urethral sphincter, any technique

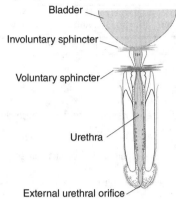

Myography is the electronic measurement of muscle activity of sphincter muscles of the anus or urethra

Bladder

Involuntary sphincter

Voluntary sphincter

Urethra

External urethral orifice

Explanation

In 51784, the physician places a pad in the anal or urethral sphincter and measures the electrical activity with the bladder filled and during emptying. In 51785, the physician places a pad or needle in the anal or urethral sphincter and measures the electrical activity with the bladder filled and during emptying.

Coding Tips

These codes imply that the service is performed by, or under the direct supervision of, a physician or other qualified health care professional, and that all instruments, equipment, fluids, gases, probes, catheters, technician's fee, medications, gloves, trays, tubing, and other sterile supplies be provided by the provider. These codes have both a technical and professional component. To claim only the professional component, append modifier 26. To claim only the technical component, append modifier TC. To claim the complete procedure (i.e., both the professional and technical components), submit without a modifier. When 51784 or 51785 is performed with another separately identifiable procedure, the highest dollar value code is listed as the primary procedure and subsequent procedures are appended with modifier 51. Code 51784 should not be reported with 51792.

ICD-10-CM Diagnostic Codes

N32.81	Overactive bladder
N35.010	Post-traumatic urethral stricture, male, meatal ♂
N35.011	Post-traumatic bulbous urethral stricture ♂
N35.012	Post-traumatic membranous urethral stricture ♂
N35.013	Post-traumatic anterior urethral stricture ♂
N35.021	Urethral stricture due to childbirth ♀
N35.028	Other post-traumatic urethral stricture, female ♀
N35.111	Postinfective urethral stricture, not elsewhere classified, male, meatal ♂
N35.112	Postinfective bulbous urethral stricture, not elsewhere classified, male ♂
N35.113	Postinfective membranous urethral stricture, not elsewhere classified, male ♂

N35.114	Postinfective anterior urethral stricture, not elsewhere classified, male ♂
N35.12	Postinfective urethral stricture, not elsewhere classified, female ♀
N35.811	Other urethral stricture, male, meatal ♂
N35.812	Other urethral bulbous stricture, male ♂
N35.813	Other membranous urethral stricture, male ♂
N35.814	Other anterior urethral stricture, male ♂
N36.41	Hypermobility of urethra
N36.42	Intrinsic sphincter deficiency (ISD)
N36.43	Combined hypermobility of urethra and intrinsic sphincter deficiency
N36.44	Muscular disorders of urethra
N36.8	Other specified disorders of urethra
N37	Urethral disorders in diseases classified elsewhere
N39.0	Urinary tract infection, site not specified
N39.3	Stress incontinence (female) (male)
N39.41	Urge incontinence
N39.42	Incontinence without sensory awareness
N39.43	Post-void dribbling
N39.46	Mixed incontinence
N39.490	Overflow incontinence
N39.491	Coital incontinence
N39.492	Postural (urinary) incontinence
N39.498	Other specified urinary incontinence
N99.110	Postprocedural urethral stricture, male, meatal ♂
N99.111	Postprocedural bulbous urethral stricture, male ♂
N99.112	Postprocedural membranous urethral stricture, male ♂
N99.113	Postprocedural anterior bulbous urethral stricture, male ♂
N99.115	Postprocedural fossa navicularis urethral stricture ♂
N99.12	Postprocedural urethral stricture, female ♀
Q64.79	Other congenital malformations of bladder and urethra
R30.1	Vesical tenesmus
R35.0	Frequency of micturition
R35.8	Other polyuria
R39.16	Straining to void
R39.82	Chronic bladder pain

AMA: **51784** 2018,Jan,8; 2017,Jan,8; 2016,Jan,13; 2015,Jan,16; 2014,Sep,13; 2014,Jan,11; 2014,Feb,11 **51785** 2018,Jan,8; 2017,Jan,8; 2016,Jan,13; 2015,Jan,16; 2014,Jan,11

Relative Value Units/Medicare Edits

Non-Facility RVU	Work	PE	MP	Total
51784	0.75	1.08	0.09	1.92
51785	1.53	8.65	0.46	10.64
Facility RVU	**Work**	**PE**	**MP**	**Total**
51784	0.75	1.08	0.09	1.92
51785	1.53	8.65	0.46	10.64

	FUD	Status	MUE	Modifiers				IOM Reference
51784	N/A	A	1(3)	51	N/A	N/A	N/A	None
51785	N/A	A	1(3)	51	N/A	N/A	80*	

* with documentation

Bladder

51792

51792   Stimulus evoked response (eg, measurement of bulbocavernosus reflex latency time)

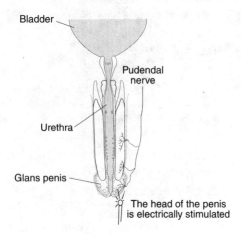

Bladder

Pudendal nerve

Urethra

Glans penis

The head of the penis is electrically stimulated

Measurement of the nerve pathways to the pudendal nerve are assessed

Explanation

The physician electrically stimulates the head of the penis. The physician measures the delay time for travel of stimulation through the pelvic nerves to the pudendal nerve.

Coding Tips

This code implies that the service is performed by, or under the direct supervision of, a physician or other qualified health care professional, and that all instruments, equipment, fluids, gases, probes, catheters, technician's fee, medications, gloves, trays, tubing, and other sterile supplies be provided by the provider. Procedure 51792 has both a technical and professional component. To claim only the professional component, append modifier 26. To claim only the technical component, append modifier TC. To claim the complete procedure (i.e., both the professional and technical components), submit without a modifier. When 51792 is performed with another separately identifiable procedure, the highest dollar value code is listed as the primary procedure and subsequent procedures are appended with modifier 51. This code should not be reported with 51784.

ICD-10-CM Diagnostic Codes

N52.01	Erectile dysfunction due to arterial insufficiency 🅰 ♂
N52.02	Corporo-venous occlusive erectile dysfunction 🅰 ♂
N52.03	Combined arterial insufficiency and corporo-venous occlusive erectile dysfunction 🅰 ♂
N52.1	Erectile dysfunction due to diseases classified elsewhere 🅰 ♂
N52.2	Drug-induced erectile dysfunction 🅰 ♂
N52.31	Erectile dysfunction following radical prostatectomy 🅰 ♂
N52.32	Erectile dysfunction following radical cystectomy 🅰 ♂
N52.33	Erectile dysfunction following urethral surgery 🅰 ♂
N52.34	Erectile dysfunction following simple prostatectomy 🅰 ♂
N52.35	Erectile dysfunction following radiation therapy 🅰 ♂
N52.36	Erectile dysfunction following interstitial seed therapy 🅰 ♂
N52.37	Erectile dysfunction following prostate ablative therapy 🅰 ♂
N52.39	Other and unspecified postprocedural erectile dysfunction 🅰 ♂
N52.8	Other male erectile dysfunction 🅰 ♂

AMA: **51792** 2018,Jan,8; 2017,Jan,8; 2016,Jan,13; 2015,Jan,16; 2014,Jan,11; 2014,Feb,11

Relative Value Units/Medicare Edits

Non-Facility RVU	Work	PE	MP	Total
51792	1.1	5.83	0.11	7.04
Facility RVU	**Work**	**PE**	**MP**	**Total**
51792	1.1	5.83	0.11	7.04

	FUD	Status	MUE	Modifiers				IOM Reference
51792	0	A	1(3)	51	N/A	N/A	80*	None

* with documentation

Terms To Know

cyst. Elevated encapsulated mass containing fluid, semisolid, or solid material with a membranous lining.

dysfunction. Abnormal or impaired function of an organ, part, or system.

hyperplasia. Abnormal proliferation in the number of normal cells in regular tissue arrangement.

hypertonicity. Excessive muscle tone and augmented resistance to normal muscle stretching.

impotence. Psychosexual or organic dysfunction in which there is partial or complete failure to attain or maintain erection until completion of the sexual act.

insufficiency. Inadequate closure of the valve that allows abnormal backward blood flow.

latency. Hidden, concealed, or dormant.

male stress incontinence. Involuntary escape of urine in men at times of minor stress against the bladder, such as coughing, sneezing, or laughing.

occlusion. Constriction, closure, or blockage of a passage.

prostate. Male gland surrounding the bladder neck and urethra that secretes a substance into the seminal fluid.

reflex. Involuntary action, movement, or activity brought about by triggering the corresponding stimulus.

Bladder

51798

51798   Measurement of post-voiding residual urine and/or bladder capacity by ultrasound, non-imaging

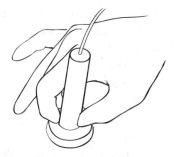

Ultrasound equipment is used to measure bladder urine volume following urination or to measure bladder capacity

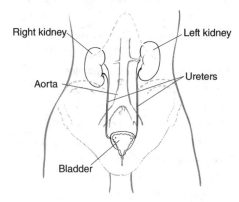

Explanation

Residual urine and/or bladder capacity is measured by ultrasound after the patient has voided. A portable ultrasound scanner is used for this purpose. Operation of the scanner is done simply by directing the scanning head over the suprapubic area while the patient is lying down in the supine position. The software built in to the scanner calculates the post-void residual urine volume immediately and also does calculations for the bladder capacity based on the individual's bladder shape and not on fixed geometric formulas.

Coding Tips

This code represents the technical component only with no associated physician work involvement.

ICD-10-CM Diagnostic Codes

N32.0	Bladder-neck obstruction
N32.3	Diverticulum of bladder
N32.81	Overactive bladder
N35.010	Post-traumatic urethral stricture, male, meatal ♂
N35.011	Post-traumatic bulbous urethral stricture ♂
N35.012	Post-traumatic membranous urethral stricture ♂
N35.013	Post-traumatic anterior urethral stricture ♂
N35.021	Urethral stricture due to childbirth ♀
N35.028	Other post-traumatic urethral stricture, female ♀
N35.111	Postinfective urethral stricture, not elsewhere classified, male, meatal ♂
N35.112	Postinfective bulbous urethral stricture, not elsewhere classified, male ♂
N35.113	Postinfective membranous urethral stricture, not elsewhere classified, male ♂
N35.114	Postinfective anterior urethral stricture, not elsewhere classified, male ♂
N35.12	Postinfective urethral stricture, not elsewhere classified, female ♀
N35.811	Other urethral stricture, male, meatal ♂
N35.812	Other urethral bulbous stricture, male ♂
N36.42	Intrinsic sphincter deficiency (ISD)
N36.43	Combined hypermobility of urethra and intrinsic sphincter deficiency
N36.44	Muscular disorders of urethra
N39.3	Stress incontinence (female) (male)
N39.41	Urge incontinence
N39.42	Incontinence without sensory awareness
N39.43	Post-void dribbling
N39.46	Mixed incontinence
N39.490	Overflow incontinence
N39.491	Coital incontinence
N39.492	Postural (urinary) incontinence
N40.1	Benign prostatic hyperplasia with lower urinary tract symptoms 🅰 ♂
N99.110	Postprocedural urethral stricture, male, meatal ♂
N99.111	Postprocedural bulbous urethral stricture, male ♂
N99.112	Postprocedural membranous urethral stricture, male ♂
N99.113	Postprocedural anterior bulbous urethral stricture, male ♂
Q64.31	Congenital bladder neck obstruction
Q64.32	Congenital stricture of urethra
Q64.33	Congenital stricture of urinary meatus
Q64.39	Other atresia and stenosis of urethra and bladder neck
Q64.6	Congenital diverticulum of bladder
R33.0	Drug induced retention of urine
R33.8	Other retention of urine
R39.12	Poor urinary stream
R39.13	Splitting of urinary stream
R39.14	Feeling of incomplete bladder emptying
R39.15	Urgency of urination
R39.16	Straining to void
R39.191	Need to immediately re-void
R39.192	Position dependent micturition
R39.198	Other difficulties with micturition
R39.81	Functional urinary incontinence

AMA: **51798** 2018,Jun,11; 2018,Jan,8; 2017,Jan,8; 2016,Jan,13; 2015,Jan,16; 2014,Jan,11

Relative Value Units/Medicare Edits

Non-Facility RVU	Work	PE	MP	Total
51798	0.0	0.28	0.01	0.29
Facility RVU	Work	PE	MP	Total
51798	0.0	0.28	0.01	0.29

	FUD	Status	MUE	Modifiers				IOM Reference
51798	N/A	A	1(3)	N/A	N/A	N/A	80*	None

* with documentation

CPT © 2020 American Medical Association. All Rights Reserved.   ● New   ▲ Revised   + Add On   ★ Telemedicine   AMA: CPT Assist   [Resequenced]   ☑ Laterality   © 2020 Optum360, LLC

51800

51800 Cystoplasty or cystourethroplasty, plastic operation on bladder and/or vesical neck (anterior Y-plasty, vesical fundus resection), any procedure, with or without wedge resection of posterior vesical neck

The physician clears a blockage in the bladder neck through one of a number of methods

Blockage in bladder neck

Explanation

The physician uses plastic surgery to correct an obstruction or defect in the bladder or vesical neck and urethra. The bladder is distended using a Foley catheter. To access the bladder, the physician makes an incision in the skin of the lower abdomen and cuts the corresponding muscles, fat, and fibrous membranes (fascia). The physician incises, trims, and shapes the bladder or vesical neck and urethra, using absorbable sutures or soft rubber drains for traction. The physician may insert a catheter through the urethra to provide support during healing. In anterior Y-plasty, the physician makes a Y-shaped flap of the bladder extending the vertical incision into the vesical neck. The vertical part of this incision is pulled up into the V-shaped incision, which becomes a straight line when sutured. The physician may remove a portion of the vesical neck. The physician places a drain tube, bringing it out through a separate stab incision in the skin, and performs a layered closure.

Coding Tips

For plastic reconstruction on the bladder and urethra (cystourethroplasty), combined with reimplantation of the ureter into the bladder (ureteroneocystostomy), see 51820. For plastic repair and reconstruction of the urethra only, see 53400–53431.

ICD-10-CM Diagnostic Codes

N32.0	Bladder-neck obstruction
N32.89	Other specified disorders of bladder
N35.010	Post-traumatic urethral stricture, male, meatal ♂
N35.011	Post-traumatic bulbous urethral stricture ♂
N35.012	Post-traumatic membranous urethral stricture ♂
N35.013	Post-traumatic anterior urethral stricture ♂
N35.016	Post-traumatic urethral stricture, male, overlapping sites ♂
N35.021	Urethral stricture due to childbirth ♀
N35.028	Other post-traumatic urethral stricture, female ♀
N35.111	Postinfective urethral stricture, not elsewhere classified, male, meatal ♂
N35.112	Postinfective bulbous urethral stricture, not elsewhere classified, male ♂
N35.113	Postinfective membranous urethral stricture, not elsewhere classified, male ♂
N35.114	Postinfective anterior urethral stricture, not elsewhere classified, male ♂
N35.12	Postinfective urethral stricture, not elsewhere classified, female ♀
N35.811	Other urethral stricture, male, meatal ♂
N35.812	Other urethral bulbous stricture, male ♂
N35.813	Other membranous urethral stricture, male ♂
N35.814	Other anterior urethral stricture, male ♂
N35.82	Other urethral stricture, female ♀
N37	Urethral disorders in diseases classified elsewhere
N39.3	Stress incontinence (female) (male)
N39.41	Urge incontinence
N39.42	Incontinence without sensory awareness
N39.46	Mixed incontinence
N99.110	Postprocedural urethral stricture, male, meatal ♂
N99.111	Postprocedural bulbous urethral stricture, male ♂
N99.112	Postprocedural membranous urethral stricture, male ♂
N99.113	Postprocedural anterior bulbous urethral stricture, male ♂
N99.115	Postprocedural fossa naviculariss urethral stricture ♂
N99.12	Postprocedural urethral stricture, female ♀
Q64.11	Supravesical fissure of urinary bladder
Q64.12	Cloacal exstrophy of urinary bladder
Q64.19	Other exstrophy of urinary bladder
Q64.31	Congenital bladder neck obstruction
Q64.39	Other atresia and stenosis of urethra and bladder neck
Q64.6	Congenital diverticulum of bladder
Q64.71	Congenital prolapse of urethra
Q64.73	Congenital urethrorectal fistula
Q64.79	Other congenital malformations of bladder and urethra
S37.23XA	Laceration of bladder, initial encounter
S37.29XA	Other injury of bladder, initial encounter
S37.33XA	Laceration of urethra, initial encounter
S37.39XA	Other injury of urethra, initial encounter

AMA: **51800** 2014,Jan,11

Relative Value Units/Medicare Edits

Non-Facility RVU	Work	PE	MP	Total
51800	18.89	8.98	2.25	30.12
Facility RVU	**Work**	**PE**	**MP**	**Total**
51800	18.89	8.98	2.25	30.12

	FUD	Status	MUE	Modifiers				IOM Reference
51800	90	A	1(2)	51	N/A	62*	80	None

* with documentation

Bladder

51820

51820   Cystourethroplasty with unilateral or bilateral ureteroneocystostomy

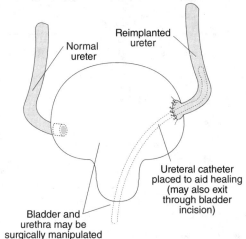

A defect in the urethra and/or bladder is repaired; one or both lower ureters are reimplanted

Normal ureter

Reimplanted ureter

Ureteral catheter placed to aid healing (may also exit through bladder incision)

Bladder and urethra may be surgically manipulated

Explanation

The physician uses plastic surgery to correct a defect in the bladder and urethra, and reimplants one or both ureters into the bladder (ureteroneocystostomy). To access the bladder, urethra, and ureters, the physician makes a midline incision in the skin of the abdomen and cuts the corresponding muscles, fat, and fibrous membranes (fascia). The physician incises, trims, and shapes the bladder and urethra, using absorbable sutures or soft rubber drains for traction. The physician brings the cut end of one or both ureters through a stab wound in the bladder and sutures the ureter(s) to the bladder. To provide support during healing, the physician inserts a ureteral catheter, bringing the tube end out through the urethra or bladder incision. The physician inserts a drain tube and performs a layered closure.

Coding Tips

If significant, additional time and effort is documented, append modifier 22 and submit a cover letter and operative report. If the physician implants the ureter into the bladder without removal of diseased or damaged bladder tissue, see 50780–50785. If the physician performs a ureteroneocystostomy to restore ureteral continuity after surgical diversion, see 50830. For ureteroneocystostomy following removal of diseased or damaged bladder tissue, see 51565. For cystourethroplasty without reimplantation of the ureter, see 51800. For plastic repair and reconstruction of the urethra only, see 53400–53431.

ICD-10-CM Diagnostic Codes

N32.0	Bladder-neck obstruction
N32.89	Other specified disorders of bladder
N35.010	Post-traumatic urethral stricture, male, meatal ♂
N35.011	Post-traumatic bulbous urethral stricture ♂
N35.012	Post-traumatic membranous urethral stricture ♂
N35.013	Post-traumatic anterior urethral stricture ♂
N35.021	Urethral stricture due to childbirth ♀
N35.028	Other post-traumatic urethral stricture, female ♀
N35.111	Postinfective urethral stricture, not elsewhere classified, male, meatal ♂
N35.112	Postinfective bulbous urethral stricture, not elsewhere classified, male ♂
N35.113	Postinfective membranous urethral stricture, not elsewhere classified, male ♂
N35.114	Postinfective anterior urethral stricture, not elsewhere classified, male ♂
N35.12	Postinfective urethral stricture, not elsewhere classified, female ♀
N35.811	Other urethral stricture, male, meatal ♂
N35.812	Other urethral bulbous stricture, male ♂
N35.813	Other membranous urethral stricture, male ♂
N35.814	Other anterior urethral stricture, male ♂
N39.3	Stress incontinence (female) (male)
N39.41	Urge incontinence
N39.42	Incontinence without sensory awareness
N39.46	Mixed incontinence
N99.110	Postprocedural urethral stricture, male, meatal ♂
N99.111	Postprocedural bulbous urethral stricture, male ♂
N99.112	Postprocedural membranous urethral stricture, male ♂
N99.113	Postprocedural anterior bulbous urethral stricture, male ♂
N99.115	Postprocedural fossa navicularis urethral stricture ♂
N99.12	Postprocedural urethral stricture, female ♀
Q64.11	Supravesical fissure of urinary bladder
Q64.12	Cloacal exstrophy of urinary bladder
Q64.19	Other exstrophy of urinary bladder
Q64.31	Congenital bladder neck obstruction
Q64.39	Other atresia and stenosis of urethra and bladder neck
Q64.6	Congenital diverticulum of bladder
Q64.71	Congenital prolapse of urethra
Q64.73	Congenital urethrorectal fistula
Q64.79	Other congenital malformations of bladder and urethra
S37.23XA	Laceration of bladder, initial encounter
S37.29XA	Other injury of bladder, initial encounter
S37.33XA	Laceration of urethra, initial encounter
S37.39XA	Other injury of urethra, initial encounter

AMA: **51820** 2014,Jan,11

Relative Value Units/Medicare Edits

Non-Facility RVU	Work	PE	MP	Total
51820	19.59	9.48	2.23	31.3
Facility RVU	**Work**	**PE**	**MP**	**Total**
51820	19.59	9.48	2.23	31.3

	FUD	Status	MUE	Modifiers				IOM Reference
51820	90	A	1(2)	51	N/A	62*	80	None

* with documentation

Bladder

51840-51841

51840 Anterior vesicourethropexy, or urethropexy (eg, Marshall-Marchetti-Krantz, Burch); simple

51841 complicated (eg, secondary repair)

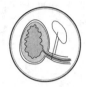 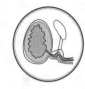

1. A common approach involves placing sutures from pubic bone to paraurethral tissues

2. The urethrovesical angle is elevated and continence restored

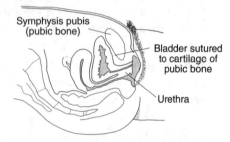

Symphysis pubis (pubic bone)

Bladder sutured to cartilage of pubic bone

Urethra

Explanation

The physician performs a vesicourethropexy or urethropexy in the Marshall-Marchetti-Krantz or Burch style. The physician makes a small horizontal incision in the abdomen above the symphysis pubis, which is the midline junction of the pubic bones at the front. The bladder is suspended by placing several sutures through the tissue surrounding the urethra and into the vaginal wall. The sutures are pulled tight so that the tissues are tacked to the symphysis pubis and the urethra is moved forward. The incision is closed by suturing. 51841 is used when the procedure is performed for the second time or if some other factor increases the time or level of complexity.

Coding Tips

When reporting 51841, the operative and diagnostic documentation should support the complicated procedure. For plastic repair and reconstruction of the bladder neck and urethra, see 51800–51820. For plastic repair and reconstruction of the urethra only, see 53400–53431. Report urethropexy (Pereyra type) with 57289.

ICD-10-CM Diagnostic Codes

N39.3   Stress incontinence (female) (male)

AMA: 51840 2018,Jan,8; 2017,Jan,8; 2016,Jan,13; 2015,Jan,16; 2014,Jan,11
51841 2018,Jan,8; 2017,Jan,8; 2016,Jan,13; 2015,Jan,16; 2014,Jan,11

Relative Value Units/Medicare Edits

Non-Facility RVU	Work	PE	MP	Total
51840	11.36	6.87	1.47	19.7
51841	13.68	7.56	1.57	22.81
Facility RVU	Work	PE	MP	Total
51840	11.36	6.87	1.47	19.7
51841	13.68	7.56	1.57	22.81

	FUD	Status	MUE	Modifiers				IOM Reference
51840	90	A	1(2)	51	N/A	62*	80	None
51841	90	A	1(2)	51	N/A	62*	80	

* with documentation

Terms To Know

anterior. Situated in the front area or toward the belly surface of the body.

Burch procedure. Surgical procedure to correct urinary stress incontinence in which the bladder is suspended by placing several sutures through the tissue surrounding the urethra and into the vaginal wall. The sutures are pulled tight so that the tissues are tacked up to the symphysis pubis and the urethra is moved forward.

Marshall-Marchetti-Krantz. Surgical procedure to correct urinary stress incontinence in which the bladder is suspended by placing several sutures through the tissue surrounding the urethra and into the vaginal wall. The sutures are pulled tight so that the tissues are tacked up to the symphysis pubis and the urethra is moved forward.

secondary repair. Delayed repair of a wound performed 10 or more days out from the initial injury or a subsequent repair done after the first procedure failed to restore function or achieve the desired results.

stress incontinence. Involuntary escape of urine at times of minor stress against the bladder, such as coughing, sneezing, or laughing.

tissue. Group of similar cells with a similar function that form definite structures and organs. Tissue types include epithelial tissue, muscle tissue, connective tissue, and nervous tissue.

urethropexy. Surgical suspension of the urethra, often with a bladder suspension or vaginal repair. Sutures may be placed within the fascial tissues along each side of the urethra to the urethrovesical junction and then elevated by pulling up on special ligatures placed above the pubis and around the supporting muscles. Sutures may also be placed in tissue surrounding the urethra into the vaginal wall and pulled tight to the symphysis pubis.

© 2020 Optum360, LLC   **N** Newborn: 0   **P** Pediatric: 0-17   **M** Maternity: 9-64   **A** Adult: 15-124   ♂ Male Only   ♀ Female Only   CPT © 2020 American Medical Association. All Rights Reserved.

Bladder

51845

51845 Abdomino-vaginal vesical neck suspension, with or without endoscopic control (eg, Stamey, Raz, modified Pereyra)

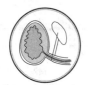

1. A common approach involves placing sutures from the pubic bone on both sides of the bladder neck through the vagina

2. The bladder neck and continence are restored, vagina is suspended

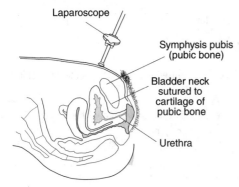

Laparoscope

Symphysis pubis (pubic bone)

Bladder neck sutured to cartilage of pubic bone

Urethra

Explanation

The physician surgically suspends the bladder neck by suturing surrounding tissue to the fibrous membranes (fascia) of the abdomen in a female patient. After inserting a catheter through the urethra to visualize the bladder neck, the physician makes an incision in the vagina, extending it upward toward the base of the bladder. On both sides of the vesical neck, the physician passes a needle through a small incision in the skin above the pubic bone down through the vaginal incision. The physician threads the needle in the vagina and pulls the needle back through the suprapubic incision. Dacron tubing may be threaded onto the sutures to provide extra periurethral support. The physician repeats this process, using an endoscope to ensure proper placement of the suspending sutures. After placing sutures on both sides of the bladder neck, the physician uses moderate upward traction to tighten the bladder neck. The physician inserts a drain tube, bringing it out through a stab incision in the skin, and performs a layered closure.

Coding Tips

This code applies exclusively to females. Report 51840–51841 if the urethra is suspended from the pubic bone by sutures through the vaginal wall and pubic bone. Use 57289 if a Pereyra type operation is used to suspend the urethra. See 51800–51820 for plastic repair and reconstruction of the bladder neck and urethra. See 53431 and 53440 for correction of male urinary incontinence.

ICD-10-CM Diagnostic Codes

N39.3   Stress incontinence (female) (male)

AMA: 51845 2018,Jan,8; 2017,Jan,8; 2016,Jan,13; 2015,Jan,16; 2014,Jan,11

Relative Value Units/Medicare Edits

Non-Facility RVU	Work	PE	MP	Total
51845	10.15	5.49	1.16	16.8
Facility RVU	**Work**	**PE**	**MP**	**Total**
51845	10.15	5.49	1.16	16.8

	FUD	Status	MUE	Modifiers				IOM Reference
51845	90	A	1(2)	51	N/A	62*	80	None

* with documentation

Terms To Know

catheter. Flexible tube inserted into an area of the body for introducing or withdrawing fluid.

drain. Device that creates a channel to allow fluid from a cavity, wound, or infected area to exit the body.

endoscopy. Visual inspection of the body using a fiberoptic scope.

fascia. Fibrous sheet or band of tissue that envelops organs, muscles, and groupings of muscles.

Pereyra procedure. Technique used for surgical correction of stress incontinence in which a suture ligature or loop is used to lift the bladder by connecting the paraurethral tissue to the abdominal muscle.

prolapse. Falling, sliding, or sinking of an organ from its normal location in the body.

Raz procedure. Abdominovaginal vesicle neck suspension procedure to control female urinary stress incontinence. The bladder neck is suspended by suturing surrounding tissue through an incision in the vagina near the base of the bladder to the fibrous membranes (fascia) of the abdomen.

Stamey procedure. Abdomino-vaginal vesicle neck suspension procedure to control female urinary stress incontinence. The bladder neck is suspended by suturing surrounding tissue through an incision in the vagina near the base of the bladder to the fibrous membranes (fascia) of the abdomen.

stress incontinence. Involuntary escape of urine at times of minor stress against the bladder, such as coughing, sneezing, or laughing.

suspension. Fixation of an organ for support; temporary state of cessation of an activity, process, or experience.

tube. Long, hollow cylindrical instrument or body structure.

51860-51865

51860 Cystorrhaphy, suture of bladder wound, injury or rupture; simple
51865 complicated

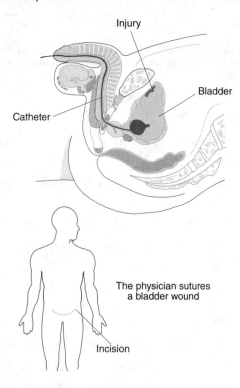

Injury

Bladder

Catheter

The physician sutures
a bladder wound

Incision

Explanation

The physician sutures a wound, injury, or rupture in the bladder. To access the bladder, urethra, and ureters, the physician makes an incision in the skin of the abdomen and cuts the corresponding muscles, fat, and fibrous membranes (fascia). To provide support during healing, the physician may insert a catheter through the urethra. The physician inserts a drain tube and performs a layered closure. Constant irrigation is provided to help prevent infection. Report 51865 if the procedure is complicated due to a previous surgery, congenital defect, or other reason.

Coding Tips

For closure of a congenital gap (exstrophy), see 51940. For closure of an opening into the bladder (cystostomy), see 51880. For closure of an opening (fistula) between the bladder and the vagina or uterus, see 51900–51925.

ICD-10-CM Diagnostic Codes

N32.89	Other specified disorders of bladder
N99.71	Accidental puncture and laceration of a genitourinary system organ or structure during a genitourinary system procedure
N99.72	Accidental puncture and laceration of a genitourinary system organ or structure during other procedure
O03.34	Damage to pelvic organs following incomplete spontaneous abortion M ♀
O03.84	Damage to pelvic organs following complete or unspecified spontaneous abortion M ♀
O04.84	Damage to pelvic organs following (induced) termination of pregnancy M ♀
O07.34	Damage to pelvic organs following failed attempted termination of pregnancy M ♀

S37.23XA	Laceration of bladder, initial encounter
S37.29XA	Other injury of bladder, initial encounter

AMA: **51860** 2014,Jan,11 **51865** 2014,Jan,11

Relative Value Units/Medicare Edits

Non-Facility RVU	Work	PE	MP	Total
51860	12.6	7.09	1.86	21.55
51865	15.8	8.05	2.12	25.97
Facility RVU	**Work**	**PE**	**MP**	**Total**
51860	12.6	7.09	1.86	21.55
51865	15.8	8.05	2.12	25.97

	FUD	Status	MUE	Modifiers				IOM Reference
51860	90	A	1(3)	51	N/A	62*	80	None
51865	90	A	1(3)	51	N/A	62*	80	

* with documentation

Terms To Know

catheter. Flexible tube inserted into an area of the body for introducing or withdrawing fluid.

congenital. Present at birth, occurring through heredity or an influence during gestation up to the moment of birth.

cysto. Cystoscopy.

defect. Imperfection, flaw, or absence.

drain. Device that creates a channel to allow fluid from a cavity, wound, or infected area to exit the body.

fascia. Fibrous sheet or band of tissue that envelops organs, muscles, and groupings of muscles.

irrigation. To wash out or cleanse a body cavity, wound, or tissue with water or other fluid.

laceration. Tearing injury; a torn, ragged-edged wound.

puncture. Creating a hole.

rupture. Tearing or breaking open of tissue.

tube. Long, hollow cylindrical instrument or body structure.

wound. Injury to living tissue often involving a cut or break in the skin.

© 2020 Optum360, LLC
N Newborn: 0   **P** Pediatric: 0-17   **M** Maternity: 9-64   **A** Adult: 15-124   ♂ Male Only   ♀ Female Only   CPT © 2020 American Medical Association. All Rights Reserved.

Coding Companion for Urology/Nephrology

Bladder

51880

51880 Closure of cystostomy (separate procedure)

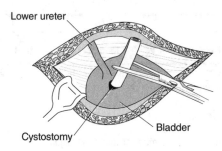

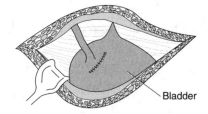

Physician removes a cystostomy tube

Explanation

The physician closes an artificial opening into the bladder (cystostomy). To access the cystostomy, the physician uses the original incision creating the cystostomy or makes an incision in the skin of the lower abdomen. After removing the sutures securing the cystostomy tube to the skin and bladder, the physician removes the cystostomy tube and sutures the bladder musculature to repair the opening. The physician places a drain tube, bringing it out through a separate stab incision in the skin, and performs a layered closure of the abdominal cystostomy incision.

Coding Tips

This separate procedure by definition is usually a component of a more complex service and is not identified separately. When performed alone or with other unrelated procedures/services it may be reported. If performed alone, list the code; if performed with other procedures/services, list the code and append modifier 59 or an X{EPSU} modifier. For creation of a cystostomy through an incision in the bladder, see 51040. For closure of an opening (fistula) between the bladder and the vagina or uterus, see 51900–51925. For suture closure of a rupture, tear, or laceration injury to the bladder, see 51860 or 51865.

ICD-10-CM Diagnostic Codes

N99.510	Cystostomy hemorrhage
N99.511	Cystostomy infection
N99.512	Cystostomy malfunction
N99.518	Other cystostomy complication
Z43.5	Encounter for attention to cystostomy

AMA: 51880 2014,Jan,11

Relative Value Units/Medicare Edits

Non-Facility RVU	Work	PE	MP	Total
51880	7.87	4.58	1.0	13.45
Facility RVU	**Work**	**PE**	**MP**	**Total**
51880	7.87	4.58	1.0	13.45

	FUD	Status	MUE	Modifiers				IOM Reference
51880	90	A	1(2)	51	N/A	62*	80	None

* with documentation

Terms To Know

closure. Repairing an incision or wound by suture or other means.

complication. Condition arising after the beginning of observation and treatment that modifies the course of the patient's illness or the medical care required, or an undesired result or misadventure in medical care.

cystostomy. Formation of an opening through the abdominal wall into the bladder.

drainage. Releasing, taking, or letting out fluids and/or gases from a body part.

hemorrhage. Internal or external bleeding with loss of significant amounts of blood.

incision. Act of cutting into tissue or an organ.

infection. Presence of microorganisms in body tissues that may result in cellular damage.

musculature. Entire muscle tissue apparatus of the body or a specific part of the body.

separate procedures. Services commonly carried out as a fundamental part of a total service and, as such, do not usually warrant separate identification. These services are identified in CPT with the parenthetical phrase (separate procedure) at the end of the description and are payable only when performed alone.

51900

51900   Closure of vesicovaginal fistula, abdominal approach

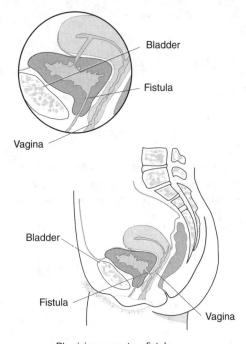

Physician corrects a fistula
between the bladder and vagina

Explanation

The physician closes a vesicovaginal fistula, which is an abnormal passage
between the bladder and the vagina. This procedure is done through the
abdomen. The fistula and surrounding scar tissue of the vaginal wall are usually
excised. The physician makes an incision in the skin, muscle, and fascia of the
abdomen. The bladder wall is opened and the bladder explored. The fistula
is excised along with the surrounding tissue. The resulting defect is closed
with sutures in multiple layers. In some cases, a pedicle graft of tissue may be
sutured between the bladder and the vagina. A urethral or suprapubic catheter
is left in the bladder to prevent distension of the bladder and tension to the
sutured areas.

Coding Tips

This code applies exclusively to females. Note that this procedure is for an
abdominal approach; a vaginal approach is coded with 57320–57330. For
closure of a vesicouterine fistula, see 51920–51925.

ICD-10-CM Diagnostic Codes

N82.0   Vesicovaginal fistula ♀

AMA: 51900 2014,Jan,11

Relative Value Units/Medicare Edits

Non-Facility RVU	Work	PE	MP	Total
51900	14.63	7.49	1.68	23.8
Facility RVU	Work	PE	MP	Total
51900	14.63	7.49	1.68	23.8

	FUD	Status	MUE	Modifiers				IOM Reference
51900	90	A	1(3)	51	N/A	62*	80	None

* with documentation

Terms To Know

approach. Method or anatomical location used to gain access to a body organ
or specific area for procedures.

catheter. Flexible tube inserted into an area of the body for introducing or
withdrawing fluid.

defect. Imperfection, flaw, or absence.

distention. Enlarged or expanded due to pressure from inside.

exploration. Examination for diagnostic purposes.

fascia. Fibrous sheet or band of tissue that envelops organs, muscles, and
groupings of muscles.

incision. Act of cutting into tissue or an organ.

pedicle graft. Mass of flesh and skin partially excised from the donor location,
retaining its blood supply through intact blood vessels, and grafted onto
another site to repair adjacent or distant defects.

scar tissue. Fibrous connective tissue that forms around a wounded area or
injury, composed mainly of fibroblasts or collagenous fibers.

tissue. Group of similar cells with a similar function that form definite
structures and organs. Tissue types include epithelial tissue, muscle tissue,
connective tissue, and nervous tissue.

vesicovaginal fistula. Abnormal communication between the bladder and
the vagina that is the most common genital fistula, often with urinary leakage
causing skin irritation of the vulva and thighs, or total incontinence.

Bladder

51920-51925

51920 Closure of vesicouterine fistula;
51925 with hysterectomy

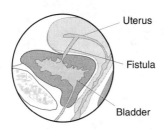

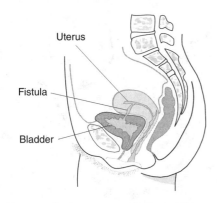

The physician corrects a fistula
between the uterus and the bladder

Explanation

The physician excises an abnormal opening between the uterus and the bladder, then sutures the clean tissues together closing the resulting defect and creating a smooth surface. In 51920, the procedure is done through the bladder with a small abdominal incision or during a laparotomy. In 51925, the physician completes the fistula closure and also removes the uterus through a small horizontal incision just above the pubic hairline. To remove the uterus, the supporting pedicles containing the tubes, ligaments, and arteries are clamped and cut free. The uterus and cervix are removed along with a narrow rim or cuff of vaginal lining. The vaginal defect may be left open for drainage. The abdominal incision is closed by suturing.

Coding Tips

These codes apply exclusively to females. For the closure of a fistula between the bladder and the vagina by abdominal approach, see 51900. For closure of a vesicoenteric fistula, see 44660–44661.

ICD-10-CM Diagnostic Codes

N82.1   Other female urinary-genital tract fistulae ♀

AMA: **51920** 2014,Jan,11 **51925** 2014,Jan,11

Relative Value Units/Medicare Edits

Non-Facility RVU	Work	PE	MP	Total
51920	13.41	7.09	1.53	22.03
51925	17.53	10.45	2.75	30.73
Facility RVU	**Work**	**PE**	**MP**	**Total**
51920	13.41	7.09	1.53	22.03
51925	17.53	10.45	2.75	30.73

	FUD	Status	MUE	Modifiers				IOM Reference
51920	90	A	1(3)	51	N/A	62*	80	None
51925	90	A	1(2)	51	N/A	62*	80	

* with documentation

Terms To Know

clamp. Tool used to grip, compress, join, or fasten body parts.

defect. Imperfection, flaw, or absence.

drainage. Releasing, taking, or letting out fluids and/or gases from a body part.

endometrial cystic hyperplasia. Abnormal cyst-forming overgrowth of the endometrium.

endometriosis. Aberrant uterine mucosal tissue appearing in areas of the pelvic cavity outside of its normal location, lining the uterus, and inflaming surrounding tissues often resulting in infertility or spontaneous abortion.

endometrium. Lining of the uterus, which thickens in preparation for fertilization. A fertilized ovum embeds into the thickened endometrium. When no fertilization takes place, the endometrial lining sheds during the process of menstruation.

fistula. Abnormal tube-like passage between two body cavities or organs or from an organ to the outside surface.

hysterectomy. Surgical removal of the uterus. A complete hysterectomy may also include removal of tubes and ovaries.

laparotomy. Incision through the flank or abdomen for therapeutic or diagnostic purposes.

malignant neoplasm. Any cancerous tumor or lesion exhibiting uncontrolled tissue growth that can progressively invade other parts of the body with its disease-generating cells.

pedicle. Stem-like, narrow base or stalk attached to a new growth.

Bladder

CPT © 2020 American Medical Association. All Rights Reserved.   ● New   ▲ Revised   + Add On   ★ Telemedicine   AMA: CPT Assist   [Resequenced]   ☑ Laterality   © 2020 Optum360, LLC

51940

51940   Closure, exstrophy of bladder

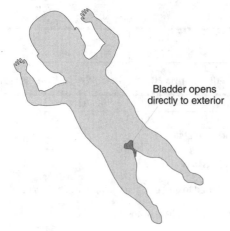

Bladder opens
directly to exterior

Exstrophy repair may include repair of the penis or vulva

Explanation

The physician repairs a congenital defect in the front of the bladder wall, which is associated with lack of closure of the pubic bone at the symphysis pubis. The physician makes an incision around the exposed bladder and around the urethra to develop thick skin flaps. The physician brings the skin flaps together in the midline to close the roof of the urethra and allow the bladder and prostatic urethra to drop back beneath the bony pelvis (male patients), or lengthen the urethra (female patients). To invert the bladder and establish a functional vesical neck, the physician dissects the edge of the bladder from the rectus muscle, and divides the fibromuscular bar that unites the pubic bone to the bladder base. To support the urethra and bladder neck, the physician brings the muscles of the urogenital diaphragm toward the midline. The physician places drain tubes and performs a layered closure.

Coding Tips

For plastic repair of the penis with exstrophy of the bladder, see 54390.

ICD-10-CM Diagnostic Codes

Q64.12   Cloacal exstrophy of urinary bladder
Q64.19   Other exstrophy of urinary bladder

AMA: 51940 2014,Jan,11

Relative Value Units/Medicare Edits

Non-Facility RVU	Work	PE	MP	Total
51940	30.66	13.25	3.49	47.4
Facility RVU	Work	PE	MP	Total
51940	30.66	13.25	3.49	47.4

	FUD	Status	MUE	Modifiers				IOM Reference
51940	90	A	1(2)	51	N/A	62*	80	None

* with documentation

Terms To Know

exstrophy. Congenital defect in the front of the bladder wall, associated with lack of closure of the pubic bone at the symphysis pubis.

51960

51960   Enterocystoplasty, including intestinal anastomosis

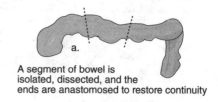

a.

A segment of bowel is
isolated, dissected, and the
ends are anastomosed to restore continuity

Top portion of bladder is removed

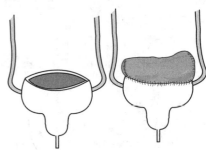

Segment of colon is attached to the top of the bladder

Explanation

The physician reconstructs or enlarges a bladder with a segment of intestine. To access the intestine and bladder, the physician makes a transverse or longitudinal incision on the lower abdomen and cuts the corresponding muscles, fat, and fibrous membranes (fascia). After dissecting an isolated segment of colonic intestine, the physician reconnects (anastomosis) the ileum end-to-end to the ascending colon, restoring continuity to the bowel. The dissected segment of colon is opened and the distal ends are sutured. An incision is made at the bladder dome, a portion of the top of the bladder is removed in preparation, and the colonic segment is sutured to the bladder. After controlling bleeding, the physician inserts a catheter and closes the abdomen in layers over the catheter for support.

Coding Tips

If significant additional time and effort is documented, append modifier 22 and submit a cover letter and operative report. If the vermiform appendix is connected to the bladder to create an opening between the bladder and skin, see 50845. For reconstruction of the bladder or bladder and urethra, see 51800–51820.

ICD-10-CM Diagnostic Codes

N30.10   Interstitial cystitis (chronic) without hematuria
N30.11   Interstitial cystitis (chronic) with hematuria
N31.0   Uninhibited neuropathic bladder, not elsewhere classified
N31.1   Reflex neuropathic bladder, not elsewhere classified
N31.2   Flaccid neuropathic bladder, not elsewhere classified
N31.8   Other neuromuscular dysfunction of bladder
N32.81   Overactive bladder
N32.89   Other specified disorders of bladder
N33   Bladder disorders in diseases classified elsewhere
Q64.0   Epispadias ♂
Q64.11   Supravesical fissure of urinary bladder
Q64.12   Cloacal exstrophy of urinary bladder

Bladder

Q64.19   Other exstrophy of urinary bladder

Q64.2   Congenital posterior urethral valves

AMA: 51960 2014,Jan,11

Relative Value Units/Medicare Edits

Non-Facility RVU	Work	PE	MP	Total
51960	25.4	11.68	2.92	40.0
Facility RVU	**Work**	**PE**	**MP**	**Total**
51960	25.4	11.68	2.92	40.0

	FUD	Status	MUE	Modifiers				IOM Reference
51960	90	A	1(2)	51	N/A	62*	80	None

* with documentation

Terms To Know

anastomosis. Surgically created connection between ducts, blood vessels, or bowel segments to allow flow from one to the other.

catheter. Flexible tube inserted into an area of the body for introducing or withdrawing fluid.

cloacal anomaly. Congenital anomaly resulting from the failure of one common urinary, anal, and reproductive vaginal passage of the early embryonic stage to develop into the properly divided rectal and urogenital sections.

dissect. Cut apart or separate tissue for surgical purposes or for visual or microscopic study.

distal. Located farther away from a specified reference point or the trunk.

exstrophy. Congenital defect in the front of the bladder wall, associated with lack of closure of the pubic bone at the symphysis pubis.

exstrophy of bladder. Congenital anomaly occurring when the bladder everts itself, or turns inside out, through an absent part of the lower abdominal and anterior bladder walls with incomplete closure of the pubic bone.

hematuria. Blood in urine, which may present as gross visible blood or as the presence of red blood cells visible only under a microscope.

hypertonicity. Excessive muscle tone and augmented resistance to normal muscle stretching.

neurogenic bladder. Dysfunctional bladder due to a central or peripheral nervous system lesion that may result in incontinence, residual urine retention, infection, stones, and renal failure.

transverse. Crosswise at right angles to the long axis of a structure or part.

51980

51980   Cutaneous vesicostomy

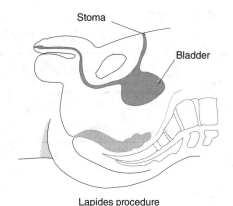

Lapides procedure

Blocksom technique is usually performed on infants; Lapides technique is performed on adults

Explanation

The physician connects the bladder to the skin (cutaneous vesicostomy) for direct urinary drainage. The Blocksom technique is usually performed on newborns. To access the bladder, the physician makes a suprapubic incision in the abdomen and cuts the corresponding muscles, fat, and fibrous membranes (fascia). After securing the bladder dome to the rectus fascia, the physician incises the bladder to create an opening that is sutured to a small incision in the skin. To support the opening during healing, the physician inserts a catheter or stent into the bladder. The physician inserts a drain tube and performs a layered closure. In adults, the Lapides technique passes a flap of bladder beneath the skin to replace a retracted section of abdominal skin. The abdominal skin is passed below the abdominal surface and sutured to the opening in the bladder, making a long-term tubular passage for urine. A catheter is placed through the stoma for two or three days.

Coding Tips

If significant additional time and effort is documented, append modifier 22 and submit a cover letter and operative report. If the vermiform appendix is connected to the bladder to create an opening between the bladder and skin, see 50845. For reconstruction of the bladder or bladder and urethra, see 51800–51820.

ICD-10-CM Diagnostic Codes

N13.71	Vesicoureteral-reflux without reflux nephropathy
N13.721	Vesicoureteral-reflux with reflux nephropathy without hydroureter, unilateral
N13.722	Vesicoureteral-reflux with reflux nephropathy without hydroureter, bilateral
N13.731	Vesicoureteral-reflux with reflux nephropathy with hydroureter, unilateral
N13.732	Vesicoureteral-reflux with reflux nephropathy with hydroureter, bilateral
N13.8	Other obstructive and reflux uropathy
N31.0	Uninhibited neuropathic bladder, not elsewhere classified
N31.1	Reflex neuropathic bladder, not elsewhere classified
N31.2	Flaccid neuropathic bladder, not elsewhere classified
N31.8	Other neuromuscular dysfunction of bladder
Q64.11	Supravesical fissure of urinary bladder

Bladder

Q64.12   Cloacal exstrophy of urinary bladder

Q64.19   Other exstrophy of urinary bladder

AMA: 51980 2014,Jan,11

Relative Value Units/Medicare Edits

Non-Facility RVU	Work	PE	MP	Total
51980	12.57	6.59	1.43	20.59
Facility RVU	**Work**	**PE**	**MP**	**Total**
51980	12.57	6.59	1.43	20.59

	FUD	Status	MUE	Modifiers				IOM Reference
51980	90	A	1(2)	51	N/A	62*	80	None

* with documentation

Terms To Know

atresia. Congenital closure or absence of a tubular organ or an opening to the body surface.

catheter. Flexible tube inserted into an area of the body for introducing or withdrawing fluid.

chordee. Ventral (downward) curvature of the penis due to a fibrous band along the corpus spongiosum seen congenitally with hypospadias, or a downward curvature seen on erection in disease conditions, causing a lack of distensibility in the tissues.

congenital. Present at birth, occurring through heredity or an influence during gestation up to the moment of birth.

epispadias. Male anomaly in which the urethral opening is abnormally located on the dorsum of the penis, appearing as a groove with no upper urethral wall covering.

fascia. Fibrous sheet or band of tissue that envelops organs, muscles, and groupings of muscles.

flap. Mass of flesh and skin partially excised from its location but retaining its blood supply that is moved to another site to repair adjacent or distant defects.

hypertonicity. Excessive muscle tone and augmented resistance to normal muscle stretching.

hypospadias. Fairly common birth defect in males in which the meatus, or urinary opening, is abnormally positioned on the underside of the penile shaft or in the perineum, requiring early surgical correction.

stenosis. Narrowing or constriction of a passage.

stent. Tube to provide support in a body cavity or lumen.

51990-51992

51990   Laparoscopy, surgical; urethral suspension for stress incontinence

51992   sling operation for stress incontinence (eg, fascia or synthetic)

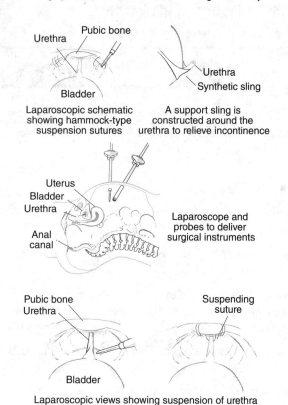

Laparoscopic schematic showing hammock-type suspension sutures

A support sling is constructed around the urethra to relieve incontinence

Laparoscope and probes to deliver surgical instruments

Laparoscopic views showing suspension of urethra

Explanation

The physician treats stress incontinence in the male or female patient. In 51990, the physician makes a 1 cm incision just below the umbilicus through which a fiberoptic laparoscope is inserted. A second incision is made on the left or right side of the abdomen and a second instrument is passed into the abdomen. The physician then manipulates the tools so that the pelvic organs can be observed through the laparoscope. The bladder is suspended by placing several sutures through the tissue surrounding the urethra and into support structures. The sutures are pulled tight so that the urethra is elevated and moved forward. In 51992, the physician inserts an instrument through the cervix into the uterus to manipulate the uterus. Next, the physician makes a 1 cm incision just below the umbilicus through which a fiberoptic laparoscope is inserted. A second incision is made and a second instrument is passed into the abdomen. The physician manipulates the tools so that the pelvic organs can be observed through the laparoscope. The physician places a sling under the junction of the urethra and bladder. The physician places a catheter in the bladder, makes an incision in the anterior wall of the vagina, and folds and tacks the tissues around the urethra. A sling is formed out of synthetic material or from fascia harvested from the sheath of the rectus abdominis muscle. The loop end of the sling is sutured around the junction of the urethra. An incision is made in the lower abdomen and the ends of the sling are grasped with a clamp and pulled into the incision and sutured to the rectus abdominis sheath. The instruments are removed and incisions are closed with sutures.

Coding Tips

Surgical laparoscopy always includes diagnostic laparoscopy. For open sling operation for stress incontinence, see 57288. For open procedures with the urethra suspended from the pubic bone by sutures through the vaginal wall

© 2020 Optum360, LLC   **N Newborn: 0**   **P Pediatric: 0-17**   **M Maternity: 9-64**   **A Adult: 15-124**   ♂ **Male Only**   ♀ **Female Only**   CPT © 2020 American Medical Association. All Rights Reserved.

Coding Companion for Urology/Nephrology

Bladder

and pubic bone, see 51840–51841. For a Pereyra type operation to suspend the urethra, see 57289. For plastic repair and reconstruction of the bladder or bladder and urethra, see 51800–51820. For plastic repair and reconstruction of the urethra, see 53400–53431. For reversal or removal of sling operation for stress incontinence, see 57287. For sling operation to correct male urinary incontinence, see 53440.

ICD-10-CM Diagnostic Codes

N39.3   Stress incontinence (female) (male)
N39.46   Mixed incontinence

AMA: 51990 2019,Feb,10; 2018,Jan,8; 2017,Jan,8; 2016,Jan,13; 2015,Jan,16; 2014,Jan,11 **51992** 2019,Feb,10; 2018,Jan,8; 2017,Jan,8; 2016,Jan,13; 2015,Jan,16; 2014,Jan,11

Relative Value Units/Medicare Edits

Non-Facility RVU	Work	PE	MP	Total
51990	13.36	6.62	1.61	21.59
51992	14.87	7.31	2.12	24.3
Facility RVU	Work	PE	MP	Total
51990	13.36	6.62	1.61	21.59
51992	14.87	7.31	2.12	24.3

	FUD	Status	MUE	Modifiers				IOM Reference
51990	90	A	1(2)	51	N/A	62*	80	100-03,230.10
51992	90	A	1(2)	51	N/A	62*	80	

* with documentation

Terms To Know

catheter. Flexible tube inserted into an area of the body for introducing or withdrawing fluid.

fascia. Fibrous sheet or band of tissue that envelops organs, muscles, and groupings of muscles.

laparoscopy. Direct visualization utilizing a thin, flexible, fiberoptic tube.

sling operation. Procedure to correct urinary incontinence. A sling of fascia or synthetic material is placed under the junction of the urethra and bladder in females, or across the muscles surrounding the urethra in males.

stress incontinence. Involuntary escape of urine at times of minor stress against the bladder, such as coughing, sneezing, or laughing.

suspension. Fixation of an organ for support; temporary state of cessation of an activity, process, or experience.

tissue. Group of similar cells with a similar function that form definite structures and organs. Tissue types include epithelial tissue, muscle tissue, connective tissue, and nervous tissue.

52000

52000   Cystourethroscopy (separate procedure)

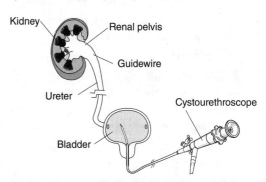

The physician examines the ureter, bladder, and urethra

Explanation

The physician examines the urethra, bladder, and ureteric openings into the bladder with a cystourethroscope passed through the urethra and bladder. No other procedure is performed at this time. After examination, the physician removes the cystourethroscope.

Coding Tips

This separate procedure by definition is usually a component of a more complex service and is not identified separately. When performed alone or with other unrelated procedures/services it may be reported. If performed alone, list the code; if performed with other procedures/services, list the code and append modifier 59 or an X{EPSU} modifier. When 52000 is performed with another separately identifiable procedure, the highest dollar value code is listed as the primary procedure and subsequent procedures are appended with modifier 51. If a microscope is attached to the cystourethroscope, it is not reported separately. Do not report 52000 with 52001, 52320, 52325, 52327, 52330, 52332, 52334, 52341, 52342, 52343, 52356, 53850-53854, 57240, 57260, or 57265 when the services are performed together on the same side. Local anesthesia is included in this service. However, this procedure may be performed under general anesthesia, depending on the age and/or condition of the patient.

ICD-10-CM Diagnostic Codes

C67.0   Malignant neoplasm of trigone of bladder
C67.1   Malignant neoplasm of dome of bladder
C67.2   Malignant neoplasm of lateral wall of bladder
C67.3   Malignant neoplasm of anterior wall of bladder
C67.4   Malignant neoplasm of posterior wall of bladder
C67.5   Malignant neoplasm of bladder neck
C67.6   Malignant neoplasm of ureteric orifice
C67.8   Malignant neoplasm of overlapping sites of bladder
C68.0   Malignant neoplasm of urethra
C79.11   Secondary malignant neoplasm of bladder
C79.19   Secondary malignant neoplasm of other urinary organs
D09.0   Carcinoma in situ of bladder
D09.19   Carcinoma in situ of other urinary organs
D30.3   Benign neoplasm of bladder
D30.4   Benign neoplasm of urethra
D41.3   Neoplasm of uncertain behavior of urethra
D41.4   Neoplasm of uncertain behavior of bladder

Bladder

D49.4	Neoplasm of unspecified behavior of bladder
D49.59	Neoplasm of unspecified behavior of other genitourinary organ
N11.0	Nonobstructive reflux-associated chronic pyelonephritis
N11.8	Other chronic tubulo-interstitial nephritis
N13.0	Hydronephrosis with ureteropelvic junction obstruction
N13.2	Hydronephrosis with renal and ureteral calculous obstruction
N21.0	Calculus in bladder
N30.10	Interstitial cystitis (chronic) without hematuria
N30.11	Interstitial cystitis (chronic) with hematuria
N30.20	Other chronic cystitis without hematuria
N30.21	Other chronic cystitis with hematuria
N30.30	Trigonitis without hematuria
N30.31	Trigonitis with hematuria
N30.40	Irradiation cystitis without hematuria
N30.41	Irradiation cystitis with hematuria
N30.80	Other cystitis without hematuria
N30.81	Other cystitis with hematuria
N32.0	Bladder-neck obstruction
N32.1	Vesicointestinal fistula
N32.2	Vesical fistula, not elsewhere classified
N32.3	Diverticulum of bladder
N32.81	Overactive bladder
N34.0	Urethral abscess
N34.1	Nonspecific urethritis
N35.010	Post-traumatic urethral stricture, male, meatal ♂
N35.011	Post-traumatic bulbous urethral stricture ♂
N35.012	Post-traumatic membranous urethral stricture ♂
N35.013	Post-traumatic anterior urethral stricture ♂
N35.021	Urethral stricture due to childbirth ♀
N35.111	Postinfective urethral stricture, not elsewhere classified, male, meatal ♂
N35.112	Postinfective bulbous urethral stricture, not elsewhere classified, male ♂
N35.113	Postinfective membranous urethral stricture, not elsewhere classified, male ♂
N35.114	Postinfective anterior urethral stricture, not elsewhere classified, male ♂
N36.0	Urethral fistula
N36.1	Urethral diverticulum
N36.2	Urethral caruncle
N36.41	Hypermobility of urethra
N36.42	Intrinsic sphincter deficiency (ISD)
N36.43	Combined hypermobility of urethra and intrinsic sphincter deficiency
N36.44	Muscular disorders of urethra
N36.5	Urethral false passage
N39.3	Stress incontinence (female) (male)
N39.41	Urge incontinence
N39.42	Incontinence without sensory awareness
N39.43	Post-void dribbling
N39.44	Nocturnal enuresis
N39.45	Continuous leakage
N39.46	Mixed incontinence

N39.490	Overflow incontinence
N40.0	Benign prostatic hyperplasia without lower urinary tract symptoms 🅐 ♂
N40.1	Benign prostatic hyperplasia with lower urinary tract symptoms 🅐 ♂
N40.2	Nodular prostate without lower urinary tract symptoms 🅐 ♂
N40.3	Nodular prostate with lower urinary tract symptoms 🅐 ♂
N41.0	Acute prostatitis 🅐 ♂
N41.1	Chronic prostatitis 🅐 ♂
N41.4	Granulomatous prostatitis 🅐 ♂
N42.0	Calculus of prostate 🅐 ♂
N42.1	Congestion and hemorrhage of prostate 🅐 ♂
N42.31	Prostatic intraepithelial neoplasia ♂
N42.32	Atypical small acinar proliferation of prostate ♂
N42.39	Other dysplasia of prostate ♂
N42.81	Prostatodynia syndrome 🅐 ♂
N42.82	Prostatosis syndrome 🅐 ♂
N42.83	Cyst of prostate 🅐 ♂
N42.89	Other specified disorders of prostate 🅐 ♂
N82.0	Vesicovaginal fistula ♀
N99.110	Postprocedural urethral stricture, male, meatal ♂
N99.111	Postprocedural bulbous urethral stricture, male ♂
N99.112	Postprocedural membranous urethral stricture, male ♂
N99.113	Postprocedural anterior bulbous urethral stricture, male ♂
N99.12	Postprocedural urethral stricture, female ♀
Q64.11	Supravesical fissure of urinary bladder
Q64.12	Cloacal exstrophy of urinary bladder
Q64.2	Congenital posterior urethral valves
Q64.31	Congenital bladder neck obstruction
Q64.32	Congenital stricture of urethra
Q64.33	Congenital stricture of urinary meatus
Q64.5	Congenital absence of bladder and urethra
Q64.6	Congenital diverticulum of bladder
Q64.71	Congenital prolapse of urethra
Q64.72	Congenital prolapse of urinary meatus
Q64.73	Congenital urethrorectal fistula
Q64.74	Double urethra
Q64.75	Double urinary meatus

AMA: **52000** 2019,Feb,10; 2018,Nov,10; 2018,Jan,8; 2017,Oct,9; 2017,Jan,8; 2016,Jan,13; 2015,Jan,16; 2014,May,3; 2014,Jan,11

Relative Value Units/Medicare Edits

Non-Facility RVU	Work	PE	MP	Total
52000	1.53	4.28	0.18	5.99
Facility RVU	Work	PE	MP	Total
52000	1.53	0.62	0.18	2.33

	FUD	Status	MUE	Modifiers				IOM Reference
52000	0	A	1(3)	51	N/A	N/A	N/A	None

* with documentation

© 2020 Optum360, LLC 🅝 Newborn: 0 🅟 Pediatric: 0-17 🅜 Maternity: 9-64 🅐 Adult: 15-124 ♂ Male Only ♀ Female Only CPT © 2020 American Medical Association. All Rights Reserved.

52001

52001 Cystourethroscopy with irrigation and evacuation of multiple obstructing clots

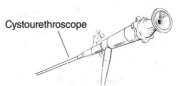

Cystourethroscope

Cystourethroscopy is employed to irrigate and evacuate multiple obstructing clots

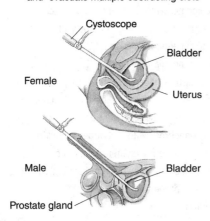

Explanation

Using a rigid or flexible cystoscope, the physician removes clots and examines the urethra, bladder, and ureteric openings into the bladder. The cystoscope is introduced into the meatus and the urethra is inspected before proceeding to the bladder. When the bladder is entered, the urine is evacuated using a syringe; the cystoscope is advanced further through the bladder and deflected upward. Following cystoscopic examination, and localization of the area of interest, the physician inserts a suction and irrigation probe with laser guide to evacuate multiple obstructing clots and to automatically remove any tissue from the operative site. The operative site is irrigated. Following completion of the procedure, the instrument is removed.

Coding Tips

Diagnostic cystourethroscopic examination is included; do not report 52000 together with 52001. For cystourethroscopy with catheterization, irrigation, instillation, or ureteropyelography, report 52005.

ICD-10-CM Diagnostic Codes

N30.01	Acute cystitis with hematuria
N30.11	Interstitial cystitis (chronic) with hematuria
N30.21	Other chronic cystitis with hematuria
N30.31	Trigonitis with hematuria
N30.41	Irradiation cystitis with hematuria
N30.81	Other cystitis with hematuria
N32.89	Other specified disorders of bladder
N36.8	Other specified disorders of urethra
R31.0	Gross hematuria
R31.1	Benign essential microscopic hematuria
R31.21	Asymptomatic microscopic hematuria
R31.29	Other microscopic hematuria
R33.0	Drug induced retention of urine
R33.8	Other retention of urine

AMA: **52001** 2014,Jan,11

Relative Value Units/Medicare Edits

Non-Facility RVU	Work	PE	MP	Total
52001	5.44	5.83	0.62	11.89
Facility RVU	**Work**	**PE**	**MP**	**Total**
52001	5.44	2.21	0.62	8.27

	FUD	Status	MUE	Modifiers				IOM Reference
52001	0	A	1(3)	51	N/A	N/A	N/A	None

* with documentation

Terms To Know

blood clot. Semisolidified, coagulated mass of mainly platelets and fibrin in the bloodstream.

evacuation. Removal or purging of waste material.

irrigation. To wash out or cleanse a body cavity, wound, or tissue with water or other fluid.

meatus. Opening or passage into the body.

obstruction. Blockage that prevents normal function of the valve or structure.

suction. Vacuum evacuation of fluid or tissue.

tissue. Group of similar cells with a similar function that form definite structures and organs. Tissue types include epithelial tissue, muscle tissue, connective tissue, and nervous tissue.

ureter. Tube leading from the kidney to the urinary bladder made up of three layers of tissue: the mucous lining of the inner layer; the smooth, muscular middle layer that propels the urine from the kidney to the bladder by peristalsis; and the outer layer made of fibrous connective tissue. Each ureter leaves the kidney from the hilum, a concave notch on the middle surface, and enters the bladder through a narrow valve-like orifice that prevents the backflow of urine to the kidney.

urethra. Small tube lined with mucous membrane that leads from the bladder to the exterior of the body.

Bladder

52005-52007

52005 Cystourethroscopy, with ureteral catheterization, with or without irrigation, instillation, or ureteropyelography, exclusive of radiologic service;

52007 with brush biopsy of ureter and/or renal pelvis

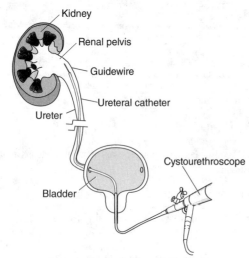

The physician passes a bristled catheter for obtaining a brush biopsy

Explanation

The physician passes the cystourethroscope through the urethra into the bladder. After insertion of a catheter into the ureter, the physician may flush (irrigate) or introduce by drops (instillate) a saline solution to better view structures, and/or may introduce contrast medium for radiologic study of the renal pelvis and ureter (ureteropyelogram, retrograde pyelogram). The physician removes the cystourethroscope. If a brush biopsy of the ureter or renal pelvis is also performed, report 52007.

Coding Tips

Report 52005 if the physician uses the cystourethroscope for examination and catheterization only. The physician usually performs this procedure with local anesthesia. However, general anesthesia may be administered depending on the age or condition of the patient. When 52005 is performed with another separately identifiable procedure, the highest dollar value code is listed as the primary procedure and subsequent procedures are appended with modifier 51. Report 52010 for catheterization of the ejaculatory duct. Supplies used when providing these procedures may be reported with the appropriate HCPCS Level II code. Check with the specific payer to determine coverage.

ICD-10-CM Diagnostic Codes

C61	Malignant neoplasm of prostate ♂
C65.1	Malignant neoplasm of right renal pelvis ☑
C65.2	Malignant neoplasm of left renal pelvis ☑
C66.1	Malignant neoplasm of right ureter ☑
C66.2	Malignant neoplasm of left ureter ☑
C67.0	Malignant neoplasm of trigone of bladder
C67.1	Malignant neoplasm of dome of bladder
C67.2	Malignant neoplasm of lateral wall of bladder
C67.3	Malignant neoplasm of anterior wall of bladder
C67.4	Malignant neoplasm of posterior wall of bladder
C67.5	Malignant neoplasm of bladder neck
C67.6	Malignant neoplasm of ureteric orifice
C67.8	Malignant neoplasm of overlapping sites of bladder
C68.0	Malignant neoplasm of urethra
C79.01	Secondary malignant neoplasm of right kidney and renal pelvis ☑
C79.02	Secondary malignant neoplasm of left kidney and renal pelvis ☑
C79.11	Secondary malignant neoplasm of bladder
D09.0	Carcinoma in situ of bladder
D29.1	Benign neoplasm of prostate ♂
D30.01	Benign neoplasm of right kidney ☑
D30.02	Benign neoplasm of left kidney ☑
D30.11	Benign neoplasm of right renal pelvis ☑
D30.12	Benign neoplasm of left renal pelvis ☑
D30.3	Benign neoplasm of bladder
D30.4	Benign neoplasm of urethra
D40.0	Neoplasm of uncertain behavior of prostate ♂
D41.4	Neoplasm of uncertain behavior of bladder
N11.1	Chronic obstructive pyelonephritis
N13.0	Hydronephrosis with ureteropelvic junction obstruction
N13.1	Hydronephrosis with ureteral stricture, not elsewhere classified
N13.2	Hydronephrosis with renal and ureteral calculous obstruction
N13.39	Other hydronephrosis
N13.4	Hydroureter
N13.5	Crossing vessel and stricture of ureter without hydronephrosis
N13.71	Vesicoureteral-reflux without reflux nephropathy
N13.721	Vesicoureteral-reflux with reflux nephropathy without hydroureter, unilateral
N13.722	Vesicoureteral-reflux with reflux nephropathy without hydroureter, bilateral
N13.731	Vesicoureteral-reflux with reflux nephropathy with hydroureter, unilateral
N13.732	Vesicoureteral-reflux with reflux nephropathy with hydroureter, bilateral
N13.8	Other obstructive and reflux uropathy
N20.0	Calculus of kidney
N20.1	Calculus of ureter
N20.2	Calculus of kidney with calculus of ureter
N21.0	Calculus in bladder
N21.1	Calculus in urethra
N21.8	Other lower urinary tract calculus
N28.0	Ischemia and infarction of kidney
N28.1	Cyst of kidney, acquired
N28.81	Hypertrophy of kidney
N28.82	Megaloureter
N28.83	Nephroptosis
N28.89	Other specified disorders of kidney and ureter
N30.10	Interstitial cystitis (chronic) without hematuria
N30.11	Interstitial cystitis (chronic) with hematuria
N30.20	Other chronic cystitis without hematuria
N30.21	Other chronic cystitis with hematuria
N30.30	Trigonitis without hematuria
N30.31	Trigonitis with hematuria
N30.40	Irradiation cystitis without hematuria

Bladder

N30.41	Irradiation cystitis with hematuria
N30.80	Other cystitis without hematuria
N30.81	Other cystitis with hematuria
N32.0	Bladder-neck obstruction
N32.1	Vesicointestinal fistula
N32.2	Vesical fistula, not elsewhere classified
N32.3	Diverticulum of bladder
N32.81	Overactive bladder
N35.010	Post-traumatic urethral stricture, male, meatal ♂
N35.011	Post-traumatic bulbous urethral stricture ♂
N35.012	Post-traumatic membranous urethral stricture ♂
N35.013	Post-traumatic anterior urethral stricture ♂
N35.021	Urethral stricture due to childbirth ♀
N39.3	Stress incontinence (female) (male)
N39.41	Urge incontinence
N39.42	Incontinence without sensory awareness
N39.43	Post-void dribbling
N39.44	Nocturnal enuresis
N39.45	Continuous leakage
N39.46	Mixed incontinence
N39.490	Overflow incontinence
N40.0	Benign prostatic hyperplasia without lower urinary tract symptoms 🅐 ♂
N40.1	Benign prostatic hyperplasia with lower urinary tract symptoms 🅐 ♂
N40.2	Nodular prostate without lower urinary tract symptoms 🅐 ♂
N40.3	Nodular prostate with lower urinary tract symptoms 🅐 ♂
N41.0	Acute prostatitis 🅐 ♂
N41.1	Chronic prostatitis 🅐 ♂
N41.4	Granulomatous prostatitis 🅐 ♂
N42.83	Cyst of prostate 🅐 ♂
N99.110	Postprocedural urethral stricture, male, meatal ♂
N99.111	Postprocedural bulbous urethral stricture, male ♂
N99.112	Postprocedural membranous urethral stricture, male ♂
N99.113	Postprocedural anterior bulbous urethral stricture, male ♂
N99.115	Postprocedural fossa navicularis urethral stricture ♂
N99.12	Postprocedural urethral stricture, female ♀
Q60.0	Renal agenesis, unilateral
Q60.1	Renal agenesis, bilateral
Q60.3	Renal hypoplasia, unilateral
Q60.4	Renal hypoplasia, bilateral
Q60.6	Potter's syndrome
Q61.01	Congenital single renal cyst
Q61.02	Congenital multiple renal cysts
Q61.11	Cystic dilatation of collecting ducts
Q61.2	Polycystic kidney, adult type
Q61.4	Renal dysplasia
Q61.5	Medullary cystic kidney
Q62.0	Congenital hydronephrosis
Q62.11	Congenital occlusion of ureteropelvic junction
Q62.12	Congenital occlusion of ureterovesical orifice
Q62.2	Congenital megaureter
Q62.31	Congenital ureterocele, orthotopic

Q62.32	Cecoureterocele
Q62.4	Agenesis of ureter
Q62.5	Duplication of ureter
Q62.61	Deviation of ureter
Q62.62	Displacement of ureter
Q62.63	Anomalous implantation of ureter
Q62.7	Congenital vesico-uretero-renal reflux
Q63.0	Accessory kidney
Q63.1	Lobulated, fused and horseshoe kidney
Q63.2	Ectopic kidney
Q63.3	Hyperplastic and giant kidney
Q64.11	Supravesical fissure of urinary bladder
Q64.12	Cloacal exstrophy of urinary bladder
Q64.2	Congenital posterior urethral valves
Q64.31	Congenital bladder neck obstruction
Q64.32	Congenital stricture of urethra
Q64.33	Congenital stricture of urinary meatus
Q64.5	Congenital absence of bladder and urethra
Q64.6	Congenital diverticulum of bladder
Q64.71	Congenital prolapse of urethra
Q64.72	Congenital prolapse of urinary meatus
Q64.73	Congenital urethrorectal fistula
Q64.74	Double urethra
Q64.75	Double urinary meatus
R30.0	Dysuria
R30.1	Vesical tenesmus
R31.0	Gross hematuria
R31.1	Benign essential microscopic hematuria
R31.21	Asymptomatic microscopic hematuria
R31.29	Other microscopic hematuria

AMA: 52005 2019,Mar,10; 2018,Jan,8; 2017,Jan,8; 2016,Jan,13; 2015,Jan,16; 2014,Jan,11 **52007** 2018,Jan,8; 2017,Jan,8; 2016,Jan,13; 2016,Jan,3; 2015,Jan,16; 2014,Jan,11

Relative Value Units/Medicare Edits

Non-Facility RVU	Work	PE	MP	Total
52005	2.37	5.73	0.27	8.37
52007	3.02	10.14	0.35	13.51
Facility RVU	Work	PE	MP	Total
52005	2.37	1.17	0.27	3.81
52007	3.02	1.39	0.35	4.76

	FUD	Status	MUE	Modifiers				IOM Reference
52005	0	A	2(3)	51	N/A	N/A	N/A	100-04,12,30.2
52007	0	A	1(2)	51	50	N/A	N/A	

* with documentation

52010

52010 Cystourethroscopy, with ejaculatory duct catheterization, with or without irrigation, instillation, or duct radiography, exclusive of radiologic service

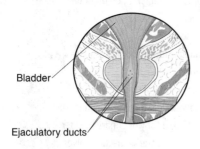

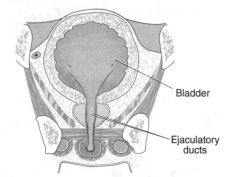

The physician checks the bladder and ejaculatory ducts

Explanation

The physician examines the urinary collecting system with a cystourethroscope passed through the urethra and bladder, and inserts a catheter into the ejaculatory duct. The physician may flush (irrigate) or introduce by drops (instillate) a saline solution to better view structures, and may introduce contrast medium for radiologic study of ejaculatory duct (duct radiography). The physician removes the cystourethroscope.

Coding Tips

When 52010 is performed with another separately identifiable procedure, the highest dollar value code is listed as the primary procedure and subsequent procedures are appended with modifier 51. If significant additional time and effort is documented, append modifier 22 and submit a cover letter and operative report. The physician usually performs this procedure with local anesthesia. However, general anesthesia may be administered depending on the age or condition of the patient. For cystourethroscopy with catheterization of the ureters, see 52005–52007. For radiological supervision and interpretation, see 74440. Supplies used when providing this procedure may be reported with the appropriate HCPCS Level II code. Check with the specific payer to determine coverage.

ICD-10-CM Diagnostic Codes

N42.89	Other specified disorders of prostate 🅰 ♂
N46.01	Organic azoospermia 🅰 ♂
N46.021	Azoospermia due to drug therapy 🅰 ♂
N46.022	Azoospermia due to infection 🅰 ♂
N46.023	Azoospermia due to obstruction of efferent ducts 🅰 ♂
N46.024	Azoospermia due to radiation 🅰 ♂
N46.025	Azoospermia due to systemic disease 🅰 ♂
N46.029	Azoospermia due to other extratesticular causes 🅰 ♂

N46.11	Organic oligospermia 🅰 ♂
N46.121	Oligospermia due to drug therapy 🅰 ♂
N46.122	Oligospermia due to infection 🅰 ♂
N46.123	Oligospermia due to obstruction of efferent ducts 🅰 ♂
N46.124	Oligospermia due to radiation 🅰 ♂
N46.125	Oligospermia due to systemic disease 🅰 ♂
N46.129	Oligospermia due to other extratesticular causes 🅰 ♂
N46.8	Other male infertility 🅰 ♂
N50.89	Other specified disorders of the male genital organs ♂
N53.11	Retarded ejaculation ♂
N53.12	Painful ejaculation ♂
N53.13	Anejaculatory orgasm ♂
N53.14	Retrograde ejaculation ♂
N53.19	Other ejaculatory dysfunction ♂
Q55.4	Other congenital malformations of vas deferens, epididymis, seminal vesicles and prostate ♂
R36.0	Urethral discharge without blood
R36.1	Hematospermia ♂

AMA: **52010** 2018,Jan,8; 2017,Jan,8; 2016,Jan,13; 2015,Jan,16; 2014,Jan,11

Relative Value Units/Medicare Edits

Non-Facility RVU	Work	PE	MP	Total
52010	3.02	7.96	0.35	11.33
Facility RVU	**Work**	**PE**	**MP**	**Total**
52010	3.02	1.39	0.35	4.76

	FUD	Status	MUE	Modifiers			IOM Reference
52010	0	A	1(2)	51	N/A	N/A	N/A	None

* with documentation

Terms To Know

catheter. Flexible tube inserted into an area of the body for introducing or withdrawing fluid.

cyst. Elevated encapsulated mass containing fluid, semisolid, or solid material with a membranous lining.

hyperplasia. Abnormal proliferation in the number of normal cells in regular tissue arrangement.

impotence. Psychosexual or organic dysfunction in which there is partial or complete failure to attain or maintain erection until completion of the sexual act.

instillation. Administering a liquid slowly over time, drop by drop.

irrigation. To wash out or cleanse a body cavity, wound, or tissue with water or other fluid.

prostate. Male gland surrounding the bladder neck and urethra that secretes a substance into the seminal fluid.

prostatic hypertrophy. Overgrowth of the normal prostate tissue.

© 2020 Optum360, LLC   **N** Newborn: 0   **P** Pediatric: 0-17   **M** Maternity: 9-64   🅰 Adult: 15-124   ♂ Male Only   ♀ Female Only   CPT © 2020 American Medical Association. All Rights Reserved.

Coding Companion for Urology/Nephrology

Bladder

52204

52204   Cystourethroscopy, with biopsy(s)

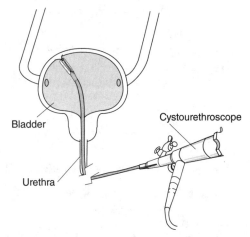

The physician extracts tissue for examination

Explanation

The physician examines the urinary collecting system with a cystourethroscope passed through the urethra and bladder, and extracts biopsy tissue from the bladder or urethra. To do so, the physician passes a cutting instrument through the endoscope to the suspect tissue and traps a specimen of tissue. Multiple samples may be collected. The physician removes the instrument and cystourethroscope.

Coding Tips

When 52204 is performed with another separately identifiable procedure, the highest dollar value code is listed as the primary procedure and subsequent procedures are appended with modifier 51. The physician usually performs this procedure with local anesthesia. However, general anesthesia may be administered depending on the age or condition of the patient. Report 53200 for open biopsy of the urethra. Report any radiological guidance separately. Supplies used when providing this procedure may be reported with the appropriate HCPCS Level II code. Check with the specific payer to determine coverage.

ICD-10-CM Diagnostic Codes

C67.0	Malignant neoplasm of trigone of bladder
C67.1	Malignant neoplasm of dome of bladder
C67.2	Malignant neoplasm of lateral wall of bladder
C67.3	Malignant neoplasm of anterior wall of bladder
C67.4	Malignant neoplasm of posterior wall of bladder
C67.5	Malignant neoplasm of bladder neck
C67.6	Malignant neoplasm of ureteric orifice
C67.8	Malignant neoplasm of overlapping sites of bladder
C68.0	Malignant neoplasm of urethra
C79.11	Secondary malignant neoplasm of bladder
C79.19	Secondary malignant neoplasm of other urinary organs
D09.0	Carcinoma in situ of bladder
D09.19	Carcinoma in situ of other urinary organs
D30.3	Benign neoplasm of bladder
D30.4	Benign neoplasm of urethra
D41.3	Neoplasm of uncertain behavior of urethra

D41.4	Neoplasm of uncertain behavior of bladder
D49.4	Neoplasm of unspecified behavior of bladder
D49.511	Neoplasm of unspecified behavior of right kidney ☑
D49.512	Neoplasm of unspecified behavior of left kidney ☑
D49.59	Neoplasm of unspecified behavior of other genitourinary organ
N21.0	Calculus in bladder
N22	Calculus of urinary tract in diseases classified elsewhere
N30.00	Acute cystitis without hematuria
N30.01	Acute cystitis with hematuria
N30.10	Interstitial cystitis (chronic) without hematuria
N30.11	Interstitial cystitis (chronic) with hematuria
N30.20	Other chronic cystitis without hematuria
N30.21	Other chronic cystitis with hematuria
N30.30	Trigonitis without hematuria
N30.31	Trigonitis with hematuria
N30.40	Irradiation cystitis without hematuria
N30.41	Irradiation cystitis with hematuria
N30.80	Other cystitis without hematuria
N30.81	Other cystitis with hematuria
N32.89	Other specified disorders of bladder
N33	Bladder disorders in diseases classified elsewhere
N34.0	Urethral abscess
N34.1	Nonspecific urethritis
N34.2	Other urethritis
N36.2	Urethral caruncle
N36.8	Other specified disorders of urethra
N37	Urethral disorders in diseases classified elsewhere
T19.0XXA	Foreign body in urethra, initial encounter
T19.1XXA	Foreign body in bladder, initial encounter

AMA: 52204 2018,Jan,8; 2017,Jan,8; 2016,May,12; 2016,Jan,13; 2015,Jan,16; 2014,Jan,11

Relative Value Units/Medicare Edits

Non-Facility RVU	Work	PE	MP	Total
52204	2.59	8.08	0.3	10.97
Facility RVU	**Work**	**PE**	**MP**	**Total**
52204	2.59	1.18	0.3	4.07

	FUD	Status	MUE	Modifiers				IOM Reference
52204	0	A	1(2)	51	N/A	N/A	N/A	None

* with documentation

Terms To Know

biopsy. Tissue or fluid removed for diagnostic purposes through analysis of the cells in the biopsy material.

specimen. Tissue cells or sample of fluid taken for analysis, pathologic examination, and diagnosis.

tissue. Group of similar cells with a similar function that form definite structures and organs. Tissue types include epithelial tissue, muscle tissue, connective tissue, and nervous tissue.

Bladder

52214

52214 Cystourethroscopy, with fulguration (including cryosurgery or laser surgery) of trigone, bladder neck, prostatic fossa, urethra, or periurethral glands

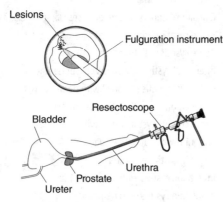

Physician uses several methods to destroy lesions in bladder

Explanation

The physician examines the urinary collecting system with a cystourethroscope passed through the urethra and bladder, and destroys tissue of the trigone, bladder neck prostatic fossa, urethra, or periurethral glands. The physician passes through the endoscope an instrument that uses electric current to destroy lesions on the urethra, periurethral glands, bladder neck, depression below the prostate surface (prostatic fossa), and triangular area at the base of the bladder (trigone). The physician may employ endoscopic use of liquid nitrogen or carbon dioxide (cryosurgery) or lasers to destroy lesions. The physician removes the instruments and cystourethroscope.

Coding Tips

When 52214 is performed with another separately identifiable procedure, the highest dollar value code is listed as the primary procedure and subsequent procedures are appended with modifier 51. The physician usually performs this procedure with local anesthesia. However, general anesthesia may be administered depending on the age or condition of the patient. For treatment of female urethral syndrome, with fulguration of polyp of the urethra, bladder neck, and/or trigone, see 52285. For fulguration of minor vesical lesions, see 52224. For fulguration and/or resection of bladder tumors, see 52234–52240. For treatment of lesions by insertion of radioactive substance, see 52250. For fulguration or cryosurgical destruction of bladder lesions through an incision, see 51020–51030. For fulguration of a ureteral or renal pelvic lesion through a cystourethroscope, ureteroscope, and/or pyeloscope, see 52354. Append modifier 78 for transurethral fulguration of prostatic tissue performed during the global period to 52601 or 52630, with a related procedure or for postoperative hemorrhage by the same physician. Report radiological guidance separately. Supplies used when providing this procedure may be reported with the appropriate HCPCS Level II code. Check with the specific payer to determine coverage.

ICD-10-CM Diagnostic Codes

C61	Malignant neoplasm of prostate ♂
C67.0	Malignant neoplasm of trigone of bladder
C67.1	Malignant neoplasm of dome of bladder
C67.5	Malignant neoplasm of bladder neck
C68.0	Malignant neoplasm of urethra
C79.11	Secondary malignant neoplasm of bladder
D09.0	Carcinoma in situ of bladder
D30.3	Benign neoplasm of bladder
D30.4	Benign neoplasm of urethra
D41.3	Neoplasm of uncertain behavior of urethra
D41.4	Neoplasm of uncertain behavior of bladder
D49.4	Neoplasm of unspecified behavior of bladder
N30.10	Interstitial cystitis (chronic) without hematuria
N30.11	Interstitial cystitis (chronic) with hematuria
N32.89	Other specified disorders of bladder
N36.1	Urethral diverticulum
N36.2	Urethral caruncle
N36.8	Other specified disorders of urethra

AMA: 52214 2018,Jan,8; 2017,Jan,8; 2016,May,12; 2016,Jan,13; 2015,Jan,16; 2014,Jan,11

Relative Value Units/Medicare Edits

Non-Facility RVU	Work	PE	MP	Total
52214	3.5	16.9	0.41	20.81
Facility RVU	**Work**	**PE**	**MP**	**Total**
52214	3.5	1.18	0.41	5.09

	FUD	Status	MUE	Modifiers				IOM Reference
52214	0	A	1(2)	51	N/A	N/A	N/A	None

* with documentation

Terms To Know

benign lesion. Neoplasm or change in tissue that is not cancerous (nonmalignant).

carcinoma in situ. Malignancy that arises from the cells of the vessel, gland, or organ of origin that remains confined to that site or has not invaded neighboring tissue.

cryosurgery. Application of intense cold, usually produced using liquid nitrogen, to locally freeze diseased or unwanted tissue and induce tissue necrosis without causing harm to adjacent tissue.

fulguration. Destruction of living tissue by using sparks from a high-frequency electric current.

laser surgery. Use of concentrated, sharply defined light beams to cut, cauterize, coagulate, seal, or vaporize tissue.

malignant neoplasm. Any cancerous tumor or lesion exhibiting uncontrolled tissue growth that can progressively invade other parts of the body with its disease-generating cells.

Bladder

52224

52224 Cystourethroscopy, with fulguration (including cryosurgery or laser surgery) or treatment of MINOR (less than 0.5 cm) lesion(s) with or without biopsy

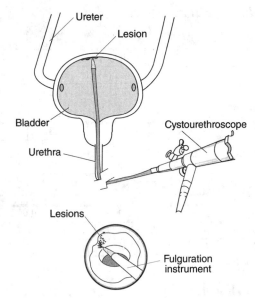

Physician destroys minor lesions in the bladder

Explanation

The physician examines the urinary collecting system with a cystourethroscope passed through the urethra and bladder, and uses electric current (fulguration) to destroy lesions smaller than 0.5 cm. The physician may also employ endoscopic use of liquid nitrogen or carbon dioxide (cryosurgery) or lasers to destroy lesions. The physician may insert an instrument to extract biopsy tissue from the bladder. The physician removes the instruments and cystourethroscope.

Coding Tips

When 52224 is performed with another separately identifiable procedure, the highest dollar value code is listed as the primary procedure and subsequent procedures are appended with modifier 51. The physician usually performs this procedure with local anesthesia. However, general anesthesia may be administered depending on the age or condition of the patient. Report 52214 for fulguration of lesions on the urethra, periurethral glands, bladder neck, depression below the prostate surface (prostatic fossa), and triangular area at the base of the bladder (trigone). For fulguration and/or resection of bladder tumors, see 52234–52240. For excision of bladder tumors through an incision in the bladder, see 51530. See 51020–51030 for fulguration or cryosurgical destruction of bladder lesions through an incision. Supplies used when providing this procedure may be reported with the appropriate HCPCS Level II code. Check with the specific payer to determine coverage.

ICD-10-CM Diagnostic Codes

C67.0	Malignant neoplasm of trigone of bladder
C67.1	Malignant neoplasm of dome of bladder
C67.2	Malignant neoplasm of lateral wall of bladder
C67.3	Malignant neoplasm of anterior wall of bladder
C67.4	Malignant neoplasm of posterior wall of bladder
C67.5	Malignant neoplasm of bladder neck
C67.6	Malignant neoplasm of ureteric orifice
C67.7	Malignant neoplasm of urachus
C67.8	Malignant neoplasm of overlapping sites of bladder
C79.11	Secondary malignant neoplasm of bladder
D09.0	Carcinoma in situ of bladder
D30.3	Benign neoplasm of bladder
D41.4	Neoplasm of uncertain behavior of bladder
D49.4	Neoplasm of unspecified behavior of bladder
N30.10	Interstitial cystitis (chronic) without hematuria
N30.11	Interstitial cystitis (chronic) with hematuria
N32.3	Diverticulum of bladder
N32.89	Other specified disorders of bladder

AMA: **52224** 2018,Jan,8; 2017,Jan,8; 2016,May,12; 2016,Jan,13; 2015,Jan,16; 2014,Jan,11

Relative Value Units/Medicare Edits

Non-Facility RVU	Work	PE	MP	Total
52224	4.05	17.22	0.47	21.74
Facility RVU	**Work**	**PE**	**MP**	**Total**
52224	4.05	1.37	0.47	5.89

	FUD	Status	MUE	Modifiers				IOM Reference
52224	0	A	1(2)	51	N/A	N/A	N/A	None

* with documentation

Terms To Know

biopsy. Tissue or fluid removed for diagnostic purposes through analysis of the cells in the biopsy material.

cryosurgery. Application of intense cold, usually produced using liquid nitrogen, to locally freeze diseased or unwanted tissue and induce tissue necrosis without causing harm to adjacent tissue.

fulguration. Destruction of living tissue by using sparks from a high-frequency electric current.

laser surgery. Use of concentrated, sharply defined light beams to cut, cauterize, coagulate, seal, or vaporize tissue. The color and wavelength of the laser light is produced by its active medium, such as argon, CO2, potassium titanyl phosphate (KTP), Krypton, and Nd:YAG, which determines the type of tissues it can best treat.

malignant neoplasm. Any cancerous tumor or lesion exhibiting uncontrolled tissue growth that can progressively invade other parts of the body with its disease-generating cells.

tissue. Group of similar cells with a similar function that form definite structures and organs. Tissue types include epithelial tissue, muscle tissue, connective tissue, and nervous tissue.

Bladder

52234-52240

52234 Cystourethroscopy, with fulguration (including cryosurgery or laser surgery) and/or resection of; SMALL bladder tumor(s) (0.5 up to 2.0 cm)

52235 MEDIUM bladder tumor(s) (2.0 to 5.0 cm)

52240 LARGE bladder tumor(s)

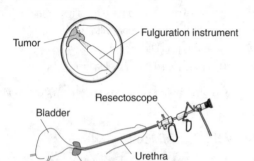

Physician excises a bladder tumor on male or female (male shown)

Explanation

The physician examines the urinary collecting system with a cystourethroscope passed through the urethra and bladder, and removes tumors of the bladder by electric current (fulguration) or excision. The physician passes an instrument through the endoscope to destroy or remove tumors of the bladder by electric current (fulguration) or excision. The physician may also use liquid nitrogen or carbon dioxide (cryosurgery) or lasers to destroy lesions. The physician removes the instruments and cystourethroscope. For small tumor(s) that are 0.5 up to 2 cm in size, report 52234. For medium bladder tumor(s) that are 2 to 5 cm in size, report 52235. For large tumor(s) that are larger than 5 cm, report 52240.

Coding Tips

If significant additional time and effort is documented, append modifier 22 and submit a cover letter and operative report. Use 52224 for fulguration of minor lesions on the bladder. Report 51530 for excision of bladder tumors through an incision in the bladder. Use 52250 for treatment of lesions by insertion of a radioactive substance. See 51020–51030 for fulguration or cryosurgical destruction of bladder lesions through an incision. Supplies used when providing these procedures may be reported with the appropriate HCPCS Level II code. Check with the specific payer to determine coverage.

ICD-10-CM Diagnostic Codes

C67.0	Malignant neoplasm of trigone of bladder
C67.1	Malignant neoplasm of dome of bladder
C67.2	Malignant neoplasm of lateral wall of bladder
C67.3	Malignant neoplasm of anterior wall of bladder
C67.4	Malignant neoplasm of posterior wall of bladder
C67.5	Malignant neoplasm of bladder neck
C67.6	Malignant neoplasm of ureteric orifice
C67.7	Malignant neoplasm of urachus
C67.8	Malignant neoplasm of overlapping sites of bladder
C79.11	Secondary malignant neoplasm of bladder
D09.0	Carcinoma in situ of bladder
D30.3	Benign neoplasm of bladder
D41.4	Neoplasm of uncertain behavior of bladder
D49.4	Neoplasm of unspecified behavior of bladder

AMA: **52234** 2018,Jan,8; 2017,Jan,8; 2016,May,12; 2016,Jan,13; 2015,Jan,16; 2014,Jan,11 **52235** 2018,Jan,8; 2017,Jan,8; 2016,May,12; 2016,Jan,13; 2015,Jan,16; 2014,Jan,11 **52240** 2018,Jan,8; 2017,Jan,8; 2016,May,12; 2016,Jan,13; 2015,Jan,16; 2014,Jan,11

Relative Value Units/Medicare Edits

Non-Facility RVU	Work	PE	MP	Total
52234	4.62	1.93	0.53	7.08
52235	5.44	2.25	0.62	8.31
52240	7.5	2.95	0.86	11.31
Facility RVU	**Work**	**PE**	**MP**	**Total**
52234	4.62	1.93	0.53	7.08
52235	5.44	2.25	0.62	8.31
52240	7.5	2.95	0.86	11.31

	FUD	Status	MUE	Modifiers				IOM Reference
52234	0	A	1(2)	51	N/A	N/A	N/A	100-04,12,30.2
52235	0	A	1(2)	51	N/A	N/A	N/A	
52240	0	A	1(2)	51	N/A	N/A	N/A	

* with documentation

Terms To Know

chronic interstitial cystitis. Persistently inflamed lesion of the bladder wall, usually accompanied by urinary frequency, pain, nocturia, and a distended bladder.

cryosurgery. Application of intense cold, usually produced using liquid nitrogen, to locally freeze diseased or unwanted tissue and induce tissue necrosis without causing harm to adjacent tissue.

cystitis cystica. Inflammation of the bladder characterized by the formation of multiple cysts.

excision. Surgical removal of an organ or tissue.

fulguration. Destruction of living tissue by using sparks from a high-frequency electric current.

resection. Surgical removal of a part or all of an organ or body part.

tumor. Pathological swelling or enlargement; a neoplastic growth of uncontrolled, abnormal multiplication of cells.

Bladder

52250

52250 Cystourethroscopy with insertion of radioactive substance, with or without biopsy or fulguration

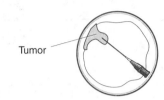

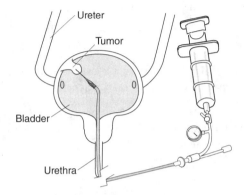

Physician injects radioactive substance

Explanation

The physician examines the urinary collecting system with a cystourethroscope passed through the urethra and bladder, and inserts a radioactive substance. To release a radioactive substance, the physician passes an instrument through the endoscope. The physician may insert instruments through the endoscope to remove lesions or extract biopsy tissue from the bladder. The physician removes the instruments and cystourethroscope.

Coding Tips

When 52250 is performed with another separately identifiable procedure, the highest dollar value code is listed as the primary procedure and subsequent procedures are appended with modifier 51. For excision of bladder tumors, see 52234–52240. See 51020–51030 for fulguration or cryosurgical destruction of bladder lesions through an incision. Use 52354 for fulguration of a ureteral or renal pelvic lesion through a cystourethroscope, ureteroscope, and/or pyeloscope. Report radiological guidance separately.

ICD-10-CM Diagnostic Codes

C67.0	Malignant neoplasm of trigone of bladder
C67.1	Malignant neoplasm of dome of bladder
C67.2	Malignant neoplasm of lateral wall of bladder
C67.3	Malignant neoplasm of anterior wall of bladder
C67.4	Malignant neoplasm of posterior wall of bladder
C67.5	Malignant neoplasm of bladder neck
C67.6	Malignant neoplasm of ureteric orifice
C67.7	Malignant neoplasm of urachus
D09.0	Carcinoma in situ of bladder

AMA: **52250** 2018,Jan,8; 2017,Jan,8; 2016,Jan,13; 2015,Jan,16; 2014,Jan,11

Relative Value Units/Medicare Edits

Non-Facility RVU	Work	PE	MP	Total
52250	4.49	1.89	0.52	6.9
Facility RVU	**Work**	**PE**	**MP**	**Total**
52250	4.49	1.89	0.52	6.9

	FUD	Status	MUE	Modifiers				IOM Reference
52250	0	A	1(2)	51	N/A	N/A	N/A	None

* with documentation

Terms To Know

biopsy. Tissue or fluid removed for diagnostic purposes through analysis of the cells in the biopsy material.

carcinoma in situ. Malignancy that arises from the cells of the vessel, gland, or organ of origin that remains confined to that site or has not invaded neighboring tissue.

fulguration. Destruction of living tissue by using sparks from a high-frequency electric current.

malignant. Any condition tending to progress toward death, specifically an invasive tumor with a loss of cellular differentiation that has the ability to spread or metastasize to other body areas.

neoplasm. New abnormal growth, tumor.

tissue. Group of similar cells with a similar function that form definite structures and organs. Tissue types include epithelial tissue, muscle tissue, connective tissue, and nervous tissue.

trigone. Triangular, smooth area of mucous membrane at the base of the bladder, located between the ureteric openings in back and the urethral opening in front.

urachus. Embryonic tube connecting the urinary bladder to the umbilicus during development of the fetus that normally closes before birth, generally in the fourth or fifth month of gestation.

Bladder

CPT © 2020 American Medical Association. All Rights Reserved.   ● **New**   ▲ **Revised**   + **Add On**   ★ **Telemedicine**   **AMA: CPT Assist**   **[Resequenced]**   ☑ **Laterality**   © 2020 Optum360, LLC

52260-52265

52260   Cystourethroscopy, with dilation of bladder for interstitial cystitis; general or conduction (spinal) anesthesia

52265   local anesthesia

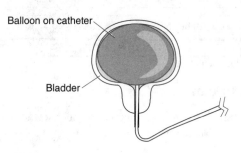

Balloon on catheter

Bladder

Cystourethroscope

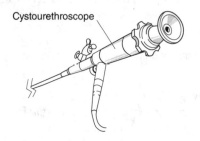

Physician uses balloon to distend bladder,
relieving chronic inflammation

Explanation

The physician examines the urinary collecting system with a cystourethroscope passed through the urethra and bladder and dilates the bladder with a balloon to relieve chronic inflammation of the bladder (interstitial cystitis). The physician removes the instrument and cystourethroscope. If general or spinal anesthesia is administered to the patient, use 52260. If the procedure is performed using local anesthesia, use 52265.

Coding Tips

When 52260 or 52265 is performed with another separately identifiable procedure, the highest dollar value code is listed as the primary procedure and subsequent procedures are appended with modifier 51. Note that 52260 is for dilation of the bladder under general or spinal anesthesia and 52265 is for local anesthesia. Supplies used when providing these procedures may be reported with the appropriate HCPCS Level II code. Check with the specific payer to determine coverage.

ICD-10-CM Diagnostic Codes

N30.10   Interstitial cystitis (chronic) without hematuria
N30.11   Interstitial cystitis (chronic) with hematuria

AMA: **52260** 2018,Jan,8; 2017,Jan,8; 2016,Jan,13; 2015,Jan,16; 2014,Jan,11
52265 2018,Jan,8; 2017,Jan,8; 2016,Jan,13; 2015,Jan,16; 2014,Jan,11

Relative Value Units/Medicare Edits

Non-Facility RVU	Work	PE	MP	Total
52260	3.91	1.69	0.48	6.08
52265	2.94	7.53	0.39	10.86
Facility RVU	**Work**	**PE**	**MP**	**Total**
52260	3.91	1.69	0.48	6.08
52265	2.94	1.37	0.39	4.7

	FUD	Status	MUE	Modifiers				IOM Reference
52260	0	A	1(2)	51	N/A	N/A	N/A	100-03,230.12
52265	0	A	1(2)	51	N/A	N/A	N/A	

* with documentation

Terms To Know

chronic interstitial cystitis. Persistently inflamed lesion of the bladder wall, usually accompanied by urinary frequency, pain, nocturia, and a distended bladder.

dilation. Artificial increase in the diameter of an opening or lumen made by medication or by instrumentation.

dysuria. Pain upon urination.

hematuria. Blood in urine, which may present as gross visible blood or as the presence of red blood cells visible only under a microscope.

inflammation. Cytologic and chemical reactions that occur in affected blood vessels and adjacent tissues in response to injury or abnormal stimulation from a physical, chemical, or biologic agent.

urethra. Small tube lined with mucous membrane that leads from the bladder to the exterior of the body.

© 2020 Optum360, LLC   **N** Newborn: 0   **P** Pediatric: 0-17   **M** Maternity: 9-64   **A** Adult: 15-124   ♂ Male Only   ♀ Female Only   CPT © 2020 American Medical Association. All Rights Reserved.

Coding Companion for Urology/Nephrology

Bladder

52270-52276

52270 Cystourethroscopy, with internal urethrotomy; female
52275   male
52276 Cystourethroscopy with direct vision internal urethrotomy

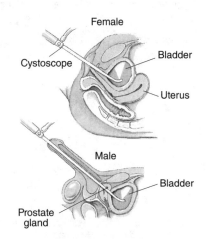

The physician inspects the urinary system and incises a constriction in the urethra

Explanation

The physician examines the urinary collecting system with a cystourethroscope passed through the urethra and bladder. With a cutting instrument introduced through the cystourethroscope, the physician incises the inside of the urethral constriction. The physician removes the instrument and cystourethroscope. For incision of a female urethra, report 52270; for a male urethra, report 52275. If the physician incises the scar tissue or stricture within the urethra to open the lumen diameter while maintaining direct vision of the urethral lumen in either sex, report 52276.

Coding Tips

When 52270, 52275, or 52276 is performed with another separately identifiable procedure, the highest dollar value code is listed as the primary procedure and subsequent procedures are appended with modifier 51. For dilation of a urethral stricture with a cystourethroscope, with or without an incision in the meatus, see 52281 and 52285. For cystourethroscopy with injection of a steroid into a urethral stricture, see 52283. Supplies used when providing these procedures may be reported with the appropriate HCPCS Level II code. Check with the specific payer to determine coverage.

ICD-10-CM Diagnostic Codes

N35.010	Post-traumatic urethral stricture, male, meatal ♂
N35.011	Post-traumatic bulbous urethral stricture ♂
N35.012	Post-traumatic membranous urethral stricture ♂
N35.013	Post-traumatic anterior urethral stricture ♂
N35.016	Post-traumatic urethral stricture, male, overlapping sites ♂
N35.021	Urethral stricture due to childbirth ♀
N35.028	Other post-traumatic urethral stricture, female ♀
N35.111	Postinfective urethral stricture, not elsewhere classified, male, meatal ♂
N35.112	Postinfective bulbous urethral stricture, not elsewhere classified, male ♂
N35.113	Postinfective membranous urethral stricture, not elsewhere classified, male ♂
N35.114	Postinfective anterior urethral stricture, not elsewhere classified, male ♂
N35.12	Postinfective urethral stricture, not elsewhere classified, female ♀
N35.811	Other urethral stricture, male, meatal ♂
N35.812	Other urethral bulbous stricture, male ♂
N35.813	Other membranous urethral stricture, male ♂
N35.814	Other anterior urethral stricture, male ♂
N35.816	Other urethral stricture, male, overlapping sites ♂
N35.82	Other urethral stricture, female ♀
N99.110	Postprocedural urethral stricture, male, meatal ♂
N99.111	Postprocedural bulbous urethral stricture, male ♂
N99.112	Postprocedural membranous urethral stricture, male ♂
N99.113	Postprocedural anterior bulbous urethral stricture, male ♂
N99.115	Postprocedural fossa navicularis urethral stricture ♂
N99.116	Postprocedural urethral stricture, male, overlapping sites ♂
N99.12	Postprocedural urethral stricture, female ♀
Q64.32	Congenital stricture of urethra
Q64.33	Congenital stricture of urinary meatus
Q64.39	Other atresia and stenosis of urethra and bladder neck

AMA: **52270** 2018,Jan,8; 2017,Jan,8; 2016,Jan,13; 2015,Jan,16; 2014,Jan,11 **52275** 2018,Jan,8; 2017,Jan,8; 2016,Jan,13; 2015,Jan,16; 2014,Jan,11 **52276** 2019,Feb,10; 2018,Jan,8; 2017,Jan,8; 2016,Jan,13; 2015,Jan,16; 2014,Jan,11

Relative Value Units/Medicare Edits

Non-Facility RVU	Work	PE	MP	Total
52270	3.36	7.72	0.39	11.47
52275	4.69	9.82	0.54	15.05
52276	4.99	2.06	0.57	7.62
Facility RVU	**Work**	**PE**	**MP**	**Total**
52270	3.36	1.48	0.39	5.23
52275	4.69	1.93	0.54	7.16
52276	4.99	2.06	0.57	7.62

	FUD	Status	MUE	Modifiers				IOM Reference
52270	0	A	1(2)	51	N/A	N/A	N/A	None
52275	0	A	1(2)	51	N/A	N/A	N/A	
52276	0	A	1(2)	51	N/A	N/A	N/A	

* with documentation

CPT © 2020 American Medical Association. All Rights Reserved.   ● New   ▲ Revised   + Add On   ★ Telemedicine   AMA: CPT Assist   [Resequenced]   ☑ Laterality   © 2020 Optum360, LLC

Bladder

52277

52277   Cystourethroscopy, with resection of external sphincter
(sphincterotomy)

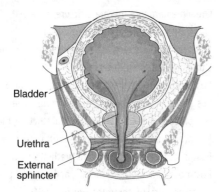

Physician resects external sphincter
Male and female procedure (male shown)

Explanation

The physician examines the urinary collecting system with a cystourethroscope
passed through the urethra and bladder, and makes an incision
(sphincterotomy) in the musculature of the urethral closure (urethral sphincter).
The physician passes a cutting instrument through the cystourethroscope for
resection of the external sphincter. After the sphincterectomy, the physician
removes the instrument and cystourethroscope.

Coding Tips

When 52277 is performed with another separately identifiable procedure, the
highest dollar value code is listed as the primary procedure and subsequent
procedures are appended with modifier 51. The physician usually performs
this procedure with local anesthesia. However, general anesthesia may be
administered depending on the age or condition of the patient. Report 57220
for plastic repair of a female urethral sphincter by vaginal approach. For needle
electromyography studies (EMG) of the urethral sphincter, see 51785. For
insertion, removal, replacement, or repair of an artificial urethral sphincter,
see 53445–53449. Supplies used when providing this procedure may be
reported with the appropriate HCPCS Level II code. Check with the specific
payer to determine coverage.

ICD-10-CM Diagnostic Codes

G83.4	Cauda equina syndrome
N31.0	Uninhibited neuropathic bladder, not elsewhere classified
N31.1	Reflex neuropathic bladder, not elsewhere classified
N31.8	Other neuromuscular dysfunction of bladder

AMA: **52277** 2018,Jan,8; 2017,Jan,8; 2016,Jan,13; 2015,Jan,16; 2014,Jan,11

Relative Value Units/Medicare Edits

Non-Facility RVU	Work	PE	MP	Total
52277	6.16	2.46	0.68	9.3
Facility RVU	Work	PE	MP	Total
52277	6.16	2.46	0.68	9.3

	FUD	Status	MUE	Modifiers				IOM Reference
52277	0	A	1(2)	51	N/A	N/A	80*	None

* with documentation

52281-52282

52281   Cystourethroscopy, with calibration and/or dilation of urethral
stricture or stenosis, with or without meatotomy, with or without
injection procedure for cystography, male or female
52282   Cystourethroscopy, with insertion of permanent urethral stent

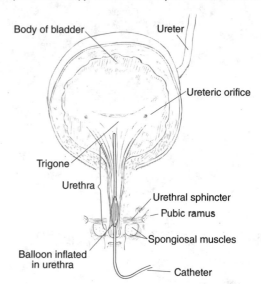

A balloon catheter is introduced into the bladder
and a stricture or stenosis of the urethra is expanded

Explanation

The physician examines the urinary collecting system with a cystourethroscope
passed through the urethra and bladder. The physician inserts progressively
larger urethral sounds, French Bougies, or filiforms and followers to dilate or
calibrate a urethral stricture or stenosis. Alternatively, a balloon dilator may
be used. The physician may pass a cutting instrument through the
cystourethroscope to make an incision (meatotomy) in the opening of the
urethra or inject radiocontrast for radiologic study of the bladder. In 52282,
using an instrument passed through the cystourethroscope, the physician
inserts a permanent stent to dilate the urethral stricture or stenosis. The
physician removes any instrument(s) and the cystourethroscope.

Coding Tips

The endoscopic descriptions in this CPT category are listed so the main
procedure can be identified without listing the minor related functions
performed at the same time. For placement of a temporary prostatic urethral
stent, see 53855. Report cystourethroscopy with urethral therapeutic drug
delivery with 0499T. Supplies used when providing this procedure may be
reported with the appropriate HCPCS Level II code. Check with the specific
payer to determine coverage.

ICD-10-CM Diagnostic Codes

N35.010	Post-traumatic urethral stricture, male, meatal ♂
N35.011	Post-traumatic bulbous urethral stricture ♂
N35.012	Post-traumatic membranous urethral stricture ♂
N35.013	Post-traumatic anterior urethral stricture ♂
N35.021	Urethral stricture due to childbirth ♀
N35.028	Other post-traumatic urethral stricture, female ♀
N35.111	Postinfective urethral stricture, not elsewhere classified, male, meatal ♂
N35.112	Postinfective bulbous urethral stricture, not elsewhere classified, male ♂

© 2020 Optum360, LLC   **N** Newborn: 0   **P** Pediatric: 0-17   **M** Maternity: 9-64   **A** Adult: 15-124   ♂ Male Only   ♀ Female Only   CPT © 2020 American Medical Association. All Rights Reserved.

Bladder

N35.113	Postinfective membranous urethral stricture, not elsewhere classified, male ♂
N35.114	Postinfective anterior urethral stricture, not elsewhere classified, male ♂
N35.12	Postinfective urethral stricture, not elsewhere classified, female ♀
N35.811	Other urethral stricture, male, meatal ♂
N35.812	Other urethral bulbous stricture, male ♂
N35.813	Other membranous urethral stricture, male ♂
N35.814	Other anterior urethral stricture, male ♂
N35.816	Other urethral stricture, male, overlapping sites ♂
N35.82	Other urethral stricture, female ♀
N40.0	Benign prostatic hyperplasia without lower urinary tract symptoms 🅰 ♂
N40.1	Benign prostatic hyperplasia with lower urinary tract symptoms 🅰 ♂
N40.2	Nodular prostate without lower urinary tract symptoms 🅰 ♂
N40.3	Nodular prostate with lower urinary tract symptoms 🅰 ♂
N99.110	Postprocedural urethral stricture, male, meatal ♂
N99.111	Postprocedural bulbous urethral stricture, male ♂
N99.112	Postprocedural membranous urethral stricture, male ♂
N99.113	Postprocedural anterior bulbous urethral stricture, male ♂
N99.115	Postprocedural fossa navicularis urethral stricture ♂
N99.12	Postprocedural urethral stricture, female ♀
Q64.32	Congenital stricture of urethra
Q64.33	Congenital stricture of urinary meatus
Q64.39	Other atresia and stenosis of urethra and bladder neck

AMA: 52281 2018,Jan,8; 2017,Oct,9; 2017,Jan,8; 2016,Jan,13; 2015,Jan,16; 2014,Jan,11 **52282** 2018,Jan,8; 2017,Jan,8; 2016,Jan,13; 2015,Jun,5; 2015,Jan,16; 2014,Jan,11

Relative Value Units/Medicare Edits

Non-Facility RVU	Work	PE	MP	Total
52281	2.75	6.09	0.32	9.16
52282	6.39	2.56	0.79	9.74
Facility RVU	Work	PE	MP	Total
52281	2.75	1.3	0.32	4.37
52282	6.39	2.56	0.79	9.74

	FUD	Status	MUE	Modifiers				IOM Reference
52281	0	A	1(2)	51	N/A	N/A	N/A	None
52282	0	A	1(2)	51	N/A	N/A	N/A	

* with documentation

Terms To Know

bougie. Probe used to dilate or calibrate a body part.

dilation. Artificial increase in the diameter of an opening or lumen made by medication or by instrumentation.

filiform. Probe with woven-thread end.

stent. Tube to provide support in a body cavity or lumen.

52283

52283 Cystourethroscopy, with steroid injection into stricture

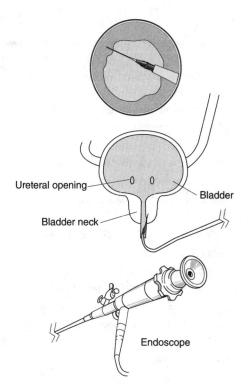

Physician injects urethra stricture with steroid

Explanation

The physician treats a stricture with steroids. The physician examines the urinary collecting system with a cystourethroscope passed through the urethra and bladder, injecting material into a stricture. The physician passes an instrument through the cystourethroscope to inject the steroid into the urethral stricture. The physician removes the instrument and cystourethroscope.

Coding Tips

When 52283 is performed with another separately identifiable procedure, the highest dollar value code is listed as the primary procedure and subsequent procedures are appended with modifier 51. The physician usually performs this procedure with local anesthesia. However, general anesthesia may be administered depending on the age or condition of the patient. Report 52281 for dilation of a urethral stricture with or without an incision in the urethral opening. Use 52270–52275 if the physician makes an internal incision to correct a urethral stricture. See 53600–53665 for other dilation procedures for the urethra. Supplies used when providing this procedure may be reported with the appropriate HCPCS Level II code. Check with the specific payer to determine coverage.

ICD-10-CM Diagnostic Codes

N35.010	Post-traumatic urethral stricture, male, meatal ♂
N35.011	Post-traumatic bulbous urethral stricture ♂
N35.012	Post-traumatic membranous urethral stricture ♂
N35.013	Post-traumatic anterior urethral stricture ♂
N35.021	Urethral stricture due to childbirth ♀
N35.028	Other post-traumatic urethral stricture, female ♀

Bladder

N35.111	Postinfective urethral stricture, not elsewhere classified, male, meatal ♂
N35.112	Postinfective bulbous urethral stricture, not elsewhere classified, male ♂
N35.113	Postinfective membranous urethral stricture, not elsewhere classified, male ♂
N35.114	Postinfective anterior urethral stricture, not elsewhere classified, male ♂
N35.116	Postinfective urethral stricture, not elsewhere classified, male, overlapping sites ♂
N35.12	Postinfective urethral stricture, not elsewhere classified, female ♀
N35.811	Other urethral stricture, male, meatal ♂
N35.812	Other urethral bulbous stricture, male ♂
N35.813	Other membranous urethral stricture, male ♂
N35.814	Other anterior urethral stricture, male ♂
N35.816	Other urethral stricture, male, overlapping sites ♂
N35.82	Other urethral stricture, female ♀
N37	Urethral disorders in diseases classified elsewhere
N99.110	Postprocedural urethral stricture, male, meatal ♂
N99.111	Postprocedural bulbous urethral stricture, male ♂
N99.112	Postprocedural membranous urethral stricture, male ♂
N99.113	Postprocedural anterior bulbous urethral stricture, male ♂
N99.115	Postprocedural fossa navicularis urethral stricture ♂
N99.116	Postprocedural urethral stricture, male, overlapping sites ♂
N99.12	Postprocedural urethral stricture, female ♀
Q64.32	Congenital stricture of urethra
Q64.33	Congenital stricture of urinary meatus
Q64.39	Other atresia and stenosis of urethra and bladder neck

AMA: 52283 2019,Feb,10; 2018,Jan,8; 2017,Jan,8; 2016,Jan,13; 2015,Mar,9; 2015,Jan,16; 2014,Jan,11

Relative Value Units/Medicare Edits

Non-Facility RVU	Work	PE	MP	Total
52283	3.73	5.14	0.44	9.31
Facility RVU	**Work**	**PE**	**MP**	**Total**
52283	3.73	1.64	0.44	5.81

	FUD	Status	MUE	Modifiers				IOM Reference
52283	0	A	1(2)	51	N/A	N/A	N/A	None

* with documentation

Terms To Know

steroids. Hormonal substances with a similar basic chemical structure, produced mainly in the adrenal cortex and gonads.

stricture. Narrowing of an anatomical structure.

52285

52285 Cystourethroscopy for treatment of the female urethral syndrome with any or all of the following: urethral meatotomy, urethral dilation, internal urethrotomy, lysis of urethrovaginal septal fibrosis, lateral incisions of the bladder neck, and fulguration of polyp(s) of urethra, bladder neck, and/or trigone

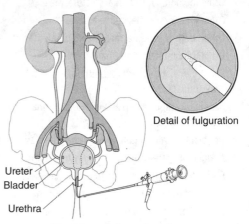

Detail of fulguration

Ureter
Bladder
Urethra

Physician repairs any number of problems with the urethra

Explanation

The physician passes a cystourethroscope through the urethra and bladder to treat female urethral syndrome. The physician may pass instruments through the cystourethroscope to incise the opening of the urethra (urethral meatotomy), dilate the urethra, incise the inside the urethra, treat septal fibrosis of the urethra and vagina, incise the bladder neck, or destroy polyps of the urethra in the bladder neck or trigone with electric current (fulguration). The physician removes the instruments and cystourethroscope.

Coding Tips

The endoscopic descriptions in this CPT category are listed so the main procedure can be identified without listing the minor related functions performed at the same time. If significant additional time and effort is documented, append modifier 22 and submit a cover letter and operative report.

ICD-10-CM Diagnostic Codes

N32.0	Bladder-neck obstruction
N34.0	Urethral abscess
N34.1	Nonspecific urethritis
N34.2	Other urethritis
N36.2	Urethral caruncle
N36.8	Other specified disorders of urethra
N37	Urethral disorders in diseases classified elsewhere

AMA: 52285 2018,Jan,8; 2017,Jan,8; 2016,Jan,13; 2015,Jan,16; 2014,Jan,11

© 2020 Optum360, LLC   **N Newborn:** 0   **P Pediatric:** 0-17   **M Maternity:** 9-64   **A Adult:** 15-124   ♂ **Male Only**   ♀ **Female Only**   CPT © 2020 American Medical Association. All Rights Reserved.

Bladder

Relative Value Units/Medicare Edits

Non-Facility RVU	Work	PE	MP	Total
52285	3.6	5.23	0.44	9.27
Facility RVU	**Work**	**PE**	**MP**	**Total**
52285	3.6	1.6	0.44	5.64

	FUD	Status	MUE	Modifiers				IOM Reference
52285	0	A	1(2)	51	N/A	N/A	N/A	None

* with documentation

Terms To Know

chronic interstitial cystitis. Persistently inflamed lesion of the bladder wall, usually accompanied by urinary frequency, pain, nocturia, and a distended bladder.

dilation. Artificial increase in the diameter of an opening or lumen made by medication or by instrumentation.

fibrosis. Formation of fibrous tissue as part of the restorative process.

fulguration. Destruction of living tissue by using sparks from a high-frequency electric current.

incise. To cut open or into.

lysis. Destruction, breakdown, dissolution, or decomposition of cells or substances by a specific catalyzing agent.

polyp. Small growth on a stalk-like attachment projecting from a mucous membrane.

trigone. Triangular, smooth area of mucous membrane at the base of the bladder, located between the ureteric openings in back and the urethral opening in front.

urethra. Small tube lined with mucous membrane that leads from the bladder to the exterior of the body.

urethral caruncle. Small, polyp-like growth of a deep red color found in women on the mucous membrane of the urethral opening.

52287

52287 Cystourethroscopy, with injection(s) for chemodenervation of the bladder

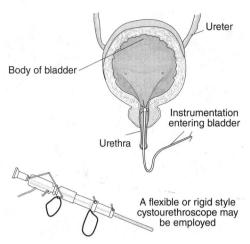

A flexible or rigid style cystourethroscope may be employed

Injections are made into the bladder for chemodenervation

Explanation

Botulinum toxin A (BTX-A) injections are used to treat an overactive bladder (OAB). The physician examines the urinary collecting system with a cystourethroscope passed through the urethra and bladder. Injections are made into multiple sites of the bladder wall. All instruments and the cystourethroscope are removed.

Coding Tips

For cystourethroscopy with steroid injection into a stricture, see 52283. Report the supply of the chemodenervation agent separately with the appropriate HCPCS Level II code.

ICD-10-CM Diagnostic Codes

N31.1	Reflex neuropathic bladder, not elsewhere classified
N31.8	Other neuromuscular dysfunction of bladder
N32.81	Overactive bladder
N39.41	Urge incontinence
N39.46	Mixed incontinence

AMA: 52287 2019,Apr,9; 2014,Jan,11

Relative Value Units/Medicare Edits

Non-Facility RVU	Work	PE	MP	Total
52287	3.2	6.68	0.39	10.27
Facility RVU	**Work**	**PE**	**MP**	**Total**
52287	3.2	1.3	0.39	4.89

	FUD	Status	MUE	Modifiers				IOM Reference
52287	0	A	1(2)	51	N/A	N/A	N/A	None

* with documentation

Terms To Know

overactive bladder. Sudden involuntary contractions of the muscular wall of the bladder that results in a sudden, strong urge to urinate.

52290

52290 Cystourethroscopy; with ureteral meatotomy, unilateral or bilateral

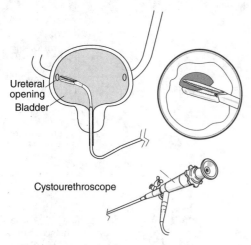

Ureteral opening
Bladder

Cystourethroscope

Physician may incise the openings of the ureters

Explanation

The physician examines the urinary collecting system with a cystourethroscope passed through the urethra and bladder, and makes an incision in the opening of the ureter(s) into the bladder (ureteral meatotomy). The physician passes the cystourethroscope through the urethra into the bladder, and inserts a cutting instrument through the cystourethroscope to incise the opening of one or both ureters into the bladder. The physician removes the instrument and cystourethroscope.

Coding Tips

When 52290 is performed with another separately identifiable procedure, the highest dollar value code is listed as the primary procedure and subsequent procedures are appended with modifier 51. For cystourethroscopic procedures with urethral meatotomy, see 52281 and 52285. For excision or fulguration of a saccular dilation of the ureteral end (ureterocele) through the cystourethroscope, see 52300–52301. For cystourethroscopy with incision or resection of a bladder diverticulum orifice, see 52305.

ICD-10-CM Diagnostic Codes

N11.1	Chronic obstructive pyelonephritis
N13.0	Hydronephrosis with ureteropelvic junction obstruction
N13.1	Hydronephrosis with ureteral stricture, not elsewhere classified
N13.2	Hydronephrosis with renal and ureteral calculous obstruction
N13.5	Crossing vessel and stricture of ureter without hydronephrosis
Q62.11	Congenital occlusion of ureteropelvic junction
Q62.12	Congenital occlusion of ureterovesical orifice
Q62.31	Congenital ureterocele, orthotopic
Q62.32	Cecoureterocele
Q62.39	Other obstructive defects of renal pelvis and ureter

AMA: 52290 2018,Jan,8; 2017,Jan,8; 2016,Jan,13; 2015,Jan,16; 2014,Jan,11

Relative Value Units/Medicare Edits

Non-Facility RVU	Work	PE	MP	Total
52290	4.58	1.92	0.53	7.03
Facility RVU	**Work**	**PE**	**MP**	**Total**
52290	4.58	1.92	0.53	7.03

	FUD	Status	MUE	Modifiers				IOM Reference
52290	0	A	1(2)	51	N/A	N/A	N/A	100-04,12,40.7

* with documentation

Terms To Know

calculus. Abnormal, stone-like concretion of calcium, cholesterol, mineral salts, or other substances that forms in any part of the body.

chronic. Persistent, continuing, or recurring.

congenital. Present at birth, occurring through heredity or an influence during gestation up to the moment of birth.

defect. Imperfection, flaw, or absence.

hydronephrosis. Distension of the kidney caused by an accumulation of urine that cannot flow out due to an obstruction that may be caused by conditions such as kidney stones or vesicoureteral reflux.

obstruction. Blockage that prevents normal function of the valve or structure.

occlusion. Constriction, closure, or blockage of a passage.

pyelonephritis. Infection of the renal pelvis and ureters that may be acute or chronic, often occurring as a result of a urinary tract infection, particularly in instances of vesicoureteric reflux, the backflow of urine from the bladder into the kidney pelvis or ureters.

stricture. Narrowing of an anatomical structure.

ureterocele. Saccular formation of the lower part of the ureter, protruding into the bladder.

52300-52305

52300 Cystourethroscopy; with resection or fulguration of orthotopic ureterocele(s), unilateral or bilateral

52301 with resection or fulguration of ectopic ureterocele(s), unilateral or bilateral

52305 with incision or resection of orifice of bladder diverticulum, single or multiple

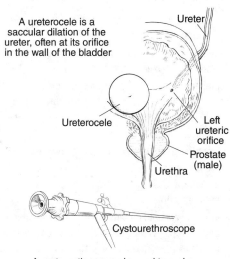

A ureterocele is a saccular dilation of the ureter, often at its orifice in the wall of the bladder

Ureter

Ureterocele

Left ureteric orifice

Prostate (male)

Urethra

Cystourethroscope

A cystourethroscope is used to make incisions within the ureters

Explanation

The physician passes the cystourethroscope through the urethra into the bladder and examines the urinary collecting system. An instrument is inserted through the cystourethroscope allowing the physician to excise the ureterocele or destroy the ureterocele with electric current (fulguration). In 52300, the physician corrects an orthotopic (normally positioned) intravesical ureterocele. A ureterocele is a saccular dilation generally associated with single ureters. The physician usually performs this procedure with local anesthesia. When an open procedure is necessary, the surgical site is chosen based on the anatomical location of the ureteral meatus, the position of the ureterocele, and the impairment of renal function. In 52301, the physician corrects an ectopic (abnormally positioned) ureterocele. An ectopic ureterocele is a saccular dilation generally located, in part, at the bladder neck or in the urethra. This type of ureterocele most often involves the upper pole of duplicated ureters. An ectopic ureterocele is four times more common than an intravesical, or orthotopic, ureterocele (52300), and, in females, the ectopic ureterocele may prolapse through the urethra. In 52305, the physician corrects a diverticulum in the bladder. The physician examines the urinary collecting system with a cystourethroscope passed through the urethra and bladder, and removes a saccular opening of the bladder (diverticulum) by excision or fulguration. The physician removes the instrument and cystourethroscope.

Coding Tips

When 52300, 52301, or 52305 is performed with another separately identifiable procedure, the highest dollar value code is listed as the primary procedure and subsequent procedures are appended with modifier 51. Note that 52300 and 52301 are unilateral or bilateral procedures and as such are reported once even if the procedure is performed on both sides. Report 51535 for excision, incision, or repair of a ureterocele through a bladder incision. Report 51525 for excision of a bladder diverticulum through an incision in the bladder.

ICD-10-CM Diagnostic Codes

N28.82   Megaloureter

N28.89   Other specified disorders of kidney and ureter

N32.3   Diverticulum of bladder

Q62.31   Congenital ureterocele, orthotopic

Q62.32   Cecoureterocele

AMA: 52300 2018,Jan,8; 2017,Jan,8; 2016,Jan,13; 2015,Jan,16; 2014,Jan,11 **52301** 2018,Jan,8; 2017,Jan,8; 2016,Jan,13; 2015,Jan,16; 2014,Jan,11 **52305** 2018,Jan,8; 2017,Jan,8; 2016,Jan,13; 2015,Jan,16; 2014,Jan,11

Relative Value Units/Medicare Edits

Non-Facility RVU	Work	PE	MP	Total
52300	5.3	2.16	0.6	8.06
52301	5.5	2.23	0.62	8.35
52305	5.3	2.12	0.62	8.04
Facility RVU	Work	PE	MP	Total
52300	5.3	2.16	0.6	8.06
52301	5.5	2.23	0.62	8.35
52305	5.3	2.12	0.62	8.04

	FUD	Status	MUE	Modifiers				IOM Reference
52300	0	A	1(2)	51	N/A	N/A	80*	None
52301	0	A	1(2)	51	N/A	N/A	80*	
52305	0	A	1(2)	51	N/A	N/A	N/A	

* with documentation

Terms To Know

diverticulum. Pouch or sac in the walls of an organ or canal.

ectopic. *1)* Fertilized ovum that implants and develops outside the uterus. The ovum may implant itself in different sites, such as the fallopian tube, the ovary, the abdomen, or the cervix. *2)* Organ or other structure that is aberrant or out of place.

fulguration. Destruction of living tissue by using sparks from a high-frequency electric current.

impairment. Loss or abnormality of anatomical, physiological, mental, or psychological structure or function. Secondary impairment originates from other, preexisting impairments.

orthotopic. Natural, normal site or proper body position.

prolapse. Falling, sliding, or sinking of an organ from its normal location in the body.

ureterocele. Saccular formation of the lower part of the ureter, protruding into the bladder.

CPT © 2020 American Medical Association. All Rights Reserved.   ● New   ▲ Revised   + Add On   ★ Telemedicine   AMA: CPT Assist   [Resequenced]   ☑ Laterality   © 2020 Optum360, LLC

52310-52315

52310 Cystourethroscopy, with removal of foreign body, calculus, or ureteral stent from urethra or bladder (separate procedure); simple
52315 complicated

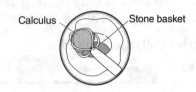

Calculus   Stone basket

The physician uses an endoscope to
remove a calculus, foreign body, or
ureteral stent from the urethra or bladder

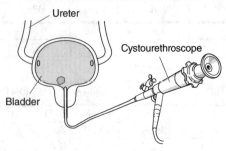

Ureter

Cystourethroscope

Bladder

Explanation

The physician examines the urinary collecting system with a cystourethroscope passed through the urethra and bladder, and removes a foreign body, calculus, or ureteral stent from the urethra or bladder. The physician passes the cystourethroscope through the urethra into the bladder, and inserts an instrument through the cystourethroscope to extract a foreign body, calculus, or ureteral stent from the urethra or bladder. The physician removes the instrument and cystourethroscope. Report 52315 if the procedure is complicated due to previous surgery or the size or condition of the foreign body, calculus, or ureteral stent.

Coding Tips

These separate procedures by definition are usually a component of a more complex service and are not identified separately. When performed alone or with other unrelated procedures/services they may be reported. If performed alone, list the code; if performed with other procedures/services, list the code and append modifier 59 or an X{EPSU} modifier. The physician usually performs these procedures with local anesthesia. However, general anesthesia may be administered depending on the age or condition of the patient. Use 52352–52353 for removal, manipulation, or lithotripsy of a calculus through a cystourethroscope with ureteroscopy and/or pyeloscopy. See 52320–52330 for removal, fragmentation, or manipulation of a ureteral calculus with a cystourethroscope. For removal of a bladder or ureteral calculus through an incision in the bladder, see 51050–51065. Supplies used when providing these procedures may be reported with the appropriate HCPCS Level II code. Check with the specific payer to determine coverage.

ICD-10-CM Diagnostic Codes

N21.0	Calculus in bladder
N21.1	Calculus in urethra
T19.0XXA	Foreign body in urethra, initial encounter
T19.1XXA	Foreign body in bladder, initial encounter
T83.112A	Breakdown (mechanical) of indwelling ureteral stent, initial encounter
T83.113A	Breakdown (mechanical) of other urinary stents, initial encounter
T83.122A	Displacement of indwelling ureteral stent, initial encounter
T83.123A	Displacement of other urinary stents, initial encounter
T83.192A	Other mechanical complication of indwelling ureteral stent, initial encounter
T83.193A	Other mechanical complication of other urinary stent, initial encounter
T83.510A	Infection and inflammatory reaction due to cystostomy catheter, initial encounter
T83.511A	Infection and inflammatory reaction due to indwelling urethral catheter, initial encounter
T83.518A	Infection and inflammatory reaction due to other urinary catheter, initial encounter
T83.590A	Infection and inflammatory reaction due to implanted urinary neurostimulation device, initial encounter
T83.591A	Infection and inflammatory reaction due to implanted urinary sphincter, initial encounter
T83.592A	Infection and inflammatory reaction due to indwelling ureteral stent, initial encounter
T83.593A	Infection and inflammatory reaction due to other urinary stents, initial encounter
T83.598A	Infection and inflammatory reaction due to other prosthetic device, implant and graft in urinary system, initial encounter
T83.81XA	Embolism due to genitourinary prosthetic devices, implants and grafts, initial encounter
T83.82XA	Fibrosis due to genitourinary prosthetic devices, implants and grafts, initial encounter
T83.83XA	Hemorrhage due to genitourinary prosthetic devices, implants and grafts, initial encounter
T83.84XA	Pain due to genitourinary prosthetic devices, implants and grafts, initial encounter
T83.85XA	Stenosis due to genitourinary prosthetic devices, implants and grafts, initial encounter
T83.86XA	Thrombosis due to genitourinary prosthetic devices, implants and grafts, initial encounter
T83.89XA	Other specified complication of genitourinary prosthetic devices, implants and grafts, initial encounter

AMA: 52310 2018,Jan,8; 2017,Jan,8; 2016,Jan,13; 2015,Jun,5; 2015,Jan,16; 2014,Jan,11 **52315** 2018,Jan,8; 2017,Jan,8; 2016,Jan,13; 2015,Jan,16; 2014,Jan,11

Relative Value Units/Medicare Edits

Non-Facility RVU	Work	PE	MP	Total
52310	2.81	5.13	0.32	8.26
52315	5.2	7.48	0.6	13.28
Facility RVU	**Work**	**PE**	**MP**	**Total**
52310	2.81	1.22	0.32	4.35
52315	5.2	2.11	0.6	7.91

	FUD	Status	MUE	Modifiers				IOM Reference
52310	0	A	1(3)	51	N/A	N/A	N/A	None
52315	0	A	2(3)	51	N/A	N/A	N/A	

* with documentation

© 2020 Optum360, LLC   **N Newborn: 0**   **P Pediatric: 0-17**   **M Maternity: 9-64**   **A Adult: 15-124**   ♂ Male Only   ♀ Female Only   CPT © 2020 American Medical Association. All Rights Reserved.

Bladder

52317-52318

52317 Litholapaxy: crushing or fragmentation of calculus by any means in bladder and removal of fragments; simple or small (less than 2.5 cm)

52318 complicated or large (over 2.5 cm)

The physician uses an endoscope
to remove, fragment, or manipulate a
calculus from the urinary collecting system

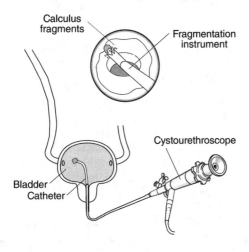

Explanation

The physician uses ultrasound to smash a calculus. The physician examines the urinary collecting system with a cystourethroscope passed through the urethra and bladder to remove a foreign body. The physician inserts an instrument that generates shock waves through the cystourethroscope. The physician crushes the calculus in the bladder (litholapaxy) and washes out the fragments through a catheter. Post-shockwave fragments too large to be easily suctioned may require manual crushing. For a calculus smaller than 2.5 cm, report 52317. For a calculus larger than 2.5 cm, report 52318.

Coding Tips

When 52317 or 52318 is performed with another separately identifiable procedure, the highest dollar value code is listed as the primary procedure and subsequent procedures are appended with modifier 51. Report 52310–52315 for removal of a foreign body, calculus, or ureteral stent from the urethra or bladder. Use 52352–52353 for removal, manipulation, or lithotripsy of a calculus through a cystourethroscope with ureteroscopy and/or pyeloscopy. Report radiological guidance separately.

ICD-10-CM Diagnostic Codes

N21.0   Calculus in bladder

AMA: 52317 2018,Jan,8; 2017,Jan,8; 2016,Jan,13; 2015,Jan,16; 2014,Jan,11
52318 2018,Jan,8; 2017,Jan,8; 2016,Jan,13; 2015,Jan,16; 2014,Jan,11

Relative Value Units/Medicare Edits

Non-Facility RVU	Work	PE	MP	Total
52317	6.71	17.48	0.78	24.97
52318	9.18	3.43	1.05	13.66
Facility RVU	**Work**	**PE**	**MP**	**Total**
52317	6.71	2.55	0.78	10.04
52318	9.18	3.43	1.05	13.66

	FUD	Status	MUE	Modifiers				IOM Reference
52317	0	A	1(3)	51	N/A	N/A	N/A	None
52318	0	A	1(3)	51	N/A	N/A	N/A	

* with documentation

Terms To Know

calculus. Abnormal, stone-like concretion of calcium, cholesterol, mineral salts, or other substances that forms in any part of the body.

catheter. Flexible tube inserted into an area of the body for introducing or withdrawing fluid.

diverticulum. Pouch or sac in the walls of an organ or canal.

foreign body. Any object or substance found in an organ and tissue that does not belong under normal circumstances.

fragment. Small piece broken off a larger whole; to divide into pieces.

52320-52330

52320 Cystourethroscopy (including ureteral catheterization); with removal of ureteral calculus
52325 with fragmentation of ureteral calculus (eg, ultrasonic or electro-hydraulic technique)
52327 with subureteric injection of implant material
52330 with manipulation, without removal of ureteral calculus

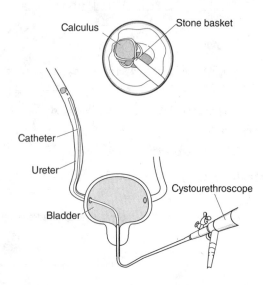

The physician uses an endoscope to remove, fragment, or manipulate a calculus from the urinary and renal collecting system

Explanation

The physician examines the urinary collecting system with a cystourethroscope passed through the urethra and bladder, and removes, fragments, or manipulates a calculus in the ureter. The physician passes the cystourethroscope through the urethra into the bladder, and inserts an instrument through the cystourethroscope to extract, fragment, or manipulate a calculus in the ureter. The physician inserts a ureteral catheter and removes the cystourethroscope. Report 52320 if the physician uses a stone basket or other instrument to remove the calculus. Report 52325 if the physician uses ultrasound or electrohydraulics to fragment the calculus. Report 52327 if the physician uses a subureteric injection of implant material. Report 52330 if the physician uses an instrument to manipulate, not remove, the calculus.

Coding Tips

Insertion and removal of a temporary ureteral catheter (52005) is included in these procedures and should not be reported separately. For removal, manipulation, or lithotripsy of a calculus through a cystourethroscope with ureteroscopy and/or pyeloscopy, see 52352–52353. For other calculus removal and/or manipulation procedures performed through a renal or ureteral endoscope, see 50561, 50580, 50961, and 50980. For other ureteral calculus removal procedures, see 50610–50630 and 51060–51065. For insertion of a self-retaining, indwelling stent performed during cystourethroscopic procedures, report 52332 in addition to the primary procedure performed (52320-52330, 52334-52352, 52354, 52355) and append modifier 51. Do not report these codes with 52000.

ICD-10-CM Diagnostic Codes

N11.1   Chronic obstructive pyelonephritis
N13.0   Hydronephrosis with ureteropelvic junction obstruction
N13.1   Hydronephrosis with ureteral stricture, not elsewhere classified
N13.2   Hydronephrosis with renal and ureteral calculous obstruction
N13.39   Other hydronephrosis
N13.4   Hydroureter
N13.5   Crossing vessel and stricture of ureter without hydronephrosis
N13.71   Vesicoureteral-reflux without reflux nephropathy
N13.8   Other obstructive and reflux uropathy
N20.1   Calculus of ureter
N20.2   Calculus of kidney with calculus of ureter
N28.82   Megaloureter
N28.89   Other specified disorders of kidney and ureter
R31.0   Gross hematuria
R31.1   Benign essential microscopic hematuria
R31.21   Asymptomatic microscopic hematuria
R31.29   Other microscopic hematuria

AMA: 52320 2018,Jan,8; 2017,Jan,8; 2016,Jan,13; 2015,Jan,16; 2014,Jan,11 **52325** 2018,Jan,8; 2017,Jan,8; 2016,Jan,13; 2015,Jan,16; 2014,Jan,11 **52327** 2018,Jan,8; 2017,Jan,8; 2016,Jan,13; 2015,Jan,16; 2014,Jan,11 **52330** 2018,Jan,8; 2017,Jan,8; 2016,Jan,13; 2015,Jan,16; 2014,May,3; 2014,Jan,11

Relative Value Units/Medicare Edits

Non-Facility RVU	Work	PE	MP	Total
52320	4.69	1.88	0.54	7.11
52325	6.15	2.39	0.68	9.22
52327	5.18	1.79	0.62	7.59
52330	5.03	10.98	0.57	16.58
Facility RVU	Work	PE	MP	Total
52320	4.69	1.88	0.54	7.11
52325	6.15	2.39	0.68	9.22
52327	5.18	1.79	0.62	7.59
52330	5.03	2.0	0.57	7.6

	FUD	Status	MUE	Modifiers				IOM Reference
52320	0	A	1(2)	51	50	N/A	N/A	100-03,230.10
52325	0	A	1(3)	51	50	N/A	N/A	
52327	0	A	1(2)	51	50	N/A	N/A	
52330	0	A	1(2)	51	50	N/A	N/A	

* with documentation

Terms To Know

calculus. Abnormal, stone-like concretion of calcium, cholesterol, mineral salts, or other substances that forms in any part of the body.

catheter. Flexible tube inserted into an area of the body for introducing or withdrawing fluid.

fragment. Small piece broken off a larger whole; to divide into pieces.

hematuria. Blood in urine, which may present as gross visible blood or as the presence of red blood cells visible only under a microscope.

hydroureter. Abnormal enlargement or distension of the ureter with water or urine caused by an obstruction.

ultrasound. Imaging using ultra-high sound frequency bounced off body structures.

© 2020 Optum360, LLC   **N** Newborn: 0   **P** Pediatric: 0-17   **M** Maternity: 9-64   **A** Adult: 15-124   ♂ Male Only   ♀ Female Only   CPT © 2020 American Medical Association. All Rights Reserved.

Coding Companion for Urology/Nephrology

Bladder

52332

52332 Cystourethroscopy, with insertion of indwelling ureteral stent (eg, Gibbons or double-J type)

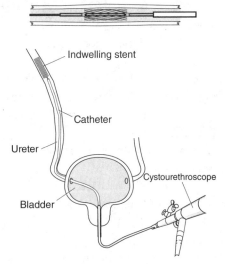

The physician uses a cystourethroscope to examine the urinary system and insert an indwelling ureteral stent

Indwelling stent

Catheter

Ureter

Cystourethroscope

Bladder

Explanation

The physician examines the urinary collecting system with a cystourethroscope passed through the urethra and bladder, and inserts an indwelling catheter (stent) in the ureter. The physician passes the cystourethroscope through the urethra into the bladder, and inserts an instrument through the cystourethroscope to insert an indwelling stent in the ureter. The stent provides support of the ureter. The physician removes the instrument and cystourethroscope.

Coding Tips

This is a unilateral procedure. If performed bilaterally, some payers require that the service be reported twice with modifier 50 appended to the second code while others require identification of the service only once with modifier 50 appended. Check with individual payers. Modifier 50 identifies a procedure performed identically on the opposite side of the body (mirror image). For insertion of a self-retaining, indwelling stent performed during cystourethroscopic procedures, report 52332 in addition to the primary procedure performed (52320-52330, 52334-52352, 52354, 52355) and append modifier 51.When 52332 is performed with another separately identifiable procedure, the highest dollar value code is listed as the primary procedure and subsequent procedures are appended with modifier 51. Do not report 52332 with 52000, 52353, or 52356 when performed together on the same side. For cystourethroscopic removal of an indwelling ureteral stent, see 52310–52315. Supplies used when providing this procedure may be reported with the appropriate HCPCS Level II code. Check with the specific payer to determine coverage.

ICD-10-CM Diagnostic Codes

C66.1	Malignant neoplasm of right ureter ☑
C66.2	Malignant neoplasm of left ureter ☑
D30.21	Benign neoplasm of right ureter ☑
D30.22	Benign neoplasm of left ureter ☑
D41.21	Neoplasm of uncertain behavior of right ureter ☑
D41.22	Neoplasm of uncertain behavior of left ureter ☑
N11.1	Chronic obstructive pyelonephritis
N13.0	Hydronephrosis with ureteropelvic junction obstruction
N13.1	Hydronephrosis with ureteral stricture, not elsewhere classified
N13.2	Hydronephrosis with renal and ureteral calculous obstruction
N13.39	Other hydronephrosis
N13.5	Crossing vessel and stricture of ureter without hydronephrosis
N13.8	Other obstructive and reflux uropathy
N20.1	Calculus of ureter
N20.2	Calculus of kidney with calculus of ureter
N28.82	Megaloureter
N28.89	Other specified disorders of kidney and ureter
Q62.11	Congenital occlusion of ureteropelvic junction
Q62.12	Congenital occlusion of ureterovesical orifice
Q62.2	Congenital megaureter
Q62.39	Other obstructive defects of renal pelvis and ureter
Q62.7	Congenital vesico-uretero-renal reflux
Q62.8	Other congenital malformations of ureter

AMA: 52332 2019,Dec,12; 2018,Jan,8; 2017,Jan,8; 2016,Jan,13; 2015,Jan,16; 2014,May,3; 2014,Jan,11

Relative Value Units/Medicare Edits

Non-Facility RVU	Work	PE	MP	Total
52332	2.82	9.81	0.32	12.95
Facility RVU	**Work**	**PE**	**MP**	**Total**
52332	2.82	1.32	0.32	4.46

	FUD	Status	MUE	Modifiers				IOM Reference
52332	0	A	1(2)	51	50	N/A	N/A	None

* with documentation

Terms To Know

fistula. Abnormal tube-like passage between two body cavities or organs or from an organ to the outside surface.

hematuria. Blood in urine, which may present as gross visible blood or as the presence of red blood cells visible only under a microscope.

stent. Tube to provide support in a body cavity or lumen.

stricture. Narrowing of an anatomical structure.

Bladder

52334

52334 Cystourethroscopy with insertion of ureteral guide wire through kidney to establish a percutaneous nephrostomy, retrograde

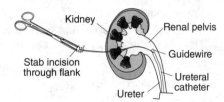

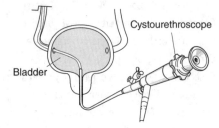

The physician passes a guidewire through a cystourethroscope, ureter, and kidney to establish a retrograde nephrostomy

Explanation

The physician examines the urinary collecting system, and creates an opening through the kidney to the exterior of the body (nephrostomy) by inserting a guidewire through a cystourethroscope. After examining the urinary collecting system through a cystourethroscope inserted through the urethra into the bladder, the physician inserts a catheter through the cystourethroscope into the ureter. The physician passes a guidewire through the ureteral catheter into the kidney and through a small incision in the skin of the flank. The physician removes the cystourethroscope and enlarges (dilates) the percutaneous opening by passing tubes with increasingly larger diameters through the skin incision over the guidewire to the kidney. The physician passes a nephrostomy tube over the guide, removes the guide, and sutures the tube to the skin. The physician usually withdraws the ureteral catheter at the end of the procedure.

Coding Tips

For cystourethroscopy with ureteroscopy and/or pyeloscopy, see 52351–52356. For percutaneous nephrostolithotomy, see 50080–50081; for establishment of a percutaneous nephrostomy, see 50432-50433. For dilation of an existing tract for an endourologic procedure, percutaneous, see 50436; including new access into the renal collecting system, see 50437. For creation of an open nephrostomy, see 50040. For nephrostomy or pyelostomy tube change, see 50435. For cystourethroscopy with incision, fulguration, or resection of congenital posterior urethral valves or obstructive hypertrophic mucosal folds, see 52400. Do not report 52334 with 50437, 52000, or 52351. For insertion of a self-retaining, indwelling stent performed during cystourethroscopic procedures, report 52332 in addition to the primary procedure performed (52320-52330, 52334-52352, 52354, 52355) and append modifier 51.

ICD-10-CM Diagnostic Codes

C64.1	Malignant neoplasm of right kidney, except renal pelvis ☑
C64.2	Malignant neoplasm of left kidney, except renal pelvis ☑
C65.1	Malignant neoplasm of right renal pelvis ☑
C65.2	Malignant neoplasm of left renal pelvis ☑
C66.1	Malignant neoplasm of right ureter ☑
C66.2	Malignant neoplasm of left ureter ☑
C67.0	Malignant neoplasm of trigone of bladder
C67.1	Malignant neoplasm of dome of bladder
C67.2	Malignant neoplasm of lateral wall of bladder
C67.3	Malignant neoplasm of anterior wall of bladder
C67.4	Malignant neoplasm of posterior wall of bladder
C67.5	Malignant neoplasm of bladder neck
C67.6	Malignant neoplasm of ureteric orifice
C67.8	Malignant neoplasm of overlapping sites of bladder
C7A.093	Malignant carcinoid tumor of the kidney
D41.4	Neoplasm of uncertain behavior of bladder
N11.1	Chronic obstructive pyelonephritis
N13.0	Hydronephrosis with ureteropelvic junction obstruction
N13.1	Hydronephrosis with ureteral stricture, not elsewhere classified
N13.2	Hydronephrosis with renal and ureteral calculous obstruction
N13.39	Other hydronephrosis
N13.5	Crossing vessel and stricture of ureter without hydronephrosis
N13.6	Pyonephrosis
N13.8	Other obstructive and reflux uropathy
N15.1	Renal and perinephric abscess
N20.0	Calculus of kidney
N20.1	Calculus of ureter
N20.2	Calculus of kidney with calculus of ureter
N28.82	Megaloureter
N28.84	Pyelitis cystica
N28.85	Pyeloureteritis cystica
N28.86	Ureteritis cystica
N28.89	Other specified disorders of kidney and ureter
N32.89	Other specified disorders of bladder
Q62.0	Congenital hydronephrosis
Q62.11	Congenital occlusion of ureteropelvic junction
Q62.12	Congenital occlusion of ureterovesical orifice
Q62.2	Congenital megaureter
Q62.39	Other obstructive defects of renal pelvis and ureter

AMA: **52334** 2018,Jan,8; 2017,Jan,8; 2016,Jan,13; 2015,Jan,16; 2014,May,3; 2014,Jan,11

Relative Value Units/Medicare Edits

Non-Facility RVU	Work	PE	MP	Total
52334	3.37	1.51	0.39	5.27
Facility RVU	**Work**	**PE**	**MP**	**Total**
52334	3.37	1.51	0.39	5.27

	FUD	Status	MUE	Modifiers				IOM Reference
52334	0	A	1(2)	51	N/A	N/A	N/A	None

* with documentation

Terms To Know

catheter. Flexible tube inserted into an area of the body for introducing or withdrawing fluid.

guidewire. Flexible metal instrument designed to lead another instrument in its proper course.

52341-52343

52341 Cystourethroscopy; with treatment of ureteral stricture (eg, balloon dilation, laser, electrocautery, and incision)
52342 with treatment of ureteropelvic junction stricture (eg, balloon dilation, laser, electrocautery, and incision)
52343 with treatment of intra-renal stricture (eg, balloon dilation, laser, electrocautery, and incision)

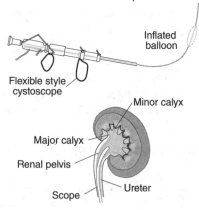

The instrument is inserted deep into the ureter

Inflated balloon

Flexible style cystoscope

Minor calyx

Major calyx

Renal pelvis

Scope

Ureter

Cystourethroscopy is performed with any of several treatments for a ureteral stricture

Explanation

The physician treats a ureteral stricture by balloon dilation, laser, electrocautery, or incision through a cystourethroscope. Under direct vision, the physician passes a flexible or rigid cystourethroscope through the urethra into the bladder. A balloon catheter is placed into the ureteral stricture, and the balloon is gently inflated. After approximately five minutes, the balloon is deflated and removed. In laser treatment of a ureteral stricture, probes, in combination with laser fibers, are used to apply laser energy to the stricture. In electrocautery, heat is applied to eliminate the stricture. The ureteral stricture may be incised alone or in combination with balloon dilation, laser, or electrocautery to open the blocked ureter. Report 52341 when a ureteral stricture is treated, 52342 when a ureteropelvic junction stricture is treated, or 52343 when an intra-renal stricture is treated.

Coding Tips

Insertion and removal of a temporary stent is included in these procedures. For insertion of a self-retaining, indwelling stent performed during cystourethroscopic procedures, report 52332 in addition to the primary procedure performed (52320-52330, 52334-52352, 52354, 52355) and append modifier 51. If significant additional time and effort is documented, append modifier 22 and submit a cover letter and operative report. For cystourethroscopy with ureteroscopy for treatment of a ureteral stricture, see 52344. For cystourethroscopy with ureteroscopy for treatment of a ureteropelvic junction stricture, see 52345. For cystourethroscopy with ureteroscopy for treatment of an intrarenal stricture, see 52346. Do not report these codes with 52000 or 52351.

ICD-10-CM Diagnostic Codes

A18.11	Tuberculosis of kidney and ureter
N11.1	Chronic obstructive pyelonephritis
N13.0	Hydronephrosis with ureteropelvic junction obstruction
N13.1	Hydronephrosis with ureteral stricture, not elsewhere classified
N13.5	Crossing vessel and stricture of ureter without hydronephrosis
N13.6	Pyonephrosis
N28.89	Other specified disorders of kidney and ureter
Q62.11	Congenital occlusion of ureteropelvic junction
Q62.12	Congenital occlusion of ureterovesical orifice

AMA: 52341 2018,Jan,8; 2017,Jan,8; 2016,Jan,3; 2016,Jan,13; 2015,Jan,16; 2014,Jan,11 **52342** 2018,Jan,8; 2017,Jan,8; 2016,Jan,13; 2015,Jan,16; 2014,Jan,11 **52343** 2018,Jan,8; 2017,Jan,8; 2016,Jan,13; 2015,Jan,16; 2014,May,3; 2014,Jan,11

Relative Value Units/Medicare Edits

Non-Facility RVU	Work	PE	MP	Total
52341	5.35	2.22	0.62	8.19
52342	5.85	2.39	0.65	8.89
52343	6.55	2.62	0.76	9.93
Facility RVU	**Work**	**PE**	**MP**	**Total**
52341	5.35	2.22	0.62	8.19
52342	5.85	2.39	0.65	8.89
52343	6.55	2.62	0.76	9.93

	FUD	Status	MUE	Modifiers				IOM Reference
52341	0	A	1(2)	51	50	N/A	N/A	None
52342	0	A	1(2)	51	50	N/A	N/A	
52343	0	A	1(2)	51	50	N/A	N/A	

* with documentation

Terms To Know

anomaly. Irregularity in the structure or position of an organ or tissue.

congenital. Present at birth, occurring through heredity or an influence during gestation up to the moment of birth.

dilation. Artificial increase in the diameter of an opening or lumen made by medication or by instrumentation.

electrocautery. Division or cutting of tissue using high-frequency electrical current to produce heat, which destroys cells.

hydronephrosis. Distension of the kidney caused by an accumulation of urine that cannot flow out due to an obstruction that may be caused by conditions such as kidney stones or vesicoureteral reflux.

hydroureter. Abnormal enlargement or distension of the ureter with water or urine caused by an obstruction.

incision. Act of cutting into tissue or an organ.

laser surgery. Use of concentrated, sharply defined light beams to cut, cauterize, coagulate, seal, or vaporize tissue.

Bladder

52344-52346

52344 Cystourethroscopy with ureteroscopy; with treatment of ureteral stricture (eg, balloon dilation, laser, electrocautery, and incision)

52345 with treatment of ureteropelvic junction stricture (eg, balloon dilation, laser, electrocautery, and incision)

52346 with treatment of intra-renal stricture (eg, balloon dilation, laser, electrocautery, and incision)

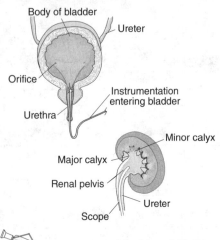

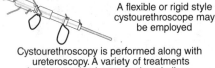

A flexible or rigid style cystourethroscope may be employed

Cystourethroscopy is performed along with ureteroscopy. A variety of treatments for a ureteral stricture, such as balloon dilation or laser treatment, are performed

Explanation

The physician treats a ureteral stricture by balloon dilation, laser, electrocautery, or incision through a cystourethroscope and ureteroscope. Under direct vision, the physician passes a flexible or rigid cystourethroscope through the urethra into the bladder and a ureteroscope into the ureter and examines the urinary collecting system. In balloon dilation, a balloon catheter is placed into the ureteral stricture, and the balloon is gently inflated. After approximately five minutes, the balloon is deflated and removed. In laser treatment of a ureteral stricture, probes, in combination with laser fibers, are used to apply laser energy to the stricture. In electrocautery, heat is applied to eliminate the stricture. Alternately, the ureteral stricture may be incised alone or in combination with balloon dilation, laser, or electrocautery to open the blocked ureter. Report 52344 when a ureteral stricture is treated, 52345 when a ureteropelvic junction stricture is treated, or 52346 when an intra-renal stricture is treated.

Coding Tips

Insertion and removal of a temporary stent is included in these procedures. For insertion of a self-retaining, indwelling stent performed during cystourethroscopic procedures, report 52332 in addition to the primary procedure performed (52320-52330, 52334-52352, 52354, 52355) and append modifier 51. If significant additional time and effort is documented, append modifier 22 and submit a cover letter and operative report. For cystourethroscopy without ureteroscopy for treatment of a ureteral stricture, see 52341. For cystourethroscopy without ureteroscopy for treatment of a ureteropelvic junction stricture, see 52342. For cystourethroscopy without ureteroscopy for treatment of an intrarenal stricture, see 52343. Report image-guided dilation of the ureter and/or ureteropelvic junction stricture,

without endoscopic guidance, with 50706. Do not report these codes with 52351.

ICD-10-CM Diagnostic Codes

A18.11	Tuberculosis of kidney and ureter
N11.1	Chronic obstructive pyelonephritis
N13.0	Hydronephrosis with ureteropelvic junction obstruction
N13.1	Hydronephrosis with ureteral stricture, not elsewhere classified
N13.5	Crossing vessel and stricture of ureter without hydronephrosis
N13.6	Pyonephrosis
N28.89	Other specified disorders of kidney and ureter
Q62.11	Congenital occlusion of ureteropelvic junction
Q62.12	Congenital occlusion of ureterovesical orifice

AMA: 52344 2018,Jan,8; 2017,Jan,8; 2016,Jan,3; 2016,Jan,13; 2015,Jan,16; 2014,Jan,11 **52345** 2018,Jan,8; 2017,Jan,8; 2016,Jan,13; 2016,Jan,3; 2015,Jan,16; 2014,Jan,11 **52346** 2018,Jan,8; 2017,Jan,8; 2016,Jan,13; 2015,Jan,16; 2014,May,3; 2014,Jan,11

Relative Value Units/Medicare Edits

Non-Facility RVU	Work	PE	MP	Total
52344	7.05	2.79	0.79	10.63
52345	7.55	2.96	0.86	11.37
52346	8.58	3.32	0.96	12.86
Facility RVU	**Work**	**PE**	**MP**	**Total**
52344	7.05	2.79	0.79	10.63
52345	7.55	2.96	0.86	11.37
52346	8.58	3.32	0.96	12.86

	FUD	Status	MUE	Modifiers				IOM Reference
52344	0	A	1(2)	51	50	N/A	N/A	100-03,230.3
52345	0	A	1(2)	51	50	N/A	80*	
52346	0	A	1(2)	51	50	N/A	80*	

* with documentation

Terms To Know

congenital. Present at birth, occurring through heredity or an influence during gestation up to the moment of birth.

dilation. Artificial increase in the diameter of an opening or lumen made by medication or by instrumentation.

electrocautery. Division or cutting of tissue using high-frequency electrical current to produce heat, which destroys cells.

hydronephrosis. Distension of the kidney caused by an accumulation of urine that cannot flow out due to an obstruction that may be caused by conditions such as kidney stones or vesicoureteral reflux.

hydroureter. Abnormal enlargement or distension of the ureter with water or urine caused by an obstruction.

laser surgery. Use of concentrated, sharply defined light beams to cut, cauterize, coagulate, seal, or vaporize tissue.

Bladder

52351

52351 Cystourethroscopy, with ureteroscopy and/or pyeloscopy; diagnostic

Instrumentation is inserted first into the urethra
and bladder and then deep into the ureter

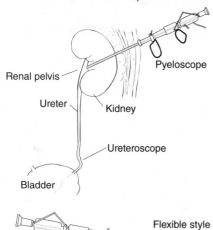

A cystourethroscopy with ureteroscopy and/or
pyeloscopy is performed for diagnostic purposes

Explanation

The physician examines the urinary collecting system for diagnostic purposes with endoscopes passed through the urethra into the bladder (cystourethroscope), ureter (ureteroscope), and renal pelvis (pyeloscope). After examination, the physician removes the endoscopes.

Coding Tips

Surgical cystourethroscopy always includes a diagnostic cystourethroscopy. To report imaging done in combination with this service, see 74485. Do not report 52351 with 52341–52346 or 52352–52356. For insertion of a self-retaining, indwelling stent performed during cystourethroscopic procedures, report 52332 in addition to the primary procedure performed (52320-52330, 52334-52352, 52354, 52355) and append modifier 51.

ICD-10-CM Diagnostic Codes

C65.1	Malignant neoplasm of right renal pelvis ☑
C65.2	Malignant neoplasm of left renal pelvis ☑
C66.1	Malignant neoplasm of right ureter ☑
C66.2	Malignant neoplasm of left ureter ☑
C67.0	Malignant neoplasm of trigone of bladder
C67.1	Malignant neoplasm of dome of bladder
C67.2	Malignant neoplasm of lateral wall of bladder
C67.3	Malignant neoplasm of anterior wall of bladder
C67.4	Malignant neoplasm of posterior wall of bladder
C67.5	Malignant neoplasm of bladder neck
C67.6	Malignant neoplasm of ureteric orifice
C67.7	Malignant neoplasm of urachus
C67.8	Malignant neoplasm of overlapping sites of bladder
C79.01	Secondary malignant neoplasm of right kidney and renal pelvis ☑
C79.02	Secondary malignant neoplasm of left kidney and renal pelvis ☑
C79.11	Secondary malignant neoplasm of bladder
C79.19	Secondary malignant neoplasm of other urinary organs
D09.0	Carcinoma in situ of bladder
D09.19	Carcinoma in situ of other urinary organs
D30.11	Benign neoplasm of right renal pelvis ☑
D30.12	Benign neoplasm of left renal pelvis ☑
D30.21	Benign neoplasm of right ureter ☑
D30.22	Benign neoplasm of left ureter ☑
D30.3	Benign neoplasm of bladder
D41.11	Neoplasm of uncertain behavior of right renal pelvis ☑
D41.12	Neoplasm of uncertain behavior of left renal pelvis ☑
D41.21	Neoplasm of uncertain behavior of right ureter ☑
D41.22	Neoplasm of uncertain behavior of left ureter ☑
D41.4	Neoplasm of uncertain behavior of bladder
D49.4	Neoplasm of unspecified behavior of bladder
N11.0	Nonobstructive reflux-associated chronic pyelonephritis
N11.1	Chronic obstructive pyelonephritis
N11.8	Other chronic tubulo-interstitial nephritis
N13.0	Hydronephrosis with ureteropelvic junction obstruction
N13.1	Hydronephrosis with ureteral stricture, not elsewhere classified
N13.2	Hydronephrosis with renal and ureteral calculous obstruction
N13.39	Other hydronephrosis
N13.4	Hydroureter
N13.5	Crossing vessel and stricture of ureter without hydronephrosis
N13.8	Other obstructive and reflux uropathy
N20.0	Calculus of kidney
N20.1	Calculus of ureter
N20.2	Calculus of kidney with calculus of ureter
N21.0	Calculus in bladder
N22	Calculus of urinary tract in diseases classified elsewhere
N28.82	Megaloureter
N28.89	Other specified disorders of kidney and ureter
N30.10	Interstitial cystitis (chronic) without hematuria
N30.11	Interstitial cystitis (chronic) with hematuria
N30.20	Other chronic cystitis without hematuria
N30.21	Other chronic cystitis with hematuria
N30.30	Trigonitis without hematuria
N30.31	Trigonitis with hematuria
N30.40	Irradiation cystitis without hematuria
N30.41	Irradiation cystitis with hematuria
N30.80	Other cystitis without hematuria
N30.81	Other cystitis with hematuria
N31.0	Uninhibited neuropathic bladder, not elsewhere classified
N31.1	Reflex neuropathic bladder, not elsewhere classified
N31.2	Flaccid neuropathic bladder, not elsewhere classified
N31.8	Other neuromuscular dysfunction of bladder
N32.0	Bladder-neck obstruction
N32.1	Vesicointestinal fistula
N32.2	Vesical fistula, not elsewhere classified
N32.3	Diverticulum of bladder
N32.81	Overactive bladder
N32.89	Other specified disorders of bladder
N33	Bladder disorders in diseases classified elsewhere

Bladder

N39.3	Stress incontinence (female) (male)	
N39.41	Urge incontinence	
N39.42	Incontinence without sensory awareness	
N39.43	Post-void dribbling	
N39.44	Nocturnal enuresis	
N39.45	Continuous leakage	
N39.46	Mixed incontinence	
N39.490	Overflow incontinence	
N39.491	Coital incontinence	
N39.492	Postural (urinary) incontinence	
N39.498	Other specified urinary incontinence	
N39.8	Other specified disorders of urinary system	
N82.0	Vesicovaginal fistula ♀	
N82.1	Other female urinary-genital tract fistulae ♀	
Q62.0	Congenital hydronephrosis	
Q62.11	Congenital occlusion of ureteropelvic junction	
Q62.12	Congenital occlusion of ureterovesical orifice	
Q62.2	Congenital megaureter	
Q62.31	Congenital ureterocele, orthotopic	
Q62.32	Cecoureterocele	
Q62.39	Other obstructive defects of renal pelvis and ureter	
Q64.11	Supravesical fissure of urinary bladder	
Q64.12	Cloacal exstrophy of urinary bladder	
Q64.19	Other exstrophy of urinary bladder	
Q64.31	Congenital bladder neck obstruction	
Q64.33	Congenital stricture of urinary meatus	
Q64.39	Other atresia and stenosis of urethra and bladder neck	
Q64.5	Congenital absence of bladder and urethra	
Q64.6	Congenital diverticulum of bladder	
Q64.72	Congenital prolapse of urinary meatus	
Q64.73	Congenital urethrorectal fistula	
Q64.79	Other congenital malformations of bladder and urethra	
R82.71	Bacteriuria	
R82.79	Other abnormal findings on microbiological examination of urine	
S37.19XA	Other injury of ureter, initial encounter	
S37.29XA	Other injury of bladder, initial encounter	
T19.1XXA	Foreign body in bladder, initial encounter	

AMA: **52351** 2018,Jan,8; 2017,Jan,8; 2016,Jan,13; 2015,Jan,16; 2014,May,3; 2014,Jan,11

Relative Value Units/Medicare Edits

Non-Facility RVU	Work	PE	MP	Total
52351	5.75	2.32	0.64	8.71
Facility RVU	Work	PE	MP	Total
52351	5.75	2.32	0.64	8.71

	FUD	Status	MUE	Modifiers				IOM Reference
52351	0	A	1(3)	51	N/A	N/A	N/A	None

* with documentation

Bladder

52352-52353

52352	Cystourethroscopy, with ureteroscopy and/or pyeloscopy; with removal or manipulation of calculus (ureteral catheterization is included)
52353	with lithotripsy (ureteral catheterization is included)

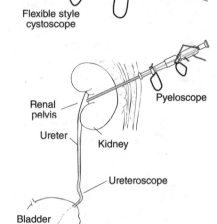

Instrumentation is inserted first into the urethra and bladder and then deep into the ureter

Flexible style cystoscope

Pyeloscope

Renal pelvis

Ureter

Kidney

Ureteroscope

Bladder

A cystourethroscopy with ureteroscopy and/or pyeloscopy is performed for diagnostic purposes along with removal or manipulation of a calculus or lithotripsy

Explanation

The physician examines the urinary collecting system with endoscopes passed through the urethra into the bladder (cystourethroscope), ureter (ureteroscope), and renal pelvis (pyeloscope), and removes or manipulates a stone (calculus). To extract or manipulate a calculus, the physician passes the appropriate surgical instruments through an endoscope to perform the procedure. A ureteral catheter is inserted and the endoscope and instruments are removed. Report 52352 if the physician passes a stone basket through an endoscope to extract or manipulate a calculus. Report 52353 if the physician uses an ultrasonic, electrohydraulic, or laser technique to fragment the calculus.

Coding Tips

Surgical cystourethroscopy always includes a diagnostic cystourethroscopy. Do not report 52351 with 52352-52353. Insertion and removal of a temporary stent is included in these procedures. For insertion of a self-retaining, indwelling stent performed during cystourethroscopic procedures, report 52332 in addition to the primary procedure performed (52320-52330, 52334-52352, 52354, 52355) and append modifier 51. Do not report 52353 with 52332 or 52356 when performed together on the same side.

ICD-10-CM Diagnostic Codes

N13.2	Hydronephrosis with renal and ureteral calculous obstruction
N20.0	Calculus of kidney
N20.1	Calculus of ureter
N20.2	Calculus of kidney with calculus of ureter
N21.0	Calculus in bladder
N21.1	Calculus in urethra
N21.8	Other lower urinary tract calculus

AMA: 52352 2018,Jan,8; 2017,Jan,8; 2016,Jan,13; 2015,Jan,16; 2014,Jan,11
52353 2019,Dec,12; 2018,Jan,8; 2017,Jan,8; 2016,Jan,13; 2015,Jan,16;
2014,May,3; 2014,Jan,11

Relative Value Units/Medicare Edits

Non-Facility RVU	Work	PE	MP	Total
52352	6.75	2.69	0.79	10.23
52353	7.5	2.95	0.86	11.31
Facility RVU	**Work**	**PE**	**MP**	**Total**
52352	6.75	2.69	0.79	10.23
52353	7.5	2.95	0.86	11.31

	FUD	Status	MUE	Modifiers				IOM Reference
52352	0	A	1(2)	51	50	N/A	N/A	100-03,230.1
52353	0	A	1(2)	51	50	N/A	N/A	

* with documentation

Terms To Know

calculus. Abnormal, stone-like concretion of calcium, cholesterol, mineral salts, or other substances that forms in any part of the body.

catheterization. Use or insertion of a tubular device into a duct, blood vessel, hollow organ, or body cavity for injecting or withdrawing fluids for diagnostic or therapeutic purposes.

hematuria. Blood in urine, which may present as gross visible blood or as the presence of red blood cells visible only under a microscope.

hydronephrosis. Distension of the kidney caused by an accumulation of urine that cannot flow out due to an obstruction that may be caused by conditions such as kidney stones or vesicoureteral reflux.

hydroureter. Abnormal enlargement or distension of the ureter with water or urine caused by an obstruction.

lithotripsy. Destruction of calcified substances in the gallbladder or urinary system by smashing the concretion into small particles to be washed out. This may be done by surgical or noninvasive methods, such as ultrasound.

manipulate. Treatment by hand.

[52356]

52356 Cystourethroscopy, with ureteroscopy and/or pyeloscopy; with lithotripsy including insertion of indwelling ureteral stent (eg, Gibbons or double-J type)

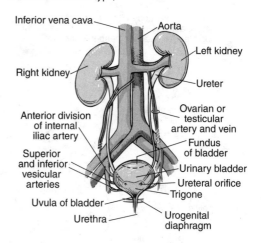

Explanation

The physician examines the urinary collecting system with endoscopes passed through the urethra into the bladder (cystourethroscope), ureter (ureteroscope), and renal pelvis (pyeloscope) and removes or manipulates a stone (calculus). To extract or manipulate a calculus, the physician passes the appropriate surgical instruments through an endoscope to fragment the calculus. An ultrasonic, electrohydraulic, or laser technique is used. A ureteral stent is inserted and the endoscope and instruments are removed.

Coding Tips

Surgical cystourethroscopy always includes a diagnostic cystourethroscopy. Do not report 52356 with 52332 or 52353 when performed together on the same side.

ICD-10-CM Diagnostic Codes

N13.2	Hydronephrosis with renal and ureteral calculous obstruction
N20.0	Calculus of kidney
N20.1	Calculus of ureter
N20.2	Calculus of kidney with calculus of ureter
N21.0	Calculus in bladder
N21.1	Calculus in urethra
N21.8	Other lower urinary tract calculus

AMA: 52356 2019,Dec,12; 2018,Jan,8; 2017,Jan,8; 2016,Jan,13; 2015,Jan,16; 2014,May,3; 2014,Jan,11

Relative Value Units/Medicare Edits

Non-Facility RVU	Work	PE	MP	Total
52356	8.0	3.08	0.9	11.98
Facility RVU	**Work**	**PE**	**MP**	**Total**
52356	8.0	3.08	0.9	11.98

	FUD	Status	MUE	Modifiers				IOM Reference
52356	0	A	1(2)	51	50	N/A	N/A	None

* with documentation

Bladder

52354-52355

52354 Cystourethroscopy, with ureteroscopy and/or pyeloscopy; with biopsy and/or fulguration of ureteral or renal pelvic lesion

52355 with resection of ureteral or renal pelvic tumor

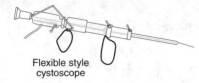

For cystourethroscopy with ureteroscopy and/or pyeloscopy, a scope is inserted first into the urethra and bladder and then deep into the ureter

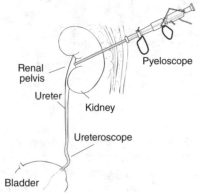

Flexible style cystoscope

Renal pelvis
Ureter
Kidney
Pyeloscope
Ureteroscope
Bladder

Explanation

The physician examines the urinary collecting system with endoscopes passed through the urethra into the bladder (cystourethroscope), ureter (ureteroscope), and renal pelvis (pyeloscope), and takes a biopsy and/or uses electric current (fulguration) to destroy a ureteral or renal pelvic lesion in 52354 and excises a ureteral or renal pelvic tumor in 52355. The physician passes instruments through the endoscope to take a biopsy of suspect tissue and/or destroys a lesion with electric current. To resect a tumor after examination, the physician inserts a cutting instrument through the endoscope and excises the tumor. After flushing the area with saline solution, the physician may insert a ureteral stent. The physician removes the cutting instrument and endoscopes.

Coding Tips

Surgical cystourethroscopy always includes a diagnostic cystourethroscopy. Do not report 52351 with 52354–52355. Insertion and removal of a temporary stent is included in these procedures. For insertion of a self-retaining, indwelling stent performed during cystourethroscopic procedures, report 52332 in addition to the primary procedure performed (52320-52330, 52334-52352, 52354, 52355) and append modifier 51. Report image-guided biopsy of the ureter and/or renal pelvis, without endoscopic guidance, with 50606.

ICD-10-CM Diagnostic Codes

C65.1	Malignant neoplasm of right renal pelvis ☑
C65.2	Malignant neoplasm of left renal pelvis ☑
C66.1	Malignant neoplasm of right ureter ☑
C66.2	Malignant neoplasm of left ureter ☑
C67.6	Malignant neoplasm of ureteric orifice
C79.01	Secondary malignant neoplasm of right kidney and renal pelvis ☑
C79.02	Secondary malignant neoplasm of left kidney and renal pelvis ☑
C79.19	Secondary malignant neoplasm of other urinary organs

D09.19	Carcinoma in situ of other urinary organs
D30.11	Benign neoplasm of right renal pelvis ☑
D30.12	Benign neoplasm of left renal pelvis ☑
D30.21	Benign neoplasm of right ureter ☑
D30.22	Benign neoplasm of left ureter ☑
D30.3	Benign neoplasm of bladder
D3A.093	Benign carcinoid tumor of the kidney
D41.11	Neoplasm of uncertain behavior of right renal pelvis ☑
D41.12	Neoplasm of uncertain behavior of left renal pelvis ☑
D41.21	Neoplasm of uncertain behavior of right ureter ☑
D41.22	Neoplasm of uncertain behavior of left ureter ☑
N28.89	Other specified disorders of kidney and ureter

AMA: 52354 2018,Jan,8; 2017,Jan,8; 2016,Jan,13; 2015,Jan,16; 2014,May,3; 2014,Jan,11 **52355** 2018,Jan,8; 2017,Jan,8; 2016,Jan,13; 2015,Jan,16; 2014,May,3; 2014,Jan,11

Relative Value Units/Medicare Edits

Non-Facility RVU	Work	PE	MP	Total
52354	8.0	3.12	0.91	12.03
52355	9.0	3.45	1.03	13.48
Facility RVU	**Work**	**PE**	**MP**	**Total**
52354	8.0	3.12	0.91	12.03
52355	9.0	3.45	1.03	13.48

	FUD	Status	MUE	Modifiers				IOM Reference
52354	0	A	1(3)	51	50	N/A	N/A	None
52355	0	A	1(3)	51	50	N/A	N/A	

* with documentation

Terms To Know

biopsy. Tissue or fluid removed for diagnostic purposes through analysis of the cells in the biopsy material.

excise. Remove or cut out.

fulguration. Destruction of living tissue by using sparks from a high-frequency electric current.

lesion. Area of damaged tissue that has lost continuity or function, due to disease or trauma.

resection. Surgical removal of a part or all of an organ or body part.

stent. Tube to provide support in a body cavity or lumen.

tissue. Group of similar cells with a similar function that form definite structures and organs. Tissue types include epithelial tissue, muscle tissue, connective tissue, and nervous tissue.

tumor. Pathological swelling or enlargement; a neoplastic growth of uncontrolled, abnormal multiplication of cells.

ureteroscopy. Examination of the interior of the ureter by means of a ureteroscope.

Bladder

52400

52400   Cystourethroscopy with incision, fulguration, or resection of congenital posterior urethral valves, or congenital obstructive hypertrophic mucosal folds

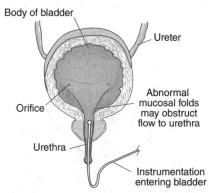

Abnormal urethral valves or mucosal folds are accessed by cystourethroscopy with incision, fulguration, or resection of obstructing tissues

Explanation

The physician examines the urinary collecting system with a cystourethroscope passed through the urethra and bladder, and incises, excises, or uses electric current (fulguration) to correct defects of the bladder neck or the back of the urethra.

Coding Tips

For transurethral resection of the bladder neck, see 52500. For simple excision of the bladder neck through an incision in the bladder, see 51520. For fulguration of trigone, bladder neck, prostatic fossa, urethra, or periurethral glands with cystourethroscopy, see 52214.

ICD-10-CM Diagnostic Codes

N32.89	Other specified disorders of bladder
Q64.11	Supravesical fissure of urinary bladder
Q64.2	Congenital posterior urethral valves
Q64.31	Congenital bladder neck obstruction
Q64.32	Congenital stricture of urethra
Q64.39	Other atresia and stenosis of urethra and bladder neck
Q64.6	Congenital diverticulum of bladder
Q64.71	Congenital prolapse of urethra
Q64.79	Other congenital malformations of bladder and urethra

AMA: 52400 2018,Jan,8; 2017,Jan,8; 2016,Jan,13; 2015,Jan,16; 2014,Jan,11

Relative Value Units/Medicare Edits

Non-Facility RVU	Work	PE	MP	Total
52400	8.69	4.09	1.0	13.78
Facility RVU	**Work**	**PE**	**MP**	**Total**
52400	8.69	4.09	1.0	13.78

	FUD	Status	MUE	Modifiers				IOM Reference
52400	90	A	1(2)	51	N/A	N/A	N/A	None

* with documentation

52402

52402   Cystourethroscopy with transurethral resection or incision of ejaculatory ducts

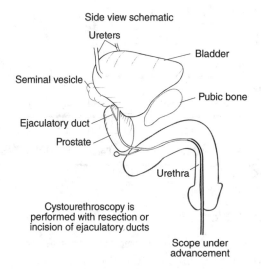

Side view schematic

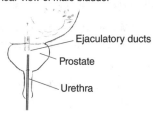

Rear view of male bladder

Explanation

Through the urethra, the physician performs a transurethral resection or a transurethral incision of the ejaculatory ducts (TUIED). The cystourethroscope is introduced into the meatus and the urethra is inspected. Instruments are inserted through the cystourethroscope to the region of the ejaculatory ducts. The seminal vesicles are compressed and the ejaculatory ducts are incised with a hook electrode or resected in one "bite" with a loop electrode. The seminal vesicles are again compressed. The area is observed through the scope and the instruments and cystourethroscope are removed.

Coding Tips

Surgical cystourethroscopy always includes a diagnostic cystourethroscopy. Insertion and removal of a temporary stent is included in this procedure. This code is specific to males. For incision into the seminal vesicle, see 55600–55605.

ICD-10-CM Diagnostic Codes

C63.7	Malignant neoplasm of other specified male genital organs ♂
C79.82	Secondary malignant neoplasm of genital organs
D07.69	Carcinoma in situ of other male genital organs ♂
D29.8	Benign neoplasm of other specified male genital organs ♂
D40.8	Neoplasm of uncertain behavior of other specified male genital organs ♂
D49.511	Neoplasm of unspecified behavior of right kidney ☑
D49.512	Neoplasm of unspecified behavior of left kidney ☑

Urethra

D49.59	Neoplasm of unspecified behavior of other genitourinary organ
N50.89	Other specified disorders of the male genital organs ♂
N51	Disorders of male genital organs in diseases classified elsewhere ♂
Q55.4	Other congenital malformations of vas deferens, epididymis, seminal vesicles and prostate ♂

AMA: **52402** 2014,Jan,11

Relative Value Units/Medicare Edits

Non-Facility RVU	Work	PE	MP	Total
52402	5.27	1.83	0.6	7.7
Facility RVU	Work	PE	MP	Total
52402	5.27	1.83	0.6	7.7

	FUD	Status	MUE	Modifiers				IOM Reference
52402	0	A	1(2)	51	N/A	N/A	N/A	None

* with documentation

Terms To Know

azoospermia. Failure of the development of sperm or the absence of sperm in semen; one of the most common factors in male infertility.

benign. Mild or nonmalignant in nature.

carcinoma in situ. Malignancy that arises from the cells of the vessel, gland, or organ of origin that remains confined to that site or has not invaded neighboring tissue.

congenital. Present at birth, occurring through heredity or an influence during gestation up to the moment of birth.

hyperplasia. Abnormal proliferation in the number of normal cells in regular tissue arrangement.

malignant neoplasm. Any cancerous tumor or lesion exhibiting uncontrolled tissue growth that can progressively invade other parts of the body with its disease-generating cells.

meatus. Opening or passage into the body.

oligospermia. Insufficient production of sperm in semen, a common factor in male infertility.

resection. Surgical removal of a part or all of an organ or body part.

seminal vesicles. Paired glands located at the base of the bladder in males that release the majority of fluid into semen through ducts that join with the vas deferens forming the ejaculatory duct.

stent. Tube to provide support in a body cavity or lumen.

52441-52442

| 52441 | Cystourethroscopy, with insertion of permanent adjustable transprostatic implant; single implant |
| + 52442 | each additional permanent adjustable transprostatic implant (List separately in addition to code for primary procedure) |

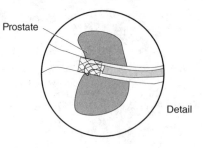

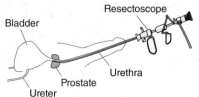

Using a scope inserted through the urethra a transprostatic implant is deployed

Explanation

The physician passes the cystourethroscope through the urethra into the bladder to evaluate the urethra and the bladder and ensure that no obstructions are present in the median lobe of the prostate. After assessment, the physician identifies the exact location in the lateral lobes where the permanent adjustable transprostatic implant will be deployed. The implant is assembled, tailored, and inserted via the use of an implant delivery device. Once inserted, the implant draws back and constricts the obstructing prostatic lobes while expanding the urethral lumen. The physician removes the delivery device and sheath and the lateral prostatic lobes remain retracted. The number of implants is determined by the physician and based on the individual patient's anatomy, prostate size, and shape of the prostatic lobes. Cystourethroscopy may be repeated to allow the physician to evaluate the final results and ensure the urethral lumen remains open without complications. An obstruction of the urethral lumen may require the insertion of multiple implants. Report 52441 for insertion of a single implant for the treatment of lower urinary tract symptoms (LUTS) associated with benign prostatic hyperplasia (BPH). Report 52442 for each additional implant inserted.

Coding Tips

Report 52442 in addition to 52441. For removal of an implant, see 52310. For insertion of a urethral stent, permanent, see 52282; prostatic, urethral stent, temporary, see 53855.

ICD-10-CM Diagnostic Codes

C61	Malignant neoplasm of prostate ♂
C63.8	Malignant neoplasm of overlapping sites of male genital organs ♂
C79.82	Secondary malignant neoplasm of genital organs
D07.5	Carcinoma in situ of prostate ♂
D09.19	Carcinoma in situ of other urinary organs
D29.1	Benign neoplasm of prostate ♂
D29.8	Benign neoplasm of other specified male genital organs ♂

D40.0	Neoplasm of uncertain behavior of prostate ♂		
D40.8	Neoplasm of uncertain behavior of other specified male genital organs ♂		
D49.511	Neoplasm of unspecified behavior of right kidney ☑		
D49.512	Neoplasm of unspecified behavior of left kidney ☑		
D49.59	Neoplasm of unspecified behavior of other genitourinary organ		
N32.0	Bladder-neck obstruction		
N40.0	Benign prostatic hyperplasia without lower urinary tract symptoms 🅰 ♂		
N40.1	Benign prostatic hyperplasia with lower urinary tract symptoms 🅰 ♂		
N40.2	Nodular prostate without lower urinary tract symptoms 🅰 ♂		
N40.3	Nodular prostate with lower urinary tract symptoms 🅰 ♂		
N41.1	Chronic prostatitis 🅰 ♂		
N41.2	Abscess of prostate 🅰 ♂		
N41.3	Prostatocystitis 🅰 ♂		
N41.4	Granulomatous prostatitis 🅰 ♂		
N41.8	Other inflammatory diseases of prostate 🅰 ♂		
N42.83	Cyst of prostate 🅰 ♂		
N42.89	Other specified disorders of prostate 🅰 ♂		
N50.89	Other specified disorders of the male genital organs ♂		
R33.8	Other retention of urine		
R39.14	Feeling of incomplete bladder emptying		

AMA: 52441 2018,Jan,8; 2017,Jan,8; 2016,Jan,13; 2015,Jun,5 **52442** 2018,Jan,8; 2017,Jan,8; 2016,Jan,13; 2015,Jun,5

Relative Value Units/Medicare Edits

Non-Facility RVU	Work	PE	MP	Total
52441	4.0	34.23	0.47	38.7
52442	1.01	27.06	0.11	28.18
Facility RVU	**Work**	**PE**	**MP**	**Total**
52441	4.0	1.6	0.47	6.07
52442	1.01	0.34	0.11	1.46

	FUD	Status	MUE	Modifiers				IOM Reference
52441	0	A	1(2)	51	N/A	N/A	N/A	None
52442	N/A	A	6(3)	N/A	N/A	N/A	N/A	
* with documentation								

Terms To Know

benign prostatic hyperplasia. Enlargement of the prostate caused by proliferation of fibrostromal elements of the gland commonly affecting men older than age 50. BPH is often characterized by urination difficulties, such as slow start, weak stream, dribbling, nocturia (night-time urination), and urinary obstruction due to compression of the urethra as the gland enlarges.

implant. Material or device inserted or placed within the body for therapeutic, reconstructive, or diagnostic purposes.

prostate. Male gland surrounding the bladder neck and urethra that secretes a substance into the seminal fluid.

UroLift® System. Brand name system indicated for minimally invasive treatment of benign prostatic hypertrophy.

52450

52450	Transurethral incision of prostate

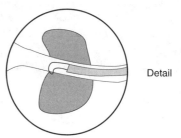

Detail

Physician incises the prostate internally

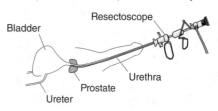

Explanation

Through a cystourethroscope, the physician incises the capsule of the prostate gland and into but not through the true prostate to create a larger passage for urine. A small transurethral tissue sample from the prostate is often collected at the same time. The bladder is catheterized for the immediate postoperative period.

Coding Tips

For transurethral resection of the prostate, first stage, see 52601; for partial resection, second stage, see 52601 and append modifier 58. For transurethral resection, residual or regrowth of obstructive prostate tissue, see 52630. For complete laser vaporization of prostate, see 52648. For drainage of a prostate abscess through a urethral endoscope, see 52700. For transurethral waterjet ablation of prostate, see 0421T. If significant additional time and effort is documented, append modifier 22 and submit a cover letter and operative report.

ICD-10-CM Diagnostic Codes

N40.0	Benign prostatic hyperplasia without lower urinary tract symptoms 🅰 ♂
N40.1	Benign prostatic hyperplasia with lower urinary tract symptoms 🅰 ♂
N40.2	Nodular prostate without lower urinary tract symptoms 🅰 ♂
N40.3	Nodular prostate with lower urinary tract symptoms 🅰 ♂
N41.1	Chronic prostatitis 🅰 ♂
N42.89	Other specified disorders of prostate 🅰 ♂

AMA: 52450 2018,Jan,8; 2017,Jan,8; 2016,Jan,13; 2015,Jun,5; 2015,Jan,16; 2014,Jan,11

CPT © 2020 American Medical Association. All Rights Reserved. ● New ▲ Revised + Add On ★ Telemedicine AMA: CPT Assist [Resequenced] ☑ Laterality © 2020 Optum360, LLC

Relative Value Units/Medicare Edits

Non-Facility RVU	Work	PE	MP	Total
52450	7.78	4.92	0.89	13.59
Facility RVU	Work	PE	MP	Total
52450	7.78	4.92	0.89	13.59

	FUD	Status	MUE	Modifiers				IOM Reference
52450	90	A	1(2)	51	N/A	N/A	N/A	None

* with documentation

Terms To Know

benign prostatic hyperplasia. Enlargement of the prostate caused by proliferation of fibrostromal elements of the gland commonly affecting men older than age 50. BPH is often characterized by urination difficulties, such as slow start, weak stream, dribbling, nocturia (night-time urination), and urinary obstruction due to compression of the urethra as the gland enlarges.

catheterization. Use or insertion of a tubular device into a duct, blood vessel, hollow organ, or body cavity for injecting or withdrawing fluids for diagnostic or therapeutic purposes.

chronic. Persistent, continuing, or recurring.

incision. Act of cutting into tissue or an organ.

LUTS. Lower urinary tract symptoms.

nodular prostate. Small mass of tissue that swells, knots, or is a protuberance in the prostate.

prostate. Male gland surrounding the bladder neck and urethra that secretes a substance into the seminal fluid.

prostatitis. Inflammation of the prostate that may be acute or chronic.

specimen. Tissue cells or sample of fluid taken for analysis, pathologic examination, and diagnosis.

tissue. Group of similar cells with a similar function that form definite structures and organs. Tissue types include epithelial tissue, muscle tissue, connective tissue, and nervous tissue.

52500

52500   Transurethral resection of bladder neck (separate procedure)

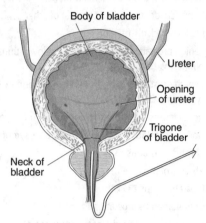

An obstruction in the neck of the bladder is approached using a cystourethroscope and the intervening tissues are resected

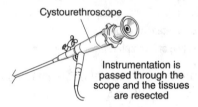

Instrumentation is passed through the scope and the tissues are resected

Explanation

The physician relieves an obstruction of the outlet of the bladder. After the scope is passed through the urethra, instruments are inserted through the cystourethroscope to the target region. The physician excises the tissue responsible for the obstruction of urine flow.

Coding Tips

This is a male only procedure. This separate procedure by definition is usually a component of a more complex service and is not identified separately. When performed alone or with other unrelated procedures/ services it may be reported. If performed alone, list the code; if performed with other procedures/services, list the code and append modifier 59 or an X{EPSU} modifier. For transurethral resection of the prostate, first stage, see 52601; for partial resection, second stage, see 52601 and append modifier 58. For transurethral resection, residual or regrowth of obstructive prostate tissue, see 52630. For complete laser vaporization of prostate, see 52648. For transurethral waterjet ablation of prostate, see 0421T. Other approaches may be reported with 55801-55845.

ICD-10-CM Diagnostic Codes

C67.5	Malignant neoplasm of bladder neck
C79.11	Secondary malignant neoplasm of bladder
D09.0	Carcinoma in situ of bladder
D30.3	Benign neoplasm of bladder
D30.8	Benign neoplasm of other specified urinary organs
D41.4	Neoplasm of uncertain behavior of bladder
D49.4	Neoplasm of unspecified behavior of bladder
N32.0	Bladder-neck obstruction

© 2020 Optum360, LLC   N Newborn: 0   P Pediatric: 0-17   M Maternity: 9-64   A Adult: 15-124   ♂ Male Only   ♀ Female Only   CPT © 2020 American Medical Association. All Rights Reserved.

N32.89	Other specified disorders of bladder	
N33	Bladder disorders in diseases classified elsewhere	
N40.0	Benign prostatic hyperplasia without lower urinary tract symptoms 🅰 ♂	
N40.1	Benign prostatic hyperplasia with lower urinary tract symptoms 🅰 ♂	
N40.2	Nodular prostate without lower urinary tract symptoms 🅰 ♂	
N40.3	Nodular prostate with lower urinary tract symptoms 🅰 ♂	
Q64.31	Congenital bladder neck obstruction	
Q64.39	Other atresia and stenosis of urethra and bladder neck	
Q64.6	Congenital diverticulum of bladder	

AMA: 52500 2018,Jan,8; 2017,Jan,8; 2016,Jan,13; 2015,Jan,16; 2014,Jan,11

Relative Value Units/Medicare Edits

Non-Facility RVU	Work	PE	MP	Total
52500	8.14	5.04	0.92	14.1
Facility RVU	Work	PE	MP	Total
52500	8.14	5.04	0.92	14.1

	FUD	Status	MUE	Modifiers				IOM Reference
52500	90	A	1(2)	51	N/A	N/A	N/A	None

* with documentation

Terms To Know

benign prostatic hyperplasia. Enlargement of the prostate caused by proliferation of fibrostromal elements of the gland commonly affecting men older than age 50. BPH is often characterized by urination difficulties, such as slow start, weak stream, dribbling, nocturia (night-time urination), and urinary obstruction due to compression of the urethra as the gland enlarges.

carcinoma in situ. Malignancy that arises from the cells of the vessel, gland, or organ of origin that remains confined to that site or has not invaded neighboring tissue.

congenital. Present at birth, occurring through heredity or an influence during gestation up to the moment of birth.

excise. Remove or cut out.

LUTS. Lower urinary tract symptoms.

malignant neoplasm. Any cancerous tumor or lesion exhibiting uncontrolled tissue growth that can progressively invade other parts of the body with its disease-generating cells.

nodular prostate. Small mass of tissue that swells, knots, or is a protuberance in the prostate.

obstruction. Blockage that prevents normal function of the valve or structure.

resection. Surgical removal of a part or all of an organ or body part.

tissue. Group of similar cells with a similar function that form definite structures and organs. Tissue types include epithelial tissue, muscle tissue, connective tissue, and nervous tissue.

52601

52601	Transurethral electrosurgical resection of prostate, including control of postoperative bleeding, complete (vasectomy, meatotomy, cystourethroscopy, urethral calibration and/or dilation, and internal urethrotomy are included)

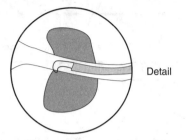

Detail

The physician resects the prostate using a resectoscope

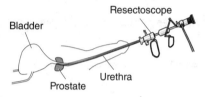

Explanation

After preliminary cystourethroscopy, the physician passes the resectoscope under direct vision up the urethra to the region of the prostate. Meatotomy, cutting to enlarge the opening of the urethra, and/or dilatation of the urethra may be necessary to allow the passage of the resectoscope. The prostate gland is removed in a systematic fashion by using a series of small cuts into the glandular tissue with an electrocautery knife. The resected tissue is removed and the area is keep clear by irrigation through the resectoscope. Bleeding is controlled by fulguration. A catheter is passed into the bladder and left in place for the postoperative period.

Coding Tips

During this procedure, the physician may need to perform a vasectomy, meatotomy, cystourethroscopy, urethral calibration/ dilation, and an internal urethrotomy in any combination. These procedures are included in 52601 and are not separately reported. For transurethral resection of the prostate, first stage, see 52601; for partial resection, second stage, see 52601 and append modifier 58. For transurethral resection, residual or regrowth of obstructive prostate tissue, see 52630. Report 52647 for non-contact laser coagulation of the prostate; 52648 for contact laser vaporization of the prostate, with or without transurethral resection (endoscopic). For open excisional procedures on the prostate gland, see 55801–55845. Report transurethral waterjet ablation of the prostate with 0421T.

ICD-10-CM Diagnostic Codes

C61	Malignant neoplasm of prostate ♂	
D07.5	Carcinoma in situ of prostate ♂	
D29.1	Benign neoplasm of prostate ♂	
D40.0	Neoplasm of uncertain behavior of prostate ♂	
N40.0	Benign prostatic hyperplasia without lower urinary tract symptoms 🅰 ♂	
N40.1	Benign prostatic hyperplasia with lower urinary tract symptoms 🅰 ♂	
N40.2	Nodular prostate without lower urinary tract symptoms 🅰 ♂	
N40.3	Nodular prostate with lower urinary tract symptoms 🅰 ♂	

Urethra

AMA: **52601** 2018,Jan,8; 2017,Jan,8; 2016,Jan,13; 2015,Jun,5; 2015,Jan,16; 2014,Jan,11

Relative Value Units/Medicare Edits

Non-Facility RVU	Work	PE	MP	Total
52601	13.16	6.39	1.5	21.05
Facility RVU	**Work**	**PE**	**MP**	**Total**
52601	13.16	6.39	1.5	21.05

	FUD	Status	MUE	Modifiers			IOM Reference
52601	90	A	1(2)	51	N/A	N/A	N/A	None

* with documentation

Terms To Know

catheter. Flexible tube inserted into an area of the body for introducing or withdrawing fluid.

dissect. Cut apart or separate tissue for surgical purposes or for visual or microscopic study.

fulguration. Destruction of living tissue by using sparks from a high-frequency electric current.

gland. Group of cells that secrete or excrete chemicals called hormones.

irrigation. To wash out or cleanse a body cavity, wound, or tissue with water or other fluid.

prostate. Male gland surrounding the bladder neck and urethra that secretes a substance into the seminal fluid.

resection. Surgical removal of a part or all of an organ or body part.

tissue. Group of similar cells with a similar function that form definite structures and organs. Tissue types include epithelial tissue, muscle tissue, connective tissue, and nervous tissue.

urethra. Small tube lined with mucous membrane that leads from the bladder to the exterior of the body.

52630

52630 Transurethral resection; residual or regrowth of obstructive prostate tissue including control of postoperative bleeding, complete (vasectomy, meatotomy, cystourethroscopy, urethral calibration and/or dilation, and internal urethrotomy are included)

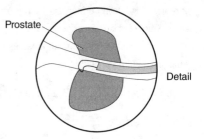

Using a scope inserted through the urethra, the physician removes residual tissues from the prostate

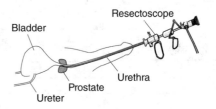

Explanation

The physician inserts an endoscope through the urethra to remove residual or regrowth obstructive tissue from a previous surgical procedure. After preliminary cystourethroscopy, the physician passes the resectoscope into the urethra to the prostate. Meatotomy, cutting to enlarge the external opening of the urethra, and dilatation of the urethra may be necessary to allow the passage of the resectoscope. The physician removes residual tissue of the prostate gland through a series of small cuts. The resected tissue is removed, and the area is kept clear by irrigation through the resectoscope. Bleeding is controlled by fulguration. A catheter is passed into the bladder and left in place.

Coding Tips

For removal of residual obstructive tissue within the postoperative period of a related procedure performed by the same physician, report with modifier 78. If significant additional time and effort is documented, append modifier 22 and submit a cover letter and operative report. For transurethral resection of a postoperative bladder neck contracture, see 52640. For initial endoscopic transurethral prostate resection procedures, see 52601 and 52648. For open excisional procedures on the prostate gland, see 55801–55845. For transurethral waterjet ablation of the prostate, see 0421T.

ICD-10-CM Diagnostic Codes

C61	Malignant neoplasm of prostate ♂
D07.5	Carcinoma in situ of prostate ♂
D29.1	Benign neoplasm of prostate ♂
D40.0	Neoplasm of uncertain behavior of prostate ♂
N40.0	Benign prostatic hyperplasia without lower urinary tract symptoms 🅰 ♂
N40.1	Benign prostatic hyperplasia with lower urinary tract symptoms 🅰 ♂
N40.2	Nodular prostate without lower urinary tract symptoms 🅰 ♂

AMA: 52630 2018,Jan,8; 2017,Jan,8; 2016,Jan,13; 2015,Jan,16; 2014,Jan,11

Relative Value Units/Medicare Edits

Non-Facility RVU	Work	PE	MP	Total
52630	6.55	4.29	0.76	11.6
Facility RVU	**Work**	**PE**	**MP**	**Total**
52630	6.55	4.29	0.76	11.6

	FUD	Status	MUE	Modifiers				IOM Reference
52630	90	A	1(2)	51	N/A	N/A	N/A	None

* with documentation

Terms To Know

catheter. Flexible tube inserted into an area of the body for introducing or withdrawing fluid.

fulguration. Destruction of living tissue by using sparks from a high-frequency electric current.

irrigation. To wash out or cleanse a body cavity, wound, or tissue with water or other fluid.

obstruction. Blockage that prevents normal function of the valve or structure.

resect. Cutting out or removing a portion or all of a bone, organ, or other structure.

TURP. Transurethral resection of the prostate. A TURP is performed to reduce the size of an enlarged prostate. Enlargement presses against the urethra, and causes difficulties in urination. Similar procedures include TEVAP, done with electrovaporization; TULIP, with ultrasound guided laser ablation; TUNA, with needle ablation; or TUMT, microwave thermotherapy.

52640

52640	Transurethral resection; of postoperative bladder neck contracture

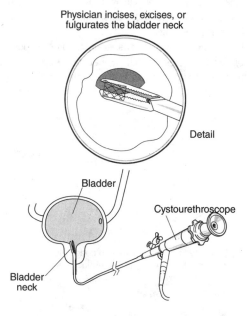

Explanation

Contracture of the bladder neck outlet usually results from scarring after a transurethral resection of the prostate gland. After preliminary cystourethroscopy, the physician passes the resectoscope under direct vision up the urethra to the region of the bladder neck contracture. Meatotomy, cutting to enlarge the opening of the urethra, and dilation of the urethra may be necessary to allow the passage of the resectoscope. The scar tissue is incised at one to three sites or resected, using a cutting electrocautery knife. The operative site is inspected for bleeding, which is controlled by fulguration. A catheter is passed into the bladder at the end of the procedure and left in place for the postoperative period.

Coding Tips

For transurethral resection of obstructive prostate tissue, residual or regrowth, see 52630. For transurethral waterjet ablation of prostate, see 0421T. For transurethral resection of the bladder neck, see 52500.

ICD-10-CM Diagnostic Codes

N32.0	Bladder-neck obstruction

AMA: 52640 2018,Jan,8; 2017,Jan,8; 2016,Jan,13; 2015,Jan,16; 2014,Jan,11

Relative Value Units/Medicare Edits

Non-Facility RVU	Work	PE	MP	Total
52640	4.79	3.79	0.54	9.12
Facility RVU	**Work**	**PE**	**MP**	**Total**
52640	4.79	3.79	0.54	9.12

	FUD	Status	MUE	Modifiers				IOM Reference
52640	90	A	1(2)	51	N/A	N/A	N/A	None

* with documentation

Urethra

52647-52648

52647   Laser coagulation of prostate, including control of postoperative bleeding, complete (vasectomy, meatotomy, cystourethroscopy, urethral calibration and/or dilation, and internal urethrotomy are included if performed)

52648   Laser vaporization of prostate, including control of postoperative bleeding, complete (vasectomy, meatotomy, cystourethroscopy, urethral calibration and/or dilation, internal urethrotomy and transurethral resection of prostate are included if performed)

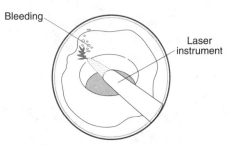

The physician uses a laser to coagulate prostatic tissue and stop postoperative bleeding

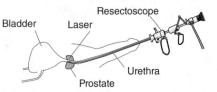

Explanation

The physician uses a laser to coagulate or vaporize the prostate through an endoscope or resectoscope inserted through the urethra. Dilation of the urethra may be necessary to permit endoscope insertion. The entire prostate is treated. To accomplish this, vasectomy, meatotomy, cystourethroscopy, and internal urethrotomy may be necessary. Once the laser treatment is complete, a urinary catheter is inserted. Report 52647 if prostatic tissue is coagulated and 52648 if it is vaporized.

Coding Tips

During these procedures, the physician may need to perform a vasectomy, meatotomy, cystourethroscopy, urethral calibration/dilation, and an internal urethrotomy in any combination. These procedures are included in 52647 and 52648 and are not separately reported. For transurethral resection of the prostate by an electrocautery knife, also including vasectomy, meatotomy, cystourethroscopy, urethral calibration/dilation, and an internal urethrotomy, see 52601. For open excisional procedures on the prostate gland, see 55801–55845.

ICD-10-CM Diagnostic Codes

N40.0   Benign prostatic hyperplasia without lower urinary tract symptoms 🄰 ♂

N40.1   Benign prostatic hyperplasia with lower urinary tract symptoms 🄰 ♂

N40.2   Nodular prostate without lower urinary tract symptoms 🄰 ♂

N40.3   Nodular prostate with lower urinary tract symptoms 🄰 ♂

AMA: **52647** 2018,Jan,8; 2017,Jan,8; 2016,Jan,13; 2015,Jan,16; 2014,Jan,11 **52648** 2018,Jan,8; 2017,Jan,8; 2016,Jan,13; 2015,Jun,5; 2015,Jan,16; 2014,Jan,11

Relative Value Units/Medicare Edits

Non-Facility RVU	Work	PE	MP	Total
52647	11.3	33.77	1.28	46.35
52648	12.15	34.28	1.39	47.82
Facility RVU	**Work**	**PE**	**MP**	**Total**
52647	11.3	6.11	1.28	18.69
52648	12.15	6.4	1.39	19.94

	FUD	Status	MUE	Modifiers				IOM Reference
52647	90	A	1(2)	51	N/A	N/A	N/A	None
52648	90	A	1(2)	51	N/A	N/A	N/A	

* with documentation

Terms To Know

Coaguloop. Brand name resection electrode designed for use with a resectoscope for prostate operations, used in transurethral electrosurgical prostate resection.

laser surgery. Use of concentrated, sharply defined light beams to cut, cauterize, coagulate, seal, or vaporize tissue.

LUTS. Lower urinary tract symptoms.

prostate. Male gland surrounding the bladder neck and urethra that secretes a substance into the seminal fluid.

tissue. Group of similar cells with a similar function that form definite structures and organs. Tissue types include epithelial tissue, muscle tissue, connective tissue, and nervous tissue.

TURP. Transurethral resection of the prostate. A TURP is performed to reduce the size of an enlarged prostate. Enlargement presses against the urethra, and causes difficulties in urination. Similar procedures include TEVAP, done with electrovaporization; TULIP, with ultrasound guided laser ablation; TUNA, with needle ablation; or TUMT, microwave thermotherapy.

52649

52649 Laser enucleation of the prostate with morcellation, including control of postoperative bleeding, complete (vasectomy, meatotomy, cystourethroscopy, urethral calibration and/or dilation, internal urethrotomy and transurethral resection of prostate are included if performed)

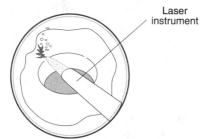

The prostate is morselized for enucleation

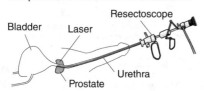

Explanation

The physician uses a laser to enucleate the prostate through an endoscope or resectoscope inserted through the urethra. Dilation of the urethra may be necessary to permit endoscope insertion. The entire prostate is treated. To accomplish this, vasectomy, meatotomy, cystourethroscopy, and internal urethrotomy may be necessary. The damaged or diseased tissue is divided and removed in small pieces (morcellation). Once the laser treatment is complete, a urinary catheter is inserted.

Coding Tips

The physician may need to perform a vasectomy, meatotomy, cystourethroscopy, urethral calibration/dilation, and an internal urethrotomy in any combination. For transurethral resection of the prostate by an electrocautery knife, also including vasectomy, meatotomy, cystourethroscopy, urethral calibration/dilation, and an internal urethrotomy, see 52601. For laser coagulation of the prostate, see 52647; laser vaporization, see 52648. For open excisional procedures on the prostate gland, see 55801–55845. Do not report 52649 with 52000, 52276, 52281, 52601, 52647, 52648, 53020, or 55250.

ICD-10-CM Diagnostic Codes

N40.0   Benign prostatic hyperplasia without lower urinary tract symptoms 🅰 ♂

N40.1   Benign prostatic hyperplasia with lower urinary tract symptoms 🅰 ♂

N40.2   Nodular prostate without lower urinary tract symptoms 🅰 ♂

N40.3   Nodular prostate with lower urinary tract symptoms 🅰 ♂

AMA: **52649** 2018,Jan,8; 2017,Jan,8; 2016,Jan,13; 2015,Jun,5; 2014,Jan,11

Relative Value Units/Medicare Edits

Non-Facility RVU	Work	PE	MP	Total
52649	14.56	7.59	1.68	23.83
Facility RVU	**Work**	**PE**	**MP**	**Total**
52649	14.56	7.59	1.68	23.83

	FUD	Status	MUE	Modifiers				IOM Reference
52649	90	A	1(2)	51	N/A	N/A	80*	None

* with documentation

Terms To Know

benign prostatic hyperplasia. Enlargement of the prostate caused by proliferation of fibrostromal elements of the gland commonly affecting men older than age 50. BPH is often characterized by urination difficulties, such as slow start, weak stream, dribbling, nocturia (night-time urination), and urinary obstruction due to compression of the urethra as the gland enlarges.

catheter. Flexible tube inserted into an area of the body for introducing or withdrawing fluid.

enucleation. Removal of a growth or organ cleanly so as to extract it in one piece.

laser. Concentrated light used to cut or seal tissue.

LUTS. Lower urinary tract symptoms.

nodular prostate. Small mass of tissue that swells, knots, or is a protuberance in the prostate.

prostate. Male gland surrounding the bladder neck and urethra that secretes a substance into the seminal fluid.

resection. Surgical removal of a part or all of an organ or body part.

tissue. Group of similar cells with a similar function that form definite structures and organs. Tissue types include epithelial tissue, muscle tissue, connective tissue, and nervous tissue.

TURP. Transurethral resection of the prostate. A TURP is performed to reduce the size of an enlarged prostate. Enlargement presses against the urethra, and causes difficulties in urination. Similar procedures include TEVAP, done with electrovaporization; TULIP, with ultrasound guided laser ablation; TUNA, with needle ablation; or TUMT, microwave thermotherapy.

urethra. Small tube lined with mucous membrane that leads from the bladder to the exterior of the body.

CPT © 2020 American Medical Association. All Rights Reserved.   ● New   ▲ Revised   + Add On   ★ Telemedicine   AMA: CPT Assist   [Resequenced]   ☑ Laterality   © 2020 Optum360, LLC

52700

52700   Transurethral drainage of prostatic abscess

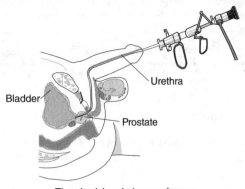

The physician drains an abscess
in and around the prostate

Explanation

The physician inserts an endoscope through the urethra to drain an abscess on or near the prostate. The physician passes a cystourethroscope through the penile urethra to the region of the prostate and identifies the area of the abscess. A needle is passed into the abscess and purulent matter is removed by aspiration. The cystourethroscope is removed.

Coding Tips

For drainage of a prostate abscess through an open incision, see 55720 or 55725; biopsy, see 55700–55705. For transurethral resection of obstructive prostate tissue, residual or regrowth, see 52630. Report litholapaxy with 52317 and 52318.

ICD-10-CM Diagnostic Codes

A54.22	Gonococcal prostatitis ♂
N41.2	Abscess of prostate A ♂
N41.3	Prostatocystitis A ♂

AMA: 52700 2018,Jan,8; 2017,Jan,8; 2016,Jan,13; 2015,Jan,16; 2014,Jan,11

Relative Value Units/Medicare Edits

Non-Facility RVU	Work	PE	MP	Total
52700	7.49	4.39	0.85	12.73
Facility RVU	**Work**	**PE**	**MP**	**Total**
52700	7.49	4.39	0.85	12.73

	FUD	Status	MUE	Modifiers				IOM Reference
52700	90	A	1(3)	51	N/A	N/A	80*	None

* with documentation

Terms To Know

abscess. Circumscribed collection of pus resulting from bacteria, frequently associated with swelling and other signs of inflammation.

aspiration. Drawing fluid out by suction.

purulent. Cyst, wound, or any other sore or condition full of or discharging pus.

53000-53010

53000   Urethrotomy or urethrostomy, external (separate procedure); pendulous urethra
53010   perineal urethra, external

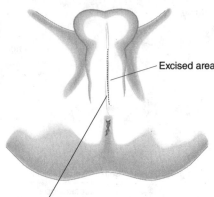

Physician removes contracture via perineal
urethra by passing sound into stricture

Explanation

The physician makes an external incision in the urethra or creates an opening between the urethra and the skin. The physician passes a sound into the urethra until it meets the obstructing stricture. A longitudinal incision is made directly over the sound. After the stricture is identified, the urethra is incised the length of the stricture so defects may be removed. The sound is removed and a catheter is passed through the urethra into the area of the incision and guided past it into the bladder. The urethra is repaired over the catheter, using sutures. Occasionally, the urethra is not repaired by suturing but is simply allowed to grow epithelial cells (epithelialize) around the catheter. In 53010, the physician meets the stricture in the perineal part of the urethra.

Coding Tips

These separate procedures by definition are usually a component of a more complex service and are not identified separately. When performed alone or with other unrelated procedures/services they may be reported. If performed alone, list the code; if performed with other procedures/services, list the code and append modifier 59 or an X{EPSU} modifier. Report 53020–53025 if the physician makes an incision in the urethral opening (urethral meatus). Report 52270–52276 if the physician uses a cystourethroscope to make an incision inside the urethra. Urethral dilation or manipulation for this procedure is not separately identified. For cystoscopy, urethroscopy, or cystourethroscopy, see 52000-52700. Report injection procedures for urethrocystography with 51600-51610.

ICD-10-CM Diagnostic Codes

N35.010	Post-traumatic urethral stricture, male, meatal ♂
N35.011	Post-traumatic bulbous urethral stricture ♂
N35.012	Post-traumatic membranous urethral stricture ♂
N35.013	Post-traumatic anterior urethral stricture ♂
N35.016	Post-traumatic urethral stricture, male, overlapping sites ♂
N35.111	Postinfective urethral stricture, not elsewhere classified, male, meatal ♂
N35.112	Postinfective bulbous urethral stricture, not elsewhere classified, male ♂
N35.113	Postinfective membranous urethral stricture, not elsewhere classified, male ♂

© 2020 Optum360, LLC   N Newborn: 0   P Pediatric: 0-17   M Maternity: 9-64   A Adult: 15-124   ♂ Male Only   ♀ Female Only   CPT © 2020 American Medical Association. All Rights Reserved.

N35.114	Postinfective anterior urethral stricture, not elsewhere classified, male ♂	
N35.116	Postinfective urethral stricture, not elsewhere classified, male, overlapping sites ♂	
N35.811	Other urethral stricture, male, meatal ♂	
N35.812	Other urethral bulbous stricture, male ♂	
N35.813	Other membranous urethral stricture, male ♂	
N35.814	Other anterior urethral stricture, male ♂	
N35.816	Other urethral stricture, male, overlapping sites ♂	
N35.82	Other urethral stricture, female ♀	
N36.8	Other specified disorders of urethra	
N37	Urethral disorders in diseases classified elsewhere	
N99.110	Postprocedural urethral stricture, male, meatal ♂	
N99.111	Postprocedural bulbous urethral stricture, male ♂	
N99.112	Postprocedural membranous urethral stricture, male ♂	
N99.113	Postprocedural anterior bulbous urethral stricture, male ♂	
N99.115	Postprocedural fossa navicularis urethral stricture ♂	
N99.116	Postprocedural urethral stricture, male, overlapping sites ♂	
Q64.32	Congenital stricture of urethra	
Q64.39	Other atresia and stenosis of urethra and bladder neck	

AMA: 53000 2014,Jan,11 **53010** 2014,Jan,11

Relative Value Units/Medicare Edits

Non-Facility RVU	Work	PE	MP	Total
53000	2.33	1.67	0.27	4.27
53010	4.45	3.53	0.51	8.49
Facility RVU	Work	PE	MP	Total
53000	2.33	1.67	0.27	4.27
53010	4.45	3.53	0.51	8.49

	FUD	Status	MUE	Modifiers				IOM Reference
53000	10	A	1(2)	51	N/A	N/A	N/A	None
53010	90	A	1(2)	51	N/A	N/A	N/A	

* with documentation

Terms To Know

dilation. Artificial increase in the diameter of an opening or lumen made by medication or by instrumentation.

perineal. Pertaining to the pelvic floor area between the thighs; the diamond-shaped area bordered by the pubic symphysis in front, the ischial tuberosities on the sides, and the coccyx in back.

sound. Long, slender tool with a type of curved, flat probe at the end for dilating strictures or detecting foreign bodies.

53020-53025

53020	Meatotomy, cutting of meatus (separate procedure); except infant
53025	infant

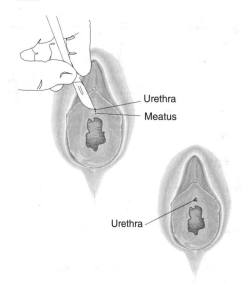

Physician makes an opening in the urethra, male or female, to remove stricture in opening

Explanation

The physician makes an incision in the opening of the urethra (urethral meatus) using a small pointed knife and a meatotomy clamp. The meatus is opened on the ventral surface and the meatus may be dilated. Sutures may be required on the mucosa of the meatus. The physician often uses a hemostat to separate the tissue in the urethra prior to making his incision. Report 53020 if the patient is older than one year, or 53025 if the patient is younger than 1 year.

Coding Tips

These separate procedures by definition are usually a component of a more complex service and are not identified separately. When performed alone or with other unrelated procedures/services they may be reported. If performed alone, list the code; if performed with other procedures/services, list the code and append modifier 59 or an X{EPSU} modifier. The physician usually performs these procedures with local anesthesia. However, general anesthesia may be administered depending on the age or condition of the patient. Report 53000–53010 if the physician makes an incision in the external urethra or creates an opening between the urethra and the skin. For cystourethroscopic procedures with urethral meatotomy, see 52281 and 52285. For cystourethroscopy with an internal incision in the urethra, see 52270–52276. For cystoscopy, urethroscopy, or cystourethroscopy, see 52000-52700. Report injection procedures for urethrocystography with 51600-51610.

ICD-10-CM Diagnostic Codes

N35.010	Post-traumatic urethral stricture, male, meatal ♂	
N35.111	Postinfective urethral stricture, not elsewhere classified, male, meatal ♂	
N99.110	Postprocedural urethral stricture, male, meatal ♂	
N99.115	Postprocedural fossa navicularis urethral stricture ♂	
Q64.33	Congenital stricture of urinary meatus	

AMA: 53020 2014,Jan,11 **53025** 2014,Jan,11

Urethra

Relative Value Units/Medicare Edits

Non-Facility RVU	Work	PE	MP	Total
53020	1.77	0.82	0.21	2.8
53025	1.13	0.7	0.12	1.95
Facility RVU	Work	PE	MP	Total
53020	1.77	0.82	0.21	2.8
53025	1.13	0.7	0.12	1.95

	FUD	Status	MUE	Modifiers				IOM Reference
53020	0	A	1(2)	51	N/A	N/A	N/A	None
53025	0	A	1(2)	51	N/A	N/A	80*	

* with documentation

Terms To Know

atresia. Congenital closure or absence of a tubular organ or an opening to the body surface.

balanoposthitis. Inflammation and/or infection of the glans penis and prepuce.

chordee. Ventral (downward) curvature of the penis due to a fibrous band along the corpus spongiosum seen congenitally with hypospadias, or a downward curvature seen on erection in disease conditions, causing a lack of distensibility in the tissues.

epispadias. Male anomaly in which the urethral opening is abnormally located on the dorsum of the penis, appearing as a groove with no upper urethral wall covering.

hemostat. Tool for clamping vessels and arresting hemorrhaging.

hypospadias. Fairly common birth defect in males in which the meatus, or urinary opening, is abnormally positioned on the underside of the penile shaft or in the perineum, requiring early surgical correction.

meatus. Opening or passage into the body.

mucosa. Moist tissue lining the mouth (buccal mucosa), stomach (gastric mucosa), intestines, and respiratory tract.

tissue. Group of similar cells with a similar function that form definite structures and organs. Tissue types include epithelial tissue, muscle tissue, connective tissue, and nervous tissue.

ventral. Pertaining or relating on, to, or toward the lower abdominal plane of the body; located on, near, or toward the front area of the body.

53040-53060

53040   Drainage of deep periurethral abscess
53060   Drainage of Skene's gland abscess or cyst

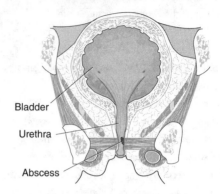

The physician inserts a needle to remove an abscess

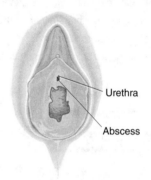

Explanation

The physician drains an abscess in the urethra resulting from a urethral infection or traumatic injury. The physician makes an incision through the skin, subcutaneous tissue, and overlying layers of muscle, fat, and tissue (fascia) over the site of the abscess. By blunt or sharp dissection, the incision is carried into the abscess. Several drains are inserted and the incision is closed in layers. Report 53040 for drainage of a deep periurethral abscess. For an abscess or cyst in Skene's or paraurethral glands in the female, report 53060.

Coding Tips

For subcutaneous abscess, simple or single, see 10060; complicated or multiple, see 10061. The physician usually performs these services under local anesthesia. However, these procedures may be performed under general anesthesia, depending on the age and/or condition of the patient. Report 53080–53085 if the physician makes an incision to drain urinary leakage in the surrounding perineal tissue. For excision or destruction of the Skene's gland by electric current (fulguration), see 53270.

ICD-10-CM Diagnostic Codes

N34.0   Urethral abscess
N36.8   Other specified disorders of urethra

AMA: **53040** 2014,Jan,11 **53060** 2014,Jan,11

Relative Value Units/Medicare Edits

Non-Facility RVU	Work	PE	MP	Total
53040	6.55	4.01	0.76	11.32
53060	2.68	2.27	0.43	5.38
Facility RVU	Work	PE	MP	Total
53040	6.55	4.01	0.76	11.32
53060	2.68	1.69	0.43	4.8

	FUD	Status	MUE	Modifiers				IOM Reference
53040	90	A	1(3)	51	N/A	N/A	80*	None
53060	10	A	1(3)	51	N/A	N/A	N/A	

* with documentation

Terms To Know

abscess. Circumscribed collection of pus resulting from bacteria, frequently associated with swelling and other signs of inflammation.

blunt dissection. Surgical technique used to expose an underlying area by separating along natural cleavage lines of tissue, without cutting.

cyst. Elevated encapsulated mass containing fluid, semisolid, or solid material with a membranous lining.

drain. Device that creates a channel to allow fluid from a cavity, wound, or infected area to exit the body.

fascia. Fibrous sheet or band of tissue that envelops organs, muscles, and groupings of muscles.

incision and drainage. Cutting open body tissue for the removal of tissue fluids or infected discharge from a wound or cavity.

infection. Presence of microorganisms in body tissues that may result in cellular damage.

Skene's gland. Paraurethral ducts that drain a group of the female urethral glands into the vestibule.

subcutaneous tissue. Sheet or wide band of adipose (fat) and areolar connective tissue in two layers attached to the dermis.

vulva. Area on the female external genitalia that includes the labia majora and minora, mons pubis, clitoris, bulb of the vestibule, vaginal vestibule and orifice, and the greater and lesser vestibular glands.

53080-53085

53080	Drainage of perineal urinary extravasation; uncomplicated (separate procedure)
53085	complicated

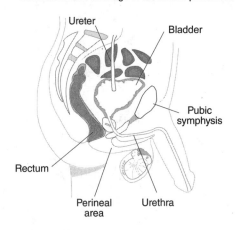

A leak in the urethral lining, or possibly a ureter, has caused urine to collect in the perineal cavity. An incision and drainage of the fluid is performed

Explanation

The physician drains urine that has passed out of the urethra (extravasation) into the perineal tissue. The physician makes an incision through the skin over the site. The incision is carried to the extravasation for drainage. Following drainage, the incision is closed with sutures. Report 53080 for uncomplicated extravasation and 53085 for complicated extravasation.

Coding Tips

Note that 53080 is a separate procedure by definition and is a component of a more complex service and is not identified separately. When performed alone or with other related procedures/services it may be reported. If performed alone, list the code; if performed with other procedures/services, list the code and append modifier 59 or an X{EPSU} modifier.

ICD-10-CM Diagnostic Codes

R39.0	Extravasation of urine

AMA: **53080** 2014,Jan,11 **53085** 2014,Jan,11

Relative Value Units/Medicare Edits

Non-Facility RVU	Work	PE	MP	Total
53080	6.92	4.4	0.79	12.11
53085	11.18	6.28	1.27	18.73
Facility RVU	Work	PE	MP	Total
53080	6.92	4.4	0.79	12.11
53085	11.18	6.28	1.27	18.73

	FUD	Status	MUE	Modifiers				IOM Reference
53080	90	A	1(3)	51	N/A	N/A	N/A	None
53085	90	A	1(3)	51	N/A	62*	80	

* with documentation

Urethra

53200

53200   Biopsy of urethra

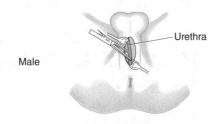

Male

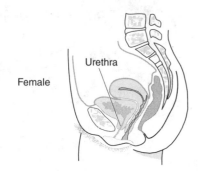

Female

The physician excises urethra tissue for biopsy

Explanation

Using an open approach, the physician excises a specimen of tissue from the urethra for biopsy. At the site to be analyzed, a portion of the suspect tissue is excised by blunt or sharp dissection. The incision is closed in layers.

Coding Tips

An excisional biopsy is not reported separately when a therapeutic excision is performed during the same surgical session. For removal of biopsy tissue from the urethra or bladder through a cystourethroscope, see 52204. For other procedures performed through a cystourethroscope that may include urethral biopsy, see 52224, 52250, and 52354. Dilation or manipulation of the urethra is not identified separately. Report 99000 for conveyance of the specimen.

ICD-10-CM Diagnostic Codes

C67.5	Malignant neoplasm of bladder neck
C68.0	Malignant neoplasm of urethra
C79.11	Secondary malignant neoplasm of bladder
C79.19	Secondary malignant neoplasm of other urinary organs
D09.0	Carcinoma in situ of bladder
D09.19	Carcinoma in situ of other urinary organs
D30.3	Benign neoplasm of bladder
D30.4	Benign neoplasm of urethra
D41.3	Neoplasm of uncertain behavior of urethra
D41.4	Neoplasm of uncertain behavior of bladder
D49.4	Neoplasm of unspecified behavior of bladder
D49.59	Neoplasm of unspecified behavior of other genitourinary organ
N34.0	Urethral abscess
N34.1	Nonspecific urethritis
N34.2	Other urethritis
N36.2	Urethral caruncle
N36.8	Other specified disorders of urethra
N37	Urethral disorders in diseases classified elsewhere

T19.0XXA   Foreign body in urethra, initial encounter

AMA: **53200** 2014,Jan,11

Relative Value Units/Medicare Edits

Non-Facility RVU	Work	PE	MP	Total
53200	2.59	1.63	0.32	4.54
Facility RVU	**Work**	**PE**	**MP**	**Total**
53200	2.59	1.18	0.32	4.09

	FUD	Status	MUE	Modifiers				IOM Reference
53200	0	A	1(3)	51	N/A	N/A	N/A	None

* with documentation

Terms To Know

abscess. Circumscribed collection of pus resulting from bacteria, frequently associated with swelling and other signs of inflammation.

approach. Method or anatomical location used to gain access to a body organ or specific area for procedures.

benign. Mild or nonmalignant in nature.

biopsy. Tissue or fluid removed for diagnostic purposes through analysis of the cells in the biopsy material.

blunt dissection. Surgical technique used to expose an underlying area by separating along natural cleavage lines of tissue, without cutting.

carcinoma in situ. Malignancy that arises from the cells of the vessel, gland, or organ of origin that remains confined to that site or has not invaded neighboring tissue.

malignant. Any condition tending to progress toward death, specifically an invasive tumor with a loss of cellular differentiation that has the ability to spread or metastasize to other body areas.

specimen. Tissue cells or sample of fluid taken for analysis, pathologic examination, and diagnosis.

stricture. Narrowing of an anatomical structure.

tissue. Group of similar cells with a similar function that form definite structures and organs. Tissue types include epithelial tissue, muscle tissue, connective tissue, and nervous tissue.

Urethra

53210-53220

53210 Urethrectomy, total, including cystostomy; female
53215   male
53220 Excision or fulguration of carcinoma of urethra

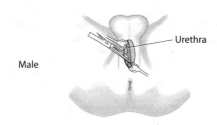

Male

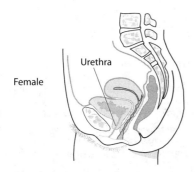

Female

The physician removes the entire urethra

Explanation

The physician removes the urethra and creates an opening between the bladder and skin for drainage of urine. The physician makes a slightly curved, suprapubic (Cherney) incision down to the ureter and bladder. The bladder is opened and the urethral orifice is circumcised and usually tied off with sutures. Tumors of the urethra are removed by partial or complete urethrectomy or by electric current (fulguration). If the bladder has been opened, it is closed in two layers or more. Report 53210 for females; use 53215 for male-specific procedure. Report 53220 for removal of malignant tumor from the urethra.

Coding Tips

If significant additional time and effort is documented, append modifier 22 and submit a cover letter and operative report. For excision or fulguration of urethral polyps, caruncle, prolapse, or Skene's glands, see 53260–53275. For fulguration of urethral tissue, lesion, or tumor through a cystourethroscope, see 52214, 52224, and 52285. Report a biopsy of the urethra with 53200.

ICD-10-CM Diagnostic Codes

C67.5	Malignant neoplasm of bladder neck
C68.0	Malignant neoplasm of urethra
C79.11	Secondary malignant neoplasm of bladder
C79.19	Secondary malignant neoplasm of other urinary organs
D09.0	Carcinoma in situ of bladder
D09.19	Carcinoma in situ of other urinary organs
D41.3	Neoplasm of uncertain behavior of urethra
D41.4	Neoplasm of uncertain behavior of bladder
D49.4	Neoplasm of unspecified behavior of bladder
D49.59	Neoplasm of unspecified behavior of other genitourinary organ

AMA: 53210 2014,Jan,11 **53215** 2014,Jan,11 **53220** 2014,Jan,11

Relative Value Units/Medicare Edits

Non-Facility RVU	Work	PE	MP	Total
53210	13.72	7.14	1.69	22.55
53215	16.85	8.01	1.96	26.82
53220	7.63	4.53	0.87	13.03
Facility RVU	**Work**	**PE**	**MP**	**Total**
53210	13.72	7.14	1.69	22.55
53215	16.85	8.01	1.96	26.82
53220	7.63	4.53	0.87	13.03

	FUD	Status	MUE	Modifiers				IOM Reference
53210	90	A	1(2)	51	N/A	62*	80	None
53215	90	A	1(2)	51	N/A	62*	80	
53220	90	A	1(3)	51	N/A	N/A	80*	

* with documentation

Terms To Know

carcinoma in situ. Malignancy that arises from the cells of the vessel, gland, or organ of origin that remains confined to that site or has not invaded neighboring tissue.

cystostomy. Formation of an opening through the abdominal wall into the bladder.

drainage. Releasing, taking, or letting out fluids and/or gases from a body part.

excision. Surgical removal of an organ or tissue.

fulguration. Destruction of living tissue by using sparks from a high-frequency electric current.

incision. Act of cutting into tissue or an organ.

malignant. Any condition tending to progress toward death, specifically an invasive tumor with a loss of cellular differentiation that has the ability to spread or metastasize to other body areas.

neoplasm. New abnormal growth, tumor.

prostate. Male gland surrounding the bladder neck and urethra that secretes a substance into the seminal fluid.

secondary. Second in order of occurrence or importance, or appearing during the course of another disease or condition.

tumor. Pathological swelling or enlargement; a neoplastic growth of uncontrolled, abnormal multiplication of cells.

urethra. Small tube lined with mucous membrane that leads from the bladder to the exterior of the body.

Urethra

CPT © 2020 American Medical Association. All Rights Reserved.   ● New   ▲ Revised   + Add On   ★ Telemedicine   AMA: CPT Assist   [Resequenced]   ☑ Laterality   © 2020 Optum360, LLC

53230-53240

53230 Excision of urethral diverticulum (separate procedure); female
53235   male
53240 Marsupialization of urethral diverticulum, male or female

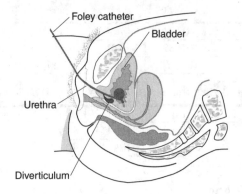

Explanation

The physician removes a urethral diverticulum. In a female patient, a longitudinal incision is made in the anterior vaginal wall and the urethral diverticulum is separated from the vaginal wall by a combination of blunt and sharp dissection. The urethra may be opened back to the orifice of the diverticulum in order to facilitate identification. A balloon catheter may be inserted and inflated. Once the diverticulum has been excised, the urethra is closed over a catheter and the vaginal wall is repaired with a layered closure. In a male patient, a cystourethroscope is inserted into the urethra and the diverticulum is excised through a transurethral incision. The physician may inject fluid or pass a balloon catheter into the diverticulum to allow it to be easily found and dissected. The diverticulum is isolated down to the neck and transected. The physician closes the urethra, leaving a catheter in the urethra. Report 53230 if performed on a female and 53235 if performed on a male. In 53240, the physician repairs a urethral diverticulum by creating a pouch (marsupialization). A longitudinal incision is made in the anterior vaginal wall of the female and the borders of the urethral diverticulum are raised and sutured to create a pouch. The interior of the sac separates and gradually closes by granulation. The urethra is closed over a catheter and the vaginal wall is repaired with a layered closure. In the male, a cystourethroscope is inserted into the urethra and the diverticulum treated in the same manner, but through the perineum.

Coding Tips

Note that 53230 and 53235, separate procedures by definition, are usually components of a more complex service and are not identified separately. When performed alone or with other unrelated procedures/services they may be reported. If performed alone, list the code; if performed with other procedures/services, list the code and append modifier 59 or an X{EPSU} modifier. Dilation or manipulation of the urethra or vagina is not reported separately. For urethroplasty for fistula or diverticulum, see 53400–53405. Report excision or fulguration of a urethra malignancy with 53220.

ICD-10-CM Diagnostic Codes

N36.1   Urethral diverticulum

AMA: **53230** 2014,Jan,11 **53235** 2014,Jan,11 **53240** 2014,Jan,11

Relative Value Units/Medicare Edits

Non-Facility RVU	Work	PE	MP	Total
53230	10.44	5.86	1.28	17.58
53235	10.99	6.03	1.25	18.27
53240	7.08	4.35	0.79	12.22
Facility RVU	Work	PE	MP	Total
53230	10.44	5.86	1.28	17.58
53235	10.99	6.03	1.25	18.27
53240	7.08	4.35	0.79	12.22

	FUD	Status	MUE	Modifiers				IOM Reference
53230	90	A	1(3)	51	N/A	62*	80	None
53235	90	A	1(3)	51	N/A	62*	80	
53240	90	A	1(3)	51	N/A	N/A	N/A	

* with documentation

Terms To Know

anterior. Situated in the front area or toward the belly surface of the body.

blunt dissection. Surgical technique used to expose an underlying area by separating along natural cleavage lines of tissue, without cutting.

catheter. Flexible tube inserted into an area of the body for introducing or withdrawing fluid.

diverticulum. Pouch or sac in the walls of an organ or canal.

excision. Surgical removal of an organ or tissue.

granulation. Formation of small, bead-like masses of cytoplasm or granules on the surface of healing wounds of an organ, membrane, or tissue.

marsupialization. Creation of a pouch in surgical treatment of a cyst in which one wall is resected and the remaining cut edges are sutured to adjacent tissue creating an open pouch of the previously enclosed cyst.

perineal. Pertaining to the pelvic floor area between the thighs; the diamond-shaped area bordered by the pubic symphysis in front, the ischial tuberosities on the sides, and the coccyx in back.

urethra. Small tube lined with mucous membrane that leads from the bladder to the exterior of the body.

53250

53250   Excision of bulbourethral gland (Cowper's gland)

The physician removes the Cowper's gland with
a transurethral incision or segmental incision

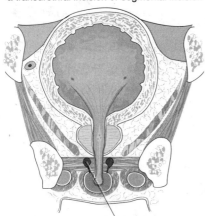

Bulbourethral gland (Cowper's gland)

Explanation

The physician excises a bulbourethral gland. A bulbourethral gland is located on each side of the prostate gland near the external sphincter and is connected to the urethra with a one-inch duct. The gland secretes what becomes part of the seminal fluid. The physician completes this procedure through transurethral or segmental resection with end-to-end sutures (anastomosis).

Coding Tips

This code is specific to males. Biopsy of the surgical site is incidental to the therapeutic procedure and not reported separately.

ICD-10-CM Diagnostic Codes

C68.0	Malignant neoplasm of urethra
C79.19	Secondary malignant neoplasm of other urinary organs
D09.19	Carcinoma in situ of other urinary organs
D30.4	Benign neoplasm of urethra
D41.3	Neoplasm of uncertain behavior of urethra
D49.59	Neoplasm of unspecified behavior of other genitourinary organ
N34.0	Urethral abscess
N34.2	Other urethritis
N36.8	Other specified disorders of urethra

AMA: 53250 2014,Jan,11

Relative Value Units/Medicare Edits

Non-Facility RVU	Work	PE	MP	Total
53250	6.52	4.14	0.76	11.42
Facility RVU	**Work**	**PE**	**MP**	**Total**
53250	6.52	4.14	0.76	11.42

	FUD	Status	MUE	Modifiers				IOM Reference
53250	90	A	1(3)	51	N/A	N/A	N/A	None

* with documentation

53260-53275

53260   Excision or fulguration; urethral polyp(s), distal urethra
53265   urethral caruncle
53270   Skene's glands
53275   urethral prolapse

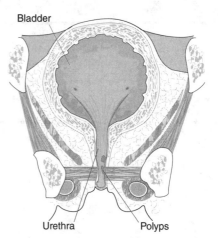

Bladder

Urethra   Polyps

The physician uses fulguration or
excision to remove a polyp

Explanation

The physician removes urethral polyps or caruncles in either sex, or in a female, removes Skene's glands or treats urethral prolapse. In a female, the physician separates the urethra from the vaginal wall. The urethra is incised. A circular excision is made around the lesion and the targeted tissue is resected. The urethra and vaginal mucosa are reattached in layers. In a male, the physician uses a transurethral approach to similarly excise the defect. Report 53260 if removing distal urethral polyps; 53265 if removing a urethral caruncle; 53270 if removing the Skene's glands; or 53275 if treating urethral prolapse.

Coding Tips

Report 52285 if fulguration of urethral polyps is part of treatment for female urethral syndrome. For drainage of an abscess of Skene's gland, see 53060. For fulguration of urethral tissue, a lesion, or a tumor through a cystourethroscope, see 52214, 52224, and 52285.

ICD-10-CM Diagnostic Codes

C68.1	Malignant neoplasm of paraurethral glands
C79.19	Secondary malignant neoplasm of other urinary organs
D09.19	Carcinoma in situ of other urinary organs
D30.8	Benign neoplasm of other specified urinary organs
D41.8	Neoplasm of uncertain behavior of other specified urinary organs
D49.59	Neoplasm of unspecified behavior of other genitourinary organ
N34.0	Urethral abscess
N36.2	Urethral caruncle
N36.8	Other specified disorders of urethra
Q64.71	Congenital prolapse of urethra

AMA: 53260 2014,Jan,11 **53265** 2014,Jan,11 **53270** 2014,Jan,11 **53275** 2014,Jan,11

Relative Value Units/Medicare Edits

Non-Facility RVU	Work	PE	MP	Total
53260	3.03	2.45	0.39	5.87
53265	3.17	2.87	0.41	6.45
53270	3.14	2.49	0.35	5.98
53275	4.57	2.47	0.54	7.58
Facility RVU	**Work**	**PE**	**MP**	**Total**
53260	3.03	1.8	0.39	5.22
53265	3.17	1.84	0.41	5.42
53270	3.14	1.81	0.35	5.3
53275	4.57	2.47	0.54	7.58

	FUD	Status	MUE	Modifiers				IOM Reference
53260	10	A	1(2)	51	N/A	N/A	N/A	None
53265	10	A	1(3)	51	N/A	N/A	N/A	
53270	10	A	1(2)	51	N/A	N/A	N/A	
53275	10	A	1(2)	51	N/A	N/A	N/A	

* with documentation

Terms To Know

abscess. Circumscribed collection of pus resulting from bacteria, frequently associated with swelling and other signs of inflammation.

anomaly. Irregularity in the structure or position of an organ or tissue.

approach. Method or anatomical location used to gain access to a body organ or specific area for procedures.

congenital. Present at birth, occurring through heredity or an influence during gestation up to the moment of birth.

defect. Imperfection, flaw, or absence.

distal. Located farther away from a specified reference point or the trunk.

excision. Surgical removal of an organ or tissue.

fulguration. Destruction of living tissue by using sparks from a high-frequency electric current.

lesion. Area of damaged tissue that has lost continuity or function, due to disease or trauma.

mucosa. Moist tissue lining the mouth (buccal mucosa), stomach (gastric mucosa), intestines, and respiratory tract.

polyp. Small growth on a stalk-like attachment projecting from a mucous membrane.

prolapse. Falling, sliding, or sinking of an organ from its normal location in the body.

resect. Cutting out or removing a portion or all of a bone, organ, or other structure.

Skene's gland. Paraurethral ducts that drain a group of the female urethral glands into the vestibule.

urethral caruncle. Small, polyp-like growth of a deep red color found in women on the mucous membrane of the urethral opening.

53400-53405

53400   Urethroplasty; first stage, for fistula, diverticulum, or stricture (eg, Johannsen type)

53405   second stage (formation of urethra), including urinary diversion

Physician reconstructs the urethra

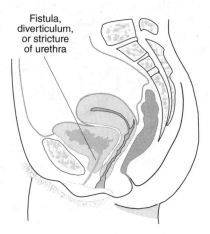

Fistula, diverticulum, or stricture of urethra

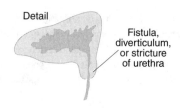

Detail

Fistula, diverticulum, or stricture of urethra

Explanation

The physician reconstructs the urethra in two stages. In the first stage (53400), the area of the stricture is identified by a catheter and urethrography and its location is marked with ink or dye. The incision is made over the stricture area and targeted tissue is removed. Otherwise, the stricture is opened widely and the normal skin of the male or female is sutured to the edge of the mucosa on each side. In those areas in which mucosa had to be removed, the skin is sutured edge-to-edge. Six to eight weeks are required for complete healing of this stage. In the second stage (53405), the physician makes parallel incisions around the defect and continues around the urethral opening both proximally and distally. The lateral skin edges are closed over an indwelling catheter to create a new urethra. The corpora and muscles are closed, respectively, becoming the new urethra structure.

Coding Tips

Report 53410 for reconstruction of the male anterior urethra in one stage. Report 53430 for reconstruction of the female urethra in one stage. See 54300–54352 for repair of hypospadias. Supplies used when providing these procedures may be reported with the appropriate HCPCS Level II code. Check with the specific payer to determine coverage.

ICD-10-CM Diagnostic Codes

N35.010	Post-traumatic urethral stricture, male, meatal ♂
N35.011	Post-traumatic bulbous urethral stricture ♂
N35.012	Post-traumatic membranous urethral stricture ♂
N35.013	Post-traumatic anterior urethral stricture ♂
N35.016	Post-traumatic urethral stricture, male, overlapping sites ♂
N35.111	Postinfective urethral stricture, not elsewhere classified, male, meatal ♂

N35.112	Postinfective bulbous urethral stricture, not elsewhere classified, male ♂	
N35.113	Postinfective membranous urethral stricture, not elsewhere classified, male ♂	
N35.114	Postinfective anterior urethral stricture, not elsewhere classified, male ♂	
N35.116	Postinfective urethral stricture, not elsewhere classified, male, overlapping sites ♂	
N35.811	Other urethral stricture, male, meatal ♂	
N35.812	Other urethral bulbous stricture, male ♂	
N35.813	Other membranous urethral stricture, male ♂	
N35.814	Other anterior urethral stricture, male ♂	
N35.816	Other urethral stricture, male, overlapping sites ♂	
N35.82	Other urethral stricture, female ♀	
N36.0	Urethral fistula	
N36.1	Urethral diverticulum	
N37	Urethral disorders in diseases classified elsewhere	
N99.110	Postprocedural urethral stricture, male, meatal ♂	
N99.111	Postprocedural bulbous urethral stricture, male ♂	
N99.112	Postprocedural membranous urethral stricture, male ♂	
N99.113	Postprocedural anterior bulbous urethral stricture, male ♂	
N99.115	Postprocedural fossa navicularis urethral stricture ♂	
N99.116	Postprocedural urethral stricture, male, overlapping sites ♂	
Q64.32	Congenital stricture of urethra	
Q64.39	Other atresia and stenosis of urethra and bladder neck	

AMA: 53400 2014,Jan,11 **53405** 2014,Jan,11

Relative Value Units/Medicare Edits

Non-Facility RVU	Work	PE	MP	Total
53400	14.13	7.39	1.64	23.16
53405	15.66	7.76	1.8	25.22
Facility RVU	Work	PE	MP	Total
53400	14.13	7.39	1.64	23.16
53405	15.66	7.76	1.8	25.22

	FUD	Status	MUE	Modifiers				IOM Reference
53400	90	A	1(2)	51	N/A	62*	80	None
53405	90	A	1(2)	51	N/A	62*	80	

* with documentation

Terms To Know

abscess. Circumscribed collection of pus resulting from bacteria, frequently associated with swelling and other signs of inflammation.

diverticulum. Pouch or sac in the walls of an organ or canal.

fistula. Abnormal tube-like passage between two body cavities or organs or from an organ to the outside surface.

stricture. Narrowing of an anatomical structure.

53410

53410 Urethroplasty, 1-stage reconstruction of male anterior urethra

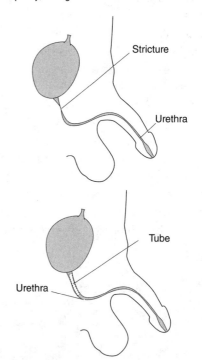

Physician repairs urethra by removing stricture through anterior incision, one-stage procedure

Explanation

The physician reconstructs the urethra of a male patient. The area of the urethral stricture is identified by catheterization. The physician cuts over the stricture area through the skin, fascia, corpus, and urethra. When the stricture is so severe that the urethral lumen cannot be identified, the physician removes the area involved. Otherwise, the stricture is opened widely and the normal skin is sutured to the edge of the mucosa on each side. In those areas in which the mucosa had to be removed, the skin is sutured edge-to-edge.

Coding Tips

This code is specific to males. Report 53400 for first-stage reconstruction for repair of a fistula, diverticulum, or stricture of the urethra. Report 53405 for second-stage reconstruction, including formation of the urethra and diversion of urine. Report 53430 for reconstruction of the female urethra in one stage. See 54300–54352 for repair of hypospadias. Urethral dilation or manipulation is not identified separately.

ICD-10-CM Diagnostic Codes

N35.010	Post-traumatic urethral stricture, male, meatal ♂	
N35.011	Post-traumatic bulbous urethral stricture ♂	
N35.012	Post-traumatic membranous urethral stricture ♂	
N35.013	Post-traumatic anterior urethral stricture ♂	
N35.016	Post-traumatic urethral stricture, male, overlapping sites ♂	
N35.111	Postinfective urethral stricture, not elsewhere classified, male, meatal ♂	
N35.112	Postinfective bulbous urethral stricture, not elsewhere classified, male ♂	
N35.113	Postinfective membranous urethral stricture, not elsewhere classified, male ♂	

CPT © 2020 American Medical Association. All Rights Reserved.   ● New   ▲ Revised   + Add On   ★ Telemedicine   AMA: CPT Assist   [Resequenced]   ☑ Laterality   © 2020 Optum360, LLC

N35.114	Postinfective anterior urethral stricture, not elsewhere classified, male ♂
N35.116	Postinfective urethral stricture, not elsewhere classified, male, overlapping sites ♂
N35.811	Other urethral stricture, male, meatal ♂
N35.812	Other urethral bulbous stricture, male ♂
N35.813	Other membranous urethral stricture, male ♂
N35.814	Other anterior urethral stricture, male ♂
N35.816	Other urethral stricture, male, overlapping sites ♂
N99.110	Postprocedural urethral stricture, male, meatal ♂
N99.111	Postprocedural bulbous urethral stricture, male ♂
N99.112	Postprocedural membranous urethral stricture, male ♂
N99.113	Postprocedural anterior bulbous urethral stricture, male ♂
N99.115	Postprocedural fossa navicularis urethral stricture ♂
N99.116	Postprocedural urethral stricture, male, overlapping sites ♂
Q64.32	Congenital stricture of urethra
Q64.39	Other atresia and stenosis of urethra and bladder neck

AMA: **53410** 2014,Jan,11

Relative Value Units/Medicare Edits

Non-Facility RVU	Work	PE	MP	Total
53410	17.68	8.56	2.02	28.26
Facility RVU	**Work**	**PE**	**MP**	**Total**
53410	17.68	8.56	2.02	28.26

	FUD	Status	MUE	Modifiers				IOM Reference
53410	90	A	1(2)	51	N/A	62*	80	None

* with documentation

Terms To Know

abscess. Circumscribed collection of pus resulting from bacteria, frequently associated with swelling and other signs of inflammation.

catheter. Flexible tube inserted into an area of the body for introducing or withdrawing fluid.

diverticulum. Pouch or sac in the walls of an organ or canal.

fascia. Fibrous sheet or band of tissue that envelops organs, muscles, and groupings of muscles.

fistula. Abnormal tube-like passage between two body cavities or organs or from an organ to the outside surface.

stricture. Narrowing of an anatomical structure.

53415

53415 Urethroplasty, transpubic or perineal, 1-stage, for reconstruction or repair of prostatic or membranous urethra

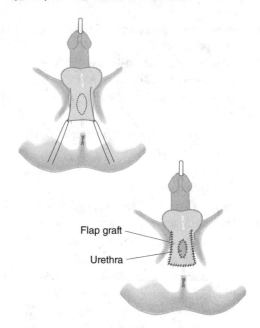

Flap graft
Urethra

Physician will use flap graft to complete repair

Explanation

The physician repairs the urethra. The stricture of the male perineal urethra is opened through a midline perineal or transpubic incision extending from the base of the scrotum to the anal margins. The physician makes an incision into the normal urethra distal to the stricture and opens the stricture on its ventral surface. From here a wide-based skin flap is developed by a U-shaped incision in the scrotum and advanced until it can be approximated to the posterior angle of the perineal incision without tension. The ends of the proximal and distal urethra are connected (anastomosis) to the extremities of the scrotal incision and anchored to the midline of the urethral bed to provide a stable urethral roof. When the urethra stricture has been opened but not excised, the edges of the longitudinal incision in the scrotal flap are sutured to the edges of the urethral wall. The outer edges of the flap are sutured to the edges of the original perineal skin incision.

Coding Tips

This code is specific to males. For two-stage reconstruction of prostatic or membranous urethra, see 53420–53425. Report 53410 for one-stage reconstruction of the male anterior urethra. Use 53430 for one-stage reconstruction of the female urethra. See 54300–54352 for repair of hypospadias. Dilation or manipulation of the urethra, prostate, and surrounding tissues is not separately identified. Free grafts are reported separately.

ICD-10-CM Diagnostic Codes

N35.010	Post-traumatic urethral stricture, male, meatal ♂
N35.011	Post-traumatic bulbous urethral stricture ♂
N35.012	Post-traumatic membranous urethral stricture ♂
N35.013	Post-traumatic anterior urethral stricture ♂
N35.016	Post-traumatic urethral stricture, male, overlapping sites ♂
N35.111	Postinfective urethral stricture, not elsewhere classified, male, meatal ♂

N35.112	Postinfective bulbous urethral stricture, not elsewhere classified, male ♂
N35.113	Postinfective membranous urethral stricture, not elsewhere classified, male ♂
N35.114	Postinfective anterior urethral stricture, not elsewhere classified, male ♂
N35.116	Postinfective urethral stricture, not elsewhere classified, male, overlapping sites ♂
N35.811	Other urethral stricture, male, meatal ♂
N35.812	Other urethral bulbous stricture, male ♂
N35.813	Other membranous urethral stricture, male ♂
N35.814	Other anterior urethral stricture, male ♂
N35.816	Other urethral stricture, male, overlapping sites ♂
N99.110	Postprocedural urethral stricture, male, meatal ♂
N99.111	Postprocedural bulbous urethral stricture, male ♂
N99.112	Postprocedural membranous urethral stricture, male ♂
N99.113	Postprocedural anterior bulbous urethral stricture, male ♂
N99.115	Postprocedural fossa navicularis urethral stricture ♂
N99.116	Postprocedural urethral stricture, male, overlapping sites ♂
Q64.32	Congenital stricture of urethra
Q64.39	Other atresia and stenosis of urethra and bladder neck

AMA: **53415** 2014,Jan,11

Relative Value Units/Medicare Edits

Non-Facility RVU	Work	PE	MP	Total
53415	20.7	9.57	2.37	32.64
Facility RVU	**Work**	**PE**	**MP**	**Total**
53415	20.7	9.57	2.37	32.64

	FUD	Status	MUE	Modifiers				IOM Reference
53415	90	A	1(2)	51	N/A	62*	80	None

* with documentation

Terms To Know

anastomosis. Surgically created connection between ducts, blood vessels, or bowel segments to allow flow from one to the other.

perineal. Pertaining to the pelvic floor area between the thighs; the diamond-shaped area bordered by the pubic symphysis in front, the ischial tuberosities on the sides, and the coccyx in back.

prostatic hypertrophy. Overgrowth of the normal prostate tissue.

reconstruction. Recreating, restoring, or rebuilding a body part or organ.

53420-53425

| 53420 | Urethroplasty, 2-stage reconstruction or repair of prostatic or membranous urethra; first stage |
| 53425 | second stage |

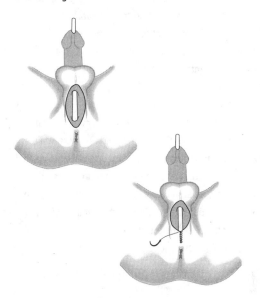

Two-stage urethroplasty requires
extensive reconstruction

Explanation

Urethroplasties are performed to open a stricture, repair trauma, or correct a prolapse. In the first stage, the physician identifies the injured area using a catheter or a urethrograph. The incision is made over the injury and carried through the skin, fat, and other tissues (fascia). If a urethral prolapse is involved, other incisions may be involved. The problem is repaired or excised and layered sutures are made to provide adequate support. A catheter is placed and left for at least six to 12 days. In the second stage, to close the urethra, the physician cuts around the urethral defect, using skin from the scrotal flap to make a urethra. The right size urethra must be constructed to allow a catheter and prevent obstructions. The physician pulls the loose skin around the urethra and closes the incisions. The first stage is 53420; report 53425 for the second stage.

Coding Tips

These codes are specific to males. Report 53415 for one-stage reconstruction of prostatic or membranous urethra. Report 53410 for one-stage reconstruction of the male anterior urethra. See 54300–54352 for repair of hypospadias. Report 53430 for reconstruction of the female urethra in one stage. Dilation or manipulation of the urethra is not reported separately.

ICD-10-CM Diagnostic Codes

N35.010	Post-traumatic urethral stricture, male, meatal ♂
N35.011	Post-traumatic bulbous urethral stricture ♂
N35.012	Post-traumatic membranous urethral stricture ♂
N35.013	Post-traumatic anterior urethral stricture ♂
N35.016	Post-traumatic urethral stricture, male, overlapping sites ♂
N35.111	Postinfective urethral stricture, not elsewhere classified, male, meatal ♂
N35.112	Postinfective bulbous urethral stricture, not elsewhere classified, male ♂

Urethra

N35.113	Postinfective membranous urethral stricture, not elsewhere classified, male ♂	
N35.114	Postinfective anterior urethral stricture, not elsewhere classified, male ♂	
N35.116	Postinfective urethral stricture, not elsewhere classified, male, overlapping sites ♂	
N35.811	Other urethral stricture, male, meatal ♂	
N35.812	Other urethral bulbous stricture, male ♂	
N35.813	Other membranous urethral stricture, male ♂	
N35.814	Other anterior urethral stricture, male ♂	
N35.816	Other urethral stricture, male, overlapping sites ♂	
N36.8	Other specified disorders of urethra	
N99.110	Postprocedural urethral stricture, male, meatal ♂	
N99.111	Postprocedural bulbous urethral stricture, male ♂	
N99.112	Postprocedural membranous urethral stricture, male ♂	
N99.113	Postprocedural anterior bulbous urethral stricture, male ♂	
N99.115	Postprocedural fossa navicularis urethral stricture ♂	
N99.116	Postprocedural urethral stricture, male, overlapping sites ♂	
Q64.32	Congenital stricture of urethra	
Q64.39	Other atresia and stenosis of urethra and bladder neck	

AMA: 53420 2014,Jan,11 **53425** 2014,Jan,11

Relative Value Units/Medicare Edits

Non-Facility RVU	Work	PE	MP	Total
53420	15.17	7.4	1.73	24.3
53425	17.07	8.03	1.95	27.05
Facility RVU	Work	PE	MP	Total
53420	15.17	7.4	1.73	24.3
53425	17.07	8.03	1.95	27.05

	FUD	Status	MUE	Modifiers				IOM Reference
53420	90	A	1(2)	51	N/A	62*	N/A	None
53425	90	A	1(2)	51	N/A	62*	80	

* with documentation

Terms To Know

catheter. Flexible tube inserted into an area of the body for introducing or withdrawing fluid.

defect. Imperfection, flaw, or absence.

fascia. Fibrous sheet or band of tissue that envelops organs, muscles, and groupings of muscles.

prolapse. Falling, sliding, or sinking of an organ from its normal location in the body.

stricture. Narrowing of an anatomical structure.

53430

53430   Urethroplasty, reconstruction of female urethra

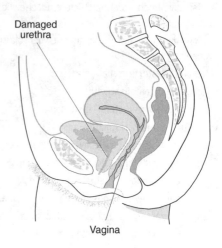

The physician, via a vaginal approach, constructs a new urethra using a flap of vaginal tissue

Explanation

The physician uses perineal or vaginal tissue to reconstruct the female urethra. With the patient in the lithotomy position and a catheter in the urethra, the physician cuts an inverted U-shaped flap above the urethral meatus and extending on the anterior vaginal wall. This flap is undermined with sharp dissection and spreading of the scissors around the upper portion of the urethral meatus, leaving a strip attached. The flap is sutured into a tube shape, reconstructing the distal urethra. The vaginal wall on each side is brought together in several layers to cover the new urethra. Small submucosal vessels are cauterized and a drain may be placed for one to two days.

Coding Tips

This code is specific to females. Report 53400 for first-stage reconstruction for repair of fistula, diverticulum, or stricture of the urethra. Report 53405 for second-stage reconstruction, including formation of the urethra and diversion of urine. For one-stage reconstruction of the male anterior urethra, see 53410. See 53415–53425 for reconstruction of prostatic or membranous urethra.

ICD-10-CM Diagnostic Codes

N35.021	Urethral stricture due to childbirth ♀	
N35.028	Other post-traumatic urethral stricture, female ♀	
N35.12	Postinfective urethral stricture, not elsewhere classified, female ♀	
N35.82	Other urethral stricture, female ♀	
N99.12	Postprocedural urethral stricture, female ♀	

AMA: 53430 2014,Jan,11

Relative Value Units/Medicare Edits

Non-Facility RVU	Work	PE	MP	Total
53430	17.43	8.41	2.23	28.07
Facility RVU	**Work**	**PE**	**MP**	**Total**
53430	17.43	8.41	2.23	28.07

	FUD	Status	MUE	Modifiers				IOM Reference
53430	90	A	1(2)	51	N/A	62*	80	None

* with documentation

Terms To Know

approach. Method or anatomical location used to gain access to a body organ or specific area for procedures.

catheter. Flexible tube inserted into an area of the body for introducing or withdrawing fluid.

cauterize. Heat or chemicals used to burn or cut.

dissection. Separating by cutting tissue or body structures apart.

distal. Located farther away from a specified reference point or the trunk.

drain. Device that creates a channel to allow fluid from a cavity, wound, or infected area to exit the body.

flap. Mass of flesh and skin partially excised from its location but retaining its blood supply that is moved to another site to repair adjacent or distant defects.

lithotomy position. Common position patients may be placed in for some surgical procedures and examinations involving the pelvis and/or lower abdomen. The patient is placed supine (on their back), hips and knees flexed, thighs apart, with feet supported in raised stirrups.

malignant. Any condition tending to progress toward death, specifically an invasive tumor with a loss of cellular differentiation that has the ability to spread or metastasize to other body areas.

meatus. Opening or passage into the body.

perineal. Pertaining to the pelvic floor area between the thighs; the diamond-shaped area bordered by the pubic symphysis in front, the ischial tuberosities on the sides, and the coccyx in back.

reconstruction. Recreating, restoring, or rebuilding a body part or organ.

stricture. Narrowing of an anatomical structure.

tissue. Group of similar cells with a similar function that form definite structures and organs. Tissue types include epithelial tissue, muscle tissue, connective tissue, and nervous tissue.

urethra. Small tube lined with mucous membrane that leads from the bladder to the exterior of the body.

53431

53431	Urethroplasty with tubularization of posterior urethra and/or lower bladder for incontinence (eg, Tenago, Leadbetter procedure)

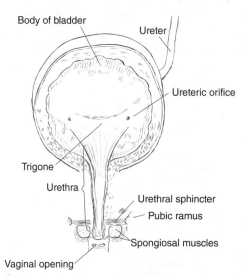

Frontal section of the female bladder, urethra, and select bone and musculature

The back wall of the urethra and/or the neck of the bladder are tubularized to address incontinence

Explanation

In the Tenago, Leadbetter procedure, the physician elongates the urethra by using bladder musculature. Continence is achieved due to contraction of the bladder musculature. The physician exposes the bladder through a suprapubic incision. The bladder is opened and the bladder neck incision is made 2 cm lateral to the urethra on each side. The musculature is drawn together in a tube and attached to the urethra. The urethral canal is closed in a two-layer technique. For the Tenago procedure, they are moved laterally.

Coding Tips

Report 53440 for a sling operation for correction of male urinary incontinence. Report 53445 if correction of urinary incontinence includes placement of inflatable urethral or bladder neck sphincter, pump, reservoir, and cuff. Free grafts are separately reported. Dilation and manipulation are not separately identified.

ICD-10-CM Diagnostic Codes

N35.010	Post-traumatic urethral stricture, male, meatal ♂
N35.011	Post-traumatic bulbous urethral stricture ♂
N35.012	Post-traumatic membranous urethral stricture ♂
N35.013	Post-traumatic anterior urethral stricture ♂
N35.016	Post-traumatic urethral stricture, male, overlapping sites ♂
N35.021	Urethral stricture due to childbirth ♀
N35.028	Other post-traumatic urethral stricture, female ♀
N35.111	Postinfective urethral stricture, not elsewhere classified, male, meatal ♂
N35.112	Postinfective bulbous urethral stricture, not elsewhere classified, male ♂
N35.113	Postinfective membranous urethral stricture, not elsewhere classified, male ♂
N35.114	Postinfective anterior urethral stricture, not elsewhere classified, male ♂

N35.116	Postinfective urethral stricture, not elsewhere classified, male, overlapping sites ♂
N35.12	Postinfective urethral stricture, not elsewhere classified, female ♀
N35.811	Other urethral stricture, male, meatal ♂
N35.812	Other urethral bulbous stricture, male ♂
N35.813	Other membranous urethral stricture, male ♂
N35.814	Other anterior urethral stricture, male ♂
N35.816	Other urethral stricture, male, overlapping sites ♂
N35.82	Other urethral stricture, female ♀
N37	Urethral disorders in diseases classified elsewhere
N39.3	Stress incontinence (female) (male)
N39.41	Urge incontinence
N39.42	Incontinence without sensory awareness
N39.43	Post-void dribbling
N39.44	Nocturnal enuresis
N39.45	Continuous leakage
N39.46	Mixed incontinence
N39.490	Overflow incontinence
N39.491	Coital incontinence
N39.492	Postural (urinary) incontinence
N39.498	Other specified urinary incontinence

AMA: 53431 2014,Jan,11

Relative Value Units/Medicare Edits

Non-Facility RVU	Work	PE	MP	Total
53431	21.18	9.72	2.42	33.32
Facility RVU	**Work**	**PE**	**MP**	**Total**
53431	21.18	9.72	2.42	33.32

	FUD	Status	MUE	Modifiers				IOM Reference
53431	90	A	1(2)	51	N/A	62*	80	100-03,230.10

* with documentation

Terms To Know

musculature. Entire muscle tissue apparatus of the body or a specific part of the body.

nocturnal enuresis. Bed-wetting.

posterior. Located in the back part or caudal end of the body.

urge incontinence. Involuntary escape of urine coming from sudden, uncontrollable impulses.

53440-53442

| 53440 | Sling operation for correction of male urinary incontinence (eg, fascia or synthetic) |
| 53442 | Removal or revision of sling for male urinary incontinence (eg, fascia or synthetic) |

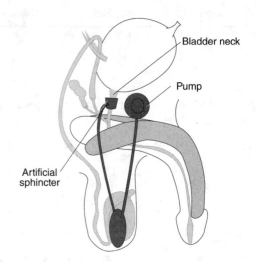

Physician removes artificial sphincter

Explanation

The physician produces a mechanical obstruction in the urethra or at the bladder neck to put pressure on the muscles, which will prevent leakage but still allows the patient to force urine. A small midline scrotal or penile incision is made to introduce a sling composed of fascia or synthetic material. The sling is placed across the muscles surrounding the urethra and anchored. Three screws on each side of the pelvic bone secure the sling. Tension of the sling is adjusted to obtain a stress pressure optimal for the patient. With the procedure completed, the incision is closed with layered sutures. Report 53442 when the physician removes the previously placed sling or accesses the site again for revision of the sling.

Coding Tips

These codes are specific to males. Report 53431 for tubularization of posterior urethra and/or lower bladder for correction of incontinence. For placement of inflatable urethral or bladder neck sphincter, pump, reservoir, and cuff, see 53445. For hypospadias repair, see 54300–54352. Dilation and manipulation of the urethra are necessary for this surgical procedure, although not separately identified. Supplies used when providing these procedures may be reported with the appropriate HCPCS Level II code. Check with the specific payer to determine coverage.

ICD-10-CM Diagnostic Codes

N39.3	Stress incontinence (female) (male)
N39.41	Urge incontinence
N39.42	Incontinence without sensory awareness
N39.43	Post-void dribbling
N39.44	Nocturnal enuresis
N39.45	Continuous leakage
N39.46	Mixed incontinence
N39.490	Overflow incontinence
N39.492	Postural (urinary) incontinence
N39.498	Other specified urinary incontinence

T83.111A	Breakdown (mechanical) of implanted urinary sphincter, initial encounter
T83.121A	Displacement of implanted urinary sphincter, initial encounter
T83.191A	Other mechanical complication of implanted urinary sphincter, initial encounter
T83.81XA	Embolism due to genitourinary prosthetic devices, implants and grafts, initial encounter
T83.82XA	Fibrosis due to genitourinary prosthetic devices, implants and grafts, initial encounter
T83.83XA	Hemorrhage due to genitourinary prosthetic devices, implants and grafts, initial encounter
T83.84XA	Pain due to genitourinary prosthetic devices, implants and grafts, initial encounter
T83.85XA	Stenosis due to genitourinary prosthetic devices, implants and grafts, initial encounter
T83.86XA	Thrombosis due to genitourinary prosthetic devices, implants and grafts, initial encounter
T83.89XA	Other specified complication of genitourinary prosthetic devices, implants and grafts, initial encounter

AMA: 53440 2020,Aug,6; 2014,Jan,11 **53442** 2020,Aug,6; 2014,Jan,11

Relative Value Units/Medicare Edits

Non-Facility RVU	Work	PE	MP	Total
53440	13.36	6.85	1.53	21.74
53442	13.49	7.58	1.55	22.62
Facility RVU	Work	PE	MP	Total
53440	13.36	6.85	1.53	21.74
53442	13.49	7.58	1.55	22.62

	FUD	Status	MUE	Modifiers				IOM Reference
53440	90	A	1(2)	51	N/A	62*	80	100-03,230.10
53442	90	A	1(2)	51	N/A	N/A	80	

* with documentation

Terms To Know

fascia. Fibrous sheet or band of tissue that envelops organs, muscles, and groupings of muscles.

incision. Act of cutting into tissue or an organ.

male stress incontinence. Involuntary escape of urine in men at times of minor stress against the bladder, such as coughing, sneezing, or laughing.

nocturnal enuresis. Bed-wetting.

revision. Reordering or rearrangement of tissue to suit a particular need or function.

sling operation. Procedure to correct urinary incontinence. A sling of fascia or synthetic material is placed under the junction of the urethra and bladder in females, or across the muscles surrounding the urethra in males.

stricture. Narrowing of an anatomical structure.

urge incontinence. Involuntary escape of urine coming from sudden, uncontrollable impulses.

53444

53444   Insertion of tandem cuff (dual cuff)

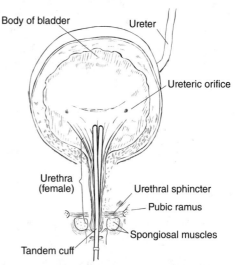

A tandem cuff is inserted into the urethra. The cuff may be used for a variety of treatment strategies

Explanation

A urethral retention catheter is placed in the bladder and a midline lower abdominal incision is made to gain access to the space of Retzius. The bladder neck and urethra are exposed and the plane between the bladder neck and urethra is dissected and the urethrovaginal septum is dissected at the midline attachment at the distance required for accommodating the tandem cuff. Having freed the bladder neck, the physician measures its circumference and the tandem cuff is placed in position around the bladder neck and the tubing brought up to the suprapubic area.

Coding Tips

Use this code for the placement of dual cuffs that are connected to existing tubing to replace an old cuff. For insertion of an inflatable urethral/bladder neck sphincter, including pump, reservoir, and cuff, see 53445. Supplies used when providing this procedure may be reported with the appropriate HCPCS Level II code. Check with the specific payer to determine coverage.

ICD-10-CM Diagnostic Codes

N39.3	Stress incontinence (female) (male)
N39.41	Urge incontinence
N39.42	Incontinence without sensory awareness
N39.43	Post-void dribbling
N39.44	Nocturnal enuresis
N39.45	Continuous leakage
N39.46	Mixed incontinence
N39.490	Overflow incontinence
N39.491	Coital incontinence
N39.492	Postural (urinary) incontinence
N39.498	Other specified urinary incontinence

AMA: 53444 2014,Jan,11

Urethra

CPT © 2020 American Medical Association. All Rights Reserved. ● New ▲ Revised + Add On ★ Telemedicine AMA: CPT Assist [Resequenced] ☑ Laterality © 2020 Optum360, LLC

Relative Value Units/Medicare Edits

Non-Facility RVU	Work	PE	MP	Total
53444	14.19	7.1	1.63	22.92
Facility RVU	Work	PE	MP	Total
53444	14.19	7.1	1.63	22.92

	FUD	Status	MUE	Modifiers				IOM Reference
53444	90	A	1(3)	51	N/A	62*	80	None

* with documentation

Terms To Know

atresia. Congenital closure or absence of a tubular organ or an opening to the body surface.

catheter. Flexible tube inserted into an area of the body for introducing or withdrawing fluid.

congenital. Present at birth, occurring through heredity or an influence during gestation up to the moment of birth.

dissection. Separating by cutting tissue or body structures apart.

male stress incontinence. Involuntary escape of urine in men at times of minor stress against the bladder, such as coughing, sneezing, or laughing.

mixed incontinence. Type of incontinence that reflects a combination of symptoms from two different types of incontinence: stress and urge incontinence. Stress urinary incontinence results from an increase of pressure on the bladder from actions such as coughing, laughing, or sneezing and urge incontinence is characterized by a sudden and strong need to urinate.

nocturnal enuresis. Bed-wetting.

septum. Anatomical partition or dividing wall.

stenosis. Narrowing or constriction of a passage.

stress incontinence. Involuntary escape of urine at times of minor stress against the bladder, such as coughing, sneezing, or laughing.

urge incontinence. Involuntary escape of urine coming from sudden, uncontrollable impulses.

53445

53445 Insertion of inflatable urethral/bladder neck sphincter, including placement of pump, reservoir, and cuff

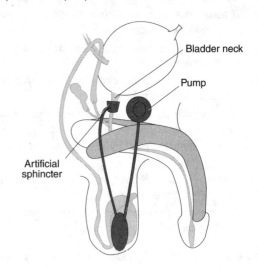

Explanation

The physician implants an artificial sphincter to stem urinary incontinence. In male patients, for whom the incontinence is caused by anything other than prostatic surgery, the prosthesis is inserted through a subpubic incision. For those patients who have undergone previous prostate surgery, the most common approach is perineal with the cuff typically placed around the urethra. In female patients, the sphincter is inserted through a suprapubic incision. The space of Retzius (between the bladder and the pubis) is opened and the bladder neck is cut free, making space for the device. The bladder neck circumference is measured and a cuff of slightly larger size is chosen and sutured around the bladder neck. A space is created below the skin low in the scrotum, and the control pump passed into this position from the subpubic incision. The pressure balloon is placed in a pocket behind the rectus muscle on the same side as the control pump. The physician injects fluid into the pressure balloon. In females, the plane between the bladder neck and vagina is dissected to provide access for reservoir placement. The pump is placed in the scrotum for male patients and in the labia or inner thigh for female patients.

Coding Tips

If significant additional time and effort is documented, append modifier 22 and submit a cover letter and operative report. For removal of inflatable urethral/bladder neck sphincter, pump, reservoir, and cuff, see 53446. For removal and replacement of inflatable urethral/bladder neck sphincter, pump, reservoir, and cuff, see 53447. For repair of inflatable urethral/bladder neck sphincter, pump, reservoir, and cuff, see 53449. Use 53440 for a sling operation for correction of male urinary incontinence. Use 53431 for tubularization of the posterior urethra and/or lower bladder for correction of incontinence. Supplies used when providing this procedure may be reported with the appropriate HCPCS Level II code. Check with the specific payer to determine coverage.

ICD-10-CM Diagnostic Codes

N39.3	Stress incontinence (female) (male)
N39.41	Urge incontinence
N39.42	Incontinence without sensory awareness
N39.43	Post-void dribbling
N39.44	Nocturnal enuresis

Urethra

© 2020 Optum360, LLC **N** Newborn: 0 **P** Pediatric: 0-17 **M** Maternity: 9-64 **A** Adult: 15-124 ♂ Male Only ♀ Female Only CPT © 2020 American Medical Association. All Rights Reserved.

Coding Companion for Urology/Nephrology

N39.45	Continuous leakage	
N39.46	Mixed incontinence	
N39.490	Overflow incontinence	
N39.491	Coital incontinence	
N39.492	Postural (urinary) incontinence	
N39.498	Other specified urinary incontinence	

AMA: 53445 2020,Aug,6; 2014,Jan,11

Relative Value Units/Medicare Edits

Non-Facility RVU	Work	PE	MP	Total
53445	13.0	7.29	1.48	21.77
Facility RVU	Work	PE	MP	Total
53445	13.0	7.29	1.48	21.77

	FUD	Status	MUE	Modifiers				IOM Reference
53445	90	A	1(2)	51	N/A	62*	80	100-03,230.10

* with documentation

Terms To Know

dissect. Cut apart or separate tissue for surgical purposes or for visual or microscopic study.

exstrophy of bladder. Congenital anomaly occurring when the bladder everts itself, or turns inside out, through an absent part of the lower abdominal and anterior bladder walls with incomplete closure of the pubic bone.

male stress incontinence. Involuntary escape of urine in men at times of minor stress against the bladder, such as coughing, sneezing, or laughing.

mixed incontinence. Type of incontinence that reflects a combination of symptoms from two different types of incontinence: stress and urge incontinence. Stress urinary incontinence results from an increase of pressure on the bladder from actions such as coughing, laughing, or sneezing and urge incontinence is characterized by a sudden and strong need to urinate.

nocturnal enuresis. Bed-wetting.

reservoir. Space or body cavity for storage of liquid.

urge incontinence. Involuntary escape of urine coming from sudden, uncontrollable impulses.

53446

53446	Removal of inflatable urethral/bladder neck sphincter, including pump, reservoir, and cuff

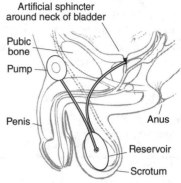

An inflatable urethral/bladder neck sphincter is removed, including pump, reservoir, and cuff

Explanation

In female patients, the physician makes a midline lower abdominal incision to gain access to the space of Retzius. The artificial urinary sphincter is exposed and the plane between the bladder neck and vagina is dissected. The device is removed and the opening is closed using suture for the rectus fascia. The subcutaneous tissues are closed and staples are used for skin closure. In male patients, the urethral bulb is exposed and the bulbospongiosus muscles are left intact over the urethra. The strap of the prosthesis is grasped under the crus and the muscle and the procedure is repeated distally to grasp the second lateral strap. The same maneuvers are repeated on the opposite site. The proximal straps are untied, as are the lateral straps. The incision is closed and a Foley catheter remains for several days.

Coding Tips

Report this code for removal of an entire artificial urethral/bladder neck incontinence system, including sphincter, pump, reservoir, and cuff, without replacement. For removal and replacement at the same operative session, see 53447. For removal and replacement through an infected operative field at the same session, see 53448. For repair of the inflatable urethral/bladder neck sphincter, pump, reservoir, and/or cuff, see 53449.

ICD-10-CM Diagnostic Codes

N99.81	Other intraoperative complications of genitourinary system
N99.89	Other postprocedural complications and disorders of genitourinary system
T83.111A	Breakdown (mechanical) of implanted urinary sphincter, initial encounter
T83.121A	Displacement of implanted urinary sphincter, initial encounter
T83.191A	Other mechanical complication of implanted urinary sphincter, initial encounter
T83.591A	Infection and inflammatory reaction due to implanted urinary sphincter, initial encounter
T83.598A	Infection and inflammatory reaction due to other prosthetic device, implant and graft in urinary system, initial encounter
T83.81XA	Embolism due to genitourinary prosthetic devices, implants and grafts, initial encounter
T83.82XA	Fibrosis due to genitourinary prosthetic devices, implants and grafts, initial encounter

Urethra

T83.83XA	Hemorrhage due to genitourinary prosthetic devices, implants and grafts, initial encounter
T83.84XA	Pain due to genitourinary prosthetic devices, implants and grafts, initial encounter
T83.85XA	Stenosis due to genitourinary prosthetic devices, implants and grafts, initial encounter
T83.86XA	Thrombosis due to genitourinary prosthetic devices, implants and grafts, initial encounter
T83.89XA	Other specified complication of genitourinary prosthetic devices, implants and grafts, initial encounter

AMA: 53446 2020,Aug,6; 2014,Jan,11

Relative Value Units/Medicare Edits

Non-Facility RVU	Work	PE	MP	Total
53446	11.02	6.25	1.26	18.53
Facility RVU	**Work**	**PE**	**MP**	**Total**
53446	11.02	6.25	1.26	18.53

	FUD	Status	MUE	Modifiers				IOM Reference
53446	90	A	1(2)	51	N/A	62*	80	None

* with documentation

Terms To Know

dissection. Separating by cutting tissue or body structures apart.

fascia. Fibrous sheet or band of tissue that envelops organs, muscles, and groupings of muscles.

Foley catheter. Temporary indwelling urethral catheter held in place in the bladder by an inflated balloon containing fluid or air.

subcutaneous tissue. Sheet or wide band of adipose (fat) and areolar connective tissue in two layers attached to the dermis.

53447

| 53447 | Removal and replacement of inflatable urethral/bladder neck sphincter including pump, reservoir, and cuff at the same operative session |

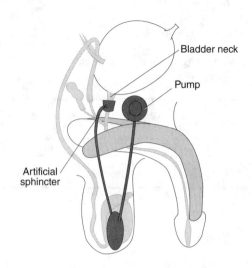

Explanation

The physician removes and replaces an artificial sphincter (including pump, reservoir, and cuff) used to stem urinary incontinence. In male patients for whom the incontinence is caused by anything other than prostatic surgery, the prosthesis is accessed through a subpubic incision. In female patients, the sphincter is accessed through a suprapubic incision. The sphincter and pump are examined, removed, and replaced. The bladder neck circumference is measured and a cuff of slightly larger size is chosen and positioned around the bladder neck. A space is created below the skin low in the scrotum and the control pump passed into this position from the subpubic incision. The pressure balloon is placed in a pocket behind the rectus muscle on the same side as the control pump. The physician injects fluid into the pressure balloon and the connections are permanently established. In females, the plane between the bladder neck and vagina is dissected.

Coding Tips

For initial insertion of inflatable urethral/bladder neck sphincter, pump, reservoir, and cuff, see 53445. For removal of inflatable urethral/bladder neck sphincter, pump, reservoir, and cuff, without replacement, see 53446. For removal and replacement of inflatable urethral/bladder neck sphincter, pump, reservoir, and cuff, through an infected operative field, see 53448. For repair of inflatable urethral/bladder neck sphincter, pump, reservoir, and cuff, see 53449.

ICD-10-CM Diagnostic Codes

N39.3	Stress incontinence (female) (male)
N39.41	Urge incontinence
N39.42	Incontinence without sensory awareness
N39.43	Post-void dribbling
N39.44	Nocturnal enuresis
N39.45	Continuous leakage
N39.46	Mixed incontinence
N39.490	Overflow incontinence
N39.491	Coital incontinence
N39.492	Postural (urinary) incontinence

Urethra

© 2020 Optum360, LLC   **N** Newborn: 0   **P** Pediatric: 0-17   **M** Maternity: 9-64   **A** Adult: 15-124   ♂ Male Only   ♀ Female Only   CPT © 2020 American Medical Association. All Rights Reserved.

N39.498	Other specified urinary incontinence
N99.81	Other intraoperative complications of genitourinary system
N99.89	Other postprocedural complications and disorders of genitourinary system
T83.111A	Breakdown (mechanical) of implanted urinary sphincter, initial encounter
T83.121A	Displacement of implanted urinary sphincter, initial encounter
T83.191A	Other mechanical complication of implanted urinary sphincter, initial encounter
T83.591A	Infection and inflammatory reaction due to implanted urinary sphincter, initial encounter
T83.598A	Infection and inflammatory reaction due to other prosthetic device, implant and graft in urinary system, initial encounter
T83.81XA	Embolism due to genitourinary prosthetic devices, implants and grafts, initial encounter
T83.82XA	Fibrosis due to genitourinary prosthetic devices, implants and grafts, initial encounter
T83.83XA	Hemorrhage due to genitourinary prosthetic devices, implants and grafts, initial encounter
T83.84XA	Pain due to genitourinary prosthetic devices, implants and grafts, initial encounter
T83.85XA	Stenosis due to genitourinary prosthetic devices, implants and grafts, initial encounter
T83.86XA	Thrombosis due to genitourinary prosthetic devices, implants and grafts, initial encounter
T83.89XA	Other specified complication of genitourinary prosthetic devices, implants and grafts, initial encounter
Z46.6	Encounter for fitting and adjustment of urinary device

AMA: 53447 2020,Aug,6; 2014,Jan,11

Relative Value Units/Medicare Edits

Non-Facility RVU	Work	PE	MP	Total
53447	14.28	7.41	1.64	23.33
Facility RVU	Work	PE	MP	Total
53447	14.28	7.41	1.64	23.33

	FUD	Status	MUE	Modifiers				IOM Reference
53447	90	A	1(2)	51	N/A	62*	80	100-03,230.10

* with documentation

Terms To Know

nocturnal enuresis. Bed-wetting.

prosthesis. Man-made substitute for a missing body part.

stress incontinence. Involuntary escape of urine at times of minor stress against the bladder, such as coughing, sneezing, or laughing.

urge incontinence. Involuntary escape of urine coming from sudden, uncontrollable impulses.

53448

53448 Removal and replacement of inflatable urethral/bladder neck sphincter including pump, reservoir, and cuff through an infected field at the same operative session including irrigation and debridement of infected tissue

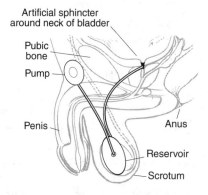

An inflatable urethral/bladder neck sphincter is removed due to infection caused by the apparatus (including pump, reservoir, and cuff). A new unit is placed during the same operative session

Explanation

In females, the vagina is prepared preoperatively and a urethral retention catheter is placed in the bladder. The patient is administered general anesthesia and placed supine. The physician makes a midline lower abdominal incision to gain access to the space of Retzius. The artificial urinary sphincter is exposed and the plane between the bladder neck and vagina is dissected. The device is removed. The area is irrigated with antibiotics and the physician debrides the infected tissue. Antibiotics are again used to flush the area. The tubing of the balloon of the replacement device is brought into the suprapubic area through a separate stab incision laterally in the rectus fascia. The control pump is passed through the suprapubic area through a subcutaneous track into the subcutaneous tissue of the ipsilateral labium. The device is emptied of fluid and a Hypaque solution is injected into the pressure balloon, using a 14-gauge blunt needle. The device components are connected, the pressure balloon is aspirated until empty, and the Hypaque solution is re-injected. Connections are completed between the control pump and cuff and reinforced by suture. The device is activated. The opening is closed using suture for the rectus fascia. The subcutaneous tissues are closed and staples are used for skin closure. In males, the patient is placed under general anesthesia in the lithotomy position. The urethral bulb is exposed and the bulbospongiosus muscles are left intact over the urethra. The strap of the prosthesis is grasped under the crus and the muscle and the procedure is repeated distally to grasp the second lateral strap. The same maneuvers are repeated on the opposite site. The proximal straps are untied, as are the lateral straps. The area is irrigated by antibiotic, and the infected tissue is debrided. The area is again flushed by antibiotic and the physician inserts the replacement pump using the same steps in the procedure for placement of the artificial sphincter described. The incision is closed and a Foley catheter is left indwelling for several days.

Coding Tips

Report this code for removal and replacement of an entire artificial urethral/bladder neck incontinence system, including sphincter, pump, reservoir, and cuff, through an infected operative field at the same session. For removal and replacement during the same operative session, not through an infected field, report 53447. For repair of the inflatable urethral/bladder neck sphincter, pump, reservoir, and/or cuff, report 53449. Do not report this code with 11042–11043.

Urethra

ICD-10-CM Diagnostic Codes

N39.3	Stress incontinence (female) (male)
N39.41	Urge incontinence
N39.42	Incontinence without sensory awareness
N39.43	Post-void dribbling
N39.44	Nocturnal enuresis
N39.45	Continuous leakage
N39.46	Mixed incontinence
N39.490	Overflow incontinence
N39.491	Coital incontinence
N39.492	Postural (urinary) incontinence
N39.498	Other specified urinary incontinence
N99.81	Other intraoperative complications of genitourinary system
N99.89	Other postprocedural complications and disorders of genitourinary system
T83.591A	Infection and inflammatory reaction due to implanted urinary sphincter, initial encounter
T83.598A	Infection and inflammatory reaction due to other prosthetic device, implant and graft In urinary system, initial encounter
T83.81XA	Embolism due to genitourinary prosthetic devices, implants and grafts, initial encounter
T83.82XA	Fibrosis due to genitourinary prosthetic devices, implants and grafts, initial encounter
T83.83XA	Hemorrhage due to genitourinary prosthetic devices, implants and grafts, initial encounter
T83.84XA	Pain due to genitourinary prosthetic devices, implants and grafts, initial encounter
T83.85XA	Stenosis due to genitourinary prosthetic devices, implants and grafts, initial encounter
T83.86XA	Thrombosis due to genitourinary prosthetic devices, implants and grafts, initial encounter
T83.89XA	Other specified complication of genitourinary prosthetic devices, implants and grafts, initial encounter

AMA: 53448 2020,Aug,6; 2014,Jan,11

Relative Value Units/Medicare Edits

Non-Facility RVU	Work	PE	MP	Total
53448	23.44	10.8	2.7	36.94
Facility RVU	Work	PE	MP	Total
53448	23.44	10.8	2.7	36.94

	FUD	Status	MUE	Modifiers				IOM Reference
53448	90	A	1(2)	51	N/A	62*	80	None

* with documentation

Terms To Know

debridement. Removal of dead or contaminated tissue and foreign matter from a wound.

irrigation. To wash out or cleanse a body cavity, wound, or tissue with water or other fluid.

tissue. Group of similar cells with a similar function that form definite structures and organs. Tissue types include epithelial tissue, muscle tissue, connective tissue, and nervous tissue.

53449

53449 Repair of inflatable urethral/bladder neck sphincter, including pump, reservoir, and cuff

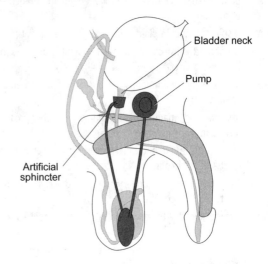

Bladder neck

Pump

Artificial sphincter

Explanation

The physician repairs an inability of an inflatable sphincter device to stem incontinence. In male patients the prosthesis is accessed through a subpubic incision. In female patients, the sphincter is accessed through a suprapubic incision. The space of Retzius (between the bladder and the pubis) is opened and the device is located. The physician checks the cuff and sutures around the bladder neck. The physician locates reservoir and checks for any malfunctions or abnormalities. The pressure balloon, usually located in a pocket behind the rectus muscle on the same side as the control pump, is evaluated for patency and function. Any necessary repairs are completed. The physician closes the incisions. The reservoir is filled and all connections are made. Several test inflations and deflations are performed during closure. The physician places a catheter in the bladder for about one day.

Coding Tips

For initial insertion of inflatable urethral/bladder neck sphincter, pump, reservoir, and cuff, see 53445. For removal of inflatable urethral/bladder neck sphincter, pump, reservoir, and cuff, without replacement, see 53446. For removal and replacement of inflatable urethral/bladder neck sphincter, pump, reservoir, and cuff, see 53447. For removal and replacement of inflatable urethral/bladder neck sphincter, pump, reservoir, and cuff, through an infected operative field, see 53448.

ICD-10-CM Diagnostic Codes

T83.111A	Breakdown (mechanical) of implanted urinary sphincter, initial encounter
T83.121A	Displacement of implanted urinary sphincter, initial encounter
T83.191A	Other mechanical complication of implanted urinary sphincter, initial encounter
T83.591A	Infection and inflammatory reaction due to implanted urinary sphincter, initial encounter
T83.598A	Infection and inflammatory reaction due to other prosthetic device, implant and graft in urinary system, initial encounter
T83.89XA	Other specified complication of genitourinary prosthetic devices, implants and grafts, initial encounter

AMA: 53449 2020,Aug,6; 2014,Jan,11

Urethra

Relative Value Units/Medicare Edits

Non-Facility RVU	Work	PE	MP	Total
53449	10.56	5.89	1.22	17.67
Facility RVU	**Work**	**PE**	**MP**	**Total**
53449	10.56	5.89	1.22	17.67

	FUD	Status	MUE	Modifiers				IOM Reference
53449	90	A	1(2)	51	N/A	62*	80	100-03,230.10

* with documentation

Terms To Know

catheter. Flexible tube inserted into an area of the body for introducing or withdrawing fluid.

male stress incontinence. Involuntary escape of urine in men at times of minor stress against the bladder, such as coughing, sneezing, or laughing.

nocturnal enuresis. Bed-wetting.

reservoir. Space or body cavity for storage of liquid.

stress incontinence. Involuntary escape of urine at times of minor stress against the bladder, such as coughing, sneezing, or laughing.

urge incontinence. Involuntary escape of urine coming from sudden, uncontrollable impulses.

53450-53460

53450 Urethromeatoplasty, with mucosal advancement
53460 Urethromeatoplasty, with partial excision of distal urethral segment (Richardson type procedure)

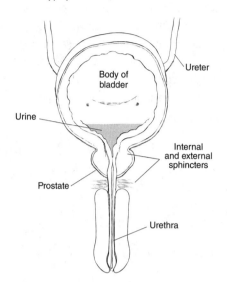

Explanation

The physician performs this surgery to open or reconstruct the urethra, improving voiding or allowing insertion of an instrument. The meatus, which may be congenitally small or narrowed as the result of infection, is opened and a mucosal flap is advanced and sutured to the glans in 53450. In 53460, the physician widens the meatus to enhance voiding. The physician makes an incision on the ventral surface of the penis and skin is freed from the shaft. Fibrous tissue is removed. An erection is artificially induced to confirm all fibrous tissue has been removed.

Coding Tips

Report 53020–53025 for incision of meatus (meatotomy) if performed as a separate procedure. Free grafts are reported separately. Any manipulation or dilation is not separately identified. For urethroplasty for hypospadias repair, see 54308–54318, 54324–54336, and 54344–54352.

ICD-10-CM Diagnostic Codes

N35.010	Post-traumatic urethral stricture, male, meatal ♂
N35.011	Post-traumatic bulbous urethral stricture ♂
N35.012	Post-traumatic membranous urethral stricture ♂
N35.013	Post-traumatic anterior urethral stricture ♂
N35.016	Post-traumatic urethral stricture, male, overlapping sites ♂
N35.021	Urethral stricture due to childbirth ♀
N35.028	Other post-traumatic urethral stricture, female ♀
N35.111	Postinfective urethral stricture, not elsewhere classified, male, meatal ♂
N35.112	Postinfective bulbous urethral stricture, not elsewhere classified, male ♂
N35.113	Postinfective membranous urethral stricture, not elsewhere classified, male ♂
N35.114	Postinfective anterior urethral stricture, not elsewhere classified, male ♂
N35.116	Postinfective urethral stricture, not elsewhere classified, male, overlapping sites ♂

CPT © 2020 American Medical Association. All Rights Reserved.   ● New   ▲ Revised   + Add On   ★ Telemedicine   AMA: CPT Assist   [Resequenced]   ☑ Laterality   © 2020 Optum360, LLC

N35.12	Postinfective urethral stricture, not elsewhere classified, female ♀
N35.811	Other urethral stricture, male, meatal ♂
N35.812	Other urethral bulbous stricture, male ♂
N35.813	Other membranous urethral stricture, male ♂
N35.814	Other anterior urethral stricture, male ♂
N35.816	Other urethral stricture, male, overlapping sites ♂
N35.82	Other urethral stricture, female ♀
N37	Urethral disorders in diseases classified elsewhere
N99.110	Postprocedural urethral stricture, male, meatal ♂
N99.111	Postprocedural bulbous urethral stricture, male ♂
N99.112	Postprocedural membranous urethral stricture, male ♂
N99.113	Postprocedural anterior bulbous urethral stricture, male ♂
N99.115	Postprocedural fossa navicularis urethral stricture ♂
N99.116	Postprocedural urethral stricture, male, overlapping sites ♂
N99.12	Postprocedural urethral stricture, female ♀
Q64.32	Congenital stricture of urethra
Q64.33	Congenital stricture of urinary meatus
Q64.39	Other atresia and stenosis of urethra and bladder neck

AMA: 53450 2018,Jan,8; 2017,Jan,8; 2016,Jan,13; 2015,Jan,16; 2014,Jan,11
53460 2014,Jan,11

Relative Value Units/Medicare Edits

Non-Facility RVU	Work	PE	MP	Total
53450	6.77	4.24	0.79	11.8
53460	7.75	4.57	0.88	13.2
Facility RVU	Work	PE	MP	Total
53450	6.77	4.24	0.79	11.8
53460	7.75	4.57	0.88	13.2

	FUD	Status	MUE	Modifiers				IOM Reference
53450	90	A	1(2)	51	N/A	N/A	N/A	None
53460	90	A	1(2)	51	N/A	N/A	80*	

* with documentation

Terms To Know

atresia. Congenital closure or absence of a tubular organ or an opening to the body surface.

balanoposthitis. Inflammation and/or infection of the glans penis and prepuce.

meatus. Opening or passage into the body.

stenosis. Narrowing or constriction of a passage.

urethral caruncle. Small, polyp-like growth of a deep red color found in women on the mucous membrane of the urethral opening.

53500

53500	Urethrolysis, transvaginal, secondary, open, including cystourethroscopy (eg, postsurgical obstruction, scarring)

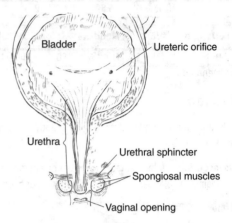

Scarring or obstructions along the urethra are addressed via vaginal approach

Explanation

Transvaginal, secondary, open urethrolysis is performed in cases when voiding is obstructed due to excessive periurethral scarring caused by previous surgical repair of stress incontinence, procedures such as bladder neck suspension. Urethrolysis involves cutting obstructive adhesions or bands of fibrous tissue that have grown to fix the urethra to the pubic bone. An incision is made through the vagina. The adhering fibrous bands and periurethral scar tissue are visualized and dissected. Lysis and removal continues until the urethra is mobilized away from the surrounding fibrous tissue. Some correction to vaginal abnormalities may be accomplished before closure of the incision. Postsurgical cystourethroscopy is included in this procedure to examine the urethra following urethrolysis.

Coding Tips

Postsurgical diagnostic cystourethroscopy is included in this procedure to examine the urethra following urethrolysis. For urethrolysis by retropubic approach, see 53899. Do not report 53500 with 52000.

ICD-10-CM Diagnostic Codes

N35.021	Urethral stricture due to childbirth ♀
N35.028	Other post-traumatic urethral stricture, female ♀
N35.12	Postinfective urethral stricture, not elsewhere classified, female ♀
N36.8	Other specified disorders of urethra
N37	Urethral disorders in diseases classified elsewhere
N99.12	Postprocedural urethral stricture, female ♀

AMA: 53500 2018,Jan,8; 2017,Jan,8; 2016,Jan,13; 2015,Jan,16; 2014,Jan,11

Relative Value Units/Medicare Edits

Non-Facility RVU	Work	PE	MP	Total
53500	13.0	6.96	1.69	21.65
Facility RVU	**Work**	**PE**	**MP**	**Total**
53500	13.0	6.96	1.69	21.65

	FUD	Status	MUE	Modifiers				IOM Reference
53500	90	A	1(2)	51	N/A	62*	80	None

* with documentation

Terms To Know

adhesion. Abnormal fibrous connection between two structures, soft tissue or bony structures, that may occur as the result of surgery, infection, or trauma.

connective tissue. Body tissue made from fibroblasts, collagen, and elastic fibrils that connects, supports, and holds together other tissues and cells and includes cartilage, collagenous, fibrous, elastic, and osseous tissue.

dissect. Cut apart or separate tissue for surgical purposes or for visual or microscopic study.

fibrous tissue. Connective tissues.

lysis. Destruction, breakdown, dissolution, or decomposition of cells or substances by a specific catalyzing agent.

obstruction. Blockage that prevents normal function of the valve or structure.

scar tissue. Fibrous connective tissue that forms around a wounded area or injury, composed mainly of fibroblasts or collagenous fibers.

secondary. Second in order of occurrence or importance, or appearing during the course of another disease or condition.

stricture. Narrowing of an anatomical structure.

urethra. Small tube lined with mucous membrane that leads from the bladder to the exterior of the body.

urethrolysis. Procedure performed to cut obstructive adhesions, fibrous bands, or periurethral scar tissue that affix the urethra to the pubic bone, obstructing voiding. This is often caused by previous surgical repair of stress incontinence, such as bladder neck suspension.

53502-53515

53502　Urethrorrhaphy, suture of urethral wound or injury, female
53505　Urethrorrhaphy, suture of urethral wound or injury; penile
53510　　perineal
53515　　prostatomembranous

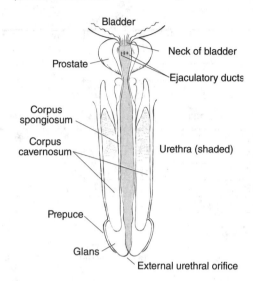

Explanation

The physician repairs a urethral wound or injury, including the skin and even more traumatic wounds requiring more than a layered closure. Examples include debridement of cuts (lacerations) or tears (avulsion). Suturing of the urethra is done in layers to prevent later complications and fistula formations. The tissue can be constructed around a catheter. Report 53502 if the patient is female; 53505 if the patient is male; 53510 if the wound in either sex is perineal; or 53515 if repair involves the prostate.

Coding Tips

Report 53020 if meatotomy is performed. For plastic repair and reconstruction of the female urethra, see 53430.

ICD-10-CM Diagnostic Codes

N99.71	Accidental puncture and laceration of a genitourinary system organ or structure during a genitourinary system procedure
N99.72	Accidental puncture and laceration of a genitourinary system organ or structure during other procedure
O71.5	Other obstetric injury to pelvic organs ⓜ ♀
S37.32XA	Contusion of urethra, initial encounter
S37.33XA	Laceration of urethra, initial encounter
S37.39XA	Other injury of urethra, initial encounter

AMA: **53502** 2014,Jan,11 **53505** 2014,Jan,11 **53510** 2014,Jan,11 **53515** 2014,Jan,11

Urethra

Relative Value Units/Medicare Edits

Non-Facility RVU	Work	PE	MP	Total
53502	8.26	4.82	0.93	14.01
53505	8.26	4.81	0.93	14.0
53510	10.96	6.02	1.25	18.23
53515	14.22	7.13	1.63	22.98
Facility RVU	Work	PE	MP	Total
53502	8.26	4.82	0.93	14.01
53505	8.26	4.81	0.93	14.0
53510	10.96	6.02	1.25	18.23
53515	14.22	7.13	1.63	22.98

	FUD	Status	MUE	Modifiers				IOM Reference
53502	90	A	1(3)	51	N/A	N/A	N/A	None
53505	90	A	1(3)	51	N/A	N/A	80	
53510	90	A	1(3)	51	N/A	62*	80	
53515	90	A	1(3)	51	N/A	62*	80	

* with documentation

Terms To Know

avulsion. Forcible tearing away of a part, by surgical means or traumatic injury.

catheter. Flexible tube inserted into an area of the body for introducing or withdrawing fluid.

debridement. Removal of dead or contaminated tissue and foreign matter from a wound.

injury. Harm or damage sustained by the body.

laceration. Tearing injury; a torn, ragged-edged wound.

perineal. Pertaining to the pelvic floor area between the thighs; the diamond-shaped area bordered by the pubic symphysis in front, the ischial tuberosities on the sides, and the coccyx in back.

suture. Numerous stitching techniques employed in wound closure.

tissue. Group of similar cells with a similar function that form definite structures and organs. Tissue types include epithelial tissue, muscle tissue, connective tissue, and nervous tissue.

urethrorrhaphy. Suture of urethral wound or injury.

wound. Injury to living tissue often involving a cut or break in the skin.

53520

53520   Closure of urethrostomy or urethrocutaneous fistula, male (separate procedure)

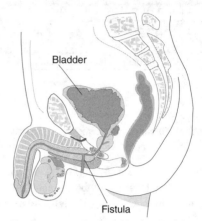

Bladder

Fistula

Fistula or stoma is closed by the physician

Explanation

The physician closes a urethrostomy or urethrocutaneous fistula. An elliptical incision is made around the opening of the urocutaneous fistula and carried deeper into the supporting tissue toward the urethra. The entire tract is freed and excised unless it involves other important structures, such as the external sphincters. When the tract cannot be completely removed, the remaining part is cut. The defect of the urethra is closed in layers over a catheter.

Coding Tips

This code is specific to males. This separate procedure by definition is usually a component of a more complex service and is not identified separately. When performed alone or with other unrelated procedures/services it may be reported. If performed alone, list the code; if performed with other procedures/services, list the code and append modifier 59 or an X{EPSU} modifier. Report 57310 for closure of a urethrovaginal fistula. Report 45820 or 45825 for closure or urethrorectal fistula.

ICD-10-CM Diagnostic Codes

N36.0   Urethral fistula

AMA: **53520** 2014,Jan,11

Relative Value Units/Medicare Edits

Non-Facility RVU	Work	PE	MP	Total
53520	9.48	5.52	1.08	16.08
Facility RVU	Work	PE	MP	Total
53520	9.48	5.52	1.08	16.08

	FUD	Status	MUE	Modifiers				IOM Reference
53520	90	A	1(3)	51	N/A	N/A	N/A	None

* with documentation

Terms To Know

defect. Imperfection, flaw, or absence.

fistula. Abnormal tube-like passage between two body cavities or organs or from an organ to the outside surface.

53600-53605

53600 Dilation of urethral stricture by passage of sound or urethral dilator, male; initial
53601   subsequent
53605 Dilation of urethral stricture or vesical neck by passage of sound or urethral dilator, male, general or conduction (spinal) anesthesia

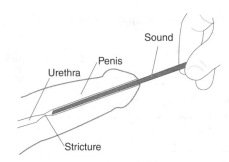

Physician passes sound past stricture

Explanation

When the physician examines the male patient, a soft rubbery urethral catheter is passed and the stricture is noted. If a stricture is found, a dilator is used. Report 53600 for the first visit and 53601 for subsequent visits. Report 53605 if spinal anesthesia is administered.

Coding Tips

These codes are specific to males. For dilation of the male urethral stricture by passage of filiform and follower, see 53620–53621. Report 74485 for radiological supervision and interpretation.

ICD-10-CM Diagnostic Codes

N35.010	Post-traumatic urethral stricture, male, meatal ♂
N35.011	Post-traumatic bulbous urethral stricture ♂
N35.012	Post-traumatic membranous urethral stricture ♂
N35.013	Post-traumatic anterior urethral stricture ♂
N35.016	Post-traumatic urethral stricture, male, overlapping sites ♂
N35.111	Postinfective urethral stricture, not elsewhere classified, male, meatal ♂
N35.112	Postinfective bulbous urethral stricture, not elsewhere classified, male ♂
N35.113	Postinfective membranous urethral stricture, not elsewhere classified, male ♂
N35.114	Postinfective anterior urethral stricture, not elsewhere classified, male ♂
N35.116	Postinfective urethral stricture, not elsewhere classified, male, overlapping sites ♂
N35.811	Other urethral stricture, male, meatal ♂
N35.812	Other urethral bulbous stricture, male ♂
N35.813	Other membranous urethral stricture, male ♂
N35.814	Other anterior urethral stricture, male ♂
N35.816	Other urethral stricture, male, overlapping sites ♂
N37	Urethral disorders in diseases classified elsewhere
N99.110	Postprocedural urethral stricture, male, meatal ♂
N99.111	Postprocedural bulbous urethral stricture, male ♂
N99.112	Postprocedural membranous urethral stricture, male ♂
N99.113	Postprocedural anterior bulbous urethral stricture, male ♂
N99.115	Postprocedural fossa navicularis urethral stricture ♂
N99.116	Postprocedural urethral stricture, male, overlapping sites ♂
Q64.32	Congenital stricture of urethra
Q64.39	Other atresia and stenosis of urethra and bladder neck

AMA: **53600** 2014,Jan,11 **53601** 2014,Jan,11 **53605** 2014,Jan,11

Relative Value Units/Medicare Edits

Non-Facility RVU	Work	PE	MP	Total
53600	1.21	1.09	0.13	2.43
53601	0.98	1.22	0.11	2.31
53605	1.28	0.44	0.15	1.87
Facility RVU	**Work**	**PE**	**MP**	**Total**
53600	1.21	0.49	0.13	1.83
53601	0.98	0.45	0.11	1.54
53605	1.28	0.44	0.15	1.87

	FUD	Status	MUE	Modifiers				IOM Reference
53600	0	A	1(3)	51	N/A	N/A	N/A	None
53601	0	A	1(3)	51	N/A	N/A	N/A	
53605	0	A	1(3)	51	N/A	N/A	N/A	

* with documentation

Terms To Know

catheter. Flexible tube inserted into an area of the body for introducing or withdrawing fluid.

congenital. Present at birth, occurring through heredity or an influence during gestation up to the moment of birth.

dilation. Artificial increase in the diameter of an opening or lumen made by medication or by instrumentation.

stricture. Narrowing of an anatomical structure.

urethra. Small tube lined with mucous membrane that leads from the bladder to the exterior of the body.

Urethra

CPT © 2020 American Medical Association. All Rights Reserved.   ● New   ▲ Revised   + Add On   ★ Telemedicine   AMA: CPT Assist   [Resequenced]   ☑ Laterality   © 2020 Optum360, LLC

53620-53621

53620 Dilation of urethral stricture by passage of filiform and follower, male; initial

53621 subsequent

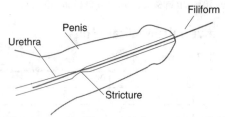

Physician passes a filiform and follower past a stricture

Explanation

The physician uses fine tools to dilate the male urethra. A filiform (a small silk-like instrument with woven spiral tips, to which followers made of a similar material can be attached by a screw-like mechanism) is used when a stricture cannot be passed. With a filiform as a guide, the follower is passed through the urethra. Increasing sizes of followers are introduced, dilating the stricture. The filiform is manipulated up a lubricated urethra to the stricture. The physician attaches a follower to the filiform and the stricture is widened. Report 53621 if it is a subsequent procedure.

Coding Tips

These codes are specific to males. The physician usually performs the procedures with local anesthesia. See 53600–53605 for dilation of the male urethral stricture by passage of sound or urethral dilator. Report 53660–53665 for dilation of the female urethra. Report 74485 for radiological supervision and interpretation.

ICD-10-CM Diagnostic Codes

N35.010	Post-traumatic urethral stricture, male, meatal ♂
N35.011	Post-traumatic bulbous urethral stricture ♂
N35.012	Post-traumatic membranous urethral stricture ♂
N35.013	Post-traumatic anterior urethral stricture ♂
N35.016	Post-traumatic urethral stricture, male, overlapping sites ♂
N35.111	Postinfective urethral stricture, not elsewhere classified, male, meatal ♂
N35.112	Postinfective bulbous urethral stricture, not elsewhere classified, male ♂
N35.113	Postinfective membranous urethral stricture, not elsewhere classified, male ♂
N35.114	Postinfective anterior urethral stricture, not elsewhere classified, male ♂
N35.116	Postinfective urethral stricture, not elsewhere classified, male, overlapping sites ♂
N35.811	Other urethral stricture, male, meatal ♂
N35.812	Other urethral bulbous stricture, male ♂
N35.813	Other membranous urethral stricture, male ♂
N35.814	Other anterior urethral stricture, male ♂
N35.816	Other urethral stricture, male, overlapping sites ♂
N37	Urethral disorders in diseases classified elsewhere
N99.110	Postprocedural urethral stricture, male, meatal ♂
N99.111	Postprocedural bulbous urethral stricture, male ♂
N99.112	Postprocedural membranous urethral stricture, male ♂
N99.113	Postprocedural anterior bulbous urethral stricture, male ♂
N99.115	Postprocedural fossa navicularis urethral stricture ♂
N99.116	Postprocedural urethral stricture, male, overlapping sites ♂
Q64.32	Congenital stricture of urethra
Q64.39	Other atresia and stenosis of urethra and bladder neck

AMA: 53620 2014,Jan,11 **53621** 2014,Jan,11

Relative Value Units/Medicare Edits

Non-Facility RVU	Work	PE	MP	Total
53620	1.62	2.42	0.18	4.22
53621	1.35	2.48	0.15	3.98
Facility RVU	**Work**	**PE**	**MP**	**Total**
53620	1.62	0.71	0.18	2.51
53621	1.35	0.57	0.15	2.07

	FUD	Status	MUE	Modifiers				IOM Reference
53620	0	A	1(2)	51	N/A	N/A	N/A	None
53621	0	A	1(3)	51	N/A	N/A	N/A	

* with documentation

Terms To Know

anterior. Situated in the front area or toward the belly surface of the body.

congenital. Present at birth, occurring through heredity or an influence during gestation up to the moment of birth.

dilation. Artificial increase in the diameter of an opening or lumen made by medication or by instrumentation.

filiform. Probe with woven-thread end.

fossa. Indentation or shallow depression.

stricture. Narrowing of an anatomical structure.

urethra. Small tube lined with mucous membrane that leads from the bladder to the exterior of the body.

Urethra

53660-53665

53660 Dilation of female urethra including suppository and/or instillation; initial

53661   subsequent

53665 Dilation of female urethra, general or conduction (spinal) anesthesia

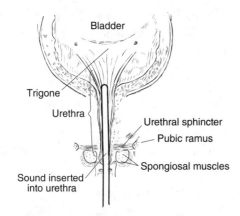

A urethral stricture in a female patient is dilated using a sound. A suppository may be inserted at the same time

Explanation

The physician uses dilators of increasing size to widen the female urethra. A suppository or instillation of a saline solution may be used. Report 53660 for initial dilation, and 53661 for subsequent dilation. Use 53665 if general or spinal anesthesia is administered for dilation of female urethral stricture.

Coding Tips

These codes are specific to females. The procedures include insertion of a suppository and/or instillation of a saline solution and are usually performed with local anesthesia. Report 53665 if dilation is done under general anesthesia. For dilation of urethra under local anesthesia, female, see 53660, 53661. For dilation of a male urethral stricture, see 53600–53621. For urethral catheterization, see 51701-51703.

ICD-10-CM Diagnostic Codes

N35.021	Urethral stricture due to childbirth ♀
N35.028	Other post-traumatic urethral stricture, female ♀
N35.12	Postinfective urethral stricture, not elsewhere classified, female ♀
N35.82	Other urethral stricture, female ♀
N99.12	Postprocedural urethral stricture, female ♀
Q64.31	Congenital bladder neck obstruction
Q64.32	Congenital stricture of urethra
Q64.39	Other atresia and stenosis of urethra and bladder neck

AMA: **53660** 2014,Jan,11 **53661** 2014,Jan,11 **53665** 2014,Jan,11

Relative Value Units/Medicare Edits

Non-Facility RVU	Work	PE	MP	Total
53660	0.71	1.22	0.09	2.02
53661	0.72	1.18	0.09	1.99
53665	0.76	0.26	0.09	1.11
Facility RVU	**Work**	**PE**	**MP**	**Total**
53660	0.71	0.4	0.09	1.2
53661	0.72	0.36	0.09	1.17
53665	0.76	0.26	0.09	1.11

	FUD	Status	MUE	Modifiers				IOM Reference
53660	0	A	1(2)	51	N/A	N/A	N/A	None
53661	0	A	1(3)	51	N/A	N/A	N/A	
53665	0	A	1(3)	51	N/A	N/A	N/A	

* with documentation

Terms To Know

atresia. Congenital closure or absence of a tubular organ or an opening to the body surface.

chronic interstitial cystitis. Persistently inflamed lesion of the bladder wall, usually accompanied by urinary frequency, pain, nocturia, and a distended bladder.

congenital. Present at birth, occurring through heredity or an influence during gestation up to the moment of birth.

dilation. Artificial increase in the diameter of an opening or lumen made by medication or by instrumentation.

instillation. Administering a liquid slowly over time, drop by drop.

obstruction. Blockage that prevents normal function of the valve or structure.

stenosis. Narrowing or constriction of a passage.

stricture. Narrowing of an anatomical structure.

suppository. Medication in the form of a solid mass at room temperature that dissolves at body temperature, for insertion into a body orifice such as the rectal, vaginal, or urethral opening.

urethra. Small tube lined with mucous membrane that leads from the bladder to the exterior of the body.

Urethra

53850-53852

53850 Transurethral destruction of prostate tissue; by microwave thermotherapy
53852 by radiofrequency thermotherapy

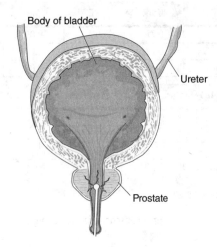

Body of bladder

Ureter

Prostate

A probe is extended up the urethra
and the prostate is treated

Explanation

In 53850, the physician performs transurethral destruction of prostate tissue by microwave thermotherapy. The physician inserts an endoscope in the penile urethra. Prior to endoscope placement, the urethra may need to be dilated to allow instrument passage. After the endoscope is passed, a microwave thermotherapy stylet is inserted in the urethra and the diseased prostate is treated with electromagnetic radiation. In 53852, the physician performs the same procedure using radiofrequency thermotherapy. An endoscope is inserted in the penile urethra. The urethra may be dilated to allow instrument passage. After the endoscope is placed, a radiofrequency thermotherapy stylet is inserted in the urethra and the diseased prostate is treated with radiant energy. In both procedures, the treated prostate is examined for evidence of bleeding, which may be controlled with electrocoagulation. The endoscope and instruments are removed. A urinary catheter is inserted into the bladder and left in place postoperatively.

Coding Tips

Although generally used to treat benign prostatic hypertrophy (BPH), these procedures may also be used to treat prostate cancer. For transurethral destruction of prostate tissue using radiofrequency generated water vapor thermotherapy, see 53854. For insertion of a temporary prostatic urethral stent with urethral measurement, see 53855; permanent, see 52282. For resection of the prostate through a cystourethroscope in one session, see 52601. For a two-stage transurethral resection of the prostate, report 52601 with modifier 58. For transurethral resection of obstructive prostate tissue, residual or regrowth, see 52630. For transurethral waterjet ablation of the prostate, see 0421T. For noncontact laser coagulation of the prostate, see 52647; contact laser vaporization of the prostate, with or without transurethral resection (endoscopic), see 52648. For open excisional procedures on the prostate gland, see 55801–55845.

ICD-10-CM Diagnostic Codes

C61	Malignant neoplasm of prostate ♂
C79.82	Secondary malignant neoplasm of genital organs
D07.5	Carcinoma in situ of prostate ♂
D29.1	Benign neoplasm of prostate ♂
D40.0	Neoplasm of uncertain behavior of prostate ♂
D49.59	Neoplasm of unspecified behavior of other genitourinary organ
N40.0	Benign prostatic hyperplasia without lower urinary tract symptoms 🄰 ♂
N40.1	Benign prostatic hyperplasia with lower urinary tract symptoms 🄰 ♂
N40.2	Nodular prostate without lower urinary tract symptoms 🄰 ♂
N40.3	Nodular prostate with lower urinary tract symptoms 🄰 ♂
N42.31	Prostatic intraepithelial neoplasia ♂
N42.32	Atypical small acinar proliferation of prostate ♂
N42.39	Other dysplasia of prostate ♂
N42.83	Cyst of prostate 🄰 ♂
N42.89	Other specified disorders of prostate 🄰 ♂

AMA: 53850 2018,Nov,10; 2018,Jan,8; 2017,Jan,8; 2016,Jan,13; 2015,Jun,5; 2015,Jan,16; 2014,Jan,11 **53852** 2018,Nov,10; 2018,Jan,8; 2017,Jan,8; 2016,Jan,13; 2015,Jun,5; 2015,Jan,16; 2014,Jan,11

Relative Value Units/Medicare Edits

Non-Facility RVU	Work	PE	MP	Total
53850	5.42	38.3	0.62	44.34
53852	5.93	36.41	0.66	43.0
Facility RVU	**Work**	**PE**	**MP**	**Total**
53850	5.42	4.06	0.62	10.1
53852	5.93	4.23	0.66	10.82

	FUD	Status	MUE	Modifiers				IOM Reference
53850	90	A	1(2)	51	N/A	N/A	N/A	None
53852	90	A	1(2)	51	N/A	N/A	N/A	

* with documentation

Terms To Know

catheter. Flexible tube inserted into an area of the body for introducing or withdrawing fluid.

coagulation. Clot formation.

destruction. Ablation or eradication of a structure or tissue.

dilation. Artificial increase in the diameter of an opening or lumen made by medication or by instrumentation.

endoscopy. Visual inspection of the body using a fiberoptic scope.

prostate. Male gland surrounding the bladder neck and urethra that secretes a substance into the seminal fluid.

radiofrequency ablation. To destroy by electromagnetic wave frequencies.

thermotherapy. Therapeutic elevation of body temperature between 107.6 and 113.0 degrees Fahrenheit.

urethra. Small tube lined with mucous membrane that leads from the bladder to the exterior of the body.

Urethra

53854

53854   Transurethral destruction of prostate tissue; by radiofrequency
         generated water vapor thermotherapy

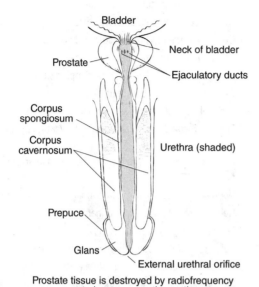

Prostate tissue is destroyed by radiofrequency
generated water vapor thermotherapy

Explanation

The physician performs transurethral destruction of prostate tissue by
radiofrequency generated water vapor thermotherapy. The physician inserts
an endoscope in the penile urethra. The urethra may be dilated to allow
instrument passage. After the endoscope is placed, a radiofrequency generated
water vapor thermotherapy stylet is inserted in the urethra and the diseased
prostate is treated with steam. The treated prostate is examined for evidence
of bleeding, which may be controlled with electrocoagulation. The endoscope
and instruments are removed. A urinary catheter is inserted into the bladder
and left in place postoperatively.

Coding Tips

Although generally used to treat benign prostatic hypertrophy (BPH), this
procedure may also be used to treat prostate cancer. Do not report 53854
with 52000, 64450, or 76872. For transurethral destruction of prostate tissue
using microwave thermotherapy, see 53850; radiofrequency thermotherapy,
see 53852. For insertion of a temporary prostatic urethral stent with urethral
measurement, see 53855; permanent, see 52282. For resection of the prostate
through a cystourethroscope in one session, see 52601. For a two-stage
transurethral resection of the prostate, report 52601 with modifier 58. For
transurethral resection of obstructive prostate tissue, residual or regrowth,
see 52630. For transurethral waterjet ablation of the prostate, see 0421T. For
transurethral ablation of malignant prostate tissue by high-energy water vapor
thermotherapy, see 0582T. For noncontact laser coagulation of the prostate,
see 52647; contact laser vaporization of the prostate, with or without
transurethral resection (endoscopic), see 52648. For open excisional procedures
on the prostate gland, see 55801–55845.

ICD-10-CM Diagnostic Codes

C61	Malignant neoplasm of prostate ♂
C79.82	Secondary malignant neoplasm of genital organs
D07.5	Carcinoma in situ of prostate ♂
D29.1	Benign neoplasm of prostate ♂
D40.0	Neoplasm of uncertain behavior of prostate ♂
D49.59	Neoplasm of unspecified behavior of other genitourinary organ
N40.0	Benign prostatic hyperplasia without lower urinary tract symptoms 🄰 ♂
N40.1	Benign prostatic hyperplasia with lower urinary tract symptoms 🄰 ♂
N40.2	Nodular prostate without lower urinary tract symptoms 🄰 ♂
N40.3	Nodular prostate with lower urinary tract symptoms 🄰 ♂
N42.30	Unspecified dysplasia of prostate ♂
N42.31	Prostatic intraepithelial neoplasia ♂
N42.32	Atypical small acinar proliferation of prostate ♂
N42.39	Other dysplasia of prostate ♂
N42.83	Cyst of prostate 🄰 ♂
N42.89	Other specified disorders of prostate 🄰 ♂

AMA: **53854** 2018,Nov,10

Relative Value Units/Medicare Edits

Non-Facility RVU	Work	PE	MP	Total
53854	5.93	44.6	0.65	51.18
Facility RVU	**Work**	**PE**	**MP**	**Total**
53854	5.93	4.23	0.65	10.81

	FUD	Status	MUE	Modifiers				IOM Reference
53854	90	A	1(2)	51	N/A	N/A	N/A	None

* with documentation

Terms To Know

benign. Mild or nonmalignant in nature.

carcinoma in situ. Malignancy that arises from the cells of the vessel, gland,
or organ of origin that remains confined to that site or has not invaded
neighboring tissue.

destruction. Ablation or eradication of a structure or tissue.

dysplasia. Abnormality or alteration in the size, shape, and organization of
cells from their normal pattern of development.

endoscopy. Visual inspection of the body using a fiberoptic scope.

malignant neoplasm. Any cancerous tumor or lesion exhibiting uncontrolled
tissue growth that can progressively invade other parts of the body with its
disease-generating cells.

prostate. Male gland surrounding the bladder neck and urethra that secretes
a substance into the seminal fluid.

thermotherapy. Therapeutic elevation of body temperature between 107.6
and 113.0 degrees Fahrenheit.

tissue. Group of similar cells with a similar function that form definite
structures and organs. Tissue types include epithelial tissue, muscle tissue,
connective tissue, and nervous tissue.

urethra. Small tube lined with mucous membrane that leads from the bladder
to the exterior of the body.

CPT © 2020 American Medical Association. All Rights Reserved.   ● New   ▲ Revised   + Add On   ★ Telemedicine   AMA: CPT Assist   [Resequenced]   ☑ Laterality   © 2020 Optum360, LLC

Urethra

53855

53855   Insertion of a temporary prostatic urethral stent, including urethral measurement

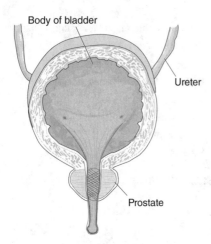

Body of bladder

Ureter

Prostate

A temporary stent is placed in the urethra at the prostate level

Explanation

A physician inserts a temporary urethral stent in a patient with prostatic urethral obstruction to improve voiding function. The stent system consists of a proximal balloon to prevent distal displacement, a urine port situated above the balloon, and the stent. Topical anesthesia is administered and the physician inserts the probe to locate the external sphincter. Once the external sphincter is located, a measurement is taken and the proper size stent selected. The stent device is mounted on a single-use insertion tool and standard catheter insertion technique is used to insert it. The proximal tip, balloon, and urine port are positioned in the bladder and the balloon is inflated with 5 cc of water. The insertion device is removed. A distal anchor mechanism is secured by sutures. A retrieval suture that extends to the meatus and deflates the balloon when pulled is also secured. The stent is typically left in place for up to 30 days.

Coding Tips

For insertion of a permanent urethral stent, see 52282. When this code is performed with another separately identifiable procedure, the highest dollar value code is listed as the primary procedure and the subsequent procedures are appended with modifier 51.

ICD-10-CM Diagnostic Codes

N32.0	Bladder-neck obstruction
N35.010	Post-traumatic urethral stricture, male, meatal ♂
N35.011	Post-traumatic bulbous urethral stricture ♂
N35.012	Post-traumatic membranous urethral stricture ♂
N35.013	Post-traumatic anterior urethral stricture ♂
N35.016	Post-traumatic urethral stricture, male, overlapping sites ♂
N35.111	Postinfective urethral stricture, not elsewhere classified, male, meatal ♂
N35.112	Postinfective bulbous urethral stricture, not elsewhere classified, male ♂
N35.113	Postinfective membranous urethral stricture, not elsewhere classified, male ♂
N35.114	Postinfective anterior urethral stricture, not elsewhere classified, male ♂
N35.116	Postinfective urethral stricture, not elsewhere classified, male, overlapping sites ♂
N35.811	Other urethral stricture, male, meatal ♂
N35.812	Other urethral bulbous stricture, male ♂
N35.813	Other membranous urethral stricture, male ♂
N35.814	Other anterior urethral stricture, male ♂
N35.816	Other urethral stricture, male, overlapping sites ♂
N36.8	Other specified disorders of urethra
N37	Urethral disorders in diseases classified elsewhere
N40.0	Benign prostatic hyperplasia without lower urinary tract symptoms 🅰 ♂
N40.1	Benign prostatic hyperplasia with lower urinary tract symptoms 🅰 ♂
N40.2	Nodular prostate without lower urinary tract symptoms 🅰 ♂
N40.3	Nodular prostate with lower urinary tract symptoms 🅰 ♂
N99.110	Postprocedural urethral stricture, male, meatal ♂
N99.111	Postprocedural bulbous urethral stricture, male ♂
N99.112	Postprocedural membranous urethral stricture, male ♂
N99.113	Postprocedural anterior bulbous urethral stricture, male ♂
N99.115	Postprocedural fossa navicularis urethral stricture ♂
N99.116	Postprocedural urethral stricture, male, overlapping sites ♂
Q64.31	Congenital bladder neck obstruction
Q64.32	Congenital stricture of urethra
Q64.33	Congenital stricture of urinary meatus
Q64.39	Other atresia and stenosis of urethra and bladder neck

AMA: **53855** 2018,Nov,10; 2018,Jan,8; 2017,Jan,8; 2016,Jan,13; 2015,Jun,5; 2015,Jan,16; 2014,Jan,11

Relative Value Units/Medicare Edits

Non-Facility RVU	Work	PE	MP	Total
53855	1.64	19.26	0.19	21.09
Facility RVU	**Work**	**PE**	**MP**	**Total**
53855	1.64	0.56	0.19	2.39

	FUD	Status	MUE	Modifiers				IOM Reference
53855	0	A	1(2)	51	N/A	N/A	80*	None

* with documentation

Terms To Know

distal. Located farther away from a specified reference point or the trunk.

meatus. Opening or passage into the body.

obstruction. Blockage that prevents normal function of the valve or structure.

stent. Tube to provide support in a body cavity or lumen.

stricture. Narrowing of an anatomical structure.

© 2020 Optum360, LLC   **N Newborn: 0**   **P Pediatric: 0-17**   **M Maternity: 9-64**   **A Adult: 15-124**   ♂ **Male Only**   ♀ **Female Only**   CPT © 2020 American Medical Association. All Rights Reserved.

Urethra

53860

53860   Transurethral radiofrequency micro-remodeling of the female bladder neck and proximal urethra for stress urinary incontinence

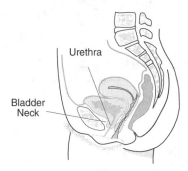

Urethra

Bladder Neck

Explanation

The physician uses radiofrequency energy to treat female stress urinary incontinence, the involuntary loss of urine from the urethra due to increased intra-abdominal pressure. Using a small transurethral probe, the physician applies low temperature radiofrequency energy to targeted submucosal areas of the bladder neck and urethra. This results in minute structural alterations to the collagen that, upon healing, makes the tissues firmer and increases the resistance to involuntary leakage.

Coding Tips

When this code is performed with another separately identifiable procedure, the highest dollar value code is listed as the primary procedure and the subsequent procedures are appended with modifier 51.

ICD-10-CM Diagnostic Codes

N39.3   Stress incontinence (female) (male)
N39.46   Mixed incontinence

AMA: **53860** 2014,Jan,11

Relative Value Units/Medicare Edits

Non-Facility RVU	Work	PE	MP	Total
53860	3.97	55.34	0.46	59.77
Facility RVU	**Work**	**PE**	**MP**	**Total**
53860	3.97	2.02	0.46	6.45

	FUD	Status	MUE	Modifiers				IOM Reference
53860	90	A	1(2)	51	N/A	N/A	80*	None

* with documentation

Terms To Know

female stress incontinence. Involuntary escape of urine at times of minor stress against the female bladder, such as coughing, sneezing, or laughing.

mixed incontinence. Type of incontinence that reflects a combination of symptoms from two different types of incontinence: stress and urge incontinence. Stress urinary incontinence results from an increase of pressure on the bladder from actions such as coughing, laughing, or sneezing and urge incontinence is characterized by a sudden and strong need to urinate.

Urethra

54000-54001

54000 Slitting of prepuce, dorsal or lateral (separate procedure); newborn
54001 except newborn

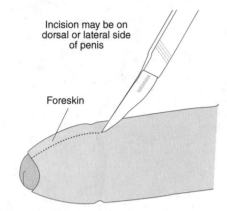

Incision may be on dorsal or lateral side of penis

Foreskin

The physician makes a cut in the foreskin to relieve constriction

Relative Value Units/Medicare Edits

Non-Facility RVU	Work	PE	MP	Total
54000	1.59	2.72	0.18	4.49
54001	2.24	3.04	0.27	5.55
Facility RVU	Work	PE	MP	Total
54000	1.59	1.35	0.18	3.12
54001	2.24	1.51	0.27	4.02

	FUD	Status	MUE	Modifiers				IOM Reference
54000	10	A	1(2)	51	N/A	N/A	80*	None
54001	10	A	1(2)	51	N/A	N/A	N/A	

* with documentation

Terms To Know

adhesion. Abnormal fibrous connection between two structures, soft tissue or bony structures, that may occur as the result of surgery, infection, or trauma.

constriction. Narrowed or squeezed portion of a tubular or luminal structure, such as a duct, vessel, or tube (e.g., esophagus). The narrowing can be a defect that is occurring naturally, or one that is surgically induced for therapeutic reasons.

dorsal. Pertaining to the back or posterior aspect.

forceps. Tool used for grasping or compressing tissue.

foreskin. Prepuce.

phimosis. Condition in which the foreskin is contracted and cannot be drawn back behind the glans penis.

prepuce. Fold of penile skin covering the glans.

retraction. Act of holding tissue or a structure back away from its normal position or the field of interest.

tissue. Group of similar cells with a similar function that form definite structures and organs. Tissue types include epithelial tissue, muscle tissue, connective tissue, and nervous tissue.

Explanation

The prepuce is the fold of penile skin commonly called the foreskin. The physician makes a cut or slit in the prepuce to relieve a constriction that prevents the retraction of the foreskin back over the head of the penis. A segment of foreskin on the dorsal or the side of the penis is crushed with forceps. Using scissors, the physician makes a cut through the crushed tissue and sutures the divided skin to control bleeding. The prepuce of a newborn is slit in 54000, while 54001 reports the slitting of the prepuce of any male other than a newborn.

Coding Tips

These separate procedures by definition are a component of a more complex service and usually are not identified separately. When performed alone or with other unrelated procedures/services they may be reported. If performed alone, list the code; if performed with other procedures/services, list the code and append modifier 59 or an X{EPSU} modifier. Do not append modifier 63 to 54000 as the description or nature of the procedure includes infants up to 4 kg. For plastic operation on the penis for chordee correction with prepuce transplantation, see 54304. For a circumcision using a clamp or other device, see 54150. For a circumcision, other than clamp, device, or dorsal slit, other than newborn, see 54161. For foreskin manipulation and lysis of adhesions, see 54450. Local or regional anesthesia is included in these services. Surgical trays, A4550, are not separately reimbursed by Medicare; however, other third-party payers may cover them. Check with the specific payer to determine coverage.

ICD-10-CM Diagnostic Codes

N47.0 Adherent prepuce, newborn ⬛ ♂
N47.1 Phimosis ♂
N47.2 Paraphimosis ♂
N47.5 Adhesions of prepuce and glans penis ♂
N47.8 Other disorders of prepuce ♂

AMA: 54000 2014,Jan,11 **54001** 2014,Jan,11

54015

54015   Incision and drainage of penis, deep

Sutures are required to repair the operative site

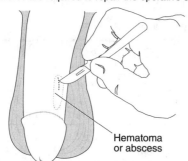

Hematoma
or abscess

A postoperative drain may be placed

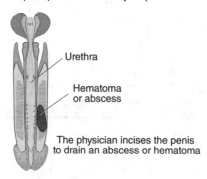

Urethra

Hematoma
or abscess

The physician incises the penis
to drain an abscess or hematoma

Explanation

The physician drains a deep abscess or hematoma (pocket of blood) by incising penile tissue. After instilling a local anesthesia, the physician makes an incision through the skin and deeper tissues into the abscessed cavity. The urethra and the main arteries and nerves are avoided. Often a drain is left in place to assure adequate drainage.

Coding Tips

Local or regional anesthesia is included in this service. However, general anesthesia may be administered depending on the age or condition of the patient. Report incision and drainage of a subcutaneous abscess, simple or single, with 10060; complicated or multiple, see 10061; hematoma, seroma, or fluid collection, see 10140; puncture aspiration for abscess, hematoma, bulla, or cyst, see 10160. For incision and removal of a subcutaneous foreign body, simple, see 10120; complicated, see 10121. If a specimen is transported to an outside laboratory, report 99000 for handling or conveyance. Surgical trays, A4550, are not separately reimbursed by Medicare; however, other third-party payers may cover them. Check with the specific payer to determine coverage.

ICD-10-CM Diagnostic Codes

A54.1	Gonococcal infection of lower genitourinary tract with periurethral and accessory gland abscess
N48.21	Abscess of corpus cavernosum and penis ♂
N48.22	Cellulitis of corpus cavernosum and penis ♂
N48.29	Other inflammatory disorders of penis ♂
N48.5	Ulcer of penis ♂

AMA: **54015** 2014,Jan,11

Relative Value Units/Medicare Edits

Non-Facility RVU	Work	PE	MP	Total
54015	5.36	2.85	0.62	8.83
Facility RVU	**Work**	**PE**	**MP**	**Total**
54015	5.36	2.85	0.62	8.83

	FUD	Status	MUE	Modifiers				IOM Reference
54015	10	A	1(3)	51	N/A	N/A	80*	None

* with documentation

Terms To Know

abscess. Circumscribed collection of pus resulting from bacteria, frequently associated with swelling and other signs of inflammation.

balanoposthitis. Inflammation and/or infection of the glans penis and prepuce.

drain. Device that creates a channel to allow fluid from a cavity, wound, or infected area to exit the body.

hematoma. Tumor-like collection of blood in some part of the body caused by a break in a blood vessel wall, usually as a result of trauma.

incision and drainage. Cutting open body tissue for the removal of tissue fluids or infected discharge from a wound or cavity.

suture. Numerous stitching techniques employed in wound closure.

tissue. Group of similar cells with a similar function that form definite structures and organs. Tissue types include epithelial tissue, muscle tissue, connective tissue, and nervous tissue.

54050-54065

54050 Destruction of lesion(s), penis (eg, condyloma, papilloma, molluscum contagiosum, herpetic vesicle), simple; chemical
54055 electrodesiccation
54056 cryosurgery
54057 laser surgery
54060 surgical excision
54065 Destruction of lesion(s), penis (eg, condyloma, papilloma, molluscum contagiosum, herpetic vesicle), extensive (eg, laser surgery, electrosurgery, cryosurgery, chemosurgery)

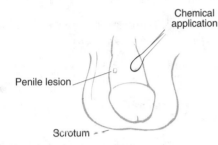

Penile lesions are destroyed

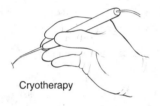

Cryotherapy

Explanation

The physician treats skin lesions of the penis by local application of a chemical (54050) or local electrodesiccation (54055) to kill the diseased tissue or organism. Using a cotton-tipped applicator soaked in the chemical or an electrodesiccator, the physician applies the treatment to the specific lesions only, taking care to avoid touching normal skin with the chemical or the electrodesiccator. Using either method, no tissue is removed and no closure is required.

Coding Tips

Local or regional anesthesia is included in the service. However, general anesthesia may be administered depending on the age or condition of the patient. If a specimen is transported to an outside laboratory, report 99000 for handling or conveyance. Surgical trays, A4550, are not separately reimbursed by Medicare; however, other third-party payers may cover them. Check with the specific payer to determine coverage.

ICD-10-CM Diagnostic Codes

A60.01	Herpesviral infection of penis ♂
A63.0	Anogenital (venereal) warts
B08.1	Molluscum contagiosum
C60.0	Malignant neoplasm of prepuce ♂
C60.1	Malignant neoplasm of glans penis ♂
C60.2	Malignant neoplasm of body of penis ♂
C60.8	Malignant neoplasm of overlapping sites of penis ♂
C63.8	Malignant neoplasm of overlapping sites of male genital organs ♂
C79.82	Secondary malignant neoplasm of genital organs
D07.69	Carcinoma in situ of other male genital organs ♂
D29.0	Benign neoplasm of penis ♂

AMA: **54050** 2014,Jan,11 **54055** 2014,Jan,11 **54056** 2014,Jan,11 **54057** 2014,Jan,11 **54060** 2014,Jan,11 **54065** 2014,Jan,11

Relative Value Units/Medicare Edits

Non-Facility RVU	Work	PE	MP	Total
54050	1.29	2.41	0.13	3.83
54055	1.25	2.21	0.13	3.59
54056	1.29	2.58	0.12	3.99
54057	1.29	2.52	0.13	3.94
54060	1.98	3.15	0.24	5.37
54065	2.47	3.54	0.26	6.27
Facility RVU	**Work**	**PE**	**MP**	**Total**
54050	1.29	1.57	0.13	2.99
54055	1.25	1.29	0.13	2.67
54056	1.29	1.71	0.12	3.12
54057	1.29	1.3	0.13	2.72
54060	1.98	1.52	0.24	3.74
54065	2.47	2.17	0.26	4.9

	FUD	Status	MUE	Modifiers				IOM Reference
54050	10	A	1(2)	51	N/A	N/A	N/A	100-03,140.5
54055	10	A	1(2)	51	N/A	N/A	N/A	
54056	10	A	1(2)	51	N/A	N/A	N/A	
54057	10	A	1(2)	51	N/A	N/A	N/A	
54060	10	A	1(2)	51	N/A	N/A	N/A	
54065	10	A	1(2)	51	N/A	N/A	N/A	

* with documentation

Terms To Know

condyloma. Infectious tumor-like growth caused by the human papilloma virus, with a branching connective tissue core and epithelial covering that occurs on the skin and mucous membranes of the perianal region and external genitalia.

cryosurgery. Application of intense cold, usually produced using liquid nitrogen, to locally freeze diseased or unwanted tissue and induce tissue necrosis without causing harm to adjacent tissue.

destruction. Ablation or eradication of a structure or tissue.

excision. Surgical removal of an organ or tissue.

laser surgery. Use of concentrated, sharply defined light beams to cut, cauterize, coagulate, seal, or vaporize tissue.

molluscum contagiosum. Common, benign, viral skin infection, usually self-limiting, that appears as a gray or flesh-colored umbilicated lesion by itself or in groups, and later becomes white with an expulsable core containing the replication bodies. It is often transmitted sexually in adults, by autoinoculation, or close contact in children.

54100-54105

54100 Biopsy of penis; (separate procedure)
54105   deep structures

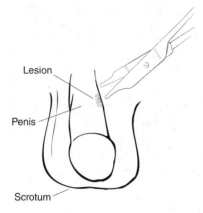

A biopsy of the penis is performed

Explanation

In 54100, the physician removes a portion of a skin lesion on the penis by punch biopsy or by excising a small portion of the lesion with scalpel or scissors. The resulting defect may require simple repair with sutures. In 54105, the physician removes a portion of a penile mass by deep punch biopsy or by making an incision in the penis and dissecting tissues to the deep mass and excising a portion of the lesion. The incision may be repaired with layered sutures.

Coding Tips

Note that 54100, a separate procedure by definition, is usually a component of a more complex service and is not identified separately. When performed alone or with other unrelated procedures/services it may be reported. If performed alone, list the code; if performed with other procedures/services, list the code and append modifier 59 or an X{EPSU} modifier. When these procedures are performed with another separately identifiable procedure, the highest dollar value code is listed as the primary procedure and subsequent procedures are appended with modifier 51. If the entire lesion is removed by surgical excision, see 54060. Local anesthesia is included in these services. However, these procedures may be performed under general anesthesia, depending on the age and/or condition of the patient. If a specimen is transported to an outside laboratory, report 99000 for handling or conveyance. Surgical trays, A4550, are not separately reimbursed by Medicare; however, other third-party payers may cover them. Check with the specific payer to determine coverage.

ICD-10-CM Diagnostic Codes

C60.0	Malignant neoplasm of prepuce ♂
C60.1	Malignant neoplasm of glans penis ♂
C60.2	Malignant neoplasm of body of penis ♂
C79.82	Secondary malignant neoplasm of genital organs
D07.4	Carcinoma in situ of penis ♂
D29.0	Benign neoplasm of penis ♂
D40.8	Neoplasm of uncertain behavior of other specified male genital organs ♂
D49.59	Neoplasm of unspecified behavior of other genitourinary organ
L40.8	Other psoriasis
N48.0	Leukoplakia of penis ♂

N48.5	Ulcer of penis ♂
N48.6	Induration penis plastica ♂
N48.81	Thrombosis of superficial vein of penis ♂
N48.82	Acquired torsion of penis ♂
N48.83	Acquired buried penis ♂
N48.89	Other specified disorders of penis ♂

AMA: **54100** 2019,Jan,9; 2018,Jan,8; 2017,Jan,8; 2016,Jan,13; 2015,Jan,16; 2014,Jan,11 **54105** 2014,Jan,11

Relative Value Units/Medicare Edits

Non-Facility RVU	Work	PE	MP	Total
54100	1.9	3.58	0.19	5.67
54105	3.54	3.79	0.41	7.74
Facility RVU	**Work**	**PE**	**MP**	**Total**
54100	1.9	1.41	0.19	3.5
54105	3.54	2.18	0.41	6.13

	FUD	Status	MUE	Modifiers				IOM Reference
54100	0	A	2(3)	51	N/A	N/A	N/A	None
54105	10	A	2(3)	51	N/A	N/A	N/A	

* with documentation

Terms To Know

benign lesion. Neoplasm or change in tissue that is not cancerous (nonmalignant).

biopsy. Tissue or fluid removed for diagnostic purposes through analysis of the cells in the biopsy material.

defect. Imperfection, flaw, or absence.

dissection. Separating by cutting tissue or body structures apart.

granuloma. Abnormal, dense collections or cells forming a mass or nodule of chronically inflamed tissue with granulations that is usually associated with an infective process.

lesion. Area of damaged tissue that has lost continuity or function, due to disease or trauma.

leukoplakia. Thickened white patches or lesions appearing on a mucous membrane, such as oral mucosa or tongue.

neoplasm. New abnormal growth, tumor.

pyogenic granuloma. Small, erythematous papule on the skin and oral or gingival mucosa that increases in size and may become pendulum-like, infected, and/or ulcerated.

thrombosis. Condition arising from the presence or formation of blood clots within a blood vessel that may cause vascular obstruction and insufficient oxygenation.

CPT © 2020 American Medical Association. All Rights Reserved.   ● **New**   ▲ **Revised**   + **Add On**   ★ **Telemedicine**   **AMA: CPT Assist**   [**Resequenced**]   ☑ **Laterality**   © 2020 Optum360, LLC

54110-54112

54110 Excision of penile plaque (Peyronie disease);
54111   with graft to 5 cm in length
54112   with graft greater than 5 cm in length

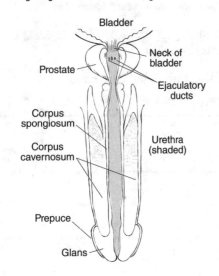

Explanation

Peyronie's disease is an induration and severe curvature of the erect penis due to fibrosis of the cavernous sheaths. The physician corrects Peyronie's disease by excising abnormal fibrous tissue on the dorsal aspect of the penis. After an incision is made around the penis, the physician retracts the skin to expose the abnormal tissue on the underlying normal spongy tissue. Avoiding critical nerves and blood vessels, with the penis erect, the defective tissue is excised. The skin is closed by suturing. Report 54111 if a graft measuring 5 cm or less in length is required; report 54112 if a graft greater than 5 cm is required.

Coding Tips

When 54110, 54111, or 54112 is performed with another separately identifiable procedure, the highest dollar value code is listed as the primary procedure and subsequent procedures are appended with modifier 51. The removal of multiple plaques is common practice and is included in 54110–54112.

ICD-10-CM Diagnostic Codes

N48.6   Induration penis plastica ♂

AMA: 54110 2014,Jan,11 **54111** 2018,Jan,8; 2017,Jan,8; 2016,Jan,13; 2015,Jan,16; 2014,Jan,11 **54112** 2014,Jan,11

Relative Value Units/Medicare Edits

Non-Facility RVU	Work	PE	MP	Total
54110	10.92	5.85	1.25	18.02
54111	14.42	7.04	1.65	23.11
54112	16.98	8.15	1.94	27.07
Facility RVU	**Work**	**PE**	**MP**	**Total**
54110	10.92	5.85	1.25	18.02
54111	14.42	7.04	1.65	23.11
54112	16.98	8.15	1.94	27.07

	FUD	Status	MUE	Modifiers				IOM Reference
54110	90	A	1(2)	51	N/A	N/A	80	None
54111	90	A	1(2)	51	N/A	62*	80	
54112	90	A	1(3)	51	N/A	62*	80	

* with documentation

Terms To Know

dorsal. Pertaining to the back or posterior aspect.

excision. Surgical removal of an organ or tissue.

fibrosis. Formation of fibrous tissue as part of the restorative process.

graft. Tissue implant from another part of the body or another person.

implant. Material or device inserted or placed within the body for therapeutic, reconstructive, or diagnostic purposes.

Peyronie's disease. Development of fibrotic hardened tissue or plaque in the cavernosal sheaths in the penis. This causes pain and a severe chordee or curvature in the penis, typically during erection.

retraction. Act of holding tissue or a structure back away from its normal position or the field of interest.

tissue. Group of similar cells with a similar function that form definite structures and organs. Tissue types include epithelial tissue, muscle tissue, connective tissue, and nervous tissue.

54115

54115 Removal foreign body from deep penile tissue (eg, plastic implant)

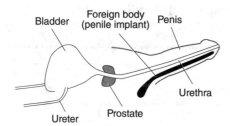

The physician removes a foreign body from deep tissues of the penis

Explanation

The physician removes a foreign body from deep within the shaft of the penis by making an incision and dissecting the tissues. The foreign body, usually a penile implant, is localized and removed. The resulting defect is closed with layered sutures.

Coding Tips

Code 54115 is used for removal of any foreign body from the deep penile tissue, such as a plastic implant or prosthesis. When 54115 is performed with another separately identifiable procedure, the highest dollar value code is listed as the primary procedure and subsequent procedures are appended with modifier 51. If significant additional time and effort is documented, append modifier 22 and submit a cover letter and operative report. For removal, repair, or replacement of a permanent inflatable, noninflatable, or multi-component prosthesis, see 54406–54417. Any manipulation or dilation is not reported separately. Local or regional anesthesia is included in the service. However, general anesthesia may be administered depending on the age or condition of the patient.

ICD-10-CM Diagnostic Codes

T19.4XXA	Foreign body in penis, initial encounter ♂
T83.410A	Breakdown (mechanical) of implanted penile prosthesis, initial encounter ♂
T83.411A	Breakdown (mechanical) of implanted testicular prosthesis, initial encounter
T83.420A	Displacement of implanted penile prosthesis, initial encounter ♂
T83.421A	Displacement of implanted testicular prosthesis, initial encounter
T83.490A	Other mechanical complication of implanted penile prosthesis, initial encounter ♂
T83.491A	Other mechanical complication of implanted testicular prosthesis, initial encounter
T83.61XA	Infection and inflammatory reaction due to implanted penile prosthesis, initial encounter
T83.62XA	Infection and inflammatory reaction due to implanted testicular prosthesis, initial encounter
T83.69XA	Infection and inflammatory reaction due to other prosthetic device, implant and graft in genital tract, initial encounter

AMA: 54115 2014,Jan,11

Relative Value Units/Medicare Edits

Non-Facility RVU	Work	PE	MP	Total
54115	6.95	5.34	0.79	13.08
Facility RVU	**Work**	**PE**	**MP**	**Total**
54115	6.95	4.5	0.79	12.24

	FUD	Status	MUE	Modifiers				IOM Reference
54115	90	A	1(3)	51	N/A	N/A	80	None

* with documentation

Terms To Know

defect. Imperfection, flaw, or absence.

dissection. Separating by cutting tissue or body structures apart.

foreign body. Any object or substance found in an organ and tissue that does not belong under normal circumstances.

implant. Material or device inserted or placed within the body for therapeutic, reconstructive, or diagnostic purposes.

infection. Presence of microorganisms in body tissues that may result in cellular damage.

inflammation. Cytologic and chemical reactions that occur in affected blood vessels and adjacent tissues in response to injury or abnormal stimulation from a physical, chemical, or biologic agent.

prosthesis. Man-made substitute for a missing body part.

tissue. Group of similar cells with a similar function that form definite structures and organs. Tissue types include epithelial tissue, muscle tissue, connective tissue, and nervous tissue.

54120-54125

54120   Amputation of penis; partial
54125   complete

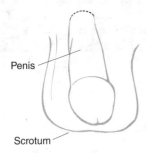

Penis

Scrotum

The penis is partially or completely amputated

Explanation

In both procedures, a portion of the penis (54120) or the complete penis (54125) is removed due to disease or mutilating injury. In 54120, the distal penis is enclosed in a rubber glove and a tourniquet is applied at the base of the penis. An incision is made completely around the penile shaft. The various structures of the penis are isolated and divided with care to leave enough of the urethra to form an opening for the passage of urine. The remaining tissues and skin are closed with layered sutures. In 54125, the distal penis is enclosed in a rubber glove and an incision is made from above the penis and carried around the base of the penile shaft and down through the midline of the scrotum. The various structures of the penis are isolated and divided with care to leave enough of the urethra for drainage. The urethra is brought through the perineum below the scrotum and an opening is created for the passage of urine. The remaining tissue and skin are closed in layered sutures with drains placed in the scrotum and a catheter in the bladder.

Coding Tips

Ligation, dissection, or debridement is not reported separately. For radical amputation or the penis, see 54130–54135. Report any free grafts or flaps separately.

ICD-10-CM Diagnostic Codes

C60.0   Malignant neoplasm of prepuce ♂
C60.1   Malignant neoplasm of glans penis ♂
C60.2   Malignant neoplasm of body of penis ♂
C60.8   Malignant neoplasm of overlapping sites of penis ♂
C79.82   Secondary malignant neoplasm of genital organs
D07.4   Carcinoma in situ of penis ♂
D29.0   Benign neoplasm of penis ♂
D40.8   Neoplasm of uncertain behavior of other specified male genital organs ♂
D49.59   Neoplasm of unspecified behavior of other genitourinary organ
S31.21XA   Laceration without foreign body of penis, initial encounter ♂
S31.22XA   Laceration with foreign body of penis, initial encounter ♂
S31.23XA   Puncture wound without foreign body of penis, initial encounter ♂
S31.24XA   Puncture wound with foreign body of penis, initial encounter ♂
S31.25XA   Open bite of penis, initial encounter ♂
S38.222A   Partial traumatic amputation of penis, initial encounter ♂
T21.36XA   Burn of third degree of male genital region, initial encounter ♂

T21.76XA   Corrosion of third degree of male genital region, initial encounter ♂

AMA: **54120** 2014,Jan,11 **54125** 2014,Jan,11

Relative Value Units/Medicare Edits

Non-Facility RVU	Work	PE	MP	Total
54120	11.01	5.95	1.27	18.23
54125	14.56	7.24	1.73	23.53
Facility RVU	Work	PE	MP	Total
54120	11.01	5.95	1.27	18.23
54125	14.56	7.24	1.73	23.53

	FUD	Status	MUE	Modifiers			IOM Reference
54120	90	A	1(2)	51	N/A	62*	80	None
54125	90	A	1(2)	51	N/A	62*	80	

* with documentation

Terms To Know

benign. Mild or nonmalignant in nature.

carcinoma in situ. Malignancy that arises from the cells of the vessel, gland, or organ of origin that remains confined to that site or has not invaded neighboring tissue.

dissection. Separating by cutting tissue or body structures apart.

distal. Located farther away from a specified reference point or the trunk.

drainage. Releasing, taking, or letting out fluids and/or gases from a body part.

ligation. Tying off a blood vessel or duct with a suture or a soft, thin wire.

malignant. Any condition tending to progress toward death, specifically an invasive tumor with a loss of cellular differentiation that has the ability to spread or metastasize to other body areas.

necrosis. Death of cells or tissue within a living organ or structure.

suture. Numerous stitching techniques employed in wound closure.

buried suture. Continuous or interrupted suture placed under the skin for a layered closure.

continuous suture. Running stitch with tension evenly distributed across a single strand to provide a leakproof closure line.

interrupted suture. Series of single stitches with tension isolated at each stitch, in which all stitches are not affected if one becomes loose, and the isolated sutures cannot act as a wick to transport an infection.

purse-string suture. Continuous suture placed around a tubular structure and tightened, to reduce or close the lumen.

retention suture. Secondary stitching that bridges the primary suture, providing support for the primary repair; a plastic or rubber bolster may be placed over the primary repair and under the retention sutures.

tissue. Group of similar cells with a similar function that form definite structures and organs. Tissue types include epithelial tissue, muscle tissue, connective tissue, and nervous tissue.

tourniquet. Device used to apply compressive force to a blood vessel in a limb and slow or prevent blood flow to and from the area.

54130-54135

54130   Amputation of penis, radical; with bilateral inguinofemoral lymphadenectomy

54135   in continuity with bilateral pelvic lymphadenectomy, including external iliac, hypogastric and obturator nodes

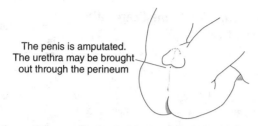

The penis is amputated. The urethra may be brought out through the perineum

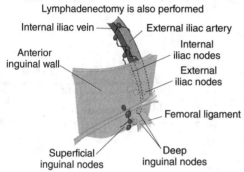

Lymphadenectomy is also performed

Internal iliac vein

External iliac artery

Internal iliac nodes

Anterior inguinal wall

External iliac nodes

Femoral ligament

Superficial inguinal nodes

Deep inguinal nodes

Explanation

The physician removes the entire penis and surrounding lymph nodes to treat invasive cancer. The distal penis is enclosed in a rubber glove. An incision is made from above the base of the penis and carried around the base of the penile shaft and down through the midline of the scrotum. The various structures of the penis are isolated and divided with care to leave enough of the urethra for drainage. The urethra is brought through the perineum below the scrotum and an opening is created for the passage of urine. The remaining tissues and skin are closed in layered sutures with drains placed in the scrotum and a catheter in the bladder. The physician also removes the lymph nodes in the groin areas. An incision is made from the pubic bone to the lateral pelvic bone exposing the area for dissection. The fatty tissues bearing the lymph nodes are removed. The defect is covered by rotating one of the thigh muscles over the area and suturing it in place. The subcutaneous tissues and the skin are closed in layered sutures over drains placed in the region. In 54135, a lower midline abdominal incision is made and the pelvic cavity is entered and the lymph nodes deep in the pelvis are removed. The abdominal incision is also closed in multiple layers of sutures.

Coding Tips

For amputation of the penis without lymphadenectomy, partial, see 54120; complete, see 54125. Lymphadenectomy procedures are reported with 38760–38770.

ICD-10-CM Diagnostic Codes

C60.0   Malignant neoplasm of prepuce ♂

C60.1   Malignant neoplasm of glans penis ♂

C60.2   Malignant neoplasm of body of penis ♂

C60.8   Malignant neoplasm of overlapping sites of penis ♂

C79.82   Secondary malignant neoplasm of genital organs

D40.8   Neoplasm of uncertain behavior of other specified male genital organs ♂

AMA: 54130 2014,Jan,11 54135 2014,Jan,11

Relative Value Units/Medicare Edits

Non-Facility RVU	Work	PE	MP	Total
54130	21.84	10.12	2.5	34.46
54135	28.17	12.27	3.24	43.68
Facility RVU	Work	PE	MP	Total
54130	21.84	10.12	2.5	34.46
54135	28.17	12.27	3.24	43.68

	FUD	Status	MUE	Modifiers				IOM Reference
54130	90	A	1(2)	51	N/A	62*	80	None
54135	90	A	1(2)	51	N/A	N/A	80	

* with documentation

Terms To Know

amputation. Removal of all or part of a limb or digit through the shaft or body of a bone.

carcinoma in situ. Malignancy that arises from the cells of the vessel, gland, or organ of origin that remains confined to that site or has not invaded neighboring tissue.

defect. Imperfection, flaw, or absence.

dissection. Separating by cutting tissue or body structures apart.

distal. Located farther away from a specified reference point or the trunk.

drain. Device that creates a channel to allow fluid from a cavity, wound, or infected area to exit the body.

lymph nodes. Bean-shaped structures along the lymphatic vessels that intercept and destroy foreign materials in the tissue and bloodstream.

lymphadenectomy. Dissection of lymph nodes free from the vessels and removal for examination by frozen section in a separate procedure to detect early-stage metastases.

malignant neoplasm. Any cancerous tumor or lesion exhibiting uncontrolled tissue growth that can progressively invade other parts of the body with its disease-generating cells.

prepuce. Fold of penile skin covering the glans.

radical. Extensive surgery.

secondary. Second in order of occurrence or importance, or appearing during the course of another disease or condition.

subcutaneous tissue. Sheet or wide band of adipose (fat) and areolar connective tissue in two layers attached to the dermis.

54150-54161

54150 Circumcision, using clamp or other device with regional dorsal penile or ring block
54160 Circumcision, surgical excision other than clamp, device, or dorsal slit; neonate (28 days of age or less)
54161   older than 28 days of age

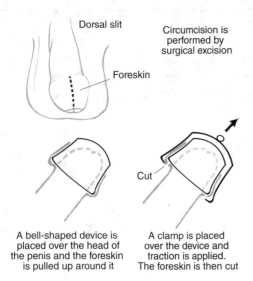

Dorsal slit

Circumcision is performed by surgical excision

Foreskin

Cut

A bell-shaped device is placed over the head of the penis and the foreskin is pulled up around it

A clamp is placed over the device and traction is applied. The foreskin is then cut

Explanation

After the administration of a local anesthetic by injection(s), the physician removes the foreskin of the penis by clamping the foreskin in a plastic device and trimming the excess protruding skin. A segment of foreskin on the dorsal or the side of the penis is crushed with forceps. A cut is made through the crushed tissue with scissors, and the divided foreskin is fitted in a plastic bell-shaped clamp. The clamp crushes a ring of the foreskin and holds the skin edges together while the excess skin is trimmed from the top of the device. The clamp is left in place and simply falls off when healing has finished days later. Alternately, the physician removes the foreskin of the penis in the baby up to 28 days of age (54160) or in a male older than 28 days (54161) by excision of the skin. A segment of foreskin on the dorsal or the side of the penis is crushed with forceps. A cut is made through the crushed tissue with scissors, and the divided foreskin is pulled down over the head of the penis while the excess skin is trimmed from around the head of the penis. Bleeding is controlled by chemical cautery or suture ligatures. The skin edges created are sutured together with absorbable suture material.

Coding Tips

Since these procedures usually are not done out of medical necessity, the patient may be responsible for charges. Verify with the insurance carrier for coverage. Append modifier 52 when the procedure is performed without a dorsal penile block or a ring block. Do not append modifier 63 to 54150 or 54160 as the description or nature of the procedure includes infants up to 4 kg. Any manipulation or dilation is not reported separately. Since these procedures usually are not done out of medical necessity, the patient may be responsible for charges. Verify with the insurance carrier for coverage. Local or regional anesthesia is included in these services. Do not report foreskin manipulation or lysis of adhesions (54450) with 54161.

ICD-10-CM Diagnostic Codes

N47.0   Adherent prepuce, newborn **N** ♂
N47.1   Phimosis ♂
N47.2   Paraphimosis ♂
N47.5   Adhesions of prepuce and glans penis ♂
N47.8   Other disorders of prepuce ♂
Z41.2   Encounter for routine and ritual male circumcision ♂

AMA: **54150** 2018,Jan,8; 2017,Jan,8; 2016,Jan,13; 2015,Jan,16; 2014,Jan,11 **54160** 2018,Jan,8; 2017,Jan,8; 2016,Jan,13; 2015,Jan,16; 2014,Jan,11 **54161** 2018,Jan,8; 2017,Jan,8; 2016,Jan,13; 2015,Jan,16; 2014,Jan,11

Relative Value Units/Medicare Edits

Non-Facility RVU	Work	PE	MP	Total
54150	1.9	2.25	0.25	4.4
54160	2.53	3.48	0.28	6.29
54161	3.32	1.97	0.39	5.68
Facility RVU	**Work**	**PE**	**MP**	**Total**
54150	1.9	0.69	0.25	2.84
54160	2.53	1.36	0.28	4.17
54161	3.32	1.97	0.39	5.68

	FUD	Status	MUE	Modifiers				IOM Reference
54150	0	A	1(2)	51	N/A	N/A	80ˣ	None
54160	10	A	1(2)	51	N/A	N/A	N/A	
54161	10	A	1(2)	51	N/A	N/A	N/A	

* with documentation

Terms To Know

absorbable sutures. Strands used for suture or repair of tissue prepared from collagen or a synthetic polymer and capable of being absorbed by tissue over time.

circumcise. Circular cutting around the genitals to remove the prepuce or foreskin.

clamp. Tool used to grip, compress, join, or fasten body parts.

dorsal. Pertaining to the back or posterior aspect.

forceps. Tool used for grasping or compressing tissue.

phimosis. Condition in which the foreskin is contracted and cannot be drawn back behind the glans penis.

prepuce. Fold of penile skin covering the glans.

tissue. Group of similar cells with a similar function that form definite structures and organs. Tissue types include epithelial tissue, muscle tissue, connective tissue, and nervous tissue.

54162

54162   Lysis or excision of penile post-circumcision adhesions

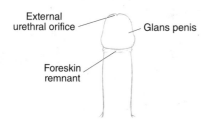

Adhesions of foreskin tissue are
lysed following circumcision

Explanation

The physician retracts the foreskin, releases the preputial post-circumcision adhesions, and cleanses the glans in a patient who is under general anesthesia. If retraction of the foreskin reveals a fibrous ring, the physician places two vertical incisions directly over the fibrous ring and the transversely running fibrous bands are divided to expose the underlying Bucks' fascia. With the foreskin retracted, the defect is closed horizontally with interrupted sutures.

Coding Tips

Use this code for post-circumcision adhesions only. For initial circumcision, see 54150–54161. For repair of an incomplete circumcision, report 54163. For lysis of preputial adhesions and stretching, see 54450.

ICD-10-CM Diagnostic Codes

N47.5   Adhesions of prepuce and glans penis ♂

AMA: 54162 2014,Jan,11

Relative Value Units/Medicare Edits

Non-Facility RVU	Work	PE	MP	Total
54162	3.32	3.68	0.39	7.39
Facility RVU	Work	PE	MP	Total
54162	3.32	2.04	0.39	5.75

	FUD	Status	MUE	Modifiers				IOM Reference
54162	10	A	1(2)	51	N/A	N/A	N/A	None

* with documentation

Terms To Know

adhesion. Abnormal fibrous connection between two structures, soft tissue or bony structures, that may occur as the result of surgery, infection, or trauma.

fibrosis. Formation of fibrous tissue as part of the restorative process.

lysis. Destruction, breakdown, dissolution, or decomposition of cells or substances by a specific catalyzing agent.

phimosis. Condition in which the foreskin is contracted and cannot be drawn back behind the glans penis.

prepuce. Fold of penile skin covering the glans.

54163

54163   Repair incomplete circumcision

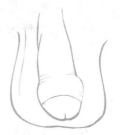

An unacceptable amount of foreskin
remains following circumcision

Foreskin tissues are excised following
an incomplete or partial circumcision

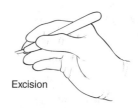

Excision

Explanation

A repeat circumcision may be performed if there is circumferential scarring of excessive residual skin or incomplete removal of the preputial skin during the initial circumcision. First, the skin at the base of the penis is cleansed with alcohol and allowed to dry. The physician uses an index finger to palpate the lateral side of the penis to determine the position of the root of the penis. With a tuberculin syringe and needle, the anesthetic is injected parallel to the root of the penis. While the penis is stabilized by gentle downward or ventral traction, the needle is inserted at the base of the penis and inserted beneath the skin surface. The anesthetic is injected and the needle withdrawn. An incision is made around the base of the foreskin, the foreskin is pulled back, and it is cut away from the penis. Stitches are usually used to close the skin edges.

Coding Tips

Report this code when a failed circumcision needs plastic correction or completion of the excision. For initial circumcision, see 54150–54161. For lysis or excision of post-circumcision adhesions, see 54162.

ICD-10-CM Diagnostic Codes

N47.0   Adherent prepuce, newborn 🅽 ♂
N47.5   Adhesions of prepuce and glans penis ♂
N47.7   Other inflammatory diseases of prepuce ♂
N47.8   Other disorders of prepuce ♂
Z41.1   Encounter for cosmetic surgery
Z41.2   Encounter for routine and ritual male circumcision ♂

AMA: 54163 2014,Jan,11

Relative Value Units/Medicare Edits

Non-Facility RVU	Work	PE	MP	Total
54163	3.32	2.56	0.39	6.27
Facility RVU	**Work**	**PE**	**MP**	**Total**
54163	3.32	2.56	0.39	6.27

	FUD	Status	MUE	Modifiers				IOM Reference
54163	10	A	1(2)	51	N/A	N/A	N/A	None

* with documentation

Terms To Know

adhesion. Abnormal fibrous connection between two structures, soft tissue or bony structures, that may occur as the result of surgery, infection, or trauma.

balanoposthitis. Inflammation and/or infection of the glans penis and prepuce.

circumcise. Circular cutting around the genitals to remove the prepuce or foreskin.

phimosis. Condition in which the foreskin is contracted and cannot be drawn back behind the glans penis.

prepuce. Fold of penile skin covering the glans.

scar tissue. Fibrous connective tissue that forms around a wounded area or injury, composed mainly of fibroblasts or collagenous fibers.

traction. Drawing out or holding tension on an area by applying a direct therapeutic pulling force.

54164

54164   Frenulotomy of penis

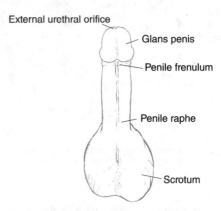

External urethral orifice

Glans penis

Penile frenulum

Penile raphe

Scrotum

The penile frenulum is the distal extension of the raphe. Excess tissues of the frenulum may interfere with retraction of the foreskin

Explanation

The physician performs an incision of the membrane that attaches the foreskin to the glans and shaft of the penis (frenulum). A dorsal penile nerve block is administered with a needle directed through the fascia of the symphysis pubis and into the frenum space where the anesthetic is deposited to block the dorsal nerves of the penis. A longitudinal incision is made ventrally though the outer layer of the prepuce. After retracting the prepuce, the physician extends the incision along the inner layer. Bleeding is controlled with an electrocoagulator. The resultant wound is closed.

Coding Tips

Do not report frenulotomy with circumcision codes, 54150–54163. Surgical trays, A4550, are not separately reimbursed by Medicare; however, other third-party payers may cover them. Check with the specific payer to determine coverage.

ICD-10-CM Diagnostic Codes

N48.89   Other specified disorders of penis ♂

AMA: 54164 2014,Jan,11

Relative Value Units/Medicare Edits

Non-Facility RVU	Work	PE	MP	Total
54164	2.82	2.4	0.32	5.54
Facility RVU	**Work**	**PE**	**MP**	**Total**
54164	2.82	2.4	0.32	5.54

	FUD	Status	MUE	Modifiers				IOM Reference
54164	10	A	1(2)	51	N/A	N/A	N/A	None

* with documentation

Terms To Know

membrane. Thin, flexible tissue layer that covers or functions to separate or connect anatomic areas, structures, or organs. May also be described as having the characteristic of allowing certain substances to permeate or pass through but not others (semipermeable).

54200, 54205

54200 Injection procedure for Peyronie disease;
54205   with surgical exposure of plaque

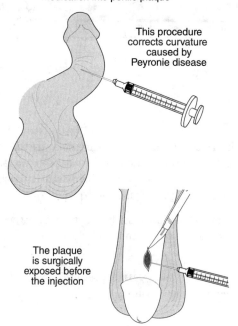

The physician injects medication into penile plaque

This procedure corrects curvature caused by Peyronie disease

The plaque is surgically exposed before the injection

Explanation

Peyronie's disease is an induration and severe curvature of the erect penis due to fibrosis of the cavernous sheaths. The physician injects medication into the abnormal fibrous tissue of the penis to correct painful curvature of the penis caused by Peyronie's disease. In 54200, no incision is made. The medication is injected into the dorsal area of the penis through the skin. In 54205, the physician makes an incision in the dorsum of the penis and identifies the abnormal fibrous tissue. An injection is made directly into the abnormal fibrous tissue under direct visualization through the incision.

Coding Tips

For more severe cases of Peyronie's disease with surgical excision of plaque and/or a graft, see 54110–54112. For injection for corpora cavernosography, see 54230–54235. Surgical trays, A4550, are not separately reimbursed by Medicare; however, other third-party payers may cover them. Check with the specific payer to determine coverage.

ICD-10-CM Diagnostic Codes

N48.6   Induration penis plastica ♂

AMA: **54200** 2014,Jan,11 **54205** 2014,Jan,11

Relative Value Units/Medicare Edits

Non-Facility RVU	Work	PE	MP	Total
54200	1.11	1.94	0.12	3.17
54205	8.97	5.36	1.03	15.36
Facility RVU	**Work**	**PE**	**MP**	**Total**
54200	1.11	1.18	0.12	2.41
54205	8.97	5.36	1.03	15.36

	FUD	Status	MUE	Modifiers				IOM Reference
54200	10	A	1(2)	51	N/A	N/A	N/A	None
54205	90	A	1(2)	51	N/A	N/A	80	

* with documentation

Terms To Know

connective tissue. Body tissue made from fibroblasts, collagen, and elastic fibrils that connects, supports, and holds together other tissues and cells and includes cartilage, collagenous, fibrous, elastic, and osseous tissue.

dorsal. Pertaining to the back or posterior aspect.

fibrosis. Formation of fibrous tissue as part of the restorative process.

fibrous tissue. Connective tissues.

incise. To cut open or into.

injection. Forcing a liquid substance into a body part such as a joint or muscle.

Peyronie's disease. Development of fibrotic hardened tissue or plaque in the cavernosal sheaths in the penis. This causes pain and a severe chordee or curvature in the penis, typically during erection.

procedure. Diagnostic or therapeutic service provided for the care and treatment of a patient, usually conforming to a specific set of steps or instructions.

sheath. Covering enclosing an organ or part.

54220

54220   Irrigation of corpora cavernosa for priapism

Cross section of penis

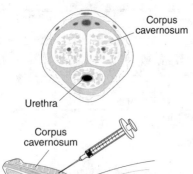

Corpus cavernosum

Urethra

Corpus cavernosum

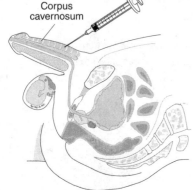

The physician irrigates and aspirates the engorged penis; the process may be repeated several times

Explanation

The corpora cavernosa are the spongy bodies of the penis, the dual columns of erectile tissue that form the back and sides of the penis. In priapism, this spongy tissue is in a state of persistent erection. The physician treats priapism by irrigating the corpora cavernosa. After adequate local anesthesia, the physician passes a large bore needle into the body of the penis and aspirates a quantity of blood and irrigates the space with 20 ml to 30 ml of saline solution. This may be accompanied by injecting medication into the same region, repeating it several times to get the abnormal erection to resolve.

Coding Tips

For injection for corpora cavernosography, see 54230. For intracavernosal injection of vasoactive drugs for dynamic cavernosometry, see 54231. For injection of corpora cavernosa with pharmacologic agent, see 54235.

ICD-10-CM Diagnostic Codes

N48.31   Priapism due to trauma ♂
N48.32   Priapism due to disease classified elsewhere ♂
N48.33   Priapism, drug-induced ♂
N48.39   Other priapism ♂

AMA: **54220** 2014,Jan,11

Relative Value Units/Medicare Edits

Non-Facility RVU	Work	PE	MP	Total
54220	2.42	3.3	0.35	6.07
Facility RVU	**Work**	**PE**	**MP**	**Total**
54220	2.42	1.09	0.35	3.86

	FUD	Status	MUE	Modifiers			IOM Reference
54220	0	A	1(3)	51	N/A	N/A	N/A	None

* with documentation

Terms To Know

aspirate. To withdraw fluid or air from a body cavity by suction.

irrigate. Washing out, lavage.

penis. Male reproductive and urinary excretion organ, the body of which is composed of three structures enclosed by fascia and skin: two parallel cylindrical bodies--the corpora cavernosa--and the corpus spongiosum lying underneath them, through which the urethra passes.

priapism. Persistent, painful erection lasting more than four hours and unrelated to sexual stimulation, causing pain and tenderness.

tissue. Group of similar cells with a similar function that form definite structures and organs. Tissue types include epithelial tissue, muscle tissue, connective tissue, and nervous tissue.

54230-54235

54230 Injection procedure for corpora cavernosography
54231 Dynamic cavernosometry, including intracavernosal injection of vasoactive drugs (eg, papaverine, phentolamine)
54235 Injection of corpora cavernosa with pharmacologic agent(s) (eg, papaverine, phentolamine)

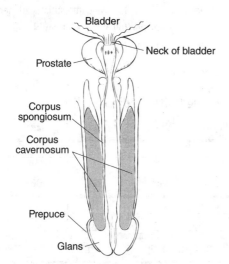

The penis is injected with contrast to highlight the corpora cavernosa

Explanation

The corpora cavernosa are the spongy bodies of the penis, the dual columns of erectile tissue that form the back and sides of the penis. The physician injects medication into the penis for x-ray studies to evaluate erectile dysfunction in 54230. After placing a constricting rubber band around the penis, the physician passes a needle into the body of the penis and aspirates a small quantity of blood. X-ray contrast medication is injected directly into the body of the penis. The constricting band is removed and x-rays are taken to demonstrate the function and integrity of the corpora cavernosa and the blood flow of the penis. In 54231, the physician injects vasoactive drugs into the corpora cavernosa for studies to evaluate erectile dysfunction. A rubber band is placed around the base of the penis and the intracavernous pressure is measured using instrumentation. The physician evaluates the penis for leakage between the diastolic and the systolic pressures. A swift rate of decay between the two indicates arterial and/or venous insufficiency of the penis. After the test, the band is removed and the instrumentation removed. In 54235, the physician injects medication into the penis to treat erectile dysfunction. After placing a constricting rubber band around the penis, the physician passes a needle into the body of the penis and aspirates a small quantity of blood. The selected medication is injected directly into the body of the penis. This produces an erection in most patients that may last from minutes to hours.

Coding Tips

For injection procedure for Peyronie's disease, see 54200. For irrigation procedure for priapism, see 54220. For radiological supervision and interpretation, see 74445.

ICD-10-CM Diagnostic Codes

F52.21	Male erectile disorder ♂
F52.4	Premature ejaculation ♂
N48.31	Priapism due to trauma ♂
N48.32	Priapism due to disease classified elsewhere ♂
N48.33	Priapism, drug-induced ♂
N48.39	Other priapism ♂
N48.6	Induration penis plastica ♂
N48.82	Acquired torsion of penis ♂
N48.89	Other specified disorders of penis ♂
N50.1	Vascular disorders of male genital organs ♂
N52.01	Erectile dysfunction due to arterial insufficiency 🅰 ♂
N52.02	Corporo-venous occlusive erectile dysfunction 🅰 ♂
N52.03	Combined arterial insufficiency and corporo-venous occlusive erectile dysfunction 🅰 ♂
N52.1	Erectile dysfunction due to diseases classified elsewhere 🅰 ♂
N52.2	Drug-induced erectile dysfunction 🅰 ♂
N52.31	Erectile dysfunction following radical prostatectomy 🅰 ♂
N52.32	Erectile dysfunction following radical cystectomy 🅰 ♂
N52.33	Erectile dysfunction following urethral surgery 🅰 ♂
N52.34	Erectile dysfunction following simple prostatectomy 🅰 ♂
N52.35	Erectile dysfunction following radiation therapy 🅰 ♂
N52.36	Erectile dysfunction following interstitial seed therapy 🅰 ♂
N52.37	Erectile dysfunction following prostate ablative therapy 🅰 ♂
N52.8	Other male erectile dysfunction 🅰 ♂
Q55.69	Other congenital malformation of penis ♂
S30.842A	External constriction of penis, initial encounter ♂
S30.842D	External constriction of penis, subsequent encounter ♂
S31.21XA	Laceration without foreign body of penis, initial encounter ♂
S31.22XA	Laceration with foreign body of penis, initial encounter ♂
S31.23XA	Puncture wound without foreign body of penis, initial encounter ♂
S31.24XA	Puncture wound with foreign body of penis, initial encounter ♂
S31.25XA	Open bite of penis, initial encounter ♂
S38.01XA	Crushing injury of penis, initial encounter ♂

AMA: **54230** 2014,Jan,11 **54231** 2014,Jan,11 **54235** 2018,Jan,8; 2017,Jan,8; 2016,Jan,13; 2015,Jan,16; 2014,Jan,11

Relative Value Units/Medicare Edits

Non-Facility RVU	Work	PE	MP	Total
54230	1.34	1.38	0.15	2.87
54231	2.04	1.79	0.24	4.07
54235	1.19	1.21	0.13	2.53
Facility RVU	**Work**	**PE**	**MP**	**Total**
54230	1.34	0.79	0.15	2.28
54231	2.04	1.06	0.24	3.34
54235	1.19	0.78	0.13	2.1

	FUD	Status	MUE	Modifiers				IOM Reference
54230	0	A	1(3)	51	N/A	N/A	N/A	None
54231	0	A	1(3)	51	N/A	N/A	N/A	
54235	0	A	1(3)	51	N/A	N/A	N/A	

* with documentation

CPT © 2020 American Medical Association. All Rights Reserved.   ● New   ▲ Revised   + Add On   ★ Telemedicine   AMA: CPT Assist   [Resequenced]   ☑ Laterality   © 2020 Optum360, LLC

Penis

54240-54250

54240 Penile plethysmography
54250 Nocturnal penile tumescence and/or rigidity test

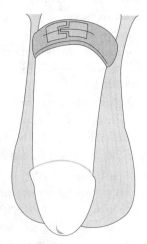

This procedure helps diagnose the cause of impotence

A gauge placed on the patient's penis monitors erections

Explanation

A plethysmograph is an instrument that measures variations in the volume of an organ and in the amount of blood in it or passing through it. The physician measures the physiological potential of the penis to attain and maintain an erection using plethysmography. The volume change of the penis is measured in response to external stimuli in 54240. In 54250, the physician monitors nighttime erections in impotent patients during rapid eye movement sleep. Testing can be performed in a sleep center or in the patient's home. During the test, the patient's penis is wired to a strain gauge monitor and recordings are made of the strength and duration of any erections occurring while the patient sleeps.

Coding Tips

For penile revascularization, see 37788; penile occlusive procedure, see 37790. For penile prostheses, inflatable, see 54410-54411; semi-rigid, see 54416-54417.

ICD-10-CM Diagnostic Codes

F52.21	Male erectile disorder ♂
F52.32	Male orgasmic disorder ♂
F52.8	Other sexual dysfunction not due to a substance or known physiological condition
F65.4	Pedophilia
F65.51	Sexual masochism
F65.52	Sexual sadism
F65.81	Frotteurism
F65.89	Other paraphilias
N48.6	Induration penis plastica ♂
N48.89	Other specified disorders of penis ♂
N52.01	Erectile dysfunction due to arterial insufficiency 🅰 ♂
N52.02	Corporo-venous occlusive erectile dysfunction 🅰 ♂
N52.03	Combined arterial insufficiency and corporo-venous occlusive erectile dysfunction 🅰 ♂
N52.1	Erectile dysfunction due to diseases classified elsewhere 🅰 ♂
N52.2	Drug-induced erectile dysfunction 🅰 ♂
N52.31	Erectile dysfunction following radical prostatectomy 🅰 ♂
N52.32	Erectile dysfunction following radical cystectomy 🅰 ♂
N52.33	Erectile dysfunction following urethral surgery 🅰 ♂
N52.34	Erectile dysfunction following simple prostatectomy 🅰 ♂
N52.35	Erectile dysfunction following radiation therapy 🅰 ♂
N52.36	Erectile dysfunction following interstitial seed therapy 🅰 ♂
N52.37	Erectile dysfunction following prostate ablative therapy 🅰 ♂
N52.8	Other male erectile dysfunction 🅰 ♂

AMA: **54240** 2014,Jan,11 **54250** 2014,Jan,11

Relative Value Units/Medicare Edits

Non-Facility RVU	Work	PE	MP	Total
54240	1.31	1.49	0.14	2.94
54250	2.22	1.1	0.19	3.51
Facility RVU	**Work**	**PE**	**MP**	**Total**
54240	1.31	1.49	0.14	2.94
54250	2.22	1.1	0.19	3.51

	FUD	Status	MUE	Modifiers				IOM Reference
54240	0	A	1(2)	N/A	N/A	N/A	80*	None
54250	0	A	1(2)	N/A	N/A	N/A	80*	

* with documentation

Terms To Know

dysfunction. Abnormal or impaired function of an organ, part, or system.

edema. Swelling due to fluid accumulation in the intercellular spaces.

impotence. Psychosexual or organic dysfunction in which there is partial or complete failure to attain or maintain erection until completion of the sexual act.

plethysmography. Recording of the volume changes in an organ or body part, particularly related to the amount of blood circulating through it.

priapism. Persistent, painful erection lasting more than four hours and unrelated to sexual stimulation, causing pain and tenderness.

54300-54304

54300   Plastic operation of penis for straightening of chordee (eg, hypospadias), with or without mobilization of urethra

54304   Plastic operation on penis for correction of chordee or for first stage hypospadias repair with or without transplantation of prepuce and/or skin flaps

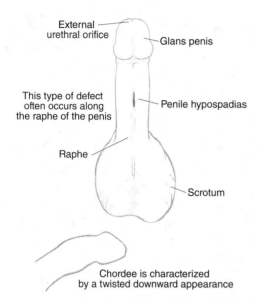

External urethral orifice

Glans penis

This type of defect often occurs along the raphe of the penis

Penile hypospadias

Raphe

Scrotum

Chordee is characterized by a twisted downward appearance

ICD-10-CM Diagnostic Codes

Q54.0	Hypospadias, balanic ♂
Q54.1	Hypospadias, penile ♂
Q54.2	Hypospadias, penoscrotal ♂
Q54.3	Hypospadias, perineal ♂
Q54.4	Congenital chordee ♂
Q54.8	Other hypospadias ♂
Q55.61	Curvature of penis (lateral) ♂

AMA: 54300 2018,Jan,8; 2017,Jan,8; 2016,Jan,13; 2015,Jan,16; 2014,Jan,11; 2014,Dec,16; 2014,Dec,16 **54304** 2014,Jan,11

Relative Value Units/Medicare Edits

Non-Facility RVU	Work	PE	MP	Total
54300	11.2	6.13	1.29	18.62
54304	13.28	6.84	1.51	21.63
Facility RVU	Work	PE	MP	Total
54300	11.2	6.13	1.29	18.62
54304	13.28	6.84	1.51	21.63

	FUD	Status	MUE	Modifiers				IOM Reference
54300	90	A	1(2)	51	N/A	62*	80	None
54304	90	A	1(2)	51	N/A	N/A	80	

* with documentation

Terms To Know

absorbable sutures. Strands used for suture or repair of tissue prepared from collagen or a synthetic polymer and capable of being absorbed by tissue over time.

chordee. Ventral (downward) curvature of the penis due to a fibrous band along the corpus spongiosum seen congenitally with hypospadias, or a downward curvature seen on erection in disease conditions, causing a lack of distensibility in the tissues.

defect. Imperfection, flaw, or absence.

dissect. Cut apart or separate tissue for surgical purposes or for visual or microscopic study.

epispadias. Male anomaly in which the urethral opening is abnormally located on the dorsum of the penis, appearing as a groove with no upper urethral wall covering.

flap graft. Mass of flesh and skin partially excised from its location but retaining its blood supply, grafted onto another site to repair adjacent or distant defects.

hypospadias. Fairly common birth defect in males in which the meatus, or urinary opening, is abnormally positioned on the underside of the penile shaft or in the perineum, requiring early surgical correction.

Explanation

In 54300, the physician corrects and repairs chordee, which is the abnormal curvature of the penis. To assist in planning the surgery, an artificial erection may be produced by placing a band around the base of the penis and injecting saline into the body of the penis. The area of deformity is determined and by using a combination of incisions and excisions of abnormal fibrous tissue and sometimes normal tissue, the defect is corrected. Care is taken to dissect around nerves and blood vessels. Sometimes the urethra is dissected free of its position and retracted temporarily away from the operative site. The separate tissues of the penis are closed in layers with absorbable suture material. An artificial erection may again be produced to test and demonstrate the adequacy of the repair. In 54304, the physician corrects and repairs chordee and also prepares the penis for correction of hypospadias, an abnormal opening of the urethra on the underside of the penis or on the perineum. To assist in planning the surgery, an artificial erection may be produced by placing a band around the base of the penis and injecting saline into the body of the penis. The area of deformity is determined and the defect is corrected using a combination of incisions and excisions of the prepuce (foreskin). Care is taken to dissect around the nerves and blood vessels. Often the foreskin is used in either a free graft or a flap graft to cover the ventral skin defects created to correct the chordee. The separate tissues of the penis are closed in layers with absorbable suture material. An artificial erection may again be produced to test and demonstrate the adequacy of the repair. The urethral opening is left on the ventral shaft of the penis for repair during a later stage.

Coding Tips

This procedure is a plastic repair specifically for chordee. For other penile angulation repairs, see 54360. For other male urethroplasties, see 53410–53425. For penile revascularization, see 37788. Any manipulation or dilation is not reported separately.

CPT © 2020 American Medical Association. All Rights Reserved.   ● New   ▲ Revised   + Add On   ★ Telemedicine   AMA: CPT Assist   [Resequenced]   ☑ Laterality   © 2020 Optum360, LLC

54308-54312

54308   Urethroplasty for second stage hypospadias repair (including urinary diversion); less than 3 cm
54312   greater than 3 cm

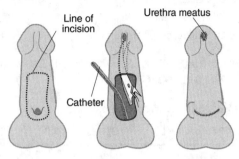

Line of incision
Urethra meatus
Catheter

The physician creates a urethra from penile skin formed into a tube; a catheter helps retain the shape of the newly created urethra

Explanation

The physician completes the repair of chordee (abnormal curvature of the penis) and hypospadias (an abnormal opening of the urethra on the underside of the penis or on the perineum) by creating a urethral opening in the end of the penis. The urethra is dissected free of the surrounding tissues to mobilize it. A distal urethra, less than 3.0 cm in 54308 or greater than 3.0 cm in 54312, is formed from the prepuce (foreskin) and an opening is created at or near the tip of the head of the penis. Urine may be diverted by the use of a catheter in the bladder. The skin is closed with sutures.

Coding Tips

This procedure is a plastic repair specific to hypospadias and the completion of chordee correction. For other penile angulation repairs, see 54360. For other male urethroplasties, see 53410–53425. For penile revascularization, see 37788. For other plastic repair of chordee with second stage hypospadias repair using a free skin graft, see 54316. Any manipulation or dilation is not reported separately. Supplies used when providing these procedures may be reported with the appropriate HCPCS Level II code. Check with the specific payer to determine coverage.

ICD-10-CM Diagnostic Codes

Q54.0   Hypospadias, balanic ♂
Q54.1   Hypospadias, penile ♂
Q54.2   Hypospadias, penoscrotal ♂
Q54.3   Hypospadias, perineal ♂
Q54.4   Congenital chordee ♂
Q54.8   Other hypospadias ♂

AMA: **54308** 2014,Jan,11 **54312** 2014,Jan,11

Relative Value Units/Medicare Edits

Non-Facility RVU	Work	PE	MP	Total
54308	12.62	6.61	1.43	20.66
54312	14.51	7.46	1.67	23.64
Facility RVU	Work	PE	MP	Total
54308	12.62	6.61	1.43	20.66
54312	14.51	7.46	1.67	23.64

	FUD	Status	MUE	Modifiers				IOM Reference
54308	90	A	1(2)	51	N/A	62*	80	None
54312	90	A	1(2)	51	N/A	62*	80	

* with documentation

Terms To Know

anomaly. Irregularity in the structure or position of an organ or tissue.

catheter. Flexible tube inserted into an area of the body for introducing or withdrawing fluid.

chordee. Ventral (downward) curvature of the penis due to a fibrous band along the corpus spongiosum seen congenitally with hypospadias, or a downward curvature seen on erection in disease conditions, causing a lack of distensibility in the tissues.

congenital. Present at birth, occurring through heredity or an influence during gestation up to the moment of birth.

dissect. Cut apart or separate tissue for surgical purposes or for visual or microscopic study.

distal. Located farther away from a specified reference point or the trunk.

epispadias. Male anomaly in which the urethral opening is abnormally located on the dorsum of the penis, appearing as a groove with no upper urethral wall covering.

hypospadias. Fairly common birth defect in males in which the meatus, or urinary opening, is abnormally positioned on the underside of the penile shaft or in the perineum, requiring early surgical correction.

perineal. Pertaining to the pelvic floor area between the thighs; the diamond-shaped area bordered by the pubic symphysis in front, the ischial tuberosities on the sides, and the coccyx in back.

prepuce. Fold of penile skin covering the glans.

urethra. Small tube lined with mucous membrane that leads from the bladder to the exterior of the body.

urethroplasty. Surgical repair or reconstruction of the urethra to correct a stricture or problem caused congenitally, from previous surgical repair, trauma, or prolapse. There are many different types of urethroplasty performed on both males and females.

54316

54316 Urethroplasty for second stage hypospadias repair (including urinary diversion) with free skin graft obtained from site other than genitalia

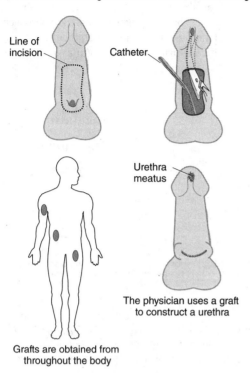

Grafts are obtained from throughout the body

The physician uses a graft to construct a urethra

Explanation

The physician completes the repair of chordee (abnormal curvature of the penis) and hypospadias (abnormal opening of the urethra on the underside of the penis or on the perineum) by creating a urethral opening in the end of the penis. The urethra is mobilized by dissecting it free from the surrounding tissues. A distal urethra is formed from skin obtained from a site other than the genitalia and sutured to the existing urethra and to an opening created at or near the tip of the head of the penis. Urine may be diverted using a catheter in the bladder. The skin and tissues are closed with fine absorbable sutures.

Coding Tips

This procedure is a plastic repair specific to hypospadias and the completion of chordee correction. For other penile angulation repairs, see 54360. For other male urethroplasty codes, see 53410–53425. For penile revascularization, see 37788. Any manipulation or dilation is not reported separately. Supplies used when providing this procedure may be reported with the appropriate HCPCS Level II code. Check with the specific payer to determine coverage.

ICD-10-CM Diagnostic Codes

Q54.0	Hypospadias, balanic ♂
Q54.1	Hypospadias, penile ♂
Q54.2	Hypospadias, penoscrotal ♂
Q54.3	Hypospadias, perineal ♂
Q54.4	Congenital chordee ♂
Q54.8	Other hypospadias ♂

AMA: 54316 2014,Jan,11

Relative Value Units/Medicare Edits

Non-Facility RVU	Work	PE	MP	Total
54316	18.05	8.66	2.06	28.77
Facility RVU	Work	PE	MP	Total
54316	18.05	8.66	2.06	28.77

	FUD	Status	MUE	Modifiers				IOM Reference
54316	90	A	1(2)	51	N/A	62*	80	None

* with documentation

Terms To Know

anomaly. Irregularity in the structure or position of an organ or tissue.

catheter. Flexible tube inserted into an area of the body for introducing or withdrawing fluid.

chordee. Ventral (downward) curvature of the penis due to a fibrous band along the corpus spongiosum seen congenitally with hypospadias, or a downward curvature seen on erection in disease conditions, causing a lack of distensibility in the tissues.

dissection. Separating by cutting tissue or body structures apart.

distal. Located farther away from a specified reference point or the trunk.

epispadias. Male anomaly in which the urethral opening is abnormally located on the dorsum of the penis, appearing as a groove with no upper urethral wall covering.

graft. Tissue implant from another part of the body or another person.

hypospadias. Fairly common birth defect in males in which the meatus, or urinary opening, is abnormally positioned on the underside of the penile shaft or in the perineum, requiring early surgical correction.

meatus. Opening or passage into the body.

perineal. Pertaining to the pelvic floor area between the thighs; the diamond-shaped area bordered by the pubic symphysis in front, the ischial tuberosities on the sides, and the coccyx in back.

urethroplasty. Surgical repair or reconstruction of the urethra to correct a stricture or problem caused congenitally, from previous surgical repair, trauma, or prolapse. There are many different types of urethroplasty performed on both males and females.

54318

54318 Urethroplasty for third stage hypospadias repair to release penis from scrotum (eg, third stage Cecil repair)

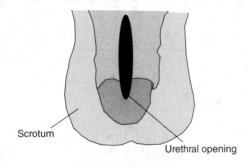

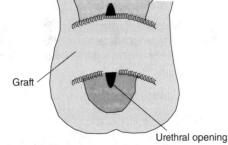

Physician uses scrotal graft to complete hypospadias repair

Explanation

The physician completes the repair of chordee (abnormal curvature of the penis) and hypospadias (an abnormal opening of the urethra on the underside of the penis or on the perineum) by separating the temporary attachments sutured between the penis and scrotum during a previous stage of the repair. Urine may be diverted using a catheter in the bladder. The skin is closed with fine sutures.

Coding Tips

This plastic repair is specifically for third stage hypospadias repair. For other male urethroplasties, see 53410–53425. For penile revascularization, see 37788. A simple scrotoplasty (55175) is not identified separately. However, a complicated scrotoplasty (55180) is identified separately. For first and second stage hypospadias repair, see 54304–54316. Any manipulation or dilation is not reported separately.

ICD-10-CM Diagnostic Codes

Q54.2   Hypospadias, penoscrotal ♂

AMA: 54318 2014,Jan,11

Relative Value Units/Medicare Edits

Non-Facility RVU	Work	PE	MP	Total
54318	12.43	6.69	1.42	20.54
Facility RVU	Work	PE	MP	Total
54318	12.43	6.69	1.42	20.54

	FUD	Status	MUE	Modifiers				IOM Reference
54318	90	A	1(2)	51	N/A	62*	80	None

* with documentation

54322-54328

54322 1-stage distal hypospadias repair (with or without chordee or circumcision); with simple meatal advancement (eg, Magpi, V-flap)
54324   with urethroplasty by local skin flaps (eg, flip-flap, prepucial flap)
54326   with urethroplasty by local skin flaps and mobilization of urethra
54328   with extensive dissection to correct chordee and urethroplasty with local skin flaps, skin graft patch, and/or island flap

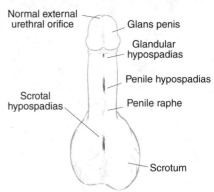

Distal hypospadias repair (near the glans penis) is performed as a single stage

Explanation

In a one-stage procedure, the physician corrects hypospadias, which is an abnormal opening of the urethra on the underside of the penis, in the distal or end portion of the penile shaft. The physician may also correct and repair a chordee, which is an abnormal curvature of the penis. An incision is made around the shaft of the penis next to the glans (head) and the skin is dissected from the penile shaft taking care to avoid injury to the urethra. An erection is artificially produced to evaluate any chordee before and after the correction. Any chordee present is corrected by excising the responsible fibrous band. In 54322, a second incision is made in the groove on the underside of the glans. Skin in the area is pulled up to the glans and fashioned into an opening by suturing in the head of the penis. A circumcision, or excision of some foreskin, may be performed. The original incision around the penis is closed by suturing. In 54324, a flap is created from the skin below the urethral opening and flipped up and over the opening of the urethra and sutured together forming a tube extension of the urethra. The foreskin is divided and sutured over the defect left by the flap on the ventral surface of the penis. In 54326, the urethra is dissected free of the shaft to mobilize it. A flap of skin is created from the foreskin and sutured together to form a tube to be used as a segment of urethra. The foreskin is further divided and sutured over the defect left by the flap on the ventral surface of the penis. In 54328, the chordee is corrected by excising the responsible fibrous band. The urethra is dissected free of the shaft to mobilize it. An island flap of skin is created from the foreskin and sutured together to form a tube to be used as a segment of urethra. This formed urethral tube flap is sutured in place between the urethral opening in the shaft of the penis and an opening created in the head of the penis. The foreskin is further divided and sutured over the defect left by the flap on the ventral surface of the penis. Foreskin removal (circumcision) may be part of this procedure.

Coding Tips

If significant additional time and effort is documented, append modifier 22 and submit a cover letter and operative report. These repairs are specifically for hypospadias repair. For other male urethroplasties, see 53410–53425. For staged hypospadias and chordee repairs, see 54304–54318.

© 2020 Optum360, LLC   N Newborn: 0   P Pediatric: 0-17   M Maternity: 9-64   A Adult: 15-124   ♂ Male Only   ♀ Female Only   CPT © 2020 American Medical Association. All Rights Reserved.

ICD-10-CM Diagnostic Codes

Q54.0   Hypospadias, balanic ♂
Q54.1   Hypospadias, penile ♂

AMA: **54322** 2014,Jan,11 **54324** 2014,Jan,11 **54326** 2014,Jan,11 **54328** 2018,Jan,8; 2017,Jan,8; 2016,Jan,13; 2015,Jan,16; 2014,Jan,11

Relative Value Units/Medicare Edits

Non-Facility RVU	Work	PE	MP	Total
54322	13.98	6.99	1.61	22.58
54324	17.55	8.42	1.99	27.96
54326	17.02	8.3	1.95	27.27
54328	16.89	8.27	1.93	27.09
Facility RVU	Work	PE	MP	Total
54322	13.98	6.99	1.61	22.58
54324	17.55	8.42	1.99	27.96
54326	17.02	8.3	1.95	27.27
54328	16.89	8.27	1.93	27.09

	FUD	Status	MUE	Modifiers				IOM Reference
54322	90	A	1(2)	51	N/A	N/A	80	None
54324	90	A	1(2)	51	N/A	62*	80	
54326	90	A	1(2)	51	N/A	62*	80	
54328	90	A	1(2)	51	N/A	62*	80	

* with documentation

Terms To Know

chordee. Ventral (downward) curvature of the penis due to a fibrous band along the corpus spongiosum seen congenitally with hypospadias, or a downward curvature seen on erection in disease conditions, causing a lack of distensibility in the tissues.

circumcision. Procedure involving the surgical removal of the foreskin, the tissue covering the head of the penis. The procedure involves the freeing of the foreskin from the head of the penis (glans), and removing the excess foreskin. When performed on a newborn, the procedure takes approximately five to 10 minutes; adults may take one hour. Healing is usually within five to seven days.

congenital. Present at birth, occurring through heredity or an influence during gestation up to the moment of birth.

defect. Imperfection, flaw, or absence.

dissection. Separating by cutting tissue or body structures apart.

distal. Located farther away from a specified reference point or the trunk.

flap. Mass of flesh and skin partially excised from its location but retaining its blood supply that is moved to another site to repair adjacent or distant defects.

hypospadias. Fairly common birth defect in males in which the meatus, or urinary opening, is abnormally positioned on the underside of the penile shaft or in the perineum, requiring early surgical correction.

prepuce. Fold of penile skin covering the glans.

ventral. Pertaining or relating on, to, or toward the lower abdominal plane of the body; located on, near, or toward the front area of the body.

54332-54336

54332   1-stage proximal penile or penoscrotal hypospadias repair requiring extensive dissection to correct chordee and urethroplasty by use of skin graft tube and/or island flap

54336   1-stage perineal hypospadias repair requiring extensive dissection to correct chordee and urethroplasty by use of skin graft tube and/or island flap

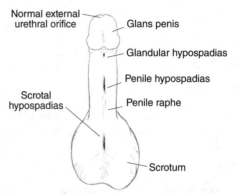

Proximal or perineal hypospadias repair is performed

Explanation

Hypospadias is an abnormal opening of the urethra on the underside of the penis or on the perineum. The physician corrects hypospadias in the base portion of the penis in a one-stage procedure. An incision is made on the ventral surface of the penis and around the urethral opening. An erection is artificially produced to evaluate the chordee before and after the correction. Chordee is corrected by excising the responsible fibrous band. Considerable dissection is required to mobilize the urethra. An island flap of skin is created from the foreskin and sutured together to form a tube to be used as a segment of urethra. This formed urethral tube flap is sutured in place between the urethral opening at the base of the shaft of the penis and an opening created in the head of the penis, in 54332. In 54336, the formed urethral tube flap is sutured in place between the urethral opening at the base of the scrotum in the perineum and an opening created in the head of the penis. The foreskin and skin overlying the shaft are further divided and dissected free and sutured over the defect left by the flap and dissections on the ventral surface of the penis. Circumcision is usually the result of the procedure.

Coding Tips

If significant additional time and effort is documented, append modifier 22 and submit a cover letter and operative report. For other one-stage distal hypospadias repairs, see 54322–54328. Plastic repair for straightening of chordee, circumcision, and simple meatotomy are included and are not reported separately. Any manipulation or dilation is not reported separately.

ICD-10-CM Diagnostic Codes

Q54.1   Hypospadias, penile ♂
Q54.2   Hypospadias, penoscrotal ♂
Q54.3   Hypospadias, perineal ♂

AMA: **54332** 2018,Jan,8; 2017,Jan,8; 2016,Jan,13; 2015,Jan,16; 2014,Jan,11 **54336** 2018,Jan,8; 2017,Jan,8; 2016,Jan,13; 2015,Jan,16; 2014,Jan,11

CPT © 2020 American Medical Association. All Rights Reserved.   ● New   ▲ Revised   + Add On   ★ Telemedicine   AMA: CPT Assist   [Resequenced]   ☑ Laterality   © 2020 Optum360, LLC

Relative Value Units/Medicare Edits

Non-Facility RVU	Work	PE	MP	Total
54332	18.37	8.77	2.1	29.24
54336	21.62	10.25	2.48	34.35
Facility RVU	**Work**	**PE**	**MP**	**Total**
54332	18.37	8.77	2.1	29.24
54336	21.62	10.25	2.48	34.35

	FUD	Status	MUE	Modifiers				IOM Reference
54332	90	A	1(2)	51	N/A	62*	80	None
54336	90	A	1(2)	51	N/A	62*	80	

* with documentation

Terms To Know

chordee. Ventral (downward) curvature of the penis due to a fibrous band along the corpus spongiosum seen congenitally with hypospadias, or a downward curvature seen on erection in disease conditions, causing a lack of distensibility in the tissues.

congenital. Present at birth, occurring through heredity or an influence during gestation up to the moment of birth.

defect. Imperfection, flaw, or absence.

dissection. Separating by cutting tissue or body structures apart.

flap. Mass of flesh and skin partially excised from its location but retaining its blood supply that is moved to another site to repair adjacent or distant defects.

free graft. Unattached piece of skin and tissue moved to another part of the body and sutured into place to repair a defect.

hypospadias. Fairly common birth defect in males in which the meatus, or urinary opening, is abnormally positioned on the underside of the penile shaft or in the perineum, requiring early surgical correction.

perineal. Pertaining to the pelvic floor area between the thighs; the diamond-shaped area bordered by the pubic symphysis in front, the ischial tuberosities on the sides, and the coccyx in back.

urethra. Small tube lined with mucous membrane that leads from the bladder to the exterior of the body.

ventral. Pertaining or relating on, to, or toward the lower abdominal plane of the body; located on, near, or toward the front area of the body.

54340-54348

54340 Repair of hypospadias complications (ie, fistula, stricture, diverticula); by closure, incision, or excision, simple

54344   requiring mobilization of skin flaps and urethroplasty with flap or patch graft

54348   requiring extensive dissection and urethroplasty with flap, patch or tubed graft (includes urinary diversion)

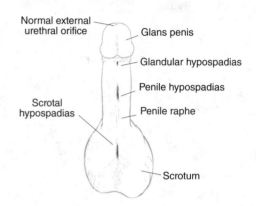

Explanation

Hypospadias is an abnormal opening of the urethra on the underside of the penis or on the perineum. The physician repairs a fistula, stricture, and/or diverticula resulting from a former hypospadias repair. The fistula (abnormal passage) or diverticula (pouch or sac) is identified and excised, often using microsurgical techniques. In 54340, the defect in the urethra is repaired by suturing and the skin is also closed with sutures. A stricture (narrowing) is corrected by dilating the area with dilating catheters or by incision and suture closure. In 54344, the defect in the urethra is repaired by closure with a free patch graft or flap graft. The skin defect is closed by simple suturing or by the use of a flap skin graft. In 54348, the defect in the urethra is repaired by closure with a free patch graft or a flap graft that both require extensive dissection, mobilization of tissues, and the creation of complicated grafts such as a tube graft. The skin defect is closed by simple suturing or by use of a flap skin graft. A stricture (narrowing) is corrected by dilating the area with dilating catheters or by incision and suture repair. The urine may be diverted through a catheter left in the bladder. The catheter can be passed through the urethra or placed directly in the bladder through the lower abdominal wall just above the pubic bone.

Coding Tips

For initial hypospadias repair, see 54300–54336. Excision of urethral diverticulum (53235, 53240) and urethroplasty for fistula, stricture, or diverticula (53400) are included. Local skin flaps or patch grafts to reconstruct the urethral area are included in 54344 and 54348. Any free vascular grafts or flaps are reported separately.

ICD-10-CM Diagnostic Codes

N99.110	Postprocedural urethral stricture, male, meatal ♂
N99.111	Postprocedural bulbous urethral stricture, male ♂
N99.112	Postprocedural membranous urethral stricture, male ♂
N99.113	Postprocedural anterior bulbous urethral stricture, male ♂
N99.115	Postprocedural fossa naviularis urethral stricture ♂
N99.116	Postprocedural urethral stricture, male, overlapping sites ♂
N99.89	Other postprocedural complications and disorders of genitourinary system

Relative Value Units/Medicare Edits

Non-Facility RVU	Work	PE	MP	Total
54340	9.71	5.61	1.12	16.44
54344	17.06	8.32	1.95	27.33
54348	18.32	8.82	2.08	29.22
Facility RVU	Work	PE	MP	Total
54340	9.71	5.61	1.12	16.44
54344	17.06	8.32	1.95	27.33
54348	18.32	8.82	2.08	29.22

	FUD	Status	MUE	Modifiers				IOM Reference
54340	90	A	1(2)	51	N/A	62*	80	None
54344	90	A	1(2)	51	N/A	62*	80	
54348	90	A	1(2)	51	N/A	62*	80	

* with documentation

Terms To Know

anomaly. Irregularity in the structure or position of an organ or tissue.

defect. Imperfection, flaw, or absence.

dissection. Separating by cutting tissue or body structures apart.

diverticulum. Pouch or sac in the walls of an organ or canal.

fistula. Abnormal tube-like passage between two body cavities or organs or from an organ to the outside surface.

flap graft. Mass of flesh and skin partially excised from its location but retaining its blood supply, grafted onto another site to repair adjacent or distant defects.

hypospadias. Fairly common birth defect in males in which the meatus, or urinary opening, is abnormally positioned on the underside of the penile shaft or in the perineum, requiring early surgical correction.

stricture. Narrowing of an anatomical structure.

urethroplasty. Surgical repair or reconstruction of the urethra to correct a stricture or problem caused congenitally, from previous surgical repair, trauma, or prolapse. There are many different types of urethroplasty performed on both males and females.

54352

Penis

54352	Repair of hypospadias cripple requiring extensive dissection and excision of previously constructed structures including re-release of chordee and reconstruction of urethra and penis by use of local skin as grafts and island flaps and skin brought in as flaps or grafts

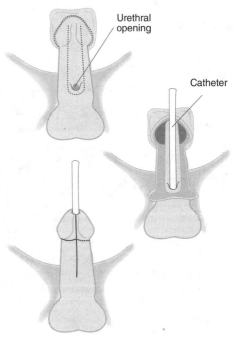

Urethral opening

Catheter

Repair includes previous corrections
to urethra and chordee

Explanation

Hypospadias is an abnormal opening of the urethra on the underside of the penis or on the perineum. The physician repairs severe, disabling complications from former hypospadias repairs. Often using microsurgical techniques and considerable excision of scarred and damaged tissues, the deformities and malfunctions of the urethra and penis are corrected. Two or three stages may be necessary to complete this complicated task. A new urethral segment is created with a free patch graft, a flap graft, or by the use of a tube graft. Extensive dissection and mobilization of tissues are generally required to complete the process. Skin defects are closed using flap or free skin grafts. Any strictures (narrowing of hollow structures) are corrected by dilating the area with dilating catheters or by incision and suture repair. Urine may be diverted through a catheter left in the bladder. The catheter can be passed through the urethra or placed in the bladder through an incision in the lower abdominal wall just above the pubic bone.

Coding Tips

For other repair of hypospadias complications, see 54340–54348. Excision of urethral diverticulum (53235, 53240) and urethroplasty for fistula, stricture, and diverticula (53400) are included in this procedure and are not reported separately. For penile revascularization, see 37788. This procedure includes local skin grafts or flaps to reconstruct the urethral area. However, any free vascular grafts or flaps are reported separately. If full or split thickness grafts are performed, see 15240–15241 and 15120–15121. Any manipulation or dilation is not reported separately.

ICD-10-CM Diagnostic Codes

N99.110   Postprocedural urethral stricture, male, meatal ♂

N99.111	Postprocedural bulbous urethral stricture, male ♂	
N99.112	Postprocedural membranous urethral stricture, male ♂	
N99.113	Postprocedural anterior bulbous urethral stricture, male ♂	
N99.115	Postprocedural fossa naviculais urethral stricture ♂	
N99.116	Postprocedural urethral stricture, male, overlapping sites ♂	
N99.89	Other postprocedural complications and disorders of genitourinary system	

AMA: 54352 2014,Jan,11

Relative Value Units/Medicare Edits

Non-Facility RVU	Work	PE	MP	Total
54352	26.13	11.78	3.0	40.91
Facility RVU	**Work**	**PE**	**MP**	**Total**
54352	26.13	11.78	3.0	40.91

	FUD	Status	MUE	Modifiers				IOM Reference
54352	90	A	1(2)	51	N/A	62*	80	None

* with documentation

Terms To Know

chordee. Ventral (downward) curvature of the penis due to a fibrous band along the corpus spongiosum seen congenitally with hypospadias, or a downward curvature seen on erection in disease conditions, causing a lack of distensibility in the tissues.

dissection. (dis. apart; -section, act of cutting) Separating by cutting tissue or body structures apart.

flap graft. Mass of flesh and skin partially excised from its location but retaining its blood supply, grafted onto another site to repair adjacent or distant defects.

hypospadias. Fairly common birth defect in males in which the meatus, or urinary opening, is abnormally positioned on the underside of the penile shaft or in the perineum, requiring early surgical correction.

microsurgery. Surgical procedures performed under magnification using a surgical microscope.

scar tissue. Fibrous connective tissue that forms around a wounded area or injury, composed mainly of fibroblasts or collagenous fibers.

54360

54360	Plastic operation on penis to correct angulation

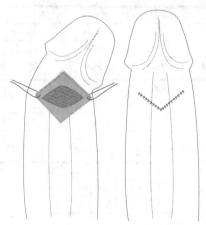

The incisions are closed with sutures

The physician repairs a curvature of the penis using a series of excisions

Explanation

The physician corrects an abnormal curvature of the penis using a series of excisions of tissue on the side of the penis. To assist in planning the surgery, an erection may be artificially produced by placing a band around the base of the penis and injecting saline into the body of the penis. The area of deformity is determined and using a combination of incisions and excisions of tissue, the defect is corrected. An incision is made in the skin of the penis just proximal to the glans (head of the penis) and the skin is pulled to the base of the penis, exposing the underlying tissues. Further dissection is done to expose the thick connective tissue on one side of the shaft. A series of parallel excisions are made and the resulting defects are closed by suturing. The separate tissues and the skin of the penis are closed in a layered fashion with absorbable suture material. An erection may again be induced to test the adequacy of the repair.

Coding Tips

For plastic operation for straightening chordee specifically, see 54300. Use 54360 for all other angulation abnormalities. Any manipulation or dilation is not reported separately.

ICD-10-CM Diagnostic Codes

N48.82	Acquired torsion of penis ♂	
Q55.61	Curvature of penis (lateral) ♂	
Q55.63	Congenital torsion of penis ♂	

AMA: 54360 2014,Jan,11

Relative Value Units/Medicare Edits

Non-Facility RVU	Work	PE	MP	Total
54360	12.78	6.58	1.46	20.82
Facility RVU	**Work**	**PE**	**MP**	**Total**
54360	12.78	6.58	1.46	20.82

	FUD	Status	MUE	Modifiers				IOM Reference
54360	90	A	1(2)	51	N/A	62*	80	None

* with documentation

Terms To Know

absorbable sutures. Strands used for suture or repair of tissue prepared from collagen or a synthetic polymer and capable of being absorbed by tissue over time.

anomaly. Irregularity in the structure or position of an organ or tissue.

chordee. Ventral (downward) curvature of the penis due to a fibrous band along the corpus spongiosum seen congenitally with hypospadias, or a downward curvature seen on erection in disease conditions, causing a lack of distensibility in the tissues.

congenital. Present at birth, occurring through heredity or an influence during gestation up to the moment of birth.

defect. Imperfection, flaw, or absence.

deformity. Irregularity or malformation of the body.

dissection. Separating by cutting tissue or body structures apart.

proximal. Located closest to a specified reference point, usually the midline or trunk.

tissue. Group of similar cells with a similar function that form definite structures and organs. Tissue types include epithelial tissue, muscle tissue, connective tissue, and nervous tissue.

54380-54390

54380	Plastic operation on penis for epispadias distal to external sphincter;
54385	with incontinence
54390	with exstrophy of bladder

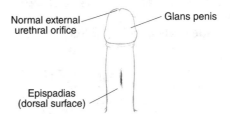

Epispadias repair for cases where the openings occur distal to the external sphincter

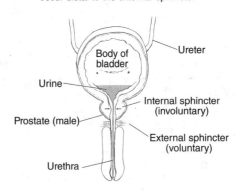

Explanation

In 54380, the physician corrects epispadias, which is the congenital absence of the upper wall of the urethra. The urethra has its opening anywhere on the top surface of the penis. A closed urethra is created by reapproximating the tissues, and by using skin grafts, tube grafts, free tissue grafts, or a combination of techniques depending on the extent of the defect. In 54385, the physician corrects epispadias and associated urinary incontinence in one or more stages. Epispadias with incontinence is the congenital absence of the upper wall of the urethra and the lack of function of the muscles that control the bladder neck. Through an incision in the lower abdomen, the surgeon reconstructs the bladder neck and reimplants the ureters from the kidneys away from the bladder neck outlet. A closed urethra is created by reapproximating the tissues and by using skin grafts, tube grafts, free tissue grafts, or a combination of techniques depending on the extent of the defect. In 54390, the physician corrects epispadias and exstrophy of the bladder in stages. Bladder exstrophy is the turning inside out of the bladder so that the bladder is open directly to the outside and as such, urine does not collect in the bladder but simply drains without any control to the outside onto the lower abdomen. The first stage is to close the bladder through incisions in the lower abdomen. The surgeon frees the bladder from the abdominal wall and proceeds to close the bladder and reimplant the ureters from the kidneys away from the bladder neck outlet. In the second stage, a closed urethra is created by reapproximating the tissues and by using skin grafts, tube grafts, free tissue grafts, or a combination of techniques depending on the extent of the defect. In the following stages, the physician reconstructs the bladder neck to provide urinary control and, if necessary, does additional surgery on the penis and urethra.

Coding Tips

If significant additional time and effort is documented, append modifier 22 and submit a cover letter and operative report. Palpation of the dorsal shaft may reveal fibrous plaque. Excision of this plaque (54110–54112) should not be reported separately. Closure of bladder exstrophy (51940) is included in 54390 and should not be reported separately. Report any free grafts or flaps separately.

ICD-10-CM Diagnostic Codes

Q64.0   Epispadias ♂

AMA: **54380** 2014,Jan,11 **54385** 2014,Jan,11 **54390** 2014,Jan,11

Relative Value Units/Medicare Edits

Non-Facility RVU	Work	PE	MP	Total
54380	14.18	7.28	1.63	23.09
54385	16.56	8.39	1.89	26.84
54390	22.77	10.49	2.6	35.86
Facility RVU	Work	PE	MP	Total
54380	14.18	7.28	1.63	23.09
54385	16.56	8.39	1.89	26.84
54390	22.77	10.49	2.6	35.86

	FUD	Status	MUE	Modifiers				IOM Reference
54380	90	A	1(2)	51	N/A	62*	80	100-03,230.10
54385	90	A	1(2)	51	N/A	62*	80	
54390	90	A	1(2)	51	N/A	62*	80	

* with documentation

Terms To Know

defect. Imperfection, flaw, or absence.

epispadias. Male anomaly in which the urethral opening is abnormally located on the dorsum of the penis, appearing as a groove with no upper urethral wall covering.

exstrophy of bladder. Congenital anomaly occurring when the bladder everts itself, or turns inside out, through an absent part of the lower abdominal and anterior bladder walls with incomplete closure of the pubic bone.

incontinence. Inability to control urination or defecation.

tissue. Group of similar cells with a similar function that form definite structures and organs. Tissue types include epithelial tissue, muscle tissue, connective tissue, and nervous tissue.

54400-54401

54400	Insertion of penile prosthesis; non-inflatable (semi-rigid)
54401	inflatable (self-contained)

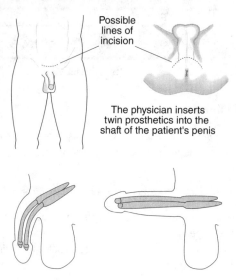

Inflatable prosthesis, shown in both states

Explanation

The physician inserts a semi-rigid penile prosthesis in 54400, which is a hinged or malleable device, or a self-contained inflatable penile prosthesis in 54401, which is a one piece, paired hydraulic device that allows fluid to be pumped from one portion of the device to another. A transverse incision is made just above the penis over the pubic bone. With care to avoid important nerves and blood vessels, dissection is carried down to the erectile tissues at the base of the penis. Incisions are made in the thick fibrous membranes surrounding the two main erectile tissues to allow the insertion of dilators to create space for the prostheses. The paired prosthetic devices are inserted one at a time into the two erectile tissue compartments down the length of the penis. The incisions and tissues are closed by suturing. The operation can also be done in similar fashion using an incision just below the scrotum in the perineum to enter the erectile tissue or in the upper scrotum at the base of the penis.

Coding Tips

If significant additional time and effort is documented, append modifier 22 and submit a cover letter and operative report. These procedures are not used for plastic implants that are inserted for healing purposes at the time of another surgery. The insertion of plastic implants for healing is included in the surgery performed. For insertion of a multi-component, inflatable penile prosthesis, see 54405. For removal, repair, or replacement of a permanent inflatable, non-inflatable, or multicomponent prosthesis, see 54406–54417. Supplies used when providing these procedures may be reported with the appropriate HCPCS Level II code(s). Check with the specific payer to determine coverage.

ICD-10-CM Diagnostic Codes

F52.21	Male erectile disorder ♂
N52.01	Erectile dysfunction due to arterial insufficiency 🄰 ♂
N52.02	Corporo-venous occlusive erectile dysfunction 🄰 ♂
N52.03	Combined arterial insufficiency and corporo-venous occlusive erectile dysfunction 🄰 ♂
N52.2	Drug-induced erectile dysfunction 🄰 ♂
N52.31	Erectile dysfunction following radical prostatectomy 🄰 ♂

N52.32	Erectile dysfunction following radical cystectomy △ ♂
N52.33	Erectile dysfunction following urethral surgery △ ♂
N52.34	Erectile dysfunction following simple prostatectomy △ ♂
N52.35	Erectile dysfunction following radiation therapy △ ♂
N52.36	Erectile dysfunction following interstitial seed therapy △ ♂
N52.37	Erectile dysfunction following prostate ablative therapy △ ♂
N52.8	Other male erectile dysfunction △ ♂

AMA: 54400 2014,Jan,11 **54401** 2014,Jan,11

Relative Value Units/Medicare Edits

Non-Facility RVU	Work	PE	MP	Total
54400	9.17	5.13	1.04	15.34
54401	10.44	7.35	1.19	18.98
Facility RVU	**Work**	**PE**	**MP**	**Total**
54400	9.17	5.13	1.04	15.34
54401	10.44	7.35	1.19	18.98

	FUD	Status	MUE	Modifiers				IOM Reference
54400	90	A	1(2)	51	N/A	62*	N/A	100-03,230.4
54401	90	A	1(2)	51	N/A	62*	N/A	

* with documentation

Terms To Know

dissection. Separating by cutting tissue or body structures apart.

insertion. Placement or implantation into a body part.

membrane. Thin, flexible tissue layer that covers or functions to separate or connect anatomic areas, structures, or organs. May also be described as having the characteristic of allowing certain substances to permeate or pass through but not others (semipermeable).

prosthesis. Man-made substitute for a missing body part.

tissue. Group of similar cells with a similar function that form definite structures and organs. Tissue types include epithelial tissue, muscle tissue, connective tissue, and nervous tissue.

transverse. Crosswise at right angles to the long axis of a structure or part.

54405

| 54405 | Insertion of multi-component, inflatable penile prosthesis, including placement of pump, cylinders, and reservoir |

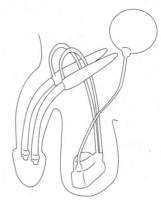

The physician inserts a multi-component penile prosthesis

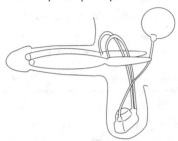

The incision or incisions are closed with sutures

Explanation

The physician inserts an inflatable penile prosthesis made of three components-the reservoir, the pump, and two inflatable cylinders. A transverse incision is made at the base of the penis in the upper scrotum. With care to avoid the urethra and important nerves and blood vessels, dissection is carried down to the erectile tissues at the base of the penis. The thick fibrous membranes surrounding the two main erectile tissues are incised and dilators are inserted to create space for the prostheses. Two prosthetic devices are inserted into the two erectile tissue compartments down the length of the penis. A pouch is made in one side of the scrotum, and the pump mechanism and tubing are inserted into the space created. Using an index finger, the surgeon creates a tunnel from the pump to the space behind the pubic bone. The reservoir is placed behind the pubic bone with tubing running from it through the tunnel to the pump in the scrotum. The incisions and tissues are closed by suturing. The operation can also be done in similar fashion using an incision just below the scrotum in the perineum to enter the erectile tissue and in the area above the pubic bone to gain access to place the reservoir.

Coding Tips

Code 54405 is not used for plastic implants that are inserted for healing purposes at the time of another surgery. The insertion of plastic implants for healing is included in the surgery performed. For insertion of a noninflatable, semirigid, or inflatable, self-contained penile prosthesis, see 54400 and 54401. For removal, repair, or replacement of a permanent inflatable, noninflatable, or multicomponent prosthesis, see 54406–54417. Any manipulation or dilation is not reported separately. Supplies used when providing this procedure may be reported with the appropriate HCPCS Level II code. Check with the specific payer to determine coverage.

ICD-10-CM Diagnostic Codes

F52.21	Male erectile disorder ♂
N52.01	Erectile dysfunction due to arterial insufficiency 🅰 ♂
N52.02	Corporo-venous occlusive erectile dysfunction 🅰 ♂
N52.03	Combined arterial insufficiency and corporo-venous occlusive erectile dysfunction 🅰 ♂
N52.2	Drug-induced erectile dysfunction 🅰 ♂
N52.31	Erectile dysfunction following radical prostatectomy 🅰 ♂
N52.32	Erectile dysfunction following radical cystectomy 🅰 ♂
N52.33	Erectile dysfunction following urethral surgery 🅰 ♂
N52.34	Erectile dysfunction following simple prostatectomy 🅰 ♂
N52.35	Erectile dysfunction following radiation therapy 🅰 ♂
N52.36	Erectile dysfunction following interstitial seed therapy 🅰 ♂
N52.37	Erectile dysfunction following prostate ablative therapy 🅰 ♂
N52.8	Other male erectile dysfunction 🅰 ♂

AMA: **54405** 2014,Jan,11

Relative Value Units/Medicare Edits

Non-Facility RVU	Work	PE	MP	Total
54405	14.52	7.18	1.67	23.37
Facility RVU	**Work**	**PE**	**MP**	**Total**
54405	14.52	7.18	1.67	23.37

	FUD	Status	MUE	Modifiers				IOM Reference
54405	90	A	1(2)	51	N/A	62*	80	None

* with documentation

Terms To Know

membrane. Thin, flexible tissue layer that covers or functions to separate or connect anatomic areas, structures, or organs. May also be described as having the characteristic of allowing certain substances to permeate or pass through but not others (semipermeable).

prosthesis. Device that replaces all or part of an internal body organ or replaces all or part of the function of a permanently inoperative or malfunctioning internal body organ.

pump. Forcing gas or liquid from a body part.

reservoir. Space or body cavity for storage of liquid.

scrotum. Skin pouch that holds the testes and supporting reproductive structures.

transverse. Crosswise at right angles to the long axis of a structure or part.

54406

54406	Removal of all components of a multi-component, inflatable penile prosthesis without replacement of prosthesis

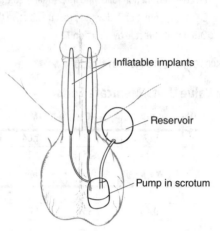

A multi-component penile implant is removed in its entirety, without replacement

Explanation

The patient is taken to the operating room, placed in a supine or lithotomy position, and the physician makes an incision using the same penoscrotal or infrapubic approach as the original procedure to remove the multicomponent, inflatable penile prosthesis. The physician makes an incision into the corpus cavernosum and the prosthesis is withdrawn. The corporotomy is closed by suture. The subcutaneous tissue is closed by suture and a dressing is applied to the incision. The bladder is emptied with a catheter. An indwelling urethral catheter, if used, is removed on the first postoperative day.

Coding Tips

If not all components are removed, report reduced services with modifier 52. For repair of components of a multicomponent, inflatable penile prosthesis, see 54408. For removal and replacement of all components of a multicomponent prosthesis, see 54410–54411. For removal without replacement of a noninflatable, or inflatable, self-contained prosthesis, report 54415. For removal and replacement of a noninflatable, or inflatable, self-contained prosthesis, see 54416–54417.

ICD-10-CM Diagnostic Codes

T83.410A	Breakdown (mechanical) of implanted penile prosthesis, initial encounter ♂
T83.411A	Breakdown (mechanical) of implanted testicular prosthesis, initial encounter
T83.420A	Displacement of implanted penile prosthesis, initial encounter ♂
T83.421A	Displacement of implanted testicular prosthesis, initial encounter
T83.490A	Other mechanical complication of implanted penile prosthesis, initial encounter ♂
T83.491A	Other mechanical complication of implanted testicular prosthesis, initial encounter
T83.61XA	Infection and inflammatory reaction due to implanted penile prosthesis, initial encounter
T83.62XA	Infection and inflammatory reaction due to implanted testicular prosthesis, initial encounter
T83.69XA	Infection and inflammatory reaction due to other prosthetic device, implant and graft in genital tract, initial encounter

Penis

Inflatable implants

Reservoir

Pump in scrotum

T85.79XA	Infection and inflammatory reaction due to other internal prosthetic devices, implants and grafts, initial encounter
T85.818A	Embolism due to other internal prosthetic devices, implants and grafts, initial encounter
T85.828A	Fibrosis due to other internal prosthetic devices, implants and grafts, initial encounter
T85.838A	Hemorrhage due to other internal prosthetic devices, implants and grafts, initial encounter
T85.848A	Pain due to other internal prosthetic devices, implants and grafts, initial encounter
T85.858A	Stenosis due to other internal prosthetic devices, implants and grafts, initial encounter
T85.868A	Thrombosis due to other internal prosthetic devices, implants and grafts, initial encounter
T85.898A	Other specified complication of other internal prosthetic devices, implants and grafts, initial encounter

AMA: 54406 2014,Jan,11

Relative Value Units/Medicare Edits

Non-Facility RVU	Work	PE	MP	Total
54406	12.89	6.74	1.48	21.11
Facility RVU	**Work**	**PE**	**MP**	**Total**
54406	12.89	6.74	1.48	21.11

	FUD	Status	MUE	Modifiers				IOM Reference
54406	90	A	1(2)	51	N/A	62*	80	None

* with documentation

Terms To Know

approach. Method or anatomical location used to gain access to a body organ or specific area for procedures.

dressing. Material applied to a wound or surgical site for protection, absorption, or drainage of the area.

epididymis. Coiled tube on the back of the testis that is the site of sperm maturation and storage and where spermatozoa are propelled into the vas deferens toward the ejaculatory duct by contraction of smooth muscle.

lithotomy position. Common position patients may be placed in for some surgical procedures and examinations involving the pelvis and/or lower abdomen. The patient is placed supine (on their back), hips and knees flexed, thighs apart, with feet supported in raised stirrups.

prosthesis. Device that replaces all or part of an internal body organ or replaces all or part of the function of a permanently inoperative or malfunctioning internal body organ.

subcutaneous tissue. Sheet or wide band of adipose (fat) and areolar connective tissue in two layers attached to the dermis.

54408

54408	Repair of component(s) of a multi-component, inflatable penile prosthesis

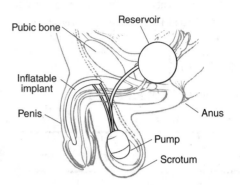

Any component of a multi-component, inflatable penile implant is repaired

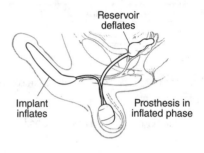

Explanation

Under general anesthesia, the patient is placed in a supine or lithotomy position and the physician makes an incision using the same penoscrotal or infrapubic approach as the original procedure to repair the previously placed multi-component, inflatable penile prosthesis. The physician makes an incision into the corpus cavernosum to inspect the previously placed prosthesis. Repairs are made. The corporotomy is closed by suture. The subcutaneous tissue is closed by suture and a dressing is applied to the incision. The bladder is emptied with a catheter. An indwelling urethral catheter, if used, is removed on the first postoperative day.

Coding Tips

For removal without replacement of all components of a multicomponent prosthesis, see 54406. For removal and replacement of all components of a multicomponent prosthesis, see 54410–54411. For removal without replacement of a noninflatable, or inflatable, self-contained prosthesis, report 54415. For removal and replacement of a noninflatable, or inflatable, self-contained prosthesis, see 54416–54417.

ICD-10-CM Diagnostic Codes

T83.410A	Breakdown (mechanical) of implanted penile prosthesis, initial encounter ♂
T83.411A	Breakdown (mechanical) of implanted testicular prosthesis, initial encounter
T83.420A	Displacement of implanted penile prosthesis, initial encounter ♂
T83.421A	Displacement of implanted testicular prosthesis, initial encounter
T83.490A	Other mechanical complication of implanted penile prosthesis, initial encounter ♂
T83.491A	Other mechanical complication of implanted testicular prosthesis, initial encounter

T83.61XA	Infection and inflammatory reaction due to implanted penile prosthesis, initial encounter
T83.62XA	Infection and inflammatory reaction due to implanted testicular prosthesis, initial encounter
T83.69XA	Infection and inflammatory reaction due to other prosthetic device, implant and graft in genital tract, initial encounter
Z44.8	Encounter for fitting and adjustment of other external prosthetic devices

AMA: 54408 2014,Jan,11

Relative Value Units/Medicare Edits

Non-Facility RVU	Work	PE	MP	Total
54408	13.91	7.31	1.61	22.83
Facility RVU	**Work**	**PE**	**MP**	**Total**
54408	13.91	7.31	1.61	22.83

	FUD	Status	MUE	Modifiers				IOM Reference
54408	90	A	1(2)	51	N/A	62*	80	None

* with documentation

Terms To Know

approach. Method or anatomical location used to gain access to a body organ or specific area for procedures.

catheter. Flexible tube inserted into an area of the body for introducing or withdrawing fluid.

dressing. Material applied to a wound or surgical site for protection, absorption, or drainage of the area.

lithotomy position. Common position patients may be placed in for some surgical procedures and examinations involving the pelvis and/or lower abdomen. The patient is placed supine (on their back), hips and knees flexed, thighs apart, with feet supported in raised stirrups.

prosthesis. Man-made substitute for a missing body part.

subcutaneous tissue. Sheet or wide band of adipose (fat) and areolar connective tissue in two layers attached to the dermis.

supine. Lying on the back.

54410

54410 Removal and replacement of all component(s) of a multi-component, inflatable penile prosthesis at the same operative session

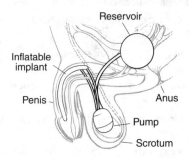

A multi-component implant is removed and a new unit is installed during the same operative session

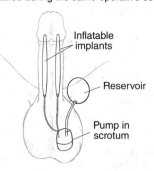

Explanation

Under general anesthesia, the patient is placed in a supine or lithotomy position and the physician makes an incision using the same penoscrotal or infrapubic approach as the original procedure to remove the previously placed multi-component, inflatable penile prosthesis and to insert a replacement during the same operative session. The physician makes an incision into the corpus cavernosum and the prosthesis is withdrawn. The replacement prosthesis is brought through the glans and the deflated cylinder is drawn into the distal corporal body for insertion into the crus of the penis. The corporotomy is closed and the cylinders are inflated and deflated several times to check the flow of the fluid to and from the cylinders. The reservoir is brought through the external inguinal ring and the bladder is emptied by catheter. The existing subfascial pocket in used to place the reservoir, as well as the pump/activator mechanism, which is placed in the existing scrotal pocket. Sutures are placed to prevent upward migration, the tubing is filled with fluid, and the physician makes the connections between the tubing of the pump and reservoir and the tubing of the pump and cylinders. Before the wound is closed, the prosthesis is cycled to check proper functioning. The corporotomy is closed by suture. The subcutaneous tissue is closed by suture and a dressing is applied to the incision. The bladder is emptied with a catheter. An indwelling urethral catheter, if used, is removed on the first postoperative day.

Coding Tips

For removal without replacement of all components of a multicomponent prosthesis, see 54406. For repair of components of a multicomponent, inflatable prosthesis, see 54408. For removal without replacement of a noninflatable, or inflatable, self-contained prosthesis, report 54415. For removal and replacement of a noninflatable, or inflatable, self-contained prosthesis, see 54416–54417. Supplies used when providing this procedure may be reported with the appropriate HCPCS Level II code. Check with the specific payer to determine coverage.

ICD-10-CM Diagnostic Codes

T83.410A	Breakdown (mechanical) of implanted penile prosthesis, initial encounter ♂
T83.411A	Breakdown (mechanical) of implanted testicular prosthesis, initial encounter
T83.420A	Displacement of implanted penile prosthesis, initial encounter ♂
T83.421A	Displacement of implanted testicular prosthesis, initial encounter
T83.490A	Other mechanical complication of implanted penile prosthesis, initial encounter ♂
T83.491A	Other mechanical complication of implanted testicular prosthesis, initial encounter
T83.61XA	Infection and inflammatory reaction due to implanted penile prosthesis, initial encounter
T83.62XA	Infection and inflammatory reaction due to implanted testicular prosthesis, initial encounter
T83.69XA	Infection and inflammatory reaction due to other prosthetic device, implant and graft in genital tract, initial encounter
T83.718A	Erosion of other implanted mesh to organ or tissue, initial encounter
T83.728A	Exposure of other implanted mesh into organ or tissue, initial encounter
T83.82XA	Fibrosis due to genitourinary prosthetic devices, implants and grafts, initial encounter
T83.83XA	Hemorrhage due to genitourinary prosthetic devices, implants and grafts, initial encounter
T83.84XA	Pain due to genitourinary prosthetic devices, implants and grafts, initial encounter
T83.85XA	Stenosis due to genitourinary prosthetic devices, implants and grafts, initial encounter
T83.86XA	Thrombosis due to genitourinary prosthetic devices, implants and grafts, initial encounter
T83.89XA	Other specified complication of genitourinary prosthetic devices, implants and grafts, initial encounter
Z44.8	Encounter for fitting and adjustment of other external prosthetic devices

AMA: **54410** 2014,Jan,11

Relative Value Units/Medicare Edits

Non-Facility RVU	Work	PE	MP	Total
54410	15.18	7.94	1.73	24.85
Facility RVU	Work	PE	MP	Total
54410	15.18	7.94	1.73	24.85

	FUD	Status	MUE	Modifiers				IOM Reference
54410	90	A	1(2)	51	N/A	62*	80	None

* with documentation

Terms To Know

prosthesis. Man-made substitute for a missing body part.

reservoir. Space or body cavity for storage of liquid.

54411

54411 Removal and replacement of all components of a multi-component inflatable penile prosthesis through an infected field at the same operative session, including irrigation and debridement of infected tissue

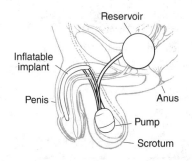

A multi-component implant that has caused infection is removed and is replaced with a new unit

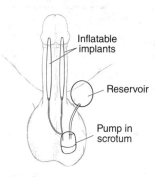

Explanation

The physician removes and replaces a multi-component inflatable penile prosthesis and irrigates and debrides infected tissue. The patient is taken to the operating room and placed under general anesthesia. The physician makes an incision using the same penoscrotal or infrapubic approach as the original procedure. The physician makes an incision into the corpus cavernosum and the prosthesis is withdrawn. Any infected tissue is debrided and irrigated with an antibiotic solution. The replacement prosthesis is brought through the glans and the deflated cylinder is drawn into the distal corporal body for insertion into the crus of the penis. The corporotomy is closed and the cylinders are inflated and deflated several times to check the flow of the fluid to and from the cylinders. The reservoir is brought through the external inguinal ring and the bladder is emptied by catheter. The existing subfascial pocket is used to place the reservoir, as well as the pump/activator mechanism, which is placed in the existing scrotal pocket. Any infected tissue is debrided and irrigated with an antibiotic solution. Sutures are placed to prevent upward migration, the tubing is filled with fluid, and the physician makes the connections between the tubing of the pump and reservoir and the tubing of the pump and cylinders. Before the wound is closed, the prosthesis is cycled to check proper functioning. The corporotomy is closed by suture. The subcutaneous tissue is closed by suture and a dressing is applied to the incision. The bladder is emptied with a catheter. An indwelling urethral catheter, if used, is removed on the first postoperative day.

Coding Tips

Do not report 11042 or 11043 in addition to 54411. If not all components are removed and replaced, report reduced services with modifier 52. For removal without replacement of all components of a multi-component prosthesis, see

CPT © 2020 American Medical Association. All Rights Reserved.   ● New   ▲ Revised   + Add On   ★ Telemedicine   AMA: CPT Assist   [Resequenced]   ☑ Laterality   © 2020 Optum360, LLC

54406. For repair of components of a multi-component, inflatable penile prosthesis, see 54408. Supplies used when providing this procedure may be reported with the appropriate HCPCS Level II code. Check with the specific payer to determine coverage.

ICD-10-CM Diagnostic Codes

T83.61XA	Infection and inflammatory reaction due to implanted penile prosthesis, initial encounter
T83.62XA	Infection and inflammatory reaction due to implanted testicular prosthesis, initial encounter
T83.69XA	Infection and inflammatory reaction due to other prosthetic device, implant and graft in genital tract, initial encounter

AMA: **54411** 2014,Jan,11

Relative Value Units/Medicare Edits

Non-Facility RVU	Work	PE	MP	Total
54411	18.35	9.25	2.12	29.72
Facility RVU	Work	PE	MP	Total
54411	18.35	9.25	2.12	29.72

	FUD	Status	MUE	Modifiers				IOM Reference
54411	90	A	1(2)	51	N/A	62*	80	None

* with documentation

Terms To Know

catheter. Flexible tube inserted into an area of the body for introducing or withdrawing fluid.

debridement. Removal of dead or contaminated tissue and foreign matter from a wound.

distal. Located farther away from a specified reference point or the trunk.

dressing. Material applied to a wound or surgical site for protection, absorption, or drainage of the area.

infection. Presence of microorganisms in body tissues that may result in cellular damage.

irrigation. To wash out or cleanse a body cavity, wound, or tissue with water or other fluid.

prosthesis. Device that replaces all or part of an internal body organ or replaces all or part of the function of a permanently inoperative or malfunctioning internal body organ.

replacement. Insertion of new tissue or material in place of old one.

reservoir. Space or body cavity for storage of liquid.

subcutaneous tissue. Sheet or wide band of adipose (fat) and areolar connective tissue in two layers attached to the dermis.

tissue. Group of similar cells with a similar function that form definite structures and organs. Tissue types include epithelial tissue, muscle tissue, connective tissue, and nervous tissue.

54415

54415	Removal of non-inflatable (semi-rigid) or inflatable (self-contained) penile prosthesis, without replacement of prosthesis

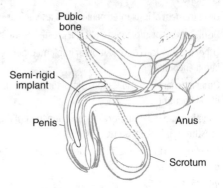

A non-inflatable or self contained inflatable implant is removed

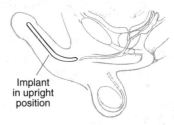

Implant in upright position

Explanation

The physician makes an incision using the same approach (i.e., penoscrotal or distal penile) as the original procedure to remove the non-inflatable or self-contained inflatable penile prosthesis in a patient who is under general anesthesia. An incision is made into the corpus cavernosum, the corporal tissue is dissected, and the prosthesis is removed from the corporal body. The wound is irrigated with antibiotics, and the corporotomy is closed by suture. The subcutaneous tissue is closed by suture and a dressing is applied to the incision. The bladder is emptied with a catheter.

Coding Tips

For removal and replacement of a noninflatable, or inflatable, self-contained prosthesis, see 54416–54417. For removal without replacement of all components of a multicomponent prosthesis, see 54406. For repair of components of a multicomponent, inflatable penile prosthesis, see 54408. For removal and replacement of all components of a multi-component prosthesis, see 54410–54411.

ICD-10-CM Diagnostic Codes

T83.410A	Breakdown (mechanical) of implanted penile prosthesis, initial encounter ♂
T83.411A	Breakdown (mechanical) of implanted testicular prosthesis, initial encounter
T83.420A	Displacement of implanted penile prosthesis, initial encounter ♂
T83.421A	Displacement of implanted testicular prosthesis, initial encounter
T83.490A	Other mechanical complication of implanted penile prosthesis, initial encounter ♂
T83.491A	Other mechanical complication of implanted testicular prosthesis, initial encounter
T83.61XA	Infection and inflammatory reaction due to implanted penile prosthesis, initial encounter

T83.62XA	Infection and inflammatory reaction due to implanted testicular prosthesis, initial encounter
T83.69XA	Infection and inflammatory reaction due to other prosthetic device, implant and graft in genital tract, initial encounter
T83.718A	Erosion of other implanted mesh to organ or tissue, initial encounter
T83.728A	Exposure of other implanted mesh into organ or tissue, initial encounter
T83.81XA	Embolism due to genitourinary prosthetic devices, implants and grafts, initial encounter
T83.82XA	Fibrosis due to genitourinary prosthetic devices, implants and grafts, initial encounter
T83.83XA	Hemorrhage due to genitourinary prosthetic devices, implants and grafts, initial encounter
T83.84XA	Pain due to genitourinary prosthetic devices, implants and grafts, initial encounter
T83.85XA	Stenosis due to genitourinary prosthetic devices, implants and grafts, initial encounter
T83.86XA	Thrombosis due to genitourinary prosthetic devices, implants and grafts, initial encounter
T83.89XA	Other specified complication of genitourinary prosthetic devices, implants and grafts, initial encounter

AMA: 54415 2014,Jan,11

Relative Value Units/Medicare Edits

Non-Facility RVU	Work	PE	MP	Total
54415	8.88	5.37	1.02	15.27
Facility RVU	Work	PE	MP	Total
54415	8.88	5.37	1.02	15.27

	FUD	Status	MUE	Modifiers				IOM Reference
54415	90	A	1(2)	51	N/A	62*	80	None

* with documentation

Terms To Know

approach. Method or anatomical location used to gain access to a body organ or specific area for procedures.

dissect. Cut apart or separate tissue for surgical purposes or for visual or microscopic study.

distal. Located farther away from a specified reference point or the trunk.

irrigate. Washing out, lavage.

seminal vesicles. Paired glands located at the base of the bladder in males that release the majority of fluid into semen through ducts that join with the vas deferens forming the ejaculatory duct.

subcutaneous tissue. Sheet or wide band of adipose (fat) and areolar connective tissue in two layers attached to the dermis.

tissue. Group of similar cells with a similar function that form definite structures and organs. Tissue types include epithelial tissue, muscle tissue, connective tissue, and nervous tissue.

54416-54417

Penis

54416	Removal and replacement of non-inflatable (semi-rigid) or inflatable (self-contained) penile prosthesis at the same operative session
54417	Removal and replacement of non-inflatable (semi-rigid) or inflatable (self-contained) penile prosthesis through an infected field at the same operative session, including irrigation and debridement of infected tissue

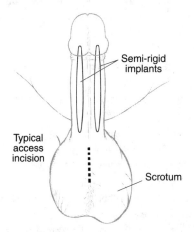

A non-inflatable or self-contained inflatable implant is removed and replaced with a similar unit

Explanation

Under general anesthesia, the patient is placed in a supine or lithotomy position, and the physician makes an incision using the same approach (i.e., penoscrotal or distal penile) as the original procedure to remove the non-inflatable (semirigid) or self-contained inflatable penile prosthesis and to insert a replacement prosthesis. An incision is made into the corpus cavernosum, the corporal tissue is dissected, and the prosthesis is removed from the corporal body. The wound is irrigated with antibiotics and the replacement prosthesis is advanced to the mid glans and introduced into the corporal space. In 54417, any infected tissue is debrided and irrigated with an antibiotic solution. The corporotomy is closed by suture. The subcutaneous tissue is closed by suture and a dressing is applied to the incision. The bladder is emptied with a catheter. An indwelling urethral catheter, if used, is removed on the first postoperative day.

Coding Tips

Do not report 11042 or 11043 with 54417. For removal without replacement of a noninflatable, or inflatable, self-contained prosthesis, report 54415. For removal without replacement of all components of a multicomponent prosthesis, see 54406. For removal and replacement of all components of a multicomponent prosthesis, not through an infected field, report 54410. Supplies used when providing these procedures may be reported with the appropriate HCPCS Level II code(s). Check with the specific payer to determine coverage.

ICD-10-CM Diagnostic Codes

T83.410A	Breakdown (mechanical) of implanted penile prosthesis, initial encounter ♂
T83.411A	Breakdown (mechanical) of implanted testicular prosthesis, initial encounter
T83.420A	Displacement of implanted penile prosthesis, initial encounter ♂
T83.421A	Displacement of implanted testicular prosthesis, initial encounter

T83.490A	Other mechanical complication of implanted penile prosthesis, initial encounter ♂		
T83.491A	Other mechanical complication of implanted testicular prosthesis, initial encounter		
T83.61XA	Infection and inflammatory reaction due to implanted penile prosthesis, initial encounter		
T83.62XA	Infection and inflammatory reaction due to implanted testicular prosthesis, initial encounter		
T83.69XA	Infection and inflammatory reaction due to other prosthetic device, implant and graft in genital tract, initial encounter		
T83.718A	Erosion of other implanted mesh to organ or tissue, initial encounter		
T83.728A	Exposure of other implanted mesh into organ or tissue, initial encounter		
T83.82XA	Fibrosis due to genitourinary prosthetic devices, implants and grafts, initial encounter		
T83.83XA	Hemorrhage due to genitourinary prosthetic devices, implants and grafts, initial encounter		
T83.84XA	Pain due to genitourinary prosthetic devices, implants and grafts, initial encounter		
T83.85XA	Stenosis due to genitourinary prosthetic devices, implants and grafts, initial encounter		
T83.86XA	Thrombosis due to genitourinary prosthetic devices, implants and grafts, initial encounter		
T83.89XA	Other specified complication of genitourinary prosthetic devices, implants and grafts, initial encounter		
Z44.8	Encounter for fitting and adjustment of other external prosthetic devices		

AMA: 54416 2014,Jan,11 **54417** 2014,Jan,11

Relative Value Units/Medicare Edits

Non-Facility RVU	Work	PE	MP	Total
54416	12.08	7.08	1.38	20.54
54417	16.1	8.01	1.85	25.96
Facility RVU	Work	PE	MP	Total
54416	12.08	7.08	1.38	20.54
54417	16.1	8.01	1.85	25.96

	FUD	Status	MUE	Modifiers				IOM Reference
54416	90	A	1(2)	51	N/A	62*	80	None
54417	90	A	1(2)	51	N/A	62*	80	

* with documentation

Terms To Know

irrigation. To wash out or cleanse a body cavity, wound, or tissue with water or other fluid.

prosthesis. Device that replaces all or part of an internal body organ or replaces all or part of the function of a permanently inoperative or malfunctioning internal body organ.

replacement. Insertion of new tissue or material in place of old one.

54420-54435

54420	Corpora cavernosa-saphenous vein shunt (priapism operation), unilateral or bilateral
54430	Corpora cavernosa-corpus spongiosum shunt (priapism operation), unilateral or bilateral
54435	Corpora cavernosa-glans penis fistulization (eg, biopsy needle, Winter procedure, rongeur, or punch) for priapism

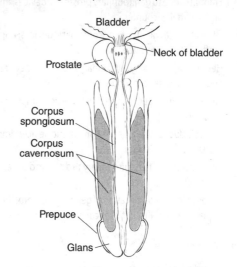

Priapism is abnormal erection and the cause may be obstruction of the outflow veins

Explanation

In 54420, the physician treats priapism, an abnormally sustained erection, by creating a shunt for the diversion of blood from the penis to the femoral vein. An incision is made in the groin area of the thigh and the saphenous vein is cut and dissected free of its attachments creating a mobile segment about 10 cm long. A second incision is made at the base of the penis and the saphenous vein is tunneled through the subcutaneous tissues to the base of the penis. A 1 cm in diameter piece of the thick fibrous tissue of the corpus cavernosum (erectile tissue) is excised and the free end of the saphenous vein is sutured to the defect. The erection resolves as blood flows from the penis to the femoral vein through this saphenous vein segment. The incisions are closed by suturing. The procedure is sometimes repeated on the opposite side. In 54430 and 54435, the physician treats priapism by creating a shunt for the diversion of blood from one region of the penis to an adjacent region. In 54430, with a catheter in the urethra into the bladder, an incision is made in the side of the penis. Dissection is carried to the thick fibrous tissues surrounding one of the corpus cavernosum (erectile tissue) and to the corpus spongiosum, which is the erectile tissue around the urethra. Oval discs of the fibrous tissue are excised from the adjacent surfaces of these two structures. The excisional defects are sutured together creating a shunt (passageway) for the flow of blood from the engorged corpus cavernosum to the corpus spongiosum thus relieving the erection. As in 54420, the tissues and the skin are sutured closed and sometimes the procedure is repeated on the opposite side. In 54435, with adequate local anesthesia, the head of the penis is punctured with a biopsy needle and advanced into the tip of the corpus cavernosum (erectile tissue). A portion of tissue from the head of the penis to the corpus cavernosum is removed as if taking a biopsy. This creates a passageway for blood trapped in the cavernosum to escape through the circulation to the head of the penis. The two puncture sites in the head of the penis are closed by suturing.

Coding Tips

Note that 54420 and 54430 are unilateral or bilateral procedures and are reported only once even if the procedure is performed on both sides. For irrigation of corpora cavernosa for priapism, see 54220. For injections of the corpora cavernosa, see 54230–54235.

ICD-10-CM Diagnostic Codes

N48.31	Priapism due to trauma ♂
N48.32	Priapism due to disease classified elsewhere ♂
N48.33	Priapism, drug-induced ♂
N48.39	Other priapism ♂

AMA: **54420** 2014,Jan,11 **54430** 2014,Jan,11 **54435** 2014,Jan,11

Relative Value Units/Medicare Edits

Non-Facility RVU	Work	PE	MP	Total
54420	12.39	6.52	1.42	20.33
54430	11.06	6.13	1.26	18.45
54435	6.81	4.38	0.79	11.98
Facility RVU	Work	PE	MP	Total
54420	12.39	6.52	1.42	20.33
54430	11.06	6.13	1.26	18.45
54435	6.81	4.38	0.79	11.98

	FUD	Status	MUE	Modifiers				IOM Reference
54420	90	A	1(2)	51	N/A	N/A	80	None
54430	90	A	1(2)	51	N/A	N/A	80	
54435	90	A	1(2)	51	N/A	N/A	N/A	

* with documentation

Terms To Know

connective tissue. Body tissue made from fibroblasts, collagen, and elastic fibrils that connects, supports, and holds together other tissues and cells and includes cartilage, collagenous, fibrous, elastic, and osseous tissue.

defect. Imperfection, flaw, or absence.

dissect. Cut apart or separate tissue for surgical purposes or for visual or microscopic study.

diversion. Rechanneling of body fluid through another conduit.

fibrous tissue. Connective tissues.

glans penis. Distal end or head of the penis.

priapism. Persistent, painful erection lasting more than four hours and unrelated to sexual stimulation, causing pain and tenderness.

shunt. Surgically created passage between blood vessels or other natural passages, such as an arteriovenous anastomosis, to divert or bypass blood flow from the normal channel.

54437

54437   Repair of traumatic corporeal tear(s)

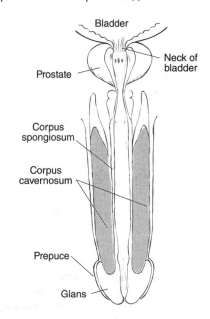

Explanation

Repair of traumatic corporeal tears vary depending on the surgeon and/or location of the tear. Typically the tears are transverse, near midline and the urethra. A tourniquet is placed at the base of the penis to restrict blood flow, leaving the operative field as clear as possible for visualization and exploration. A midline perineal incision is made to reveal the corporeal body. A Gittes test may be performed to aid in locating the tear. The injection of saline and erection simulation can flush out possible blood clots hiding the leak. The tear is repaired with sutures. The incision is closed in layers. Some surgeons may place a catheter overnight while other surgeons only utilize this when the trauma is very close to the urethra. Postoperative treatment can range from antibiotics to compression dressings to erection inhibitors.

Coding Tips

For repair of the urethra, see 53410 and/or 53415. For plastic repair of the penis due to injury, see 54440.

ICD-10-CM Diagnostic Codes

S39.840A   Fracture of corpus cavernosum penis, initial encounter ♂

Relative Value Units/Medicare Edits

Non-Facility RVU	Work	PE	MP	Total
54437	11.5	6.66	1.31	19.47
Facility RVU	Work	PE	MP	Total
54437	11.5	6.66	1.31	19.47

	FUD	Status	MUE	Modifiers			IOM Reference
54437	90	A	1(2)	51	N/A	62*	80	None

* with documentation

Terms To Know

repair. Surgical closure of a wound. The wound may be a result of injury/trauma or it may be a surgically created defect. Repairs are divided into three categories: simple, intermediate, and complex.

54438

54438   Replantation, penis, complete amputation including urethral repair

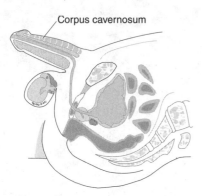

Corpus cavernosum

Amputated penis is replanted

Explanation

The penis is reattached after traumatic amputation requiring repair of the urethra. The patient is placed under general anesthesia and often given blood transfusion due to blood loss from the amputation. A tourniquet is positioned at the proximal end under the pubis. Debridement of the area using an operating microscope is performed. The amputated part is attached to a catheter that is inserted into the bladder. Urethra repair is performed by end-to-end anastomosis with the cavernosal bodies using interrupted absorbable sutures. The area is flushed with heparin saline in order to reveal the deep dorsal penile vein, and end-to-end anastomosis is completed. Other deep vasculature is repaired in a similar manner. The tunica albuginea of the cavernosal bodies and septum are secured in place with running sutures. Buck's fascia is also closed. Superficial vessels are anastomosed. The skin is adjusted to complete closure. A transurethral catheter is inserted. Heparin is administered for about a week to thin the blood during the healing process.

Coding Tips

For replantation of an incomplete penile amputation, see 54437 for corporeal tear(s) repair and 53410 and 53415 for urethra repair. For plastic repair of the penis due to injury, see 54440.

ICD-10-CM Diagnostic Codes

S38.221A   Complete traumatic amputation of penis, initial encounter ♂

Relative Value Units/Medicare Edits

Non-Facility RVU	Work	PE	MP	Total
54438	24.5	11.32	2.82	38.64
Facility RVU	Work	PE	MP	Total
54438	24.5	11.32	2.82	38.64

	FUD	Status	MUE	Modifiers				IOM Reference
54438	90	A	1(2)	51	N/A	62*	80	None

* with documentation

Terms To Know

amputation. Removal of all or part of a limb or digit through the shaft or body of a bone.

replantation. Surgical reattachment or replacement of a body part or structure to its previous site, such as a digit or tooth.

54440

54440   Plastic operation of penis for injury

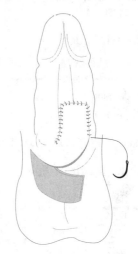

An injury to the penis is repaired
using plastic techniques

Microsurgery, debridement, urethral
repair, or grafts may be required

Explanation

The physician repairs an injury of the penis using one or more of plastic surgery techniques. The repair may require skin grafts, tissue grafts, urethral repair, extensive debridement, microsurgical repairs, or any combination.

Coding Tips

Submit a cover letter and operative report with this by-report procedure. This code includes any combination of complex repairs and closures, which are not reported separately. Report any free grafts or flaps separately. If a urethroplasty or plastic repair better describes what the physician is performing, refer to that code.

ICD-10-CM Diagnostic Codes

S31.21XA	Laceration without foreign body of penis, initial encounter ♂
S31.22XA	Laceration with foreign body of penis, initial encounter ♂
S31.23XA	Puncture wound without foreign body of penis, initial encounter ♂
S31.24XA	Puncture wound with foreign body of penis, initial encounter ♂
S31.25XA	Open bite of penis, initial encounter ♂
S38.221A	Complete traumatic amputation of penis, initial encounter ♂
S38.222A	Partial traumatic amputation of penis, initial encounter ♂
S39.840A	Fracture of corpus cavernosum penis, initial encounter ♂
S39.848A	Other specified injuries of external genitals, initial encounter

AMA: 54440 2014,Jan,11

Relative Value Units/Medicare Edits

Non-Facility RVU	Work	PE	MP	Total
54440	0.0	0.0	0.0	0.0
Facility RVU	Work	PE	MP	Total
54440	0.0	0.0	0.0	0.0

	FUD	Status	MUE	Modifiers				IOM Reference
54440	90	C	1(2)	51	N/A	62*	80	None

* with documentation

Terms To Know

amputation. Removal of all or part of a limb or digit through the shaft or body of a bone.

debridement. Removal of dead or contaminated tissue and foreign matter from a wound.

flap. Mass of flesh and skin partially excised from its location but retaining its blood supply that is moved to another site to repair adjacent or distant defects.

graft. Tissue implant from another part of the body or another person.

injury. Harm or damage sustained by the body.

laceration. Tearing injury; a torn, ragged-edged wound.

microsurgery. Surgical procedures performed under magnification using a surgical microscope.

repair. Surgical closure of a wound. The wound may be a result of injury/trauma or it may be a surgically created defect. Repairs are divided into three categories: simple, intermediate, and complex.

tissue. Group of similar cells with a similar function that form definite structures and organs. Tissue types include epithelial tissue, muscle tissue, connective tissue, and nervous tissue.

54450

54450	Foreskin manipulation including lysis of preputial adhesions and stretching

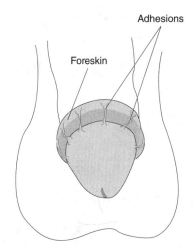

The physician treats adhesions of the foreskin

Explanation

The physician treats adhesions between the uncircumcised foreskin and the head of the penis that prevent the retraction of the foreskin. Adhesions are broken by stretching the foreskin back over the head of the penis onto the shaft or by inserting a clamp between the foreskin and the head of the penis and spreading the jaws of the clamp.

Coding Tips

For slitting prepuce, dorsal or lateral, see 54000–54001. For circumcision, see 54150–54161. For lysis or excision of penile post-circumcision adhesions, see 54162. For a frenulotomy of the penis, see 54164.

ICD-10-CM Diagnostic Codes

N47.0	Adherent prepuce, newborn N ♂
N47.1	Phimosis ♂
N47.2	Paraphimosis ♂
N47.5	Adhesions of prepuce and glans penis ♂
N47.7	Other inflammatory diseases of prepuce ♂
N47.8	Other disorders of prepuce ♂

AMA: 54450 2014,Jan,11

Relative Value Units/Medicare Edits

Non-Facility RVU	Work	PE	MP	Total
54450	1.12	0.73	0.13	1.98
Facility RVU	Work	PE	MP	Total
54450	1.12	0.41	0.13	1.66

	FUD	Status	MUE	Modifiers				IOM Reference
54450	0	A	1(2)	51	N/A	N/A	N/A	None

* with documentation

54500-54505

54500 Biopsy of testis, needle (separate procedure)
54505 Biopsy of testis, incisional (separate procedure)

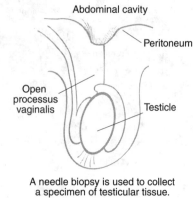

A needle biopsy is used to collect
a specimen of testicular tissue.

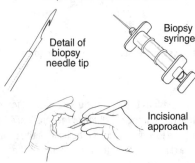

Detail of biopsy needle tip

Biopsy syringe

Incisional approach

Explanation

The physician obtains a sample of testicular tissue by needle biopsy in 54500. While the testis is held firmly with the scrotal skin stretched tightly over the testis and the epididymis positioned away from the biopsy site, a biopsy needle is inserted into the testis at the area of concern. The needle biopsy sheath is advanced over the needle and twisted to shear off the enclosed sample and then withdrawn with the sample enclosed. The scrotal wound may be closed by suturing. In 54505, the physician obtains a sample of testicular tissue by direct incisional biopsy. The procedure is done under either local or regional anesthesia. While the testis is held firmly with the scrotal skin stretched tightly over the testis and the epididymis positioned away from the biopsy site, a small incision is made through the skin of the scrotum. The underlying tissues are incised and dissected to expose the testis. The testis is stabilized by two sutures and an ellipse of tissue is removed between the two sutures. The incisions are closed by suturing.

Coding Tips

These separate procedures by definition are usually a component of a more complex service and are not identified separately. When performed alone or with other unrelated procedures/services they may be reported. If performed alone, list the code; if performed with other procedures/services, list the code and append modifier 59 or an X{EPSU} modifier. When 54500 or 54505 are performed with another separately identifiable procedure, the highest dollar value code is listed as the primary procedure and subsequent procedures are appended with modifier 51. Note that 54505 is a unilateral procedure. If performed bilaterally, some payers require that the service be reported twice with modifier 50 appended to the second code while others require identification of the service only once with modifier 50 appended. Check with individual payers. Modifier 50 identifies a procedure performed identically on the opposite side of the body (mirror image). If specimen is transported to an outside laboratory, report 99000 for handling or conveyance. For excision of

an extraparenchymal lesion of the testis, see 54512. For surgical pathology of the testis biopsy, see 88307. For fine needle aspiration biopsy, see 10004–10012 and 10021; evaluation of fine needle aspirate, see 88172–88173. When 54505 is combined with vasogram, seminal vesiculogram, or epididymogram, see 55300.

ICD-10-CM Diagnostic Codes

C62.01	Malignant neoplasm of undescended right testis ♂ ☑
C62.02	Malignant neoplasm of undescended left testis ♂ ☑
C62.11	Malignant neoplasm of descended right testis ♂ ☑
C62.12	Malignant neoplasm of descended left testis ♂ ☑
D07.61	Carcinoma in situ of scrotum ♂
D07.69	Carcinoma in situ of other male genital organs ♂
D29.21	Benign neoplasm of right testis ♂ ☑
D29.22	Benign neoplasm of left testis ♂ ☑
D40.11	Neoplasm of uncertain behavior of right testis ♂ ☑
D40.12	Neoplasm of uncertain behavior of left testis ♂ ☑
D49.59	Neoplasm of unspecified behavior of other genitourinary organ
E29.1	Testicular hypofunction ♂
N44.1	Cyst of tunica albuginea testis ♂
N44.2	Benign cyst of testis ♂
N46.01	Organic azoospermia 🅐 ♂
N46.021	Azoospermia due to drug therapy 🅐 ♂
N46.022	Azoospermia due to infection 🅐 ♂
N46.024	Azoospermia due to radiation 🅐 ♂
N46.025	Azoospermia due to systemic disease 🅐 ♂
N46.11	Organic oligospermia 🅐 ♂
N46.121	Oligospermia due to drug therapy 🅐 ♂
N46.122	Oligospermia due to infection 🅐 ♂
N46.124	Oligospermia due to radiation 🅐 ♂
N46.125	Oligospermia due to systemic disease 🅐 ♂
N46.129	Oligospermia due to other extratesticular causes 🅐 ♂
N50.0	Atrophy of testis ♂
N50.811	Right testicular pain ♂
N50.812	Left testicular pain ♂
N50.82	Scrotal pain ♂
N50.89	Other specified disorders of the male genital organs ♂
N53.8	Other male sexual dysfunction ♂

AMA: **54500** 2019,Apr,4; 2014,Jan,11 **54505** 2018,Jan,8; 2017,Jan,8; 2016,Jan,13; 2015,Jan,16; 2014,Jan,11

Relative Value Units/Medicare Edits

Non-Facility RVU	Work	PE	MP	Total
54500	1.31	0.68	0.15	2.14
54505	3.5	2.15	0.41	6.06
Facility RVU	Work	PE	MP	Total
54500	1.31	0.68	0.15	2.14
54505	3.5	2.15	0.41	6.06

	FUD	Status	MUE	Modifiers				IOM Reference
54500	0	A	1(3)	51	50	N/A	80*	None
54505	10	A	1(3)	51	50	N/A	80*	

* with documentation

© 2020 Optum360, LLC   **N Newborn: 0**   **P Pediatric: 0-17**   **M Maternity: 9-64**   **A Adult: 15-124**   ♂ Male Only   ♀ Female Only   CPT © 2020 American Medical Association. All Rights Reserved.

Testis

54512

54512   Excision of extraparenchymal lesion of testis

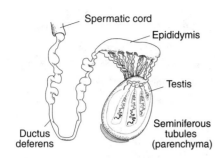

The lesion occurs in tissues outside of
the sperm producing lobules of the testes

Explanation

The physician excises an extraparenchymal lesion of the testis. The physician makes an inguinal incision, incising the skin and subcutaneous fat. The testicle is delivered through the incision, the tunica vaginalis is opened, and the lesion is excised. The incision is closed with suture.

Coding Tips

If a specimen is transported to an outside laboratory, report 99000 for handling or conveyance.

ICD-10-CM Diagnostic Codes

C62.01	Malignant neoplasm of undescended right testis ♂ ☑
C62.02	Malignant neoplasm of undescended left testis ♂ ☑
C62.11	Malignant neoplasm of descended right testis ♂ ☑
C62.12	Malignant neoplasm of descended left testis ♂ ☑
C79.82	Secondary malignant neoplasm of genital organs
D07.69	Carcinoma in situ of other male genital organs ♂
D29.21	Benign neoplasm of right testis ♂ ☑
D29.22	Benign neoplasm of left testis ♂ ☑
D40.11	Neoplasm of uncertain behavior of right testis ♂ ☑
D40.12	Neoplasm of uncertain behavior of left testis ♂ ☑
D49.59	Neoplasm of unspecified behavior of other genitourinary organ
N44.1	Cyst of tunica albuginea testis ♂
N44.2	Benign cyst of testis ♂
N44.8	Other noninflammatory disorders of the testis ♂
N45.2	Orchitis ♂
N45.3	Epididymo-orchitis ♂
N49.1	Inflammatory disorders of spermatic cord, tunica vaginalis and vas deferens ♂
N50.3	Cyst of epididymis ♂
N50.811	Right testicular pain ♂
N50.812	Left testicular pain ♂
N50.82	Scrotal pain ♂
N50.89	Other specified disorders of the male genital organs ♂

AMA: 54512 2018,Jan,8; 2017,Jan,8; 2016,Jan,13; 2015,Jan,16; 2014,Jan,11

Relative Value Units/Medicare Edits

Non-Facility RVU	Work	PE	MP	Total
54512	9.33	5.12	1.11	15.56
Facility RVU	**Work**	**PE**	**MP**	**Total**
54512	9.33	5.12	1.11	15.56

	FUD	Status	MUE	Modifiers				IOM Reference
54512	90	A	1(3)	51	50	62*	N/A	None

* with documentation

Terms To Know

benign. Mild or nonmalignant in nature.

carcinoma in situ. Malignancy that arises from the cells of the vessel, gland, or organ of origin that remains confined to that site or has not invaded neighboring tissue.

dissection. Separating by cutting tissue or body structures apart.

excision. Surgical removal of an organ or tissue.

extraparenchymal. Occurring outside of or away from the seminiferous tubules (parenchymal) tissue. The parenchymal are small tubes found in the testes where the spermatozoa develop.

lesion. Area of damaged tissue that has lost continuity or function, due to disease or trauma.

malignant. Any condition tending to progress toward death, specifically an invasive tumor with a loss of cellular differentiation that has the ability to spread or metastasize to other body areas.

neoplasm. New abnormal growth, tumor.

secondary. Second in order of occurrence or importance, or appearing during the course of another disease or condition.

seminiferous tubules. Small tubes found in the testes where the spermatozoa develop.

testes. Male gonadal paired glands located in the scrotum that secrete testosterone and contain the seminiferous tubules where sperm is produced.

tunica vaginalis. Serous membrane that partially covers the testes formed by an outpocketing of the peritoneum when the testes descend.

54520

54520 Orchiectomy, simple (including subcapsular), with or without testicular prosthesis, scrotal or inguinal approach

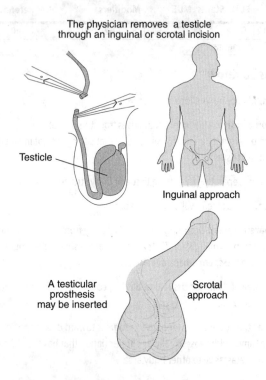

The physician removes a testicle through an inguinal or scrotal incision

Testicle

Inguinal approach

A testicular prosthesis may be inserted

Scrotal approach

Explanation

An incision is made in one side of the scrotum and the tissues are separated to expose the spermatic cord. The spermatic cord is opened and the individual bundles making up the cord are cross-clamped, cut, and secured with nonabsorbable suture material. The testis is removed through the scrotal incision. If the patient so chooses, and if no contraindications are present, a prosthetic testis is inserted into the scrotum before the wound is closed in layers by suturing. An alternative method uses an incision in the groin. The testis is pulled through the incision after cutting and tying the cord in a fashion similar to the scrotal approach.

Coding Tips

This is a unilateral procedure. If performed bilaterally, some payers require that the service be reported twice with modifier 50 appended to the second code while others require identification of the service only once with modifier 50 appended. Check with individual payers. Modifier 50 identifies a procedure performed identically on the opposite side of the body (mirror image). For a partial orchiectomy, see 54522; radical for tumor via inguinal approach, see 54530; including abdominal exploration, see 54535. For a laparoscopic orchiectomy, see 54690. For an orchiectomy with hernia repair, use 49505 or 49507 and 54520.

ICD-10-CM Diagnostic Codes

C62.01	Malignant neoplasm of undescended right testis ♂ ☑
C62.02	Malignant neoplasm of undescended left testis ♂ ☑
C62.11	Malignant neoplasm of descended right testis ♂ ☑
C62.12	Malignant neoplasm of descended left testis ♂ ☑
C79.82	Secondary malignant neoplasm of genital organs
D07.69	Carcinoma in situ of other male genital organs ♂
D29.21	Benign neoplasm of right testis ♂ ☑
D29.22	Benign neoplasm of left testis ♂ ☑
D49.59	Neoplasm of unspecified behavior of other genitourinary organ
N44.01	Extravaginal torsion of spermatic cord ♂
N44.02	Intravaginal torsion of spermatic cord ♂
N44.03	Torsion of appendix testis ♂
N44.04	Torsion of appendix epididymis ♂
N45.2	Orchitis ♂
N45.3	Epididymo-orchitis ♂
N45.4	Abscess of epididymis or testis ♂
S31.31XA	Laceration without foreign body of scrotum and testes, initial encounter ♂
S31.32XA	Laceration with foreign body of scrotum and testes, initial encounter ♂
S31.33XA	Puncture wound without foreign body of scrotum and testes, initial encounter ♂
S31.34XA	Puncture wound with foreign body of scrotum and testes, initial encounter ♂
S31.35XA	Open bite of scrotum and testes, initial encounter ♂
S38.02XA	Crushing injury of scrotum and testis, initial encounter ♂
S38.232A	Partial traumatic amputation of scrotum and testis, initial encounter ♂
Z40.09	Encounter for prophylactic removal of other organ

AMA: 54520 2018,Jan,8; 2017,Jan,8; 2016,Jan,13; 2015,Jan,16; 2014,Jan,11

Relative Value Units/Medicare Edits

Non-Facility RVU	Work	PE	MP	Total
54520	5.3	3.45	0.65	9.4
Facility RVU	**Work**	**PE**	**MP**	**Total**
54520	5.3	3.45	0.65	9.4

	FUD	Status	MUE	Modifiers				IOM Reference
54520	90	A	1(2)	51	50	N/A	N/A	100-03,230.3

* with documentation

Terms To Know

epididymo-orchitis. Inflammation of the testes and epididymis.

orchiectomy. Surgical removal of one or both testicles via a scrotal or groin incision, indicated in cases of cancer, traumatic injury, and sex reassignment surgery.

prosthesis. Man-made substitute for a missing body part.

scrotum. Skin pouch that holds the testes and supporting reproductive structures.

spermatic cord. Structure of the male reproductive organs that consists of the ductus deferens, testicular artery, nerves, and veins that drain the testes.

torsion of testis. Twisting, turning, or rotation of the testicle upon itself, so as to compromise or cut off the blood supply.

© 2020 Optum360, LLC **N Newborn: 0** **P Pediatric: 0-17** **M Maternity: 9-64** **A Adult: 15-124** ♂ **Male Only** ♀ **Female Only** CPT © 2020 American Medical Association. All Rights Reserved.

Testis

54522

54522　Orchiectomy, partial

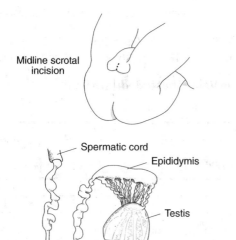

Midline scrotal incision

Spermatic cord

Epididymis

Testis

Ductus deferens

A portion of the testis is removed as necessary

A portion of a testis is removed (partial orchiectomy)

Explanation

The physician performs a partial excision of one testis or both testes. The surgeon makes a longitudinal incision midline in the scrotum to expose the testis. The tunica vaginalis is incised, and the testicular vessels and vas deferens are identified, clamped separately, and divided. The cords are ligated at a level slightly above the area of infection, abscess, neoplasm, or trauma and the spermatic cord is isolated for manipulation of the testicle. The testis is delivered to the wound and dissected below the ligated cords. The wound is closed by suture and a pressure dressing and scrotal supporter are applied.

Coding Tips

For simple orchiectomy, see 54520. For radical orchiectomy, inguinal approach for tumor, see 54530. For radical orchiectomy for tumor, with abdominal exploration, see 54535. For laparoscopic orchiectomy, see 54690. Local or regional anesthesia is included in the service. However, general anesthesia may be administered depending on the age or condition of the patient.

ICD-10-CM Diagnostic Codes

C61	Malignant neoplasm of prostate ♂
C62.01	Malignant neoplasm of undescended right testis ♂ ☑
C62.02	Malignant neoplasm of undescended left testis ♂ ☑
C62.11	Malignant neoplasm of descended right testis ♂ ☑
C62.12	Malignant neoplasm of descended left testis ♂ ☑
C79.82	Secondary malignant neoplasm of genital organs
D29.21	Benign neoplasm of right testis ♂ ☑
D29.22	Benign neoplasm of left testis ♂ ☑
D49.59	Neoplasm of unspecified behavior of other genitourinary organ
N44.01	Extravaginal torsion of spermatic cord ♂
N44.02	Intravaginal torsion of spermatic cord ♂
N44.03	Torsion of appendix testis ♂
N44.04	Torsion of appendix epididymis ♂
N44.1	Cyst of tunica albuginea testis ♂
N44.2	Benign cyst of testis ♂
N44.8	Other noninflammatory disorders of the testis ♂
N45.1	Epididymitis ♂
N45.3	Epididymo-orchitis ♂
N45.4	Abscess of epididymis or testis ♂
N50.1	Vascular disorders of male genital organs ♂
N50.811	Right testicular pain ♂
N50.812	Left testicular pain ♂
N50.82	Scrotal pain ♂
N50.89	Other specified disorders of the male genital organs ♂
S31.31XA	Laceration without foreign body of scrotum and testes, initial encounter ♂
S31.32XA	Laceration with foreign body of scrotum and testes, initial encounter ♂
S31.33XA	Puncture wound without foreign body of scrotum and testes, initial encounter ♂
S31.34XA	Puncture wound with foreign body of scrotum and testes, initial encounter ♂
S31.35XA	Open bite of scrotum and testes, initial encounter ♂
S38.02XA	Crushing injury of scrotum and testis, initial encounter ♂
S38.231A	Complete traumatic amputation of scrotum and testis, initial encounter ♂
S38.232A	Partial traumatic amputation of scrotum and testis, initial encounter ♂

AMA: **54522** 2018,Jan,8; 2017,Jan,8; 2016,Jan,13; 2015,Jan,16; 2014,Jan,11

Relative Value Units/Medicare Edits

Non-Facility RVU	Work	PE	MP	Total
54522	10.25	5.59	1.17	17.01
Facility RVU	**Work**	**PE**	**MP**	**Total**
54522	10.25	5.59	1.17	17.01

	FUD	Status	MUE	Modifiers				IOM Reference
54522	90	A	1(2)	51	50	62*	80	None

* with documentation

Terms To Know

dissection. Separating by cutting tissue or body structures apart.

ligation. Tying off a blood vessel or duct with a suture or a soft, thin wire.

malignant. Any condition tending to progress toward death, specifically an invasive tumor with a loss of cellular differentiation that has the ability to spread or metastasize to other body areas.

orchiectomy. Surgical removal of one or both testicles via a scrotal or groin incision, indicated in cases of cancer, traumatic injury, and sex reassignment surgery.

pressure dressing. Wound dressing used to apply pressure to the injured area, often used after skin grafting procedures.

tunica vaginalis. Serous membrane that partially covers the testes formed by an outpocketing of the peritoneum when the testes descend.

CPT © 2020 American Medical Association. All Rights Reserved. ● New ▲ Revised ＋ Add On ★ Telemedicine AMA: CPT Assist [Resequenced] ☑ Laterality © 2020 Optum360, LLC

54530-54535

54530   Orchiectomy, radical, for tumor; inguinal approach
54535   with abdominal exploration

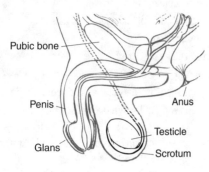

A testicle is removed

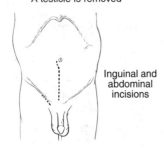

Inguinal and abdominal incisions

Explanation

The physician performs a radical orchiectomy by removing en bloc the contents of half of the scrotum. An incision is made in the inguinal area from the pubic bone toward the lateral pelvic bone. The incision made deep into the tissues and the spermatic cord is dissected free and cross-clamped. The testis and all its associated structures are pushed up from the scrotum into the incision and removed. Packing is placed in the empty scrotum. When the spermatic cord is opened and the individual bundles making up the cord are cross-clamped, cut, and secured with nonabsorbable suture material, care is taken to avoid important nerves and vessels in the area. The packing is removed and bleeding controlled. A prosthetic testis may be placed in the scrotum before the incision is closed in layers by suturing. This procedure results in complete removal of the testis. In 54535, a midline incision is made from the upper to the lower abdomen and the abdominal cavity is entered. The back wall of the abdomen is exposed and the lymph nodes are checked for spread of tumor. Some may be removed and/or biopsied and the abdominal wound is closed in layers by suturing.

Coding Tips

For orchiopexy with hernia repair, see 49505 or 49507 and 54520. For radical retroperitoneal lymphadenectomy, see 38780. For partial orchiectomy, see 54522. For simple orchiectomy, with or without testicular prosthesis, see 54520.

ICD-10-CM Diagnostic Codes

C61	Malignant neoplasm of prostate ♂
C62.01	Malignant neoplasm of undescended right testis ♂ ☑
C62.02	Malignant neoplasm of undescended left testis ♂ ☑
C62.11	Malignant neoplasm of descended right testis ♂ ☑
C62.12	Malignant neoplasm of descended left testis ♂ ☑
C79.82	Secondary malignant neoplasm of genital organs
D07.69	Carcinoma in situ of other male genital organs ♂
D29.21	Benign neoplasm of right testis ♂ ☑
D29.22	Benign neoplasm of left testis ♂ ☑
D40.11	Neoplasm of uncertain behavior of right testis ♂ ☑
D40.12	Neoplasm of uncertain behavior of left testis ♂ ☑
D49.59	Neoplasm of unspecified behavior of other genitourinary organ

AMA: 54530 2018,Jan,8; 2017,Jan,8; 2016,Jan,13; 2015,Jan,16; 2014,Jan,11
54535 2018,Jan,8; 2017,Jan,8; 2016,Jan,13; 2015,Jan,16; 2014,Jan,11

Relative Value Units/Medicare Edits

Non-Facility RVU	Work	PE	MP	Total
54530	8.46	5.17	1.0	14.63
54535	13.19	6.8	1.5	21.49
Facility RVU	Work	PE	MP	Total
54530	8.46	5.17	1.0	14.63
54535	13.19	6.8	1.5	21.49

	FUD	Status	MUE	Modifiers				IOM Reference
54530	90	A	1(2)	51	50	62*	80	100-03,230.3
54535	90	A	1(2)	51	50	N/A	80	

* with documentation

Terms To Know

approach. Method or anatomical location used to gain access to a body organ or specific area for procedures.

carcinoma in situ. Malignancy that arises from the cells of the vessel, gland, or organ of origin that remains confined to that site or has not invaded neighboring tissue.

en bloc. In total.

exploration. Examination for diagnostic purposes.

malignant neoplasm. Any cancerous tumor or lesion exhibiting uncontrolled tissue growth that can progressively invade other parts of the body with its disease-generating cells.

orchiectomy. Surgical removal of one or both testicles via a scrotal or groin incision, indicated in cases of cancer, traumatic injury, and sex reassignment surgery.

prosthesis. Man-made substitute for a missing body part.

radical. Extensive surgery.

secondary. Second in order of occurrence or importance, or appearing during the course of another disease or condition.

testes. Male gonadal paired glands located in the scrotum that secrete testosterone and contain the seminiferous tubules where sperm is produced.

tumor. Pathological swelling or enlargement; a neoplastic growth of uncontrolled, abnormal multiplication of cells.

Testis

54550-54560

54550 Exploration for undescended testis (inguinal or scrotal area)
54560 Exploration for undescended testis with abdominal exploration

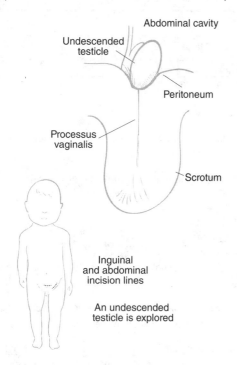

Abdominal cavity

Undescended testicle

Peritoneum

Processus vaginalis

Scrotum

Inguinal and abdominal incision lines

An undescended testicle is explored

Explanation

The physician searches for a testis that failed to descend into the scrotum during development. An incision is made in the scrotum or the inguinal area from the pubic bone to the upper lateral pelvic area in the skin fold made by the thigh and the lower abdomen. The tissues are separated by dissection to find the testis in the area. In 54560, the incision and exploration are extended into the abdominal cavity. No other procedure is performed. The incision is closed in layers by suturing.

Coding Tips

These are unilateral procedures. If performed bilaterally, some payers require that the service be reported twice with modifier 50 appended to the second code while others require identification of the service only once with modifier 50 appended. Check with individual payers. Modifier 50 identifies a procedure performed identically on the opposite side of the body (mirror image). Because fertility is seldom regained with this procedure, it may be considered cosmetic and may not be reimbursed by the insurance carrier. For laparoscopic orchiopexy for intra-abdominal testis, see 54692.

ICD-10-CM Diagnostic Codes

Q53.111	Unilateral intraabdominal testis ♂
Q53.112	Unilateral inguinal testis ♂
Q53.12	Ectopic perineal testis, unilateral ♂
Q53.13	Unilateral high scrotal testis ♂
Q53.211	Bilateral intraabdominal testes ♂
Q53.212	Bilateral inguinal testes ♂
Q53.22	Ectopic perineal testis, bilateral ♂
Q53.23	Bilateral high scrotal testes ♂
Q55.0	Absence and aplasia of testis ♂
R39.83	Unilateral non-palpable testicle ♂
R39.84	Bilateral non-palpable testicles ♂

AMA: 54550 2018,Jan,8; 2017,Mar,10; 2017,Jan,8; 2016,Jan,13; 2015,Jan,16; 2014,Jan,11 **54560** 2018,Jan,8; 2017,Jan,8; 2016,Jan,13; 2015,Jan,16; 2014,Jan,11

Relative Value Units/Medicare Edits

Non-Facility RVU	Work	PE	MP	Total
54550	8.41	4.83	0.96	14.2
54560	12.1	6.36	1.38	19.84
Facility RVU	**Work**	**PE**	**MP**	**Total**
54550	8.41	4.83	0.96	14.2
54560	12.1	6.36	1.38	19.84

	FUD	Status	MUE	Modifiers				IOM Reference
54550	90	A	1(2)	51	50	N/A	80	None
54560	90	A	1(2)	51	50	62*	80	

* with documentation

Terms To Know

aplasia. Incomplete development of an organ or tissue. Aplasia may be congenital (present at birth) or acquired.

dissection. Separating by cutting tissue or body structures apart.

ectopic. Organ or other structure that is aberrant or out of place.

exploration. Examination for diagnostic purposes.

inguinal. Within the groin region.

scrotum. Skin pouch that holds the testes and supporting reproductive structures.

testes. Male gonadal paired glands located in the scrotum that secrete testosterone and contain the seminiferous tubules where sperm is produced.

Testis

54600

54600 Reduction of torsion of testis, surgical, with or without fixation of contralateral testis

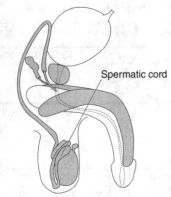

Spermatic cord

The physician untwists the spermatic cord on one side, and may anchor the testis on the other side to prevent the same problem

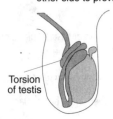

Torsion of testis

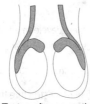

Testes after correction

Explanation

The physician treats a torsion of the testis, which is a twisting of the testis upon itself so that its blood supply is compromised. The physician makes an incision in the scrotum and exposes the twisted testis. The testis and spermatic cord is untwisted to restore blood flow to the organ. If the testis is viable, the surgeon anchors the testis to the inside wall of the scrotum with three or more sutures. The incision is closed in layers by suturing. Because the problem that allowed the testis to twist may affect the other testis (contralateral testis), a second procedure is commonly performed to anchor it in similar fashion.

Coding Tips

When 54600 is performed with another separately identifiable procedure, the highest dollar value code is listed as the primary procedure and subsequent procedures are appended with modifier 51. However, if a second step or procedure is performed to anchor the contralateral testis to the other side at the same operative session, it is included in 54600 and should not be reported separately. If significant additional time and effort is documented, append modifier 22 and submit a cover letter and operative report.

ICD-10-CM Diagnostic Codes

N44.01   Extravaginal torsion of spermatic cord ♂
N44.02   Intravaginal torsion of spermatic cord ♂

AMA: 54600 2018,Jan,8; 2017,Jan,8; 2016,Jan,13; 2015,Jan,16; 2014,Jan,11

Relative Value Units/Medicare Edits

Non-Facility RVU	Work	PE	MP	Total
54600	7.64	4.56	0.87	13.07
Facility RVU	Work	PE	MP	Total
54600	7.64	4.56	0.87	13.07

	FUD	Status	MUE	Modifiers				IOM Reference
54600	90	A	1(2)	51	50	N/A	N/A	None

* with documentation

Terms To Know

contralateral. Located on, or affecting, the opposite side of the body, usually as it relates to a bilateral body part.

extravaginal torsion of spermatic cord. Torsion of the spermatic cord just below the tunica vaginalis attachments.

intra. Within.

reduce. Restoration to normal position or alignment.

scrotum. Skin pouch that holds the testes and supporting reproductive structures.

spermatic cord. Structure of the male reproductive organs that consists of the ductus deferens, testicular artery, nerves, and veins that drain the testes.

testes. Male gonadal paired glands located in the scrotum that secrete testosterone and contain the seminiferous tubules where sperm is produced.

torsion of testis. Twisting, turning, or rotation of the testicle upon itself, so as to compromise or cut off the blood supply.

54620

54620   Fixation of contralateral testis (separate procedure)

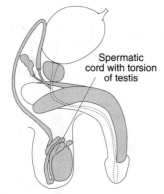

Spermatic cord with torsion of testis

The physician anchors the testis to the scrotum with sutures to prevent torsion of the testis. This is done in patients with a history of torsion

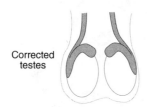

Corrected testes

Explanation

The physician makes an incision in the scrotum and exposes the testis on side opposite to the one that had previously been twisted. The surgeon anchors the testis to the inside wall of the scrotum with three or more sutures to prevent the twisting of the cord and the testis. The incision is closed in layers by suturing.

Coding Tips

This separate procedure by definition is usually a component of a more complex service and is not identified separately. When performed alone or with other unrelated procedures/ services it may be reported. If performed alone, list the code; if performed with other procedures/services, list the code and append modifier 59 or an X{EPSU} modifier. Fixation of contralateral testis (54620) performed during the same operative session as the testicle torsion reduction is included in 54600 and is not reported separately.

ICD-10-CM Diagnostic Codes

N44.01   Extravaginal torsion of spermatic cord ♂

N44.02   Intravaginal torsion of spermatic cord ♂

AMA: 54620 2014,Jan,11

Relative Value Units/Medicare Edits

Non-Facility RVU	Work	PE	MP	Total
54620	5.21	2.83	0.6	8.64
Facility RVU	Work	PE	MP	Total
54620	5.21	2.83	0.6	8.64

	FUD	Status	MUE	Modifiers				IOM Reference
54620	10	A	1(2)	51	50	N/A	N/A	None

* with documentation

54640

54640   Orchiopexy, inguinal or scrotal approach

The undescended testicle is relocated to the scrotum

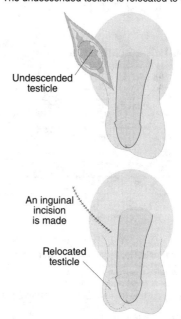

Undescended testicle

An inguinal incision is made

Relocated testicle

Any inguinal hernia is also repaired

Explanation

Orchiopexy is the surgical fixation of an undescended testicle into the scrotum. An incision is made in the scrotum or the inguinal area from the pubic bone to the upper lateral pelvic area in the skin crease made by the thigh and the lower abdomen. The physician searches for a testis that failed to descend in to the scrotum during development. The tissues are separated by dissection to find the testis in the inguinal canal area. The spermatic cord is mobilized to allow positioning of the testis in the scrotum. In the scrotum, a small pouch is created for the testis where the testis is sutured in place to prevent retraction back in to the inguinal canal. If there is a concomitant hernia it is often repaired at the same time through the same incision. The hernia present in the inguinal canal is repaired by folding and suturing of tissues to strengthen the abdominal wall and correct the weakness responsible for the hernia. The incision is closed in layers by suturing.

Coding Tips

This is a unilateral procedure. If performed bilaterally, some payers require that the service be reported twice with modifier 50 appended to the second code while others require identification of the service only once with modifier 50 appended. Check with individual payers. Modifier 50 identifies a procedure performed identically on the opposite side of the body (mirror image). When 54640 is performed with another separately identifiable procedure, the highest dollar value code is listed as the primary procedure and subsequent procedures are appended with modifier 51. When orchiopexy is performed with an inguinal hernia repair, see 49495–49525. For exploration of undescended testis only, see 54550–54560. Because fertility is seldom regained with this procedure, it may be considered cosmetic and may not be reimbursed by the insurance carrier.

ICD-10-CM Diagnostic Codes

Q53.01   Ectopic testis, unilateral ♂

Q53.02   Ectopic testes, bilateral ♂

Q53.12	Ectopic perineal testis, unilateral ♂	
Q53.22	Ectopic perineal testis, bilateral ♂	
R39.83	Unilateral non-palpable testicle ♂	
R39.84	Bilateral non-palpable testicles ♂	

AMA: 54640 2018,Jan,8; 2017,Mar,10; 2017,Jan,8; 2016,Jan,13; 2015,Jan,16; 2014,Jan,11

Relative Value Units/Medicare Edits

Non-Facility RVU	Work	PE	MP	Total
54640	7.73	3.86	0.96	12.55
Facility RVU	**Work**	**PE**	**MP**	**Total**
54640	7.73	3.86	0.96	12.55

	FUD	Status	MUE	Modifiers				IOM Reference
54640	90	A	1(2)	51	50	N/A	80*	None

* with documentation

Terms To Know

approach. Method or anatomical location used to gain access to a body organ or specific area for procedures.

dissection. Separating by cutting tissue or body structures apart.

fixation. Act or condition of being attached, secured, fastened, or held in position.

hernia. Protrusion of a body structure through tissue.

inguinal. Within the groin region.

inguinal hernia. Loop of intestine that protrudes through the abdominal peritoneum into the inguinal canal.

orchiopexy. Surgical fixation of an undescended testicle within the scrotum.

reducible hernia. Protrusion of tissue through the wall of another structure that can be manually returned to the correct anatomical position.

scrotum. Skin pouch that holds the testes and supporting reproductive structures.

spermatic cord. Structure of the male reproductive organs that consists of the ductus deferens, testicular artery, nerves, and veins that drain the testes.

testes. Male gonadal paired glands located in the scrotum that secrete testosterone and contain the seminiferous tubules where sperm is produced.

tissue. Group of similar cells with a similar function that form definite structures and organs. Tissue types include epithelial tissue, muscle tissue, connective tissue, and nervous tissue.

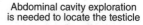

54650

54650   Orchiopexy, abdominal approach, for intra-abdominal testis (eg, Fowler-Stephens)

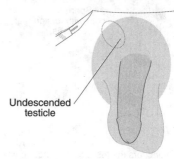

Abdominal cavity exploration is needed to locate the testicle

Undescended testicle

The testicle is then relocated to the scrotum

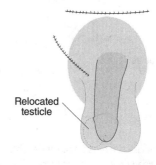

Relocated testicle

Explanation

Orchiopexy is the surgical fixation of an undescended testicle into the scrotum. An incision is made in the inguinal area from the pubic bone to the upper lateral pelvic area in the skin fold made by the thigh and the lower abdomen. The physician searches the abdominal cavity for a testis that failed to descend in to the scrotum during development. The tissues are separated by dissection and the incision is extended into the abdominal cavity to find the testis in the abdominal area. The tissues are separated by dissection to find the testis in the area. At this point several surgical options are available. The one chosen will depend on the mobility of the testis and how far it can be brought down through the inguinal canal and into the scrotum. The procedure may take two stages approximately six to 12 months apart. Eventually, the spermatic cord is mobilized sufficiently to allow positioning of the testis in the scrotum. In the scrotum a small pouch is created for the testis where the testis is sutured in place to prevent retraction back in to the inguinal canal or into the abdominal cavity. The incision is closed in layers by suturing.

Coding Tips

This is a unilateral procedure. If performed bilaterally, some payers require that the service be reported twice with modifier 50 appended to the second code while others require identification of the service only once with modifier 50 appended. Check with individual payers. Modifier 50 identifies a procedure performed identically on the opposite side of the body (mirror image). When 54650 is performed with another separately identifiable procedure, the highest dollar value code is listed as the primary procedure and subsequent procedures are appended with modifier 51. For exploration of undescended testis only, see 54550 and 54560. For laparoscopic orchiopexy for intra-abdominal testis, see 54692. For orchiopexy, inguinal approach, see 54640. Because fertility is

© 2020 Optum360, LLC   **N** Newborn: 0   **P** Pediatric: 0-17   **M** Maternity: 9-64   **A** Adult: 15-124   ♂ Male Only   ♀ Female Only   CPT © 2020 American Medical Association. All Rights Reserved.

Testis

seldom regained with this procedure, it may be considered cosmetic and may not be reimbursed by the insurance carrier.

ICD-10-CM Diagnostic Codes

Q53.111	Unilateral intraabdominal testis ♂
Q53.211	Bilateral intraabdominal testes ♂
R39.83	Unilateral non-palpable testicle ♂
R39.84	Bilateral non-palpable testicles ♂

AMA: 54650 2018,Jan,8; 2017,Jan,8; 2016,Jan,13; 2015,Jan,16; 2014,Jan,11

Relative Value Units/Medicare Edits

Non-Facility RVU	Work	PE	MP	Total
54650	12.39	6.74	1.42	20.55
Facility RVU	**Work**	**PE**	**MP**	**Total**
54650	12.39	6.74	1.42	20.55

	FUD	Status	MUE	Modifiers				IOM Reference
54650	90	A	1(2)	51	50	N/A	80	None

* with documentation

Terms To Know

approach. Method or anatomical location used to gain access to a body organ or specific area for procedures.

dissect. Cut apart or separate tissue for surgical purposes or for visual or microscopic study.

fixation. Act or condition of being attached, secured, fastened, or held in position.

intra. Within.

orchiopexy. Surgical fixation of an undescended testicle within the scrotum.

scrotum. Skin pouch that holds the testes and supporting reproductive structures.

spermatic cord. Structure of the male reproductive organs that consists of the ductus deferens, testicular artery, nerves, and veins that drain the testes.

testes. Male gonadal paired glands located in the scrotum that secrete testosterone and contain the seminiferous tubules where sperm is produced.

tissue. Group of similar cells with a similar function that form definite structures and organs. Tissue types include epithelial tissue, muscle tissue, connective tissue, and nervous tissue.

54660

54660   Insertion of testicular prosthesis (separate procedure)

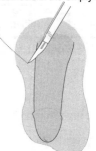

Through an inguinal incision, the physician places a prosthesis in the empty scrotal sac

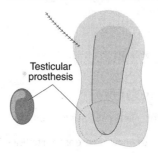

The incision is closed with sutures

Testicular prosthesis

Explanation

For cosmetic reasons, the physician places an artificial testis in the scrotum of a patient. After adequate local anesthesia, an incision is made in the inguinal area and the empty scrotal sac is dilated by passing a dissecting finger or a moist gauze sponge through the inguinal canal into the scrotum. A prosthetic testis is inserted into the scrotal sac and the neck of the scrotum is closed by suturing. The inguinal incision is closed in layers by suturing.

Coding Tips

This separate procedure by definition is usually a component of a more complex service and is not identified separately. When performed alone or with other unrelated procedures/services it may be reported. If performed alone, list the code; if performed with other procedures/services, list the code and append modifier 59 or an X{EPSU} modifier. This is a unilateral procedure. If performed bilaterally, some payers require that the service be reported twice with modifier 50 appended to the second code while others require identification of the service only once with modifier 50 appended. Check with individual payers. Modifier 50 identifies a procedure performed identically on the opposite side of the body (mirror image). When the testicular prosthesis insertion is done in the same surgical session that the testicle is removed, see 54520. Do not report 54660 together with 54520. For exploration of undescended testis, see 54550 and 54560. For orchiopexy, inguinal approach, with or without hernia repair, see 54640. For orchiopexy, abdominal approach, see 54650.

ICD-10-CM Diagnostic Codes

Q55.0	Absence and aplasia of testis ♂
Q55.1	Hypoplasia of testis and scrotum ♂
Q55.29	Other congenital malformations of testis and scrotum ♂

AMA: 54660 2018,Jan,8; 2017,Jan,8; 2016,Jan,13; 2015,Jan,16; 2014,Jan,11

Relative Value Units/Medicare Edits

Non-Facility RVU	Work	PE	MP	Total
54660	5.74	3.91	0.64	10.29
Facility RVU	Work	PE	MP	Total
54660	5.74	3.91	0.64	10.29

	FUD	Status	MUE	Modifiers				IOM Reference
54660	90	A	1(2)	51	50	N/A	80*	100-02,16,180

* with documentation

Terms To Know

anomaly. Irregularity in the structure or position of an organ or tissue.

congenital. Present at birth, occurring through heredity or an influence during gestation up to the moment of birth.

dilation. Artificial increase in the diameter of an opening or lumen made by medication or by instrumentation.

dissect. Cut apart or separate tissue for surgical purposes or for visual or microscopic study.

inguinal. Within the groin region.

insertion. Placement or implantation into a body part.

orchiectomy. Surgical removal of one or both testicles via a scrotal or groin incision, indicated in cases of cancer, traumatic injury, and sex reassignment surgery.

prosthesis. Man-made substitute for a missing body part.

scrotum. Skin pouch that holds the testes and supporting reproductive structures.

testes. Male gonadal paired glands located in the scrotum that secrete testosterone and contain the seminiferous tubules where sperm is produced.

54670

54670   Suture or repair of testicular injury

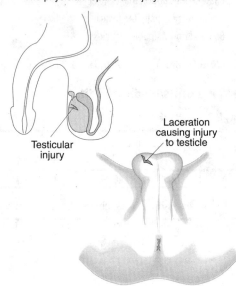

The physician repairs an injury to the testicle

Testicular injury

Laceration causing injury to testicle

Explanation

The physician repairs injury (laceration or traumatic rupture) to the testis that occurs as a result of either a blunt or penetrating injury. Often a laceration is present in the scrotum and the testis is explored and repaired through the open wound. Otherwise, an incision is made in the scrotum to expose the testis. Any devitalized testicular tissue is removed by sharp dissection and the thick tough fibrous tissue encasing the testis is closed by suturing. The scrotum is closed in layers by suturing. Often a rubber drain is placed to prevent the accumulation of fluid and blood in the scrotum.

Coding Tips

This is a general procedure. Report any more specific code that would apply for accurate reporting of the services performed.

ICD-10-CM Diagnostic Codes

S31.31XA	Laceration without foreign body of scrotum and testes, initial encounter ♂
S31.32XA	Laceration with foreign body of scrotum and testes, initial encounter ♂
S31.33XA	Puncture wound without foreign body of scrotum and testes, initial encounter ♂
S31.34XA	Puncture wound with foreign body of scrotum and testes, initial encounter ♂
S31.35XA	Open bite of scrotum and testes, initial encounter ♂
S38.02XA	Crushing injury of scrotum and testis, initial encounter ♂
S38.231A	Complete traumatic amputation of scrotum and testis, initial encounter ♂
S38.232A	Partial traumatic amputation of scrotum and testis, initial encounter ♂

AMA: **54670** 2018,Jan,8; 2017,Jan,8; 2016,Jan,13; 2015,Jan,16; 2014,Jan,11

Relative Value Units/Medicare Edits

Non-Facility RVU	Work	PE	MP	Total
54670	6.65	4.33	0.77	11.75
Facility RVU	Work	PE	MP	Total
54670	6.65	4.33	0.77	11.75

	FUD	Status	MUE	Modifiers				IOM Reference
54670	90	A	1(3)	51	50	N/A	80*	None

* with documentation

Terms To Know

connective tissue. Body tissue made from fibroblasts, collagen, and elastic fibrils that connects, supports, and holds together other tissues and cells and includes cartilage, collagenous, fibrous, elastic, and osseous tissue.

devitalized. Deprivation of vital necessities or of life itself.

dissection. (dis. apart; -section, act of cutting) Separating by cutting tissue or body structures apart.

drain. Device that creates a channel to allow fluid from a cavity, wound, or infected area to exit the body.

fibrous tissue. Connective tissues.

laceration. Tearing injury; a torn, ragged-edged wound.

rupture. Tearing or breaking open of tissue.

scrotum. Skin pouch that holds the testes and supporting reproductive structures.

testes. Male gonadal paired glands located in the scrotum that secrete testosterone and contain the seminiferous tubules where sperm is produced.

wound. Injury to living tissue often involving a cut or break in the skin.

54680

54680   Transplantation of testis(es) to thigh (because of scrotal destruction)

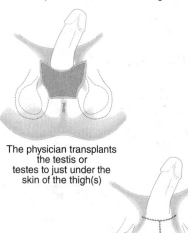

The patient's scrotum is no longer viable

The physician transplants the testis or testes to just under the skin of the thigh(s)

This procedure can be unilateral or bilateral

Explanation

The physician transplants the testis(es) under the skin of the thigh to preserve function and viability following massive injury or surgical loss of the scrotal skin. The thigh is chosen because the temperature just under the skin is approximately the same as in the scrotum, a condition to normal testicular function. Incisions are made in the skin of the thigh adjacent to the scrotum and the testis is sutured in place with attention to preserving blood flow to the organ. The thigh incisions are closed in layers over a rubber drain brought out through the skin. In four to six weeks scrotal reconstruction is begun.

Coding Tips

This is the first stage of a complex four- to six-week reconstruction. Complex closures of the thigh region are not identified separately. This is a unilateral or bilateral procedure and is reported once even if the procedure is performed on both sides; modifier 50 is not applicable. For scrotal reconstruction, see 55175–55180.

ICD-10-CM Diagnostic Codes

C63.2	Malignant neoplasm of scrotum ♂
C79.82	Secondary malignant neoplasm of genital organs
D29.4	Benign neoplasm of scrotum ♂
S31.31XA	Laceration without foreign body of scrotum and testes, initial encounter ♂
S31.32XA	Laceration with foreign body of scrotum and testes, initial encounter ♂
S31.33XA	Puncture wound without foreign body of scrotum and testes, initial encounter ♂
S31.34XA	Puncture wound with foreign body of scrotum and testes, initial encounter ♂
S31.35XA	Open bite of scrotum and testes, initial encounter ♂
S38.02XA	Crushing injury of scrotum and testis, initial encounter ♂

CPT © 2020 American Medical Association. All Rights Reserved.   ● New   ▲ Revised   + Add On   ★ Telemedicine   AMA: CPT Assist   [Resequenced]   ☑ Laterality   © 2020 Optum360, LLC

S38.232A	Partial traumatic amputation of scrotum and testis, initial encounter ♂	
S39.848A	Other specified injuries of external genitals, initial encounter	
T21.36XA	Burn of third degree of male genital region, initial encounter ♂	
T21.76XA	Corrosion of third degree of male genital region, initial encounter ♂	

AMA: 54680 2018,Jan,8; 2017,Jan,8; 2016,Jan,13; 2015,Jan,16; 2014,Jan,11

Relative Value Units/Medicare Edits

Non-Facility RVU	Work	PE	MP	Total
54680	14.04	7.1	1.61	22.75
Facility RVU	**Work**	**PE**	**MP**	**Total**
54680	14.04	7.1	1.61	22.75

	FUD	Status	MUE	Modifiers				IOM Reference
54680	90	A	1(2)	51	50	62*	80	None

* with documentation

Terms To Know

benign lesion. Neoplasm or change in tissue that is not cancerous (nonmalignant).

carcinoma in situ. Malignancy that arises from the cells of the vessel, gland, or organ of origin that remains confined to that site or has not invaded neighboring tissue.

destruction. Ablation or eradication of a structure or tissue.

drain. Device that creates a channel to allow fluid from a cavity, wound, or infected area to exit the body.

malignant neoplasm. Any cancerous tumor or lesion exhibiting uncontrolled tissue growth that can progressively invade other parts of the body with its disease-generating cells.

reconstruction. Recreating, restoring, or rebuilding a body part or organ.

scrotum. Skin pouch that holds the testes and supporting reproductive structures.

secondary. Second in order of occurrence or importance, or appearing during the course of another disease or condition.

testes. Male gonadal paired glands located in the scrotum that secrete testosterone and contain the seminiferous tubules where sperm is produced.

transplantation. Grafting or movement of an organ or tissue from one site or person to another.

54690

54690	Laparoscopy, surgical; orchiectomy

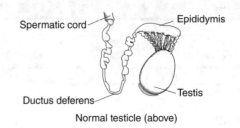

Spermatic cord / Epididymis / Ductus deferens / Testis

Normal testicle (above)

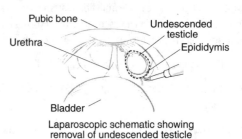

Pubic bone / Undescended testicle / Urethra / Epididymis / Bladder

Laparoscopic schematic showing removal of undescended testicle

Explanation

The physician removes one or both testicles, which may be undescended, injured or diseased using a laparoscope. The physician places a trocar at the umbilicus into the abdominal or retroperitoneal space and insufflates the abdominal cavity. The physician places a laparoscope through the umbilical incision and additional trocars are placed into the abdomen. The testis and all its associated structures are pushed up from the scrotum or freed from their undescended intra-abdominal location and removed through the abdominal or retroperitoneal space via the trocar port. Packing may be placed in the empty scrotum. Care is taken to avoid important nerves and vessels in the area. A prosthetic testis may be placed in the scrotum before the incision is closed in layers by suturing. The trocars are removed and the incisions are closed with sutures.

Coding Tips

Surgical laparoscopy always includes a diagnostic laparoscopy; the diagnostic laparoscopy should not be reported separately. For open removal of a testicle, see 54520; radical for tumor via an inguinal approach, see 54530; including abdominal exploration, see 54535. For surgical pathology, see 88305.

ICD-10-CM Diagnostic Codes

C62.01	Malignant neoplasm of undescended right testis ♂ ☑
C62.02	Malignant neoplasm of undescended left testis ♂ ☑
C62.11	Malignant neoplasm of descended right testis ♂ ☑
C62.12	Malignant neoplasm of descended left testis ♂ ☑
C79.82	Secondary malignant neoplasm of genital organs
D07.69	Carcinoma in situ of other male genital organs ♂
D29.21	Benign neoplasm of right testis ♂ ☑
D29.22	Benign neoplasm of left testis ♂ ☑
D40.11	Neoplasm of uncertain behavior of right testis ♂ ☑
D40.12	Neoplasm of uncertain behavior of left testis ♂ ☑
D49.59	Neoplasm of unspecified behavior of other genitourinary organ
Z40.09	Encounter for prophylactic removal of other organ

AMA: **54690** 2019,Feb,10; 2018,Jan,8; 2017,Jan,8; 2016,Jan,13; 2015,Jan,16; 2014,Jan,11

Relative Value Units/Medicare Edits

Non-Facility RVU	Work	PE	MP	Total
54690	11.7	5.92	1.32	18.94
Facility RVU	**Work**	**PE**	**MP**	**Total**
54690	11.7	5.92	1.32	18.94

	FUD	Status	MUE	Modifiers				IOM Reference
54690	90	A	1(2)	51	50	62*	80	None

* with documentation

Terms To Know

atrophy. Reduction in size or activity in an anatomic structure, due to wasting away from disease or other factors.

insufflation. Blowing air or gas into a body cavity.

laparoscopy. Direct visualization of the peritoneal cavity, outer fallopian tubes, uterus, and ovaries utilizing a laparoscope, a thin, flexible fiberoptic tube.

orchiectomy. Surgical removal of one or both testicles via a scrotal or groin incision, indicated in cases of cancer, traumatic injury, and sex reassignment surgery.

packing. Material placed into a cavity or wound, such as gels, gauze, pads, and sponges.

retroperitoneal. Located behind the peritoneum, the membrane that lines the abdominopelvic walls and forms a covering for the internal organs.

scrotum. Skin pouch that holds the testes and supporting reproductive structures.

torsion of testis. Twisting, turning, or rotation of the testicle upon itself, so as to compromise or cut off the blood supply.

trocar. Cannula or a sharp pointed instrument used to puncture and aspirate fluid from cavities.

vas deferens. Duct that arises in the tail of the epididymis that stores and carries sperm from the epididymis toward the urethra.

54692

54692   Laparoscopy, surgical; orchiopexy for intra-abdominal testis

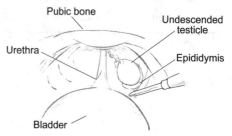

Laparoscopic schematic showing manipulation of undescended testicle

The testis is freed of its attachments in the abdominal cavity and mobilized into the scrotum where it is fixed

Explanation

The physician performs an orchiopexy (surgical fixation of an undescended testicle into the scrotum) with the assistance of a fiberoptic laparoscope. A paraumbilical port is created by placing a trocar at the level of the umbilicus. The abdominal wall is insufflated. The laparoscope is placed through the umbilical port and additional trocars are placed into the abdominal cavity. The physician uses the laparoscope fitted with a fiberoptic camera and/or an operating instrument to search the abdominal cavity for the undescended testis. The physician may have several surgical options depending on the mobility of the testis and how far it can be brought down through the inguinal canal and into the scrotum. The procedure may take two stages approximately three to 12 months apart. The spermatic cord is mobilized sufficiently to allow positioning of the testis in the scrotum, which often occurs during the first and perhaps only operative session. A small pouch is created for the testis where the testis is sutured in place to prevent retraction back into the inguinal canal or into the abdominal cavity. The small abdominal incisions are closed by staple or suture in the usual fashion.

Coding Tips

For open orchiopexy for intra-abdominal testis, see 54650. For exploration for undescended testis only, see 54550–54560. Because fertility is seldom regained with this procedure, it may be considered cosmetic and may not be reimbursed by the insurance carrier.

ICD-10-CM Diagnostic Codes

Q53.111	Unilateral intraabdominal testis ♂
Q53.211	Bilateral intraabdominal testes ♂
R39.83	Unilateral non-palpable testicle ♂
R39.84	Bilateral non-palpable testicles ♂

AMA: **54692** 2018,Jan,8; 2017,Jan,8; 2016,Jan,13; 2015,Jan,16; 2014,Jan,11

Testis

CPT © 2020 American Medical Association. All Rights Reserved.   ● New   ▲ Revised   + Add On   ★ Telemedicine   AMA: CPT Assist   [Resequenced]   ☑ Laterality   © 2020 Optum360, LLC

Relative Value Units/Medicare Edits

Non-Facility RVU	Work	PE	MP	Total
54692	13.74	6.58	1.58	21.9
Facility RVU	**Work**	**PE**	**MP**	**Total**
54692	13.74	6.58	1.58	21.9

	FUD	Status	MUE	Modifiers				IOM Reference
54692	90	A	1(2)	51	50	N/A	N/A	None

* with documentation

Terms To Know

fixation. Act or condition of being attached, secured, fastened, or held in position.

fixation. Act or condition of being attached, secured, fastened, or held in position.

intra. Within.

laparoscopy. Direct visualization utilizing a thin, flexible, fiberoptic tube.

orchiopexy. Surgical fixation of an undescended testicle within the scrotum.

scrotum. Skin pouch that holds the testes and supporting reproductive structures.

spermatic cord. Structure of the male reproductive organs that consists of the ductus deferens, testicular artery, nerves, and veins that drain the testes.

testes. Male gonadal paired glands located in the scrotum that secrete testosterone and contain the seminiferous tubules where sperm is produced.

trocar. Cannula or a sharp pointed instrument used to puncture and aspirate fluid from cavities.

54700

54700 Incision and drainage of epididymis, testis and/or scrotal space (eg, abscess or hematoma)

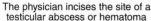

The physician incises the site of a testicular abscess or hematoma

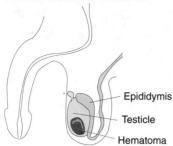

Epididymis
Testicle
Hematoma

The problem may affect the testicle, epididymis, or scrotal space

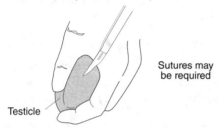

Sutures may be required

Testicle

Explanation

The physician drains a collection of blood or an abscess within the scrotum. If the testis is the target of the drainage, it is held firmly with the scrotal skin stretched tightly over the testis and the epididymis positioned away from the site. A small incision is made through the skin of the scrotum. The underlying tissues are incised and dissected to expose the testis and the site to be drained. The testis may be stabilized by two sutures as an incision is made into the abscess or hematoma and fluid is expressed. Packing or a rubber drain may be placed to promote drainage. The incisions are usually not closed by suturing. Similar procedures are followed if the target is the epididymis or the scrotal space.

Coding Tips

When 54700 is performed with another separately identifiable procedure, the highest dollar value code is listed as the primary procedure and subsequent procedures are appended with modifier 51. When 54700 is used for a procedure on the testis, it is a unilateral procedure. If performed bilaterally, some payers require that the service be reported twice with modifier 50 appended to the second code while others require identification of the service only once with modifier 50 appended. Check with individual payers. Modifier 50 identifies a procedure performed identically on the opposite side of the body (mirror image). For drainage of a scrotal wall abscess, see 55100. For debridement of necrotizing soft tissue infection of external genitalia, see 11004-11006. Local or regional anesthesia is included in this service. However, general anesthesia may be administered depending on the age or condition of the patient.

ICD-10-CM Diagnostic Codes

N45.4	Abscess of epididymis or testis ♂
N49.2	Inflammatory disorders of scrotum ♂
N49.8	Inflammatory disorders of other specified male genital organs ♂
N99.820	Postprocedural hemorrhage of a genitourinary system organ or structure following a genitourinary system procedure
N99.821	Postprocedural hemorrhage of a genitourinary system organ or structure following other procedure
N99.840	Postprocedural hematoma of a genitourinary system organ or structure following a genitourinary system procedure
N99.841	Postprocedural hematoma of a genitourinary system organ or structure following other procedure
N99.842	Postprocedural seroma of a genitourinary system organ or structure following a genitourinary system procedure
N99.843	Postprocedural seroma of a genitourinary system organ or structure following other procedure
R36.1	Hematospermia ♂
S30.21XA	Contusion of penis, initial encounter ♂
S30.22XA	Contusion of scrotum and testes, initial encounter ♂

AMA: 54700 2018,Jan,8; 2017,Jan,8; 2016,Jan,13; 2015,Jan,16; 2014,Jan,11

Relative Value Units/Medicare Edits

Non-Facility RVU	Work	PE	MP	Total
54700	3.47	2.24	0.47	6.18
Facility RVU	**Work**	**PE**	**MP**	**Total**
54700	3.47	2.24	0.47	6.18

	FUD	Status	MUE	Modifiers				IOM Reference
54700	10	A	1(3)	51	50	N/A	N/A	None

* with documentation

Terms To Know

abscess. Circumscribed collection of pus resulting from bacteria, frequently associated with swelling and other signs of inflammation.

contusion. Superficial injury (bruising) produced by impact without a break in the skin.

dissect. Cut apart or separate tissue for surgical purposes or for visual or microscopic study.

drainage. Releasing, taking, or letting out fluids and/or gases from a body part.

epididymis. Coiled tube on the back of the testis that is the site of sperm maturation and storage and where spermatozoa are propelled into the vas deferens toward the ejaculatory duct by contraction of smooth muscle.

epididymo-orchitis. Inflammation of the testes and epididymis.

hematoma. Tumor-like collection of blood in some part of the body caused by a break in a blood vessel wall, usually as a result of trauma.

incision and drainage. Cutting open body tissue for the removal of tissue fluids or infected discharge from a wound or cavity.

orchitis. Testicular inflammation.

packing. Material placed into a cavity or wound, such as gels, gauze, pads, and sponges.

scrotum. Skin pouch that holds the testes and supporting reproductive structures.

54800

54800   Biopsy of epididymis, needle

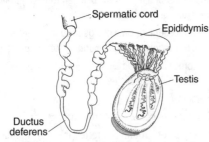

The epididymis is a structure just posterior to the testis that contain ducts to store spermatozoa and allow for maturation before entry into the ductus deferens

Explanation

The physician obtains a sample of epididymal tissues by needle biopsy. While the testis is held firmly with the scrotal skin stretched tightly over the testis and the epididymis positioned just under the taut skin, a biopsy needle is inserted into the area of concern in the epididymis. The needle biopsy sheath is advanced over the needle and twisted to shear off the enclosed sample and withdrawn containing the sample. The scrotal wound may be closed by suturing.

Coding Tips

If a biopsy of the epididymis is performed on both sides, some payers require that the service be reported twice with modifier 50 appended to the second code while others require identification of the service only once with modifier 50 appended. Check with individual payers. Modifier 50 identifies a procedure performed identically on the opposite side of the body (mirror image). If a specimen is transported to an outside laboratory, report 99000 for handling or conveyance. For excision of a local lesion of the epididymis, see 54830. For fine needle aspiration biopsy, see 10004–10012 and 10021. For evaluation of fine needle aspirate, see 88172 and 88173.

ICD-10-CM Diagnostic Codes

C63.01	Malignant neoplasm of right epididymis ♂ ☑
C63.02	Malignant neoplasm of left epididymis ♂ ☑
C79.82	Secondary malignant neoplasm of genital organs
D07.69	Carcinoma in situ of other male genital organs ♂
D29.31	Benign neoplasm of right epididymis ♂ ☑
D29.32	Benign neoplasm of left epididymis ♂ ☑
D40.8	Neoplasm of uncertain behavior of other specified male genital organs ♂
D49.59	Neoplasm of unspecified behavior of other genitourinary organ
N45.1	Epididymitis ♂
N45.3	Epididymo-orchitis ♂
N50.811	Right testicular pain ♂
N50.812	Left testicular pain ♂
N50.82	Scrotal pain ♂
N50.89	Other specified disorders of the male genital organs ♂

AMA: 54800 2019,Apr,4; 2018,Jan,8; 2017,Jan,8; 2016,Jan,13; 2015,Jan,16; 2014,Jan,11

Relative Value Units/Medicare Edits

Non-Facility RVU	Work	PE	MP	Total
54800	2.33	1.03	0.27	3.63
Facility RVU	Work	PE	MP	Total
54800	2.33	1.03	0.27	3.63

	FUD	Status	MUE	Modifiers				IOM Reference
54800	0	A	1(2)	51	50	N/A	80*	None

* with documentation

Terms To Know

benign. Mild or nonmalignant in nature.

biopsy. Tissue or fluid removed for diagnostic purposes through analysis of the cells in the biopsy material.

carcinoma in situ. Malignancy that arises from the cells of the vessel, gland, or organ of origin that remains confined to that site or has not invaded neighboring tissue.

dissection. Separating by cutting tissue or body structures apart.

epididymis. Coiled tube on the back of the testis that is the site of sperm maturation and storage and where spermatozoa are propelled into the vas deferens toward the ejaculatory duct by contraction of smooth muscle.

spermatic cord. Structure of the male reproductive organs that consists of the ductus deferens, testicular artery, nerves, and veins that drain the testes.

suture. Numerous stitching techniques employed in wound closure.

vas deferens. Duct that arises in the tail of the epididymis that stores and carries sperm from the epididymis toward the urethra.

wound. Injury to living tissue often involving a cut or break in the skin.

54830

54830   Excision of local lesion of epididymis

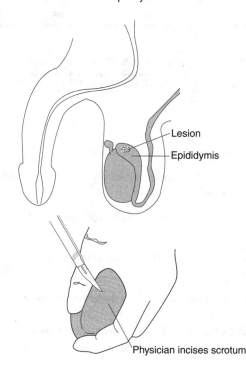

Lesion
Epididymis

Physician incises scrotum

Explanation

The physician removes a local lesion of the epididymis by direct incision. The procedure is done under local or regional anesthesia. While the testis is held firmly with the scrotal skin stretched tightly over the testis and the epididymis positioned just under the taut skin, a small incision is made through the skin of the scrotum. The underlying tissues are incised and dissected to expose the epididymis and the area of concern. The epididymis may be stabilized by two sutures placed on each side of the lesion and an ellipse of tissue is removed from the epididymis containing the lesion between the two sutures. The stabilizing sutures are tied across the excision site to close it. The scrotal incision is closed by suturing.

Coding Tips

For biopsy of the epididymis, see 54800. For exploration of the epididymis, see 54865. For incision and drainage of the epididymis, see 54700. Local or regional anesthesia is included in the service. If a specimen is transported to an outside laboratory, report 99000 for handling or conveyance.

ICD-10-CM Diagnostic Codes

C63.01	Malignant neoplasm of right epididymis ♂ ☑
C63.02	Malignant neoplasm of left epididymis ♂ ☑
C79.82	Secondary malignant neoplasm of genital organs
D07.69	Carcinoma in situ of other male genital organs ♂
D29.31	Benign neoplasm of right epididymis ♂ ☑
D29.32	Benign neoplasm of left epididymis ♂ ☑
D40.8	Neoplasm of uncertain behavior of other specified male genital organs ♂
D49.59	Neoplasm of unspecified behavior of other genitourinary organ
N50.3	Cyst of epididymis ♂
N50.811	Right testicular pain ♂
N50.812	Left testicular pain ♂

N50.82	Scrotal pain ♂
N50.89	Other specified disorders of the male genital organs ♂

AMA: 54830 2018,Jan,8; 2017,Jan,8; 2016,Jan,13; 2015,Jan,16; 2014,Jan,11

Relative Value Units/Medicare Edits

Non-Facility RVU	Work	PE	MP	Total
54830	6.01	4.03	0.68	10.72
Facility RVU	**Work**	**PE**	**MP**	**Total**
54830	6.01	4.03	0.68	10.72

	FUD	Status	MUE	Modifiers				IOM Reference
54830	90	A	1(2)	51	50	N/A	80*	None

* with documentation

Terms To Know

benign lesion. Neoplasm or change in tissue that is not cancerous (nonmalignant).

carcinoma in situ. Malignancy that arises from the cells of the vessel, gland, or organ of origin that remains confined to that site or has not invaded neighboring tissue.

dissection. Separating by cutting tissue or body structures apart.

epididymis. Coiled tube on the back of the testis that is the site of sperm maturation and storage and where spermatozoa are propelled into the vas deferens toward the ejaculatory duct by contraction of smooth muscle.

lesion. Area of damaged tissue that has lost continuity or function, due to disease or trauma.

malignant. Any condition tending to progress toward death, specifically an invasive tumor with a loss of cellular differentiation that has the ability to spread or metastasize to other body areas.

scrotum. Skin pouch that holds the testes and supporting reproductive structures.

secondary. Second in order of occurrence or importance, or appearing during the course of another disease or condition.

tissue. Group of similar cells with a similar function that form definite structures and organs. Tissue types include epithelial tissue, muscle tissue, connective tissue, and nervous tissue.

54840

54840   Excision of spermatocele, with or without epididymectomy

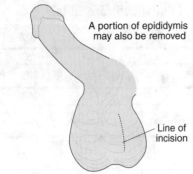

A portion of epididymis may also be removed

Line of incision

The spermatocele is excised through a scrotal incision

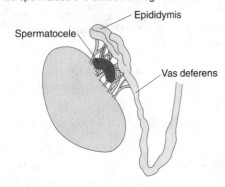

Epididymis

Spermatocele

Vas deferens

Explanation

The physician removes a spermatocele, which is a small cyst, filled with fluid and spermatozoa, between the body of the testis and the epididymis. After adequate local anesthesia, an incision is made in the scrotum and the testis with its attached epididymis is brought out of the wound. The cyst is dissected free of the testis and excised. The involved area of the epididymis is sutured to the underlying testis and the scrotal wound is closed by suturing. Alternately the epididymis may be dissected free of all of its attachments to the testis. The blood vessels involved are tied and cut and/or cauterized to control bleeding. The freed epididymis is thus removed, a rubber drain is placed in the scrotum and the incision is closed by suturing.

Coding Tips

This is a unilateral procedure. If performed bilaterally, some payers require that the service be reported twice with modifier 50 appended to the second code while others require identification of the service only once with modifier 50 appended. Check with individual payers. Modifier 50 identifies a procedure performed identically on the opposite side of the body (mirror image). For epididymectomy without spermatocele excision, unilateral, see 54860; bilateral, see 54861.

ICD-10-CM Diagnostic Codes

N43.41   Spermatocele of epididymis, single ♂
N43.42   Spermatocele of epididymis, multiple ♂

AMA: **54840** 2018,Jan,8; 2017,Jan,8; 2016,Jan,13; 2015,Jan,16; 2014,Jan,11

Relative Value Units/Medicare Edits

Non-Facility RVU	Work	PE	MP	Total
54840	5.27	3.4	0.6	9.27
Facility RVU	**Work**	**PE**	**MP**	**Total**
54840	5.27	3.4	0.6	9.27

	FUD	Status	MUE	Modifiers				IOM Reference
54840	90	A	1(2)	51	50	N/A	N/A	None

* with documentation

Terms To Know

cauterize. Heat or chemicals used to burn or cut.

cyst. Elevated encapsulated mass containing fluid, semisolid, or solid material with a membranous lining.

dissect. Cut apart or separate tissue for surgical purposes or for visual or microscopic study.

drain. Device that creates a channel to allow fluid from a cavity, wound, or infected area to exit the body.

epididymis. Coiled tube on the back of the testis that is the site of sperm maturation and storage and where spermatozoa are propelled into the vas deferens toward the ejaculatory duct by contraction of smooth muscle.

excise. Remove or cut out.

scrotum. Skin pouch that holds the testes and supporting reproductive structures.

spermatic cord. Structure of the male reproductive organs that consists of the ductus deferens, testicular artery, nerves, and veins that drain the testes.

spermatocele. Noncancerous accumulation of fluid and dead sperm cells normally located at the head of the epididymis that exhibits itself as a hard, smooth scrotal mass and does not normally require treatment unless it becomes enlarged or causes pain.

54860-54861

54860 Epididymectomy; unilateral
54861   bilateral

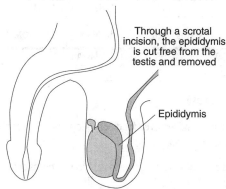

Through a scrotal incision, the epididymis is cut free from the testis and removed

Epididymis

The operative incision is closed with sutures

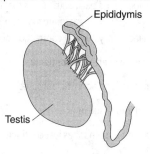

Epididymis

Testis

Explanation

The physician removes the epididymis. After adequate local anesthesia, an incision is made in the scrotum and the testis, with its attached epididymis, is brought out of the wound. The epididymis is dissected free of all of its attachments to the testis. The blood vessels involved are tied and cut and/or cauterized to control bleeding. The freed epididymis is thus removed, a rubber drain is left in the scrotum, and the incision is closed by suturing. The epididymectomy is performed on one side in 54860 or both sides in 54861.

Coding Tips

If a spermatocele is excised with the epididymectomy, see 54840.

ICD-10-CM Diagnostic Codes

C63.01	Malignant neoplasm of right epididymis ♂ ☑
C63.02	Malignant neoplasm of left epididymis ♂ ☑
C79.82	Secondary malignant neoplasm of genital organs
D07.69	Carcinoma in situ of other male genital organs ♂
D29.31	Benign neoplasm of right epididymis ♂ ☑
D29.32	Benign neoplasm of left epididymis ♂ ☑
D40.8	Neoplasm of uncertain behavior of other specified male genital organs ♂
N45.1	Epididymitis ♂
N50.811	Right testicular pain ♂
N50.812	Left testicular pain ♂
N50.82	Scrotal pain ♂
N50.89	Other specified disorders of the male genital organs ♂

AMA: **54860** 2014,Jan,11 **54861** 2014,Jan,11

Relative Value Units/Medicare Edits

Non-Facility RVU	Work	PE	MP	Total
54860	6.95	4.33	0.79	12.07
54861	9.7	5.56	1.12	16.38
Facility RVU	**Work**	**PE**	**MP**	**Total**
54860	6.95	4.33	0.79	12.07
54861	9.7	5.56	1.12	16.38

	FUD	Status	MUE	Modifiers				IOM Reference
54860	90	A	1(2)	51	N/A	N/A	N/A	None
54861	90	A	1(2)	51	N/A	N/A	80*	

* with documentation

Terms To Know

blood vessel. Tubular channel consisting of arteries, veins, and capillaries that transports blood throughout the body.

carcinoma in situ. Malignancy that arises from the cells of the vessel, gland, or organ of origin that remains confined to that site or has not invaded neighboring tissue.

cauterize. Heat or chemicals used to burn or cut.

dissect. Cut apart or separate tissue for surgical purposes or for visual or microscopic study.

drain. Device that creates a channel to allow fluid from a cavity, wound, or infected area to exit the body.

epididymis. Coiled tube on the back of the testis that is the site of sperm maturation and storage and where spermatozoa are propelled into the vas deferens toward the ejaculatory duct by contraction of smooth muscle.

epididymo-orchitis. Inflammation of the testes and epididymis.

lipoma. Benign tumor containing fat cells and the most common of soft tissue lesions, which are usually painless and asymptomatic, with the exception of an angiolipoma.

malignant. Any condition tending to progress toward death, specifically an invasive tumor with a loss of cellular differentiation that has the ability to spread or metastasize to other body areas.

orchitis. Testicular inflammation.

scrotum. Skin pouch that holds the testes and supporting reproductive structures.

testes. Male gonadal paired glands located in the scrotum that secrete testosterone and contain the seminiferous tubules where sperm is produced.

wound. Injury to living tissue often involving a cut or break in the skin.

54865

54865   Exploration of epididymis, with or without biopsy

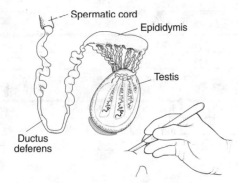

Spermatic cord
Epididymis
Testis
Ductus deferens

The epididymis is a structure just posterior to the testis that contain ducts to store spermatozoa and allow for maturation before entry into the ductus deferens

This is an open procedure on the epididymis

Explanation

The physician explores the epididymis by making an incision in the scrotum. The procedure is done under local or regional anesthesia. While the testis is held firmly with the scrotal skin stretched tightly over the testis and the epididymis positioned just under the taught skin, a small incision is made through the skin of the scrotum. The underlying tissues are incised and dissected to expose the epididymis. The epididymis may be biopsied by placing two sutures on each side of the area of concern and an ellipse of tissue is removed from the epididymis containing the lesion between the two sutures. The stabilizing sutures are tied across the excision site to close it. The scrotal incision is closed by suturing. Alternatively, a biopsy may be done by needle puncture under direct vision.

Coding Tips

If a biopsy of the epididymis is performed on both sides, some payers require that the service be reported twice with modifier 50 appended to the second code while others require identification of the service only once with modifier 50 appended. Check with individual payers. Modifier 50 identifies a procedure performed identically on the opposite side of the body (mirror image). For excision of a local lesion of epididymis, see 54830. For evaluation of fine needle aspirate, see 88172 and 88173. If a specimen is transported to an outside laboratory, report 99000 for handling or conveyance.

ICD-10-CM Diagnostic Codes

C63.01	Malignant neoplasm of right epididymis ♂ ☑
C63.02	Malignant neoplasm of left epididymis ♂ ☑
C79.82	Secondary malignant neoplasm of genital organs
D07.69	Carcinoma in situ of other male genital organs ♂
D29.31	Benign neoplasm of right epididymis ♂ ☑
D29.32	Benign neoplasm of left epididymis ♂ ☑
D40.8	Neoplasm of uncertain behavior of other specified male genital organs ♂
D49.59	Neoplasm of unspecified behavior of other genitourinary organ
N45.1	Epididymitis ♂

AMA: **54865** 2014,Jan,11

Relative Value Units/Medicare Edits

Non-Facility RVU	Work	PE	MP	Total
54865	5.77	3.92	0.64	10.33
Facility RVU	**Work**	**PE**	**MP**	**Total**
54865	5.77	3.92	0.64	10.33

	FUD	Status	MUE	Modifiers				IOM Reference
54865	90	A	1(3)	51	N/A	N/A	80*	None

* with documentation

Terms To Know

biopsy. Tissue or fluid removed for diagnostic purposes through analysis of the cells in the biopsy material.

dissect. Cut apart or separate tissue for surgical purposes or for visual or microscopic study.

epididymis. Coiled tube on the back of the testis that is the site of sperm maturation and storage and where spermatozoa are propelled into the vas deferens toward the ejaculatory duct by contraction of smooth muscle.

excision. Surgical removal of an organ or tissue.

exploration. Examination for diagnostic purposes.

incision. Act of cutting into tissue or an organ.

lesion. Area of damaged tissue that has lost continuity or function, due to disease or trauma.

scrotum. Skin pouch that holds the testes and supporting reproductive structures.

testes. Male gonadal paired glands located in the scrotum that secrete testosterone and contain the seminiferous tubules where sperm is produced.

tissue. Group of similar cells with a similar function that form definite structures and organs. Tissue types include epithelial tissue, muscle tissue, connective tissue, and nervous tissue.

54900-54901

54900 Epididymovasostomy, anastomosis of epididymis to vas deferens; unilateral
54901 bilateral

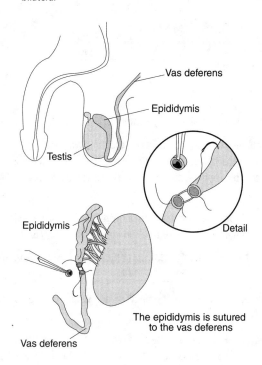

Vas deferens

Epididymis

Testis

Epididymis

Detail

Epididymis

The epididymis is sutured to the vas deferens

Vas deferens

Explanation

The physician treats obstruction of the flow of spermatozoa from the epididymis to vas deferens, the tube that carries the semen. After adequate anesthesia, an incision is made in the scrotum and the testis with its attached epididymis and the vas deferens is brought out of the wound. The vas deferens is transected and the selected area of the epididymis is opened and the appropriate tubule in the area is brought out of the surrounding tissues and transected. The cut ends of these two tubes are sutured together and the vas deferens is sutured to the epididymis. A rubber drain is often placed in the scrotum and the incision is closed by suturing. In 54900, the procedure is performed on one side; in 54901, the procedure is bilateral.

Coding Tips

For epididymectomy, unilateral, see 54840; bilateral, see 54861. If an operating microscope is utilized during anastomosis, report 69990 in addition to the primary procedure. However, head gear (e.g., loupes, binoculars) is considered an integral part of this procedure.

ICD-10-CM Diagnostic Codes

N46.023   Azoospermia due to obstruction of efferent ducts ▲ ♂
N46.123   Oligospermia due to obstruction of efferent ducts ▲ ♂
Z31.0   Encounter for reversal of previous sterilization

AMA: **54900** 2018,Jan,8; 2017,Jan,8; 2016,Jan,13; 2015,Jan,16; 2014,Jan,11
54901 2018,Jan,8; 2017,Jan,8; 2016,Jan,13; 2015,Jan,16; 2014,Jan,11

Relative Value Units/Medicare Edits

Non-Facility RVU	Work	PE	MP	Total
54900	14.2	7.3	1.63	23.13
54901	19.1	9.26	2.19	30.55
Facility RVU	**Work**	**PE**	**MP**	**Total**
54900	14.2	7.3	1.63	23.13
54901	19.1	9.26	2.19	30.55

	FUD	Status	MUE	Modifiers				IOM Reference
54900	90	A	1(2)	51	N/A	N/A	80*	None
54901	90	A	1(2)	51	N/A	N/A	80*	

* with documentation

Terms To Know

anastomosis. Surgically created connection between ducts, blood vessels, or bowel segments to allow flow from one to the other.

anomaly. Irregularity in the structure or position of an organ or tissue.

congenital. Present at birth, occurring through heredity or an influence during gestation up to the moment of birth.

drain. Device that creates a channel to allow fluid from a cavity, wound, or infected area to exit the body.

epididymis. Coiled tube on the back of the testis that is the site of sperm maturation and storage and where spermatozoa are propelled into the vas deferens toward the ejaculatory duct by contraction of smooth muscle.

obstruction. Blockage that prevents normal function of the valve or structure.

oligospermia. Insufficient production of sperm in semen, a common factor in male infertility.

scrotum. Skin pouch that holds the testes and supporting reproductive structures.

tissue. Group of similar cells with a similar function that form definite structures and organs. Tissue types include epithelial tissue, muscle tissue, connective tissue, and nervous tissue.

transection. Transverse dissection; to cut across a long axis; cross section.

vas deferens. Duct that arises in the tail of the epididymis that stores and carries sperm from the epididymis toward the urethra.

wound. Injury to living tissue often involving a cut or break in the skin.

55000

55000 Puncture aspiration of hydrocele, tunica vaginalis, with or without injection of medication

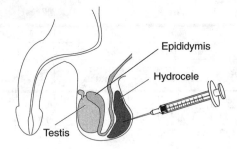

The physician aspirates fluid from a hydrocele by inserting a needle into the testis

After the aspiration of fluid, medication may be injected into the hydrocele

Explanation

A hydrocele is a sac of fluid in the tunica vaginalis or along the spermatic cord. The physician treats a hydrocele by aspirating the fluid. After injecting a small area with local anesthetic, the physician inserts a needle on an aspirating syringe into the fluid filled hydrocele sac and withdraws the fluid into the syringe. After the aspiration and with the needle still in place, the sac may be injected with sclerosing medication to prevent accumulation of new fluid by stimulating scarring and hardening of the empty sac.

Coding Tips

This is a unilateral procedure. If performed bilaterally, some payers require that the service be reported twice with modifier 50 appended to the second code while others require identification of the service only once with modifier 50 appended. Check with individual payers. Modifier 50 identifies a procedure performed identically on the opposite side of the body (mirror image). For excision of a hydrocele, see 55040–55041. This code includes injection of medication. If a specimen is transported to an outside laboratory, report 99000 for handling or conveyance.

ICD-10-CM Diagnostic Codes

N43.0	Encysted hydrocele ♂
N43.1	Infected hydrocele ♂
N43.2	Other hydrocele ♂
N50.811	Right testicular pain ♂
N50.812	Left testicular pain ♂
N50.82	Scrotal pain ♂
N50.89	Other specified disorders of the male genital organs ♂
P83.5	Congenital hydrocele ♂

AMA: **55000** 2014,Jan,11

Relative Value Units/Medicare Edits

Non-Facility RVU	Work	PE	MP	Total
55000	1.43	1.78	0.18	3.39
Facility RVU	**Work**	**PE**	**MP**	**Total**
55000	1.43	0.83	0.18	2.44

	FUD	Status	MUE	Modifiers				IOM Reference
55000	0	A	1(3)	51	50	N/A	N/A	None

* with documentation

Terms To Know

aspiration. Drawing fluid out by suction.

hydrocele. Serous fluid that collects in the tunica vaginalis, the spermatic cord, or the canal of Nuck. Hydroceles may be congenital, due to a defect in the tunica vaginalis, or secondary, due to fluid accumulation, injury, infection, or radiotherapy.

puncture aspiration. Use of a knife or needle to pierce a fluid-filled cavity and then withdraw the fluid using a syringe or suction device.

sclerose. To become hard or firm and indurated from increased formation of connective tissue or disease.

scrotum. Skin pouch that holds the testes and supporting reproductive structures.

spermatic cord. Structure of the male reproductive organs that consists of the ductus deferens, testicular artery, nerves, and veins that drain the testes.

testes. Male gonadal paired glands located in the scrotum that secrete testosterone and contain the seminiferous tubules where sperm is produced.

tunica vaginalis. Serous membrane that partially covers the testes formed by an outpocketing of the peritoneum when the testes descend.

Tunical Vaginalis

55040-55041

55040   Excision of hydrocele; unilateral
55041   bilateral

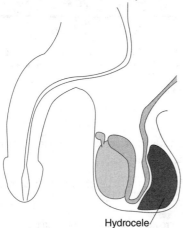

The physician makes a scrotal or inguinal
incision and excises the hydrocele

Hydrocele

Explanation

A hydrocele is a sac of fluid in the tunica vaginalis or along the spermatic cord. The physician treats a hydrocele by removing it. After injecting an area with local anesthetic and using aseptic techniques, the physician makes an incision in the scrotum or in the inguinal area. Care is taken to keep the hydrocele intact while it is dissected free of its attachments to the testis and other structures. The sac is opened, drained and partially excised leaving a remnant of tissue. The remaining tissue is swung back behind the epididymis and the spermatic cord and closed by suturing the edges together. The testis is anchored to the inside of the scrotum with three sutures to prevent later torsion or twisting of the testis. A rubber drain may be left in the scrotum and the incision closed in layers by suturing. The hydrocele is on one side in 55040. In 55041, each side is treated for hydrocele.

Coding Tips

To report excision of hydrocele with hernia repair, see 49495–49501. For puncture aspiration of a hydrocele, see 55000. For excision of a spermatic cord hydrocele, see 55500.

ICD-10-CM Diagnostic Codes

N43.0   Encysted hydrocele ♂
N43.1   Infected hydrocele ♂
N43.2   Other hydrocele ♂
P83.5   Congenital hydrocele ♂

AMA: 55040 2018,Jan,8; 2017,Nov,10; 2017,Jan,8; 2016,Jan,13; 2015,Jan,16; 2014,Jan,11 55041 2014,Jan,11

Relative Value Units/Medicare Edits

Non-Facility RVU	Work	PE	MP	Total
55040	5.45	3.63	0.64	9.72
55041	8.54	5.19	1.02	14.75
Facility RVU	Work	PE	MP	Total
55040	5.45	3.63	0.64	9.72
55041	8.54	5.19	1.02	14.75

	FUD	Status	MUE		Modifiers			IOM Reference
55040	90	A	1(2)	51	N/A	N/A	N/A	None
55041	90	A	1(2)	51	N/A	N/A	N/A	

* with documentation

Terms To Know

congenital. Present at birth, occurring through heredity or an influence during gestation up to the moment of birth.

dissect. Cut apart or separate tissue for surgical purposes or for visual or microscopic study.

drain. Device that creates a channel to allow fluid from a cavity, wound, or infected area to exit the body.

epididymis. Coiled tube on the back of the testis that is the site of sperm maturation and storage and where spermatozoa are propelled into the vas deferens toward the ejaculatory duct by contraction of smooth muscle.

excision. Surgical removal of an organ or tissue.

hydrocele. Serous fluid that collects in the tunica vaginalis, the spermatic cord, or the canal of Nuck. Hydroceles may be congenital, due to a defect in the tunica vaginalis, or secondary, due to fluid accumulation, injury, infection, or radiotherapy.

inguinal. Within the groin region.

scrotum. Skin pouch that holds the testes and supporting reproductive structures.

spermatic cord. Structure of the male reproductive organs that consists of the ductus deferens, testicular artery, nerves, and veins that drain the testes.

testes. Male gonadal paired glands located in the scrotum that secrete testosterone and contain the seminiferous tubules where sperm is produced.

tissue. Group of similar cells with a similar function that form definite structures and organs. Tissue types include epithelial tissue, muscle tissue, connective tissue, and nervous tissue.

torsion of testis. Twisting, turning, or rotation of the testicle upon itself, so as to compromise or cut off the blood supply.

tunica vaginalis. Serous membrane that partially covers the testes formed by an outpocketing of the peritoneum when the testes descend.

CPT © 2020 American Medical Association. All Rights Reserved.   ● New   ▲ Revised   + Add On   ★ Telemedicine   AMA: CPT Assist   [Resequenced]   ☑ Laterality   © 2020 Optum360, LLC

55060

55060 Repair of tunica vaginalis hydrocele (Bottle type)

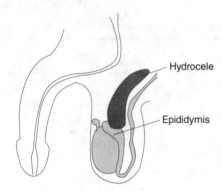

Hydrocele

Epididymis

The physician mobilizes the testis to excise a hydrocele from the epididymis or testis

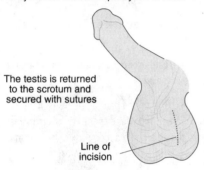

The testis is returned to the scrotum and secured with sutures

Line of incision

Explanation

The physician treats a hydrocele by removing the abnormal fluid filled sac in the scrotum or in the inguinal canal. After injecting an area with local anesthetic and using aseptic techniques, the physician makes an incision in the scrotum or in the inguinal area. Care is taken to keep the hydrocele intact while it is dissected free of its attachments to the testis and other structures. The sac is opened high along its front surface and the testis is pushed up through the sac and out through the incision. This inverts the hydrocele sac which is tacked by suturing to the spermatic cord structures behind the testis. The testis is returned to the scrotum and is anchored to the inside of the scrotum with three sutures to prevent later torsion or twisting of the testis. A rubber drain may be left in the scrotum and the incision closed in layers by suturing.

Coding Tips

This is a unilateral procedure. If performed bilaterally, some payers require that the service be reported twice with modifier 50 appended to the second code while others require identification of the service only once with modifier 50 appended. Check with individual payers. Modifier 50 identifies a procedure performed identically on the opposite side of the body (mirror image). For puncture aspiration of a hydrocele, see 55000. For excision of a hydrocele, see 55040–55041.

ICD-10-CM Diagnostic Codes

N43.0	Encysted hydrocele ♂
N43.1	Infected hydrocele ♂
N43.2	Other hydrocele ♂
P83.5	Congenital hydrocele ♂

AMA: **55060** 2018,Jan,8; 2017,Jan,8; 2016,Jan,13; 2015,Jan,16; 2014,Nov,14; 2014,Jan,11

Relative Value Units/Medicare Edits

Non-Facility RVU	Work	PE	MP	Total
55060	6.15	4.08	0.74	10.97
Facility RVU	**Work**	**PE**	**MP**	**Total**
55060	6.15	4.08	0.74	10.97

	FUD	Status	MUE	Modifiers				IOM Reference
55060	90	A	1(2)	51	50	N/A	80*	None

* with documentation

Terms To Know

congenital. Present at birth, occurring through heredity or an influence during gestation up to the moment of birth.

dissect. Cut apart or separate tissue for surgical purposes or for visual or microscopic study.

drain. Device that creates a channel to allow fluid from a cavity, wound, or infected area to exit the body.

hydrocele. Serous fluid that collects in the tunica vaginalis, the spermatic cord, or the canal of Nuck. Hydroceles may be congenital, due to a defect in the tunica vaginalis, or secondary, due to fluid accumulation, injury, infection, or radiotherapy.

infection. Presence of microorganisms in body tissues that may result in cellular damage.

inguinal. Within the groin region.

scrotum. Skin pouch that holds the testes and supporting reproductive structures.

spermatic cord. Structure of the male reproductive organs that consists of the ductus deferens, testicular artery, nerves, and veins that drain the testes.

testes. Male gonadal paired glands located in the scrotum that secrete testosterone and contain the seminiferous tubules where sperm is produced.

torsion of testis. Twisting, turning, or rotation of the testicle upon itself, so as to compromise or cut off the blood supply.

Tunical Vaginalis

55100

55100   Drainage of scrotal wall abscess

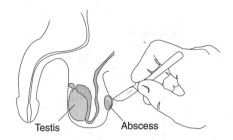

Testis   Abscess

The physician incises and drains
an abscess of the scrotal wall

Explanation

After adequate local anesthesia, the physician makes an incision directly into the abscess of the scrotal wall. Pus is expressed and a drain or medicated gauze packing placed in the abscess cavity.

Coding Tips

For incision and drainage of the scrotal space (e.g., for abscess or hematoma), see 54700. Local or regional anesthesia is included in the service. If a specimen is transported to an outside laboratory, report 99000 for handling or conveyance.

ICD-10-CM Diagnostic Codes

N49.1   Inflammatory disorders of spermatic cord, tunica vaginalis and vas deferens ♂

N49.2   Inflammatory disorders of scrotum ♂

N49.8   Inflammatory disorders of other specified male genital organs ♂

AMA: 55100 2014,Jan,11

Relative Value Units/Medicare Edits

Non-Facility RVU	Work	PE	MP	Total
55100	2.45	3.63	0.35	6.43
Facility RVU	**Work**	**PE**	**MP**	**Total**
55100	2.45	2.0	0.35	4.8

	FUD	Status	MUE	Modifiers			IOM Reference
55100	10	A	2(3)	51	N/A	N/A	N/A	None

* with documentation

Terms To Know

abscess. Circumscribed collection of pus resulting from bacteria, frequently associated with swelling and other signs of inflammation.

incision and drainage. Cutting open body tissue for the removal of tissue fluids or infected discharge from a wound or cavity.

packing. Material placed into a cavity or wound, such as gels, gauze, pads, and sponges.

scrotum. Skin pouch that holds the testes and supporting reproductive structures.

55110

55110   Scrotal exploration

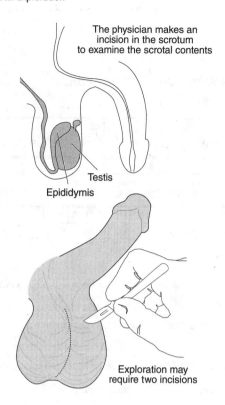

The physician makes an
incision in the scrotum
to examine the scrotal contents

Testis
Epididymis

Exploration may
require two incisions

Explanation

The physician makes an incision in the scrotum for the purpose of direct visual inspection of the contents of the scrotum. This may involve one or both sides of the scrotum and may be done through one or two incisions and require incisions through the various layers of tissues to expose the testis and other structures. A drain may be left in the scrotum and the incisions closed in successive layers of sutures.

Coding Tips

This is a bilateral code and is reported once even if the procedure is performed on both sides. Local or regional anesthesia is included in this service. However, general anesthesia may be administered depending on the age or condition of the patient. If a specimen is transported to an outside laboratory, report 99000 for handling or conveyance.

ICD-10-CM Diagnostic Codes

C79.82   Secondary malignant neoplasm of genital organs

D29.4   Benign neoplasm of scrotum ♂

D40.8   Neoplasm of uncertain behavior of other specified male genital organs ♂

N44.01   Extravaginal torsion of spermatic cord ♂

N44.02   Intravaginal torsion of spermatic cord ♂

N44.03   Torsion of appendix testis ♂

N44.04   Torsion of appendix epididymis ♂

N49.2   Inflammatory disorders of scrotum ♂

N49.8   Inflammatory disorders of other specified male genital organs ♂

N50.811   Right testicular pain ♂

N50.812   Left testicular pain ♂

N50.82   Scrotal pain ♂

N50.89	Other specified disorders of the male genital organs ♂
Q55.0	Absence and aplasia of testis ♂
Q55.21	Polyorchism ♂
Q55.8	Other specified congenital malformations of male genital organs ♂

AMA: 55110 2014,Jan,11

Relative Value Units/Medicare Edits

Non-Facility RVU	Work	PE	MP	Total
55110	6.33	4.08	0.78	11.19
Facility RVU	**Work**	**PE**	**MP**	**Total**
55110	6.33	4.08	0.78	11.19

	FUD	Status	MUE	Modifiers				IOM Reference
55110	90	A	1(2)	51	N/A	N/A	N/A	None

* with documentation

Terms To Know

aplasia. Incomplete development of an organ or tissue. Aplasia may be congenital (present at birth) or acquired.

drain. Device that creates a channel to allow fluid from a cavity, wound, or infected area to exit the body.

epididymo-orchitis. Inflammation of the testes and epididymis.

exploration. Examination for diagnostic purposes.

extravaginal torsion of spermatic cord. Torsion of the spermatic cord just below the tunica vaginalis attachments.

malignant neoplasm. Any cancerous tumor or lesion exhibiting uncontrolled tissue growth that can progressively invade other parts of the body with its disease-generating cells.

polyorchism. Congenital anomaly in which there are more than two testes.

scrotum. Skin pouch that holds the testes and supporting reproductive structures.

secondary. Second in order of occurrence or importance, or appearing during the course of another disease or condition.

tissue. Group of similar cells with a similar function that form definite structures and organs. Tissue types include epithelial tissue, muscle tissue, connective tissue, and nervous tissue.

varices. Enlarged, dilated, or twisted turning veins.

55120

55120 Removal of foreign body in scrotum

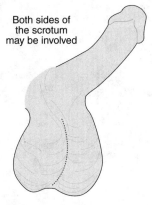

Both sides of the scrotum may be involved

The physician makes an incision in the scrotum to remove a foreign body

Explanation

The physician makes an incision in the scrotum for the purpose of foreign body removal. This may involve one or both sides of the scrotum and may be done through one or two incisions and may require incisions through the various layers of tissues to expose and locate the object. The foreign body is identified and isolated and removed with care to avoid damaging tissues in the scrotum. A drain may be placed in the scrotum and the incisions closed in successive layers of sutures.

Coding Tips

If significant additional time and effort is documented, append modifier 22 and submit a cover letter and operative report. This code includes any complex closures the physician may perform. For scrotoplasty, see 55175–55180. For other foreign body removal except scrotum, see the appropriate anatomical site. Local or regional anesthesia is included in this service. However, general anesthesia may be administered depending on the age or condition of the patient.

ICD-10-CM Diagnostic Codes

S30.853A	Superficial foreign body of scrotum and testes, initial encounter ♂
S31.32XA	Laceration with foreign body of scrotum and testes, initial encounter ♂
S31.34XA	Puncture wound with foreign body of scrotum and testes, initial encounter ♂
T81.510A	Adhesions due to foreign body accidentally left in body following surgical operation, initial encounter
T81.518A	Adhesions due to foreign body accidentally left in body following other procedure, initial encounter
T81.520A	Obstruction due to foreign body accidentally left in body following surgical operation, initial encounter
T81.590A	Other complications of foreign body accidentally left in body following surgical operation, initial encounter

AMA: 55120 2014,Jan,11

Scrotum

Relative Value Units/Medicare Edits

Non-Facility RVU	Work	PE	MP	Total
55120	5.72	3.83	0.64	10.19
Facility RVU	**Work**	**PE**	**MP**	**Total**
55120	5.72	3.83	0.64	10.19

	FUD	Status	MUE	Modifiers				IOM Reference
55120	90	A	1(3)	51	N/A	N/A	80*	None

* with documentation

Terms To Know

adhesion. Abnormal fibrous connection between two structures, soft tissue or bony structures, that may occur as the result of surgery, infection, or trauma.

drain. Device that creates a channel to allow fluid from a cavity, wound, or infected area to exit the body.

foreign body. Any object or substance found in an organ and tissue that does not belong under normal circumstances.

laceration. Tearing injury; a torn, ragged-edged wound.

obstruction. Blockage that prevents normal function of the valve or structure.

scrotum. Skin pouch that holds the testes and supporting reproductive structures.

superficial. On the skin surface or near the surface of any involved structure or field of interest.

tissue. Group of similar cells with a similar function that form definite structures and organs. Tissue types include epithelial tissue, muscle tissue, connective tissue, and nervous tissue.

55150

55150   Resection of scrotum

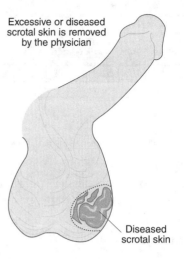

Excessive or diseased scrotal skin is removed by the physician

Diseased scrotal skin

Explanation

The physician removes excessive or diseased scrotal skin by excision. The extent of the procedure is dependent upon the disease process and the degree of involvement. The physician makes incisions in the scrotal skin, taking care to avoid injury to the underlying scrotal contents. In the simple case, the excess skin is removed and the defects closed in layers by suturing. In the more involved cases the testes and spermatic cords must be mobilized and removed from the scrotum and swung out of the way by making incisions in the inguinal areas. The affected scrotal skin is excised and the testes and cord structures returned to their anatomic positions. If not enough scrotal skin remains, flaps of skin are raised from the adjacent thighs and rotated to cover the testes. These grafts or flaps are separately reported. Rubber drains may be left in the scrotum and the operative site closed in layers by suturing.

Coding Tips

When 55150 is performed with another separately identifiable procedure, the highest dollar value code is listed as the primary procedure and subsequent procedures are appended with modifier 51. For excision of a lesion of the testis, see 54512. For complicated plastic repair of the scrotum (scrotoplasty), see 55180. This code includes any basic closure or repair the physician may perform. Report any free grafts or flaps separately.

ICD-10-CM Diagnostic Codes

C63.2	Malignant neoplasm of scrotum ♂
C79.82	Secondary malignant neoplasm of genital organs
D07.61	Carcinoma in situ of scrotum ♂
D29.4	Benign neoplasm of scrotum ♂
D40.8	Neoplasm of uncertain behavior of other specified male genital organs ♂
N50.811	Right testicular pain ♂
N50.812	Left testicular pain ♂
N50.82	Scrotal pain ♂
N50.89	Other specified disorders of the male genital organs ♂

AMA: 55150 2014,Jan,11

Scrotum

Relative Value Units/Medicare Edits

Non-Facility RVU	Work	PE	MP	Total
55150	8.14	5.07	0.99	14.2
Facility RVU	Work	PE	MP	Total
55150	8.14	5.07	0.99	14.2

	FUD	Status	MUE	Modifiers				IOM Reference
55150	90	A	1(2)	51	N/A	62*	80	None

* with documentation

Terms To Know

benign lesion. Neoplasm or change in tissue that is not cancerous (nonmalignant).

carcinoma in situ. Malignancy that arises from the cells of the vessel, gland, or organ of origin that remains confined to that site or has not invaded neighboring tissue.

defect. Imperfection, flaw, or absence.

drain. Device that creates a channel to allow fluid from a cavity, wound, or infected area to exit the body.

inguinal. Within the groin region.

malignant. Any condition tending to progress toward death, specifically an invasive tumor with a loss of cellular differentiation that has the ability to spread or metastasize to other body areas.

resection. Surgical removal of a part or all of an organ or body part.

scrotum. Skin pouch that holds the testes and supporting reproductive structures.

spermatic cord. Structure of the male reproductive organs that consists of the ductus deferens, testicular artery, nerves, and veins that drain the testes.

testes. Male gonadal paired glands located in the scrotum that secrete testosterone and contain the seminiferous tubules where sperm is produced.

55175-55180

55175	Scrotoplasty; simple
55180	complicated

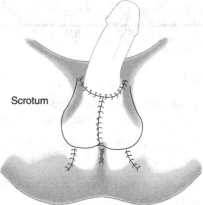

Skin of the scrotum is revised

Scrotum

The scrotal defect may be congenital or acquired

Explanation

The physician repairs defects and developmental abnormalities of the scrotum by wound revisions or the creation and suturing of simple scrotal skin flaps in 55175. In 55180, the reconstruction is more complex and the physician uses free skin grafts, mesh grafts, and/or the extensive use of rotational pedicle grafts from adjacent skin. These flaps or grafts are separately reported.

Coding Tips

These codes include any closures or repairs. Resection of the scrotum (55150) and simple scrotoplasty are mutually exclusive of each other and should not be reported together. Scrotoplasty may be done as a reconstruction stage of a more complicated procedure, such as transplantation of the testis to the thigh because of scrotal destruction (54680). To indicate that this is a staged or related procedure performed during the postoperative period by the same physician, append modifier 58. Report any free grafts or flaps separately.

ICD-10-CM Diagnostic Codes

C63.2	Malignant neoplasm of scrotum ♂
C79.82	Secondary malignant neoplasm of genital organs
D29.4	Benign neoplasm of scrotum ♂
D40.8	Neoplasm of uncertain behavior of other specified male genital organs ♂
Q55.29	Other congenital malformations of testis and scrotum ♂
S31.31XA	Laceration without foreign body of scrotum and testes, initial encounter ♂
S31.32XA	Laceration with foreign body of scrotum and testes, initial encounter ♂
S31.33XA	Puncture wound without foreign body of scrotum and testes, initial encounter ♂
S31.34XA	Puncture wound with foreign body of scrotum and testes, initial encounter ♂
S31.35XA	Open bite of scrotum and testes, initial encounter ♂
S38.231A	Complete traumatic amputation of scrotum and testis, initial encounter ♂
S38.232A	Partial traumatic amputation of scrotum and testis, initial encounter ♂

Scrotum

AMA: 55175 2018,Jan,8; 2017,Jan,8; 2016,Jan,13; 2015,Jan,16; 2014,Jan,11; 2014,Dec,16; 2014,Dec,16 **55180** 2014,Jan,11

Relative Value Units/Medicare Edits

Non-Facility RVU	Work	PE	MP	Total
55175	5.87	3.92	0.67	10.46
55180	11.78	6.78	1.44	20.0
Facility RVU	Work	PE	MP	Total
55175	5.87	3.92	0.67	10.46
55180	11.78	6.78	1.44	20.0

	FUD	Status	MUE	Modifiers				IOM Reference
55175	90	A	1(2)	51	N/A	N/A	80*	None
55180	90	A	1(2)	51	N/A	N/A	80*	

* with documentation

Terms To Know

anomaly. Irregularity in the structure or position of an organ or tissue.

benign lesion. Neoplasm or change in tissue that is not cancerous (nonmalignant).

carcinoma in situ. Malignancy that arises from the cells of the vessel, gland, or organ of origin that remains confined to that site or has not invaded neighboring tissue.

congenital. Present at birth, occurring through heredity or an influence during gestation up to the moment of birth.

defect. Imperfection, flaw, or absence.

fistula. Abnormal tube-like passage between two body cavities or organs or from an organ to the outside surface.

flap. Mass of flesh and skin partially excised from its location but retaining its blood supply that is moved to another site to repair adjacent or distant defects.

flap graft. Mass of flesh and skin partially excised from its location but retaining its blood supply, grafted onto another site to repair adjacent or distant defects.

free flap. Tissue that is completely detached from the donor site and transplanted to the recipient site, receiving its blood supply from capillary ingrowth at the recipient site.

malignant. Any condition tending to progress toward death, specifically an invasive tumor with a loss of cellular differentiation that has the ability to spread or metastasize to other body areas.

pedicle graft. Mass of flesh and skin partially excised from the donor location, retaining its blood supply through intact blood vessels, and grafted onto another site to repair adjacent or distant defects.

reconstruction. Recreating, restoring, or rebuilding a body part or organ.

scrotum. Skin pouch that holds the testes and supporting reproductive structures.

tunica vaginalis. Serous membrane that partially covers the testes formed by an outpocketing of the peritoneum when the testes descend.

Scrotum

55200

55200   Vasotomy, cannulization with or without incision of vas, unilateral or bilateral (separate procedure)

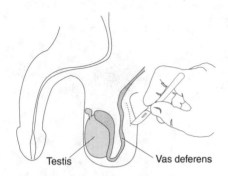

Testis   Vas deferens

The physician makes an incision in the scrotal skin overlying the vas deferens; a needle withdraws fluid samples from the vas deferens
This checks for patency of the vas deferens

Explanation

The physician enters the vas deferens (the tube that carries spermatozoa from the testis) for purpose of obtaining a sample of semen or testing the patency of the tubes. Under local anesthesia, an incision is made in the upper outer scrotum overlying the spermatic cord. The tissues are dissected to expose the vas deferens. The tube is entered by puncturing with a small needle and fluid samples removed or solution injected to check for blockages. An alternate method involves the tube being cut open with a scalpel. A blunt needle is placed in the tube under direct vision and fluid samples removed or the tube checked for patency. If an incision is made in the tube, the tube must be repaired using microsurgical techniques before the scrotal incisions are closed in layers by suturing.

Coding Tips

This separate procedure by definition is usually a component of a more complex service and is not identified separately. When performed alone or with other unrelated procedures/services it may be reported. If performed alone, list the code; if performed with other procedures/services, list the code and append modifier 59 or an X{EPSU} modifier. This is a unilateral or bilateral code and is reported once even if the procedure is performed on both sides. For vasectomy, see 55250. For vasotomy for vasograms, seminal vesiculograms, or epididymograms, see 55300. For vasovasostomy and vasovasorrhaphy, see 55400. Local or regional anesthesia is included in the service. However, general anesthesia may be administered depending on the age or condition of the patient.

ICD-10-CM Diagnostic Codes

N46.023	Azoospermia due to obstruction of efferent ducts ▲ ♂
N46.123	Oligospermia due to obstruction of efferent ducts ▲ ♂
N49.0	Inflammatory disorders of seminal vesicle ♂
N50.89	Other specified disorders of the male genital organs ♂

AMA: **55200** 2014,Jan,11

Relative Value Units/Medicare Edits

Non-Facility RVU	Work	PE	MP	Total
55200	4.55	6.72	0.52	11.79
Facility RVU	Work	PE	MP	Total
55200	4.55	2.93	0.52	8.0

	FUD	Status	MUE	Modifiers				IOM Reference
55200	90	A	1(2)	51	N/A	N/A	80*	None

* with documentation

Terms To Know

azoospermia. Failure of the development of sperm or the absence of sperm in semen; one of the most common factors in male infertility.

dissect. Cut apart or separate tissue for surgical purposes or for visual or microscopic study.

efferent. Conveying away from the center.

hematospermia. Blood in the seminal fluid, often caused by inflammation of the prostate or seminal vesicles, or prostate cancer. In primary hematospermia, the presence of blood in the seminal fluid is the only symptom.

impotence. Psychosexual or organic dysfunction in which there is partial or complete failure to attain or maintain erection until completion of the sexual act.

microsurgery. Surgical procedures performed under magnification using a surgical microscope.

obstruction. Blockage that prevents normal function of the valve or structure.

oligospermia. Insufficient production of sperm in semen, a common factor in male infertility.

patency. State of a tube-like structure or conduit being open and unobstructed.

scrotum. Skin pouch that holds the testes and supporting reproductive structures.

spermatic cord. Structure of the male reproductive organs that consists of the ductus deferens, testicular artery, nerves, and veins that drain the testes.

tissue. Group of similar cells with a similar function that form definite structures and organs. Tissue types include epithelial tissue, muscle tissue, connective tissue, and nervous tissue.

vas deferens. Duct that arises in the tail of the epididymis that stores and carries sperm from the epididymis toward the urethra.

Vas Deferens

55250

55250 Vasectomy, unilateral or bilateral (separate procedure), including postoperative semen examination(s)

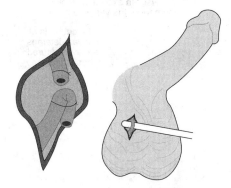

The physician cuts the vas deferens and ties the ends with sutures

Explanation

The physician grasps the upper scrotum near the inguinal area and holds the spermatic cord between the thumb and the index finger. The skin overlying the immobilized cord is injected with local anesthetic and an incision is made through the scrotal wall to expose the tubular structures. Another incision is made to expose the vas deferens (spermatic tube) and the tissues dissected to free it from the adjacent vessels and supporting tissues. The isolated vas deferens is cut in two places and the intervening section of tube is removed. The cut ends of the vas deferens are cauterized and tied with suture material. The incisions are closed in layers by suturing. The procedure is usually repeated on the opposite side.

Coding Tips

This code is appropriate for reporting when any technique or a combination of techniques (clamps and hot cautery) is used. This separate procedure by definition is usually a component of a more complex service and is not identified separately. When performed alone or with other unrelated procedures/services it may be reported. If performed alone, list the code; if performed with other procedures/services, list the code and append modifier 59 or an X{EPSU} modifier.

ICD-10-CM Diagnostic Codes

Z30.2   Encounter for sterilization

AMA: 55250 2018,Jan,8; 2017,Jan,8; 2016,Jan,13; 2015,Jan,16; 2014,Jan,11

Relative Value Units/Medicare Edits

Non-Facility RVU	Work	PE	MP	Total
55250	3.37	6.56	0.39	10.32
Facility RVU	**Work**	**PE**	**MP**	**Total**
55250	3.37	2.79	0.39	6.55

	FUD	Status	MUE	Modifiers				IOM Reference
55250	90	A	1(2)	51	N/A	N/A	N/A	100-03,230.3

* with documentation

55300

55300 Vasotomy for vasograms, seminal vesiculograms, or epididymograms, unilateral or bilateral

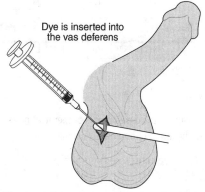

Dye is inserted into the vas deferens

The vas deferens is exposed before the dye is injected. This procedure may be repeated on the other side. The incision is repaired with sutures

Explanation

The physician enters the vas deferens (the tube that carries spermatozoa from the testis) for purpose of testing the patency of the spermatozoa collecting system. An incision is made in the upper outer scrotum overlying the spermatic cord and the tissues dissected to expose the vas deferens.

Coding Tips

When 55300 is performed with another separately identifiable procedure, the highest dollar value code is listed as the primary procedure and subsequent procedures are appended with modifier 51. This is a unilateral or bilateral code and is reported once even if the procedure is performed on both sides. When combined with a biopsy of the testis, see 54505 and append modifier 51. For vasotomy cannulization, see 55200. For radiological supervision and interpretation, see 74440.

ICD-10-CM Diagnostic Codes

N46.01	Organic azoospermia 🅰 ♂
N46.021	Azoospermia due to drug therapy 🅰 ♂
N46.022	Azoospermia due to infection 🅰 ♂
N46.023	Azoospermia due to obstruction of efferent ducts 🅰 ♂
N46.024	Azoospermia due to radiation 🅰 ♂
N46.025	Azoospermia due to systemic disease 🅰 ♂
N46.029	Azoospermia due to other extratesticular causes 🅰 ♂
N46.11	Organic oligospermia 🅰 ♂
N46.121	Oligospermia due to drug therapy 🅰 ♂
N46.122	Oligospermia due to infection 🅰 ♂
N46.123	Oligospermia due to obstruction of efferent ducts 🅰 ♂
N46.124	Oligospermia due to radiation 🅰 ♂
N46.125	Oligospermia due to systemic disease 🅰 ♂
N46.129	Oligospermia due to other extratesticular causes 🅰 ♂
N46.8	Other male infertility 🅰 ♂
N50.89	Other specified disorders of the male genital organs ♂
Q55.3	Atresia of vas deferens ♂
Z31.41	Encounter for fertility testing

AMA: 55300 2014,Jan,11

Relative Value Units/Medicare Edits

Non-Facility RVU	Work	PE	MP	Total
55300	3.5	1.48	0.41	5.39
Facility RVU	**Work**	**PE**	**MP**	**Total**
55300	3.5	1.48	0.41	5.39

	FUD	Status	MUE	Modifiers				IOM Reference
55300	0	A	1(2)	51	N/A	N/A	80*	None

* with documentation

Terms To Know

azoospermia. Failure of the development of sperm or the absence of sperm in semen; one of the most common factors in male infertility.

dissect. Cut apart or separate tissue for surgical purposes or for visual or microscopic study.

epididymis. Coiled tube on the back of the testis that is the site of sperm maturation and storage and where spermatozoa are propelled into the vas deferens toward the ejaculatory duct by contraction of smooth muscle.

oligospermia. Insufficient production of sperm in semen, a common factor in male infertility.

patency. State of a tube-like structure or conduit being open and unobstructed.

scrotum. Skin pouch that holds the testes and supporting reproductive structures.

seminal vesicles. Paired glands located at the base of the bladder in males that release the majority of fluid into semen through ducts that join with the vas deferens forming the ejaculatory duct.

tissue. Group of similar cells with a similar function that form definite structures and organs. Tissue types include epithelial tissue, muscle tissue, connective tissue, and nervous tissue.

vas deferens. Duct that arises in the tail of the epididymis that stores and carries sperm from the epididymis toward the urethra.

55400

55400   Vasovasostomy, vasovasorrhaphy

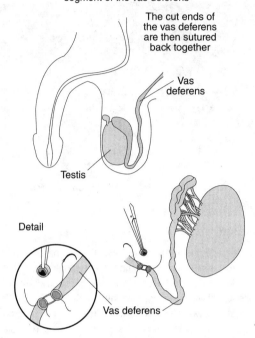

The physician excises a blocked segment of the vas deferens

The cut ends of the vas deferens are then sutured back together

Vas deferens

Testis

Detail

Vas deferens

Explanation

The physician treats a blockage in the vas deferens, the tube that carries semen. After anesthesia, an incision is made in the scrotum. The testis with its attached epididymis and the vas deferens are brought out of the wound. Dye injection studies and semen sampling is often done during the operation to determine the site of the blockage and to accurately choose the segment of tube for excision. The vas deferens is transected in two places, one on each side of the blocked area and the abnormal segment removed. The created cut ends are sutured together in one or two layers with care to align accurately the lumens of the tubes. The testis and associated structures are returned to the scrotum. A rubber drain is often placed in the scrotum and the incisions closed by suturing.

Coding Tips

This is a unilateral procedure. If performed bilaterally, some payers require that the service be reported twice with modifier 50 appended to the second code while others require identification of the service only once with modifier 50 appended. Check with individual payers. Modifier 50 identifies a procedure performed identically on the opposite side of the body (mirror image). Use of an operating microscope is reported separately, see 69990.

ICD-10-CM Diagnostic Codes

N46.023	Azoospermia due to obstruction of efferent ducts 🄰 ♂
N46.123	Oligospermia due to obstruction of efferent ducts 🄰 ♂
N49.0	Inflammatory disorders of seminal vesicle ♂
N50.89	Other specified disorders of the male genital organs ♂
Q55.3	Atresia of vas deferens ♂
Z31.0	Encounter for reversal of previous sterilization

AMA: 55400 2018,Jan,8; 2017,Jan,8; 2016,Jan,13; 2015,Jan,16; 2014,Jan,11

Relative Value Units/Medicare Edits

Non-Facility RVU	Work	PE	MP	Total
55400	8.61	4.82	0.99	14.42
Facility RVU	**Work**	**PE**	**MP**	**Total**
55400	8.61	4.82	0.99	14.42

	FUD	Status	MUE	Modifiers				IOM Reference
55400	90	A	1(2)	51	50	62*	80	None

* with documentation

Terms To Know

atresia. Congenital closure or absence of a tubular organ or an opening to the body surface.

drain. Device that creates a channel to allow fluid from a cavity, wound, or infected area to exit the body.

epididymis. Coiled tube on the back of the testis that is the site of sperm maturation and storage and where spermatozoa are propelled into the vas deferens toward the ejaculatory duct by contraction of smooth muscle.

lumen. Space inside an intestine, artery, vein, duct, or tube.

scrotum. Skin pouch that holds the testes and supporting reproductive structures.

testes. Male gonadal paired glands located in the scrotum that secrete testosterone and contain the seminiferous tubules where sperm is produced.

transection. Transverse dissection; to cut across a long axis; cross section.

vas deferens. Duct that arises in the tail of the epididymis that stores and carries sperm from the epididymis toward the urethra.

Vas Deferens

55500

55500   Excision of hydrocele of spermatic cord, unilateral (separate procedure)

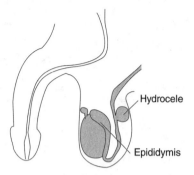

The physician excises a hydrocele of the spermatic cord

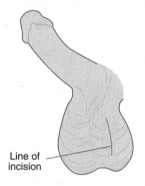

Line of incision

Explanation

A hydrocele is an abnormal fluid-filled sac. The physician treats a hydrocele of the spermatic cord by removing from the spermatic cord above the testis in the scrotum or in the inguinal canal. After injecting the area with local anesthetic, the physician makes an incision in the scrotum or in the inguinal area. The hydrocele is kept intact while it is freed of its attachments to the spermatic cord. The sac is opened, drained, and excised all the way to the internal inguinal ring in the upper groin area. The remaining tissues are repaired and closed by suturing. The testis is anchored to the inside of the scrotum with three sutures to prevent later torsion or twisting of the testis. A rubber drain may be placed in the scrotum and the incision closed in layers by suturing.

Coding Tips

This separate procedure by definition is usually a component of a more complex service and is not identified separately. When performed alone or with other unrelated procedures/services it may be reported. If performed alone, list the code; if performed with other procedures/services, list the code and append modifier 59 or an X{EPSU} modifier. This is a unilateral procedure. If performed bilaterally, some payers require that the service be reported twice with modifier 50 appended to the second code while others require identification of the service only once with modifier 50 appended. Check with individual payers. Modifier 50 identifies a procedure performed identically on the opposite side of the body (mirror image). For aspiration, excision, or repair of a hydrocele of the tunic vaginalis, see 55000–55060. For excision of a lesion of the spermatic cord, see 55520. Local or regional anesthesia is included in the service. If a specimen is transported to an outside laboratory, report 99000 for handling or conveyance.

ICD-10-CM Diagnostic Codes

N43.0	Encysted hydrocele ♂
N43.1	Infected hydrocele ♂
N43.2	Other hydrocele ♂
P83.5	Congenital hydrocele ♂

AMA: 55500 2018,Jan,8; 2017,Jan,8; 2016,Jan,13; 2015,Jan,16; 2014,Jan,11

Relative Value Units/Medicare Edits

Non-Facility RVU	Work	PE	MP	Total
55500	6.22	4.23	0.9	11.35
Facility RVU	**Work**	**PE**	**MP**	**Total**
55500	6.22	4.23	0.9	11.35

	FUD	Status	MUE	Modifiers				IOM Reference
55500	90	A	1(2)	51	50	N/A	80*	None

* with documentation

Terms To Know

congenital. Present at birth, occurring through heredity or an influence during gestation up to the moment of birth.

drain. Device that creates a channel to allow fluid from a cavity, wound, or infected area to exit the body.

excise. Remove or cut out.

hydrocele. Serous fluid that collects in the tunica vaginalis, the spermatic cord, or the canal of Nuck. Hydroceles may be congenital, due to a defect in the tunica vaginalis, or secondary, due to fluid accumulation, injury, infection, or radiotherapy.

inguinal. Within the groin region.

scrotum. Skin pouch that holds the testes and supporting reproductive structures.

spermatic cord. Structure of the male reproductive organs that consists of the ductus deferens, testicular artery, nerves, and veins that drain the testes.

testes. Male gonadal paired glands located in the scrotum that secrete testosterone and contain the seminiferous tubules where sperm is produced.

tissue. Group of similar cells with a similar function that form definite structures and organs. Tissue types include epithelial tissue, muscle tissue, connective tissue, and nervous tissue.

torsion of testis. Twisting, turning, or rotation of the testicle upon itself, so as to compromise or cut off the blood supply.

© 2020 Optum360, LLC   **N** Newborn: 0   **P** Pediatric: 0-17   **M** Maternity: 9-64   **A** Adult: 15-124   ♂ Male Only   ♀ Female Only   CPT © 2020 American Medical Association. All Rights Reserved.

Spermatic Cord

55520

55520   Excision of lesion of spermatic cord (separate procedure)

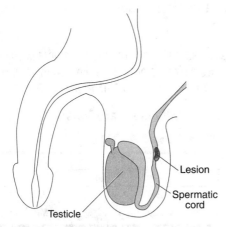

Through a scrotal or inguinal incision, the physician excises a lesion on the spermatic cord

A drain may be placed following surgery

Explanation

The physician removes a lesion of the spermatic cord by dissection and excision. After injecting the area with local anesthetic, the physician makes an incision in the scrotum or in the inguinal area and dissects the tissues to expose the lesion. Care is taken to keep the lesion intact while it is dissected free of its attachments to the spermatic cord. This may involve mobilization of the testis. The lesion is removed by cutting all of its attachments. The tissues damaged during the dissection are repaired and closed by suturing. If the testis has been mobilized, it is anchored to the inside of the scrotum with three sutures to prevent later torsion or twisting. A drain may be placed in the scrotum and the incision is closed in layers by suturing.

Coding Tips

This separate procedure by definition is usually a component of a more complex service and is not identified separately. When performed alone or with other unrelated procedures/ services it may be reported. If performed alone, list the code; if performed with other procedures/services, list the code and append modifier 59 or an X{EPSU} modifier. This is a unilateral procedure. If performed bilaterally, some payers require that the service be reported twice with modifier 50 appended to the second code while others require identification of the service only once with modifier 50 appended. Check with individual payers. Modifier 50 identifies a procedure performed identically on the opposite side of the body (mirror image). If a specimen is transported to an outside laboratory, report 99000 for handling or conveyance. For excision of a local lesion of the epididymis, see 54830.

ICD-10-CM Diagnostic Codes

C63.11	Malignant neoplasm of right spermatic cord ♂ ☑
C63.12	Malignant neoplasm of left spermatic cord ♂ ☑
C79.82	Secondary malignant neoplasm of genital organs
D07.69	Carcinoma in situ of other male genital organs ♂
D17.6	Benign lipomatous neoplasm of spermatic cord ♂
D40.8	Neoplasm of uncertain behavior of other specified male genital organs ♂
N49.1	Inflammatory disorders of spermatic cord, tunica vaginalis and vas deferens ♂

AMA: 55520 2018,Jan,8; 2017,Jan,8; 2016,Jan,13; 2015,Jan,16; 2014,Jan,11

Relative Value Units/Medicare Edits

Non-Facility RVU	Work	PE	MP	Total
55520	6.66	5.03	1.51	13.2
Facility RVU	Work	PE	MP	Total
55520	6.66	5.03	1.51	13.2

	FUD	Status	MUE	Modifiers				IOM Reference
55520	90	A	1(2)	51	50	62*	80	None

* with documentation

Terms To Know

benign lesion. Neoplasm or change in tissue that is not cancerous (nonmalignant).

carcinoma in situ. Malignancy that arises from the cells of the vessel, gland, or organ of origin that remains confined to that site or has not invaded neighboring tissue.

dissection. Separating by cutting tissue or body structures apart.

excision. Surgical removal of an organ or tissue.

lesion. Area of damaged tissue that has lost continuity or function, due to disease or trauma.

lipoma. Benign tumor containing fat cells and the most common of soft tissue lesions, which are usually painless and asymptomatic, with the exception of an angiolipoma.

malignant. Any condition tending to progress toward death, specifically an invasive tumor with a loss of cellular differentiation that has the ability to spread or metastasize to other body areas.

scrotum. Skin pouch that holds the testes and supporting reproductive structures.

spermatic cord. Structure of the male reproductive organs that consists of the ductus deferens, testicular artery, nerves, and veins that drain the testes.

tissue. Group of similar cells with a similar function that form definite structures and organs. Tissue types include epithelial tissue, muscle tissue, connective tissue, and nervous tissue.

torsion of testis. Twisting, turning, or rotation of the testicle upon itself, so as to compromise or cut off the blood supply.

Spermatic Cord

55530-55540

55530   Excision of varicocele or ligation of spermatic veins for varicocele; (separate procedure)
55535   abdominal approach
55540   with hernia repair

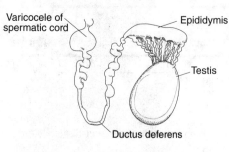

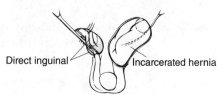

A hernia may also be present

Explanation

In 55530, a varicocele is an abnormal dilation of the veins of the spermatic cord in the scrotum. The physician ligates the spermatic veins and/or excises a varicocele. An incision is made in the pubic area on the affected side and carried down to the spermatic cord as it passes through the inguinal canal. The cord is brought up into the incision and the structures of the cord are dissected, the veins identified, and ligated with suture material. Alternately, an incision is made in the scrotum and the dilated veins ligated separately may be removed. The operative incision is closed in layers by suturing. In 55535, the same procedure is carried out, via an abdominal approach. The physician ligates the spermatic veins and/or excises a varicocele, which is an abnormal dilation of the veins of the spermatic cord in the scrotum. An incision is made in the lateral lower abdomen just medial to the bony prominence of the pelvic bone on the affected side and carried down through the abdominal musculature to the spermatic vein and artery. The vein is identified and ligated (tied off) with suture material. The abdominal incision is closed in layers by suturing. In 55540, the physician repairs an inguinal hernia and ligates the spermatic veins or excises a varicocele (an abnormal dilation of the veins of the spermatic cord in the scrotum). An incision is made in the pubic area on the affected side to expose the spermatic cord as it passes through the inguinal canal. The cord is brought into the incision, the structures of the cord are dissected, and the veins identified and ligated. The hernia is repaired through the same incision by folding and suturing of tissues to strengthen the abdominal wall and correct the weakness responsible for the hernia. Alternately, an incision is made in the scrotum and the dilated veins ligated separately and may be removed (excision) and a second incision made for hernia repair. All incisions are closed in layers by suturing.

Coding Tips

Note that 55530, a separate procedure by definition, is usually a component of a more complex service and is not identified separately. When performed alone or with other unrelated procedures/ services it may be reported. If performed alone, list the code; if performed with other procedures/services, list the code and append modifier 59 or an X{EPSU} modifier. These are unilateral procedures. If performed bilaterally, some payers require that the service be reported twice with modifier 50 appended to the second code while others require identification of the service only once with modifier 50 appended. Check with individual payers. Modifier 50 identifies a procedure performed identically on the opposite side of the body (mirror image). For laparoscopic ligation of spermatic veins for varicocele, see 55550.

ICD-10-CM Diagnostic Codes

I86.1   Scrotal varices ♂

AMA: **55530** 2018,Jan,8; 2017,Jan,8; 2016,Jan,13; 2015,Jan,16; 2014,Jan,11 **55535** 2018,Jan,8; 2017,Jan,8; 2016,Jan,13; 2015,Jan,16; 2014,Jan,11 **55540** 2018,Jan,8; 2017,Jan,8; 2016,Jan,13; 2015,Jan,16; 2014,Jan,11

Relative Value Units/Medicare Edits

Non-Facility RVU	Work	PE	MP	Total
55530	5.75	3.73	0.65	10.13
55535	7.19	4.4	0.82	12.41
55540	8.3	5.76	2.0	16.06
Facility RVU	Work	PE	MP	Total
55530	5.75	3.73	0.65	10.13
55535	7.19	4.4	0.82	12.41
55540	8.3	5.76	2.0	16.06

	FUD	Status	MUE	Modifiers				IOM Reference
55530	90	A	1(2)	51	50	62*	N/A	None
55535	90	A	1(2)	51	50	62*	80	
55540	90	A	1(2)	51	50	62*	N/A	

* with documentation

Terms To Know

approach. Method or anatomical location used to gain access to a body organ or specific area for procedures.

dissect. Cut apart or separate tissue for surgical purposes or for visual or microscopic study.

hernia. Protrusion of a body structure through tissue.

inguinal hernia. Loop of intestine that protrudes through the abdominal peritoneum into the inguinal canal.

ligation. Tying off a blood vessel or duct with a suture or a soft, thin wire.

scrotum. Skin pouch that holds the testes and supporting reproductive structures.

spermatic cord. Structure of the male reproductive organs that consists of the ductus deferens, testicular artery, nerves, and veins that drain the testes.

varices. Enlarged, dilated, or twisted turning veins.

varicocele. Abnormal dilation of the veins of the spermatic cord in the scrotum.

© 2020 Optum360, LLC   N Newborn: 0   P Pediatric: 0-17   M Maternity: 9-64   A Adult: 15-124   ♂ Male Only   ♀ Female Only   CPT © 2020 American Medical Association. All Rights Reserved.

Spermatic Cord

55550

55550 Laparoscopy, surgical, with ligation of spermatic veins for varicocele

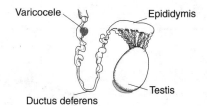

Testicle showing varicocele along spermatic vein

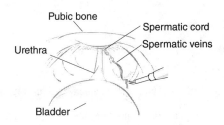

Laparoscopic schematic showing approach to spermatic veins

Explanation

The physician ligates (ties or binds with suture) the spermatic veins and/or excises a varicocele which is an abnormal dilation of the veins of the spermatic cord in the scrotum. An umbilical port is created by placing a trocar at the level of the umbilicus. The abdominal wall is insufflated. The laparoscope is placed through the umbilical port and additional trocars are placed into the abdominal or pelvic cavity. The physician uses the laparoscope fitted with a fiberoptic camera and/or an operating instrument to explore and surgically ligate the spermatic veins to repair or remove the varicocele. The structures of the cord are dissected, the veins identified, and ligated with suture. The abdomen is deflated, the trocars removed, and the incisions are closed with sutures.

Coding Tips

Surgical laparoscopy always includes diagnostic laparoscopy. For open ligation of a varicocele, see 55530–55540.

ICD-10-CM Diagnostic Codes

I86.1	Scrotal varices ♂

AMA: **55550** 2018,Jan,8; 2017,Jan,8; 2016,Jan,13; 2015,Jan,16; 2014,Jan,11

Relative Value Units/Medicare Edits

Non-Facility RVU	Work	PE	MP	Total
55550	7.2	4.35	0.82	12.37
Facility RVU	Work	PE	MP	Total
55550	7.2	4.35	0.82	12.37

	FUD	Status	MUE	Modifiers				IOM Reference
55550	90	A	1(2)	51	50	62*	80	None

* with documentation

Spermatic Cord

CPT © 2020 American Medical Association. All Rights Reserved.   ● New   ▲ Revised   + Add On   ★ Telemedicine   AMA: CPT Assist   [Resequenced]   ☑ Laterality   © 2020 Optum360, LLC

55600-55605

55600 Vesiculotomy;
55605   complicated

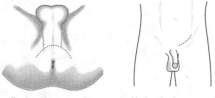

Perineal approach   Abdominal approach

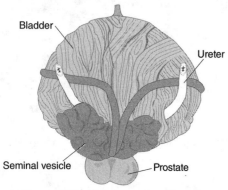

The seminal vesicle is punctured through
an abdominal or perineal approach

Explanation

The physician incises or punctures one of the seminal vesicles, paired glands that lie behind the urinary bladder and produce fluid that is mixed with the semen produced in the testis. The seminal vesicle is approached through an incision in the lower abdomen or an incision in the perineum (area between the base of the scrotum and the anus). In the abdominal method, the physician either retracts the bladder forward toward the pubic bone to expose the back of the bladder where the seminal vesicles are positioned, or the surgeon cuts through the front and back walls to gain access to the gland. The operative wounds are closed in layers by suturing. If the procedure does not require extensive dissection, report 55600; if extensive, report 55605.

Coding Tips

When 55600 or 55605 is performed with another separately identifiable procedure, the highest dollar value code is listed as the primary procedure and subsequent procedures are appended with modifier 51. These are unilateral procedures. If performed bilaterally, some payers require that the service be reported twice with modifier 50 appended to the second code while others require identification of the service only once with modifier 50 appended. Check with individual payers. Modifier 50 identifies a procedure performed identically on the opposite side of the body (mirror image).

ICD-10-CM Diagnostic Codes

N49.0   Inflammatory disorders of seminal vesicle ♂
N50.89   Other specified disorders of the male genital organs ♂
N53.8   Other male sexual dysfunction ♂
R36.1   Hematospermia ♂

AMA: **55600** 2014,Jan,11 **55605** 2014,Jan,11

Relative Value Units/Medicare Edits

Non-Facility RVU	Work	PE	MP	Total
55600	7.01	4.35	0.79	12.15
55605	8.76	5.31	1.0	15.07
Facility RVU	Work	PE	MP	Total
55600	7.01	4.35	0.79	12.15
55605	8.76	5.31	1.0	15.07

	FUD	Status	MUE	Modifiers				IOM Reference
55600	90	A	1(2)	51	50	N/A	80*	None
55605	90	A	1(2)	51	50	N/A	80*	

* with documentation

Terms To Know

approach. Method or anatomical location used to gain access to a body organ or specific area for procedures.

dissection. Separating by cutting tissue or body structures apart.

perineal. Pertaining to the pelvic floor area between the thighs; the diamond-shaped area bordered by the pubic symphysis in front, the ischial tuberosities on the sides, and the coccyx in back.

seminal vesicles. Paired glands located at the base of the bladder in males that release the majority of fluid into semen through ducts that join with the vas deferens forming the ejaculatory duct.

testes. Male gonadal paired glands located in the scrotum that secrete testosterone and contain the seminiferous tubules where sperm is produced.

wound. Injury to living tissue often involving a cut or break in the skin.

Seminal Vesicles

55650

55650   Vesiculectomy, any approach

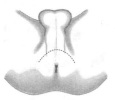
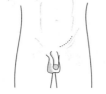

Perineal approach   Abdominal approach

Perineal or abdominal approach may be used

The physician removes a seminal vesicle

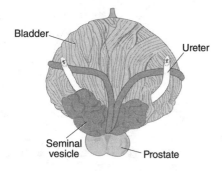

Bladder

Ureter

Seminal vesicle   Prostate

Explanation

The physician removes one of the seminal vesicles, paired glands that lie behind the urinary bladder and produce a fluid that is mixed with semen from the testis. Through an incision in the lower abdomen or an incision in the perineum (area between the base of the scrotum and the anus) the seminal vesicle is approached. If the abdominal method is used, the surgeon retracts the bladder forward toward the pubic bone to expose the back of the bladder where the seminal vesicles are positioned or the surgeon cuts through the front and back walls to gain access to the glands. The surgeon dissects the gland free of its attachments and clips it at its joint with the ejaculatory duct and removes it. The operative wounds are closed in layers by suturing.

Coding Tips

If significant additional time and effort is documented, append modifier 22 and submit a cover letter and operative report. This is a unilateral procedure. If performed bilaterally, some payers require that the service be reported twice with modifier 50 appended to the second code while others require identification of the service only once with modifier 50 appended. Check with individual payers. Modifier 50 identifies a procedure performed identically on the opposite side of the body (mirror image). Any major procedures performed on the urinary bladder are reported separately. For vesiculotomy, see 55600–55605.

ICD-10-CM Diagnostic Codes

C63.7	Malignant neoplasm of other specified male genital organs ♂
C79.82	Secondary malignant neoplasm of genital organs
D07.69	Carcinoma in situ of other male genital organs ♂
D29.8	Benign neoplasm of other specified male genital organs ♂
D40.8	Neoplasm of uncertain behavior of other specified male genital organs ♂
D49.59	Neoplasm of unspecified behavior of other genitourinary organ
N49.0	Inflammatory disorders of seminal vesicle ♂

N50.89	Other specified disorders of the male genital organs ♂

AMA: 55650 2014,Jan,11

Relative Value Units/Medicare Edits

Non-Facility RVU	Work	PE	MP	Total
55650	12.65	6.63	1.44	20.72
Facility RVU	**Work**	**PE**	**MP**	**Total**
55650	12.65	6.63	1.44	20.72

	FUD	Status	MUE	Modifiers				IOM Reference
55650	90	A	1(2)	51	50	62*	80	None

* with documentation

Terms To Know

approach. Method or anatomical location used to gain access to a body organ or specific area for procedures.

benign. Mild or nonmalignant in nature.

carcinoma in situ. Malignancy that arises from the cells of the vessel, gland, or organ of origin that remains confined to that site or has not invaded neighboring tissue.

dissection. Separating by cutting tissue or body structures apart.

malignant. Any condition tending to progress toward death, specifically an invasive tumor with a loss of cellular differentiation that has the ability to spread or metastasize to other body areas.

neoplasm. New abnormal growth, tumor.

perineal. Pertaining to the pelvic floor area between the thighs; the diamond-shaped area bordered by the pubic symphysis in front, the ischial tuberosities on the sides, and the coccyx in back.

secondary. Second in order of occurrence or importance, or appearing during the course of another disease or condition.

seminal vesicles. Paired glands located at the base of the bladder in males that release the majority of fluid into semen through ducts that join with the vas deferens forming the ejaculatory duct.

stricture. Narrowing of an anatomical structure.

wound. Injury to living tissue often involving a cut or break in the skin.

Seminal Vesicles

55680

55680 Excision of Mullerian duct cyst

The physician excises a Mullerian duct cyst

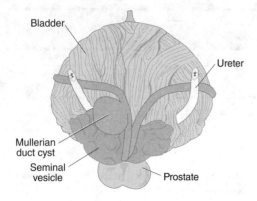

Explanation

The physician excises a Mullerian duct cyst, a remnant of the prenatal development of the seminal vesicle. The seminal vesicles are paired glands that lie behind the urinary bladder and produce a fluid that is mixed with the semen from the testis. Through an incision in the lower abdomen or an incision in the perineum (area between the base of the scrotum and the anus) the seminal vesicle is approached. If the abdominal method is used, the surgeon retracts the bladder forward toward the pubic bone to expose the back of the bladder where the seminal vesicles are positioned or the surgeon cuts through the front and back walls to gain access to the glands. The surgeon dissects the cyst free of its attachments and clips it at the attachment to the seminal vesicle and removes it. The operative wounds are closed in layers by suturing.

Coding Tips

If significant additional time and effort is documented, append modifier 22 and submit a cover letter and operative report. For injection procedures of seminal vesicles, see 52010 or 55300.

ICD-10-CM Diagnostic Codes

Q55.8   Other specified congenital malformations of male genital organs ♂

AMA: 55680 2014,Jan,11

Relative Value Units/Medicare Edits

Non-Facility RVU	Work	PE	MP	Total
55680	5.67	3.68	0.64	9.99
Facility RVU	**Work**	**PE**	**MP**	**Total**
55680	5.67	3.68	0.64	9.99

	FUD	Status	MUE	Modifiers				IOM Reference
55680	90	A	1(3)	51	50	N/A	80*	None

* with documentation

Terms To Know

Mullerian duct cyst. Atypical, congenital, cyst-like lesion that is typically small in size and often presents without any particular symptoms. This cyst is located approximately midway behind the top half of the prostatic urethra and is joined to the seminal colliculus (verumontanum) with a thin stalk.

© 2020 Optum360, LLC   N Newborn: 0   P Pediatric: 0-17   M Maternity: 9-64   A Adult: 15-124   ♂ Male Only   ♀ Female Only   CPT © 2020 American Medical Association. All Rights Reserved.

Seminal Vesicles

55700-55705

55700 Biopsy, prostate; needle or punch, single or multiple, any approach
55705   incisional, any approach

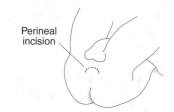

Needle or punch biopsy is
commonly performed via anal approach

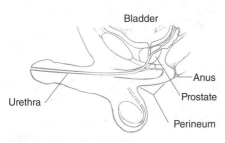

Explanation

The physician obtains tissue from the prostate for analysis by needle or punch biopsy through one or more of three approaches. The biopsy needle is passed into the suspect area of the prostate by puncturing through skin of the perineum (the area between the base of the scrotum and the anus), by advancing the needle into the rectum by guidance with the index finger and puncturing through the rectal mucosa, or by advancing a biopsy instrument through the urethra. The biopsy needle is inserted into the prostate guided by an index finger or by ultrasound and the needle biopsy sheath is advanced over the needle and twisted to shear off the enclosed sample. The needle is withdrawn, containing the sample. This may be repeated two or more times to assure adequate sampling and the puncture site is bandaged. Report 55705 if biopsy tissue from the prostate is obtained by direct incisional sampling through any of the three approaches.

Coding Tips

Code 55700 represents one of three codes (one in the male reproductive system and two in radiology 76942, 76872) used to report a standard transrectal ultrasound (TRUS) guided biopsy. Report 55700 and 76942 together to collect prostatic tissue for evaluation to assess whether cancer is present in the prostate. For MRI-TRUS fusion-guided prostate biopsy, report 76999 or 76498 with 55700. Check with the individual payer for specific reporting guidance for MRI and ultrasound imaging fusion. For fine needle aspiration biopsy, see 10004–10012 and 10021. For evaluation of fine needle aspirate, see 88172–88173. Report imaging guidance with 76942, 77002, 77012, or 77021, when performed. Note that 55700 includes multiple biopsies taken. If more than one incisional biopsy is done, report 55705 for each site incised and append modifier 51 to additional codes. For transperineal stereotactic template guided saturation prostate biopsy, see 55706. If a specimen is transported to an outside laboratory, report 99000 for handling or conveyance.

ICD-10-CM Diagnostic Codes

A18.14	Tuberculosis of prostate ⒜ ♂
C61	Malignant neoplasm of prostate ♂
C79.82	Secondary malignant neoplasm of genital organs
D07.5	Carcinoma in situ of prostate ♂

D29.1	Benign neoplasm of prostate ♂
D40.0	Neoplasm of uncertain behavior of prostate ♂
D49.59	Neoplasm of unspecified behavior of other genitourinary organ
N40.0	Benign prostatic hyperplasia without lower urinary tract symptoms ⒜ ♂
N40.1	Benign prostatic hyperplasia with lower urinary tract symptoms ⒜ ♂
N40.2	Nodular prostate without lower urinary tract symptoms ⒜ ♂
N40.3	Nodular prostate with lower urinary tract symptoms ⒜ ♂
N41.0	Acute prostatitis ⒜ ♂
N41.1	Chronic prostatitis ⒜ ♂
N41.2	Abscess of prostate ⒜ ♂
N41.3	Prostatocystitis ⒜ ♂
N41.4	Granulomatous prostatitis ⒜ ♂
N41.8	Other inflammatory diseases of prostate ⒜ ♂
N42.31	Prostatic intraepithelial neoplasia ♂
N42.32	Atypical small acinar proliferation of prostate ♂
N42.39	Other dysplasia of prostate ♂
N42.81	Prostatodynia syndrome ⒜ ♂
N42.82	Prostatosis syndrome ⒜ ♂
N42.83	Cyst of prostate ⒜ ♂
N42.89	Other specified disorders of prostate ⒜ ♂
R97.20	Elevated prostate specific antigen [PSA] ⒜ ♂
R97.21	Rising PSA following treatment for malignant neoplasm of prostate ⒜ ♂

AMA: **55700** 2018,Jul,11; 2018,Jan,8; 2017,Jan,8; 2016,Jan,13; 2015,Jan,16; 2014,Jan,11 **55705** 2014,Jan,11

Relative Value Units/Medicare Edits

Non-Facility RVU	Work	PE	MP	Total
55700	2.5	4.31	0.28	7.09
55705	4.61	2.53	0.53	7.67
Facility RVU	**Work**	**PE**	**MP**	**Total**
55700	2.5	0.99	0.28	3.77
55705	4.61	2.53	0.53	7.67

	FUD	Status	MUE	Modifiers				IOM Reference
55700	0	A	1(2)	51	N/A	N/A	N/A	None
55705	10	A	1(2)	51	N/A	62*	N/A	

* with documentation

Terms To Know

approach. Method or anatomical location used to gain access to a body organ or specific area for procedures.

biopsy. Tissue or fluid removed for diagnostic purposes.

prostate. Male gland surrounding the bladder neck and urethra that secretes a substance into the seminal fluid.

CPT © 2020 American Medical Association. All Rights Reserved.   ● New   ▲ Revised   ✛ Add On   ★ Telemedicine   AMA: CPT Assist   [Resequenced]   ☑ Laterality   © 2020 Optum360, LLC

55706

55706 Biopsies, prostate, needle, transperineal, stereotactic template guided saturation sampling, including imaging guidance

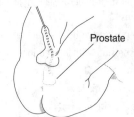

Warming catheter is inserted into urethra

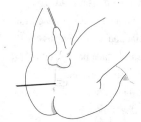

Transperineal approach for prostate biopsies

Explanation
The physician uses stereotactic template-guided saturation sampling biopsies to map prostate cancer in high-risk patients. Transrectal ultrasound is used to visualize the prostate. Zones or reference planes of the prostate are determined, and a brachytherapy grid is placed against the perineum and rectum. Using the transperineal route under ultrasonic guidance, multiple biopsies are taken of the prostate. Typically, from 20 to 40 biopsies are taken using the grid as a guide, beginning at the highest point in the prostate and moving right to left in a row, down row by row until the grid is complete. In deeper planes, both a proximal and distal biopsy may be obtained. Each biopsy sample is marked for its coordinates, and all are mapped in 3D to determine the extent and exact position of malignant cells.

Coding Tips
If specimen is transported to an outside laboratory, report 99000 for handling or conveyance. Do not report 55706 with 55700.

ICD-10-CM Diagnostic Codes
C61	Malignant neoplasm of prostate ♂
C79.82	Secondary malignant neoplasm of genital organs
D40.0	Neoplasm of uncertain behavior of prostate ♂
D49.59	Neoplasm of unspecified behavior of other genitourinary organ

AMA: 55706 2018,Jan,8; 2017,Jan,8; 2016,Jan,13; 2015,Jan,16; 2014,Jan,11

Relative Value Units/Medicare Edits
Non-Facility RVU	Work	PE	MP	Total
55706	6.28	3.8	0.67	10.75
Facility RVU	Work	PE	MP	Total
55706	6.28	3.8	0.67	10.75

	FUD	Status	MUE	Modifiers				IOM Reference
55706	10	A	1(2)	51	N/A	62*	80	None
* with documentation								

55720-55725

55720 Prostatotomy, external drainage of prostatic abscess, any approach; simple
55725   complicated

Any approach may be used

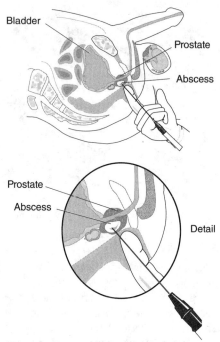

An abscess in the prostate is incised and drained

Explanation
The physician performs a simple prostatotomy (cutting or puncturing the prostate) through one of two usual approaches. An aspirating needle is passed into the abscessed area of the prostate by puncturing through skin of the perineum (the area between the base of the scrotum and the anus), or by advancing the needle into the rectum by guidance with the index finger and puncturing through the rectal mucosa. The needle is inserted into the abscess in the prostate guided by an index finger or by ultrasound and the contents of the abscess removed by aspiration. The needle is withdrawn and the puncture site bandaged. Report 55720 for simple drainage, or 55725 if the procedure is complicated by excessive bleeding, infection, or other problem.

Coding Tips
For transurethral drainage of the prostate, see 52700. For initial transurethral resection of the prostate, first stage, see 52601. For partial resection of the prostate, second stage, see 52601 and append modifier 58. For prostatectomy, other approach or method, see 55801–55845. This procedure is usually performed under local or regional anesthesia, which is included in the service. However, general anesthesia may be administered depending on the age or condition of the patient.

ICD-10-CM Diagnostic Codes
N41.2	Abscess of prostate 🅰 ♂

AMA: 55720 2014,Jan,11 **55725** 2014,Jan,11

Prostate

Relative Value Units/Medicare Edits

Non-Facility RVU	Work	PE	MP	Total
55720	7.73	4.44	0.88	13.05
55725	10.05	5.94	1.15	17.14
Facility RVU	Work	PE	MP	Total
55720	7.73	4.44	0.88	13.05
55725	10.05	5.94	1.15	17.14

	FUD	Status	MUE	Modifiers				IOM Reference
55720	90	A	1(3)	51	N/A	62*	80	None
55725	90	A	1(3)	51	N/A	62*	80	

* with documentation

Terms To Know

abscess. Circumscribed collection of pus resulting from bacteria, frequently associated with swelling and other signs of inflammation.

approach. Method or anatomical location used to gain access to a body organ or specific area for procedures.

aspiration. Drawing fluid out by suction.

incision and drainage. Cutting open body tissue for the removal of tissue fluids or infected discharge from a wound or cavity.

perineal. Pertaining to the pelvic floor area between the thighs; the diamond-shaped area bordered by the pubic symphysis in front, the ischial tuberosities on the sides, and the coccyx in back.

prostate. Male gland surrounding the bladder neck and urethra that secretes a substance into the seminal fluid.

ultrasound. Imaging using ultra-high sound frequency bounced off body structures.

55801

55801   Prostatectomy, perineal, subtotal (including control of postoperative bleeding, vasectomy, meatotomy, urethral calibration and/or dilation, and internal urethrotomy)

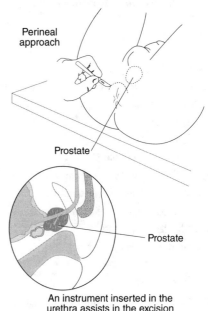

The physician excises the prostate through a perineal incision

Perineal approach

Prostate

Prostate

An instrument inserted in the urethra assists in the excision

Explanation

The physician performs a prostatectomy (removal of the prostate gland) through an incision made in the perineum. The caliber (internal diameter) of the urethra is measured and if it is not adequate, the opening of the urethra is enlarged (meatotomy) and the diameter of the penile urethra is enlarged with an instrument (internal urethrotomy). A curved instrument (Lowery Tractor) is advanced into the urethra to the prostate to help to identify the structures and aid in the dissection. Through the perineal incision and with manipulation of the tractor, the tissues are dissected to expose the prostate. The curved tractor instrument in the urethra is replaced with a straight tractor. A portion of the prostate or the entire gland is removed with care to preserve the seminal vesicles. The operation is "subtotal" because the seminal vesicles remain intact. The bladder outlet is revised and the vas deferens is ligated and may be partially removed (vasectomy). Bleeding is controlled by ligation or cautery. A Foley catheter is placed in the bladder. A rubber drain may be placed in the site of the operative wound and brought out through a separate stab wound. The dissected tissues and the skin incision are closed in layers by suturing.

Coding Tips

This code includes the control of postoperative bleeding, vasectomy, meatotomy, urethral calibration and/or dilation, and internal urethrotomy in any combination. If significant additional time and effort is documented, append modifier 22 and submit a cover letter and operative report. For suprapubic, subtotal prostatectomy, see 55821. For retropubic, subtotal prostatectomy, see 55831. For initial transurethral removal of the prostate, first stage, see 52601; for second stage partial resection of the prostate, see 52601 and append modifier 58. For transurethral resection of obstructive prostate tissue, residual or regrowth, see 52630.

Prostate

CPT © 2020 American Medical Association. All Rights Reserved.   ● **New**   ▲ **Revised**   + **Add On**   ★ **Telemedicine**   **AMA: CPT Assist**   **[Resequenced]**   ☑ **Laterality**   © 2020 Optum360, LLC

ICD-10-CM Diagnostic Codes

C61	Malignant neoplasm of prostate ♂
C79.82	Secondary malignant neoplasm of genital organs
D07.5	Carcinoma in situ of prostate ♂
D29.1	Benign neoplasm of prostate ♂
D40.0	Neoplasm of uncertain behavior of prostate ♂
D49.59	Neoplasm of unspecified behavior of other genitourinary organ
N40.0	Benign prostatic hyperplasia without lower urinary tract symptoms 🅐 ♂
N40.1	Benign prostatic hyperplasia with lower urinary tract symptoms 🅐 ♂
N40.2	Nodular prostate without lower urinary tract symptoms 🅐 ♂
N40.3	Nodular prostate with lower urinary tract symptoms 🅐 ♂
N41.0	Acute prostatitis 🅐 ♂
N41.1	Chronic prostatitis 🅐 ♂
N41.3	Prostatocystitis 🅐 ♂
N41.4	Granulomatous prostatitis 🅐 ♂
N41.8	Other inflammatory diseases of prostate 🅐 ♂
N42.31	Prostatic intraepithelial neoplasia ♂
N42.32	Atypical small acinar proliferation of prostate ♂
N42.39	Other dysplasia of prostate ♂
N42.81	Prostatodynia syndrome 🅐 ♂
N42.82	Prostatosis syndrome 🅐 ♂
N42.83	Cyst of prostate 🅐 ♂
N42.89	Other specified disorders of prostate 🅐 ♂
Z15.03	Genetic susceptibility to malignant neoplasm of prostate ♂

AMA: **55801** 2014,Jan,11

Relative Value Units/Medicare Edits

Non-Facility RVU	Work	PE	MP	Total
55801	19.8	9.55	2.27	31.62
Facility RVU	**Work**	**PE**	**MP**	**Total**
55801	19.8	9.55	2.27	31.62

	FUD	Status	MUE	Modifiers				IOM Reference
55801	90	A	1(2)	51	N/A	62*	80	None

* with documentation

Terms To Know

approach. Method or anatomical location used to gain access to a body organ or specific area for procedures.

dissection. (dis. apart; -section, act of cutting) Separating by cutting tissue or body structures apart.

perineal. Pertaining to the pelvic floor area between the thighs; the diamond-shaped area bordered by the pubic symphysis in front, the ischial tuberosities on the sides, and the coccyx in back.

prostate. Male gland surrounding the bladder neck and urethra that secretes a substance into the seminal fluid.

seminal vesicles. Paired glands located at the base of the bladder in males that release the majority of fluid into semen through ducts that join with the vas deferens forming the ejaculatory duct.

55810-55815

55810	Prostatectomy, perineal radical;
55812	with lymph node biopsy(s) (limited pelvic lymphadenectomy)
55815	with bilateral pelvic lymphadenectomy, including external iliac, hypogastric and obturator nodes

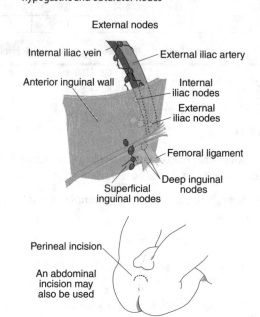

Lymph nodes may also be biopsied or removed

Explanation

The physician performs a radical prostatectomy through an incision made in the skin between the base of the scrotum and the anus. If the internal diameter of the urethra is not adequate, the opening of the urethra is enlarged (meatotomy) and the diameter of the penile urethra is enlarged with an instrument (internal urethrotomy). A curved instrument (Lowery Tractor) is advanced up the urethra to the prostate to aid in the dissection. Through the perineal incision and with manipulation of the tractor, the tissues are dissected to expose the prostate. The curved tractor instrument in the urethra is replaced with a straight tractor. The entire gland is removed along with the seminal vesicles and the vas deferens. The bladder outlet is revised and bleeding controlled by ligation or cautery. In 55812, local lymph nodes are also removed for analysis. A Foley catheter is placed and left in the bladder. A rubber drain may be placed in the site of the operative wound and brought out through a separate stab wound. The dissected tissues and the skin incision are closed in layers by suturing. In 55815, a pelvic lymphadenectomy through a separate lower abdominal incision is performed. A midline abdominal incision is made from the upper to the lower abdomen and the back wall of the abdomen is exposed. All lymph nodes along back wall of the pelvic and abdominal cavities are removed. The abdominal wound is closed in layers by suturing.

Coding Tips

For initial and postoperative transurethral resection procedures on the prostate, see 52601–52630. For limited pelvic lymphadenectomy for staging (separate procedure), see 38562. For independent node dissection, see 38770–38780. If 55815 is carried out on different days, report 38770 with modifier 50 and 55810.

ICD-10-CM Diagnostic Codes

C61	Malignant neoplasm of prostate ♂
C79.82	Secondary malignant neoplasm of genital organs

© 2020 Optum360, LLC   **N** Newborn: 0   **P** Pediatric: 0-17   **M** Maternity: 9-64   🅐 Adult: 15-124   ♂ Male Only   ♀ Female Only   CPT © 2020 American Medical Association. All Rights Reserved.

Prostate

| D40.0 | Neoplasm of uncertain behavior of prostate ♂ |
| D49.59 | Neoplasm of unspecified behavior of other genitourinary organ |

AMA: **55810** 2014,Jan,11 **55812** 2014,Jan,11 **55815** 2014,Jan,11

Relative Value Units/Medicare Edits

Non-Facility RVU	Work	PE	MP	Total
55810	24.29	10.75	2.82	37.86
55812	29.89	13.16	3.43	46.48
55815	32.95	14.19	3.78	50.92
Facility RVU	**Work**	**PE**	**MP**	**Total**
55810	24.29	10.75	2.82	37.86
55812	29.89	13.16	3.43	46.48
55815	32.95	14.19	3.78	50.92

	FUD	Status	MUE	Modifiers				IOM Reference
55810	90	A	1(2)	51	N/A	62*	80	None
55812	90	A	1(2)	51	N/A	62*	80	
55815	90	A	1(2)	51	N/A	62*	80	

* with documentation

Terms To Know

dissect. Cut apart or separate tissue for surgical purposes or for visual or microscopic study.

lymph nodes. Bean-shaped structures along the lymphatic vessels that intercept and destroy foreign materials in the tissue and bloodstream.

perineal. Pertaining to the pelvic floor area between the thighs; the diamond-shaped area bordered by the pubic symphysis in front, the ischial tuberosities on the sides, and the coccyx in back.

radical. Extensive surgery.

seminal vesicles. Paired glands located at the base of the bladder in males that release the majority of fluid into semen through ducts that join with the vas deferens forming the ejaculatory duct.

tissue. Group of similar cells with a similar function that form definite structures and organs. Tissue types include epithelial tissue, muscle tissue, connective tissue, and nervous tissue.

vas deferens. Duct that arises in the tail of the epididymis that stores and carries sperm from the epididymis toward the urethra.

55821-55831

| 55821 | Prostatectomy (including control of postoperative bleeding, vasectomy, meatotomy, urethral calibration and/or dilation, and internal urethrotomy); suprapubic, subtotal, 1 or 2 stages |
| 55831 | retropubic, subtotal |

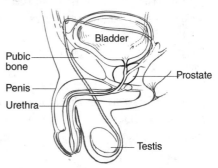

The prostate is surgically removed

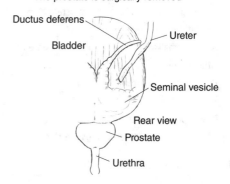

Rear view

Explanation

The physician removes the prostate gland through an incision made in the lower abdomen just above the pubic area. In preparation for removal of the prostate, the caliber (internal diameter) of the urethra is measured and if it is not adequate the opening of the urethra is enlarged (meatotomy) and the diameter of the penile urethra is enlarged with an instrument (internal urethrotomy) and a catheter is passed into the urethra into the bladder. Through the lower abdominal incision the urinary bladder is exposed and opened by an incision in the region just above the bladder neck. During the dissection to expose the bladder a vasectomy may be performed. The bladder mucosa over the prostate is removed by excision to expose the prostate. The entire gland is removed by "shelling it out" by blunt dissection with the surgeon's index finger. The bladder outlet and the bladder wall are revised and bleeding controlled by packing with rolls of gauze, by ligation or cautery of bleeding vessels. A second catheter is placed and left in the bladder through the incision in the lower abdomen. A rubber drain is placed in the space between the pubic bone and the bladder and brought out through a separate stab wound. The dissected tissues and the skin incision are closed in layers by suturing. Report 55831 for a retropubic subtotal prostatectomy.

Coding Tips

These procedures include the control of postoperative bleeding, vasectomy, meatotomy, urethral calibration and/or dilation, and internal urethrotomy in any combination. Report 55821 if the approach is suprapubic and 55831 if the approach is retropubic. Note that 55821 is performed in one or two stages and both are included. It should only be reported once even if two stages of the procedure are performed. For perineal subtotal prostatectomy, see 55801.

Prostate

ICD-10-CM Diagnostic Codes

C61	Malignant neoplasm of prostate ♂
C79.82	Secondary malignant neoplasm of genital organs
D07.5	Carcinoma in situ of prostate ♂
D29.1	Benign neoplasm of prostate ♂
D40.0	Neoplasm of uncertain behavior of prostate ♂
D49.59	Neoplasm of unspecified behavior of other genitourinary organ
N40.0	Benign prostatic hyperplasia without lower urinary tract symptoms Ⓐ ♂
N40.1	Benign prostatic hyperplasia with lower urinary tract symptoms Ⓐ ♂
N40.2	Nodular prostate without lower urinary tract symptoms Ⓐ ♂
N40.3	Nodular prostate with lower urinary tract symptoms Ⓐ ♂
N41.0	Acute prostatitis Ⓐ ♂
N41.1	Chronic prostatitis Ⓐ ♂
N41.3	Prostatocystitis Ⓐ ♂
N41.4	Granulomatous prostatitis Ⓐ ♂
N41.8	Other inflammatory diseases of prostate Ⓐ ♂
N42.31	Prostatic intraepithelial neoplasia ♂
N42.32	Atypical small acinar proliferation of prostate ♂
N42.39	Other dysplasia of prostate ♂
N42.81	Prostatodynia syndrome Ⓐ ♂
N42.82	Prostatosis syndrome Ⓐ ♂
N42.83	Cyst of prostate Ⓐ ♂
N42.89	Other specified disorders of prostate Ⓐ ♂

AMA: 55821 2014,Jan,11 **55831** 2014,Jan,11

Relative Value Units/Medicare Edits

Non-Facility RVU	Work	PE	MP	Total
55821	15.76	7.66	1.82	25.24
55831	17.19	8.15	1.98	27.32
Facility RVU	**Work**	**PE**	**MP**	**Total**
55821	15.76	7.66	1.82	25.24
55831	17.19	8.15	1.98	27.32

	FUD	Status	MUE	Modifiers			IOM Reference
55821	90	A	1(2)	51	N/A	62*	80	None
55831	90	A	1(2)	51	N/A	62*	80	

* with documentation

Terms To Know

blunt dissection. Surgical technique used to expose an underlying area by separating along natural cleavage lines of tissue, without cutting.

drain. Device that creates a channel to allow fluid from a cavity, wound, or infected area to exit the body.

packing. Material placed into a cavity or wound, such as gels, gauze, pads, and sponges.

tissue. Group of similar cells with a similar function that form definite structures and organs. Tissue types include epithelial tissue, muscle tissue, connective tissue, and nervous tissue.

55840-55842

55840   Prostatectomy, retropubic radical, with or without nerve sparing;
55842   with lymph node biopsy(s) (limited pelvic lymphadenectomy)

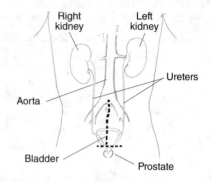

Pubic and midline incisions

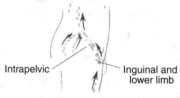

A retropubic radical prostatectomy is performed.
A limited number of lymph nodes may also be removed

Explanation

The physician performs a radical prostatectomy (removal of the prostate gland) through an incision made in the lower abdomen just above the pubic area. In preparation for removal of the prostate, a catheter is passed up the urethra into the bladder. Through a lower abdominal incision, with or without care to spare the nerves in the area, the urinary bladder is exposed and displaced backwards to enter the space behind the pubic bone and expose the area of the prostate. The gland with the capsule intact and the seminal vesicles and the portions of the vas deferens in the area are removed by freeing the prostate by blunt dissection and by transecting the urethra and by cutting through the bladder outlet. The urinary catheter is brought into the operative site and used to create traction for the dissection. A second catheter is place in the bladder after the first one is removed along with the prostate. The transected urethra is repaired by suturing to the newly created bladder outlet. A rubber drain is placed in the space between the pubic bone and the bladder and brought out through a separate stab wound. The dissected tissues and the skin incision are closed in layers by suturing. Report 55842 if a pelvic lymph node biopsy through a midline abdominal incision is done with the radical retropubic prostatectomy (this may be done in two stages within seven to 10 days). A midline incision is made from the upper to the lower abdomen and the abdominal cavity is entered. The back wall of the abdomen is exposed and the lymph nodes are checked for spread of tumor. Some may be removed and/or biopsied.

Coding Tips

For radical retropubic prostatectomy with bilateral pelvic lymphadenectomy, see 55845. For initial transurethral resection of the prostate, first stage, see 52601. For partial resection of prostate, second stage, see 52601 and append modifier 58. For transurethral resection of obstructive prostate tissue, residual or regrowth, see 52630. For exposure of the prostate for insertion of radioactive elements, see 55860–55865.

ICD-10-CM Diagnostic Codes

C61	Malignant neoplasm of prostate ♂
C79.82	Secondary malignant neoplasm of genital organs
D40.0	Neoplasm of uncertain behavior of prostate ♂
D49.59	Neoplasm of unspecified behavior of other genitourinary organ

AMA: **55840** 2014,Jan,11 **55842** 2014,Jan,11

Relative Value Units/Medicare Edits

Non-Facility RVU	Work	PE	MP	Total
55840	21.36	9.98	2.47	33.81
55842	21.36	9.98	2.49	33.83
Facility RVU	**Work**	**PE**	**MP**	**Total**
55840	21.36	9.98	2.47	33.81
55842	21.36	9.98	2.49	33.83

	FUD	Status	MUE	Modifiers				IOM Reference
55840	90	A	1(2)	51	N/A	62*	80	None
55842	90	A	1(2)	51	N/A	62*	80	

* with documentation

Terms To Know

biopsy. Tissue or fluid removed for diagnostic purposes through analysis of the cells in the biopsy material.

blunt dissection. Surgical technique used to expose an underlying area by separating along natural cleavage lines of tissue, without cutting.

catheter. Flexible tube inserted into an area of the body for introducing or withdrawing fluid.

lymph nodes. Bean-shaped structures along the lymphatic vessels that intercept and destroy foreign materials in the tissue and bloodstream.

malignant neoplasm. Any cancerous tumor or lesion exhibiting uncontrolled tissue growth that can progressively invade other parts of the body with its disease-generating cells.

radical. Extensive surgery.

retropubic space. Pelvic cavity.

secondary. Second in order of occurrence or importance, or appearing during the course of another disease or condition.

seminal vesicles. Paired glands located at the base of the bladder in males that release the majority of fluid into semen through ducts that join with the vas deferens forming the ejaculatory duct.

tissue. Group of similar cells with a similar function that form definite structures and organs. Tissue types include epithelial tissue, muscle tissue, connective tissue, and nervous tissue.

transection. Transverse dissection; to cut across a long axis; cross section.

55845

55845   Prostatectomy, retropubic radical, with or without nerve sparing; with bilateral pelvic lymphadenectomy, including external iliac, hypogastric, and obturator nodes

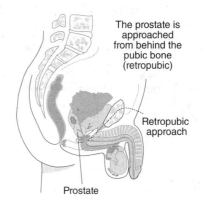

The prostate is approached from behind the pubic bone (retropubic)

Retropubic approach

Prostate

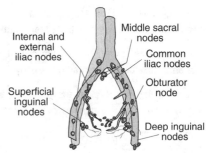

Internal and external iliac nodes

Middle sacral nodes

Common iliac nodes

Obturator node

Superficial inguinal nodes

Deep inguinal nodes

The physician removes the prostate and bilateral pelvic, external iliac, hypogastric, and obturator nodes

Explanation

The physician performs a radical prostatectomy and a pelvic lymph node biopsy through a midline abdominal incision (this may be done in two stages within seven to 10 days). A midline incision is made from the upper to the lower abdomen and the abdominal cavity is entered. The back wall of the abdomen is exposed and all of the lymph nodes along the back wall of the pelvic and abdominal cavities are removed. In preparation for removal of the prostate, a catheter is passed into the urethra and into the bladder. Through the abdominal incision, with or without care to spare the nerves in the area, the urinary bladder is exposed and displaced backwards to enter the space behind the pubic bone and expose the area of the prostate. The gland with the capsule intact, the seminal vesicles, and the portions of the vas deferens in the area are removed by freeing the prostate by blunt dissection and by transecting the urethra and cutting through the bladder outlet. The urinary catheter is brought into the operative site and used to create traction for the dissection. A second catheter is placed in the bladder after the first one is removed along with the prostate. The dissected tissues and the skin incision are closed in layers by suturing.

Coding Tips

For radical retropubic prostatectomy with lymph node biopsies, see 55842. For laparoscopic retropubic radical prostatectomy, see 55866. For initial transurethral resection of the prostate, first stage, see 52601. For partial resection of the prostate, second stage, see 52601 and append modifier 58. For transurethral resection of obstructive prostate tissue, residual or regrowth, see 52630. For exposure of the prostate for insertion of radioactive elements, see 55860–55865. If 55845 is carried out on different days, report 38770 with modifier 50 and 55840.

Prostate

ICD-10-CM Diagnostic Codes

C61 Malignant neoplasm of prostate ♂
C79.82 Secondary malignant neoplasm of genital organs

AMA: 55845 2014,Jan,11

Relative Value Units/Medicare Edits

Non-Facility RVU	Work	PE	MP	Total
55845	25.18	11.28	2.92	39.38
Facility RVU	**Work**	**PE**	**MP**	**Total**
55845	25.18	11.28	2.92	39.38

	FUD	Status	MUE	Modifiers				IOM Reference
55845	90	A	1(2)	51	N/A	62*	80	None

* with documentation

Terms To Know

blunt dissection. Surgical technique used to expose an underlying area by separating along natural cleavage lines of tissue, without cutting.

calculus. Abnormal, stone-like concretion of calcium, cholesterol, mineral salts, or other substances that forms in any part of the body.

lymph nodes. Bean-shaped structures along the lymphatic vessels that intercept and destroy foreign materials in the tissue and bloodstream.

lymphadenectomy. Dissection of lymph nodes free from the vessels and removal for examination by frozen section in a separate procedure to detect early-stage metastases.

malignant. Any condition tending to progress toward death, specifically an invasive tumor with a loss of cellular differentiation that has the ability to spread or metastasize to other body areas.

neoplasm. New abnormal growth, tumor.

prostate. Male gland surrounding the bladder neck and urethra that secretes a substance into the seminal fluid.

radical. Extensive surgery.

retropubic space. Pelvic cavity.

secondary. Second in order of occurrence or importance, or appearing during the course of another disease or condition.

55860-55865

55860 Exposure of prostate, any approach, for insertion of radioactive substance;
55862 with lymph node biopsy(s) (limited pelvic lymphadenectomy)
55865 with bilateral pelvic lymphadenectomy, including external iliac, hypogastric and obturator nodes

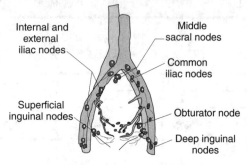

Radioactive pellets are implanted in the prostate. Lymph nodes may also be biopsied or removed

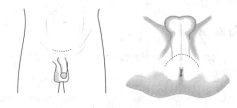

Possible lines of incision

Explanation

In 55860, through an incision made in the lower abdomen just above the pubic area, the physician inserts radioactive materials in the prostate. In preparation for the radiation treatment, a catheter is passed into the urethra into the bladder and a sheath is inserted into the rectum. Through the lower abdominal incision the urinary bladder is exposed and displaced backwards to enter the space behind the pubic bone and expose the prostate gland. With a finger in the rectum to guide the placement, the physician passes a hollow needle into the prostate through the abdominal incision. The needle is positioned in the prostate tumor and radioactive seeds are introduced into the needle and implanted in the prostate using an applicator. The needle is withdrawn a few millimeters and another seed is placed. This is repeated several times through multiple needle insertions. A rubber drain(s) is placed in the space between the pubic bone and the bladder and brought out through the incision wound. In 55862, the pelvic and abdominal lymph nodes are examined and biopsied. A midline incision is made from the upper to the lower abdomen and the abdominal cavity is entered. The back wall of the abdomen is exposed and the lymph nodes are checked for spread of tumor. Some may be removed and/or biopsied. In 55865, the pelvic lymph nodes on both sides are removed. The dissected tissues and the skin incision are closed in layers by suturing. Alternatively, other approaches may be used in a similar fashion.

Coding Tips

This code includes any approach the physician may use. For application of interstitial radioelements, see 77770–77772 and 77778.

ICD-10-CM Diagnostic Codes

C61 Malignant neoplasm of prostate ♂
C79.82 Secondary malignant neoplasm of genital organs
D07.5 Carcinoma in situ of prostate ♂

© 2020 Optum360, LLC **N Newborn: 0** **P Pediatric: 0-17** **M Maternity: 9-64** **A Adult: 15-124** ♂ **Male Only** ♀ **Female Only** CPT © 2020 American Medical Association. All Rights Reserved.

412   *Coding Companion for Urology/Nephrology*

Prostate

D40.0   Neoplasm of uncertain behavior of prostate ♂

D49.59   Neoplasm of unspecified behavior of other genitourinary organ

AMA: 55860 2014,Jan,11 55862 2014,Jan,11 55865 2014,Jan,11

Relative Value Units/Medicare Edits

Non-Facility RVU	Work	PE	MP	Total
55860	15.84	7.63	1.81	25.28
55862	20.04	9.33	2.3	31.67
55865	24.57	11.18	2.82	38.57
Facility RVU	**Work**	**PE**	**MP**	**Total**
55860	15.84	7.63	1.81	25.28
55862	20.04	9.33	2.3	31.67
55865	24.57	11.18	2.82	38.57

	FUD	Status	MUE	Modifiers				IOM Reference
55860	90	A	1(2)	51	N/A	62*	N/A	None
55862	90	A	1(2)	51	N/A	62*	80	
55865	90	A	1(2)	51	N/A	62*	80	

* with documentation

Terms To Know

approach. Method or anatomical location used to gain access to a body organ or specific area for procedures.

biopsy. Tissue or fluid removed for diagnostic purposes through analysis of the cells in the biopsy material.

carcinoma in situ. Malignancy that arises from the cells of the vessel, gland, or organ of origin that remains confined to that site or has not invaded neighboring tissue.

dissect. Cut apart or separate tissue for surgical purposes or for visual or microscopic study.

lymph nodes. Bean-shaped structures along the lymphatic vessels that intercept and destroy foreign materials in the tissue and bloodstream.

lymphadenectomy. Dissection of lymph nodes free from the vessels and removal for examination by frozen section in a separate procedure to detect early-stage metastases.

malignant. Any condition tending to progress toward death, specifically an invasive tumor with a loss of cellular differentiation that has the ability to spread or metastasize to other body areas.

radioactive substances. Materials used in the diagnosis and treatment of disease that emit high-speed particles and energy-containing rays.

secondary. Second in order of occurrence or importance, or appearing during the course of another disease or condition.

tissue. Group of similar cells with a similar function that form definite structures and organs. Tissue types include epithelial tissue, muscle tissue, connective tissue, and nervous tissue.

tumor. Pathological swelling or enlargement; a neoplastic growth of uncontrolled, abnormal multiplication of cells.

55866

55866   Laparoscopy, surgical prostatectomy, retropubic radical, including nerve sparing, includes robotic assistance, when performed

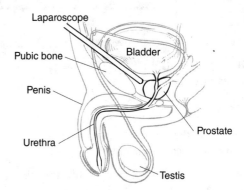

A retropubic radical prostatectomy is performed laparoscopically. The technique of sparing nerves of the region is employed

Explanation

The physician performs a laparoscopic radical prostatectomy, sometimes using robotic assistance. This cannot be done on a patient with prior open prostate surgery. The patient is positioned for laparoscopic surgery with the legs in low lithotomy position for rectal access. Five trocars are placed and the cavity is insufflated with gas. The vas deferens is divided, the seminal vesicles are mobilized, and the prostate is dissected off the rectum. The space of Retzius is developed by dividing the urachus medial to the umbilical ligaments. The endopelvic fascia is incised on both sides and the prostatic levator muscle attachments are bluntly removed. A suture is passed between the urethra and dorsal venous complex and tied. A second suture is passed through the anterior prostate. The bladder neck is opened anteriorly, the posterior margin is separated from the prostate, and the underlying seminal vesicles are exposed. The two prostatic pedicles are divided close to the prostate with the involved seminal vesicle retracted. The back surface of the prostate on each side is dissected from the neurovascular bundles until the prostate remains attached only at the apex. Between the two previously placed sutures, the dorsal vein is divided, the urethra is exposed, and the catheter is removed. The urethra is completely divided. The surgeon places a finger in the rectum for guidance and divides the muscles and remaining attachments to free the prostate completely. The vesicourethral anastomosis is done next with polyglycolic acid suture in running or interrupted simple sutures. A Foley catheter is placed and the anastomosis of the bladder to the urethra is tested. A suction drain is placed through a trocar site and the prostate is removed through a small port site incision.

Coding Tips

Surgical laparoscopy always includes a diagnostic laparoscopy; the diagnostic laparoscopy should not be reported separately. If significant additional time and effort is documented, append modifier 22 and submit a cover letter and operative report. For open radical retropubic prostatectomy, see 55840.

ICD-10-CM Diagnostic Codes

C61	Malignant neoplasm of prostate ♂
C79.82	Secondary malignant neoplasm of genital organs
D40.0	Neoplasm of uncertain behavior of prostate ♂
D49.59	Neoplasm of unspecified behavior of other genitourinary organ

AMA: 55866 2018,Jan,8; 2017,Jan,8; 2016,Jan,13; 2015,Jan,16; 2014,Jan,11

Prostate

Relative Value Units/Medicare Edits

Non-Facility RVU	Work	PE	MP	Total
55866	26.8	11.8	3.09	41.69
Facility RVU	Work	PE	MP	Total
55866	26.8	11.8	3.09	41.69

	FUD	Status	MUE	Modifiers				IOM Reference
55866	90	A	1(2)	51	N/A	62*	80	None

* with documentation

Terms To Know

anastomosis. Surgically created connection between ducts, blood vessels, or bowel segments to allow flow from one to the other.

Foley catheter. Temporary indwelling urethral catheter held in place in the bladder by an inflated balloon containing fluid or air.

laparoscopy. Direct visualization of the peritoneal cavity, outer fallopian tubes, uterus, and ovaries utilizing a laparoscope, a thin, flexible fiberoptic tube.

prostate. Male gland surrounding the bladder neck and urethra that secretes a substance into the seminal fluid.

radical. Extensive surgery.

retropubic space. Pelvic cavity.

robotic assisted surgery. Technology used to assist a surgeon that involves instrumentation combined with the use of robotic arms, devices, or systems. Through the use of a robotic system, the surgeon guides the instrumentation from a console while maintaining direct visualization. Robotic assisted surgery can be performed with many minimally invasive procedures, such as laparoscopic or thoracoscopic procedures.

urethra. Small tube lined with mucous membrane that leads from the bladder to the exterior of the body.

55870

55870   Electroejaculation

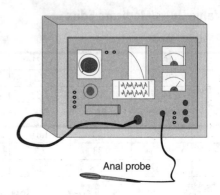

Anal probe

Explanation

The physician uses an electrovibratory device that stimulates ejaculation. The electrostimulator probe is placed in the rectum and positioned adjacent to the prostate gland and a current of electricity is passed into the region of the prostate, seminal vesicles and the vas deferens. The stimulation excites the nerves of the area, causing ejaculation. The semen is collected and used for artificial insemination.

Coding Tips

For artificial insemination, see 58321 and 58322.

ICD-10-CM Diagnostic Codes

N53.11	Retarded ejaculation ♂
N53.13	Anejaculatory orgasm ♂
N53.19	Other ejaculatory dysfunction ♂
Z31.84	Encounter for fertility preservation procedure

AMA: **55870** 2014,Jan,11

Relative Value Units/Medicare Edits

Non-Facility RVU	Work	PE	MP	Total
55870	2.58	2.15	0.3	5.03
Facility RVU	Work	PE	MP	Total
55870	2.58	1.21	0.3	4.09

	FUD	Status	MUE	Modifiers				IOM Reference
55870	0	A	1(2)	51	N/A	62*	N/A	None

* with documentation

Terms To Know

prostate. Male gland surrounding the bladder neck and urethra that secretes a substance into the seminal fluid.

seminal vesicles. Paired glands located at the base of the bladder in males that release the majority of fluid into semen through ducts that join with the vas deferens forming the ejaculatory duct.

vas deferens. Duct that arises in the tail of the epididymis that stores and carries sperm from the epididymis toward the urethra.

© 2020 Optum360, LLC   **N** Newborn: 0   **P** Pediatric: 0-17   **M** Maternity: 9-64   **A** Adult: 15-124   ♂ Male Only   ♀ Female Only   CPT © 2020 American Medical Association. All Rights Reserved.

Prostate

55873

55873 Cryosurgical ablation of the prostate (includes ultrasonic guidance and monitoring)

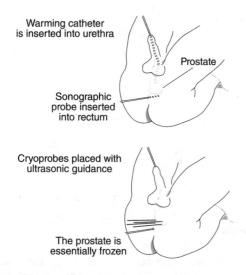

Warming catheter is inserted into urethra

Prostate

Sonographic probe inserted into rectum

Cryoprobes placed with ultrasonic guidance

The prostate is essentially frozen

Explanation

The physician performs cryosurgical ablation of the prostate with ultrasonic guidance and monitoring. The physician places a suprapubic catheter into the bladder through a stab incision just above the pubic hairline. Next, the physician inserts a warming catheter through the urethra and into the bladder. The scrotum is elevated out of the operative field using a gauze sling. An ultrasound probe is inserted into the rectum to monitor the freezing process, and to view in real-time the probe placement during the procedure. Under ultrasonic guidance, the surgeon inserts from three to eight needles into the perineum and advances the needles into the prostate. Into each needle the surgeon advances a guidewire used to facilitate instrumentation. The skin is incised and a dilator is inserted over each guidewire to dilate the channels. Saline is injected to aid visibility of the ultrasound, the guidewire is removed, and a cryoprobe (3 mm diameter) is inserted through each dilator for direct contact with the prostate tissue. The cryoprobes, which deliver super-cooled liquid nitrogen or argon gas (both inert materials) to the prostate, are turned on at -70°C. Up to five cryoprobes can be running simultaneously at any one time. The five cryoprobes are turned on, taking the temperature down to -190°C, while the warming catheter guards against freezing the ureter. If the prostate thaws, the probes may be repositioned, and a second freeze may be performed. Once the prostate gland is completely frozen (resembling an ice ball) and all of the visible prostate tissue is destroyed, the surgeon removes the probes and applies pressure to the perineum to prevent hematoma formation. The punctures are sutured shut and the urethral warming catheter is removed.

Coding Tips

For prostatectomy, perineal subtotal, see 55801. For suprapubic subtotal prostatectomy, see 55821. For retropubic subtotal prostatectomy, see 55831. Supplies used when providing this procedure may be reported with the appropriate HCPCS Level II code. Check with the specific payer to determine coverage.

ICD-10-CM Diagnostic Codes

C61	Malignant neoplasm of prostate ♂
C79.82	Secondary malignant neoplasm of genital organs
D07.5	Carcinoma in situ of prostate ♂
D29.1	Benign neoplasm of prostate ♂
D40.0	Neoplasm of uncertain behavior of prostate ♂
D49.59	Neoplasm of unspecified behavior of other genitourinary organ

AMA: 55873 2019,Sep,10; 2018,Jan,8; 2017,Jan,8; 2016,Jan,13; 2015,Sep,12; 2015,Jan,16; 2014,Jan,11

Relative Value Units/Medicare Edits

Non-Facility RVU	Work	PE	MP	Total
55873	13.6	160.37	1.56	175.53
Facility RVU	**Work**	**PE**	**MP**	**Total**
55873	13.6	6.9	1.56	22.06

	FUD	Status	MUE	Modifiers				IOM Reference
55873	90	A	1(2)	51	N/A	N/A	N/A	100-03,230.9

* with documentation

Terms To Know

ablation. Removal or destruction of a body part or tissue or its function. Ablation may be performed by surgical means, hormones, drugs, radiofrequency, heat, chemical application, or other methods.

catheter. Flexible tube inserted into an area of the body for introducing or withdrawing fluid.

cryosurgery. Application of intense cold, usually produced using liquid nitrogen, to locally freeze diseased or unwanted tissue and induce tissue necrosis without causing harm to adjacent tissue.

guidewire. Flexible metal instrument designed to lead another instrument in its proper course.

perineal. Pertaining to the pelvic floor area between the thighs; the diamond-shaped area bordered by the pubic symphysis in front, the ischial tuberosities on the sides, and the coccyx in back.

prostate. Male gland surrounding the bladder neck and urethra that secretes a substance into the seminal fluid.

real-time. Immediate imaging, with movement as it happens.

tissue. Group of similar cells with a similar function that form definite structures and organs. Tissue types include epithelial tissue, muscle tissue, connective tissue, and nervous tissue.

ultrasound. Imaging using ultra-high sound frequency bounced off body structures.

Prostate

55874

55874   Transperineal placement of biodegradable material, peri-prostatic, single or multiple injection(s), including image guidance, when performed

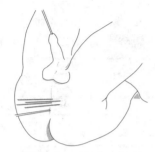

Periprostatic injection of biodegradable material

Explanation

Transperineal placement of biodegradable material is a procedure that works to position the front area (anterior) of the rectal wall away from the prostate when the patient is undergoing radiotherapy for treatment of prostate cancer and subsequently limits the radiation exposure to the anterior rectum. One proprietary system is made up of materials that break down naturally by the action of biological agents and is placed inside the patient through a needle. Imaging guidance is included in this service, when performed. The system retains its position throughout the duration of the patient's radiotherapy treatments and, because the system is biodegradable, is absorbed by the patient's body over time. This code is reported for single or multiple injections.

Coding Tips

Do not report 55874 with 76942. For transperineal placement of needles/catheters into the prostate for interstitial radioelement application, with or without cystoscopy, see 55875.

ICD-10-CM Diagnostic Codes

C61	Malignant neoplasm of prostate ♂
C79.82	Secondary malignant neoplasm of genital organs
D07.5	Carcinoma in situ of prostate ♂
D29.1	Benign neoplasm of prostate ♂
D40.0	Neoplasm of uncertain behavior of prostate ♂
D49.59	Neoplasm of unspecified behavior of other genitourinary organ

Relative Value Units/Medicare Edits

Non-Facility RVU	Work	PE	MP	Total
55874	3.03	83.79	0.27	87.09
Facility RVU	**Work**	**PE**	**MP**	**Total**
55874	3.03	1.47	0.27	4.77

	FUD	Status	MUE	Modifiers				IOM Reference
55874	0	A	1(2)	51	N/A	62*	N/A	None

* with documentation

Terms To Know

SpaceOAR® System. Brand name gel that acts as a protective spacer between the rectum and prostate. It is indicated for males undergoing radiation treatment for prostate cancer.

55875

55875   Transperineal placement of needles or catheters into prostate for interstitial radioelement application, with or without cystoscopy

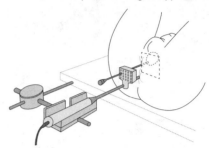

Through a needle, radioactive seeds are implanted in a tumor of the prostate using an applicator

Several seeds may be implanted at one session

Explanation

Transperineal placement of needles or catheters into the prostate gland for interstitial radioelement application is a form of brachytherapy. Brachytherapy is the application of radioactive isotopes for internal radiation. Radioactive material is encapsulated for interstitial implantation into the prostate tissue. Using separately reportable ultrasound or fluoroscopic guidance, the physician inserts the encapsulated radioactive seeds directly into the prostate tissue transperineally, using appropriate applicators (thin catheter tubes or needles). A previous transrectal ultrasound has been done on the volume of the prostate to map out the precise locations of the radioactive seeds. The radioactive isotopes, such as Iodine-125 or Palladium-103, contained within the tiny seeds are left in place and deliver their dose of radiation over a period of months. They do not cause any harm after they have become inert. This method provides radiation to the prescribed body area while minimizing exposure to normal tissue.

Coding Tips

Code 55860 should not be used in place of this code. Exposure of the prostate means that part of the prostate can be directly visualized during the procedure; it requires an incision be made (e.g., through the abdomen, suprapubic, retropubic, etc.). When 55875 is performed with another separately identifiable procedure, the highest dollar value code is listed as the primary procedure and subsequent procedures are appended with modifier 51. For interstitial radioelement application performed during this surgery, see 77770–77772 and 77778. For ultrasonic guidance for interstitial radioelement application, see 76965. Cystoscopy, when performed, is included in this procedure and should not be reported separately.

ICD-10-CM Diagnostic Codes

C61	Malignant neoplasm of prostate ♂
C79.82	Secondary malignant neoplasm of genital organs
D07.5	Carcinoma in situ of prostate ♂
D40.0	Neoplasm of uncertain behavior of prostate ♂
D49.59	Neoplasm of unspecified behavior of other genitourinary organ

AMA: **55875** 2018,Jan,8; 2017,Jan,8; 2016,Jan,13; 2015,Jan,16; 2014,Jan,11

Prostate

Relative Value Units/Medicare Edits

Non-Facility RVU	Work	PE	MP	Total
55875	13.46	7.35	1.39	22.2
Facility RVU	Work	PE	MP	Total
55875	13.46	7.35	1.39	22.2

	FUD	Status	MUE	Modifiers				IOM Reference
55875	90	A	1(2)	51	N/A	N/A	80*	None

* with documentation

Terms To Know

brachytherapy. Form of radiation therapy in which radioactive pellets or seeds are implanted directly into the tissue being treated to deliver their dose of radiation in a more directed fashion. Brachytherapy provides radiation to the prescribed body area while minimizing exposure to normal tissue.

catheter. Flexible tube inserted into an area of the body for introducing or withdrawing fluid.

fluoroscopy. Radiology technique that allows visual examination of part of the body or a function of an organ using a device that projects an x-ray image on a fluorescent screen.

interstitial. Within the small spaces or gaps occurring in tissue or organs.

interstitial radiation. Radioactive source placed into the tissue being treated.

isotope. Chemical element possessing the same atomic number (protons in the nucleus) as another, but with a different atomic weight (number of neutrons).

prostate. Male gland surrounding the bladder neck and urethra that secretes a substance into the seminal fluid.

tissue. Group of similar cells with a similar function that form definite structures and organs. Tissue types include epithelial tissue, muscle tissue, connective tissue, and nervous tissue.

ultrasound. Imaging using ultra-high sound frequency bounced off body structures.

55876

55876   Placement of interstitial device(s) for radiation therapy guidance (eg, fiducial markers, dosimeter), prostate (via needle, any approach), single or multiple

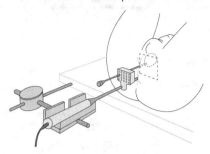

Fiducial markers or dosimeters are inserted into the prostate

The markers help target and align the therapy; the dosimeter measures radiation

Explanation

The physician places one or more interstitial devices for radiation therapy guidance into the prostate via needle, using various approaches. In one method, the patient is placed in the lithotomy position. Under guidance from a transrectal ultrasound wand, the physician injects a small capsule into the tissue of the prostate using a percutaneous needle injection device. The capsule allows for precision in targeting radiation and/or for measuring the radiation doses received. An injected capsule fiducial marker is visible by ultrasound and fluoroscopy, allowing for an accurate triangulation of the tissue to be treated. An injected capsule dosimeter relays radiation dose information so that the clinical team can monitor for any deviation between the radiation plan and the actual radiation received by the patient. The inserted capsule may act as a fiducial marker, dosimeter, or, in many cases, will serve in both roles. This code reports the needle insertion of one or more of these devices into the patient's prostate during a single surgical session.

Coding Tips

When 55876 is performed with another separately identifiable procedure, the highest dollar value code is listed as the primary procedure and subsequent procedures are appended with modifier 51. To report imaging guidance for placement of the device, see 76942, 77002, 77012, and 77021. For placement of catheters into other pelvic organs, see 55920. Report the interstitial device separately using the appropriate HCPCS Level II supply code.

ICD-10-CM Diagnostic Codes

C61	Malignant neoplasm of prostate ♂
C79.82	Secondary malignant neoplasm of genital organs
D07.5	Carcinoma in situ of prostate ♂
D40.0	Neoplasm of uncertain behavior of prostate ♂
D49.59	Neoplasm of unspecified behavior of other genitourinary organ

AMA: **55876** 2018,Jan,8; 2017,Jan,8; 2016,Jun,3; 2016,Jan,13; 2015,Jan,16; 2014,Jan,11

Prostate

CPT © 2020 American Medical Association. All Rights Reserved.   ● **New**   ▲ **Revised**   + **Add On**   ★ **Telemedicine**   **AMA: CPT Assist**   [**Resequenced**]   ☑ **Laterality**   © 2020 Optum360, LLC

Relative Value Units/Medicare Edits

Non-Facility RVU	Work	PE	MP	Total
55876	1.73	2.25	0.18	4.16
Facility RVU	Work	PE	MP	Total
55876	1.73	1.0	0.18	2.91

	FUD	Status	MUE	Modifiers				IOM Reference
55876	0	A	1(2)	51	N/A	62*	N/A	None

* with documentation

Terms To Know

approach. Method or anatomical location used to gain access to a body organ or specific area for procedures.

carcinoma in situ. Malignancy that arises from the cells of the vessel, gland, or organ of origin that remains confined to that site or has not invaded neighboring tissue.

dosimetry. Component in the administration of radiation oncology therapy in which a radiation dose is calculated to a specific site, including implant or beam orientation and exposure, isodose strengths, tissue inhomogeneities, and volume.

fiducial marker. Compact medical device or object placed in or near a tumor to serve as a landmark for the placement of radiation beams during treatment. Use of a fiducial marker allows the clinician to direct radiation to the tumor while preserving surrounding healthy tissue.

fluoroscopy. Radiology technique that allows visual examination of part of the body or a function of an organ using a device that projects an x-ray image on a fluorescent screen.

imaging. Radiologic means of producing pictures for clinical study of the internal structures and functions of the body, such as x-ray, ultrasound, magnetic resonance, or positron emission tomography.

interstitial. Within the small spaces or gaps occurring in tissue or organs.

lithotomy position. Common position patients may be placed in for some surgical procedures and examinations involving the pelvis and/or lower abdomen. The patient is placed supine (on their back), hips and knees flexed, thighs apart, with feet supported in raised stirrups.

neoplasm. New abnormal growth, tumor.

percutaneous. Through the skin.

prostate. Male gland surrounding the bladder neck and urethra that secretes a substance into the seminal fluid.

55880

- 55880   Ablation of malignant prostate tissue, transrectal, with high intensity-focused ultrasound (HIFU), including ultrasound guidance

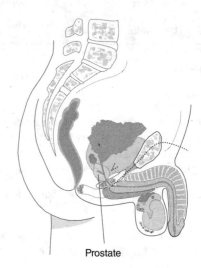

Malignant prostate tissue is ablated using a transrectal approach

Explanation

The physician destroys malignant prostate tissue using high intensity focused ultrasound (HIFU) ablation. With the patient typically under general or spinal anesthesia, the physician inserts an ultrasound probe into the patient's rectum. The probe is surrounded by a cooling balloon that protects the rectal mucosa from the high temperature. The ultrasound transducers are positioned at the level of the prostate. The probe provides ultrasound images of the prostate and then delivers timed bursts of heat to create coagulation necrosis in a targeted area. HIFU treatment may be repeated if necessary.

Coding Tips

For ablation of malignant prostate tissue using transurethral high-energy water vapor thermotherapy, see 0582T.

ICD-10-CM Diagnostic Codes

C61   Malignant neoplasm of prostate ♂
C79.82   Secondary malignant neoplasm of genital organs

Relative Value Units/Medicare Edits

Non-Facility RVU	Work	PE	MP	Total
55880				
Facility RVU	Work	PE	MP	Total
55880				

	FUD	Status	MUE	Modifiers				IOM Reference
55880	N/A		-	N/A	N/A	N/A	N/A	None

* with documentation

© 2020 Optum360, LLC   Ⓝ Newborn: 0   Ⓟ Pediatric: 0-17   Ⓜ Maternity: 9-64   Ⓐ Adult: 15-124   ♂ Male Only   ♀ Female Only   CPT © 2020 American Medical Association. All Rights Reserved.

55920

55920 Placement of needles or catheters into pelvic organs and/or genitalia (except prostate) for subsequent interstitial radioelement application

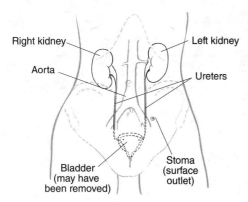

Needles or catheters are placed in the genitalia or pelvic organs

Explanation

The physician places needles or catheters into the pelvic organs and/or genitalia, excluding the prostate, for subsequent interstitial radioelement application. The radioactive isotopes that are introduced subsequently, such as iodine-125 or palladium-103, are contained within tiny seeds that are left in place to deliver radiation over a period of months. They do not cause any harm after becoming inert. This method provides radiation to the prescribed body area while minimizing exposure to normal tissue.

Coding Tips

For placement of needles or catheters into the prostate, see 55875. For insertion of uterine tandems and/or vaginal ovoids for clinical brachytherapy, see 57155. For insertion of Heyman capsules for clinical brachytherapy, see 58346.

ICD-10-CM Diagnostic Codes

C60.0	Malignant neoplasm of prepuce ♂
C60.1	Malignant neoplasm of glans penis ♂
C60.2	Malignant neoplasm of body of penis ♂
C60.8	Malignant neoplasm of overlapping sites of penis ♂
C62.01	Malignant neoplasm of undescended right testis ♂ ☑
C62.02	Malignant neoplasm of undescended left testis ♂ ☑
C62.11	Malignant neoplasm of descended right testis ♂ ☑
C62.12	Malignant neoplasm of descended left testis ♂ ☑
C63.01	Malignant neoplasm of right epididymis ♂ ☑
C63.02	Malignant neoplasm of left epididymis ♂ ☑
C63.11	Malignant neoplasm of right spermatic cord ♂ ☑
C63.12	Malignant neoplasm of left spermatic cord ♂ ☑
C63.2	Malignant neoplasm of scrotum ♂
C63.8	Malignant neoplasm of overlapping sites of male genital organs ♂
C67.0	Malignant neoplasm of trigone of bladder
C67.1	Malignant neoplasm of dome of bladder
C67.2	Malignant neoplasm of lateral wall of bladder
C67.3	Malignant neoplasm of anterior wall of bladder
C67.4	Malignant neoplasm of posterior wall of bladder
C67.5	Malignant neoplasm of bladder neck
C67.6	Malignant neoplasm of ureteric orifice
C67.7	Malignant neoplasm of urachus
C67.8	Malignant neoplasm of overlapping sites of bladder
C68.0	Malignant neoplasm of urethra
C68.1	Malignant neoplasm of paraurethral glands
C76.3	Malignant neoplasm of pelvis
C79.11	Secondary malignant neoplasm of bladder
C79.82	Secondary malignant neoplasm of genital organs

AMA: 55920 2018,Jan,8; 2017,Jan,8; 2016,Jan,13; 2015,Jan,16; 2014,Jan,11

Relative Value Units/Medicare Edits

Non-Facility RVU	Work	PE	MP	Total
55920	8.31	4.14	0.64	13.09
Facility RVU	**Work**	**PE**	**MP**	**Total**
55920	8.31	4.14	0.64	13.09

	FUD	Status	MUE	Modifiers				IOM Reference
55920	0	A	1(2)	51	N/A	N/A	80*	None

* with documentation

Terms To Know

catheter. Flexible tube inserted into an area of the body for introducing or withdrawing fluid.

epididymis. Coiled tube on the back of the testis that is the site of sperm maturation and storage and where spermatozoa are propelled into the vas deferens toward the ejaculatory duct by contraction of smooth muscle.

glans penis. Distal end or head of the penis.

interstitial. Within the small spaces or gaps occurring in tissue or organs.

isotope. Chemical element possessing the same atomic number (protons in the nucleus) as another, but with a different atomic weight (number of neutrons).

malignant neoplasm. Any cancerous tumor or lesion exhibiting uncontrolled tissue growth that can progressively invade other parts of the body with its disease-generating cells.

radioactive substances. Materials used in the diagnosis and treatment of disease that emit high-speed particles and energy-containing rays.

radioelement. Any element that emits particle or electromagnetic radiations from nuclear disintegration, occurring naturally in any element with an atomic number above 83.

scrotum. Skin pouch that holds the testes and supporting reproductive structures.

secondary. Second in order of occurrence or importance, or appearing during the course of another disease or condition.

spermatic cord. Structure of the male reproductive organs that consists of the ductus deferens, testicular artery, nerves, and veins that drain the testes.

testes. Male gonadal paired glands located in the scrotum that secrete testosterone and contain the seminiferous tubules where sperm is produced.

55970-55980

55970   Intersex surgery; male to female
55980   female to male

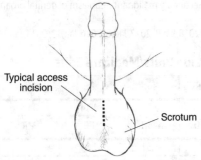

A vagina is fashioned from penile skin and tissues

Typical access incision

Scrotum

The testes are removed from the scrotum

Male sex organs are reformed in stages into female genitalia or female genitalia is refashioned into male organs

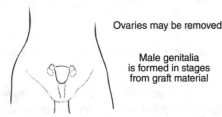

Ovaries may be removed

Male genitalia is formed in stages from graft material

Explanation

In a series of staged procedures, the physician removes portions of the male genitalia and forms female external genitals. In 55970, the penis is dissected and portions are removed with care to preserve vital nerves and vessels in order to fashion a clitoris-like structure. The urethral opening is moved to a position similar to that of a normal female. A vagina is made by dissecting and opening the perineum. This opening is lined using pedicle or split thickness grafts. Labia are created out of skin from the scrotum and adjacent tissue. A stent or obturator is usually left in place in the newly created vagina for three weeks or longer. In 55980, for female to male intersex surgery, the physician forms a penis and scrotum using pedicle flap grafts and free skin grafts. Portions of the clitoris are used as well as the adjacent skin. Prostheses are often placed in the penis in order to have a sexually functional organ. Prosthetic testicles are fixed in the scrotum. The vagina is closed or removed.

Coding Tips

This series of procedures may be indicated because of congenital defects, genital anomalies, or it may be a matter of patient preference. When performed for patient preference, the patient is generally responsible for all charges related to the procedures.

ICD-10-CM Diagnostic Codes

F64.0   Transsexualism
F64.1   Dual role transvestism
F64.2   Gender identity disorder of childhood P
F64.8   Other gender identity disorders

AMA: **55970** 2014,Jan,11 **55980** 2014,Jan,11

Relative Value Units/Medicare Edits

Non-Facility RVU	Work	PE	MP	Total
55970	0.0	0.0	0.0	0.0
55980	0.0	0.0	0.0	0.0
Facility RVU	Work	PE	MP	Total
55970	0.0	0.0	0.0	0.0
55980	0.0	0.0	0.0	0.0

	FUD	Status	MUE	Modifiers				IOM Reference
55970	N/A	C	1(2)	N/A	N/A	N/A	N/A	100-02,16,180
55980	N/A	C	1(2)	N/A	N/A	N/A	N/A	

* with documentation

Terms To Know

dissection. Separating by cutting tissue or body structures apart.

flap graft. Mass of flesh and skin partially excised from its location but retaining its blood supply, grafted onto another site to repair adjacent or distant defects.

free graft. Unattached piece of skin and tissue moved to another part of the body and sutured into place to repair a defect.

obturator. Prosthesis used to close an acquired or congenital opening in the palate that aids in speech and chewing.

pedicle graft. Mass of flesh and skin partially excised from the donor location, retaining its blood supply through intact blood vessels, and grafted onto another site to repair adjacent or distant defects.

prosthesis. Man-made substitute for a missing body part.

scrotum. Skin pouch that holds the testes and supporting reproductive structures.

split thickness skin graft. Graft using the epidermis and part of the dermis.

stent. Tube to provide support in a body cavity or lumen.

57220

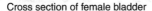

57220　Plastic operation on urethral sphincter, vaginal approach (eg, Kelly urethral plication)

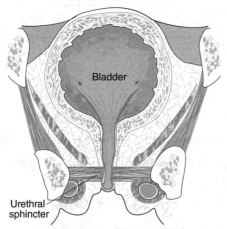

Cross section of female bladder

Bladder

Urethral sphincter

The physician accesses the sphincter through a vaginal incision

Sutures at the junction of the bladder and urethra support the urethral sphincter

Explanation

The physician accesses the urethral sphincter from the vagina. With a catheter in the urethra, the physician dissects the midline vaginal wall separating it from the bladder and the proximal urethra. Sutures are placed at the junction of the bladder and urethra on each side of the urethra. This supports the area. Excess vaginal tissue is excised and the vaginal wall is closed.

Coding Tips

This is a female only procedure. For a Marshall-Marchetti-Krantz urethral suspension, abdominal approach, see 51840 and 51841.

ICD-10-CM Diagnostic Codes

N39.3　　Stress incontinence (female) (male)

AMA: 57220 2019,Jul,6; 2014,Jan,11

Relative Value Units/Medicare Edits

Non-Facility RVU	Work	PE	MP	Total
57220	4.85	4.08	0.74	9.67
Facility RVU	Work	PE	MP	Total
57220	4.85	4.08	0.74	9.67

	FUD	Status	MUE	Modifiers				IOM Reference
57220	90	A	1(2)	51	N/A	62*	80	None

* with documentation

Terms To Know

plication. Surgical technique involving folding, tucking, or pleating to reduce the size of a hollow structure or organ.

stress incontinence. Involuntary escape of urine at times of minor stress against the bladder, such as coughing, sneezing, or laughing.

57230

57230　Plastic repair of urethrocele

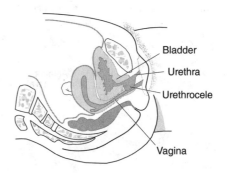

Bladder

Urethra

Urethrocele

Vagina

Physician repairs urethrocele via vagina

Explanation

The physician repairs a urethrocele, which is a sagging or prolapse of the urethra through its opening or a bulging of the posterior wall of the urethra against the vaginal canal. The prolapsed urethral tissue is excised from the meatus in a circular manner. The cut edges of urethral mucosa and vaginal mucosa are sutured.

Coding Tips

This is a female only procedure. For a Marshall-Marchetti-Krantz urethral suspension, abdominal approach, see 51840 and 51841.

ICD-10-CM Diagnostic Codes

N36.8	Other specified disorders of urethra
N81.0	Urethrocele ♀
N81.11	Cystocele, midline ♀
N81.12	Cystocele, lateral ♀
Q64.71	Congenital prolapse of urethra

AMA: 57230 2019,Jul,6; 2014,Jan,11

Relative Value Units/Medicare Edits

Non-Facility RVU	Work	PE	MP	Total
57230	6.3	4.56	0.99	11.85
Facility RVU	Work	PE	MP	Total
57230	6.3	4.56	0.99	11.85

	FUD	Status	MUE	Modifiers				IOM Reference
57230	90	A	1(2)	51	N/A	62*	80	None

* with documentation

Terms To Know

meatus. Opening or passage into the body.

posterior. Located in the back part or caudal end of the body.

prolapse. Falling, sliding, or sinking of an organ from its normal location in the body.

urethrocele. Urethral herniation into the vaginal wall.

57240

57240 Anterior colporrhaphy, repair of cystocele with or without repair of urethrocele, including cystourethroscopy, when performed

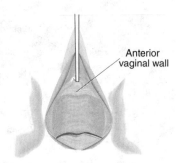

Through an incision in the anterior wall of the vagina, the physician repairs a cystocele

Anterior vaginal wall

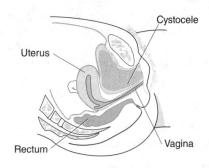

Cystocele
Uterus
Rectum
Vagina

Explanation

The physician repairs a cystocele, which is a herniation of the bladder through its support tissues and against the anterior vaginal wall causing it to bulge downward. The physician may also repair a urethrocele, which is a prolapse of the urethra. An incision is made from the apex of the vagina to within 1 cm of the urethral meatus. Plication sutures are placed along the urethral course from the meatus to the bladder neck. A suture is placed through the pubourethral ligament to the posterior symphysis pubis on each side of the urethra. The sutures are tied (ligated) and the posterior urethra is pulled upward to a retropubic position. If a cystocele is repaired, mattress sutures are placed in the mobilized paravesical tissue. The vaginal mucosa is closed. Cystourethroscopy is included when performed with this procedure.

Coding Tips

For a Marshall-Marchetti-Krantz urethral suspension, abdominal approach, see 51840 and 51841. For plastic repair of a urethrocele, see 57230. Do not report 57240 with 52000.

ICD-10-CM Diagnostic Codes

N36.8	Other specified disorders of urethra
N81.0	Urethrocele ♀
N81.11	Cystocele, midline ♀
N81.12	Cystocele, lateral ♀
Q64.71	Congenital prolapse of urethra

AMA: 57240 2019,Jul,6; 2018,Jan,8; 2017,Jan,8; 2016,Jan,13; 2015,Jan,16; 2014,Jan,11

Relative Value Units/Medicare Edits

Non-Facility RVU	Work	PE	MP	Total
57240	10.08	5.96	1.45	17.49
Facility RVU	**Work**	**PE**	**MP**	**Total**
57240	10.08	5.96	1.45	17.49

	FUD	Status	MUE	Modifiers				IOM Reference
57240	90	A	1(2)	51	N/A	62*	80	None

* with documentation

Terms To Know

anterior. Situated in the front area or toward the belly surface of the body.

apex. Highest point of a root end of a tooth, or the end of any organ.

colporrhaphy. Plastic repair or reconstruction of the vagina by suturing the vaginal wall and surrounding fibrous tissue.

cystocele. Herniation of the bladder into the vagina.

ligation. Tying off a blood vessel or duct with a suture or a soft, thin wire.

meatus. Opening or passage into the body.

plication. Surgical technique involving folding, tucking, or pleating to reduce the size of a hollow structure or organ.

posterior. Located in the back part or caudal end of the body.

prolapse. Falling, sliding, or sinking of an organ from its normal location in the body.

retropubic space. Pelvic cavity.

urethrocele. Urethral herniation into the vaginal wall.

uterovaginal prolapse. Uterus displaced downward and exposed in the external genitalia.

© 2020 Optum360, LLC   **N** Newborn: 0   **P** Pediatric: 0-17   **M** Maternity: 9-64   **A** Adult: 15-124   ♂ Male Only   ♀ Female Only   CPT © 2020 American Medical Association. All Rights Reserved.

Vagina

57260-57265

57260 Combined anteroposterior colporrhaphy, including cystourethroscopy, when performed;

57265   with enterocele repair

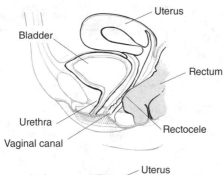

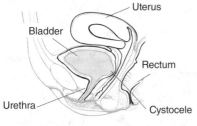

A plastic repair of the vaginal canal is performed, often to correct a herniation of the bladder (cystocele). An enterocele (herniation of the intestine) may also be repaired during the procedure

Explanation

The physician repairs a cystocele and rectocele by colporrhaphy. Colporrhaphy involves a plastic repair of the vagina and the fibrous tissue separating the bladder, vagina, and rectum. A cystocele is a herniation of the bladder through its support tissues causing the anterior vaginal wall to bulge downward. A rectocele is a protrusion of part of the rectum through its support tissues causing the posterior vaginal wall to bulge. Using a combined vaginal approach and a posterior midline incision that includes the perineum and posterior vaginal wall, the physician dissects the tissues between the bladder, urethra, vagina, and rectum. The specific tissue weaknesses are repaired and strengthened using tissue transfer techniques and layered and plication suturing. In 57260, the physician may also repair a urethrocele, which is a prolapse of the urethra, and perform a perineorrhaphy, which is plastic repair of the perineum, including midline approximation of the levator and perineal muscles. In 57265, the physician performs all of the same services and also repairs an enterocele, which is a herniation of the bowel contents of the rectouterine pouch that protrudes into the septum of tissue between the bladder and vagina or between the vagina and rectum. Through the vagina, the enterocele sac is incised and ligated and the uterosacral ligaments and endopelvic fascia anterior to the rectum are approximated. In both procedures, incisions are closed with sutures. Cystourethroscopy is included when performed with these procedures.

Coding Tips

For a Marshall-Marchetti-Krantz urethral suspension, abdominal approach, see 51840 and 51841. For plastic repair of a urethrocele, see 57230. For plastic operation of a urethral sphincter, vaginal approach, see 57220. Do not report these codes with 52000.

ICD-10-CM Diagnostic Codes

K62.3   Rectal prolapse

N36.8   Other specified disorders of urethra

N81.0   Urethrocele ♀

N81.11   Cystocele, midline ♀

N81.12   Cystocele, lateral ♀

N81.2   Incomplete uterovaginal prolapse ♀

N81.3   Complete uterovaginal prolapse ♀

N81.5   Vaginal enterocele ♀

N81.6   Rectocele ♀

N81.81   Perineocele ♀

Q64.71   Congenital prolapse of urethra

AMA: 57260 2019,Jul,6; 2018,Jan,8; 2017,Jan,8; 2016,Jan,13; 2015,Jan,16; 2014,Jan,11 **57265** 2019,Jul,6; 2018,Jan,8; 2017,Jan,8; 2016,Jan,13; 2015,Jan,16; 2014,Jan,11

Relative Value Units/Medicare Edits

Non-Facility RVU	Work	PE	MP	Total
57260	13.25	7.18	2.0	22.43
57265	15.0	7.86	2.32	25.18
Facility RVU	**Work**	**PE**	**MP**	**Total**
57260	13.25	7.18	2.0	22.43
57265	15.0	7.86	2.32	25.18

	FUD	Status	MUE	Modifiers				IOM Reference
57260	90	A	1(2)	51	N/A	62*	80	None
57265	90	A	1(2)	51	N/A	62*	80	

* with documentation

Terms To Know

anterior. Situated in the front area or toward the belly surface of the body.

approach. Method or anatomical location used to gain access to a body organ or specific area for procedures.

colporrhaphy. Plastic repair or reconstruction of the vagina by suturing the vaginal wall and surrounding fibrous tissue.

connective tissue. Body tissue made from fibroblasts, collagen, and elastic fibrils that connects, supports, and holds together other tissues and cells and includes cartilage, collagenous, fibrous, elastic, and osseous tissue.

dissect. Cut apart or separate tissue for surgical purposes or for visual or microscopic study.

enterocele. Intestinal herniation into the vaginal wall.

fibrous tissue. Connective tissues.

posterior. Located in the back part or caudal end of the body.

prolapse. Falling, sliding, or sinking of an organ from its normal location in the body.

rectocele. Rectal tissue herniation into the vaginal wall.

tissue. Group of similar cells with a similar function that form definite structures and organs. Tissue types include epithelial tissue, muscle tissue, connective tissue, and nervous tissue.

urethrocele. Urethral herniation into the vaginal wall.

Vagina

CPT © 2020 American Medical Association. All Rights Reserved. ● New   ▲ Revised   + Add On   ★ Telemedicine   AMA: CPT Assist   [Resequenced]   ☑ Laterality   © 2020 Optum360, LLC

57267

+ **57267** Insertion of mesh or other prosthesis for repair of pelvic floor defect, each site (anterior, posterior compartment), vaginal approach (List separately in addition to code for primary procedure)

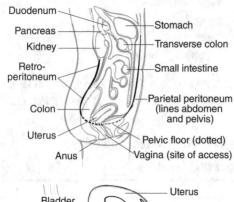

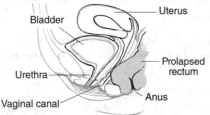

Synthetic mesh is often placed over defects of the abdominal wall and pelvic floor. The mesh provides support and structure for the healing process

Explanation

The physician inserts mesh or other prosthetic support material to repair a pelvic floor defect using a vaginal approach. Pelvic floor defects resulting in prolapse of the pelvic viscera occur when the pelvic fascia weakens or is damaged. The physician selects the appropriate type of prosthetic support material. Some mesh supports, such as horseshoe shaped mesh, are purchased preformed in the desired configuration. Other types of mesh supports, such as tension free tapes, are cut and fashioned by the physician during surgery into the required shapes and sizes. The mesh is inserted through the vagina and placed at the site requiring support. The exact placement of the mesh is determined by the type of pelvic floor defect being repaired. For example, horseshoe mesh is placed between the pubis and sacrum to close the area between the pelvic viscera and the inferior pelvic hiatus. Report 57267 in addition to the primary procedure for each site requiring insertion of mesh or other prosthesis, such as an anterior repair for cystocele or a posterior repair for a rectocele.

Coding Tips

Report 57267 in addition to the codes for the primary vaginal or rectocele repair (45560, 57240–57265, or 57285).

ICD-10-CM Diagnostic Codes

This/these CPT code(s) are add-on code(s). See the primary procedure code that this code is performed with for your ICD-10-CM code selections.

AMA: 57267 2019,Jul,6; 2018,Jan,8; 2017,Jan,8; 2016,Jan,13; 2015,Jan,16; 2014,Jan,11

Relative Value Units/Medicare Edits

Non-Facility RVU	Work	PE	MP	Total
57267	4.88	1.78	0.68	7.34
Facility RVU	Work	PE	MP	Total
57267	4.88	1.78	0.68	7.34

	FUD	Status	MUE	Modifiers				IOM Reference
57267	N/A	A	2(3)	N/A	N/A	62*	80	None

* with documentation

Terms To Know

anterior. Situated in the front area or toward the belly surface of the body.

approach. Method or anatomical location used to gain access to a body organ or specific area for procedures.

cystocele. Herniation of the bladder into the vagina.

defect. Imperfection, flaw, or absence.

fascia. Fibrous sheet or band of tissue that envelops organs, muscles, and groupings of muscles.

mesh. Synthetic fabric used as a prosthetic patch in hernia repair.

pelvis. Distal anterior portion of the trunk that lies between the hipbones, sacrum, and coccyx bones; the inferior portion of the abdominal cavity.

posterior. Located in the back part or caudal end of the body.

prolapse. Falling, sliding, or sinking of an organ from its normal location in the body.

prosthesis. Man-made substitute for a missing body part.

rectocele. Rectal tissue herniation into the vaginal wall.

viscera. Large interior organs enclosed within a cavity, generally referring to the abdominal organs.

57284-57285

57284 Paravaginal defect repair (including repair of cystocele, if performed); open abdominal approach
57285   vaginal approach

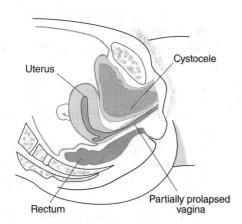

The physician repairs paravaginal defects

Explanation

The physician repairs a paravaginal defect, in which there is loss of the lateral vaginal attachment to the pelvic sidewall, by dissecting the tissues between the vagina and the bladder and urethra. The specific tissue weaknesses are found, repaired, and strengthened using tissue transfer techniques and plication suturing. The paravaginal repair may be performed alone or in conjunction with cystocele repair, in which a herniation of the bladder through its support tissues into the anterior vaginal wall causes it to bulge downward. These procedures help restore the normal anatomic relationships of the urethra, bladder, and vagina. Report 57284 if access is achieved via laparotomy (open abdominal approach) and 57285 if a vaginal approach is utilized.

Coding Tips

If only one of the components of these procedures is performed, see other codes in this section of CPT. For example, if repair of a cystocele with anterior colporrhaphy is performed by itself, report 57240. For a Marshall-Marchetti-Krantz urethral suspension, abdominal approach, see 51840 and 51841. For laparoscopic repair of stress incontinence, see 51990 and 51992. For sling operation for stress incontinence, see 57288. Do not report 57284 with 51840–51841 or 58152. Do not report 57284 or 57285 with 51990, 57240, 57260, 57265, or 58267.

ICD-10-CM Diagnostic Codes

N81.0	Urethrocele ♀
N81.11	Cystocele, midline ♀
N81.12	Cystocele, lateral ♀
N81.2	Incomplete uterovaginal prolapse ♀
N81.3	Complete uterovaginal prolapse ♀
N81.6	Rectocele ♀
N81.81	Perineocele ♀
N81.83	Incompetence or weakening of rectovaginal tissue ♀
N81.85	Cervical stump prolapse ♀
N81.89	Other female genital prolapse ♀
N99.3	Prolapse of vaginal vault after hysterectomy ♀

AMA: **57284** 2019,Jul,6; 2018,Jan,8; 2017,Jan,8; 2016,Jan,13; 2015,Jan,16; 2014,Jan,11 **57285** 2019,Jul,6; 2018,Jan,8; 2017,Jan,8; 2016,Jan,13; 2015,Jan,16; 2014,Jan,11

Relative Value Units/Medicare Edits

Non-Facility RVU	Work	PE	MP	Total
57284	14.33	7.56	1.99	23.88
57285	11.6	6.59	1.69	19.88
Facility RVU	**Work**	**PE**	**MP**	**Total**
57284	14.33	7.56	1.99	23.88
57285	11.6	6.59	1.69	19.88

	FUD	Status	MUE	Modifiers				IOM Reference
57284	90	A	1(2)	51	N/A	62	80	100-03,230.10
57285	90	A	1(2)	51	N/A	62	80	

* with documentation

Terms To Know

anterior. Situated in the front area or toward the belly surface of the body.

approach. Method or anatomical location used to gain access to a body organ or specific area for procedures.

cystocele. Herniation of the bladder into the vagina.

defect. Imperfection, flaw, or absence.

dissect. Cut apart or separate tissue for surgical purposes or for visual or microscopic study.

laparotomy. Incision through the flank or abdomen for therapeutic or diagnostic purposes.

plication. Surgical technique involving folding, tucking, or pleating to reduce the size of a hollow structure or organ.

tissue. Group of similar cells with a similar function that form definite structures and organs. Tissue types include epithelial tissue, muscle tissue, connective tissue, and nervous tissue.

Vagina

57287

57287 Removal or revision of sling for stress incontinence (eg, fascia or synthetic)

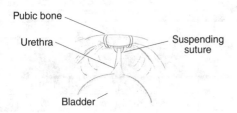

Overhead schematic showing suspension sutures (fascial suspension may also be found)

A synthetic or fascial sling for stress incontinence is revisited and revised or removed

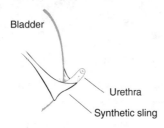

Explanation

The physician removes or revises a fascial or synthetic sling previously placed to correct urinary stress incontinence. To remove a sling, the physician makes a small abdominal skin incision to the level of the rectus fascia and releases the arm of the sling from the rectus abdominis. The physician releases the sling's attachment to the junction of the urethra via canals or tunnels formed by an instrument or a finger placed through a vertical or flap incision in the vaginal wall. In revision of a sling the physician may remove and partially or completely replace the sling using fascia or a synthetic graft through an abdominal and vaginal approach. The sling may be revised by increasing the tension on the sling using suture at one or both of the attachment sites at the junction of the urethra and/or to the rectus abdominis muscle. At the end of the procedure the area is irrigated, and hemostasis is achieved. The abdominal and/or vaginal incisions are closed with layered suture.

Coding Tips

When 57287 is performed with another separately identifiable procedure, the highest dollar value code is listed as the primary procedure and subsequent procedures are appended with modifier 51. For initial sling operation, see 57288. For laparoscopic sling operation for stress incontinence, see 51992.

ICD-10-CM Diagnostic Codes

N39.3	Stress incontinence (female) (male)
T83.118A	Breakdown (mechanical) of other urinary devices and implants, initial encounter
T83.128A	Displacement of other urinary devices and implants, initial encounter
T83.198A	Other mechanical complication of other urinary devices and implants, initial encounter
T83.21XA	Breakdown (mechanical) of graft of urinary organ, initial encounter
T83.22XA	Displacement of graft of urinary organ, initial encounter
T83.23XA	Leakage of graft of urinary organ, initial encounter
T83.24XA	Erosion of graft of urinary organ, initial encounter
T83.25XA	Exposure of graft of urinary organ, initial encounter
T83.29XA	Other mechanical complication of graft of urinary organ, initial encounter
T83.81XA	Embolism due to genitourinary prosthetic devices, implants and grafts, initial encounter
T83.82XA	Fibrosis due to genitourinary prosthetic devices, implants and grafts, initial encounter
T83.83XA	Hemorrhage due to genitourinary prosthetic devices, implants and grafts, initial encounter
T83.84XA	Pain due to genitourinary prosthetic devices, implants and grafts, initial encounter
T83.85XA	Stenosis due to genitourinary prosthetic devices, implants and grafts, initial encounter
T83.86XA	Thrombosis due to genitourinary prosthetic devices, implants and grafts, initial encounter
T83.89XA	Other specified complication of genitourinary prosthetic devices, implants and grafts, initial encounter
Z46.6	Encounter for fitting and adjustment of urinary device

AMA: 57287 2019,Jul,6; 2018,Jan,8; 2017,Jan,8; 2016,Jan,13; 2015,Jan,16; 2014,Jan,11

Relative Value Units/Medicare Edits

Non-Facility RVU	Work	PE	MP	Total
57287	11.15	8.02	1.51	20.68
Facility RVU	Work	PE	MP	Total
57287	11.15	8.02	1.51	20.68

	FUD	Status	MUE	Modifiers				IOM Reference
57287	90	A	1(2)	51	N/A	62*	80	100-03,230.10

* with documentation

Terms To Know

approach. Method or anatomical location used to gain access to a body organ or specific area for procedures.

fascia. Fibrous sheet or band of tissue that envelops organs, muscles, and groupings of muscles.

flap. Mass of flesh and skin partially excised from its location but retaining its blood supply that is moved to another site to repair adjacent or distant defects.

graft. Tissue implant from another part of the body or another person.

hemostasis. Interruption of blood flow or the cessation or arrest of bleeding.

irrigate. Washing out, lavage.

sling operation. Procedure to correct urinary incontinence. A sling of fascia or synthetic material is placed under the junction of the urethra and bladder in females, or across the muscles surrounding the urethra in males.

stress incontinence. Involuntary escape of urine at times of minor stress against the bladder, such as coughing, sneezing, or laughing.

© 2020 Optum360, LLC   **N** Newborn: 0   **P** Pediatric: 0-17   **M** Maternity: 9-64   **A** Adult: 15-124   ♂ Male Only   ♀ Female Only   CPT © 2020 American Medical Association. All Rights Reserved.

Vagina

57288

57288　Sling operation for stress incontinence (eg, fascia or synthetic)

The physician places a support sling
to eliminate stress incontinence

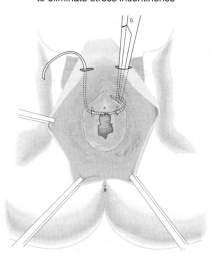

The sling can be synthetic or fascial

Explanation

Through vaginal and abdominal incisions, the physician places a sling under the junction of the urethra and bladder. The physician places a catheter in the bladder, makes an incision in the anterior wall of the vagina, and folds and tacks the tissues around the urethra. A sling is formed out of synthetic material or from fascia harvested from the sheath of the rectus abdominis muscle. The loop end of the sling is sutured around the junction of the urethra. An incision is made in the lower abdomen and the ends of the sling are grasped with a clamp and pulled into the incision and sutured to the rectus abdominis sheath. The abdominal and vaginal incisions are closed in layers by suturing.

Coding Tips

For removal or revision of sling, see 57287. For a Marshall-Marchetti-Krantz urethral suspension, abdominal approach, see 51840 and 51841. For laparoscopic sling operation for stress incontinence, see 51992. Supplies used when providing this procedure may be reported with the appropriate HCPCS Level II code. Check with the specific payer to determine coverage.

ICD-10-CM Diagnostic Codes

N39.3　　　Stress incontinence (female) (male)

AMA: 57288 2019,Jul,6; 2019,Feb,10; 2018,Jan,8; 2017,Jan,8; 2016,Jan,13; 2015,Jan,16; 2014,Jan,11

Relative Value Units/Medicare Edits

Non-Facility RVU	Work	PE	MP	Total
57288	12.13	7.37	1.69	21.19
Facility RVU	**Work**	**PE**	**MP**	**Total**
57288	12.13	7.37	1.69	21.19

	FUD	Status	MUE	Modifiers				IOM Reference
57288	90	A	1(2)	51	N/A	62*	80	None

* with documentation

57289

57289　Pereyra procedure, including anterior colporrhaphy

Pereyra ligature carrier

The physician guides the
ligature with a finger
inserted in the vagina

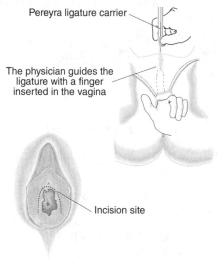

Incision site

A cystocele is also repaired

The proximal urethra is sutured
to the rectus abdominus muscle

Explanation

The physician makes an inverted U-shaped incision in the area between the vagina and the urethra. By blunt and sharp dissection, the physician creates an opening in the space on each side of the urethra as it passes into the bladder. Using a continuous suture for each side, the physician stitches the fascial tissues along the urethra to the urethrovesical junction. The physician makes an incision in the abdomen above the pubis and, doing each side in turn, drives a Pereyra ligature carrier through the tissues just lateral to the midline and takes it down to the sutured tissue. The sutures are threaded into the instrument and brought back through the abdominal incision. The urethrovesical junction is elevated by pulling on the sutures and fixing them around the rectus abdominis muscle. In addition, the physician performs an anterior colporrhaphy using a vaginal approach, which corrects a cystocele and repairs the tissues between the vagina, bladder, and urethra.

Coding Tips

When 57289 is performed with another separately identifiable procedure, the highest dollar value code is listed as the primary procedure and subsequent procedures are appended with modifier 51. For a Marshall-Marchetti-Krantz urethral suspension, abdominal approach, see 51840 and 51841.

ICD-10-CM Diagnostic Codes

N39.3　　　Stress incontinence (female) (male)
N81.11　　Cystocele, midline ♀
N81.12　　Cystocele, lateral ♀

AMA: 57289 2019,Jul,6; 2018,Jan,8; 2017,Jan,8; 2016,Jan,13; 2015,Jan,16; 2014,Jan,11

Vagina

Relative Value Units/Medicare Edits

Non-Facility RVU	Work	PE	MP	Total
57289	12.8	7.85	2.0	22.65
Facility RVU	**Work**	**PE**	**MP**	**Total**
57289	12.8	7.85	2.0	22.65

	FUD	Status	MUE	Modifiers				IOM Reference
57289	90	A	1(2)	51	N/A	62*	80	None

* with documentation

Terms To Know

anterior. Situated in the front area or toward the belly surface of the body.

approach. Method or anatomical location used to gain access to a body organ or specific area for procedures.

blunt dissection. Surgical technique used to expose an underlying area by separating along natural cleavage lines of tissue, without cutting.

colporrhaphy. Plastic repair or reconstruction of the vagina by suturing the vaginal wall and surrounding fibrous tissue.

cystocele. Herniation of the bladder into the vagina.

fascia. Fibrous sheet or band of tissue that envelops organs, muscles, and groupings of muscles.

ligation. Tying off a blood vessel or duct with a suture or a soft, thin wire.

Pereyra procedure. Technique used for surgical correction of stress incontinence in which a suture ligature or loop is used to lift the bladder by connecting the paraurethral tissue to the abdominal muscle.

prolapse. Falling, sliding, or sinking of an organ from its normal location in the body.

stress incontinence. Involuntary escape of urine at times of minor stress against the bladder, such as coughing, sneezing, or laughing.

tissue. Group of similar cells with a similar function that form definite structures and organs. Tissue types include epithelial tissue, muscle tissue, connective tissue, and nervous tissue.

uterovaginal prolapse. Uterus displaced downward and exposed in the external genitalia.

57423

57423   Paravaginal defect repair (including repair of cystocele, if performed), laparoscopic approach

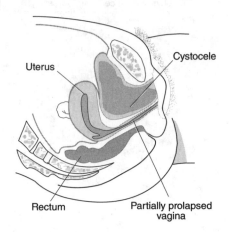

The physician repairs paravaginal defects

Explanation

The physician performs laparoscopic repair of a paravaginal defect, in which there is loss of the lateral vaginal attachment to the pelvic sidewall. Through small stab incisions in the abdomen, a fiberoptic laparoscope and trocars are inserted into the abdominal/pelvic space and the abdomen is insufflated. The bladder may be filled with sterile water to allow the surgeon to identify the superior border of the bladder's edge and then drained to prevent injury after the space of Retzius has been entered and the pubic ramus visualized. Following identification of the defect, the surgeon inserts the nondominant hand into the vagina in order to elevate the anterior vaginal wall and pubocervical fascia to their normal positions. Nonabsorbable sutures with attached needles are introduced through the laparoscopy port and grasped using a laparoscopic needle driver. A series of four to six sutures are placed and tied sequentially along the defects from the ischial spine toward the urethra. The procedure is repeated on the opposite side if a bilateral defect is present. The paravaginal defect repair may be performed alone or in conjunction with cystocele repair, in which a herniation of the bladder through its support tissues into the anterior vaginal wall causes it to bulge downward. These procedures help restore the normal anatomic relationships of the urethra, bladder, and vagina. At completion of the procedure, laparoscopic tools are removed, excess gas expelled, and fascial defects and skin edges are sutured.

Coding Tips

If only one of the components of this procedure is performed, see other codes in this section of CPT. For example, if repair of a cystocele with anterior colporrhaphy is performed by itself, report 57240. For a Marshall-Marchetti-Krantz urethral suspension, abdominal approach, see 51840 and 51841. For laparoscopic repair of stress incontinence, see 51990 and 51992. For open sling operation for stress incontinence, see 57288. Do not report 57423 with 49320, 51840–51841, 51990, 57240, 57260, 58152, or 58267.

ICD-10-CM Diagnostic Codes

N81.0	Urethrocele ♀
N81.11	Cystocele, midline ♀
N81.12	Cystocele, lateral ♀
N81.2	Incomplete uterovaginal prolapse ♀

Vagina

N81.3	Complete uterovaginal prolapse ♀
N81.6	Rectocele ♀
N81.81	Perineocele ♀
N81.83	Incompetence or weakening of rectovaginal tissue ♀
N81.85	Cervical stump prolapse ♀
N81.89	Other female genital prolapse ♀
N99.3	Prolapse of vaginal vault after hysterectomy ♀

AMA: 57423 2019,Jul,6; 2018,Jan,8; 2017,Jan,8; 2016,Jan,13; 2015,Jan,16; 2014,Jan,11

Relative Value Units/Medicare Edits

Non-Facility RVU	Work	PE	MP	Total
57423	16.08	8.33	2.42	26.83
Facility RVU	**Work**	**PE**	**MP**	**Total**
57423	16.08	8.33	2.42	26.83

	FUD	Status	MUE	Modifiers				IOM Reference
57423	90	A	1(2)	51	N/A	62	80	None

* with documentation

Terms To Know

approach. Method or anatomical location used to gain access to a body organ or specific area for procedures.

cystocele. Herniation of the bladder into the vagina.

defect. Imperfection, flaw, or absence.

fascia. Fibrous sheet or band of tissue that envelops organs, muscles, and groupings of muscles.

insufflation. Blowing air or gas into a body cavity.

laparoscopic. Minimally invasive procedure used for intraabdominal inspection; surgery that uses an endoscopic instrument inserted through small access incisions into the peritoneum for video-controlled imaging.

para-. Indicates near, similar, beside, or past.

perineocele. Uncommon condition in which herniation occurs in the perineal area between the rectum and vagina, the rectum and bladder, or beside the rectum.

prolapse. Falling, sliding, or sinking of an organ from its normal location in the body.

rectocele. Rectal tissue herniation into the vaginal wall.

repair. Surgical closure of a wound. The wound may be a result of injury/trauma or it may be a surgically created defect. Repairs are divided into three categories: simple, intermediate, and complex.

trocar. Cannula or a sharp pointed instrument used to puncture and aspirate fluid from cavities.

90935-90937

90935 Hemodialysis procedure with single evaluation by a physician or other qualified health care professional
90937 Hemodialysis procedure requiring repeated evaluation(s) with or without substantial revision of dialysis prescription

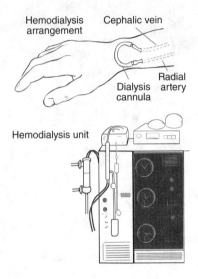

Hemodialysis arrangement
Cephalic vein
Dialysis cannula
Radial artery

Hemodialysis unit

Explanation

Hemodialysis is a process to remove toxins from the blood and to maintain fluid and electrolyte balance when the kidneys no longer function. The procedure involves using a previously placed catheter in an artery or a vein to withdraw the patient's blood, mechanically circulating the blood through a dialysis machine to remove the toxins and wastes, and transfusing the blood back to the patient. Code 90935 applies to one hemodialysis treatment that includes a single physician or other qualified health care provider's evaluation of the patient and 90937 is for a hemodialysis procedure when patient re-evaluation(s) must be done during the procedure, with or without substantial revision of the dialysis prescription.

Coding Tips

These codes include the hemodialysis procedure and all evaluation and management services provided that are related to the patient's renal disease on the day of the procedure. Any E/M services that are separately identifiable and unrelated to the dialysis or renal failure are reported separately with modifier 25. For home visit hemodialysis services performed by a nonphysician health care professional, see 99512. For prolonged physician or other qualified health care provider attendance, see 99354-99360.

ICD-10-CM Diagnostic Codes

I12.0	Hypertensive chronic kidney disease with stage 5 chronic kidney disease or end stage renal disease
I13.0	Hypertensive heart and chronic kidney disease with heart failure and stage 1 through stage 4 chronic kidney disease, or unspecified chronic kidney disease
I13.11	Hypertensive heart and chronic kidney disease without heart failure, with stage 5 chronic kidney disease, or end stage renal disease
I13.2	Hypertensive heart and chronic kidney disease with heart failure and with stage 5 chronic kidney disease, or end stage renal disease
I16.0	Hypertensive urgency
I16.1	Hypertensive emergency

N17.0	Acute kidney failure with tubular necrosis
N17.1	Acute kidney failure with acute cortical necrosis
N17.2	Acute kidney failure with medullary necrosis
N17.8	Other acute kidney failure
N18.4	Chronic kidney disease, stage 4 (severe)
N18.5	Chronic kidney disease, stage 5
N18.6	End stage renal disease
Z49.31	Encounter for adequacy testing for hemodialysis

AMA: **90935** 2018,Jan,8; 2017,Jan,8; 2016,Jan,13; 2015,Jan,16; 2014,Jan,11
90937 2018,Jan,8; 2017,Jan,8; 2016,Jan,13; 2015,Jan,16; 2014,Jan,11

Relative Value Units/Medicare Edits

Non-Facility RVU	Work	PE	MP	Total
90935	1.48	0.51	0.09	2.08
90937	2.11	0.74	0.12	2.97
Facility RVU	Work	PE	MP	Total
90935	1.48	0.51	0.09	2.08
90937	2.11	0.74	0.12	2.97

	FUD	Status	MUE	Modifiers				IOM Reference
90935	0	A	1(3)	N/A	N/A	N/A	80*	100-02,1,10;
90937	0	A	1(3)	N/A	N/A	N/A	80*	100-02,11,20;
								100-03,130.8;
								100-04,3,100.6;
								100-04,4,200.2

* with documentation

Terms To Know

cannula. Tube inserted into a blood vessel, duct, or body cavity to facilitate passage.

catheter. Flexible tube inserted into an area of the body for introducing or withdrawing fluid.

chronic kidney disease. Decreased renal efficiencies resulting in reduced ability of the kidney to filter waste. The National Kidney Foundation's classification includes five clinical stages, based on the glomerular filtration rate (GFR). The stages of CKD are as follows: stage 1, some kidney damage with normal or slightly increased GFR (> 90); stage 2, mild kidney damage with a GFR value of 60 to 89; stage 3, moderate kidney damage with a GFR value of 30 to 59; stage 4, severe kidney damage and a GFR value of 15 to 29; and stage 5, severe kidney damage that has progressed to a GFR value of less than 15. Dialysis or transplantation is required at stage 5.

ESRD. End stage renal disease. Progression of chronic renal failure to lasting and irreparable kidney damage that requires dialysis or renal transplant for survival.

hemodialysis. Cleansing of wastes and contaminating elements from the blood by virtue of different diffusion rates through a semipermeable membrane, which separates blood from a filtration solution that diffuses other elements out of the blood.

qualified health care professional. Educated, licensed or certified, and regulated professional operating under a specified scope of practice to provide patient services that are separate and distinct from other clinical staff.

© 2020 Optum360, LLC   **N** Newborn: 0   **P** Pediatric: 0-17   **M** Maternity: 9-64   **A** Adult: 15-124   ♂ Male Only   ♀ Female Only   CPT © 2020 American Medical Association. All Rights Reserved.

Medicine Services

90940

90940 Hemodialysis access flow study to determine blood flow in grafts and arteriovenous fistulae by an indicator method

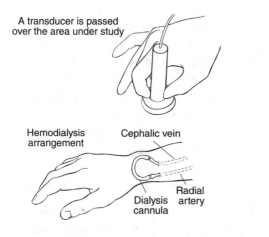

A transducer is passed over the area under study

Hemodialysis arrangement

Cephalic vein

Dialysis cannula

Radial artery

Explanation

A hemodialysis access flow study is performed to determine blood flow in a graft or arteriovenous fistula. The health care provider performs the test after approximately 30 minutes of treatment and after turning off ultrafiltration. In the direct dilution method, also known as the urea-based measurement of recirculation, arterial and venous line samples are drawn and the blood rate is reduced to 120 mL/minute. The blood pumped is turned off 10 seconds after reducing the blood flow rate and an arterial line is clamped above the sampling port. Systemic arterial samples are drawn, the line is disconnected, and dialysis is resumed. Measurements of BUN in the arterial, venous, and arterial sample are taken and the percent recirculation is calculated. This code includes the hook-up, measurement, and disconnection.

Coding Tips

For a duplex scan of hemodialysis access, see 93990. For external cannula declotting without balloon catheter, see 36860; with balloon catheter, see 36861. For declotting of an implanted vascular access device or catheter by thrombolytic agent, see 36593.

ICD-10-CM Diagnostic Codes

I12.0	Hypertensive chronic kidney disease with stage 5 chronic kidney disease or end stage renal disease
I13.0	Hypertensive heart and chronic kidney disease with heart failure and stage 1 through stage 4 chronic kidney disease, or unspecified chronic kidney disease
I13.11	Hypertensive heart and chronic kidney disease without heart failure, with stage 5 chronic kidney disease, or end stage renal disease
I13.2	Hypertensive heart and chronic kidney disease with heart failure and with stage 5 chronic kidney disease, or end stage renal disease
I16.0	Hypertensive urgency
I16.1	Hypertensive emergency
N17.0	Acute kidney failure with tubular necrosis
N17.1	Acute kidney failure with acute cortical necrosis
N17.2	Acute kidney failure with medullary necrosis
N17.8	Other acute kidney failure
N18.4	Chronic kidney disease, stage 4 (severe)
N18.5	Chronic kidney disease, stage 5
N18.6	End stage renal disease
T82.318A	Breakdown (mechanical) of other vascular grafts, initial encounter
T82.328A	Displacement of other vascular grafts, initial encounter
T82.338A	Leakage of other vascular grafts, initial encounter
T82.398A	Other mechanical complication of other vascular grafts, initial encounter
T82.41XA	Breakdown (mechanical) of vascular dialysis catheter, initial encounter
T82.42XA	Displacement of vascular dialysis catheter, initial encounter
T82.43XA	Leakage of vascular dialysis catheter, initial encounter
T82.49XA	Other complication of vascular dialysis catheter, initial encounter
T82.510A	Breakdown (mechanical) of surgically created arteriovenous fistula, initial encounter
T82.511A	Breakdown (mechanical) of surgically created arteriovenous shunt, initial encounter
T82.514A	Breakdown (mechanical) of infusion catheter, initial encounter
T82.520A	Displacement of surgically created arteriovenous fistula, initial encounter
T82.521A	Displacement of surgically created arteriovenous shunt, initial encounter
T82.524A	Displacement of infusion catheter, initial encounter
T82.528A	Displacement of other cardiac and vascular devices and implants, initial encounter
T82.530A	Leakage of surgically created arteriovenous fistula, initial encounter
T82.531A	Leakage of surgically created arteriovenous shunt, initial encounter
T82.534A	Leakage of infusion catheter, initial encounter
T82.590A	Other mechanical complication of surgically created arteriovenous fistula, initial encounter
T82.591A	Other mechanical complication of surgically created arteriovenous shunt, initial encounter
T82.594A	Other mechanical complication of infusion catheter, initial encounter
Z49.31	Encounter for adequacy testing for hemodialysis

AMA: **90940** 2018,Jan,8; 2017,Jan,8; 2016,Jan,13; 2015,Jan,16; 2014,Jan,11

Relative Value Units/Medicare Edits

Non-Facility RVU	Work	PE	MP	Total
90940	0.0	0.0	0.0	0.0
Facility RVU	**Work**	**PE**	**MP**	**Total**
90940	0.0	0.0	0.0	0.0

	FUD	Status	MUE	Modifiers				IOM Reference
90940	N/A	X	1(3)	N/A	N/A	N/A	N/A	None

* with documentation

CPT © 2020 American Medical Association. All Rights Reserved.   ● New   ▲ Revised   ＋ Add On   ★ Telemedicine   AMA: CPT Assist   [Resequenced]   ☑ Laterality   © 2020 Optum360, LLC

Medicine Services

90945-90947

90945 Dialysis procedure other than hemodialysis (eg, peritoneal dialysis, hemofiltration, or other continuous renal replacement therapies), with single evaluation by a physician or other qualified health care professional

90947 Dialysis procedure other than hemodialysis (eg, peritoneal dialysis, hemofiltration, or other continuous renal replacement therapies) requiring repeated evaluations by a physician or other qualified health care professional, with or without substantial revision of dialysis prescription

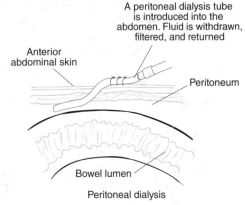

A peritoneal dialysis tube is introduced into the abdomen. Fluid is withdrawn, filtered, and returned

Anterior abdominal skin

Peritoneum

Bowel lumen

Peritoneal dialysis

The procedure may include, but is not limited to, peritoneal dialysis

Explanation

Dialysis is a process to remove toxins from the blood and to maintain fluid and electrolyte balance when the kidneys no longer function. In peritoneal dialysis, a fluid is introduced into the peritoneal cavity that removes toxins and electrolytes, which passively leach into the fluid. Hemofiltration, similar to hemodialysis, employs passing large volumes of blood over extracorporeal, adsorbent filters that remove waste products from the blood. Other continuous renal replacement therapies may be employed, such as continuous arteriovenous hemofiltration that uses small-volume, low-resistance blood filters that are powered by the patient's own arterial pressure, thus eliminating the need for a mechanical pump. Code 90945 applies to one dialysis procedure, other than hemodialysis, with a single physician or other qualified health care provider's evaluation of the patient. Code 90947 applies to a dialysis procedure, other than hemodialysis, that requires repeated provider evaluations, with or without substantial revision of a dialysis prescription.

Coding Tips

For prolonged physician or other qualified health care provider attendance, see 99354–99360. These codes include the dialysis procedure (other than hemodialysis) and all evaluation and management services provided that are related to the patient's renal disease on the day of the procedure. Any E/M services that are separately identifiable and unrelated to the dialysis or renal failure are reported separately with modifier 25. For home infusion of a peritoneal dialysis, see 99601–99602. For percutaneous insertion of an intraperitoneal tunneled catheter, see 49418; open approach, see 49421.

ICD-10-CM Diagnostic Codes

I12.0	Hypertensive chronic kidney disease with stage 5 chronic kidney disease or end stage renal disease
I13.0	Hypertensive heart and chronic kidney disease with heart failure and stage 1 through stage 4 chronic kidney disease, or unspecified chronic kidney disease
I13.11	Hypertensive heart and chronic kidney disease without heart failure, with stage 5 chronic kidney disease, or end stage renal disease
I13.2	Hypertensive heart and chronic kidney disease with heart failure and with stage 5 chronic kidney disease, or end stage renal disease
I16.0	Hypertensive urgency
I16.1	Hypertensive emergency
N17.0	Acute kidney failure with tubular necrosis
N17.1	Acute kidney failure with acute cortical necrosis
N17.2	Acute kidney failure with medullary necrosis
N17.8	Other acute kidney failure
N18.4	Chronic kidney disease, stage 4 (severe)
N18.5	Chronic kidney disease, stage 5
N18.6	End stage renal disease
Z49.31	Encounter for adequacy testing for hemodialysis

AMA: 90945 2018,Jan,8; 2017,Jan,8; 2016,Jan,13; 2015,Jan,16; 2014,Jan,11
90947 2018,Jan,8; 2017,Jan,8; 2016,Jan,13; 2015,Jan,16; 2014,Jan,11

Relative Value Units/Medicare Edits

Non-Facility RVU	Work	PE	MP	Total
90945	1.56	0.79	0.09	2.44
90947	2.52	0.87	0.15	3.54
Facility RVU	**Work**	**PE**	**MP**	**Total**
90945	1.56	0.79	0.09	2.44
90947	2.52	0.87	0.15	3.54

	FUD	Status	MUE	Modifiers				IOM Reference
90945	0	A	1(3)	N/A	N/A	N/A	80*	100-02,1,10;
90947	0	A	1(3)	N/A	N/A	N/A	80*	100-04,3,100.6; 100-04,4,200.2

* with documentation

Terms To Know

dialysis. Artificial filtering of the blood to remove contaminating waste elements and restore normal balance.

other qualified health care professional. Individual who is qualified by education, training, licensure/regulation, and facility privileging to perform a professional service within his or her scope of practice and independently (or as incident-to) report the professional service without requiring physician supervision. Payers may state exemptions in writing or state and local regulations may not follow this definition for performance of some services. Always refer to any relevant plan policies and federal and/or state laws to determine who may perform and report services.

90951-90953

★90951 End-stage renal disease (ESRD) related services monthly, for patients younger than 2 years of age to include monitoring for the adequacy of nutrition, assessment of growth and development, and counseling of parents; with 4 or more face-to-face visits by a physician or other qualified health care professional per month

★90952 with 2-3 face-to-face visits by a physician or other qualified health care professional per month

90953 with 1 face-to-face visit by a physician or other qualified health care professional per month

Explanation

These codes apply to all outpatient ESRD-related services provided during a one-month period for patients younger than 2 years of age. These codes include establishing the dialyzing cycle, all outpatient management for each dialysis visit, patient management during the dialysis treatment, any telephone calls, and evaluation and management related to the ESRD, such as assessing the patient's nutritional status, growth, and development and providing parental counseling. Dialysis treatment is not included. Code assignment is based on the number of face-to-face visits by a physician or other qualified health care provider per month. Report 90951 for four or more visits, 90952 for two or three visits, and 90953 for one visit.

Coding Tips

These codes are reported once per month and are assigned according to age and the number of face-to-face visits with the physician. These codes are reported when a complete assessment is performed regardless of when the assessment was completed relative to other episodes of care including hospitalizations. Do not report 90951-90953 with 99439, 99487-99489, or 99490-99491. Report the injection of 1 mcg of epoetin beta with HCPCS Level II code J0887. Medicare has provisionally identified code 90953 as a telehealth/telemedicine service. Current Medicare coverage guidelines should be reviewed. Commercial payers should be contacted regarding their coverage guidelines. Telemedicine services may be reported by the performing provider by adding modifier 95 to these procedure codes. Services at the origination site are reported with HCPCS Level II code Q3014.

ICD-10-CM Diagnostic Codes

I12.0	Hypertensive chronic kidney disease with stage 5 chronic kidney disease or end stage renal disease
I13.11	Hypertensive heart and chronic kidney disease without heart failure, with stage 5 chronic kidney disease, or end stage renal disease
I13.2	Hypertensive heart and chronic kidney disease with heart failure and with stage 5 chronic kidney disease, or end stage renal disease
I16.0	Hypertensive urgency
I16.1	Hypertensive emergency
N18.5	Chronic kidney disease, stage 5
N18.6	End stage renal disease
Z49.31	Encounter for adequacy testing for hemodialysis

AMA: 90951 2018,Jan,8; 2018,Feb,11; 2017,Jan,8; 2016,Jan,13; 2015,Jan,16; 2014,Oct,3; 2014,Jan,11 **90952** 2018,Jan,8; 2018,Feb,11; 2017,Jan,8; 2016,Jan,13; 2015,Jan,16; 2014,Oct,3; 2014,Jan,11 **90953** 2018,Jan,8; 2018,Feb,11; 2017,Jan,8; 2016,Jan,13; 2015,Jan,16; 2014,Oct,3; 2014,Jan,11

Relative Value Units/Medicare Edits

Non-Facility RVU	Work	PE	MP	Total
90951	18.46	6.96	1.18	26.6
90952	0.0	0.0	0.0	0.0
90953	0.0	0.0	0.0	0.0
Facility RVU	Work	PE	MP	Total
90951	18.46	6.96	1.18	26.6
90952	0.0	0.0	0.0	0.0
90953	0.0	0.0	0.0	0.0

	FUD	Status	MUE	Modifiers				IOM Reference
90951	N/A	A	1(2)	N/A	N/A	N/A	80*	None
90952	N/A	C	1(2)	N/A	N/A	N/A	80*	
90953	N/A	C	1(2)	N/A	N/A	N/A	80*	

* with documentation

Terms To Know

chronic kidney disease. Decreased renal efficiencies resulting in reduced ability of the kidney to filter waste. The National Kidney Foundation's classification includes five clinical stages, based on the glomerular filtration rate (GFR). The stages of CKD are as follows: stage 1, some kidney damage with normal or slightly increased GFR (> 90); stage 2, mild kidney damage with a GFR value of 60 to 89; stage 3, moderate kidney damage with a GFR value of 30 to 59; stage 4, severe kidney damage and a GFR value of 15 to 29; and stage 5, severe kidney damage that has progressed to a GFR value of less than 15. Dialysis or transplantation is required at stage 5.

counseling. Discussion with a patient and/or family concerning one or more of the following areas: diagnostic results, impressions, and/or recommended diagnostic studies; prognosis; risks and benefits of management (treatment) options; instructions for management (treatment) and/or follow-up; importance of compliance with chosen management (treatment) options; risk factor reduction; and patient and family education.

ESRD. End stage renal disease. Progression of chronic renal failure to lasting and irreparable kidney damage that requires dialysis or renal transplant for survival.

face to face. Interaction between two parties, usually provider and patient, that occurs in the physical presence of each other.

nutrition. Enteral and parenteral nutrition describe the administration of nutrients. Enteral nutrition: Nutrients are provided by a nasogastric or gastric tube for patients who cannot ingest, chew, or swallow food, though their bodies are able to absorb the nutrients. Parenteral nutrition: Nutrients are provided subcutaneously, intravenously, intramuscularly, or intradermally for patients during the postoperative period and in other conditions, such as shock, coma, and renal failure.

other qualified health care professional. Individual who is qualified by education, training, licensure/regulation, and facility privileging to perform a professional service within his or her scope of practice and independently (or as incident-to) report the professional service without requiring physician supervision. Payers may state exemptions in writing or state and local regulations may not follow this definition for performance of some services. Always refer to any relevant plan policies and federal and/or state laws to determine who may perform and report services.

Medicine Services

90954-90956

★90954   End-stage renal disease (ESRD) related services monthly, for patients 2-11 years of age to include monitoring for the adequacy of nutrition, assessment of growth and development, and counseling of parents; with 4 or more face-to-face visits by a physician or other qualified health care professional per month

★90955   with 2-3 face-to-face visits by a physician or other qualified health care professional per month

90956   with 1 face-to-face visit by a physician or other qualified health care professional per month

Explanation

These codes apply to all outpatient ESRD-related services provided during a one-month period for patients 2 to 11 years of age. These codes include establishing the dialyzing cycle, all outpatient management for each dialysis visit, patient management during the dialysis treatment, any telephone calls, and evaluation and management related to the ESRD, such as assessing the patient's nutritional status, growth, and development and providing parental counseling. Dialysis treatment is not included. Code assignment is based on the number of face-to-face visits by a physician or other qualified health care provider per month. Report 90954 for four or more visits, 90955 for two or three visits, and 90956 for one visit.

Coding Tips

These codes are reported once per month and are assigned according to age and the number of face-to-face visits with the physician. These codes are reported when a complete assessment is performed regardless of when the assessment was completed relative to other episodes of care including hospitalizations. Do not report 90954-90956 with 99439, 99487-99489, or 99490-99491. Report the injection of 1 mcg of epoetin beta with HCPCS Level II code J0887. Medicare has provisionally identified code 90956 as a telehealth/telemedicine service. Current Medicare coverage guidelines should be reviewed. Commercial payers should be contacted regarding their coverage guidelines. Telemedicine services may be reported by the performing provider by adding modifier 95 to these procedure codes. Services at the origination site are reported with HCPCS Level II code Q3014.

ICD-10-CM Diagnostic Codes

I12.0	Hypertensive chronic kidney disease with stage 5 chronic kidney disease or end stage renal disease
I13.11	Hypertensive heart and chronic kidney disease without heart failure, with stage 5 chronic kidney disease, or end stage renal disease
I13.2	Hypertensive heart and chronic kidney disease with heart failure and with stage 5 chronic kidney disease, or end stage renal disease
I16.0	Hypertensive urgency
I16.1	Hypertensive emergency
N18.5	Chronic kidney disease, stage 5
N18.6	End stage renal disease
Z49.31	Encounter for adequacy testing for hemodialysis

AMA: 90954 2018,Jan,8; 2018,Feb,11; 2017,Jan,8; 2016,Jan,13; 2015,Jan,16; 2014,Oct,3; 2014,Jan,11 **90955** 2018,Jan,8; 2018,Feb,11; 2017,Jan,8; 2016,Jan,13; 2015,Jan,16; 2014,Oct,3; 2014,Jan,11 **90956** 2018,Jan,8; 2018,Feb,11; 2017,Jan,8; 2016,Jan,13; 2015,Jan,16; 2014,Oct,3; 2014,Jan,11

Relative Value Units/Medicare Edits

Non-Facility RVU	Work	PE	MP	Total
90954	15.98	6.1	0.99	23.07
90955	8.79	3.69	0.52	13.0
90956	5.95	2.73	0.37	9.05
Facility RVU	Work	PE	MP	Total
90954	15.98	6.1	0.99	23.07
90955	8.79	3.69	0.52	13.0
90956	5.95	2.73	0.37	9.05

	FUD	Status	MUE	Modifiers				IOM Reference
90954	N/A	A	1(2)	N/A	N/A	N/A	80*	None
90955	N/A	A	1(2)	N/A	N/A	N/A	80*	
90956	N/A	A	1(2)	N/A	N/A	N/A	80*	

* with documentation

Terms To Know

chronic kidney disease. Decreased renal efficiencies resulting in reduced ability of the kidney to filter waste. The National Kidney Foundation's classification includes five clinical stages, based on the glomerular filtration rate (GFR). The stages of CKD are as follows: stage 1, some kidney damage with normal or slightly increased GFR (> 90); stage 2, mild kidney damage with a GFR value of 60 to 89; stage 3, moderate kidney damage with a GFR value of 30 to 59; stage 4, severe kidney damage and a GFR value of 15 to 29; and stage 5, severe kidney damage that has progressed to a GFR value of less than 15. Dialysis or transplantation is required at stage 5.

counseling. Discussion with a patient and/or family concerning one or more of the following areas: diagnostic results, impressions, and/or recommended diagnostic studies; prognosis; risks and benefits of management (treatment) options; instructions for management (treatment) and/or follow-up; importance of compliance with chosen management (treatment) options; risk factor reduction; and patient and family education.

ESRD. End stage renal disease. Progression of chronic renal failure to lasting and irreparable kidney damage that requires dialysis or renal transplant for survival.

face to face. Interaction between two parties, usually provider and patient, that occurs in the physical presence of each other.

other qualified health care professional. Individual who is qualified by education, training, licensure/regulation, and facility privileging to perform a professional service within his or her scope of practice and independently (or as incident-to) report the professional service without requiring physician supervision. Payers may state exemptions in writing or state and local regulations may not follow this definition for performance of some services. Always refer to any relevant plan policies and federal and/or state laws to determine who may perform and report services.

© 2020 Optum360, LLC   **N** Newborn: 0   **P** Pediatric: 0-17   **M** Maternity: 9-64   **A** Adult: 15-124   ♂ Male Only   ♀ Female Only   CPT © 2020 American Medical Association. All Rights Reserved.

Medicine Services

90957-90959

★**90957** End-stage renal disease (ESRD) related services monthly, for patients 12-19 years of age to include monitoring for the adequacy of nutrition, assessment of growth and development, and counseling of parents; with 4 or more face-to-face visits by a physician or other qualified health care professional per month

★**90958** with 2-3 face-to-face visits by a physician or other qualified health care professional per month

90959 with 1 face-to-face visit by a physician or other qualified health care professional per month

Explanation

These codes apply to all outpatient ESRD-related services provided during a one-month period for patients 12 to 19 years of age. These codes include establishing the dialyzing cycle, all outpatient management for each dialysis visit, patient management during the dialysis treatment, any telephone calls, and evaluation and management related to the ESRD, such as assessing the patient's nutritional status, growth, and development and providing parental counseling. Dialysis treatment is not included. Code assignment is based on the number of face-to-face visits by a physician or other qualified health care provider per month. Report 90957 for four or more visits, 90958 for two or three visits, and 90959 for one visit.

Coding Tips

These codes are reported once per month and are assigned according to age and the number of face-to-face visits with the physician. These codes are reported when a complete assessment is performed regardless of when the assessment was completed relative to other episodes of care including hospitalizations. Do not report 90957-90959 with 99439, 99487-99489, or 99490-99491. Report the injection of 1 mcg of epoetin beta with HCPCS Level II code J0887. Medicare has provisionally identified code 90959 as a telehealth/telemedicine service. Current Medicare coverage guidelines should be reviewed. Commercial payers should be contacted regarding their coverage guidelines. Telemedicine services may be reported by the performing provider by adding modifier 95 to these procedure codes. Services at the origination site are reported with HCPCS Level II code Q3014.

ICD-10-CM Diagnostic Codes

I12.0	Hypertensive chronic kidney disease with stage 5 chronic kidney disease or end stage renal disease
I13.11	Hypertensive heart and chronic kidney disease without heart failure, with stage 5 chronic kidney disease, or end stage renal disease
I13.2	Hypertensive heart and chronic kidney disease with heart failure and with stage 5 chronic kidney disease, or end stage renal disease
I16.0	Hypertensive urgency
I16.1	Hypertensive emergency
N18.5	Chronic kidney disease, stage 5
N18.6	End stage renal disease
Z49.31	Encounter for adequacy testing for hemodialysis

AMA: 90957 2018,Jan,8; 2018,Feb,11; 2017,Jan,8; 2016,Jan,13; 2015,Jan,16; 2014,Oct,3; 2014,Jan,11 **90958** 2018,Jan,8; 2018,Feb,11; 2017,Jan,8; 2016,Jan,13; 2015,Jan,16; 2014,Oct,3; 2014,Jan,11 **90959** 2018,Jan,8; 2018,Feb,11; 2017,Jan,8; 2016,Jan,13; 2015,Jan,16; 2014,Oct,3; 2014,Jan,11

Relative Value Units/Medicare Edits

Non-Facility RVU	Work	PE	MP	Total
90957	12.52	5.0	0.78	18.3
90958	8.34	3.58	0.51	12.43
90959	5.5	2.57	0.34	8.41
Facility RVU	**Work**	**PE**	**MP**	**Total**
90957	12.52	5.0	0.78	18.3
90958	8.34	3.58	0.51	12.43
90959	5.5	2.57	0.34	8.41

	FUD	Status	MUE	Modifiers				IOM Reference
90957	N/A	A	1(2)	N/A	N/A	N/A	80*	None
90958	N/A	A	1(2)	N/A	N/A	N/A	80*	
90959	N/A	A	1(2)	N/A	N/A	N/A	80*	

* with documentation

Terms To Know

chronic kidney disease. Decreased renal efficiencies resulting in reduced ability of the kidney to filter waste. The National Kidney Foundation's classification includes five clinical stages, based on the glomerular filtration rate (GFR). The stages of CKD are as follows: stage 1, some kidney damage with normal or slightly increased GFR (> 90); stage 2, mild kidney damage with a GFR value of 60 to 89; stage 3, moderate kidney damage with a GFR value of 30 to 59; stage 4, severe kidney damage and a GFR value of 15 to 29; and stage 5, severe kidney damage that has progressed to a GFR value of less than 15. Dialysis or transplantation is required at stage 5.

counseling. Discussion with a patient and/or family concerning one or more of the following areas: diagnostic results, impressions, and/or recommended diagnostic studies; prognosis; risks and benefits of management (treatment) options; instructions for management (treatment) and/or follow-up; importance of compliance with chosen management (treatment) options; risk factor reduction; and patient and family education.

ESRD. End stage renal disease. Progression of chronic renal failure to lasting and irreparable kidney damage that requires dialysis or renal transplant for survival.

face to face. Interaction between two parties, usually provider and patient, that occurs in the physical presence of each other.

nutrition. Enteral and parenteral nutrition describe the administration of nutrients. Enteral nutrition: Nutrients are provided by a nasogastric or gastric tube for patients who cannot ingest, chew, or swallow food, though their bodies are able to absorb the nutrients. Parenteral nutrition: Nutrients are provided subcutaneously, intravenously, intramuscularly, or intradermally for patients during the postoperative period and in other conditions, such as shock, coma, and renal failure.

other qualified health care professional. Individual who is qualified by education, training, licensure/regulation, and facility privileging to perform a professional service within his or her scope of practice and independently (or as incident-to) report the professional service without requiring physician supervision. Payers may state exemptions in writing or state and local regulations may not follow this definition for performance of some services. Always refer to any relevant plan policies and federal and/or state laws to determine who may perform and report services.

Medicine Services

90960-90962

★**90960** End-stage renal disease (ESRD) related services monthly, for patients 20 years of age and older; with 4 or more face-to-face visits by a physician or other qualified health care professional per month

★**90961** with 2-3 face-to-face visits by a physician or other qualified health care professional per month

90962 with 1 face-to-face visit by a physician or other qualified health care professional per month

Explanation

These codes apply to all outpatient ESRD-related services provided during a one-month period for patients 20 years of age or older. These codes include establishing the dialyzing cycle, all outpatient management for each dialysis visit, patient management during the dialysis treatment, any telephone calls, and evaluation and management related to the ESRD. Dialysis treatment is not included. Code assignment is based on the number of face-to-face visits by a physician or other qualified health care provider per month. Report 90960 for four or more visits, 90961 for two or three visits, and 90962 for one visit.

Coding Tips

These codes are reported once per month and are assigned according to age and the number of face-to-face visits with the physician. These codes are reported when a complete assessment is performed regardless of when the assessment was completed relative to other episodes of care including hospitalizations. Do not report 90960-90962 with 99439, 99487-99489, or 99490-99491. Report the injection of 1 mcg of epoetin beta with HCPCS Level II code J0887. Medicare has provisionally identified code 90962 as a telehealth/telemedicine service. Current Medicare coverage guidelines should be reviewed. Commercial payers should be contacted regarding their coverage guidelines. Telemedicine services may be reported by the performing provider by adding modifier 95 to these procedure codes. Services at the origination site are reported with HCPCS Level II code Q3014.

ICD-10-CM Diagnostic Codes

I12.0	Hypertensive chronic kidney disease with stage 5 chronic kidney disease or end stage renal disease
I13.11	Hypertensive heart and chronic kidney disease without heart failure, with stage 5 chronic kidney disease, or end stage renal disease
I13.2	Hypertensive heart and chronic kidney disease with heart failure and with stage 5 chronic kidney disease, or end stage renal disease
I16.0	Hypertensive urgency
I16.1	Hypertensive emergency
N18.5	Chronic kidney disease, stage 5
N18.6	End stage renal disease
Z49.31	Encounter for adequacy testing for hemodialysis

AMA: 90960 2018,Jan,8; 2018,Feb,11; 2017,Jan,8; 2016,Jan,13; 2015,Jan,16; 2014,Oct,3; 2014,Jan,11 **90961** 2018,Jan,8; 2018,Feb,11; 2017,Jan,8; 2016,Jan,13; 2015,Jan,16; 2014,Oct,3; 2014,Jan,11 **90962** 2018,Jan,8; 2018,Feb,11; 2017,Jan,8; 2016,Jan,13; 2015,Jan,16; 2014,Oct,3; 2014,Jan,11

Relative Value Units/Medicare Edits

Non-Facility RVU	Work	PE	MP	Total
90960	5.18	2.58	0.31	8.07
90961	4.26	2.26	0.26	6.78
90962	3.15	1.89	0.19	5.23
Facility RVU	**Work**	**PE**	**MP**	**Total**
90960	5.18	2.58	0.31	8.07
90961	4.26	2.26	0.26	6.78
90962	3.15	1.89	0.19	5.23

	FUD	Status	MUE	Modifiers				IOM Reference
90960	N/A	A	1(2)	N/A	N/A	N/A	80*	None
90961	N/A	A	1(2)	N/A	N/A	N/A	80*	
90962	N/A	A	1(2)	N/A	N/A	N/A	80*	

* with documentation

Terms To Know

chronic kidney disease. Decreased renal efficiencies resulting in reduced ability of the kidney to filter waste. The National Kidney Foundation's classification includes five clinical stages, based on the glomerular filtration rate (GFR). The stages of CKD are as follows: stage 1, some kidney damage with normal or slightly increased GFR (> 90); stage 2, mild kidney damage with a GFR value of 60 to 89; stage 3, moderate kidney damage with a GFR value of 30 to 59; stage 4, severe kidney damage and a GFR value of 15 to 29; and stage 5, severe kidney damage that has progressed to a GFR value of less than 15. Dialysis or transplantation is required at stage 5.

dialysis. Artificial filtering of the blood to remove contaminating waste elements and restore normal balance.

ESRD. End stage renal disease. Progression of chronic renal failure to lasting and irreparable kidney damage that requires dialysis or renal transplant for survival.

face to face. Interaction between two parties, usually provider and patient, that occurs in the physical presence of each other.

qualified health care professional. Educated, licensed or certified, and regulated professional operating under a specified scope of practice to provide patient services that are separate and distinct from other clinical staff.

90963-90966

90963 End-stage renal disease (ESRD) related services for home dialysis per full month, for patients younger than 2 years of age to include monitoring for the adequacy of nutrition, assessment of growth and development, and counseling of parents

90964 End-stage renal disease (ESRD) related services for home dialysis per full month, for patients 2-11 years of age to include monitoring for the adequacy of nutrition, assessment of growth and development, and counseling of parents

90965 End-stage renal disease (ESRD) related services for home dialysis per full month, for patients 12-19 years of age to include monitoring for the adequacy of nutrition, assessment of growth and development, and counseling of parents

90966 End-stage renal disease (ESRD) related services for home dialysis per full month, for patients 20 years of age and older

Explanation

These codes apply to all ESRD-related physician services provided during a one-month period to home dialysis patients of specified ages. These codes include establishing the dialyzing cycle as well as physician evaluation and management related to the ESRD. Codes 90963–90965 also include assessment of the patient's nutritional status, growth and development, and provision of parental counseling. Code assignment is based on age. Report 90963 for patients younger than 2 years of age, 90964 for patients 2 to 11 years of age, 90965 for patients 12 to 19 years of age, and 90966 for patients over the age of 20.

Coding Tips

These codes are reported once per month and are assigned according to age when dialysis services are provided in the home. These codes are reported when a complete assessment is performed regardless of when the assessment was completed relative to other episodes of care including hospitalizations. Do not report 90963-90966 with 99439, 99487-99489, or 99490-99491. Report the injection of 1 mcg of epoetin beta with HCPCS Level II code J0887. Medicare has identified these codes as telehealth/telemedicine services. Commercial payers should be contacted regarding their coverage guidelines. Telemedicine services may be reported by the performing provider by adding modifier 95 to these procedure codes. Services at the origination site are reported with HCPCS Level II code Q3014.

ICD-10-CM Diagnostic Codes

I12.0	Hypertensive chronic kidney disease with stage 5 chronic kidney disease or end stage renal disease
I13.11	Hypertensive heart and chronic kidney disease without heart failure, with stage 5 chronic kidney disease, or end stage renal disease
I13.2	Hypertensive heart and chronic kidney disease with heart failure and with stage 5 chronic kidney disease, or end stage renal disease
I16.0	Hypertensive urgency
I16.1	Hypertensive emergency
N18.5	Chronic kidney disease, stage 5
N18.6	End stage renal disease
Z49.31	Encounter for adequacy testing for hemodialysis

AMA: **90963** 2018,Jan,8; 2018,Feb,11; 2017,Jan,8; 2016,Jan,13; 2015,Jan,16; 2014,Oct,3; 2014,Jan,11 **90964** 2018,Jan,8; 2018,Feb,11; 2017,Jan,8; 2016,Jan,13; 2015,Jan,16; 2014,Oct,3; 2014,Jan,11 **90965** 2018,Jan,8; 2018,Feb,11; 2017,Jan,8;

Relative Value Units/Medicare Edits

Non-Facility RVU	Work	PE	MP	Total
90963	10.56	4.26	0.64	15.46
90964	9.14	3.82	0.56	13.52
90965	8.69	3.7	0.53	12.92
90966	4.26	2.25	0.26	6.77
Facility RVU	Work	PE	MP	Total
90963	10.56	4.26	0.64	15.46
90964	9.14	3.82	0.56	13.52
90965	8.69	3.7	0.53	12.92
90966	4.26	2.25	0.26	6.77

	FUD	Status	MUE	Modifiers				IOM Reference
90963	N/A	A	1(2)	N/A	N/A	N/A	80*	None
90964	N/A	A	1(2)	N/A	N/A	N/A	80*	
90965	N/A	A	1(2)	N/A	N/A	N/A	80*	
90966	N/A	A	1(2)	N/A	N/A	N/A	80*	

* with documentation

Terms To Know

assessment. Process of collecting and studying information and data, such as test values, signs, and symptoms.

chronic kidney disease. Decreased renal efficiencies resulting in reduced ability of the kidney to filter waste. The National Kidney Foundation's classification includes five clinical stages, based on the glomerular filtration rate (GFR). The stages of CKD are as follows: stage 1, some kidney damage with normal or slightly increased GFR (> 90); stage 2, mild kidney damage with a GFR value of 60 to 89; stage 3, moderate kidney damage with a GFR value of 30 to 59; stage 4, severe kidney damage and a GFR value of 15 to 29; and stage 5, severe kidney damage that has progressed to a GFR value of less than 15. Dialysis or transplantation is required at stage 5.

counseling. Discussion with a patient and/or family concerning one or more of the following areas: diagnostic results, impressions, and/or recommended diagnostic studies; prognosis; risks and benefits of management (treatment) options; instructions for management (treatment) and/or follow-up; importance of compliance with chosen management (treatment) options; risk factor reduction; and patient and family education.

dialysis. Artificial filtering of the blood to remove contaminating waste elements and restore normal balance.

ESRD. End stage renal disease. Progression of chronic renal failure to lasting and irreparable kidney damage that requires dialysis or renal transplant for survival.

evaluation. Dynamic process in which the physical, occupational, sports, or other therapist makes clinical judgments based on data gathered during the examination.

Medicine Services

90967-90970

90967 End-stage renal disease (ESRD) related services for dialysis less than a full month of service, per day; for patients younger than 2 years of age

90968 for patients 2-11 years of age

90969 for patients 12-19 years of age

90970 for patients 20 years of age and older

Explanation

This code range applies to all ESRD-related services provided to dialysis patients of specified ages who receive dialysis services for less than a full month. These codes are reported per day and are appropriate for use in the following circumstances: home dialysis patients who receive less than a full month of services; patients who are transient; a partial month in which one or more face-to-face visits occurred without a complete assessment; hospitalization of the patient prior to a complete assessment being made; and discontinuance of dialysis due to patient's recovery, receipt of a kidney transplant, or death. For reporting purposes, a month is considered 30 days. Code assignment is based on age. Report 90967 for patients younger than 2 years of age, 90968 for patients 2 to 11 years of age, 90969 for patients 12 to 19 years of age, and 90970 for patients over the age of 20.

Coding Tips

These codes report ESRD-related services provided for less than a full month (per day) and are age-specific. Do not report 90967-90970 with 99439, 99487-99489, or 99490-99491. Report the injection of 1 mcg of epoetin beta with HCPCS Level II code J0887. Medicare has identified these codes as telehealth/telemedicine services. Commercial payers should be contacted regarding their coverage guidelines. Telemedicine services may be reported by the performing provider by adding modifier 95 to these procedure codes. Services at the origination site are reported with HCPCS Level II code Q3014.

ICD-10-CM Diagnostic Codes

I12.0	Hypertensive chronic kidney disease with stage 5 chronic kidney disease or end stage renal disease
I13.11	Hypertensive heart and chronic kidney disease without heart failure, with stage 5 chronic kidney disease, or end stage renal disease
I13.2	Hypertensive heart and chronic kidney disease with heart failure and with stage 5 chronic kidney disease, or end stage renal disease
I16.0	Hypertensive urgency
I16.1	Hypertensive emergency
N18.5	Chronic kidney disease, stage 5
N18.6	End stage renal disease
Z49.31	Encounter for adequacy testing for hemodialysis

AMA: 90967 2018,Jan,8; 2018,Feb,11; 2017,Jan,8; 2016,Jan,13; 2015,Jan,16; 2014,Oct,3; 2014,Jan,11 **90968** 2018,Jan,8; 2018,Feb,11; 2017,Jan,8; 2016,Jan,13; 2015,Jan,16; 2014,Oct,3; 2014,Jan,11 **90969** 2018,Jan,8; 2018,Feb,11; 2017,Jan,8; 2016,Jan,13; 2015,Jan,16; 2014,Oct,3; 2014,Jan,11 **90970** 2018,Jan,8; 2018,Feb,11; 2017,Jan,8; 2016,Jan,13; 2015,Jan,16; 2014,Oct,3; 2014,Jan,11

Relative Value Units/Medicare Edits

Non-Facility RVU	Work	PE	MP	Total
90967	0.35	0.14	0.02	0.51
90968	0.3	0.13	0.02	0.45
90969	0.29	0.12	0.02	0.43
90970	0.14	0.08	0.01	0.23
Facility RVU	Work	PE	MP	Total
90967	0.35	0.14	0.02	0.51
90968	0.3	0.13	0.02	0.45
90969	0.29	0.12	0.02	0.43
90970	0.14	0.08	0.01	0.23

	FUD	Status	MUE	Modifiers				IOM Reference
90967	N/A	A	1(2)	N/A	N/A	N/A	80*	None
90968	N/A	A	1(2)	N/A	N/A	N/A	80*	
90969	N/A	A	1(2)	N/A	N/A	N/A	80*	
90970	N/A	A	1(2)	N/A	N/A	N/A	80*	

* with documentation

Terms To Know

assessment. Process of collecting and studying information and data, such as test values, signs, and symptoms.

chronic kidney disease. Decreased renal efficiencies resulting in reduced ability of the kidney to filter waste. The National Kidney Foundation's classification includes five clinical stages, based on the glomerular filtration rate (GFR). The stages of CKD are as follows: stage 1, some kidney damage with normal or slightly increased GFR (> 90); stage 2, mild kidney damage with a GFR value of 60 to 89; stage 3, moderate kidney damage with a GFR value of 30 to 59; stage 4, severe kidney damage and a GFR value of 15 to 29; and stage 5, severe kidney damage that has progressed to a GFR value of less than 15. Dialysis or transplantation is required at stage 5.

dialysis. Artificial filtering of the blood to remove contaminating waste elements and restore normal balance.

ESRD. End stage renal disease. Progression of chronic renal failure to lasting and irreparable kidney damage that requires dialysis or renal transplant for survival.

face to face. Interaction between two parties, usually provider and patient, that occurs in the physical presence of each other.

© 2020 Optum360, LLC

N Newborn: 0　**P** Pediatric: 0-17　**M** Maternity: 9-64　**A** Adult: 15-124　♂ Male Only　♀ Female Only

CPT © 2020 American Medical Association. All Rights Reserved.

90989-90993

90989 Dialysis training, patient, including helper where applicable, any mode, completed course

90993 Dialysis training, patient, including helper where applicable, any mode, course not completed, per training session

Explanation

The physician or health care provider trains the patient and/or the patient's caregiving helper to perform the dialysis procedure, any mode. Report 90989 when the course is completed; 90993 is reported per training session of the course when it is not completed.

Coding Tips

Report 90993 when only a portion of the course is completed, for each session that is given. Report 90989 one time only for the entire course when completed. It is not appropriate to report 90993 for individual sessions followed by 90989 at a later time when the entire course of self-care and treatment is completed.

ICD-10-CM Diagnostic Codes

I12.0	Hypertensive chronic kidney disease with stage 5 chronic kidney disease or end stage renal disease
I13.11	Hypertensive heart and chronic kidney disease without heart failure, with stage 5 chronic kidney disease, or end stage renal disease
I13.2	Hypertensive heart and chronic kidney disease with heart failure and with stage 5 chronic kidney disease, or end stage renal disease
I16.0	Hypertensive urgency
I16.1	Hypertensive emergency
N17.0	Acute kidney failure with tubular necrosis
N17.1	Acute kidney failure with acute cortical necrosis
N17.2	Acute kidney failure with medullary necrosis
N17.8	Other acute kidney failure
N18.4	Chronic kidney disease, stage 4 (severe)
N18.5	Chronic kidney disease, stage 5
N18.6	End stage renal disease

AMA: 90989 2018,Jan,8; 2018,Feb,11; 2017,Jan,8; 2016,Jan,13; 2015,Jan,16; 2014,Jan,11 **90993** 2018,Jan,8; 2018,Feb,11; 2017,Jan,8; 2016,Jan,13; 2015,Jan,16; 2014,Jan,11

Relative Value Units/Medicare Edits

Non-Facility RVU	Work	PE	MP	Total
90989	0.0	0.0	0.0	0.0
90993	0.0	0.0	0.0	0.0
Facility RVU	Work	PE	MP	Total
90989	0.0	0.0	0.0	0.0
90993	0.0	0.0	0.0	0.0

	FUD	Status	MUE	Modifiers				IOM Reference
90989	N/A	X	1(2)	N/A	N/A	N/A	N/A	100-04,3,100.6
90993	N/A	X	1(3)	N/A	N/A	N/A	N/A	

* with documentation

93980-93981

93980 Duplex scan of arterial inflow and venous outflow of penile vessels; complete study

93981 follow-up or limited study

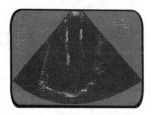

Arterial and venous flow of the penile area is studied

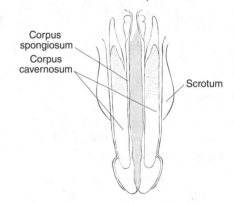

Corpus spongiosum
Corpus cavernosum
Scrotum

Explanation

The physician performs a Duplex ultrasound scan, producing real-time images integrating B-mode two-dimensional structure with Doppler mapping or imaging of motion with time, of the arteries and veins in the penis to evaluate vascular blood flow in and out of the penis in relation to blockages. Report 93980 for a complete evaluation and 93981 for a follow-up or a limited study.

Coding Tips

Use these codes to report the duplex scan of vascular inflow and outflow of the penile vessels only. For a duplex scan of the vascular inflow and outflow of scrotal contents, see 93975–93976.

ICD-10-CM Diagnostic Codes

F52.21	Male erectile disorder ♂
N50.1	Vascular disorders of male genital organs ♂
N52.01	Erectile dysfunction due to arterial insufficiency 🅰 ♂
N52.02	Corporo-venous occlusive erectile dysfunction 🅰 ♂
N52.03	Combined arterial insufficiency and corporo-venous occlusive erectile dysfunction 🅰 ♂
N52.2	Drug-induced erectile dysfunction 🅰 ♂
N52.31	Erectile dysfunction following radical prostatectomy 🅰 ♂
N52.32	Erectile dysfunction following radical cystectomy 🅰 ♂
N52.33	Erectile dysfunction following urethral surgery 🅰 ♂
N52.34	Erectile dysfunction following simple prostatectomy 🅰 ♂
N52.35	Erectile dysfunction following radiation therapy 🅰 ♂
N52.36	Erectile dysfunction following interstitial seed therapy 🅰 ♂
N52.37	Erectile dysfunction following prostate ablative therapy 🅰 ♂
N52.8	Other male erectile dysfunction 🅰 ♂
S38.01XA	Crushing injury of penis, initial encounter ♂

CPT © 2020 American Medical Association. All Rights Reserved. ● New ▲ Revised + Add On ★ Telemedicine AMA: CPT Assist [Resequenced] ☑ Laterality © 2020 Optum360, LLC

Medicine Services

S38.02XA   Crushing injury of scrotum and testis, initial encounter ♂

AMA: **93980** 2018,Jan,8; 2018,Feb,11; 2017,Jan,8; 2016,Jan,13; 2015,Jan,16; 2014,Jan,11 **93981** 2018,Jan,8; 2018,Feb,11; 2017,Jan,8; 2016,Jan,13; 2015,Jan,16; 2014,Jan,11

Relative Value Units/Medicare Edits

Non-Facility RVU	Work	PE	MP	Total
93980	1.25	2.15	0.06	3.46
93981	0.44	1.61	0.03	2.08
Facility RVU	**Work**	**PE**	**MP**	**Total**
93980	1.25	2.15	0.06	3.46
93981	0.44	1.61	0.03	2.08

	FUD	Status	MUE	Modifiers				IOM Reference
93980	N/A	A	1(3)	N/A	N/A	N/A	80*	None
93981	N/A	A	1(3)	N/A	N/A	N/A	80*	

* with documentation

Terms To Know

2-D. Two-dimensional or cross-sectional view produced by reconstructed B-mode ultrasound scanning or multiple angled x-ray images, such as from computed tomography, for diagnostic purposes.

artery. Vessel through which oxygenated blood passes away from the heart to any part of the body.

B-mode. Implies two-dimensional procedure with two-dimensional display.

doppler. Ultrasonography used to augment two-dimensional images by registering velocity. When emitted sound waves reflect back off a moving object, the frequency of the reflected sound waves varies in relation to the speed of the moving object and may be used in many different procedures.

duplex scan. Noninvasive vascular diagnostic technique that uses ultrasonic scanning to identify the pattern and direction of blood flow within arteries or veins displayed in real time images.

evaluation. Dynamic process in which the dentist makes clinical judgments based on data gathered during the examination.

real-time. Immediate imaging, with movement as it happens.

vein. Vessel through which oxygen-depleted blood passes back to the heart.

93985-93986

93985   Duplex scan of arterial inflow and venous outflow for preoperative vessel assessment prior to creation of hemodialysis access; complete bilateral study
93986   complete unilateral study

Explanation

The physician performs a Duplex ultrasound scan, producing real-time images integrating B-mode two-dimensional structure with Doppler mapping or imaging of motion with time for preoperative assessment of vascular blood flow prior to the creation of a hemodialysis access. This assessment includes the arterial inflow and venous outflow. Native arteriovenous fistula (AVF) is the preferred vascular access for hemodialysis patients, lasting longer and having fewer complications than grafts and central venous catheters. The use of the Doppler ultrasound (DUS) in preoperative vascular mapping enables identification of vessels that are most appropriate for fistula construction. Report 93985 for a complete bilateral study and 93986 for a complete unilateral study.

Coding Tips

Do not report 93985 or 93986 with 93990 for the same extremity. Do not report 93985 with 93925, 93930, or 93970 for the same extremity. Do not report 93986 with 93926, 93931, or 93971 for the same extremity.

ICD-10-CM Diagnostic Codes

E10.21	Type 1 diabetes mellitus with diabetic nephropathy
E10.22	Type 1 diabetes mellitus with diabetic chronic kidney disease
E10.29	Type 1 diabetes mellitus with other diabetic kidney complication
E11.21	Type 2 diabetes mellitus with diabetic nephropathy
E11.22	Type 2 diabetes mellitus with diabetic chronic kidney disease
E11.29	Type 2 diabetes mellitus with other diabetic kidney complication
E13.21	Other specified diabetes mellitus with diabetic nephropathy
E13.22	Other specified diabetes mellitus with diabetic chronic kidney disease
E13.29	Other specified diabetes mellitus with other diabetic kidney complication
I12.0	Hypertensive chronic kidney disease with stage 5 chronic kidney disease or end stage renal disease
I13.11	Hypertensive heart and chronic kidney disease without heart failure, with stage 5 chronic kidney disease, or end stage renal disease
I13.2	Hypertensive heart and chronic kidney disease with heart failure and with stage 5 chronic kidney disease, or end stage renal disease
N18.5	Chronic kidney disease, stage 5
N18.6	End stage renal disease
Z49.31	Encounter for adequacy testing for hemodialysis

Medicine Services

Relative Value Units/Medicare Edits

Non-Facility RVU	Work	PE	MP	Total
93985	0.8	6.61	0.12	7.53
93986	0.5	3.77	0.1	4.37
Facility RVU	Work	PE	MP	Total
93985	0.8	6.61	0.12	7.53
93986	0.5	3.77	0.1	4.37

	FUD	Status	MUE	Modifiers				IOM Reference
93985	N/A	A	1(3)	N/A	N/A	N/A	80*	None
93986	N/A	A	1(3)	N/A	N/A	N/A	80*	

* with documentation

Terms To Know

chronic kidney disease. Decreased renal efficiencies resulting in reduced ability of the kidney to filter waste. The National Kidney Foundation's classification includes five clinical stages, based on the glomerular filtration rate (GFR). The stages of CKD are as follows: stage 1, some kidney damage with normal or slightly increased GFR (> 90); stage 2, mild kidney damage with a GFR value of 60 to 89; stage 3, moderate kidney damage with a GFR value of 30 to 59; stage 4, severe kidney damage and a GFR value of 15 to 29; and stage 5, severe kidney damage that has progressed to a GFR value of less than 15. Dialysis or transplantation is required at stage 5.

duplex scan. Noninvasive vascular diagnostic technique that uses ultrasonic scanning to identify the pattern and direction of blood flow within arteries or veins displayed in real time images.

ESRD. End stage renal disease. Progression of chronic renal failure to lasting and irreparable kidney damage that requires dialysis or renal transplant for survival.

hemodialysis. Cleansing of wastes and contaminating elements from the blood by virtue of different diffusion rates through a semipermeable membrane, which separates blood from a filtration solution that diffuses other elements out of the blood.

93990

93990 Duplex scan of hemodialysis access (including arterial inflow, body of access and venous outflow)

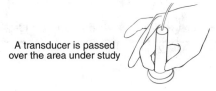
A transducer is passed over the area under study

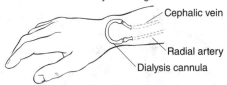
Hemodialysis arrangement
Cephalic vein
Radial artery
Dialysis cannula

A Duplex ultrasound scan is performed on a dialysis catheter

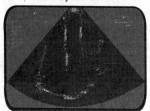
Arterial and venous flow are studied

Explanation

The physician performs a Duplex ultrasound scan, producing real-time images integrating B-mode two-dimensional structure with Doppler mapping or imaging of motion with time, of a hemodialysis access site, including the arterial inflow, body of the access site or device, and venous outflow, to evaluate vascular blood flow in relation to blockage.

Coding Tips

For hemoperfusion, see 90997. For measurement of hemodialysis access flow via indicator dilution methods, see 90940.

ICD-10-CM Diagnostic Codes

I12.0	Hypertensive chronic kidney disease with stage 5 chronic kidney disease or end stage renal disease
I13.11	Hypertensive heart and chronic kidney disease without heart failure, with stage 5 chronic kidney disease, or end stage renal disease
I13.2	Hypertensive heart and chronic kidney disease with heart failure and with stage 5 chronic kidney disease, or end stage renal disease
I16.0	Hypertensive urgency
I16.1	Hypertensive emergency
N18.5	Chronic kidney disease, stage 5
N18.6	End stage renal disease

AMA: 93990 2019,Oct,8; 2018,Jan,8; 2018,Feb,11; 2017,Jan,8; 2016,Jan,13; 2015,Jan,16; 2014,Jan,11

Relative Value Units/Medicare Edits

Non-Facility RVU	Work	PE	MP	Total
93990	0.5	3.78	0.11	4.39
Facility RVU	Work	PE	MP	Total
93990	0.5	3.78	0.11	4.39

	FUD	Status	MUE	Modifiers				IOM Reference
93990	N/A	A	2(3)	N/A	N/A	N/A	80*	None

* with documentation

Terms To Know

2-D. Two-dimensional or cross-sectional view produced by reconstructed B-mode ultrasound scanning or multiple angled x-ray images, such as from computed tomography, for diagnostic purposes.

B-mode. Implies two-dimensional procedure with two-dimensional display.

chronic kidney disease. Decreased renal efficiencies resulting in reduced ability of the kidney to filter waste. The National Kidney Foundation's classification includes five clinical stages, based on the glomerular filtration rate (GFR). The stages of CKD are as follows: stage 1, some kidney damage with normal or slightly increased GFR (> 90); stage 2, mild kidney damage with a GFR value of 60 to 89; stage 3, moderate kidney damage with a GFR value of 30 to 59; stage 4, severe kidney damage and a GFR value of 15 to 29; and stage 5, severe kidney damage that has progressed to a GFR value of less than 15. Dialysis or transplantation is required at stage 5.

doppler. Ultrasonography used to augment two-dimensional images by registering velocity. When emitted sound waves reflect back off a moving object, the frequency of the reflected sound waves varies in relation to the speed of the moving object and may be used in many different procedures.

duplex scan. Noninvasive vascular diagnostic technique that uses ultrasonic scanning to identify the pattern and direction of blood flow within arteries or veins displayed in real time images.

ESRD. End stage renal disease. Progression of chronic renal failure to lasting and irreparable kidney damage that requires dialysis or renal transplant for survival.

hemodialysis. Cleansing of wastes and contaminating elements from the blood by virtue of different diffusion rates through a semipermeable membrane, which separates blood from a filtration solution that diffuses other elements out of the blood.

imaging. Radiologic means of producing pictures for clinical study of the internal structures and functions of the body, such as x-ray, ultrasound, magnetic resonance, or positron emission tomography.

real-time. Immediate imaging, with movement as it happens.

transducer. Apparatus that transfers or translates one type of energy into another, such as converting pressure to an electrical signal.

99512

99512   Home visit for hemodialysis

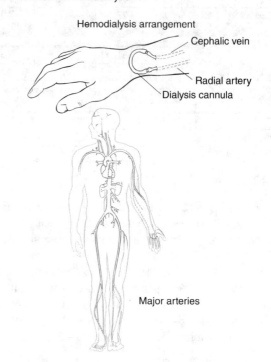

Explanation

This code reports a home visit for hemodialysis. A home health nurse commonly visits the patient three times a week to provide hemodialysis. Each treatment lasts from two to four hours. Before treatment, access is made to the bloodstream to provide a way for blood to be carried from the patient to the dialysis machine, which filters out wastes and extra fluids and returns the blood back to the patient. The access may be under the skin or outside the body. During treatment, the patient can read, write, sleep, talk, or watch television.

Coding Tips

For hemoperfusion, see 90997. For home infusion of peritoneal dialysis, see 99601–99602.

ICD-10-CM Diagnostic Codes

I12.0	Hypertensive chronic kidney disease with stage 5 chronic kidney disease or end stage renal disease
I13.0	Hypertensive heart and chronic kidney disease with heart failure and stage 1 through stage 4 chronic kidney disease, or unspecified chronic kidney disease
I13.11	Hypertensive heart and chronic kidney disease without heart failure, with stage 5 chronic kidney disease, or end stage renal disease
I13.2	Hypertensive heart and chronic kidney disease with heart failure and with stage 5 chronic kidney disease, or end stage renal disease
I16.0	Hypertensive urgency
I16.1	Hypertensive emergency
N18.4	Chronic kidney disease, stage 4 (severe)
N18.5	Chronic kidney disease, stage 5
N18.6	End stage renal disease

© 2020 Optum360, LLC   **N** Newborn: 0   **P** Pediatric: 0-17   **M** Maternity: 9-64   **A** Adult: 15-124   ♂ Male Only   ♀ Female Only   CPT © 2020 American Medical Association. All Rights Reserved.

Medicine Services

| Z49.01 | Encounter for fitting and adjustment of extracorporeal dialysis catheter |
| Z49.31 | Encounter for adequacy testing for hemodialysis |

AMA: **99512** 2018,Jan,8; 2017,Jan,8; 2016,Jan,13; 2015,Jan,16; 2014,Jan,11

Relative Value Units/Medicare Edits

Non-Facility RVU	Work	PE	MP	Total
99512	0.0	0.0	0.0	0.0
Facility RVU	**Work**	**PE**	**MP**	**Total**
99512	0.0	0.0	0.0	0.0

	FUD	Status	MUE	Modifiers				IOM Reference
99512	N/A	I	0(3)	N/A	N/A	N/A	N/A	None

* with documentation

Terms To Know

cannula. Tube inserted into a blood vessel, duct, or body cavity to facilitate passage.

chronic kidney disease. Decreased renal efficiencies resulting in reduced ability of the kidney to filter waste. The National Kidney Foundation's classification includes five clinical stages, based on the glomerular filtration rate (GFR). The stages of CKD are as follows: stage 1, some kidney damage with normal or slightly increased GFR (> 90); stage 2, mild kidney damage with a GFR value of 60 to 89; stage 3, moderate kidney damage with a GFR value of 30 to 59; stage 4, severe kidney damage and a GFR value of 15 to 29; and stage 5, severe kidney damage that has progressed to a GFR value of less than 15. Dialysis or transplantation is required at stage 5.

ESRD. End stage renal disease. Progression of chronic renal failure to lasting and irreparable kidney damage that requires dialysis or renal transplant for survival.

hemodialysis. Cleansing of wastes and contaminating elements from the blood by virtue of different diffusion rates through a semipermeable membrane, which separates blood from a filtration solution that diffuses other elements out of the blood.

home health services. Services furnished to patients in their homes under the care of physicians. These services include part-time or intermittent skilled nursing care, physical therapy, medical social services, medical supplies, and some rehabilitation equipment. Home health supplies and services must be prescribed by a physician, and the beneficiary must be confined at home in order for Medicare to pay the benefits in full.

99601-99602

| 99601 | Home infusion/specialty drug administration, per visit (up to 2 hours); |
| + 99602 | each additional hour (List separately in addition to code for primary procedure) |

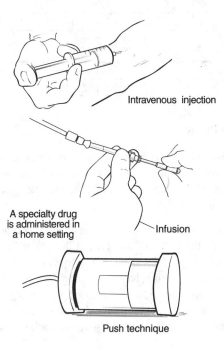

Intravenous injection

A specialty drug is administered in a home setting

Infusion

Push technique

Explanation

A home health professional visits the patient at home to perform the infusion of a specialty drug per a physician's order. The home health provider brings the supplies and medication required and administers and oversees the infusion. Each infusion takes up to two hours per visit for 99601. Report 99602 for each additional hour.

Coding Tips

Report 99602 in addition to 99601. These codes do not include the patient's self-administration of the medication. Any and all solutions, equipment, supplies, and drugs are excluded from this code and must be reported separately.

ICD-10-CM Diagnostic Codes

The application of this code is too broad to adequately present ICD-10-CM diagnostic code links here. Refer to your ICD-10-CM book.

AMA: **99601** 2005,Nov,1-9 **99602** 2005,Nov,1-9

Relative Value Units/Medicare Edits

Non-Facility RVU	Work	PE	MP	Total
99601	0.0	0.0	0.0	0.0
99602	0.0	0.0	0.0	0.0
Facility RVU	**Work**	**PE**	**MP**	**Total**
99601	0.0	0.0	0.0	0.0
99602	0.0	0.0	0.0	0.0

	FUD	Status	MUE	Modifiers				IOM Reference
99601	N/A	I	0(3)	N/A	N/A	N/A	N/A	None
99602	N/A	I	0(3)	N/A	N/A	N/A	N/A	

* with documentation

Terms To Know

add-on code. Code representing a procedure performed in addition to the primary procedure and is represented with a + in the CPT book. Add-on codes are never reported for stand-alone services but are reported secondarily in addition to the primary procedure.

drugs and biologicals. Drugs and biologicals included - or approved for inclusion - in the United States Pharmacopoeia, the National Formulary, the United States Homeopathic Pharmacopoeia, in New Drugs or Accepted Dental Remedies, or approved by the pharmacy and drug therapeutics committee of the medical staff of the hospital. Also included are medically accepted and FDA approved drugs used in an anticancer chemotherapeutic regimen. The carrier determines medical acceptance based on supportive clinical evidence.

home health. Palliative and therapeutic care and assistance in the activities of daily life to home bound Medicare and private plan members.

infusion. Introduction of a therapeutic fluid, other than blood, into the bloodstream.

intravenous. Within a vein or veins.

medications. Drugs and biologicals that an individual is already taking, that are ordered for the individual during the course of treatment, or that are ordered for an individual after treatment has been provided.

supplies. Items or accessories needed for the performance of procedures, or for the effective use of durable medical equipment, prosthetics, orthotic devices, and appliances.

G0102

G0102 Prostate cancer screening; digital rectal examination

Explanation

This code reports a prostate cancer screening performed manually by the physician as a digital rectal exam in order to palpate the prostate and check for abnormalities.

Coding Tips

This screening service is covered by Medicare once every 12 months for men who are 50 years of age or older. A minimum of 11 months must have passed following the month in which the last Medicare-covered screening digital rectal examination was performed.

ICD-10-CM Diagnostic Codes

Z12.5   Encounter for screening for malignant neoplasm of prostate ♂

Relative Value Units/Medicare Edits

Non-Facility RVU	Work	PE	MP	Total
G0102	0.17	0.46	0.01	0.64
Facility RVU	**Work**	**PE**	**MP**	**Total**
G0102	0.17	0.07	0.01	0.25

	FUD	Status	MUE	Modifiers				IOM Reference
G0102	N/A	A	1(2)	N/A	N/A	N/A	N/A	None

* with documentation

Terms To Know

malignant neoplasm. Any cancerous tumor or lesion exhibiting uncontrolled tissue growth that can progressively invade other parts of the body with its disease-generating cells.

prostate. Male gland surrounding the bladder neck and urethra that secretes a substance into the seminal fluid.

rectal. Pertaining to the rectum, the end portion of the large intestine.

screening test. Exam or study used by a physician to identify abnormalities, regardless of whether the patient exhibits symptoms.

G0168

G0168 Wound closure utilizing tissue adhesive(s) only

Explanation

Wound closure done by using tissue adhesive only, not any kind of suturing or stapling, is reported with this code. Tissue adhesives, such as Dermabond, are materials that are applied directly to the skin or tissue of an open wound to hold the margins closed for healing.

Coding Tips

This code is reported when a Medicare patient undergoes a superficial repair or closure using a tissue adhesive only. This includes instances where sutures have been used for the repair of deeper layers and tissue adhesive is used to close the superficial layer. Payment for this service is at the discretion of the carrier.

ICD-10-CM Diagnostic Codes

S30.812A   Abrasion of penis, initial encounter ♂

S30.813A   Abrasion of scrotum and testes, initial encounter ♂

S30.814A   Abrasion of vagina and vulva, initial encounter ♀

S31.010A   Laceration without foreign body of lower back and pelvis without penetration into retroperitoneum, initial encounter

S31.030A   Puncture wound without foreign body of lower back and pelvis without penetration into retroperitoneum, initial encounter

S31.050A   Open bite of lower back and pelvis without penetration into retroperitoneum, initial encounter

S31.110A   Laceration without foreign body of abdominal wall, right upper quadrant without penetration into peritoneal cavity, initial encounter ☑

S31.111A   Laceration without foreign body of abdominal wall, left upper quadrant without penetration into peritoneal cavity, initial encounter ☑

S31.112A   Laceration without foreign body of abdominal wall, epigastric region without penetration into peritoneal cavity, initial encounter

S31.113A   Laceration without foreign body of abdominal wall, right lower quadrant without penetration into peritoneal cavity, initial encounter ☑

S31.114A   Laceration without foreign body of abdominal wall, left lower quadrant without penetration into peritoneal cavity, initial encounter ☑

S31.115A   Laceration without foreign body of abdominal wall, periumbilic region without penetration into peritoneal cavity, initial encounter

S31.130A   Puncture wound of abdominal wall without foreign body, right upper quadrant without penetration into peritoneal cavity, initial encounter ☑

S31.131A   Puncture wound of abdominal wall without foreign body, left upper quadrant without penetration into peritoneal cavity, initial encounter ☑

S31.132A   Puncture wound of abdominal wall without foreign body, epigastric region without penetration into peritoneal cavity, initial encounter

S31.133A   Puncture wound of abdominal wall without foreign body, right lower quadrant without penetration into peritoneal cavity, initial encounter ☑

CPT © 2020 American Medical Association. All Rights Reserved.   ● New   ▲ Revised   + Add On   ★ Telemedicine   AMA: CPT Assist   [Resequenced]   ☑ Laterality   © 2020 Optum360, LLC

HCPCS

S31.134A	Puncture wound of abdominal wall without foreign body, left lower quadrant without penetration into peritoneal cavity, initial encounter ☑
S31.135A	Puncture wound of abdominal wall without foreign body, periumbilic region without penetration into peritoneal cavity, initial encounter
S31.150A	Open bite of abdominal wall, right upper quadrant without penetration into peritoneal cavity, initial encounter ☑
S31.151A	Open bite of abdominal wall, left upper quadrant without penetration into peritoneal cavity, initial encounter ☑
S31.152A	Open bite of abdominal wall, epigastric region without penetration into peritoneal cavity, initial encounter
S31.153A	Open bite of abdominal wall, right lower quadrant without penetration into peritoneal cavity, initial encounter ☑
S31.154A	Open bite of abdominal wall, left lower quadrant without penetration into peritoneal cavity, initial encounter ☑
S31.155A	Open bite of abdominal wall, periumbilic region without penetration into peritoneal cavity, initial encounter
S31.21XA	Laceration without foreign body of penis, initial encounter ♂
S31.23XA	Puncture wound without foreign body of penis, initial encounter ♂
S31.25XA	Open bite of penis, initial encounter ♂
S31.31XA	Laceration without foreign body of scrotum and testes, initial encounter ♂
S31.33XA	Puncture wound without foreign body of scrotum and testes, initial encounter ♂
S31.35XA	Open bite of scrotum and testes, initial encounter ♂
S31.41XA	Laceration without foreign body of vagina and vulva, initial encounter ♀
S31.43XA	Puncture wound without foreign body of vagina and vulva, initial encounter ♀
S31.45XA	Open bite of vagina and vulva, initial encounter ♀

Relative Value Units/Medicare Edits

Non-Facility RVU	Work	PE	MP	Total
G0168	0.31	2.66	0.06	3.03
Facility RVU	Work	PE	MP	Total
G0168	0.31	0.17	0.06	0.54

	FUD	Status	MUE	Modifiers			IOM Reference
G0168	0	A	2(3)	51	N/A	N/A	N/A	None

* with documentation

Terms To Know

abrasion. Removal of layers of the skin occurring as a superficial injury, or a procedure for removal of problematic skin or skin lesions.

closure. Repairing an incision or wound by suture or other means.

laceration. Tearing injury; a torn, ragged-edged wound.

superficial. On the skin surface or near the surface of any involved structure or field of interest.

wound. Injury to living tissue often involving a cut or break in the skin.

HCPCS

G0420-G0421

G0420 Face-to-face educational services related to the care of chronic kidney disease; individual, per session, per 1 hour

G0421 Face-to-face educational services related to the care of chronic kidney disease; group, per session, per 1 hour

Explanation

Face-to-face kidney disease education services provide patients with chronic kidney disease the information they need to manage concurrent health issues and to prevent complications. These services also include an explanation of the need to delay dialysis, as well as the treatment options available for renal replacement. These educational services may be done on an individual basis or in a group setting.

Relative Value Units/Medicare Edits

Non-Facility RVU	Work	PE	MP	Total
G0420	2.12	0.93	0.12	3.17
G0421	0.5	0.21	0.03	0.74
Facility RVU	**Work**	**PE**	**MP**	**Total**
G0420	2.12	0.93	0.12	3.17
G0421	0.5	0.21	0.03	0.74

76700-76705

76700 Ultrasound, abdominal, real time with image documentation; complete

76705 limited (eg, single organ, quadrant, follow-up)

Explanation

Diagnostic ultrasound is an imaging technique bouncing sound waves far above the level of human perception through interior body structures. The sound waves pass through different densities of tissue and reflect back to a receiving unit at varying speeds. The unit converts the waves to electrical pulses that are immediately displayed in picture form on screen. Real time scanning displays structure images and movement with time. Report 76700 for ultrasound and real time of the entire abdomen and 76705 for a single quadrant or organ of the abdomen.

Relative Value Units/Medicare Edits

Non-Facility RVU	Work	PE	MP	Total
76700	0.81	2.6	0.06	3.47
76705	0.59	1.94	0.04	2.57
Facility RVU	**Work**	**PE**	**MP**	**Total**
76700	0.81	2.6	0.06	3.47
76705	0.59	1.94	0.04	2.57

76770-76775

76770 Ultrasound, retroperitoneal (eg, renal, aorta, nodes), real time with image documentation; complete

76775 limited

Explanation

Diagnostic ultrasound is an imaging technique bouncing sound waves far above the level of human perception through interior body structures. The sound waves pass through different densities of tissue and reflect back to a receiving unit at varying speeds. The unit converts the waves to electrical pulses that are immediately displayed in picture form on screen. Real time scanning displays structure images and movement with time. Report 76770 for ultrasound and real time for a complete retroperitoneal exam that includes renal, aortic, and lymphatic structures and 76775 for a limited retroperitoneal exam.

Relative Value Units/Medicare Edits

Non-Facility RVU	Work	PE	MP	Total
76770	0.74	2.41	0.04	3.19
76775	0.58	1.04	0.04	1.66
Facility RVU	**Work**	**PE**	**MP**	**Total**
76770	0.74	2.41	0.04	3.19
76775	0.58	1.04	0.04	1.66

76776

76776 Ultrasound, transplanted kidney, real time and duplex Doppler with image documentation

Explanation

This code reports ultrasound of a transplanted kidney, with duplex Doppler studies. Diagnostic ultrasound is an imaging technique bouncing sound waves far above the level of human perception through interior body structures. The sound waves pass through different densities of tissue and reflect back to a receiving unit at varying speeds. The unit converts the waves to electrical pulses that are immediately displayed in picture form on screen. Duplex studies combine real time with Doppler, which uses the frequency shifts of the emitted waves against their echoes to measure velocity, such as for blood flow.

Relative Value Units/Medicare Edits

Non-Facility RVU	Work	PE	MP	Total
76776	0.76	3.58	0.07	4.41
Facility RVU	**Work**	**PE**	**MP**	**Total**
76776	0.76	3.58	0.07	4.41

76870

76870 Ultrasound, scrotum and contents

Explanation

Diagnostic ultrasound is an imaging technique bouncing sound waves far above the level of human perception through interior body structures. The sound waves pass through different densities of tissue and reflect back to a receiving unit at varying speeds. The unit converts the waves to electrical pulses that are immediately displayed in picture form on screen. This code reports ultrasonography of the scrotum and scrotal contents.

Relative Value Units/Medicare Edits

Non-Facility RVU	Work	PE	MP	Total
76870	0.64	2.28	0.04	2.96
Facility RVU	**Work**	**PE**	**MP**	**Total**
76870	0.64	2.28	0.04	2.96

76872-76873

76872 Ultrasound, transrectal;

76873 prostate volume study for brachytherapy treatment planning (separate procedure)

Explanation

Diagnostic ultrasound is an imaging technique bouncing sound waves far above the level of human perception through interior body structures. The sound waves pass through different densities of tissue and reflect back to a receiving unit at varying speeds. The unit converts the waves to electrical pulses that are immediately displayed in picture form on screen. Report 76872 for transrectal ultrasound or echography for either sex; Report 76873 for a prostate volume evaluation for planning brachytherapy treatment, which involves planting tiny radioactive elements into a treatment area.

Relative Value Units/Medicare Edits

Non-Facility RVU	Work	PE	MP	Total
76872	0.69	3.71	0.03	4.43
76873	1.55	3.35	0.06	4.96
Facility RVU	**Work**	**PE**	**MP**	**Total**
76872	0.69	3.71	0.03	4.43
76873	1.55	3.35	0.06	4.96

76981-76983

76981	Ultrasound, elastography; parenchyma (eg, organ)
76982	first target lesion
+ **76983**	each additional target lesion (List separately in addition to code for primary procedure)

Explanation

Ultrasound elastography, also known as sonoelastography, is a noninvasive imaging technique that can be used to depict relative tissue stiffness or displacement (strain) in response to an imparted force. Tumors are usually stiffer, or less elastic, than surrounding soft tissue, making the identification of tumors using this imaging modality effective. The ultrasound technician takes a normal image followed by an image while pushing down or compressing the organ area. This happens multiple times and the images are generated in real time by using algorithms to give a clearer picture of the motion of the tissue being imaged. Report 76981 for imaging of an organ; 76982 for the initial target lesion; and 76983 for each additional target lesion.

Relative Value Units/Medicare Edits

Non-Facility RVU	Work	PE	MP	Total
76981	0.59	2.41	0.04	3.04
76982	0.59	2.08	0.04	2.71
76983	0.5	1.15	0.02	1.67
Facility RVU	**Work**	**PE**	**MP**	**Total**
76981	0.59	2.41	0.04	3.04
76982	0.59	2.08	0.04	2.71
76983	0.5	1.15	0.02	1.67

80047

80047 Basic metabolic panel (Calcium, ionized) This panel must include the following: Calcium, ionized (82330) Carbon dioxide (bicarbonate) (82374) Chloride (82435) Creatinine (82565) Glucose (82947) Potassium (84132) Sodium (84295) Urea Nitrogen (BUN) (84520)

Explanation

A basic metabolic panel with ionized calcium includes the following tests: calcium (ionized) (82330), carbon dioxide (82374), chloride (82435), creatinine (82565), glucose (82947), potassium (84132), sodium (84295), and urea nitrogen (BUN) (84520). Blood specimen is obtained by venipuncture. See the specific codes for additional information about the listed tests.

Relative Value Units/Medicare Edits

Non-Facility RVU	Work	PE	MP	Total
80047	0.0	0.0	0.0	0.0
Facility RVU	**Work**	**PE**	**MP**	**Total**
80047	0.0	0.0	0.0	0.0

80048

80048 Basic metabolic panel (Calcium, total) This panel must include the following: Calcium, total (82310) Carbon dioxide (bicarbonate) (82374) Chloride (82435) Creatinine (82565) Glucose (82947) Potassium (84132) Sodium (84295) Urea nitrogen (BUN) (84520)

Explanation

A basic metabolic panel with total calcium includes the following tests: total calcium (82310), carbon dioxide (82374), chloride (82435), creatinine (82565), glucose (82947), potassium (84132), sodium (84295), and urea nitrogen (BUN) (84520). The blood specimen is obtained by venipuncture. See the specific codes for additional information about the listed tests.

Relative Value Units/Medicare Edits

Non-Facility RVU	Work	PE	MP	Total
80048	0.0	0.0	0.0	0.0
Facility RVU	**Work**	**PE**	**MP**	**Total**
80048	0.0	0.0	0.0	0.0

80050

80050 General health panel This panel must include the following: Comprehensive metabolic panel (80053) Blood count, complete (CBC), automated and automated differential WBC count (85025 or 85027 and 85004) OR Blood count, complete (CBC), automated (85027) and appropriate manual differential WBC count (85007 or 85009) Thyroid stimulating hormone (TSH) (84443)

Explanation

A general health panel includes the following tests: albumin (82040), total bilirubin (82247), calcium (82310), carbon dioxide (bicarbonate) (82374), chloride (82435), creatinine (82565), glucose (82947), alkaline phosphatase (84075), potassium (84132), total protein (84155), sodium (84295), alanine amino transferase (ALT) (SGPT) (84460), aspartate amino transferase (AST) (SGOT) (84450), urea nitrogen (BUN) (84520), and thyroid stimulating hormone (84443). In addition, this panel includes a hemogram with automated differential (85025 or 85027 and 85004) or hemogram (85027) with manual differential (85007 or 85009). Blood specimen is obtained by venipuncture. See specific codes for additional information about the listed tests.

Relative Value Units/Medicare Edits

Non-Facility RVU	Work	PE	MP	Total
80050	0.0	0.0	0.0	0.0
Facility RVU	**Work**	**PE**	**MP**	**Total**
80050	0.0	0.0	0.0	0.0

80051

80051 Electrolyte panel This panel must include the following: Carbon dioxide (bicarbonate) (82374) Chloride (82435) Potassium (84132) Sodium (84295)

Explanation

An electrolyte panel includes the following tests: carbon dioxide (82374), chloride (82435), potassium (84132), and sodium (84295). Blood specimen is obtained by venipuncture. See specific codes for additional information about the listed tests.

© 2020 Optum360, LLC
● New   ▲ Revised   + Add On   ★ Telemedicine   [Resequenced]   CPT © 2020 American Medical Association. All Rights Reserved.

Appendix

Relative Value Units/Medicare Edits

Non-Facility RVU	Work	PE	MP	Total
80051	0.0	0.0	0.0	0.0
Facility RVU	**Work**	**PE**	**MP**	**Total**
80051	0.0	0.0	0.0	0.0

80053

80053   Comprehensive metabolic panel This panel must include the following: Albumin (82040) Bilirubin, total (82247) Calcium, total (82310) Carbon dioxide (bicarbonate) (82374) Chloride (82435) Creatinine (82565) Glucose (82947) Phosphatase, alkaline (84075) Potassium (84132) Protein, total (84155) Sodium (84295) Transferase, alanine amino (ALT) (SGPT) (84460) Transferase, aspartate amino (AST) (SGOT) (84450) Urea nitrogen (BUN) (84520)

Explanation

A comprehensive metabolic panel includes the following tests: albumin (82040), total bilirubin (82247), total calcium (82310), carbon dioxide (bicarbonate) (82374), chloride (82435), creatinine (82565), glucose (82947), alkaline phosphatase (84075), potassium (84132), total protein (84155), sodium (84295), alanine amino transferase (ALT) (SGPT) (84460), aspartate amino transferase (AST) (SGOT) (84450), and urea nitrogen (BUN) (84520). Blood specimen is obtained by venipuncture. See the specific codes for additional information about the listed tests.

Relative Value Units/Medicare Edits

Non-Facility RVU	Work	PE	MP	Total
80053	0.0	0.0	0.0	0.0
Facility RVU	**Work**	**PE**	**MP**	**Total**
80053	0.0	0.0	0.0	0.0

80069

80069   Renal function panel This panel must include the following: Albumin (82040) Calcium, total (82310) Carbon dioxide (bicarbonate) (82374) Chloride (82435) Creatinine (82565) Glucose (82947) Phosphorus inorganic (phosphate) (84100) Potassium (84132) Sodium (84295) Urea nitrogen (BUN) (84520)

Explanation

A renal function panel includes the following tests: albumin (82040), total calcium (82310), carbon dioxide (bicarbonate) (82374), chloride (82435), creatinine (82565), glucose (82947), inorganic phosphorus (phosphate) (84100), potassium (84132), sodium (84295), and urea nitrogen (BUN) (84520).

Relative Value Units/Medicare Edits

Non-Facility RVU	Work	PE	MP	Total
80069	0.0	0.0	0.0	0.0
Facility RVU	**Work**	**PE**	**MP**	**Total**
80069	0.0	0.0	0.0	0.0

80158

80158   Cyclosporine

Explanation

This drug is also known as Sandimmune. It is an immunosuppressant and is often monitored. Test specimens are frequently collected at the trough period, which is typically about 12 hours after the last dose when serum concentration is at its lowest. Method is high performance liquid chromatography (HPLC) or fluorescence polarization immunoassay (FPIA).

Relative Value Units/Medicare Edits

Non-Facility RVU	Work	PE	MP	Total
80158	0.0	0.0	0.0	0.0
Facility RVU	**Work**	**PE**	**MP**	**Total**
80158	0.0	0.0	0.0	0.0

81000

81000   Urinalysis, by dip stick or tablet reagent for bilirubin, glucose, hemoglobin, ketones, leukocytes, nitrite, pH, protein, specific gravity, urobilinogen, any number of these constituents; non-automated, with microscopy

Explanation

This type of test may be ordered by the brand name product and the analytes tested. Although screens are considered to show the presence of an analyte (qualitative), some newer products are semi-quantitative. Many are plastic strips that contain sites impregnated with chemicals that react with urine when the strip is dipped into a specimen. The result is a color change that is compared against a standardized chart. Most strips will test for numerous analytes, as well as for pH and specific gravity. Tablets work in a similar fashion. A drop of urine is placed on the tablet and a chemical reaction causes a color change that is compared to a standard chart. Usually only a single analyte is under consideration, per tablet. Code 81000 involves a manual (nonautomated) test and includes a microscopic examination. Microscopy involves examination of the urine sediments or solids. The urine is first centrifuged in a graduated tube to concentrate the sediments. Samples (either wet or dry) are examined, usually under both high and low power, and abnormal constituents are noted. These may include a wide range of biological abnormalities, such as blood cells, casts, and bacteria, as well as chemical anomalies, such as crystals.

Relative Value Units/Medicare Edits

Non-Facility RVU	Work	PE	MP	Total
81000	0.0	0.0	0.0	0.0
Facility RVU	**Work**	**PE**	**MP**	**Total**
81000	0.0	0.0	0.0	0.0

81001

81001   Urinalysis, by dip stick or tablet reagent for bilirubin, glucose, hemoglobin, ketones, leukocytes, nitrite, pH, protein, specific gravity, urobilinogen, any number of these constituents; automated, with microscopy

Explanation

This type of test may be ordered by the type of processor used and the analytes tested. The testing methodology is similar to the manual strips, except that the color change caused by the chemical reaction with urine is processed and read mechanically. The strip is exposed to the urine sample and is mechanically fed through a processor that reads the colors emitted by the reaction. The unit will be calibrated according to international standards and readings have a high degree of accuracy. The result may be displayed on a monitor, but is always printed or recorded in some form. Code 81001 also includes a microscopy. Microscopy involves examination of the urine sediments or solids. The urine is first centrifuged in a graduated tube to concentrate the sediments. Samples (either wet or dry) are examined, usually under both high and low power, and abnormal constituents are noted. These may include a wide range of biological abnormalities, such as blood cells, casts, and bacteria, as well as chemical anomalies, such as crystals.

Appendix

CPT © 2020 American Medical Association. All Rights Reserved.   ● New   ▲ Revised   + Add On   ★ Telemedicine   [Resequenced]   © 2020 Optum360, LLC

Relative Value Units/Medicare Edits

Non-Facility RVU	Work	PE	MP	Total
81001	0.0	0.0	0.0	0.0
Facility RVU	**Work**	**PE**	**MP**	**Total**
81001	0.0	0.0	0.0	0.0

81002

81002   Urinalysis, by dip stick or tablet reagent for bilirubin, glucose, hemoglobin, ketones, leukocytes, nitrite, pH, protein, specific gravity, urobilinogen, any number of these constituents; non-automated, without microscopy

Explanation

This type of test may be ordered by the brand name product and the analytes tested. Although usually considered screens to show the presence of an analyte (qualitative), some newer products are semi-quantitative. Many are plastic strips that contain sites impregnated with chemicals that react with urine when the strip is dipped into a specimen. The result is a color change that is compared against a standardized chart. Most strips will test for numerous analytes, as well as for pH and specific gravity. Tablets work in a similar fashion. A drop of urine is placed on the tablet and a chemical reaction causes a color change that is compared to a standard chart. Usually only a single analyte is under consideration per tablet, however. Code 81002 does not include a microscopic examination of the urine sample or its components.

Relative Value Units/Medicare Edits

Non-Facility RVU	Work	PE	MP	Total
81002	0.0	0.0	0.0	0.0
Facility RVU	**Work**	**PE**	**MP**	**Total**
81002	0.0	0.0	0.0	0.0

81003

81003   Urinalysis, by dip stick or tablet reagent for bilirubin, glucose, hemoglobin, ketones, leukocytes, nitrite, pH, protein, specific gravity, urobilinogen, any number of these constituents; automated, without microscopy

Explanation

This type of test may be ordered by the type of processor used and the analytes tested. The testing methodology is similar to the manual strips, except that the color change caused by the chemical reaction with urine is processed and read mechanically. The strip is exposed to the urine sample and is mechanically fed through a processor that reads the colors emitted by the reaction. The unit will be calibrated according to international standards and readings have a high degree of accuracy. The result may be displayed on a monitor, but is always printed or recorded in some form. Code 81003 does not include a microscopic examination of the urine sample or its components.

Relative Value Units/Medicare Edits

Non-Facility RVU	Work	PE	MP	Total
81003	0.0	0.0	0.0	0.0
Facility RVU	**Work**	**PE**	**MP**	**Total**
81003	0.0	0.0	0.0	0.0

81005

81005   Urinalysis; qualitative or semiquantitative, except immunoassays

Explanation

This test may be ordered by the type of processor used and the analytes under examination. The method will be any type of automated analyzer, usually colorimetry. The results of a semi-quantitative test indicate the presence or absence of an analyte and may be expressed as simply positive or negative. A qualitative result may be indicated as trace, 1+, 2+, etc.

Relative Value Units/Medicare Edits

Non-Facility RVU	Work	PE	MP	Total
81005	0.0	0.0	0.0	0.0
Facility RVU	**Work**	**PE**	**MP**	**Total**
81005	0.0	0.0	0.0	0.0

81007

81007   Urinalysis; bacteriuria screen, except by culture or dipstick

Explanation

This type of test may be ordered by the brand name of the commercial kit used and the bacteria that the kit screens for. Human urine is normally free of bacteria. However, bacteria can easily be introduced upon voiding. In addition, specimens containing any amount of pathological bacteria can have the organisms rapidly multiply after collection. For this reason, specimens are often examined shortly after collection. Method includes any method except culture or dipstick. The test is often performed by commercial kit. The type of kit used should be specified in the report.

Relative Value Units/Medicare Edits

Non-Facility RVU	Work	PE	MP	Total
81007	0.0	0.0	0.0	0.0
Facility RVU	**Work**	**PE**	**MP**	**Total**
81007	0.0	0.0	0.0	0.0

81015

81015   Urinalysis; microscopic only

Explanation

This test may be ordered as a microscopic analysis. Human urine is normally free of bacteria. However, bacteria can easily be introduced upon voiding. In addition, specimens containing any amount of pathological bacteria can have the organisms rapidly multiply after collection. For this reason, specimens are often examined shortly after collection. The sample may first be centrifuged into a graduated tube to concentrate the sediments, or solid matter, held in suspension. The concentration of bacteria as well as cell types, crystals, and other elements seen is reported.

Relative Value Units/Medicare Edits

Non-Facility RVU	Work	PE	MP	Total
81015	0.0	0.0	0.0	0.0
Facility RVU	**Work**	**PE**	**MP**	**Total**
81015	0.0	0.0	0.0	0.0

82565

82565   Creatinine; blood

Explanation

Serum creatinine is the most common laboratory test for evaluating renal function. Method is enzymatic or colorimetry.

Appendix

Relative Value Units/Medicare Edits

Non-Facility RVU	Work	PE	MP	Total
82565	0.0	0.0	0.0	0.0
Facility RVU	**Work**	**PE**	**MP**	**Total**
82565	0.0	0.0	0.0	0.0

82948

82948 Glucose; blood, reagent strip

Explanation

This test is used to monitor disorders of carbohydrate metabolism. Blood specimen is obtained by finger stick. A drop of blood is placed on the reagent strip for a specified amount of time. When the prescribed amount of time has elapsed, the strip is blotted and the reagent strip is compared to a color chart. Method is reagent strip with visual comparison.

Relative Value Units/Medicare Edits

Non-Facility RVU	Work	PE	MP	Total
82948	0.0	0.0	0.0	0.0
Facility RVU	**Work**	**PE**	**MP**	**Total**
82948	0.0	0.0	0.0	0.0

83516-83518

83516 Immunoassay for analyte other than infectious agent antibody or infectious agent antigen; qualitative or semiquantitative, multiple step method
83518 qualitative or semiquantitative, single step method (eg, reagent strip)

Explanation

Immunoassay uses highly specific antigen to antibody binding to identify specific chemical substances. This code reports a number of immunoassay techniques for identifying analytes (chemical substances) that are not specifically identified elsewhere, excluding infectious agent antibody or infectious agent antigen. More specific methods reported with these codes include enzyme immunoassay (EIA) and fluoroimmunoassay (FIA). This test identifies (qualitative analysis) the substance or roughly measures (semi-quantitative analysis) the amount of the substance. Code 83516 reports multiple step method, while 83518 reports single step method.

Relative Value Units/Medicare Edits

Non-Facility RVU	Work	PE	MP	Total
83516	0.0	0.0	0.0	0.0
83518	0.0	0.0	0.0	0.0
Facility RVU	**Work**	**PE**	**MP**	**Total**
83516	0.0	0.0	0.0	0.0
83518	0.0	0.0	0.0	0.0

84152-84154

84152 Prostate specific antigen (PSA); complexed (direct measurement)
84153 total
84154 free

Explanation

The specimen is serum. Methods may include radioimmunoassay (RIA) and monoclonal two-site immunoradiometric assay. These tests may be performed to determine the presence of cancer of the prostate, benign prostatic hypertrophy (BPH), prostatitis, post prostatectomy to detect residual cancer, and to monitor therapy. There are several forms of PSA present in serum. PSA may be complexed with the protease inhibitor alpha-1 antichymotrypsin (PSA-ACT). Complexed PSA is the most measurable form. PSA is also found in a free form. Free PSA is not complexed to a protease inhibitor. Higher levels of free PSA are more often associated with benign conditions of the prostate than with prostate cancer. Total PSA measures both complexed and free levels to provide a total amount present in the serum. A percentage of each form is sometimes calculated to distinguish benign from malignant conditions. Code 84152 reports complexed PSA; 84153 is for total serum PSA; 84154 is for free (not complexed) PSA.

Relative Value Units/Medicare Edits

Non-Facility RVU	Work	PE	MP	Total
84152	0.0	0.0	0.0	0.0
84153	0.0	0.0	0.0	0.0
84154	0.0	0.0	0.0	0.0
Facility RVU	**Work**	**PE**	**MP**	**Total**
84152	0.0	0.0	0.0	0.0
84153	0.0	0.0	0.0	0.0
84154	0.0	0.0	0.0	0.0

84402-84410

84402 Testosterone; free
84403 total
84410 bioavailable, direct measurement (eg, differential precipitation)

Explanation

These tests may be used to evaluate testosterone levels. Testosterone is an androgenic hormone responsible for, among other biological activities, secondary male characteristics in women. Increased testosterone levels in women may be linked to a variety of conditions, including hirsutism. Report 84403 for total testosterone, which includes protein bound and free testosterone. Report 84402 for testosterone as a free unbound protein. This test may be ordered to assist in diagnosis of hypogonadism, hypopituitarism, and Klinefelter's syndrome, among other disorders. The specimen is serum. Method may be by radioimmunoassay (RIA) and immunoassay (non-isotopic). Report 84410 for bioavailable testosterone. The majority of circulating testosterone is bound to sex hormone-binding globulin (SHBG) or testosterone-binding globulin. Slightly less than one-third of testosterone in the blood binds to albumin and a smaller proportion circulates as free testosterone; the free testosterone and the testosterone bound to albumin is called the bioavailable testosterone, which is all non-SHBG bound testosterone. This test is performed in cases where the patient's level of SHBG is abnormal. The specimen is serum. Method may be based on the differential precipitation of SHBG by ammonium sulfate and subsequent equilibration of the specimen and trace amounts of tritium-labeled testosterone. This test may be ordered to provide more detailed information to assist in diagnosing patients presenting with decreased SHBG levels and other conditions such as obesity, hypothyroidism, androgen use, and a type of kidney disease called nephritic syndrome.

Relative Value Units/Medicare Edits

Non-Facility RVU	Work	PE	MP	Total
84402	0.0	0.0	0.0	0.0
84403	0.0	0.0	0.0	0.0
84410	0.0	0.0	0.0	0.0
Facility RVU	**Work**	**PE**	**MP**	**Total**
84402	0.0	0.0	0.0	0.0
84403	0.0	0.0	0.0	0.0
84410	0.0	0.0	0.0	0.0

Appendix

85004

85004   Blood count; automated differential WBC count

Explanation

This test may be ordered as a blood count with automated differential. The specimen is whole blood. Method is automated cell counter. The blood count typically includes a measurement of normal cell constituents including white blood cells or leukocytes, red blood cells, and platelets. In addition, this test includes a differential count of the white blood cells or "diff" in which the following leukocytes are differentiated and counted automatically: neutrophils or granulocytes, lymphocytes, monocytes, eosinophils, and basophils.

Relative Value Units/Medicare Edits

Non-Facility RVU	Work	PE	MP	Total
85004	0.0	0.0	0.0	0.0
Facility RVU	Work	PE	MP	Total
85004	0.0	0.0	0.0	0.0

85007-85008

85007   Blood count; blood smear, microscopic examination with manual differential WBC count
85008   blood smear, microscopic examination without manual differential WBC count

Explanation

These tests may be ordered as a manual blood smear examination, RBC smear, peripheral blood smear, or RBC morphology without differential parameters in 85008 and with manual WBC differential in 85007. The specimen is whole blood. The method is manual testing. A blood smear is prepared and microscopically examined for the presence of normal cell constituents, including white blood cells, red blood cells, and platelets. In 85008, the white blood cell and platelet or thrombocyte counts are estimated and red cell morphology is commented on if abnormal. In 85007, a manual differential of white blood cells is included in which the following leukocytes are differentiated: neutrophils or granulocytes, lymphocytes, monocytes, eosinophils, and basophils.

Relative Value Units/Medicare Edits

Non-Facility RVU	Work	PE	MP	Total
85007	0.0	0.0	0.0	0.0
85008	0.0	0.0	0.0	0.0
Facility RVU	Work	PE	MP	Total
85007	0.0	0.0	0.0	0.0
85008	0.0	0.0	0.0	0.0

85009

85009   Blood count; manual differential WBC count, buffy coat

Explanation

This test may be ordered as a buffy coat differential or as a differential WBC count, buffy coat. Specimen is whole blood. Other collection types (e.g., finger stick or heel stick) do not yield the volume of blood required for this test. Method is manual testing. The whole blood is centrifuged to concentrate the white blood cells, and a manual WBC differential is performed in which the following leukocytes are differentiated: neutrophils or granulocytes, lymphocytes, monocytes, eosinophils, and basophils. This test is usually performed when the number of WBCs or leukocytes is abnormally low and the presence of abnormal white cells (e.g., blasts or cancer cells) is suspected clinically.

Relative Value Units/Medicare Edits

Non-Facility RVU	Work	PE	MP	Total
85009	0.0	0.0	0.0	0.0
Facility RVU	Work	PE	MP	Total
85009	0.0	0.0	0.0	0.0

85013

85013   Blood count; spun microhematocrit

Explanation

This test may be ordered as a microhematocrit, a spun microhematocrit, or a "spun crit." The specimen (whole blood) is by finger stick or heel stick in infants. The sample is placed in a tube and into a microcentrifuge device. The vials can be read manually against a chart for the volume of packed red cells or a digital reader in the centrifuge device. A spun microhematocrit only reports the volume of packed red cells. It is typically performed at sites where limited testing is available, the patient is a very difficult blood draw, or on infants.

Relative Value Units/Medicare Edits

Non-Facility RVU	Work	PE	MP	Total
85013	0.0	0.0	0.0	0.0
Facility RVU	Work	PE	MP	Total
85013	0.0	0.0	0.0	0.0

85014

85014   Blood count; hematocrit (Hct)

Explanation

This test may be ordered as a hematocrit, Hmt, or Hct. The specimen is whole blood. Method is automated cell counter. The hematocrit or volume of packed red cells (VPRC) in the blood sample is calculated by multiplying the red blood cell count or RBC times the mean corpuscular volume or MCV.

Relative Value Units/Medicare Edits

Non-Facility RVU	Work	PE	MP	Total
85014	0.0	0.0	0.0	0.0
Facility RVU	Work	PE	MP	Total
85014	0.0	0.0	0.0	0.0

85018

85018   Blood count; hemoglobin (Hgb)

Explanation

This test may be ordered as hemoglobin, Hgb, or hemoglobin concentration. The specimen is whole blood. Method is usually automated cell counter but a manual method is seen in labs with a limited test menu and blood bank drawing stations. Hemoglobin is an index of the oxygen-carrying capacity of the blood.

Relative Value Units/Medicare Edits

Non-Facility RVU	Work	PE	MP	Total
85018	0.0	0.0	0.0	0.0
Facility RVU	Work	PE	MP	Total
85018	0.0	0.0	0.0	0.0

Appendix

85025-85027

85025 Blood count; complete (CBC), automated (Hgb, Hct, RBC, WBC and platelet count) and automated differential WBC count

85027 complete (CBC), automated (Hgb, Hct, RBC, WBC and platelet count)

Explanation

These tests may be ordered as a complete automated blood count (CBC). The specimen is whole blood. Method is automated cell counter. These codes include the measurement of erythrocytes (red blood cells or RBC), leukocytes (white blood cells or WBC), hemoglobin, hematocrit (volume of packed red blood cells or VPRC), platelet or thrombocyte count, and indices (mean corpuscular hemoglobin or MCH, mean corpuscular hemoglobin concentration or MCHC, mean corpuscular volume or MCV, and red cell distribution width or RDW). Code 85025 includes an automated differential of the white blood cells or "diff" in which the following leukocytes are differentiated: neutrophils or granulocytes, lymphocytes, monocytes, eosinophils, and basophils. Report 85027 if the complete CBC, or automated blood count, is done without the differential WBC count.

Relative Value Units/Medicare Edits

Non-Facility RVU	Work	PE	MP	Total
85025	0.0	0.0	0.0	0.0
85027	0.0	0.0	0.0	0.0
Facility RVU	**Work**	**PE**	**MP**	**Total**
85025	0.0	0.0	0.0	0.0
85027	0.0	0.0	0.0	0.0

85032

85032 Blood count; manual cell count (erythrocyte, leukocyte, or platelet) each

Explanation

This code reports a manual cell count done for red blood cells (erythrocytes), white blood cells (leukocytes), or platelets (thrombocytes), each. The specimen is whole blood. The method is manual examination and counting.

Relative Value Units/Medicare Edits

Non-Facility RVU	Work	PE	MP	Total
85032	0.0	0.0	0.0	0.0
Facility RVU	**Work**	**PE**	**MP**	**Total**
85032	0.0	0.0	0.0	0.0

85041

85041 Blood count; red blood cell (RBC), automated

Explanation

This test may be ordered as red blood cell count or RBC. The specimen is by whole blood Method is automated cell counter.

Relative Value Units/Medicare Edits

Non-Facility RVU	Work	PE	MP	Total
85041	0.0	0.0	0.0	0.0
Facility RVU	**Work**	**PE**	**MP**	**Total**
85041	0.0	0.0	0.0	0.0

85044

85044 Blood count; reticulocyte, manual

Explanation

This test may be ordered as a manual reticulocyte count or as a manual "retic." The specimen is whole blood. Method is manual. A blood smear is prepared and stained with a dye that highlights the reticulum in the immature red blood cells, or the reticulocytes. The reticulocytes are reported as a percentage of total red blood cells.

Relative Value Units/Medicare Edits

Non-Facility RVU	Work	PE	MP	Total
85044	0.0	0.0	0.0	0.0
Facility RVU	**Work**	**PE**	**MP**	**Total**
85044	0.0	0.0	0.0	0.0

85045

85045 Blood count; reticulocyte, automated

Explanation

This test may be ordered as an automated reticulocyte count, an "auto retic," or a reticulocyte by flow cytometry. The specimen is whole blood. Method is automated cell counter or flow cytometer. Reticulocytes are immature red blood cells that still contain mitochondria and ribosomes. The reticulocytes are reported as a percentage of total red blood cells.

Relative Value Units/Medicare Edits

Non-Facility RVU	Work	PE	MP	Total
85045	0.0	0.0	0.0	0.0
Facility RVU	**Work**	**PE**	**MP**	**Total**
85045	0.0	0.0	0.0	0.0

85046

85046 Blood count; reticulocytes, automated, including 1 or more cellular parameters (eg, reticulocyte hemoglobin content [CHr], immature reticulocyte fraction [IRF], reticulocyte volume [MRV], RNA content), direct measurement

Explanation

This test may be ordered as a reticulocyte count and hemoglobin concentration, "retics" and Hgb, or as an "auto retic" and hemoglobin. The specimen is whole blood. Method is automated cell counter. The blood is stained with a dye that marks the reticulum in immature red blood cells, or reticulocytes. The reticulocytes are reported as a percentage of total red blood cells. The automated reticulocyte blood count also includes one or more cellular parameters, such as the hemoglobin content of the reticulocytes (CHr), the fraction of immature reticulocytes (IRF), the RNA content, or the volume of reticulocytes.

Relative Value Units/Medicare Edits

Non-Facility RVU	Work	PE	MP	Total
85046	0.0	0.0	0.0	0.0
Facility RVU	**Work**	**PE**	**MP**	**Total**
85046	0.0	0.0	0.0	0.0

85048-85049

85048 Blood count; leukocyte (WBC), automated

85049 platelet, automated

Explanation

These tests may be ordered as an automated white blood cell or WBC count, white cell count, or leukocyte count for 85048 and as an automated platelet count in 85049. The specimen is whole blood. Method is automated cell counter. In 85048, the population of white blood cells, or WBCs in the blood sample, is counted by machine. Only the number of white blood cells or leukocytes is reported. In 85049, the population of platelets or thrombocytes in the blood sample is counted by machine. Only the number of platelets is reported.

Relative Value Units/Medicare Edits

Non-Facility RVU	Work	PE	MP	Total
85048	0.0	0.0	0.0	0.0
85049	0.0	0.0	0.0	0.0
Facility RVU	Work	PE	MP	Total
85048	0.0	0.0	0.0	0.0
85049	0.0	0.0	0.0	0.0

87081-87084

87081   Culture, presumptive, pathogenic organisms, screening only;
87084   with colony estimation from density chart

Explanation

These codes describe presumptive screening cultures for one or more pathogenic organisms. The methodology is by culture and the culture should be identified by type (e.g., anaerobic, aerobic) and specimen source (e.g., pleural, peritoneal, bronchial aspirates). If a specific organism is suspected, the person ordering the test typically uses common names, such as strep screen, staph screen, etc., to specify the organism for screening. Presumptive identification includes gram staining as well as up to three tests, such as a catalase, oxidase, or urease test. Screenings included in this code are nonmotile, catalase-positive, gram-positive rod bacteria. Report 87084 when an estimation of the number of organisms is also made, based on a density chart.

Relative Value Units/Medicare Edits

Non-Facility RVU	Work	PE	MP	Total
87081	0.0	0.0	0.0	0.0
87084	0.0	0.0	0.0	0.0
Facility RVU	Work	PE	MP	Total
87081	0.0	0.0	0.0	0.0
87084	0.0	0.0	0.0	0.0

87086-87088

87086   Culture, bacterial; quantitative colony count, urine
87088   with isolation and presumptive identification of each isolate, urine

Explanation

These codes report the performance of a urine bacterial culture with a calibrated inoculating device so that a colony count accurately correlates with the number of organisms in the urine. In 87088, isolation and presumptive identification of bacteria recovered from the sample is done by means of identifying colony morphology, subculturing organisms to selective media and the performance of a gram stain or other simple test to identify bacteria to the genus level. There are several automated systems that detect the presence of bacteria using colorimetric, radiometric, or spectrophotometric means. In 87086, quantified colony count numbers within the urine sample are measured.

Relative Value Units/Medicare Edits

Non-Facility RVU	Work	PE	MP	Total
87086	0.0	0.0	0.0	0.0
87088	0.0	0.0	0.0	0.0
Facility RVU	Work	PE	MP	Total
87086	0.0	0.0	0.0	0.0
87088	0.0	0.0	0.0	0.0

87880

▲ 87880   Infectious agent antigen detection by immunoassay with direct optical (ie, visual) observation; Streptococcus, group A

Explanation

This test may be requested as an optical immunoassay for Streptococcus A. Streptococcus A is a form of beta hemolytic streptococcus, which causes pharyngitis. Untreated infection can cause rheumatic fever or glomerulonephritis. This test reports detection using a competitive protein-binding assay where an antigen binds to an antibody, which is fixed to a reflecting surface. This change in reflection can be observed directly as a color change.

Relative Value Units/Medicare Edits

Non-Facility RVU	Work	PE	MP	Total
87880	0.0	0.0	0.0	0.0
Facility RVU	Work	PE	MP	Total
87880	0.0	0.0	0.0	0.0

90460-90461

90460   Immunization administration through 18 years of age via any route of administration, with counseling by physician or other qualified health care professional; first or only component of each vaccine or toxoid administered
+   90461   each additional vaccine or toxoid component administered (List separately in addition to code for primary procedure)

Explanation

The physician or other qualified health care professional instructs the patient or family on the benefits and risks related to the vaccine or toxoid. The physician counsels the patient or family regarding signs and symptoms of adverse effects and when to seek medical attention for any adverse effects. A physician, nurse, or medical assistant administers an immunization by any route to the patient. It may be a single vaccine or a combination vaccine/toxoid in one immunization administration (e.g., diphtheria, pertussis, and tetanus toxoids are in a single DPT immunization). Report 90460 for the first or only vaccine/toxoid component. Report 90461 for each additional component. These codes report immunization administration to patients 18 years of age or younger.

Relative Value Units/Medicare Edits

Non-Facility RVU	Work	PE	MP	Total
90460	0.17	0.22	0.01	0.4
90461	0.15	0.2	0.01	0.36
Facility RVU	Work	PE	MP	Total
90460	0.17	0.22	0.01	0.4
90461	0.15	0.2	0.01	0.36

Appendix

90473-90474

90473 Immunization administration by intranasal or oral route; 1 vaccine (single or combination vaccine/toxoid)

+ 90474 each additional vaccine (single or combination vaccine/toxoid) (List separately in addition to code for primary procedure)

Explanation

A physician, nurse, or medical assistant administers an immunization to a patient via an intranasal (e.g., nasal spray) or an oral route (e.g., a liquid that is swallowed). It may be a single vaccine or a combination vaccine/toxoid in one immunization administration (e.g., adenovirus, Rotavirus, typhoid, poliovirus). Report 90473 for one vaccine and 90474 for each additional vaccine (single or combination vaccine/toxoid).

Relative Value Units/Medicare Edits

Non-Facility RVU	Work	PE	MP	Total
90473	0.17	0.22	0.01	0.4
90474	0.15	0.2	0.01	0.36
Facility RVU	Work	PE	MP	Total
90473	0.17	0.22	0.01	0.4
90474	0.15	0.2	0.01	0.36

90997

90997 Hemoperfusion (eg, with activated charcoal or resin)

Explanation

Hemoperfusion is a technique to remove toxins from the blood and to maintain fluid and electrolyte balance when the kidneys no longer function. The physician draws the patient's blood, perfuses the blood through activated charcoal or resin, and transfuses the blood back into the patient using a needle and catheter.

Relative Value Units/Medicare Edits

Non-Facility RVU	Work	PE	MP	Total
90997	1.84	0.61	0.11	2.56
Facility RVU	Work	PE	MP	Total
90997	1.84	0.61	0.11	2.56

93975

93975 Duplex scan of arterial inflow and venous outflow of abdominal, pelvic, scrotal contents and/or retroperitoneal organs; complete study

Explanation

The physician or assistant performs a Duplex ultrasound scan, which is a combination of real-time and Doppler studies, of the arteries and veins in the abdominal, pelvic, or genitorectal areas to evaluate vascular blood flow in relation to blockage. This code applies to a complete bilateral evaluation.

Relative Value Units/Medicare Edits

Non-Facility RVU	Work	PE	MP	Total
93975	1.16	6.55	0.12	7.83
Facility RVU	Work	PE	MP	Total
93975	1.16	6.55	0.12	7.83

93976

93976 Duplex scan of arterial inflow and venous outflow of abdominal, pelvic, scrotal contents and/or retroperitoneal organs; limited study

Explanation

The physician or assistant performs a Duplex ultrasound scan, which is a combination of real-time and Doppler studies, of the arteries and veins in the abdominal, pelvic, or genitorectal areas to evaluate vascular blood flow in relation to blockage. This code applies to a limited evaluation.

Relative Value Units/Medicare Edits

Non-Facility RVU	Work	PE	MP	Total
93976	0.8	3.77	0.07	4.64
Facility RVU	Work	PE	MP	Total
93976	0.8	3.77	0.07	4.64

93985-93986

93985 Duplex scan of arterial inflow and venous outflow for preoperative vessel assessment prior to creation of hemodialysis access; complete bilateral study

93986 complete unilateral study

Explanation

The physician performs a Duplex ultrasound scan, producing real-time images integrating B-mode two-dimensional structure with Doppler mapping or imaging of motion with time for preoperative assessment of vascular blood flow prior to the creation of a hemodialysis access. This assessment includes the arterial inflow and venous outflow. Native arteriovenous fistula (AVF) is the preferred vascular access for hemodialysis patients, lasting longer and having fewer complications than grafts and central venous catheters. The use of the Doppler ultrasound (DUS) in preoperative vascular mapping enables identification of vessels that are most appropriate for fistula construction. Report 93985 for a complete bilateral study and 93986 for a complete unilateral study.

Relative Value Units/Medicare Edits

Non-Facility RVU	Work	PE	MP	Total
93985	0.8	6.61	0.12	7.53
93986	0.5	3.77	0.1	4.37
Facility RVU	Work	PE	MP	Total
93985	0.8	6.61	0.12	7.53
93986	0.5	3.77	0.1	4.37

95990-95991

95990 Refilling and maintenance of implantable pump or reservoir for drug delivery, spinal (intrathecal, epidural) or brain (intraventricular), includes electronic analysis of pump, when performed;

95991 requiring skill of a physician or other qualified health care professional

Explanation

Refilling and maintenance of an implantable spinal (intrathecal, epidural) or intraventricular (brain) pump or reservoir is done. Implantable pumps or reservoirs are placed in subcutaneous pockets at appropriate sites on the body and hold a long-term supply of the drug or medication being infused into the patient. They are refilled through the skin by a needle placed into the pump device. The patient's specific pump is identified and the required volume amount is checked. The site of the implant is prepped. The refill kit is assembled and a template is positioned over the site. A needle is inserted through the template center hole and into the pump/reservoir, which is filled with more drug infusate. The pump may have electronic analysis performed, including evaluation of reservoir status, alarm status, and drug prescription status. Report 95991 when a physician or other qualified health care provider's skill is required to perform the refill and/or maintenance.

Appendix

Relative Value Units/Medicare Edits

Non-Facility RVU	Work	PE	MP	Total
95990	0.0	2.5	0.05	2.55
95991	0.77	2.38	0.09	3.24
Facility RVU	**Work**	**PE**	**MP**	**Total**
95990	0.0	2.5	0.05	2.55
95991	0.77	0.3	0.09	1.16

96360-96361

96360 Intravenous infusion, hydration; initial, 31 minutes to 1 hour

\+ 96361 each additional hour (List separately in addition to code for primary procedure)

Explanation

A physician or an assistant under direct physician supervision infuses a hydration solution (prepackaged fluid and electrolytes) for 31 minutes to one hour through an intravenous catheter inserted by needle into a patient's vein or by infusion through an existing indwelling intravascular access catheter or port. Report 96361 for each additional hour beyond the first hour. Intravenous infusion for hydration lasting 30 minutes or less is not reported.

Relative Value Units/Medicare Edits

Non-Facility RVU	Work	PE	MP	Total
96360	0.17	0.77	0.02	0.96
96361	0.09	0.28	0.01	0.38
Facility RVU	**Work**	**PE**	**MP**	**Total**
96360	0.17	0.77	0.02	0.96
96361	0.09	0.28	0.01	0.38

96365-96368

96365 Intravenous infusion, for therapy, prophylaxis, or diagnosis (specify substance or drug); initial, up to 1 hour

\+ 96366 each additional hour (List separately in addition to code for primary procedure)

\+ 96367 additional sequential infusion of a new drug/substance, up to 1 hour (List separately in addition to code for primary procedure)

\+ 96368 concurrent infusion (List separately in addition to code for primary procedure)

Explanation

A physician or an assistant under direct physician supervision injects or infuses a therapeutic, prophylactic (preventive), or diagnostic medication other than chemotherapy or other highly complex drugs or biologic agents via intravenous route. Infusions are administered through an intravenous catheter inserted by needle into a patient's vein or by injection or infusion through an existing indwelling intravascular access catheter or port. Report 96365 for the initial hour and 96366 for each additional hour. Report 96367 for each additional sequential infusion of a different substance or drug, up to one hour, and 96368 for each concurrent infusion of substances other than chemotherapy or other highly complex drugs or biologic agents.

Relative Value Units/Medicare Edits

Non-Facility RVU	Work	PE	MP	Total
96365	0.21	1.74	0.05	2.0
96366	0.18	0.42	0.01	0.61
96367	0.19	0.66	0.02	0.87
96368	0.17	0.41	0.01	0.59
Facility RVU	**Work**	**PE**	**MP**	**Total**
96365	0.21	1.74	0.05	2.0
96366	0.18	0.42	0.01	0.61
96367	0.19	0.66	0.02	0.87
96368	0.17	0.41	0.01	0.59

96372-96376

96372 Therapeutic, prophylactic, or diagnostic injection (specify substance or drug); subcutaneous or intramuscular

96373 intra-arterial

96374 intravenous push, single or initial substance/drug

\+ 96375 each additional sequential intravenous push of a new substance/drug (List separately in addition to code for primary procedure)

\+ 96376 each additional sequential intravenous push of the same substance/drug provided in a facility (List separately in addition to code for primary procedure)

Explanation

The physician or an assistant under direct physician supervision administers a therapeutic, prophylactic, or diagnostic substance by subcutaneous or intramuscular injection (96372), intra-arterial injection (96373), or by push into an intravenous catheter or intravascular access device (96374 for a single or initial substance, 96375 for each additional sequential IV push of a new substance, and 96376 for each additional sequential IV push of the same substance after 30 minutes have elapsed). The push technique involves an infusion of less than 15 minutes. Code 96376 may be reported only by facilities.

Relative Value Units/Medicare Edits

Non-Facility RVU	Work	PE	MP	Total
96372	0.17	0.22	0.01	0.4
96373	0.17	0.34	0.01	0.52
96374	0.18	0.91	0.02	1.11
96375	0.1	0.35	0.01	0.46
96376	0.0	0.0	0.0	0.0
Facility RVU	**Work**	**PE**	**MP**	**Total**
96372	0.17	0.22	0.01	0.4
96373	0.17	0.34	0.01	0.52
96374	0.18	0.91	0.02	1.11
96375	0.1	0.35	0.01	0.46
96376	0.0	0.0	0.0	0.0

98960-98962

★98960 Education and training for patient self-management by a qualified, nonphysician health care professional using a standardized curriculum, face-to-face with the patient (could include caregiver/family) each 30 minutes; individual patient

★98961 2-4 patients

★98962 5-8 patients

Appendix

Explanation

The qualified, nonphysician health care professional provides education and training using a standard curriculum. This training is prescribed by a physician to enable the patient to concurrently self-manage established illnesses or diseases with health care providers. Report 98960 for education and training provided for an individual patient for each 30 minutes of service. Report 98961 for a group of two to four patients and 98962 for a group of five to eight patients.

Relative Value Units/Medicare Edits

Non-Facility RVU	Work	PE	MP	Total
98960	0.0	0.75	0.02	0.77
98961	0.0	0.36	0.01	0.37
98962	0.0	0.26	0.01	0.27
Facility RVU	**Work**	**PE**	**MP**	**Total**
98960	0.0	0.75	0.02	0.77
98961	0.0	0.36	0.01	0.37
98962	0.0	0.26	0.01	0.27

99051

99051   Service(s) provided in the office during regularly scheduled evening, weekend, or holiday office hours, in addition to basic service

Explanation

This code is adjunct to basic services rendered. The physician reports this code to indicate services provided during posted evening, weekend, or holiday office hours in addition to basic services.

Relative Value Units/Medicare Edits

Non-Facility RVU	Work	PE	MP	Total
99051	0.0	0.0	0.0	0.0
Facility RVU	**Work**	**PE**	**MP**	**Total**
99051	0.0	0.0	0.0	0.0

99053

99053   Service(s) provided between 10:00 PM and 8:00 AM at 24-hour facility, in addition to basic service

Explanation

This code is adjunct to basic services rendered. The physician reports this code to indicate services provided between 10 p.m. and 8 a.m. at a 24-hour facility in addition to basic services.

Relative Value Units/Medicare Edits

Non-Facility RVU	Work	PE	MP	Total
99053	0.0	0.0	0.0	0.0
Facility RVU	**Work**	**PE**	**MP**	**Total**
99053	0.0	0.0	0.0	0.0

99060

99060   Service(s) provided on an emergency basis, out of the office, which disrupts other scheduled office services, in addition to basic service

Explanation

This code is adjunct to basic services rendered. The physician reports this code to indicate services provided on an emergency basis in a location other than the physician's office that disrupt other scheduled office services.

Relative Value Units/Medicare Edits

Non-Facility RVU	Work	PE	MP	Total
99060	0.0	0.0	0.0	0.0
Facility RVU	**Work**	**PE**	**MP**	**Total**
99060	0.0	0.0	0.0	0.0

0421T

0421T   Transurethral waterjet ablation of prostate, including control of post-operative bleeding, including ultrasound guidance, complete (vasectomy, meatotomy, cystourethroscopy, urethral calibration and/or dilation, and internal urethrotomy are included when performed)

Explanation

Transurethral waterjet ablation of the prostate is a minimally invasive procedure that employs an aquablation system to destroy prostatic glandular tissue using a high-speed solution of sodium chloride in water (saline) guided with exact electromechanical control using a real-time transrectal ultrasound image. The surgeon destroys the prostatic tissue by moving along a fixed, predetermined glandular tissue map, while at the same time collecting samples of prostatic tissue to analyze after the procedure has been completed. When needed, control of bleeding (hemostasis) is performed using a low power blue laser beam contained in a water column to cause coagulation. This procedure is performed for patients with symptomatic benign prostatic hyperplasia.

0548T-0551T

0548T   Transperineal periurethral balloon continence device; bilateral placement, including cystoscopy and fluoroscopy
0549T   unilateral placement, including cystoscopy and fluoroscopy
0550T   removal, each balloon
0551T   adjustment of balloon(s) fluid volume

Explanation

These procedures describe minimally invasive, long-term, and adjustable continence therapy for stress urinary incontinence (SUI) utilizing a proprietary balloon device. Indications often include post-prostatectomy incontinence in males and intrinsic sphincter deficiency or a previously failed surgery in females. Following appropriate anesthesia (general, spinal, or local), the patient is placed in a lithotomy position that enables access to the perineum. A cystourethroscopy is performed, leaving the cystoscope sheath in place during the procedure for visualization and palpation of the ureter. Via transverse perineal incisions and under fluoroscopic guidance, implantation instruments are advanced to the area of the bladder neck and the tissue is dilated to create a space for the balloon device. The balloon is inserted to the level of the bladder neck under fluoroscopic guidance and inflated using a needle to inject an isotonic filling solution into the port. The procedure is repeated on the contralateral side. Titanium ports are placed under the skin of the scrotum in males and under the skin of the labia majora in females. Incisions are closed with resorbable sutures and a dressing is applied. The fluid-filled balloons provide support and pressure to stop urine leakages during sneezing, coughing, exercising, or other physical exertion. Once implanted, the clinician can adjust the device at any time as required to meet the patient's needs. Report 0548T for bilateral placement and 0549T for unilateral placement. For removal, report 0550T for each balloon removed. Report 0551T for balloon fluid volume adjustments.

0559T-0560T

0559T   Anatomic model 3D-printed from image data set(s); first individually prepared and processed component of an anatomic structure
+ 0560T   each additional individually prepared and processed component of an anatomic structure (List separately in addition to code for primary procedure)

Explanation

These codes describe the creation of three-dimensional (3D) printed models of individually prepared and processed elements of anatomic structures, such as bones, arteries, veins, nerves, ureters, muscles, tendons, ligaments, joints, visceral organs, and the brain. Models may be comprised of one or more distinct parts and incorporate various colors and materials. Uses of 3D-printed anatomic models are continuing to increase for a number of applications including, but not limited to, surgery planning, preparing and practicing for the procedure, training and education of health care professionals, and for patient education.

0561T-0562T

| | 0561T | Anatomic guide 3D-printed and designed from image data set(s); first anatomic guide |
| + | 0562T | each additional anatomic guide (List separately in addition to code for primary procedure) |

Explanation

Three-dimensional (3D) printed cutting or drilling guides are patient-specific surgery guides combining individualized imaging information that is used by the surgeon to navigate a procedure. Each guide is a sole, distinctive tool created to be an exact fit to the patient's natural anatomy customized to precisely match every intervention aspect, such as position and angles that mirror the actual surgery. The use of guides saves considerable time and resources; the predictability permitted by the guides allows for greater confidence in the operation room, which subsequently improves patient outcomes. In some cases, the surgery may require the use of a 3D-printed model and cutting or drilling guide for the same patient.

0582T

| 0582T | Transurethral ablation of malignant prostate tissue by high-energy water vapor thermotherapy, including intraoperative imaging and needle guidance |

Explanation

The physician performs transurethral destruction of malignant prostate tissue by radiofrequency generated water vapor thermotherapy. The physician inserts an endoscope in the penile urethra. The urethra may be dilated to allow instrument passage. After the endoscope is placed, a radiofrequency generated water vapor thermotherapy stylet is inserted in the urethra and the diseased prostate is treated with steam. The treated prostate is examined for evidence of bleeding, which may be controlled with electrocoagulation. The endoscope and instruments are removed. A urinary catheter is inserted into the bladder and left in place postoperatively.

0596T-0597T

| • | 0596T | Temporary female intraurethral valve-pump (ie, voiding prosthesis); initial insertion, including urethral measurement |
| • | 0597T | replacement |

Explanation

The physician treats permanent urinary retention due to impaired detrusor contractility (IDC) with a replaceable urinary prosthesis that mimics normal urination. This two-component system consists of a urethral insert with an internal valve-pump mechanism and a hand-held rechargeable activator that operates the valve-pump. Approximately one week prior to the insertion procedure, the correct device size is determined using a proprietary sizing tool. On the day of the procedure, the patient is placed in the lithotomy position and the meatus area is cleansed. Analgesic medical lubricant is applied to the external body of the device, after which it is inserted into the urethra using an introducer until the outer flange touches the edge of the meatus. The introducer's plunger is depressed, the device is released, and the introducer is removed. Following insertion, the physician performs a check for leakage and for proper device functioning using the activator. Holding the activator against the lower pubic

area just above the urethral opening, the button is depressed to initiate urination. Upon completion of urination, the button is released and the activator is held in place for an additional three seconds until the valve has closed, completing the urination process. Report 0596T for the initial insertion and 0597T for a replacement procedure.

0602T-0603T

| • | 0602T | Glomerular filtration rate (GFR) measurement(s), transdermal, including sensor placement and administration of a single dose of fluorescent pyrazine agent |
| • | 0603T | Glomerular filtration rate (GFR) monitoring, transdermal, including sensor placement and administration of more than one dose of fluorescent pyrazine agent, each 24 hours |

Explanation

Glomerular filtration rate (GFR) is a test that estimates the amount of blood passing through the glomeruli (the tiny filters in the kidneys that strain waste from the blood). One real-time transdermal measurement system involves a small light sensor being placed on the patient's skin and the administration of a biocompatible fluorescent tracer, such as MB-102 or Relmapirazin. The tracer is removed from the blood solely by GFR, and as it is cleared by the kidney, the measured fluorescence decreases. Algorithms in the device monitor convert these factors into a measured GFR. Intended to measure GFR in patients with normal or impaired renal function, this method can be especially beneficial in those undergoing chemotherapy. Measured GFR levels obtained just prior to drug dosing and at specific times post-infusion may be used to adjust chemotherapy dosage to ensure minimal toxicity while affording maximal efficacy. Report 0602T for transdermal GFR measurement and administration of a single dose of fluorescent pyrazine agent, and 0603T for administration of more than one dose, each 24 hours. Both codes include sensor placement.

0619T

| • | 0619T | Cystourethroscopy with transurethral anterior prostate commissurotomy and drug delivery, including transrectal ultrasound and fluoroscopy, when performed |

Explanation

The physician treats symptomatic benign prostatic hyperplasia (BPH) with transurethral delivery of therapeutic drugs. In one method, the physician utilizes a proprietary dilation catheter, the end of which has a semi-compliant inflatable double lobe balloon that is coated with the pharmaceutical paclitaxel. The cystourethroscope is introduced into the meatus and the urethra is inspected. The catheter is inserted and exerts radial force to dilate the prostatic urethra, resulting in anterior commissurotomy and localized transfer of the paclitaxel from the drug-coated balloon. The area is observed through the scope and the instruments and cystourethroscope are removed. This code includes transrectal ultrasound and fluoroscopy, when performed.

© 2020 Optum360, LLC   ● New   ▲ Revised   + Add On   ★ Telemedicine   [Resequenced]   CPT © 2020 American Medical Association. All Rights Reserved.

Coding Companion for Urology/Nephrology

Appendix

Correct Coding Initiative Update 26.3

❖Indicates Mutually Exclusive Edit

0421T 00910, 00914-00916, 0213T, 0216T, 0228T, 0230T, 0499T, 11000-11006, 11042-11047, 12001-12007, 12011-12057, 13100-13133, 13151-13153, 36000, 36400-36410, 36420-36430, 36440, 36591-36592, 36600, 36640, 43752, 51040, 51102, 51700-51703, 52000-52005, 52204-52240, 52270-52276, 52281, 52283, 52287, 52305-52315, 52400, 52441, 52500, 52630, 52700, 53000-53025, 53600-53621, 53855, 55000, 55200-55250, 55700-55705, 61650, 62320-62327, 64400, 64405-64408, 64415-64435, 64445-64454, 64461, 64463, 64479, 64483, 64486-64490, 64493, 64505, 64510-64530, 69990, 76000, 76872, 76942, 76970, 76998, 77001-77002, 92012-92014, 93000-93010, 93040-93042, 93318, 93355, 94002, 94200, 94250, 94680-94690, 94770, 95812-95816, 95819, 95822, 95829, 95955, 96360, 96365, 96372, 96374-96377, 96523, 97597-97598, 97602, 99155, 99156, 99157, 99211-99223, 99231-99255, 99291-99292, 99304-99310, 99315-99316, 99334-99337, 99347-99350, 99374-99375, 99377-99378, 99446-99449, 99451-99452, 99495-99496, G0463, G0471, J2001, P9612

0548T 0213T, 0216T, 0228T, 0230T, 0549T, 0551T, 11000-11006, 11042-11047, 12001-12007, 12011-12056, 36591-36592, 51990-51992, 52301, 53000-53025, 53080, 53444, 64450, 93318, 93355, 96365-96368, 96372, 96374-96377, 96523, 97597-97598, 97602, 99155, 99156, 99157, 99211-99223, 99231-99255, 99291-99292, 99304-99310, 99315-99316, 99334-99337, 99347-99350, 99374-99375, 99377-99378, 99446-99449, 99451-99452, 99495-99496, G0463, G0471

0549T 0213T, 0216T, 0228T, 0230T, 0551T, 11000-11006, 11042-11047, 12001-12007, 12011-12057, 13100-13133, 13151-13153, 36000, 36400-36410, 36420-36430, 36440, 36591-36592, 36600, 36640, 43752, 51701-51703, 51990-51992, 52000, 52301, 53000-53025, 53080, 53444, 62320-62327, 64400, 64405-64408, 64415-64435, 64445-64450, 64461-64463, 64479-64505, 64510-64530, 69990, 76000, 77002, 92012-92014, 93000-93010, 93040-93042, 93318, 93355, 94002, 94200, 94250, 94680-94690, 94770, 95812-95816, 95819, 95822, 95829, 95955, 96360-96368, 96372, 96374-96377, 96523, 97597-97598, 97602, 99155, 99156, 99157, 99211-99223, 99231-99255, 99291-99292, 99304-99310, 99315-99316, 99334-99337, 99347-99350, 99374-99375, 99377-99378, 99446-99449, 99451-99452, 99495-99496, G0463, G0471

0550T 0213T, 0216T, 0228T, 0230T, 0551T, 11000-11006, 11042-11047, 12001-12007, 12011-12057, 13100-13133, 13151-13153, 36000, 36400-36410, 36420-36430, 36440, 36591-36592, 36600, 36640, 43752, 51701-51703, 52000, 53000-53025, 53080, 53445, 62320-62327, 64400, 64405-64408, 64415-64435, 64445-64450, 64461-64463, 64479-64505, 64510-64530, 69990, 92012-92014, 93000-93010, 93040-93042, 93318, 93355, 94002, 94200, 94250, 94680-94690, 94770, 95812-95816, 95819, 95822, 95829, 95955, 96360-96368, 96372, 96374-96377, 96523, 97597-97598, 97602, 99155, 99156, 99157, 99211-99223, 99231-99255, 99291-99292, 99304-99310, 99315-99316, 99334-99337, 99347-99350, 99374-99375, 99377-99378, 99446-99449, 99451-99452, 99495-99496, G0463, G0471

0551T No CCI edits apply to this code.

0559T 76376-76377

0560T 76376-76377

0561T 76376-76377

0562T 76376-76377

0582T 0213T, 0216T, 0228T, 0230T, 0421T❖, 36591-36592, 51102, 51700, 52001, 52281, 52441, 52500, 52640❖, 53000-53025, 53600-53621, 53850-53852❖, 53855, 55700, 64450, 76873, 76940, 76998, 77013,

77022, 93318, 93355, 96376, 96523, 99446-99449, 99495-99496, G0463, G0471, J0670, J2001, P9612

0596T No CCI edits apply to this code.

0597T No CCI edits apply to this code.

0602T No CCI edits apply to this code.

0603T No CCI edits apply to this code.

0619T No CCI edits apply to this code.

10004 0213T, 0216T, 10012, 10035, 19281, 19283, 19285, 19287, 36000, 36410, 36591-36592, 61650, 62324-62327, 64415-64417, 64450, 64454, 64486-64490, 64493, 76000, 76380❖, 76942, 76970, 76998, 77001-77002, 77012, 77021, 96360, 96365, 96372, 96374-96377, 96523, J2001

10005 0213T, 0216T, 10004, 10008, 10010-10012, 10021, 10035, 11102-11107, 19281, 19283, 19285, 19287, 36000, 36410, 36591-36592, 61650, 62324-62327, 64415-64417, 64450, 64454, 64486-64490, 64493, 76000, 76380❖, 76942, 76970, 76998, 77001-77002, 77012, 77021, 96360, 96365, 96372, 96374-96377, 96523, J2001

10006 0213T, 0216T, 10004, 10035, 19281, 19283, 19285, 19287, 36000, 36410, 36591-36592, 61650, 62324-62327, 64415-64417, 64450, 64454, 64486-64490, 64493, 76000, 76380❖, 76942, 76970, 76998, 77001-77002, 77012, 77021, 96360, 96365, 96372, 96374-96377, 96523, J2001

10007 0213T, 0216T, 10004-10006, 10010-10012, 10021, 10035, 11102-11107, 19281, 19283, 19285, 19287, 36000, 36410, 36591-36592, 61650, 62324-62327, 64415-64417, 64450, 64454, 64486-64490, 64493, 76000, 76380❖, 76942, 76970, 76998, 77001-77002, 77012, 77021, 96360, 96365, 96372, 96374-96377, 96523, J2001

10008 0213T, 0216T, 10004, 10021, 10035, 19281, 19283, 19285, 19287, 36000, 36410, 36591-36592, 61650, 62324-62327, 64415-64417, 64450, 64454, 64486-64490, 64493, 76000, 76380❖, 76942, 76970, 76998, 77001-77002, 77012, 77021, 96360, 96365, 96372, 96374-96377, 96523, J2001

10009 0213T, 0216T, 10004-10008, 10011-10012, 10021, 10035, 11102-11106, 19281, 19283, 19285, 19287, 36000, 36410, 36591-36592, 61650, 62324-62327, 64415-64417, 64450, 64454, 64486-64490, 64493, 76000, 76380❖, 76942, 76970, 76998, 77001-77002, 77012, 77021, 96360, 96365, 96372, 96374-96377, 96523, J2001

10010 0213T, 0216T, 10004, 10021, 10035, 19281, 19283, 19285, 19287, 36000, 36410, 36591-36592, 61650, 62324-62327, 64415-64417, 64450, 64454, 64486-64490, 64493, 76000, 76380❖, 76942, 76970, 76998, 77001-77002, 77012, 77021, 96360, 96365, 96372, 96374-96377, 96523, J2001

10011 0213T, 0216T, 10004, 10006, 10008, 10010, 10035, 19281, 19283, 19285, 19287, 36000, 36410, 36591-36592, 61650, 62324-62327, 64415-64417, 64450, 64454, 64486-64490, 64493, 76000, 76380❖, 76942, 76970, 76998, 77001-77002, 77012, 77021, 96360, 96365, 96372, 96374-96377, 96523, J2001

10012 0213T, 0216T, 10035, 19281, 19283, 19285, 19287, 36000, 36410, 36591-36592, 61650, 62324-62327, 64415-64417, 64450, 64454, 64486-64490, 64493, 76000, 76380❖, 76942, 76970, 76998, 77001-77002, 77012, 77021, 96360, 96365, 96372, 96374-96377, 96523, J2001

10021 0213T, 0216T, 10006, 10011-10012, 10035, 11102-11105, 11107, 19281, 19283, 19285, 19287, 36000, 36410, 36591-36592, 61650,

62324-62327, 64415-64417, 64450, 64454, 64486-64490, 64493, 76000, 76380✦, 76942, 76970, 76998, 77001-77002, 77012, 77021, 96360, 96365, 96372, 96374-96377, 96523, J2001

10030 0213T, 0216T, 0228T, 0230T, 10060-10061✦, 10080-10081✦, 10140✦, 10160✦, 11055-11057, 11401-11406✦, 11421-11426✦, 11441-11471✦, 11600-11606✦, 11620-11646✦, 11719-11721, 11765, 12001-12007, 12011-12057, 13100-13133, 13151-13153, 20500, 29580-29581, 36000, 36400-36410, 36420-36430, 36440, 36591-36592, 36600, 36640, 43752, 51701-51703, 61650, 62320-62327, 64400, 64405-64408, 64415-64435, 64445-64454, 64461-64463, 64479-64505, 64510-64530, 69990, 75989, 76000, 76380, 76942, 76970, 76998, 77002-77003, 77012, 77021, 92012-92014, 93000-93010, 93040-93042, 93318, 93355, 94002, 94200, 94250, 94680-94690, 94770, 95812-95816, 95819, 95822, 95829, 95955, 96360-96368, 96372, 96374-96377, 96523, 97597-97598, 97602-97608, 99155, 99156, 99157, 99211-99223, 99231-99255, 99291-99292, 99304-99310, 99315-99316, 99334-99337, 99347-99350, 99374-99375, 99377-99378, 99446-99449, 99451-99452, G0127, G0463, G0471, J0670, J2001

10180 0213T, 0216T, 0228T, 0230T, 11720-11721, 12001-12007, 12011-12057, 13100-13133, 13151-13153, 20500, 36000, 36400-36410, 36420-36430, 36440, 36591-36592, 36600, 36640, 43752, 51701-51703, 62320-62327, 64400, 64405-64408, 64415-64435, 64445-64454, 64461-64463, 64479-64505, 64510-64530, 69990, 92012-92014, 93000-93010, 93040-93042, 93318, 93355, 94002, 94200, 94250, 94680-94690, 94770, 95812-95816, 95819, 95822, 95829, 95955, 96360-96368, 96372, 96374-96377, 96523, 99155, 99156, 99157, 99211-99223, 99231-99255, 99291-99292, 99304-99310, 99315-99316, 99334-99337, 99347-99350, 99374-99375, 99377-99378, 99446-99449, 99451-99452, 99495-99496, G0463, G0471, J0670, J2001

11004 0213T, 0216T, 0228T, 0230T, 0437T, 0552T, 10030, 10060-10061, 11000, 11010-11012, 11042-11044, 11102-11107, 12001-12007, 12011-12018, 12021-12057, 13100-13133, 13151-13153, 15769, 15777, 20552-20553, 20560-20561, 20700-20701, 36000, 36400-36410, 36420-36430, 36440, 36591-36592, 36600, 36640, 43752, 57267, 62320-62327, 64400, 64405-64408, 64415-64435, 64445-64454, 64461-64463, 64479-64505, 64510-64530, 66987-66988, 69990, 92012-92014, 93000-93010, 93040-93042, 93318, 93355, 94002, 94200, 94250, 94680-94690, 94770, 95812-95816, 95819, 95822, 95829, 95955, 96360-96368, 96372, 96374-96377, 96523, 97597-97598, 97610, 99155, 99156, 99157, 99211-99223, 99231-99255, 99291-99292, 99304-99310, 99315-99316, 99334-99337, 99347-99350, 99374-99375, 99377-99378, 99446-99449, 99451-99452, 99495-99496, G0463, G0471

11005 0213T, 0216T, 0228T, 0230T, 0437T, 0552T, 10030, 10060-10061, 11000, 11004, 11010-11012, 11042-11044, 11102-11107, 12001-12007, 12011-12018, 12021-12057, 13100-13133, 13151-13153, 15769, 15777, 20552-20553, 20560-20561, 20700-20701, 36000, 36400-36410, 36420-36430, 36440, 36591-36592, 36600, 36640, 43752, 57267, 62320-62327, 64400, 64405-64408, 64415-64435, 64445-64454, 64461-64463, 64479-64505, 64510-64530, 66987-66988, 69990, 92012-92014, 93000-93010, 93040-93042, 93318, 93355, 94002, 94200, 94250, 94680-94690, 94770, 95812-95816, 95819, 95822, 95829, 95955, 96360-96368, 96372, 96374-96377, 96523, 97597-97598, 97610, 99155, 99156, 99157, 99211-99223, 99231-99255, 99291-99292, 99304-99310, 99315-99316, 99334-99337, 99347-99350, 99374-99375, 99377-99378, 99446-99449, 99451-99452, 99495-99496, G0463, G0471

11006 0213T, 0216T, 0228T, 0230T, 0437T, 0552T, 10030, 10060-10061, 11000, 11004-11005, 11010-11012, 11042-11044, 11102-11107, 12001-12007, 12011-12018, 12021-12057, 13100-13133, 13151-13153, 15769, 15777, 20552-20553, 20560-20561, 20700-20701, 36000,

36400-36410, 36420-36430, 36440, 36591-36592, 36600, 36640, 43752, 57267, 62320-62327, 64400, 64405-64408, 64415-64435, 64445-64454, 64461-64463, 64479-64505, 64510-64530, 66987-66988, 69990, 92012-92014, 93000-93010, 93040-93042, 93318, 93355, 94002, 94200, 94250, 94680-94690, 94770, 95812-95816, 95819, 95822, 95829, 95955, 96360-96368, 96372, 96374-96377, 96523, 97597-97598, 97610, 99155, 99156, 99157, 99211-99223, 99231-99255, 99291-99292, 99304-99310, 99315-99316, 99334-99337, 99347-99350, 99374-99375, 99377-99378, 99446-99449, 99451-99452, 99495-99496, G0463, G0471

11008 36591-36592, 96523

12001 0213T, 0216T, 0228T, 0230T, 0543T-0544T, 0545T, 0567T-0574T, 0580T, 0581T, 0582T, 11042, 11055-11056, 11719, 11740-11750, 11900-11901, 20560-20561, 36000, 36400-36410, 36420-36430, 36440, 36591-36592, 36600, 36640, 43752, 51701-51703, 64400, 64405-64408, 64415-64435, 64445-64450, 64479-64484, 64490-64505, 64510-64530, 66987-66988, 69990, 92012-92014, 93000-93010, 93040-93042, 93318, 93355, 94002, 94200, 94250, 94680-94690, 94770, 95812-95816, 95819, 95822, 95829, 95955, 96360-96368, 96372, 96374-96377, 96523, 97597-97598, 97602-97608, 99155, 99156, 99157, 99211-99223, 99231-99255, 99291-99292, 99304-99310, 99315-99316, 99334-99337, 99347-99350, 99374-99375, 99377-99378, 99446-99449, 99451-99452, 99495-99496, G0168, G0463, G0471, J0670, J2001

12002 0213T, 0216T, 0228T, 0230T, 0543T-0544T, 0545T, 0567T-0574T, 0580T, 0581T, 0582T, 11042, 11740, 11900-11901, 12001, 12013-12014✦, 20560-20561, 20701, 36000, 36400-36410, 36420-36430, 36440, 36591-36592, 36600, 36640, 43752, 51701-51703, 64400, 64405-64408, 64415-64435, 64445-64450, 64479-64484, 64490-64505, 64510-64530, 66987-66988, 69990, 92012-92014, 93000-93010, 93040-93042, 93318, 93355, 94002, 94200, 94250, 94680-94690, 94770, 95812-95816, 95819, 95822, 95829, 95955, 96360-96368, 96372, 96374-96377, 96523, 97597-97598, 97602-97608, 99155, 99156, 99157, 99211-99223, 99231-99255, 99291-99292, 99304-99310, 99315-99316, 99334-99337, 99347-99350, 99374-99375, 99377-99378, 99446-99449, 99451-99452, 99495-99496, G0168, G0463, G0471, J0670, J2001

12004 0213T, 0216T, 0228T, 0230T, 0543T-0544T, 0545T, 0567T-0574T, 0580T, 0581T, 0582T, 11042, 11900-11901, 12001-12002, 12015✦, 20560-20561, 20701, 36000, 36400-36410, 36420-36430, 36440, 36591-36592, 36600, 36640, 43752, 51701-51703, 64400, 64405-64408, 64415-64435, 64445-64450, 64479-64484, 64490-64505, 64510-64530, 66987-66988, 69990, 92012-92014, 93000-93010, 93040-93042, 93318, 93355, 94002, 94200, 94250, 94680-94690, 94770, 95812-95816, 95819, 95822, 95829, 95955, 96360-96368, 96372, 96374-96377, 96523, 97597-97598, 97602-97608, 99155, 99156, 99157, 99211-99223, 99231-99255, 99291-99292, 99304-99310, 99315-99316, 99334-99337, 99347-99350, 99374-99375, 99377-99378, 99446-99449, 99451-99452, 99495-99496, G0168, G0463, G0471, J0670, J2001

12005 0213T, 0216T, 0228T, 0230T, 0543T-0544T, 0545T, 0567T-0574T, 0580T, 0581T, 0582T, 11042-11043, 11900-11901, 12001-12004, 12016✦, 20560-20561, 20700-20701, 36000, 36400-36410, 36420-36430, 36440, 36591-36592, 36600, 36640, 43752, 51701-51703, 64400, 64405-64408, 64415-64435, 64445-64451, 64479-64484, 64490-64505, 64510-64530, 66987-66988, 69990, 92012-92014, 93000-93010, 93040-93042, 93318, 93355, 94002, 94200, 94250, 94680-94690, 94770, 95812-95816, 95819, 95822, 95829, 95955, 96360-96368, 96372, 96374-96377, 96523, 97597-97598, 97602-97608, 99155, 99156, 99157, 99211-99223, 99231-99255, 99291-99292, 99304-99310, 99315-99316, 99334-99337, 99347-99350, 99374-99375, 99377-99378, 99446-99449, 99451-99452, 99495-99496, G0168, G0463, G0471, J0670, J2001

12006 0213T, 0216T, 0228T, 0230T, 0543T-0544T, 0545T, 0567T-0574T, 0580T, 0581T, 0582T, 11042-11043, 11900-11901, 12001-12005, 12017❖, 20560-20561, 20700-20701, 36000, 36400-36410, 36420-36430, 36440, 36591-36592, 36600, 36640, 43752, 51701-51703, 64400, 64405-64408, 64415-64435, 64445-64451, 64479-64484, 64490-64505, 64510-64530, 66987-66988, 69990, 92012-92014, 93000-93010, 93040-93042, 93318, 93355, 94002, 94200, 94250, 94680-94690, 94770, 95812-95816, 95819, 95822, 95829, 95955, 96360-96368, 96372, 96374-96377, 96523, 97597-97598, 97602-97608, 99155, 99156, 99157, 99211-99223, 99231-99255, 99291-99292, 99304-99310, 99315-99316, 99334-99337, 99347-99350, 99374-99375, 99377-99378, 99446-99449, 99451-99452, 99495-99496, G0168, G0463, G0471, J0670, J2001

12007 0213T, 0216T, 0228T, 0230T, 0543T-0544T, 0545T, 0567T-0574T, 0580T, 0581T, 0582T, 11900-11901, 12001-12006, 12018❖, 15772, 15774, 20560-20561, 20700-20701, 36000, 36400-36410, 36420-36430, 36440, 36591-36592, 36600, 36640, 43752, 51701-51703, 64400, 64405-64408, 64415-64435, 64445-64451, 64479-64484, 64490-64505, 64510-64530, 66987-66988, 69990, 92012-92014, 93000-93010, 93040-93042, 93318, 93355, 94002, 94200, 94250, 94680-94690, 94770, 95812-95816, 95819, 95822, 95829, 95955, 96360-96368, 96372, 96374-96377, 96523, 97597-97598, 97602-97608, 99155, 99156, 99157, 99211-99223, 99231-99255, 99291-99292, 99304-99310, 99315-99316, 99334-99337, 99347-99350, 99374-99375, 99377-99378, 99446-99449, 99451-99452, 99495-99496, G0168, G0463, G0471, J0670, J2001

12020 0213T, 0216T, 0228T, 0230T, 0543T-0544T, 0545T, 0567T-0574T, 0580T, 0581T, 0582T, 11000-11006, 11042-11047, 11900-11901, 12021, 15772, 15774, 20560-20561, 20700-20701, 36000, 36400-36410, 36420-36430, 36440, 36591-36592, 36600, 36640, 43752, 51701-51703, 64400, 64405-64408, 64415-64435, 64445-64451, 64479-64484, 64490-64505, 64510-64530, 66987-66988, 69990, 92012-92014, 93000-93010, 93040-93042, 93318, 93355, 94002, 94200, 94250, 94680-94690, 94770, 95812-95816, 95819, 95822, 95829, 95955, 96360-96368, 96372, 96374-96377, 96523, 97597-97598, 97602-97608, 99155, 99156, 99157, 99211-99223, 99231-99255, 99291-99292, 99304-99310, 99315-99316, 99334-99337, 99347-99350, 99374-99375, 99377-99378, 99446-99449, 99451-99452, 99495-99496, G0168, G0463, G0471, J0670, J2001

12021 0213T, 0216T, 0228T, 0230T, 0543T-0544T, 0567T-0574T, 0580T, 0581T, 0582T, 11042, 11900-11901, 20560-20561, 20700-20701, 36000, 36400-36410, 36420-36430, 36440, 36591-36592, 36600, 36640, 43752, 51701-51703, 64400, 64405-64408, 64415-64435, 64445-64451, 64479-64484, 64490-64505, 64510-64530, 66987-66988, 69990, 92012-92014, 93000-93010, 93040-93042, 93318, 93355, 94002, 94200, 94250, 94680-94690, 94770, 95812-95816, 95819, 95822, 95829, 95955, 96360-96368, 96372, 96374-96377, 96523, 97597-97598, 97602-97608, 99155, 99156, 99157, 99211-99223, 99231-99255, 99291-99292, 99304-99310, 99315-99316, 99334-99337, 99347-99350, 99374-99375, 99377-99378, 99446-99449, 99451-99452, 99495-99496, G0168, G0463, G0471, J2001

12041 0213T, 0216T, 0228T, 0230T, 0543T-0544T, 0567T-0574T, 0580T, 0581T, 0582T, 11055-11056, 11740, 11900-11901, 12031, 20560-20561, 20700-20701, 36000, 36400-36410, 36420-36430, 36440, 36591-36592, 36600, 36640, 43752, 51701-51703, 64400, 64405-64408, 64415-64435, 64445-64451, 64479-64484, 64490-64505, 64510-64530, 66987-66988, 69990, 92012-92014, 93000-93010, 93040-93042, 93318, 93355, 94002, 94200, 94250, 94680-94690, 94770, 95812-95816, 95819, 95822, 95829, 95955, 96360-96368, 96372, 96374-96377, 96523, 97597-97598, 97602-97608, 99155, 99156, 99157, 99211-99223, 99231-99255, 99291-99292, 99304-99310, 99315-99316, 99334-99337, 99347-99350,

99374-99375, 99377-99378, 99446-99449, 99451-99452, 99495-99496, G0168, G0463, G0471, J0670, J2001

12042 0213T, 0216T, 0228T, 0230T, 0567T-0574T, 0580T, 0581T, 0582T, 11042, 11740, 11900-11901, 12041, 15772, 15774, 20560-20561, 20700-20701, 36000, 36400-36410, 36420-36430, 36440, 36591-36592, 36600, 36640, 43752, 51701-51703, 64400, 64405-64408, 64415-64435, 64445-64451, 64479-64484, 64490-64505, 64510-64530, 66987-66988, 69990, 92012-92014, 93000-93010, 93040-93042, 93318, 93355, 94002, 94200, 94250, 94680-94690, 94770, 95812-95816, 95819, 95822, 95829, 95955, 96360-96368, 96372, 96374-96377, 96523, 97597-97598, 97602-97608, 99155, 99156, 99157, 99211-99223, 99231-99255, 99291-99292, 99304-99310, 99315-99316, 99334-99337, 99347-99350, 99374-99375, 99377-99378, 99446-99449, 99451-99452, 99495-99496, G0168, G0463, G0471, J0670, J2001

12044 0213T, 0216T, 0228T, 0230T, 0567T-0574T, 0580T, 0581T, 0582T, 11043-11044, 11900-11901, 12041-12042, 12054❖, 15772, 15774, 20560-20561, 20700-20701, 36000, 36400-36410, 36420-36430, 36440, 36591-36592, 36600, 36640, 43752, 51701-51703, 64400, 64405-64408, 64415-64435, 64445-64451, 64479-64484, 64490-64505, 64510-64530, 66987-66988, 69990, 92012-92014, 93000-93010, 93040-93042, 93318, 93355, 94002, 94200, 94250, 94680-94690, 94770, 95812-95816, 95819, 95822, 95829, 95955, 96360-96368, 96372, 96374-96377, 96523, 97597-97598, 97602-97608, 99155, 99156, 99157, 99211-99223, 99231-99255, 99291-99292, 99304-99310, 99315-99316, 99334-99337, 99347-99350, 99374-99375, 99377-99378, 99446-99449, 99451-99452, 99495-99496, G0168, G0463, G0471, J0670, J2001

12045 0213T, 0216T, 0228T, 0230T, 0567T-0574T, 0580T, 0581T, 0582T, 11042, 11900-11901, 12041-12044, 12055❖, 15772, 15774, 20560-20561, 20700-20701, 36000, 36400-36410, 36420-36430, 36440, 36591-36592, 36600, 36640, 43752, 51701-51703, 64400, 64405-64408, 64415-64435, 64445-64451, 64479-64484, 64490-64505, 64510-64530, 64625, 66987-66988, 69990, 92012-92014, 93000-93010, 93040-93042, 93318, 93355, 94002, 94200, 94250, 94680-94690, 94770, 95812-95816, 95819, 95822, 95829, 95955, 96360-96368, 96372, 96374-96377, 96523, 97597-97598, 97602-97608, 99155, 99156, 99157, 99211-99223, 99231-99255, 99291-99292, 99304-99310, 99315-99316, 99334-99337, 99347-99350, 99374-99375, 99377-99378, 99446-99449, 99451-99452, 99495-99496, G0168, G0463, G0471, J0670, J2001

12046 0213T, 0216T, 0228T, 0230T, 0567T-0574T, 0580T, 0581T, 0582T, 11043-11044, 11900-11901, 12041-12045, 12056❖, 15772, 15774, 20560-20561, 20700-20701, 36000, 36400-36410, 36420-36430, 36440, 36591-36592, 36600, 36640, 43752, 51701-51703, 64400, 64405-64408, 64415-64435, 64445-64451, 64479-64484, 64490-64505, 64510-64530, 64625, 66987-66988, 69990, 92012-92014, 93000-93010, 93040-93042, 93318, 93355, 94002, 94200, 94250, 94680-94690, 94770, 95812-95816, 95819, 95822, 95829, 95955, 96360-96368, 96372, 96374-96377, 96523, 97597-97598, 97602-97608, 99155, 99156, 99157, 99211-99223, 99231-99255, 99291-99292, 99304-99310, 99315-99316, 99334-99337, 99347-99350, 99374-99375, 99377-99378, 99446-99449, 99451-99452, 99495-99496, G0168, G0463, G0471, J0670, J2001

12047 0213T, 0216T, 0228T, 0230T, 0567T-0574T, 0580T, 0581T, 0582T, 11900-11901, 12037-12046, 12057❖, 15772, 15774, 20560-20561, 20700-20701, 36000, 36400-36410, 36420-36430, 36440, 36591-36592, 36600, 36640, 43752, 51701-51703, 64400, 64405-64408, 64415-64435, 64445-64451, 64479-64484, 64490-64505, 64510-64530, 64625, 66987-66988, 69990, 92012-92014, 93000-93010, 93040-93042, 93318, 93355, 94002, 94200, 94250, 94680-94690, 94770, 95812-95816, 95819, 95822, 95829, 95955, 96360-96368, 96372, 96374-96377, 96523, 97597-97598, 97602-97608, 99155, 99156, 99157, 99211-99223,

CPT © 2020 American Medical Association. All Rights Reserved.

CCI Edits

99231-99255, 99291-99292, 99304-99310, 99315-99316, 99334-99337, 99347-99350, 99374-99375, 99377-99378, 99446-99449, 99451-99452, 99495-99496, G0168, G0463, G0471, J0670, J2001

13131 0213T, 0216T, 0228T, 0230T, 0548T, 0567T-0574T, 0580T, 0581T, 0582T, 11000, 11010-11012, 11042-11044, 11900-11901, 13133, 13160❖, 15772, 15774, 20560-20561, 20700-20701, 36000, 36400-36410, 36420-36430, 36440, 36591-36592, 36600, 36640, 43752, 51701-51703, 64400, 64405-64408, 64415-64435, 64445-64451, 64479-64484, 64490-64505, 64510-64530, 64625, 66987-66988, 69990, 92012-92014, 93000-93010, 93040-93042, 93318, 93355, 94002, 94200, 94250, 94680-94690, 94770, 95812-95816, 95819, 95822, 95829, 95955, 96360-96368, 96372, 96374-96377, 96523, 97597-97598, 97602-97608, 99155, 99156, 99157, 99211-99223, 99231-99255, 99291-99292, 99304-99310, 99315-99316, 99334-99337, 99347-99350, 99374-99375, 99377-99378, 99446-99449, 99451-99452, 99495-99496, G0168, G0463, G0471, J0670, J2001

13132 0213T, 0216T, 0228T, 0230T, 0548T, 0567T-0574T, 0580T, 0581T, 0582T, 11000, 11010-11012, 11042-11044, 11056, 11900-11901, 13131, 13160❖, 15772, 15774, 20560-20561, 20700-20701, 36000, 36400-36410, 36420-36430, 36440, 36591-36592, 36600, 36640, 43752, 51701-51703, 64400, 64405-64408, 64415-64435, 64445-64451, 64479-64484, 64490-64505, 64510-64530, 64625, 66987-66988, 69990, 92012-92014, 93000-93010, 93040-93042, 93318, 93355, 94002, 94200, 94250, 94680-94690, 94770, 95812-95816, 95819, 95822, 95829, 95955, 96360-96368, 96372, 96374-96377, 96523, 97597-97598, 97602-97608, 99155, 99156, 99157, 99211-99223, 99231-99255, 99291-99292, 99304-99310, 99315-99316, 99334-99337, 99347-99350, 99374-99375, 99377-99378, 99446-99449, 99451-99452, 99495-99496, G0168, G0463, G0471, J0670, J2001

13133 0548T, 0567T-0574T, 0580T, 0581T, 0582T, 11900-11901, 13160❖, 20560-20561, 20700-20701, 36591-36592, 64451, 66987-66988, 69990, 96523, J0670, J2001

13160 0213T, 0216T, 0228T, 0230T, 10180, 11000-11006, 11010-11012, 11042-11047, 11102, 11104, 11106, 11900-11901, 12001-12007, 12011-12057, 36000, 36400-36410, 36420-36430, 36440, 36591-36592, 36600, 36640, 43752, 51701-51703, 62320-62327, 64400, 64405-64408, 64415-64435, 64445-64454, 64461-64463, 64479-64505, 64510-64530, 69990, 92012-92014, 93000-93010, 93040-93042, 93318, 93355, 94002, 94200, 94250, 94680-94690, 94770, 95812-95816, 95819, 95822, 95829, 95955, 96360-96368, 96372, 96374-96377, 96523, 97597-97598, 97602-97608, 99155, 99156, 99157, 99211-99223, 99231-99255, 99291-99292, 99304-99310, 99315-99316, 99334-99337, 99347-99350, 99374-99375, 99377-99378, 99446-99449, 99451-99452, 99495-99496, G0168, G0463, G0471

15002 01951-01952, 0213T, 0216T, 0228T, 0230T, 11000-11006, 11042-11047, 11102, 11104, 11106, 11400-11421❖, 11423-11444❖, 11450❖, 11600-11604❖, 11620-11624❖, 11640-11643❖, 12001-12007, 12011-12057, 13100-13133, 13151-13153, 36000, 36400-36410, 36420-36430, 36440, 36591-36592, 36600, 36640, 43752, 51701-51703, 62320-62327, 64400, 64405-64408, 64415-64435, 64445-64454, 64461-64463, 64479-64505, 64510-64530, 69990, 92012-92014, 93000-93010, 93040-93042, 93318, 93355, 94002, 94200, 94250, 94680-94690, 94770, 95812-95816, 95819, 95822, 95829, 95955, 96360-96368, 96372, 96374-96377, 96523, 97597-97598, 97602, 99155, 99156, 99157, 99211-99223, 99231-99255, 99291-99292, 99304-99310, 99315-99316, 99334-99337, 99347-99350, 99374-99375, 99377-99378, 99446-99449, 99451-99452, 99495-99496, G0168, G0463, G0471, J0670, J2001

15003 11000-11006, 11042-11047, 36591-36592, 96523, 97597-97598, 97602, J0670, J2001

15004 01951-01952, 0213T, 0216T, 0228T, 0230T, 11000-11006, 11042-11047, 11102, 11104, 11106, 11400-11421❖, 11423-11450❖, 11462❖, 11470❖, 11600-11604❖, 11620-11644❖, 12001-12007, 12011-12057, 13100-13133, 13151-13153, 36000, 36400-36410, 36420-36430, 36440, 36591-36592, 36600, 36640, 51701-51703, 62320-62327, 64400, 64405-64408, 64415-64435, 64445-64454, 64461-64463, 64479-64505, 64510-64530, 69990, 92012-92014, 93000-93010, 93040-93042, 93318, 93355, 94002, 94200, 94250, 94680-94690, 94770, 95812-95816, 95819, 95822, 95829, 95955, 96360-96368, 96372, 96374-96377, 96523, 97597-97598, 97602, 99155, 99156, 99157, 99211-99223, 99231-99255, 99291-99292, 99304-99310, 99315-99316, 99334-99337, 99347-99350, 99374-99375, 99377-99378, 99446-99449, 99451-99452, 99495-99496, G0168, G0463, G0471, J0670, J2001

15005 11000-11006, 11042-11047, 36591-36592, 96523, 97597-97598, 97602, J0670, J2001

15120 01951-01952, 0213T, 0216T, 0228T, 0230T, 0490T, 11000-11006, 11042-11047, 11102, 11104, 11106, 12001-12007, 12011-12057, 13100-13133, 13151-13153, 15050, 15852, 16020-16030, 20526-20553, 20560-20561, 25259, 26340, 29000-29015, 29035-29200, 29240-29450, 29505-29581, 29584, 36000, 36400-36410, 36420-36430, 36440, 36591-36592, 36600, 36640, 43752, 51701-51703, 62320-62327, 64400, 64405-64408, 64415-64435, 64445-64454, 64461-64463, 64479-64505, 64510-64530, 69990, 92012-92014, 93000-93010, 93040-93042, 93318, 93355, 94002, 94200, 94250, 94680-94690, 94770, 95812-95816, 95819, 95822, 95829, 95955, 96360-96368, 96372, 96374-96377, 96523, 97597-97598, 97602-97608, 99155, 99156, 99157, 99211-99223, 99231-99255, 99291-99292, 99304-99310, 99315-99316, 99334-99337, 99347-99350, 99374-99375, 99377-99378, 99446-99449, 99451-99452, 99495-99496, G0168, G0463, G0471, J0670, J2001

15121 11000-11006, 11042-11047, 36591-36592, 96523, 97597-97598, 97602, J0670, J2001

15240 01951-01952, 0213T, 0216T, 0228T, 0230T, 11000-11006, 11042-11047, 11102, 11104, 11106, 12001-12007, 12011-12057, 13100-13133, 13151-13153, 15852, 16020-16030, 20526, 20551-20553, 20560-20561, 25259, 26340, 29000-29015, 29035-29200, 29240-29450, 29505-29581, 29584, 36000, 36400-36410, 36420-36430, 36440, 36591-36592, 36600, 36640, 43752, 51701-51703, 62320-62327, 64400, 64405-64408, 64415-64435, 64445-64454, 64461-64463, 64479-64505, 64510-64530, 69990, 92012-92014, 93000-93010, 93040-93042, 93318, 93355, 94002, 94200, 94250, 94680-94690, 94770, 95812-95816, 95819, 95822, 95829, 95955, 96360-96368, 96372, 96374-96377, 96523, 97597-97598, 97602-97608, 99155, 99156, 99157, 99211-99223, 99231-99255, 99291-99292, 99304-99310, 99315-99316, 99334-99337, 99347-99350, 99374-99375, 99377-99378, 99446-99449, 99451-99452, 99495-99496, G0168, G0463, G0471, J0670, J2001

15241 11000-11006, 11042-11047, 36591-36592, 96523, 97597-97598, 97602, J0670, J2001

17270 0213T, 0216T, 0228T, 0230T, 0419T-0420T❖, 11102, 11104, 11106, 11600-11606❖, 11620-11646❖, 11900-11901, 12001-12007, 12011-12057, 13100-13133, 13151-13153, 17000❖, 17004❖, 17110-17111❖, 17340, 36000, 36400-36410, 36420-36430, 36440, 36591-36592, 36600, 36640, 43752, 51701-51703, 62320-62327, 64400, 64405-64408, 64415-64435, 64445-64454, 64461-64463, 64479-64505, 64510-64530, 69990, 92012-92014, 93000-93010, 93040-93042, 93318, 93355, 94002, 94200, 94250, 94680-94690, 94770, 95812-95816, 95819, 95822, 95829, 95955, 96360-96368, 96372, 96374-96377, 96523, 99155, 99156, 99157, 99211-99223, 99231-99255, 99291-99292,

99304-99310, 99315-99316, 99334-99337, 99347-99350, 99374-99375,
99377-99378, 99446-99449, 99451-99452, 99495-99496, G0463,
G0471, J0670, J2001

17271 0213T, 0216T, 0228T, 0230T, 11102, 11104, 11106, 11601-11606♦,
11621-11646♦, 11900-11901, 12001-12007, 12011-12057,
13100-13133, 13151-13153, 17000♦, 17004♦, 17110-17111♦, 17340,
36000, 36400-36410, 36420-36430, 36440, 36591-36592, 36600, 36640,
43752, 51701-51703, 62320-62327, 64400, 64405-64408, 64415-64435,
64445-64454, 64461-64463, 64479-64505, 64510-64530, 69990,
92012-92014, 93000-93010, 93040-93042, 93318, 93355, 94002, 94200,
94250, 94680-94690, 94770, 95812-95816, 95819, 95822, 95829,
95955, 96360-96368, 96372, 96374-96377, 96523, 99155, 99156,
99157, 99211-99223, 99231-99255, 99291-99292, 99304-99310,
99315-99316, 99334-99337, 99347-99350, 99374-99375, 99377-99378,
99446-99449, 99451-99452, 99495-99496, G0463, G0471, J0670, J2001

17272 0213T, 0216T, 0228T, 0230T, 11102, 11104, 11106, 11601-11606♦,
11621-11626♦, 11641-11646♦, 11900-11901, 12001-12007,
12011-12057, 13100-13133, 13151-13153, 17000♦, 17004♦,
17110-17111♦, 17340, 36000, 36400-36410, 36420-36430, 36440,
36591-36592, 36600, 36640, 43752, 51701-51703, 62320-62327, 64400,
64405-64408, 64415-64435, 64445-64454, 64461-64463, 64479-64505,
64510-64530, 69990, 92012-92014, 93000-93010, 93040-93042, 93318,
93355, 94002, 94200, 94250, 94680-94690, 94770, 95812-95816,
95819, 95822, 95829, 95955, 96360-96368, 96372, 96374-96377,
96523, 99155, 99156, 99157, 99211-99223, 99231-99255, 99291-99292,
99304-99310, 99315-99316, 99334-99337, 99347-99350, 99374-99375,
99377-99378, 99446-99449, 99451-99452, 99495-99496, G0463,
G0471, J0670, J2001

17273 0213T, 0216T, 0228T, 0230T, 11102, 11104, 11106, 11602-11606♦,
11622-11626♦, 11641-11646♦, 11900-11901, 12001-12007,
12011-12057, 13100-13133, 13151-13153, 17000♦, 17004♦,
17110-17111♦, 17340, 36000, 36400-36410, 36420-36430, 36440,
36591-36592, 36600, 36640, 43752, 51701-51703, 62320-62327, 64400,
64405-64408, 64415-64435, 64445-64454, 64461-64463, 64479-64505,
64510-64530, 69990, 92012-92014, 93000-93010, 93040-93042, 93318,
93355, 94002, 94200, 94250, 94680-94690, 94770, 95812-95816,
95819, 95822, 95829, 95955, 96360-96368, 96372, 96374-96377,
96523, 99155, 99156, 99157, 99211-99223, 99231-99255, 99291-99292,
99304-99310, 99315-99316, 99334-99337, 99347-99350, 99374-99375,
99377-99378, 99446-99449, 99451-99452, 99495-99496, G0463,
G0471, J0670, J2001

17274 0213T, 0216T, 0228T, 0230T, 11102, 11104, 11106, 11606♦,
11623-11626♦, 11642-11646♦, 11900-11901, 12001-12007,
12011-12057, 13100-13133, 13151-13153, 17000♦, 17004♦,
17110-17111♦, 17340, 36000, 36400-36410, 36420-36430, 36440,
36591-36592, 36600, 36640, 43752, 51701-51703, 62320-62327, 64400,
64405-64408, 64415-64435, 64445-64454, 64461-64463, 64479-64505,
64510-64530, 69990, 92012-92014, 93000-93010, 93040-93042, 93318,
93355, 94002, 94200, 94250, 94680-94690, 94770, 95812-95816,
95819, 95822, 95829, 95955, 96360-96368, 96372, 96374-96377,
96523, 99155, 99156, 99157, 99211-99223, 99231-99255, 99291-99292,
99304-99310, 99315-99316, 99334-99337, 99347-99350, 99374-99375,
99377-99378, 99446-99449, 99451-99452, 99495-99496, G0463,
G0471, J0670, J2001

17276 0213T, 0216T, 0228T, 0230T, 11102, 11104, 11106, 11606♦,
11624-11626♦, 11643-11646♦, 11900-11901, 12001-12007,
12011-12057, 13100-13133, 13151-13153, 17000♦, 17004♦,
17110-17111♦, 17340, 36000, 36400-36410, 36420-36430, 36440,
36591-36592, 36600, 36640, 43752, 51701-51703, 62320-62327, 64400,

64405-64408, 64415-64435, 64445-64454, 64461-64463, 64479-64505,
64510-64530, 69990, 92012-92014, 93000-93010, 93040-93042, 93318,
93355, 94002, 94200, 94250, 94680-94690, 94770, 95812-95816,
95819, 95822, 95829, 95955, 96360-96368, 96372, 96374-96377,
96523, 99155, 99156, 99157, 99211-99223, 99231-99255, 99291-99292,
99304-99310, 99315-99316, 99334-99337, 99347-99350, 99374-99375,
99377-99378, 99446-99449, 99451-99452, 99495-99496, G0463,
G0471, J0670, J2001

35840 0213T, 0216T, 0228T, 0230T, 12001-12007, 12011-12057, 13100-13133,
13151-13153, 36000, 36002, 36400-36410, 36420-36430, 36440,
36591-36592, 36595-36596♦, 36600, 36640, 43752, 49000-49002,
51701-51703, 62320-62327, 64400, 64405-64408, 64415-64435,
64445-64454, 64461-64463, 64479-64505, 64510-64530, 69990, 75625,
75630, 75635, 75726, 75731, 75733, 75810, 75825, 75831, 75833,
75840, 75842, 75885, 75887, 75889, 75891, 92012-92014,
93000-93010, 93040-93042, 93318, 93355, 94002, 94200, 94250,
94680-94690, 94770, 95812-95816, 95819, 95822, 95829, 95955,
96360-96368, 96372, 96374-96377, 96523, 99155, 99156, 99157,
99211-99223, 99231-99255, 99291-99292, 99304-99310, 99315-99316,
99334-99337, 99347-99350, 99374-99375, 99377-99378, 99446-99449,
99451-99452, 99495-99496, G0463, G0471

36415 36591-36592, 96523, 99211

36416 36591-36592, 96523

36593 35201-35206, 35226-35236, 35256-35266, 35286, 36005, 36591-36592,
69990, 96523, J1642-J1644

36598 0213T, 0216T, 0228T, 0230T, 12001-12007, 12011-12057, 13100-13133,
13151-13153, 35201-35206, 35226-35236, 35256-35266, 35286, 36000,
36005, 36400-36410, 36420-36430, 36440, 36591-36592, 36600, 36640,
43752, 51701-51703, 62320-62327, 64400, 64405-64408, 64415-64435,
64445-64454, 64461-64463, 64479-64505, 64510-64530, 76000, 77002,
92012-92014, 93000-93010, 93040-93042, 93318, 93355, 94002, 94200,
94250, 94680-94690, 94770, 95812-95816, 95819, 95822, 95829,
95955, 96360-96368, 96372, 96374-96377, 96523, 99155, 99156,
99157, 99211-99223, 99231-99255, 99291-99292, 99304-99310,
99315-99316, 99334-99337, 99347-99350, 99374-99375, 99377-99378,
99446-99449, 99451-99452, 99495-99496, G0463, G0471, J1642-J1644

36800 01844, 01924-01926, 0213T, 0216T, 0228T, 0230T, 11000-11006,
11042-11047, 12001-12007, 12011-12057, 13100-13133, 13151-13153,
35201-35206, 35226-35236, 35256-35266, 35286, 35800, 35860, 36000,
36002-36005, 36400-36410, 36420-36430, 36440, 36591-36592, 36600,
36640, 36810-36815♦, 36819♦, 36820♦, 36821♦, 36831-36833♦, 36835♦,
36861♦, 43752, 49421♦, 51701-51703, 62320-62327, 64400,
64405-64408, 64415-64435, 64445-64454, 64461-64463, 64479-64505,
64510-64530, 69990, 92012-92014, 93000-93010, 93040-93042, 93318,
93355, 94002, 94200, 94250, 94680-94690, 94770, 95812-95816,
95819, 95822, 95829, 95955, 96360-96368, 96372, 96374-96377,
96523, 97597-97598, 97602, 99155, 99156, 99157, 99211-99223,
99231-99255, 99291-99292, 99304-99310, 99315-99316, 99334-99337,
99347-99350, 99374-99375, 99377-99378, 99446-99449, 99451-99452,
99495-99496, G0463, G0471

36810 01844, 01924-01926, 0213T, 0216T, 0228T, 0230T, 11000-11006,
11042-11047, 12001-12007, 12011-12057, 13100-13133, 13151-13153,
35201-35206, 35226-35236, 35256-35266, 35286, 36000, 36002-36005,
36400-36410, 36420-36430, 36440, 36591-36592, 36600, 36640,
36819♦, 36820♦, 36821♦, 36823-36833♦, 36835♦, 43752, 51701-51703,
62320-62327, 64400, 64405-64408, 64415-64435, 64445-64454,
64461-64463, 64479-64505, 64510-64530, 69990, 92012-92014,
93000-93010, 93040-93042, 93050, 93318, 93355, 94002, 94200,
94250, 94680-94690, 94770, 95812-95816, 95819, 95822, 95829,

95955, 96360-96368, 96372, 96374-96377, 96523, 97597-97598, 97602, 99155, 99156, 99157, 99211-99223, 99231-99255, 99291-99292, 99304-99310, 99315-99316, 99334-99337, 99347-99350, 99374-99375, 99377-99378, 99446-99449, 99451-99452, 99495-99496, G0463, G0471

36815 01844, 01924-01926, 0213T, 0216T, 0228T, 0230T, 11000-11006, 11042-11047, 12001-12007, 12011-12057, 13100-13133, 13151-13153, 35201-35206, 35226-35236, 35256-35266, 35286, 36000, 36002-36005, 36400-36410, 36420-36430, 36440, 36591-36592, 36600, 36640, 36810✦, 36819✦, 36820✦, 36821✦, 36823-36833✦, 36835✦, 43752, 51701-51703, 62320-62327, 64400, 64405-64408, 64415-64435, 64445-64454, 64461-64463, 64479-64505, 64510-64530, 69990, 92012-92014, 93000-93010, 93040-93042, 93050, 93318, 93355, 94002, 94200, 94250, 94680-94690, 94770, 95812-95816, 95819, 95822, 95829, 95955, 96360-96368, 96372, 96374-96377, 96523, 97597-97598, 97602, 99155, 99156, 99157, 99211-99223, 99231-99255, 99291-99292, 99304-99310, 99315-99316, 99334-99337, 99347-99350, 99374-99375, 99377-99378, 99446-99449, 99451-99452, 99495-99496, G0463, G0471

36818 01844, 01924-01926, 0213T, 0216T, 0228T, 0230T, 12001-12007, 12011-12057, 13100-13133, 13151-13153, 33951-33954✦, 35206, 35226, 35236, 35256, 35266, 35286, 35702-35703, 35860, 36000, 36002-36005, 36400-36410, 36420-36430, 36440, 36591-36592, 36600, 36640, 36800-36815✦, 36821, 36825-36833✦, 36835✦, 36860-36861✦, 36901-36906✦, 43752, 51701-51703, 62320-62327, 64400, 64405-64408, 64415-64435, 64445-64454, 64461-64463, 64479-64505, 64510-64530, 69990, 92012-92014, 93000-93010, 93040-93042, 93318, 93355, 94002, 94200, 94250, 94680-94690, 94770, 95812-95816, 95819, 95822, 95829, 95955, 96360-96368, 96372, 96374-96377, 96523, 99155, 99156, 99157, 99211-99223, 99231-99255, 99291-99292, 99304-99310, 99315-99316, 99334-99337, 99347-99350, 99374-99375, 99377-99378, 99446-99449, 99451-99452, 99495-99496, G0463, G0471

36819 01844, 01924-01926, 0213T, 0216T, 0228T, 0230T, 12001-12007, 12011-12057, 13100-13133, 13151-13153, 33951-33954✦, 35206, 35226, 35236, 35256, 35266, 35286, 35702-35703, 35860, 36000, 36002-36005, 36400-36410, 36420-36430, 36440, 36591-36592, 36600, 36640, 36818, 36821, 36823✦, 36830, 36901-36906✦, 43752, 51701-51703, 62320-62327, 64400, 64405-64408, 64415-64435, 64445-64454, 64461-64463, 64479-64505, 64510-64530, 69990, 92012-92014, 93000-93010, 93040-93042, 93318, 93355, 94002, 94200, 94250, 94680-94690, 94770, 95812-95816, 95819, 95822, 95829, 95955, 96360-96368, 96372, 96374-96377, 96523, 99155, 99156, 99157, 99211-99223, 99231-99255, 99291-99292, 99304-99310, 99315-99316, 99334-99337, 99347-99350, 99374-99375, 99377-99378, 99446-99449, 99451-99452, 99495-99496, G0463, G0471

36820 01844, 01924-01926, 0213T, 0216T, 0228T, 0230T, 12001-12007, 12011-12057, 13100-13133, 13151-13153, 33951-33954✦, 35206, 35226, 35236, 35256, 35266, 35286, 35702-35703, 35860, 36000, 36005, 36400-36410, 36420-36430, 36440, 36591-36592, 36600, 36640, 36818-36819, 36823✦, 36901-36903, 43752, 51701-51703, 62320-62327, 64400, 64405-64408, 64415-64435, 64445-64454, 64461-64463, 64479-64505, 64510-64530, 69990, 92012-92014, 93000-93010, 93040-93042, 93318, 93355, 94002, 94200, 94250, 94680-94690, 94770, 95812-95816, 95819, 95822, 95829, 95955, 96360-96368, 96372, 96374-96377, 96523, 99155, 99156, 99157, 99211-99223, 99231-99255, 99291-99292, 99304-99310, 99315-99316, 99334-99337, 99347-99350, 99374-99375, 99377-99378, 99446-99449, 99451-99452, 99495-99496, G0463, G0471

36821 01844, 01924-01926, 0213T, 0216T, 0228T, 0230T, 12001-12007, 12011-12057, 13100-13133, 13151-13153, 35206, 35226, 35236, 35256, 35266, 35286, 35702-35703, 35860, 36000, 36002-36005, 36400-36410,

36420-36430, 36440, 36591-36592, 36600, 36640, 36820✦, 36823-36825✦, 36833✦, 36901-36903, 43752, 51701-51703, 62320-62327, 64400, 64405-64408, 64415-64435, 64445-64454, 64461-64463, 64479-64505, 64510-64530, 69990, 92012-92014, 93000-93010, 93040-93042, 93318, 93355, 94002, 94200, 94250, 94680-94690, 94770, 95812-95816, 95819, 95822, 95829, 95955, 96360-96368, 96372, 96374-96377, 96523, 99155, 99156, 99157, 99211-99223, 99231-99255, 99291-99292, 99304-99310, 99315-99316, 99334-99337, 99347-99350, 99374-99375, 99377-99378, 99446-99449, 99451-99452, 99495-99496, G0463, G0471

36825 01844, 01924-01926, 0213T, 0216T, 0228T, 0230T, 12001-12007, 12011-12057, 13100-13133, 13151-13153, 35206, 35226, 35236, 35256, 35266, 35286, 35702-35703, 35860, 36000, 36002-36005, 36400-36410, 36420-36430, 36440, 36591-36592, 36600, 36640, 36819✦, 36820✦, 36833✦, 36901-36903, 43752, 51701-51703, 62320-62327, 64400, 64405-64408, 64415-64435, 64445-64454, 64461-64463, 64479-64505, 64510-64530, 69990, 92012-92014, 93000-93010, 93040-93042, 93318, 93355, 94002, 94200, 94250, 94680-94690, 94770, 95812-95816, 95819, 95822, 95829, 95955, 96360-96368, 96372, 96374-96377, 96523, 99155, 99156, 99157, 99211-99223, 99231-99255, 99291-99292, 99304-99310, 99315-99316, 99334-99337, 99347-99350, 99374-99375, 99377-99378, 99446-99449, 99451-99452, 99495-99496, G0463, G0471

36830 01844, 01924-01926, 0213T, 0216T, 0228T, 0230T, 12001-12007, 12011-12057, 13100-13133, 13151-13153, 35206, 35226, 35236, 35256, 35266, 35286, 35702-35703, 35800, 35860, 36000, 36002-36005, 36400-36410, 36420-36430, 36440, 36591-36592, 36600, 36640, 36820✦, 36821✦, 36825✦, 36901-36903, 43752, 51701-51703, 62320-62327, 64400, 64405-64408, 64415-64435, 64445-64454, 64461-64463, 64479-64505, 64510-64530, 69990, 92012-92014, 93000-93010, 93040-93042, 93318, 93355, 94002, 94200, 94250, 94680-94690, 94770, 95812-95816, 95819, 95822, 95829, 95955, 96360-96368, 96372, 96374-96377, 96523, 99155, 99156, 99157, 99211-99223, 99231-99255, 99291-99292, 99304-99310, 99315-99316, 99334-99337, 99347-99350, 99374-99375, 99377-99378, 99446-99449, 99451-99452, 99495-99496, G0463, G0471

36831 01844, 01924-01926, 0213T, 0216T, 0228T, 0230T, 11000-11006, 11042-11047, 12001-12007, 12011-12057, 13100-13133, 13151-13153, 34001✦, 34101-34111✦, 34201-34203✦, 34421-34451✦, 35206, 35226, 35236, 35256, 35266, 35286, 35702-35703, 35800, 35860, 35875-35876✦, 36000, 36002-36005, 36400-36410, 36420-36430, 36440, 36591-36593, 36600, 36640, 36819✦, 36820✦, 36821✦, 36825-36830✦, 36832-36833✦, 36901-36906, 36909, 37211-37214, 43752, 51701-51703, 61645, 62320-62327, 64400, 64405-64408, 64415-64435, 64445-64454, 64461-64463, 64479-64505, 64510-64530, 69990, 92012-92014, 93000-93010, 93040-93042, 93318, 93355, 94002, 94200, 94250, 94680-94690, 94770, 95812-95816, 95819, 95822, 95829, 95955, 96360-96368, 96372, 96374-96377, 96523, 97597-97598, 97602, 99155, 99156, 99157, 99211-99223, 99231-99255, 99291-99292, 99304-99310, 99315-99316, 99334-99337, 99347-99350, 99374-99375, 99377-99378, 99446-99449, 99451-99452, 99495-99496, G0463, G0471

36832 01844, 01924-01926, 0213T, 0216T, 0228T, 0230T, 11000-11006, 11042-11047, 12001-12007, 12011-12057, 13100-13133, 13151-13153, 35206, 35226, 35236, 35256, 35266, 35286, 35702-35703, 35860, 36000, 36002-36005, 36400-36410, 36420-36430, 36440, 36591-36592, 36600, 36640, 36819✦, 36820✦, 36821✦, 36825-36830✦, 36833✦, 36835✦, 43752, 51701-51703, 62320-62327, 64400, 64405-64408, 64415-64435, 64445-64454, 64461-64463, 64479-64505, 64510-64530, 69990, 92012-92014, 93000-93010, 93040-93042, 93318, 93355, 94002, 94200, 94250, 94680-94690, 94770, 95812-95816, 95819, 95822, 95829, 95955, 96360-96368, 96372, 96374-96377, 96523, 97597-97598, 97602,

99155, 99156, 99157, 99211-99223, 99231-99255, 99291-99292,
99304-99310, 99315-99316, 99334-99337, 99347-99350, 99374-99375,
99377-99378, 99446-99449, 99451-99452, 99495-99496, G0463, G0471

36833 01844, 01924-01926, 0213T, 0216T, 0228T, 0230T, 11000-11006,
11042-11047, 12001-12007, 12011-12057, 13100-13133, 13151-13153,
34001, 34101-34111, 34201-34203, 34421-34451, 34490, 35206, 35226,
35236, 35256, 35266, 35286, 35800, 35860, 35876✦, 36000,
36002-36005, 36400-36410, 36420-36430, 36440, 36591-36593, 36600,
36640, 36819✦, 36820✦, 36830✦, 37211-37214, 43752, 51701-51703,
61645, 62320-62327, 64400, 64405-64408, 64415-64435, 64445-64454,
64461-64463, 64479-64505, 64510-64530, 69990, 92012-92014,
93000-93010, 93040-93042, 93318, 93355, 94002, 94200, 94250,
94680-94690, 94770, 95812-95816, 95819, 95822, 95829, 95955,
96360-96368, 96372, 96374-96377, 96523, 97597-97598, 97602, 99155,
99156, 99157, 99211-99223, 99231-99255, 99291-99292, 99304-99310,
99315-99316, 99334-99337, 99347-99350, 99374-99375, 99377-99378,
99446-99449, 99451-99452, 99495-99496, G0463, G0471

36835 01844, 01924-01926, 0213T, 0216T, 0228T, 0230T, 11000-11006,
11042-11047, 12001-12007, 12011-12057, 13100-13133, 13151-13153,
35206, 35226, 35236, 35256, 35266, 35286, 36000, 36002-36005,
36400-36410, 36420-36430, 36440, 36591-36592, 36600, 36640,
36819✦, 36820✦, 36825-36831✦, 36833✦, 43752, 51701-51703,
62320-62327, 64400, 64405-64408, 64415-64435, 64445-64454,
64461-64463, 64479-64505, 64510-64530, 69990, 92012-92014,
93000-93010, 93040-93042, 93318, 93355, 94002, 94200, 94250,
94680-94690, 94770, 95812-95816, 95819, 95822, 95829, 95955,
96360-96368, 96372, 96374-96377, 96523, 97597-97598, 97602, 99155,
99156, 99157, 99211-99223, 99231-99255, 99291-99292, 99304-99310,
99315-99316, 99334-99337, 99347-99350, 99374-99375, 99377-99378,
99446-99449, 99451-99452, 99495-99496, G0463, G0471

36860 01844, 01924-01926, 0213T, 0216T, 0228T, 0230T, 12001-12007,
12011-12057, 13100-13133, 13151-13153, 35201-35206, 35226-35236,
35256-35266, 35286, 35860, 36000, 36002-36005, 36400-36410,
36420-36430, 36440, 36591-36593, 36600, 36640, 36800-36815✦,
36819✦, 36820✦, 36821✦, 36825-36833✦, 36835✦, 36861✦, 36901-36903,
36907-36909, 37211-37214, 43752, 51701-51703, 62320-62327, 64400,
64405-64408, 64415-64435, 64445-64454, 64461-64463, 64479-64505,
64510-64530, 69990, 76942, 76970, 76998, 77001-77002, 92012-92014,
93000-93010, 93040-93042, 93318, 93355, 94002, 94200, 94250,
94680-94690, 94770, 95812-95816, 95819, 95822, 95829, 95955,
96360-96368, 96372, 96374-96377, 96523, 99155, 99156, 99157,
99211-99223, 99231-99255, 99291-99292, 99304-99310, 99315-99316,
99334-99337, 99347-99350, 99374-99375, 99377-99378, 99446-99449,
99451-99452, 99495-99496, G0463, G0471, J0670, J1642-J1644, J2001

36861 01844, 01924-01926, 0213T, 0216T, 0228T, 0230T, 12001-12007,
12011-12057, 13100-13133, 13151-13153, 35201-35206, 35226-35236,
35256-35266, 35286, 36000, 36002-36005, 36400-36410, 36420-36430,
36440, 36591-36593, 36600, 36640, 36810-36815✦, 36819✦, 36820✦,
36821✦, 36825-36833✦, 36901-36903, 36907-36909, 37211-37214,
43752, 51701-51703, 62320-62327, 64400, 64405-64408, 64415-64435,
64445-64454, 64461-64463, 64479-64505, 64510-64530, 69990, 76942,
76970, 76998, 77001-77002, 92012-92014, 93000-93010, 93040-93042,
93318, 93355, 94002, 94200, 94250, 94680-94690, 94770,
95812-95816, 95819, 95822, 95829, 95955, 96360-96368, 96372,
96374-96377, 96523, 99155, 99156, 99157, 99211-99223, 99231-99255,
99291-99292, 99304-99310, 99315-99316, 99334-99337, 99347-99350,
99374-99375, 99377-99378, 99446-99449, 99451-99452, 99495-99496,
G0463, G0471

37788 0213T, 0216T, 0228T, 0230T, 12001-12007, 12011-12057, 13100-13133,
13151-13153, 36000, 36400-36410, 36420-36430, 36440, 36591-36592,
36600, 36640, 43752, 51701-51703, 62320-62327, 64400, 64405-64408,
64415-64435, 64445-64454, 64461-64463, 64479-64505, 64510-64530,
69990, 92012-92014, 93000-93010, 93040-93042, 93318, 93355, 94002,
94200, 94250, 94680-94690, 94770, 95812-95816, 95819, 95822,
95829, 95955, 96360-96368, 96372, 96374-96377, 96523, 99155,
99156, 99157, 99211-99223, 99231-99255, 99291-99292, 99304-99310,
99315-99316, 99334-99337, 99347-99350, 99374-99375, 99377-99378,
99446-99449, 99451-99452, 99495-99496, G0463, G0471

37790 0213T, 0216T, 0228T, 0230T, 12001-12007, 12011-12057, 13100-13133,
13151-13153, 36000, 36400-36410, 36420-36430, 36440, 36591-36592,
36600, 36640, 43752, 51701-51703, 62320-62327, 64400, 64405-64408,
64415-64435, 64445-64454, 64461-64463, 64479-64505, 64510-64530,
69990, 92012-92014, 93000-93010, 93040-93042, 93318, 93355, 94002,
94200, 94250, 94680-94690, 94770, 95812-95816, 95819, 95822,
95829, 95955, 96360-96368, 96372, 96374-96377, 96523, 99155,
99156, 99157, 99211-99223, 99231-99255, 99291-99292, 99304-99310,
99315-99316, 99334-99337, 99347-99350, 99374-99375, 99377-99378,
99446-99449, 99451-99452, 99495-99496, G0463, G0471

38500 0213T, 0216T, 0228T, 0230T, 10005, 10007, 10009, 10011, 10021,
11000-11006, 11042-11047, 12001-12007, 12011-12057, 13100-13133,
13151-13153, 36000, 36400-36410, 36420-36430, 36440, 36591-36592,
36600, 36640, 38505✦, 43752, 51701-51703, 62320-62327, 64400,
64405-64408, 64415-64435, 64445-64454, 64461-64463, 64479-64505,
64510-64530, 69990, 92012-92014, 93000-93010, 93040-93042, 93318,
93355, 94002, 94200, 94250, 94680-94690, 94770, 95812-95816,
95819, 95822, 95829, 95955, 96360-96368, 96372, 96374-96377,
96523, 97597-97598, 97602, 99155, 99156, 99157, 99211-99223,
99231-99255, 99291-99292, 99304-99310, 99315-99316, 99334-99337,
99347-99350, 99374-99375, 99377-99378, 99446-99449, 99451-99452,
99495-99496, G0463, G0471, J0670, J2001

38505 0213T, 0216T, 0228T, 0230T, 10005, 10007, 10009, 10011, 10021,
11000-11006, 11042-11047, 12001-12007, 12011-12057, 13100-13133,
13151-13153, 36000, 36400-36410, 36420-36430, 36440, 36591-36592,
36600, 36640, 43752, 51701-51703, 62320-62327, 64400, 64405-64408,
64415-64435, 64445-64454, 64461-64463, 64479-64505, 64510-64530,
69990, 76000, 77001, 92012-92014, 93000-93010, 93040-93042, 93318,
93355, 94002, 94200, 94250, 94680-94690, 94770, 95812-95816,
95819, 95822, 95829, 95955, 96360-96368, 96372, 96374-96377,
96523, 97597-97598, 97602, 99155, 99156, 99157, 99211-99223,
99231-99255, 99291-99292, 99304-99310, 99315-99316, 99334-99337,
99347-99350, 99374-99375, 99377-99378, 99446-99449, 99451-99452,
99495-99496, G0463, G0471, J2001

38531 0213T, 0216T, 0228T, 0230T, 10021, 11000-11006, 11042-11047,
12001-12007, 12011-12057, 13100-13133, 13151-13153, 22902✦,
36000, 36400-36410, 36420-36430, 36440, 36591-36592, 36600, 36640,
38500-38505✦, 43752, 51701-51703, 62320-62327, 64400,
64405-64408, 64415-64435, 64445-64454, 64461-64463, 64479-64505,
64510-64530, 69990, 92012-92014, 93000-93010, 93040-93042, 93318,
93355, 94002, 94200, 94250, 94680-94690, 94770, 95812-95816,
95819, 95822, 95829, 95955, 96360-96368, 96372, 96374-96377,
96523, 97597-97598, 97602, 99155, 99156, 99157, 99211-99223,
99231-99255, 99291-99292, 99304-99310, 99315-99316, 99334-99337,
99347-99350, 99374-99375, 99377-99378, 99446-99449, 99495-99496,
G0463, G0471, J0670, J2001

38562 0213T, 0216T, 0228T, 0230T, 11000-11006, 11042-11047, 12001-12007,
12011-12057, 13100-13133, 13151-13153, 36000, 36400-36410,
36420-36430, 36440, 36591-36592, 36600, 36640, 43752, 44005,

44180, 44602-44605, 44820-44850, 44950, 44970, 49000-49010, 49255, 49320-49321, 49570, 51701-51703, 52000, 62320-62327, 64400, 64405-64408, 64415-64435, 64445-64454, 64461-64463, 64479-64505, 64510-64530, 69990, 92012-92014, 93000-93010, 93040-93042, 93318, 93355, 94002, 94200, 94250, 94680-94690, 94770, 95812-95816, 95819, 95822, 95829, 95955, 96360-96368, 96372, 96374-96377, 96523, 97597-97598, 97602, 99155, 99156, 99157, 99211-99223, 99231-99255, 99291-99292, 99304-99310, 99315-99316, 99334-99337, 99347-99350, 99374-99375, 99377-99378, 99446-99449, 99451-99452, 99495-99496, G0463, G0471

38564 0213T, 0216T, 0228T, 0230T, 11000-11006, 11042-11047, 12001-12007, 12011-12057, 13100-13133, 13151-13153, 36000, 36400-36410, 36420-36430, 36440, 36591-36592, 36600, 36640, 38570, 43752, 44602-44605, 44950, 44970, 49000-49002, 49320-49321, 51701-51703, 52000, 62320-62327, 64400, 64405-64408, 64415-64435, 64445-64454, 64461-64463, 64479-64505, 64510-64530, 69990, 92012-92014, 93000-93010, 93040-93042, 93318, 93355, 94002, 94200, 94250, 94680-94690, 94770, 95812-95816, 95819, 95822, 95829, 95955, 96360-96368, 96372, 96374-96377, 96523, 97597-97598, 97602, 99155, 99156, 99157, 99211-99223, 99231-99255, 99291-99292, 99304-99310, 99315-99316, 99334-99337, 99347-99350, 99374-99375, 99377-99378, 99446-99449, 99451-99452, 99495-99496, G0463, G0471

38570 0213T, 0216T, 0228T, 0230T, 10005, 10007, 10009, 10011, 10021, 12001-12007, 12011-12057, 13100-13133, 13151-13153, 36000, 36400-36410, 36420-36430, 36440, 36591-36592, 36600, 36640, 38562, 43752, 44602-44605, 44950, 44970, 49010, 49082-49084, 49320, 49400, 51701-51703, 57410, 62320-62327, 64400, 64405-64408, 64415-64435, 64445-64454, 64461-64463, 64479-64505, 64510-64530, 69990, 76000, 77001-77002, 92012-92014, 93000-93010, 93040-93042, 93318, 93355, 94002, 94200, 94250, 94680-94690, 94770, 95812-95816, 95819, 95822, 95829, 95955, 96360-96368, 96372, 96374-96377, 96523, 99155, 99156, 99157, 99211-99223, 99231-99255, 99291-99292, 99304-99310, 99315-99316, 99334-99337, 99347-99350, 99374-99375, 99377-99378, 99446-99449, 99451-99452, 99495-99496, G0463, G0471

38571 0213T, 0216T, 0228T, 0230T, 11000-11006, 11042-11047, 12001-12007, 12011-12057, 13100-13133, 13151-13153, 36000, 36400-36410, 36420-36430, 36440, 36591-36592, 36600, 36640, 38562, 38570, 43752, 44602-44605, 44950, 44970, 49010, 49082-49084, 49320-49321, 49400, 51701-51703, 52000, 57410, 62320-62327, 64400, 64405-64408, 64415-64435, 64445-64454, 64461-64463, 64479-64505, 64510-64530, 69990, 76000, 77001-77002, 92012-92014, 93000-93010, 93040-93042, 93318, 93355, 94002, 94200, 94250, 94680-94690, 94770, 95812-95816, 95819, 95822, 95829, 95955, 96360-96368, 96372, 96374-96377, 96523, 97597-97598, 97602, 99155, 99156, 99157, 99211-99223, 99231-99255, 99291-99292, 99304-99310, 99315-99316, 99334-99337, 99347-99350, 99374-99375, 99377-99378, 99446-99449, 99451-99452, 99495-99496, G0463, G0471

38572 0213T, 0216T, 0228T, 0230T, 10005, 10007, 10009, 10011, 10021, 11000-11006, 11042-11047, 12001-12007, 12011-12057, 13100-13133, 13151-13153, 36000, 36400-36410, 36420-36430, 36440, 36591-36592, 36600, 36640, 38562-38571, 38770, 43752, 44602-44605, 44950, 44970, 49010, 49082-49084, 49320-49321, 49400, 51701-51703, 52000, 57410, 62320-62327, 64400, 64405-64408, 64415-64435, 64445-64454, 64461-64463, 64479-64505, 64510-64530, 69990, 76000, 77001-77002, 92012-92014, 93000-93010, 93040-93042, 93318, 93355, 94002, 94200, 94250, 94680-94690, 94770, 95812-95816, 95819, 95822, 95829, 95955, 96360-96368, 96372, 96374-96377, 96523, 97597-97598, 97602, 99155, 99156, 99157, 99211-99223, 99231-99255, 99291-99292,

99304-99310, 99315-99316, 99334-99337, 99347-99350, 99374-99375, 99377-99378, 99446-99449, 99451-99452, 99495-99496, G0463, G0471

38573 0213T, 0216T, 0228T, 0230T, 10005, 10007, 10009, 10011, 10021, 11000-11006, 11042-11047, 12001-12007, 12011-12057, 13100-13133, 13151-13153, 36000, 36400-36410, 36420-36430, 36440, 36591-36592, 36600, 36640, 38562-38572, 38765, 38770, 38780, 43752, 44602-44605, 44950, 44970, 49010, 49082-49084, 49255, 49320-49321, 49326, 49400, 51701-51703, 52000, 55860-55862, 57410, 58150, 58180, 58541-58544, 58550, 58552-58553, 58950, 58960, 62320-62327, 64400, 64405-64408, 64415-64435, 64445-64454, 64461-64463, 64479-64505, 64510-64530, 69990, 76000, 77001-77002, 92012-92014, 93000-93010, 93040-93042, 93318, 93355, 94002, 94200, 94250, 94680-94690, 94770, 95812-95816, 95819, 95822, 95829, 95955, 96360-96368, 96372, 96374-96377, 96523, 97597-97598, 97602, 99155, 99156, 99157, 99211-99223, 99231-99255, 99291-99292, 99304-99310, 99315-99316, 99334-99337, 99347-99350, 99374-99375, 99377-99378, 99446-99449, 99451-99452, 99495-99496, G0463, G0471

38747 11000-11006, 11042-11047, 36591-36592, 38500, 38531, 38570, 44950, 44970, 49000-49002, 49320-49321, 96523, 97597-97598, 97602

38760 0213T, 0216T, 0228T, 0230T, 11000-11006, 11042-11047, 12001-12007, 12011-12057, 13100-13133, 13151-13153, 36000, 36400-36410, 36420-36430, 36440, 36591-36592, 36600, 36640, 38500, 38531❖, 43752, 51701-51703, 62320-62327, 64400, 64405-64408, 64415-64435, 64445-64454, 64461-64463, 64479-64505, 64510-64530, 69990, 92012-92014, 93000-93010, 93040-93042, 93318, 93355, 94002, 94200, 94250, 94680-94690, 94770, 95812-95816, 95819, 95822, 95829, 95955, 96360-96368, 96372, 96374-96377, 96523, 97597-97598, 97602, 99155, 99156, 99157, 99211-99223, 99231-99255, 99291-99292, 99304-99310, 99315-99316, 99334-99337, 99347-99350, 99374-99375, 99377-99378, 99446-99449, 99451-99452, 99495-99496, G0463, G0471

38765 0213T, 0216T, 0228T, 0230T, 11000-11006, 11042-11047, 12001-12007, 12011-12057, 13100-13133, 13151-13153, 36000, 36400-36410, 36420-36430, 36440, 36591-36592, 36600, 36640, 38500, 38531❖, 38562, 38571, 38760, 38770, 43752, 51701-51703, 52000, 62320-62327, 64400, 64405-64408, 64415-64435, 64445-64454, 64461-64463, 64479-64505, 64510-64530, 69990, 92012-92014, 93000-93010, 93040-93042, 93318, 93355, 94002, 94200, 94250, 94680-94690, 94770, 95812-95816, 95819, 95822, 95829, 95955, 96360-96368, 96372, 96374-96377, 96523, 97597-97598, 97602, 99155, 99156, 99157, 99211-99223, 99231-99255, 99291-99292, 99304-99310, 99315-99316, 99334-99337, 99347-99350, 99374-99375, 99377-99378, 99446-99449, 99451-99452, 99495-99496, G0463, G0471, J0670, J2001

38770 0213T, 0216T, 0228T, 0230T, 11000-11006, 11042-11047, 12001-12007, 12011-12057, 13100-13133, 13151-13153, 36000, 36400-36410, 36420-36430, 36440, 36591-36592, 36600, 36640, 38500, 38531, 38562-38564, 38571, 38760, 43752, 44005, 44180, 44602-44605, 44820-44850, 44950, 44970, 49000-49010, 49320-49321, 49570, 51701-51703, 52000, 62320-62327, 64400, 64405-64408, 64415-64435, 64445-64454, 64461-64463, 64479-64505, 64510-64530, 69990, 92012-92014, 93000-93010, 93040-93042, 93318, 93355, 94002, 94200, 94250, 94680-94690, 94770, 95812-95816, 95819, 95822, 95829, 95955, 96360-96368, 96372, 96374-96377, 96523, 97597-97598, 97602, 99155, 99156, 99157, 99211-99223, 99231-99255, 99291-99292, 99304-99310, 99315-99316, 99334-99337, 99347-99350, 99374-99375, 99377-99378, 99446-99449, 99451-99452, 99495-99496, G0463, G0471

38780 0213T, 0216T, 0228T, 0230T, 11000-11006, 11042-11047, 12001-12007, 12011-12057, 13100-13133, 13151-13153, 36000, 36400-36410, 36420-36430, 36440, 36591-36592, 36600, 36640, 38500, 38531, 38562-38572, 38765, 38770, 43752, 44005, 44180, 44602-44605,

CPT © 2020 American Medical Association. All Rights Reserved.

44820-44850, 44950, 44970, 49000-49010, 49320-49321, 49570, 51701-51703, 52000, 62320-62327, 64400, 64405-64408, 64415-64435, 64445-64454, 64461-64463, 64479-64505, 64510-64530, 69990, 92012-92014, 93000-93010, 93040-93042, 93318, 93355, 94002, 94200, 94250, 94680-94690, 94770, 95812-95816, 95819, 95822, 95829, 95955, 96360-96368, 96372, 96374-96377, 96523, 97597-97598, 97602, 99155, 99156, 99157, 99211-99223, 99231-99255, 99291-99292, 99304-99310, 99315-99316, 99334-99337, 99347-99350, 99374-99375, 99377-99378, 99446-99449, 99451-99452, 99495-99496, G0463, G0471

44660 0213T, 0216T, 0228T, 0230T, 11000-11006, 11042-11047, 12001-12007, 12011-12057, 13100-13133, 13151-13153, 36000, 36400-36410, 36420-36430, 36440, 36591-36592, 36600, 36640, 43752, 44005, 44120, 44140-44151, 44155-44180, 44500, 44602-44605, 44661❖, 44701, 44820-44850, 44950, 44970, 49000-49010, 49255, 49320, 49560-49566, 49570, 50715, 51550-51565, 51701-51703, 62320-62327, 64400, 64405-64408, 64415-64435, 64445-64454, 64461-64463, 64479-64505, 64510-64530, 69990, 92012-92014, 93000-93010, 93040-93042, 93318, 93355, 94002, 94200, 94250, 94680-94690, 94770, 95812-95816, 95819, 95822, 95829, 95955, 96360-96368, 96372, 96374-96377, 96523, 97597-97598, 97602, 99155, 99156, 99157, 99211-99223, 99231-99255, 99291-99292, 99304-99310, 99315-99316, 99334-99337, 99347-99350, 99374-99375, 99377-99378, 99446-99449, 99451-99452, 99495-99496, G0463, G0471

44661 0213T, 0216T, 0228T, 0230T, 11000-11006, 11042-11047, 12001-12007, 12011-12057, 13100-13133, 13151-13153, 36000, 36400-36410, 36420-36430, 36440, 36591-36592, 36600, 36640, 43752, 44005, 44021, 44120, 44140-44151, 44155-44180, 44500, 44602-44605, 44620, 44701, 44820-44850, 44950, 44970, 45380, 49000-49010, 49020, 49040, 49060, 49255, 49320, 49560-49566, 49570-49572, 49585-49587, 51550-51565, 51701-51703, 62320-62327, 64400, 64405-64408, 64415-64435, 64445-64454, 64461-64463, 64479-64505, 64510-64530, 69990, 92012-92014, 93000-93010, 93040-93042, 93318, 93355, 94002, 94200, 94250, 94680-94690, 94770, 95812-95816, 95819, 95822, 95829, 95955, 96360-96368, 96372, 96374-96377, 96523, 97597-97598, 97602, 99155, 99156, 99157, 99211-99223, 99231-99255, 99291-99292, 99304-99310, 99315-99316, 99334-99337, 99347-99350, 99374-99375, 99377-99378, 99446-99449, 99451-99452, 99495-99496, G0463, G0471

46744 00902, 0213T, 0216T, 0228T, 0230T, 11000-11006, 11042-11047, 12001-12007, 12011-12057, 13100-13133, 13151-13153, 36000, 36400-36410, 36420-36430, 36440, 36591-36592, 36600, 36640, 43752, 45900-45990, 46040, 46080, 46220, 46600-46601, 46748❖, 46940-46942, 51701-51703, 53000-53025, 62320-62327, 64400, 64405-64408, 64415-64435, 64445-64454, 64461-64463, 64479-64505, 64510-64530, 69990, 92012-92014, 93000-93010, 93040-93042, 93318, 93355, 94002, 94200, 94250, 94680-94690, 94770, 95812-95816, 95819, 95822, 95829, 95955, 96360-96368, 96372, 96374-96377, 96523, 97597-97598, 97602, 99155, 99156, 99157, 99211-99223, 99231-99255, 99291-99292, 99304-99310, 99315-99316, 99334-99337, 99347-99350, 99374-99375, 99377-99378, 99446-99449, 99451-99452, 99495-99496, G0463, G0471

46746 00902, 0213T, 0216T, 0228T, 0230T, 11000-11006, 11042-11047, 12001-12007, 12011-12057, 13100-13133, 13151-13153, 36000, 36400-36410, 36420-36430, 36440, 36591-36592, 36600, 36640, 43752, 45900-45990, 46040, 46080, 46220, 46600-46601, 46940-46942, 51701-51703, 53000-53025, 62320-62327, 64400, 64405-64408, 64415-64435, 64445-64454, 64461-64463, 64479-64505, 64510-64530, 69990, 92012-92014, 93000-93010, 93040-93042, 93318, 93355, 94002, 94200, 94250, 94680-94690, 94770, 95812-95816, 95819, 95822, 95829, 95955, 96360-96368, 96372, 96374-96377, 96523, 97597-97598, 97602, 99155, 99156, 99157, 99211-99223, 99231-99255, 99291-99292,

99304-99310, 99315-99316, 99334-99337, 99347-99350, 99374-99375, 99377-99378, 99446-99449, 99451-99452, 99495-99496, G0463, G0471

49000 0213T, 0216T, 0228T, 0230T, 10005, 10007, 10009, 10011, 10021, 11000-11006, 11042-11047, 12001-12007, 12011-12057, 13100-13133, 13151-13153, 20102, 36000, 36400-36410, 36420-36430, 36440, 36591-36592, 36600, 36640, 43752, 44015, 44180, 44950, 44970, 49013-49014, 49255, 51701-51703, 57410, 62320-62327, 64400, 64405-64408, 64415-64435, 64445-64454, 64461-64463, 64479-64505, 64510-64530, 69990, 92012-92014, 93000-93010, 93040-93042, 93318, 93355, 94002, 94200, 94250, 94680-94690, 94770, 95812-95816, 95819, 95822, 95829, 95955, 96360-96368, 96372, 96374-96377, 96523, 97597-97598, 97602, 99155, 99156, 99157, 99211-99223, 99231-99255, 99291-99292, 99304-99310, 99315-99316, 99334-99337, 99347-99350, 99374-99375, 99377-99378, 99446-99449, 99451-99452, 99495-99496, G0463, G0471

49002 0213T, 0216T, 0228T, 0230T, 11000-11006, 11042-11047, 12001-12007, 12011-12057, 13100-13133, 13151-13153, 20102, 36000, 36400-36410, 36420-36430, 36440, 36591-36592, 36600, 36640, 43752, 44005, 44180, 44820-44850, 44950, 44970, 49000, 49010-49014, 49255, 49570, 51701-51703, 62320-62327, 64400, 64405-64408, 64415-64435, 64445-64454, 64461-64463, 64479-64505, 64510-64530, 69990, 92012-92014, 93000-93010, 93040-93042, 93318, 93355, 94002, 94200, 94250, 94680-94690, 94770, 95812-95816, 95819, 95822, 95829, 95955, 96360-96368, 96372, 96374-96377, 96523, 97597-97598, 97602, 99155, 99156, 99157, 99211-99223, 99231-99255, 99291-99292, 99304-99310, 99315-99316, 99334-99337, 99347-99350, 99374-99375, 99377-99378, 99446-99449, 99451-99452, 99495-99496, G0463, G0471

49010 0213T, 0216T, 0228T, 0230T, 10005, 10007, 10009, 10011, 10021, 12001-12007, 12011-12057, 13100-13133, 13151-13153, 20102, 36000, 36400-36410, 36420-36430, 36440, 36591-36592, 36600, 36640, 43752, 44180, 44950, 44970, 49000, 49013-49014, 49255, 49320, 51701-51703, 62320-62327, 64400, 64405-64408, 64415-64435, 64445-64454, 64461-64463, 64479-64505, 64510-64530, 69990, 92012-92014, 93000-93010, 93040-93042, 93318, 93355, 94002, 94200, 94250, 94680-94690, 94770, 95812-95816, 95819, 95822, 95829, 95955, 96360-96368, 96372, 96374-96377, 96523, 99155, 99156, 99157, 99211-99223, 99231-99255, 99291-99292, 99304-99310, 99315-99316, 99334-99337, 99347-99350, 99374-99375, 99377-99378, 99446-99449, 99451-99452, 99495-99496, G0463, G0471

49020 0213T, 0216T, 0228T, 0230T, 12001-12007, 12011-12057, 13100-13133, 13151-13153, 20102, 36000, 36400-36410, 36420-36430, 36440, 36591-36592, 36600, 36640, 43752, 44005, 44180, 44602-44605, 44820-44850, 44950, 44970, 49000-49014, 49185, 49203-49204, 49255, 49320, 49402, 49406-49407, 49424, 49570, 51701-51703, 62320-62327, 64400, 64405-64408, 64415-64435, 64445-64454, 64461-64463, 64479-64505, 64510-64530, 69990, 76000, 77001-77002, 92012-92014, 93000-93010, 93040-93042, 93318, 93355, 94002, 94200, 94250, 94680-94690, 94770, 95812-95816, 95819, 95822, 95829, 95955, 96360-96368, 96372, 96374-96377, 96523, 99155, 99156, 99157, 99211-99223, 99231-99255, 99291-99292, 99304-99310, 99315-99316, 99334-99337, 99347-99350, 99374-99375, 99377-99378, 99446-99449, 99451-99452, 99495-99496, G0463, G0471

49060 0213T, 0216T, 0228T, 0230T, 12001-12007, 12011-12057, 13100-13133, 13151-13153, 20102, 36000, 36400-36410, 36420-36430, 36440, 36591-36592, 36600, 36640, 43752, 44005, 44180, 44602-44605, 44820-44850, 44950, 44970, 49000-49020❖, 49185, 49255, 49320, 49406-49407❖, 49423-49424, 49570, 51701-51703, 60540-60545, 62320-62327, 64400, 64405-64408, 64415-64435, 64445-64454, 64461-64463, 64479-64505, 64510-64530, 69990, 92012-92014,

CCI Edits

93000-93010, 93040-93042, 93318, 93355, 94002, 94200, 94250, 94680-94690, 94770, 95812-95816, 95819, 95822, 95829, 95955, 96360-96368, 96372, 96374-96377, 96523, 99155, 99156, 99157, 99211-99223, 99231-99255, 99291-99292, 99304-99310, 99315-99316, 99334-99337, 99347-99350, 99374-99375, 99377-99378, 99446-99449, 99451-99452, 99495-99496, G0463, G0471

49082 0213T, 0216T, 0228T, 0230T, 12001-12007, 12011-12057, 13100-13133, 13151-13153, 20102, 36000, 36400-36410, 36420-36430, 36440, 36591-36592, 36600, 36640, 43752, 49013-49014, 51701-51703, 62320-62327, 64400, 64405-64408, 64415-64435, 64445-64454, 64461-64463, 64479-64505, 64510-64530, 69990, 76000, 76380, 76942, 76970, 76998, 77001-77002, 77012, 77021, 92012-92014, 93000-93010, 93040-93042, 93318, 93355, 94002, 94200, 94250, 94680-94690, 94770, 95812-95816, 95819, 95822, 95829, 95955, 96360-96368, 96372, 96374-96377, 96523, 99155, 99156, 99157, 99211-99223, 99231-99255, 99291-99292, 99304-99310, 99315-99316, 99334-99337, 99347-99350, 99374-99375, 99377-99378, 99446-99449, 99451-99452, 99495-99496, G0463, G0471

49083 0213T, 0216T, 0228T, 0230T, 12001-12007, 12011-12057, 13100-13133, 13151-13153, 20102, 36000, 36400-36410, 36420-36430, 36440, 36591-36592, 36600, 36640, 43752, 49013-49014, 49082, 51701-51703, 62320-62327, 64400, 64405-64408, 64415-64435, 64445-64454, 64461-64463, 64479-64505, 64510-64530, 69990, 76000, 76380, 76942, 76970, 76998, 77001-77002, 77012, 77021, 92012-92014, 93000-93010, 93040-93042, 93318, 93355, 94002, 94200, 94250, 94680-94690, 94770, 95812-95816, 95819, 95822, 95829, 95955, 96360-96368, 96372, 96374-96377, 96523, 99155, 99156, 99157, 99211-99223, 99231-99255, 99291-99292, 99304-99310, 99315-99316, 99334-99337, 99347-99350, 99374-99375, 99377-99378, 99446-99449, 99451-99452, 99495-99496, G0463, G0471

49084 0213T, 0216T, 0228T, 0230T, 12001-12007, 12011-12057, 13100-13133, 13151-13153, 20102, 36000, 36400-36410, 36420-36430, 36440, 36591-36592, 36600, 36640, 43752, 49013-49014, 49082-49083, 51701-51703, 62320-62327, 64400, 64405-64408, 64415-64435, 64445-64454, 64461-64463, 64479-64505, 64510-64530, 69990, 76000, 76380, 76942, 76970, 76998, 77001-77002, 77012, 77021, 92012-92014, 93000-93010, 93040-93042, 93318, 93355, 94002, 94200, 94250, 94680-94690, 94770, 95812-95816, 95819, 95822, 95829, 95955, 96360-96368, 96372, 96374-96377, 96523, 99155, 99156, 99157, 99211-99223, 99231-99255, 99291-99292, 99304-99310, 99315-99316, 99334-99337, 99347-99350, 99374-99375, 99377-99378, 99446-99449, 99451-99452, 99495-99496, G0463, G0471

49180 0213T, 0216T, 0228T, 0230T, 10005, 10007, 10009, 10011, 10021, 12001-12007, 12011-12057, 13100-13133, 13151-13153, 36000, 36400-36410, 36420-36430, 36440, 36591-36592, 36600, 36640, 43752, 44950, 44970, 51701-51703, 62320-62327, 64400, 64405-64408, 64415-64435, 64445-64454, 64461-64463, 64479-64505, 64510-64530, 69990, 92012-92014, 93000-93010, 93040-93042, 93318, 93355, 94002, 94200, 94250, 94680-94690, 94770, 95812-95816, 95819, 95822, 95829, 95955, 96360-96368, 96372, 96374-96377, 96523, 99155, 99156, 99157, 99211-99223, 99231-99255, 99291-99292, 99304-99310, 99315-99316, 99334-99337, 99347-99350, 99374-99375, 99377-99378, 99446-99449, 99451-99452, 99495-99496, G0463, G0471, J0670, J1642-J1644, J2001

49185 0213T, 0216T, 0228T, 0230T, 0524T✦, 12001-12007, 12011-12057, 13100-13133, 13151-13153, 32560✦, 36000, 36400-36410, 36420-36430, 36440, 36465✦, 36468✦, 36470-36471✦, 36591-36592, 36600, 36640, 43752, 44602-44605, 49320, 49424, 51701-51703, 62320-62327, 64400, 64405-64408, 64415-64435, 64445-64454,

64461-64463, 64479-64505, 64510-64530, 69990, 76000, 76080, 76380, 76942, 76970, 76998, 77001-77002, 77012, 77021, 92012-92014, 93000-93010, 93040-93042, 93318, 93355, 94002, 94200, 94250, 94680-94690, 94770, 95812-95816, 95819, 95822, 95829, 95955, 96360-96368, 96372, 96374-96377, 96523, 99155, 99156, 99157, 99211-99223, 99231-99255, 99291-99292, 99304-99310, 99315-99316, 99334-99337, 99347-99350, 99374-99375, 99377-99378, 99446-99449, 99451-99452, 99495-99496, G0463, G0471, J0670, J2001

49320 0213T, 0216T, 0228T, 0230T, 12001-12007, 12011-12057, 13100-13133, 13151-13153, 36000, 36400-36410, 36420-36430, 36440, 36591-36592, 36600, 36640, 43752, 44005, 47001, 49082-49084, 49400, 50715, 51701-51703, 57410, 62320-62327, 64400, 64405-64408, 64415-64435, 64445-64454, 64461-64463, 64479-64505, 64510-64530, 69990, 76000, 77001-77002, 92012-92014, 93000-93010, 93040-93042, 93318, 93355, 94002, 94200, 94250, 94680-94690, 94770, 95812-95816, 95819, 95822, 95829, 95955, 96360-96368, 96372, 96374-96377, 96523, 99155, 99156, 99157, 99211-99223, 99231-99255, 99291-99292, 99304-99310, 99315-99316, 99334-99337, 99347-99350, 99374-99375, 99377-99378, 99446-99449, 99451-99452, 99495-99496, G0463, G0471

49321 0213T, 0216T, 0228T, 0230T, 10005, 10007, 10009, 10011, 10021, 12001-12007, 12011-12057, 13100-13133, 13151-13153, 36000, 36400-36410, 36420-36430, 36440, 36591-36592, 36600, 36640, 43653, 43752, 44005, 44180, 44602-44605, 44950, 47001, 49082-49084, 49320, 49400, 50715, 51701-51703, 57410, 62320-62327, 64400, 64405-64408, 64415-64435, 64445-64454, 64461-64463, 64479-64505, 64510-64530, 69990, 76000, 77001-77002, 92012-92014, 93000-93010, 93040-93042, 93318, 93355, 94002, 94200, 94250, 94680-94690, 94770, 95812-95816, 95819, 95822, 95829, 95955, 96360-96368, 96372, 96374-96377, 96523, 99155, 99156, 99157, 99211-99223, 99231-99255, 99291-99292, 99304-99310, 99315-99316, 99334-99337, 99347-99350, 99374-99375, 99377-99378, 99446-99449, 99451-99452, 99495-99496, G0463, G0471

49324 0213T, 0216T, 0228T, 0230T, 11000-11006, 11042-11047, 12001-12007, 12011-12057, 13100-13133, 13151-13153, 36000, 36400-36410, 36420-36430, 36440, 36591-36592, 36600, 36640, 43653, 43752, 44005, 44180, 44602-44605, 44950, 44970, 49000, 49082-49084, 49320, 49400, 49421-49422✦, 49436, 50715, 51701-51703, 58660, 62320-62327, 64400, 64405-64408, 64415-64435, 64445-64454, 64461-64463, 64479-64505, 64510-64530, 69990, 76000, 77001-77002, 92012-92014, 93000-93010, 93040-93042, 93318, 93355, 94002, 94200, 94250, 94680-94690, 94770, 95812-95816, 95819, 95822, 95829, 95955, 96360-96368, 96372, 96374-96377, 96523, 97597-97598, 97602, 99155, 99156, 99157, 99211-99223, 99231-99255, 99291-99292, 99304-99310, 99315-99316, 99334-99337, 99347-99350, 99374-99375, 99377-99378, 99446-99449, 99451-99452, 99495-99496, G0463, G0471

49325 0213T, 0216T, 0228T, 0230T, 11000-11006, 11042-11047, 12001-12007, 12011-12057, 13100-13133, 13151-13153, 36000, 36400-36410, 36420-36430, 36440, 36591-36592, 36600, 36640, 43653, 43752, 44005, 44180, 44602-44605, 44950, 44970, 49000, 49082-49084, 49320, 49324✦, 49400, 49421-49422✦, 50715, 51701-51703, 58660, 62320-62327, 64400, 64405-64408, 64415-64435, 64445-64454, 64461-64463, 64479-64505, 64510-64530, 69990, 76000, 77001-77002, 92012-92014, 93000-93010, 93040-93042, 93318, 93355, 94002, 94200, 94250, 94680-94690, 94770, 95812-95816, 95819, 95822, 95829, 95955, 96360-96368, 96372, 96374-96377, 96523, 97597-97598, 97602, 99155, 99156, 99157, 99211-99223, 99231-99255, 99291-99292, 99304-99310, 99315-99316, 99334-99337, 99347-99350, 99374-99375, 99377-99378, 99446-99449, 99451-99452, 99495-99496, G0463, G0471

49327 36591-36592, 43653, 44005, 44180, 44970, 49082-49084, 49320, 49400, 50715, 57410, 58660, 76000, 76380, 76942, 76970, 76998, 77002, 77012, 77021, 96523

49400 0213T, 0216T, 12001-12007, 12011-12057, 13100-13133, 13151-13153, 36000, 36400-36410, 36420-36430, 36440, 36591-36592, 36600, 36640, 43752, 51701-51703, 62320-62327, 64400, 64405-64408, 64415-64435, 64445-64454, 64461-64463, 64479-64505, 64510-64530, 69990, 76000, 76942, 76970, 76998, 77001-77002, 92012-92014, 93000-93010, 93040-93042, 93318, 93355, 94002, 94200, 94250, 94680-94690, 94770, 95812-95816, 95819, 95822, 95829, 95955, 96360-96368, 96372, 96374-96377, 96523, 99155, 99156, 99157, 99211-99223, 99231-99255, 99291-99292, 99304-99310, 99315-99316, 99334-99337, 99347-99350, 99374-99375, 99377-99378, 99446-99449, 99451-99452, 99495-99496, G0463, G0471

49402 0213T, 0216T, 11000-11006, 11042-11047, 12001-12007, 12011-12057, 13100-13133, 13151-13153, 20102, 36000, 36400-36410, 36420-36430, 36440, 36591-36592, 36600, 36640, 43752, 44005, 44180, 44602-44605, 44820-44850, 44950, 44970, 49000-49014, 49255, 49320, 49429, 49560-49566, 49570-49572, 49580, 49582-49587, 51701-51703, 62320-62327, 64400, 64405-64408, 64415-64435, 64445-64454, 64461-64463, 64479-64505, 64510-64530, 69990, 92012-92014, 93000-93010, 93040-93042, 93318, 93355, 94002, 94200, 94250, 94680-94690, 94770, 95812-95816, 95819, 95822, 95829, 95955, 96360-96368, 96372, 96374-96377, 96523, 97597-97598, 97602, 99155, 99156, 99157, 99211-99223, 99231-99255, 99291-99292, 99304-99310, 99315-99316, 99334-99337, 99347-99350, 99374-99375, 99377-99378, 99446-99449, 99451-99452, 99495-99496, G0463, G0471

49405 0213T, 0216T, 0228T, 0230T, 12001-12007, 12011-12057, 13100-13133, 13151-13153, 32551, 32554-32557✦, 32601, 32607-32609, 36000, 36400-36410, 36420-36430, 36440, 36591-36592, 36600, 36640, 43752, 44602-44605, 44950, 44970, 47000-47001, 48102, 49000-49002, 49185, 49320, 49406✦, 49423-49424, 51701-51703, 62320-62327, 64400, 64405-64408, 64415-64435, 64445-64454, 64461-64463, 64479-64505, 64510-64530, 69990, 75989, 76000, 76380, 76942, 76970, 76998, 77001-77003, 77012, 77021, 92012-92014, 93000-93010, 93040-93042, 93318, 93355, 94002, 94200, 94250, 94680-94690, 94770, 95812-95816, 95819, 95822, 95829, 95955, 96360-96368, 96372, 96374-96377, 96523, 99155, 99156, 99157, 99211-99223, 99231-99255, 99291-99292, 99304-99310, 99315-99316, 99334-99337, 99347-99350, 99374-99375, 99377-99378, 99446-99449, 99451-99452, G0463, G0471, J0670, J2001

49406 00910, 0213T, 0216T, 0228T, 0230T, 12001-12007, 12011-12057, 13100-13133, 13151-13153, 36000, 36400-36410, 36420-36430, 36440, 36591-36592, 36600, 36640, 43752, 44005, 44180, 44602-44605, 44701, 44820-44850, 44950, 44970, 49000-49010, 49082-49084✦, 49180-49185, 49255, 49320, 49322, 49400, 49402, 49423-49424, 49570, 50010, 50205, 50715, 51045, 51570, 51701-51703, 57410, 58660, 58700, 58800, 58900, 62320-62327, 64400, 64405-64408, 64415-64435, 64445-64454, 64461-64463, 64479-64505, 64510-64530, 69990, 75989, 76000, 76380, 76942, 76970, 76998, 77001-77003, 77012, 77021, 92012-92014, 93000-93010, 93040-93042, 93318, 93355, 94002, 94200, 94250, 94680-94690, 94770, 95812-95816, 95819, 95822, 95829, 95955, 96360-96368, 96372, 96374-96377, 96523, 99155, 99156, 99157, 99211-99223, 99231-99255, 99291-99292, 99304-99310, 99315-99316, 99334-99337, 99347-99350, 99374-99375, 99377-99378, 99446-99449, 99451-99452, G0463, G0471, J0670, J2001

49407 0213T, 0216T, 0228T, 0230T, 12001-12007, 12011-12057, 13100-13133, 13151-13153, 36000, 36400-36410, 36420-36430, 36440, 36591-36592, 36600, 36640, 43752, 44701, 45005, 45900-45990, 46040, 46080,

46220, 46600-46601, 46940-46942, 49082-49084✦, 49185, 49322, 49406, 49423-49424, 50715, 51701-51703, 57410, 58660, 58805, 58900, 62320-62327, 64400, 64405-64408, 64415-64435, 64445-64454, 64461-64463, 64479-64505, 64510-64530, 69990, 75989, 76000, 76380, 76942, 76970, 76998, 77001-77003, 77012, 77021, 92012-92014, 93000-93010, 93040-93042, 93318, 93355, 94002, 94200, 94250, 94680-94690, 94770, 95812-95816, 95819, 95822, 95829, 95955, 96360-96368, 96372, 96374-96377, 96523, 99155, 99156, 99157, 99211-99223, 99231-99255, 99291-99292, 99304-99310, 99315-99316, 99334-99337, 99347-99350, 99374-99375, 99377-99378, 99446-99449, 99451-99452, G0463, G0471, J0670, J2001

49412 10036✦, 36591-36592, 49327, 76000, 76380, 76942, 76970, 76998, 77002, 77012, 77021, 96523

49418 11000-11006, 11042-11047, 12001-12007, 12011-12057, 13100-13133, 13151-13153, 36000, 36400-36410, 36420-36430, 36440, 36591-36592, 36600, 36640, 43752, 49324-49325✦, 49400, 49421✦, 51701-51703, 62320-62327, 64400, 64405-64408, 64415-64435, 64445-64454, 64461-64463, 64479-64505, 64510-64530, 69990, 76000, 76380, 76942, 76970, 76998, 77001-77002, 77012, 77021, 92012-92014, 93000-93010, 93040-93042, 93318, 93355, 94002, 94200, 94250, 94680-94690, 94770, 95812-95816, 95819, 95822, 95829, 95955, 96360-96368, 96372, 96374-96377, 96523, 97597-97598, 97602, 99155, 99156, 99157, 99211-99223, 99231-99255, 99291-99292, 99304-99310, 99315-99316, 99334-99337, 99347-99350, 99374-99375, 99377-99378, 99446-99449, 99451-99452, 99495-99496, G0463, G0471, J0670, J2001

49421 0213T, 0216T, 11000-11006, 11042-11047, 12001-12007, 12011-12057, 13100-13133, 13151-13153, 36000, 36400-36410, 36420-36430, 36440, 36591-36592, 36600, 36640, 43752, 44005, 44180, 44602-44605, 44820-44850, 49000-49010, 49255, 49320, 49400, 49402, 49422✦, 49436, 49570, 51701-51703, 62320-62327, 64400, 64405-64408, 64415-64435, 64445-64454, 64461-64463, 64479-64505, 64510-64530, 69990, 92012-92014, 93000-93010, 93040-93042, 93318, 93355, 94002, 94200, 94250, 94680-94690, 94770, 95812-95816, 95819, 95822, 95829, 95955, 96360-96368, 96372, 96374-96377, 96523, 97597-97598, 97602, 99155, 99156, 99157, 99211-99223, 99231-99255, 99291-99292, 99304-99310, 99315-99316, 99334-99337, 99347-99350, 99374-99375, 99377-99378, 99446-99449, 99451-99452, 99495-99496, G0463, G0471

49422 0213T, 0216T, 11000-11006, 11042-11047, 12001-12007, 12011-12057, 13100-13133, 13151-13153, 36000, 36400-36410, 36420-36430, 36440, 36591-36592, 36600, 36640, 43752, 44005, 44180, 44602-44605, 44820-44850, 49000-49010, 49255, 49320, 49400, 49436, 49570, 51701-51703, 62320-62327, 64400, 64405-64408, 64415-64435, 64445-64454, 64461-64463, 64479-64505, 64510-64530, 69990, 92012-92014, 93000-93010, 93040-93042, 93318, 93355, 94002, 94200, 94250, 94680-94690, 94770, 95812-95816, 95819, 95822, 95829, 95955, 96360-96368, 96372, 96374-96377, 96523, 97597-97598, 97602, 99155, 99156, 99157, 99211-99223, 99231-99255, 99291-99292, 99304-99310, 99315-99316, 99334-99337, 99347-99350, 99374-99375, 99377-99378, 99446-99449, 99451-99452, 99495-99496, G0463, G0471

49435 11000-11006, 11042-11047, 36591-36592, 96523, 97597-97598, 97602

49436 0213T, 0216T, 12001-12007, 12011-12057, 13100-13133, 13151-13153, 36000, 36400-36410, 36420-36430, 36440, 36591-36592, 36600, 36640, 43752, 51701-51703, 62320-62327, 64400, 64405-64408, 64415-64435, 64445-64454, 64461-64463, 64479-64505, 64510-64530, 69990, 92012-92014, 93000-93010, 93040-93042, 93318, 93355, 94002, 94200, 94250, 94680-94690, 94770, 95812-95816, 95819, 95822, 95829, 95955, 96360-96368, 96372, 96374-96377, 96523, 99155, 99156, 99157, 99211-99223, 99231-99255, 99291-99292, 99304-99310,

99315-99316, 99334-99337, 99347-99350, 99374-99375, 99377-99378, 99446-99449, 99451-99452, 99495-99496, G0463, G0471

50010 0213T, 0216T, 0228T, 0230T, 12001-12007, 12011-12057, 13100-13133, 13151-13153, 36000, 36400-36410, 36420-36430, 36440, 36591-36592, 36600, 36640, 43752, 44602-44605, 44950, 44970, 49000-49010, 50100, 51701-51703, 60540-60545, 62320-62327, 64400, 64405-64408, 64415-64435, 64445-64454, 64461-64463, 64479-64505, 64510-64530, 69990, 92012-92014, 93000-93010, 93040-93042, 93318, 93355, 94002, 94200, 94250, 94680-94690, 94770, 95812-95816, 95819, 95822, 95829, 95955, 96360-96368, 96372, 96374-96377, 96523, 99155, 99156, 99157, 99211-99223, 99231-99255, 99291-99292, 99304-99310, 99315-99316, 99334-99337, 99347-99350, 99374-99375, 99377-99378, 99446-99449, 99451-99452, 99495-99496, G0463, G0471

50020 0213T, 0216T, 0228T, 0230T, 12001-12007, 12011-12057, 13100-13133, 13151-13153, 36000, 36400-36410, 36420-36430, 36440, 36591-36592, 36600, 36640, 43752, 44602-44605, 44950, 44970, 49000-49010, 49020✦, 49405-49406, 50010, 50205, 51701-51703, 62320-62327, 64400, 64405-64408, 64415-64435, 64445-64454, 64461-64463, 64479-64505, 64510-64530, 69990, 92012-92014, 93000-93010, 93040-93042, 93318, 93355, 94002, 94200, 94250, 94680-94690, 94770, 95812-95816, 95819, 95822, 95829, 95955, 96360-96368, 96372, 96374-96377, 96523, 99155, 99156, 99157, 99211-99223, 99231-99255, 99291-99292, 99304-99310, 99315-99316, 99334-99337, 99347-99350, 99374-99375, 99377-99378, 99446-99449, 99451-99452, 99495-99496, G0463, G0471

50040 0213T, 0216T, 0228T, 0230T, 11000-11006, 11042-11047, 12001-12007, 12011-12057, 13100-13133, 13151-13153, 36000, 36400-36410, 36420-36430, 36440, 36591-36592, 36600, 36640, 43752, 44602-44605, 44950, 44970, 49000-49010, 49406, 50010-50020, 50045✦, 50500, 50541, 51701-51703, 62320-62327, 64400, 64405-64408, 64415-64435, 64445-64454, 64461-64463, 64479-64505, 64510-64530, 69990, 92012-92014, 93000-93010, 93040-93042, 93318, 93355, 94002, 94200, 94250, 94680-94690, 94770, 95812-95816, 95819, 95822, 95829, 95955, 96360-96368, 96372, 96374-96377, 96523, 97597-97598, 97602, 99155, 99156, 99157, 99211-99223, 99231-99255, 99291-99292, 99304-99310, 99315-99316, 99334-99337, 99347-99350, 99374-99375, 99377-99378, 99446-99449, 99451-99452, 99495-99496, G0463, G0471

50045 0213T, 0216T, 0228T, 0230T, 11000-11006, 11042-11047, 12001-12007, 12011-12057, 13100-13133, 13151-13153, 36000, 36400-36410, 36420-36430, 36440, 36591-36592, 36600, 36640, 43752, 44602-44605, 44950, 44970, 49000-49010, 49406, 50010-50020, 50541, 51701-51703, 62320-62327, 64400, 64405-64408, 64415-64435, 64445-64454, 64461-64463, 64479-64505, 64510-64530, 69990, 92012-92014, 93000-93010, 93040-93042, 93318, 93355, 94002, 94200, 94250, 94680-94690, 94770, 95812-95816, 95819, 95822, 95829, 95955, 96360-96368, 96372, 96374-96377, 96523, 97597-97598, 97602, 99155, 99156, 99157, 99211-99223, 99231-99255, 99291-99292, 99304-99310, 99315-99316, 99334-99337, 99347-99350, 99374-99375, 99377-99378, 99446-99449, 99451-99452, 99495-99496, G0463, G0471

50060 0213T, 0216T, 0228T, 0230T, 11000-11006, 11042-11047, 12001-12007, 12011-12057, 13100-13133, 13151-13153, 36000, 36400-36410, 36420-36430, 36440, 36591-36592, 36600, 36640, 43752, 44602-44605, 44950, 44970, 49000-49010, 49406, 50020, 50040-50045, 50065-50075✦, 50500, 51701-51703, 62320-62327, 64400, 64405-64408, 64415-64435, 64445-64454, 64461-64463, 64479-64505, 64510-64530, 69990, 92012-92014, 93000-93010, 93040-93042, 93318, 93355, 94002, 94200, 94250, 94680-94690, 94770, 95812-95816, 95819, 95822, 95829, 95955, 96360-96368, 96372, 96374-96377, 96523, 97597-97598, 97602, 99155, 99156, 99157, 99211-99223,

99231-99255, 99291-99292, 99304-99310, 99315-99316, 99334-99337, 99347-99350, 99374-99375, 99377-99378, 99446-99449, 99451-99452, 99495-99496, G0463, G0471

50065 0213T, 0216T, 0228T, 0230T, 11000-11006, 11042-11047, 12001-12007, 12011-12057, 13100-13133, 13151-13153, 36000, 36400-36410, 36420-36430, 36440, 36591-36592, 36600, 36640, 43752, 44602-44605, 44950, 44970, 49000-49010, 49406, 50020, 50040-50045, 50075✦, 50500, 51701-51703, 62320-62327, 64400, 64405-64408, 64415-64435, 64445-64454, 64461-64463, 64479-64505, 64510-64530, 69990, 92012-92014, 93000-93010, 93040-93042, 93318, 93355, 94002, 94200, 94250, 94680-94690, 94770, 95812-95816, 95819, 95822, 95829, 95955, 96360-96368, 96372, 96374-96377, 96523, 97597-97598, 97602, 99155, 99156, 99157, 99211-99223, 99231-99255, 99291-99292, 99304-99310, 99315-99316, 99334-99337, 99347-99350, 99374-99375, 99377-99378, 99446-99449, 99451-99452, 99495-99496, G0463, G0471

50070 0213T, 0216T, 0228T, 0230T, 11000-11006, 11042-11047, 12001-12007, 12011-12057, 13100-13133, 13151-13153, 36000, 36400-36410, 36420-36430, 36440, 36591-36592, 36600, 36640, 43752, 44602-44605, 44950, 44970, 49000-49010, 49406, 50020, 50040-50045, 50065✦, 50075✦, 50500, 51701-51703, 62320-62327, 64400, 64405-64408, 64415-64435, 64445-64454, 64461-64463, 64479-64505, 64510-64530, 69990, 92012-92014, 93000-93010, 93040-93042, 93318, 93355, 94002, 94200, 94250, 94680-94690, 94770, 95812-95816, 95819, 95822, 95829, 95955, 96360-96368, 96372, 96374-96377, 96523, 97597-97598, 97602, 99155, 99156, 99157, 99211-99223, 99231-99255, 99291-99292, 99304-99310, 99315-99316, 99334-99337, 99347-99350, 99374-99375, 99377-99378, 99446-99449, 99451-99452, 99495-99496, G0463, G0471

50075 0213T, 0216T, 0228T, 0230T, 11000-11006, 11042-11047, 12001-12007, 12011-12057, 13100-13133, 13151-13153, 36000, 36400-36410, 36420-36430, 36440, 36591-36592, 36600, 36640, 43752, 44602-44605, 44950, 44970, 49000-49010, 49406, 50020, 50040-50045, 50500, 51701-51703, 62320-62327, 64400, 64405-64408, 64415-64435, 64445-64454, 64461-64463, 64479-64505, 64510-64530, 69990, 92012-92014, 93000-93010, 93040-93042, 93318, 93355, 94002, 94200, 94250, 94680-94690, 94770, 95812-95816, 95819, 95822, 95829, 95955, 96360-96368, 96372, 96374-96377, 96523, 97597-97598, 97602, 99155, 99156, 99157, 99211-99223, 99231-99255, 99291-99292, 99304-99310, 99315-99316, 99334-99337, 99347-99350, 99374-99375, 99377-99378, 99446-99449, 99451-99452, 99495-99496, G0463, G0471

50080 0213T, 0216T, 0228T, 0230T, 11000-11006, 11042-11047, 12001-12007, 12011-12057, 13100-13133, 13151-13153, 36000, 36400-36410, 36420-36430, 36440, 36591-36592, 36600, 36640, 43752, 50081, 50382, 50436-50437, 50561, 50693-50695, 50961, 50980, 51701-51703, 52320-52325, 52330, 52352-52353, 52356, 62320-62327, 64400, 64405-64408, 64415-64435, 64445-64454, 64461-64463, 64479-64505, 64510-64530, 69990, 76380, 76942, 76970, 76998, 77001-77002, 77012, 77021, 92012-92014, 93000-93010, 93040-93042, 93318, 93355, 94002, 94200, 94250, 94680-94690, 94770, 95812-95816, 95819, 95822, 95829, 95955, 96360-96368, 96372, 96374-96377, 96523, 97597-97598, 97602, 99155, 99156, 99157, 99211-99223, 99231-99255, 99291-99292, 99304-99310, 99315-99316, 99334-99337, 99347-99350, 99374-99375, 99377-99378, 99446-99449, 99451-99452, 99495-99496, G0463, G0471

50081 0213T, 0216T, 0228T, 0230T, 11000-11006, 11042-11047, 12001-12007, 12011-12057, 13100-13133, 13151-13153, 36000, 36400-36410, 36420-36430, 36440, 36591-36592, 36600, 36640, 43752, 50382, 50436-50437, 50561, 50693-50695, 50961, 50980, 51701-51703, 52320-52325, 52330, 52352-52353, 52356, 62320-62327, 64400, 64405-64408, 64415-64435, 64445-64454, 64461-64463, 64479-64505,

CPT © 2020 American Medical Association. All Rights Reserved.

64510-64530, 69990, 76380, 76942, 76970, 76998, 77001-77002, 77012, 77021, 92012-92014, 93000-93010, 93040-93042, 93318, 93355, 94002, 94200, 94250, 94680-94690, 94770, 95812-95816, 95819, 95822, 95829, 95955, 96360-96368, 96372, 96374-96377, 96523, 97597-97598, 97602, 99155, 99156, 99157, 99211-99223, 99231-99255, 99291-99292, 99304-99310, 99315-99316, 99334-99337, 99347-99350, 99374-99375, 99377-99378, 99446-99449, 99451-99452, 99495-99496, G0463, G0471

50100 0213T, 0216T, 0228T, 0230T, 12001-12007, 12011-12057, 13100-13133, 13151-13153, 36000, 36400-36410, 36420-36430, 36440, 36591-36592, 36600, 36640, 43752, 44602-44605, 44950, 44970, 49000-49010, 49406, 50020, 51701-51703, 62320-62327, 64400, 64405-64408, 64415-64435, 64445-64454, 64461-64463, 64479-64505, 64510-64530, 69990, 92012-92014, 93000-93010, 93040-93042, 93318, 93355, 94002, 94200, 94250, 94680-94690, 94770, 95812-95816, 95819, 95822, 95829, 95955, 96360-96368, 96372, 96374-96377, 96523, 99155, 99156, 99157, 99211-99223, 99231-99255, 99291-99292, 99304-99310, 99315-99316, 99334-99337, 99347-99350, 99374-99375, 99377-99378, 99446-99449, 99451-99452, 99495-99496, G0463, G0471

50120 0213T, 0216T, 0228T, 0230T, 11000-11006, 11042-11047, 12001-12007, 12011-12057, 13100-13133, 13151-13153, 36000, 36400-36410, 36420-36430, 36440, 36591-36592, 36600, 36640, 43752, 44602-44605, 44950, 44970, 49000-49010, 49406, 50020, 50544, 51701-51703, 62320-62327, 64400, 64405-64408, 64415-64435, 64445-64454, 64461-64463, 64479-64505, 64510-64530, 69990, 92012-92014, 93000-93010, 93040-93042, 93318, 93355, 94002, 94200, 94250, 94680-94690, 94770, 95812-95816, 95819, 95822, 95829, 95955, 96360-96368, 96372, 96374-96377, 96523, 97597-97598, 97602, 99155, 99156, 99157, 99211-99223, 99231-99255, 99291-99292, 99304-99310, 99315-99316, 99334-99337, 99347-99350, 99374-99375, 99377-99378, 99446-99449, 99451-99452, 99495-99496, G0463, G0471

50125 0213T, 0216T, 0228T, 0230T, 11000-11006, 11042-11047, 12001-12007, 12011-12057, 13100-13133, 13151-13153, 36000, 36400-36410, 36420-36430, 36440, 36591-36592, 36600, 36640, 43752, 44602-44605, 44950, 44970, 49000-49010, 49406, 50020, 50120, 50544, 51701-51703, 62320-62327, 64400, 64405-64408, 64415-64435, 64445-64454, 64461-64463, 64479-64505, 64510-64530, 69990, 92012-92014, 93000-93010, 93040-93042, 93318, 93355, 94002, 94200, 94250, 94680-94690, 94770, 95812-95816, 95819, 95822, 95829, 95955, 96360-96368, 96372, 96374-96377, 96523, 97597-97598, 97602, 99155, 99156, 99157, 99211-99223, 99231-99255, 99291-99292, 99304-99310, 99315-99316, 99334-99337, 99347-99350, 99374-99375, 99377-99378, 99446-99449, 99451-99452, 99495-99496, G0463, G0471

50130 0213T, 0216T, 0228T, 0230T, 11000-11006, 11042-11047, 12001-12007, 12011-12057, 13100-13133, 13151-13153, 36000, 36400-36410, 36420-36430, 36440, 36591-36592, 36600, 36640, 43752, 44602-44605, 44950, 44970, 49000-49010, 49406, 50020, 50120-50125, 50544, 51701-51703, 62320-62327, 64400, 64405-64408, 64415-64435, 64445-64454, 64461-64463, 64479-64505, 64510-64530, 69990, 92012-92014, 93000-93010, 93040-93042, 93318, 93355, 94002, 94200, 94250, 94680-94690, 94770, 95812-95816, 95819, 95822, 95829, 95955, 96360-96368, 96372, 96374-96377, 96523, 97597-97598, 97602, 99155, 99156, 99157, 99211-99223, 99231-99255, 99291-99292, 99304-99310, 99315-99316, 99334-99337, 99347-99350, 99374-99375, 99377-99378, 99446-99449, 99451-99452, 99495-99496, G0463, G0471

50135 0213T, 0216T, 0228T, 0230T, 11000-11006, 11042-11047, 12001-12007, 12011-12057, 13100-13133, 13151-13153, 36000, 36400-36410, 36420-36430, 36440, 36591-36592, 36600, 36640, 43752, 44602-44605, 44950, 44970, 49000-49010, 49406, 50020, 50120-50130, 50544,

51701-51703, 62320-62327, 64400, 64405-64408, 64415-64435, 64445-64454, 64461-64463, 64479-64505, 64510-64530, 69990, 92012-92014, 93000-93010, 93040-93042, 93318, 93355, 94002, 94200, 94250, 94680-94690, 94770, 95812-95816, 95819, 95822, 95829, 95955, 96360-96368, 96372, 96374-96377, 96523, 97597-97598, 97602, 99155, 99156, 99157, 99211-99223, 99231-99255, 99291-99292, 99304-99310, 99315-99316, 99334-99337, 99347-99350, 99374-99375, 99377-99378, 99446-99449, 99451-99452, 99495-99496, G0463, G0471

50200 0213T, 0216T, 0228T, 0230T, 10005, 10007, 10009, 10011, 10021, 12001-12007, 12011-12057, 13100-13133, 13151-13153, 36000, 36400-36410, 36420-36430, 36440, 36591-36592, 36600, 36640, 43752, 44950, 44970, 50205❖, 51701-51703, 62320-62327, 64400, 64405-64408, 64415-64435, 64445-64454, 64461-64463, 64479-64505, 64510-64530, 69990, 76000, 76970, 76998, 92012-92014, 93000-93010, 93040-93042, 93318, 93355, 94002, 94200, 94250, 94680-94690, 94770, 95812-95816, 95819, 95822, 95829, 95955, 96360-96368, 96372, 96374-96377, 96523, 99155, 99156, 99157, 99211-99223, 99231-99255, 99291-99292, 99304-99310, 99315-99316, 99334-99337, 99347-99350, 99374-99375, 99377-99378, 99446-99449, 99451-99452, 99495-99496, G0463, G0471, J0670, J1642-J1644, J2001

50205 0213T, 0216T, 0228T, 0230T, 10005, 10007, 10009, 10011, 10021, 12001-12007, 12011-12057, 13100-13133, 13151-13153, 36000, 36400-36410, 36420-36430, 36440, 36591-36592, 36600, 36640, 43752, 44950, 44970, 49010, 50500, 51701-51703, 62320-62327, 64400, 64405-64408, 64415-64435, 64445-64454, 64461-64463, 64479-64505, 64510-64530, 69990, 92012-92014, 93000-93010, 93040-93042, 93318, 93355, 94002, 94200, 94250, 94680-94690, 94770, 95812-95816, 95819, 95822, 95829, 95955, 96360-96368, 96372, 96374-96377, 96523, 99155, 99156, 99157, 99211-99223, 99231-99255, 99291-99292, 99304-99310, 99315-99316, 99334-99337, 99347-99350, 99374-99375, 99377-99378, 99446-99449, 99451-99452, 99495-99496, G0463, G0471

50220 0213T, 0216T, 0228T, 0230T, 11000-11006, 11042-11047, 12001-12007, 12011-12057, 13100-13133, 13151-13153, 32551, 32556-32557, 36000, 36400-36410, 36420-36430, 36440, 36591-36592, 36600, 36640, 38747, 43752, 44602-44605, 44950, 44970, 49000-49010, 50100, 50205, 50250-50290, 50541-50546, 50548, 50605, 50650, 51701-51703, 52005, 60540-60545, 60650, 62320-62327, 64400, 64405-64408, 64415-64435, 64445-64454, 64461-64463, 64479-64505, 64510-64530, 69990, 92012-92014, 93000-93010, 93040-93042, 93318, 93355, 94002, 94200, 94250, 94680-94690, 94770, 95812-95816, 95819, 95822, 95829, 95955, 96360-96368, 96372, 96374-96377, 96523, 97597-97598, 97602, 99155, 99156, 99157, 99211-99223, 99231-99255, 99291-99292, 99304-99310, 99315-99316, 99334-99337, 99347-99350, 99374-99375, 99377-99378, 99446-99449, 99451-99452, 99495-99496, G0463, G0471

50225 0213T, 0216T, 0228T, 0230T, 11000-11006, 11042-11047, 12001-12007, 12011-12057, 13100-13133, 13151-13153, 20650, 32556-32557, 36000, 36400-36410, 36420-36430, 36440, 36591-36592, 36600, 36640, 38747, 43752, 44602-44605, 44950, 44970, 49000-49010, 49203, 50100, 50205, 50220, 50250-50290, 50541-50546, 50548, 50605, 50650, 51701-51703, 60540-60545, 60650, 62320-62327, 64400, 64405-64408, 64415-64435, 64445-64454, 64461-64463, 64479-64505, 64510-64530, 69990, 92012-92014, 93000-93010, 93040-93042, 93318, 93355, 94002, 94200, 94250, 94680-94690, 94770, 95812-95816, 95819, 95822, 95829, 95955, 96360-96368, 96372, 96374-96377, 96523, 97597-97598, 97602, 99155, 99156, 99157, 99211-99223, 99231-99255, 99291-99292, 99304-99310, 99315-99316, 99334-99337, 99347-99350, 99374-99375, 99377-99378, 99446-99449, 99451-99452, 99495-99496, G0463, G0471

50230 0213T, 0216T, 0228T, 0230T, 11000-11006, 11042-11047, 12001-12007, 12011-12057, 13100-13133, 13151-13153, 32551, 32556-32557,

CPT © 2020 American Medical Association. All Rights Reserved.
Coding Companion for Urology/Nephrology

35702-35703, 36000, 36400-36410, 36420-36430, 36440, 36591-36592, 36600, 36640, 38100-38101, 38120, 38562-38570, 38780, 43752, 44950, 44970, 49010, 49203, 49255, 50080-50100, 50205, 50220, 50250-50290, 50526, 50541-50546, 50548, 50605, 50650, 51701-51703, 52281, 52332, 52356, 60540-60545, 60650, 62320-62327, 64400, 64405-64408, 64415-64435, 64445-64454, 64461-64463, 64479-64505, 64510-64530, 69990, 92012-92014, 93000-93010, 93040-93042, 93318, 93355, 94002, 94200, 94250, 94680-94690, 94770, 95812-95816, 95819, 95822, 95829, 95955, 96360-96368, 96372, 96374-96377, 96523, 97597-97598, 97602, 99155, 99156, 99157, 99211-99223, 99231-99255, 99291-99292, 99304-99310, 99315-99316, 99334-99337, 99347-99350, 99374-99375, 99377-99378, 99446-99449, 99451-99452, 99495-99496, G0463, G0471

50234 0213T, 0216T, 0228T, 0230T, 11000-11006, 11042-11047, 12001-12007, 12011-12057, 13100-13133, 13151-13153, 32551, 32556-32557, 36000, 36400-36410, 36420-36430, 36440, 36591-36592, 36600, 36640, 38747, 43752, 44602-44605, 44950, 44970, 49000-49010, 49203, 50100, 50236♦, 50250-50290, 50500, 50541-50546, 50548, 50650-50660, 51701-51703, 52000, 52240, 60540-60545, 60650, 62320-62327, 64400, 64405-64408, 64415-64435, 64445-64454, 64461-64463, 64479-64505, 64510-64530, 69990, 92012-92014, 93000-93010, 93040-93042, 93318, 93355, 94002, 94200, 94250, 94680-94690, 94770, 95812-95816, 95819, 95822, 95829, 95955, 96360-96368, 96372, 96374-96377, 96523, 97597-97598, 97602, 99155, 99156, 99157, 99211-99223, 99231-99255, 99291-99292, 99304-99310, 99315-99316, 99334-99337, 99347-99350, 99374-99375, 99377-99378, 99446-99449, 99451-99452, 99495-99496, G0463, G0471

50236 0213T, 0216T, 0228T, 0230T, 11000-11006, 11042-11047, 12001-12007, 12011-12057, 13100-13133, 13151-13153, 32551, 32556-32557, 36000, 36400-36410, 36420-36430, 36440, 36591-36592, 36600, 36640, 38747, 43752, 44602-44605, 44950, 44970, 49000-49010, 49203-49204, 50100, 50250-50290, 50500, 50541-50546, 50548, 50650-50660, 51701-51703, 52000, 52240, 60540-60545, 60650, 62320-62327, 64400, 64405-64408, 64415-64435, 64445-64454, 64461-64463, 64479-64505, 64510-64530, 69990, 92012-92014, 93000-93010, 93040-93042, 93318, 93355, 94002, 94200, 94250, 94680-94690, 94770, 95812-95816, 95819, 95822, 95829, 95955, 96360-96368, 96372, 96374-96377, 96523, 97597-97598, 97602, 99155, 99156, 99157, 99211-99223, 99231-99255, 99291-99292, 99304-99310, 99315-99316, 99334-99337, 99347-99350, 99374-99375, 99377-99378, 99446-99449, 99451-99452, 99495-99496, G0463, G0471

50240 0213T, 0216T, 0228T, 0230T, 11000-11006, 11042-11047, 12001-12007, 12011-12057, 13100-13133, 13151-13153, 32551, 32556-32557, 35840, 36000, 36400-36410, 36420-36430, 36440, 36591-36592, 36600, 36640, 38100-38101, 38120, 43752, 44602-44605, 44950, 44970, 49000-49010, 50100, 50250-50290, 50500, 50541-50544, 51701-51703, 60540-60545, 60650, 62320-62327, 64400, 64405-64408, 64415-64435, 64445-64454, 64461-64463, 64479-64505, 64510-64530, 69990, 92012-92014, 93000-93010, 93040-93042, 93318, 93355, 94002, 94200, 94250, 94680-94690, 94770, 95812-95816, 95819, 95822, 95829, 95955, 96360-96368, 96372, 96374-96377, 96523, 97597-97598, 97602, 99155, 99156, 99157, 99211-99223, 99231-99255, 99291-99292, 99304-99310, 99315-99316, 99334-99337, 99347-99350, 99374-99375, 99377-99378, 99446-99449, 99451-99452, 99495-99496, G0463, G0471

50250 0213T, 0216T, 0228T, 0230T, 12001-12007, 12011-12057, 13100-13133, 13151-13153, 36000, 36400-36410, 36420-36430, 36440, 36591-36592, 36600, 36640, 43653, 43752, 44820-44850, 44950, 44970, 49000-49010, 49203, 50040-50045, 50100, 50500, 50541-50542, 50544, 50592-50593♦, 50715, 51701-51703, 62320-62327, 64400, 64405-64408, 64415-64435, 64445-64454, 64461-64463, 64479-64505, 64510-64530, 69990, 76940, 76942, 76970, 76998, 92012-92014,

93000-93010, 93040-93042, 93318, 93355, 94002, 94200, 94250, 94680-94690, 94770, 95812-95816, 95819, 95822, 95829, 95955, 96360-96368, 96372, 96374-96377, 96523, 99155, 99156, 99157, 99211-99223, 99231-99255, 99291-99292, 99304-99310, 99315-99316, 99334-99337, 99347-99350, 99374-99375, 99377-99378, 99446-99449, 99451-99452, 99495-99496, G0463, G0471

50280 0213T, 0216T, 0228T, 0230T, 11000-11006, 11042-11047, 12001-12007, 12011-12057, 13100-13133, 13151-13153, 36000, 36400-36410, 36420-36430, 36440, 36591-36592, 36600, 36640, 43752, 44602-44605, 44950, 44970, 49000-49010, 50040-50045, 50100, 50500, 50541, 50544, 51701-51703, 62320-62327, 64400, 64405-64408, 64415-64435, 64445-64454, 64461-64463, 64479-64505, 64510-64530, 69990, 92012-92014, 93000-93010, 93040-93042, 93318, 93355, 94002, 94200, 94250, 94680-94690, 94770, 95812-95816, 95819, 95822, 95829, 95955, 96360-96368, 96372, 96374-96377, 96523, 97597-97598, 97602, 99155, 99156, 99157, 99211-99223, 99231-99255, 99291-99292, 99304-99310, 99315-99316, 99334-99337, 99347-99350, 99374-99375, 99377-99378, 99446-99449, 99451-99452, 99495-99496, G0463, G0471

50290 0213T, 0216T, 0228T, 0230T, 11000-11006, 11042-11047, 12001-12007, 12011-12057, 13100-13133, 13151-13153, 36000, 36400-36410, 36420-36430, 36440, 36591-36592, 36600, 36640, 43752, 44602-44605, 44950, 44970, 49000-49010, 50100, 50500, 50544, 51701-51703, 62320-62327, 64400, 64405-64408, 64415-64435, 64445-64454, 64461-64463, 64479-64505, 64510-64530, 69990, 92012-92014, 93000-93010, 93040-93042, 93318, 93355, 94002, 94200, 94250, 94680-94690, 94770, 95812-95816, 95819, 95822, 95829, 95955, 96360-96368, 96372, 96374-96377, 96523, 97597-97598, 97602, 99155, 99156, 99157, 99211-99223, 99231-99255, 99291-99292, 99304-99310, 99315-99316, 99334-99337, 99347-99350, 99374-99375, 99377-99378, 99446-99449, 99451-99452, 99495-99496, G0463, G0471

50300 0213T, 0216T, 11000-11006, 11042-11047, 36000, 36410, 36591-36592, 44602-44605, 44950, 44970, 49000-49010, 50220-50240, 50541-50546, 50548, 50605, 61650, 62324-62327, 64415-64417, 64450, 64454, 64486-64490, 64493, 69990, 96523, 97597-97598, 97602

50320 0213T, 0216T, 0228T, 0230T, 11000-11006, 11042-11047, 12001-12007, 12011-12057, 13100-13133, 13151-13153, 36000, 36400-36410, 36420-36430, 36440, 36591-36592, 36600, 36640, 43752, 44602-44605, 44950, 44970, 49000-49010, 50220-50240, 50541-50548, 50605, 50650, 51701-51703, 62320-62327, 64400, 64405-64408, 64415-64435, 64445-64454, 64461-64463, 64479-64505, 64510-64530, 69990, 92012-92014, 93000-93010, 93040-93042, 93318, 93355, 94002, 94200, 94250, 94680-94690, 94770, 95812-95816, 95819, 95822, 95829, 95955, 96360-96368, 96372, 96374-96377, 96523, 97597-97598, 97602, 99155, 99156, 99157, 99211-99223, 99231-99255, 99291-99292, 99304-99310, 99315-99316, 99334-99337, 99347-99350, 99374-99375, 99377-99378, 99446-99449, 99451-99452, 99495-99496, G0463, G0471

50323 11000-11006, 11042-11047, 36591-36592, 60540-60545, 69990, 96523, 97597-97598, 97602

50325 11000-11006, 11042-11047, 36591-36592, 49400, 50323♦, 69990, 96523, 97597-97598, 97602

50327 36591-36592, 69990, 96523

50328 36591-36592, 69990, 96523

50329 36591-36592, 69990, 96523

50340 0213T, 0216T, 0228T, 0230T, 11000-11006, 11042-11047, 12001-12007, 12011-12057, 13100-13133, 13151-13153, 36000, 36400-36410, 36420-36430, 36440, 36591-36592, 36600, 36640, 38100-38101, 38120, 43752, 44602-44605, 44950, 44970, 49000-49010, 50220-50240, 50541-50546, 50548, 50605, 50650, 51701-51703, 62320-62327, 64400,

© 2020 Optum360, LLC
CPT © 2020 American Medical Association. All Rights Reserved.

64405-64408, 64415-64435, 64445-64454, 64461-64463, 64479-64505, 64510-64530, 69990, 92012-92014, 93000-93010, 93040-93042, 93318, 93355, 94002, 94200, 94250, 94680-94690, 94770, 95812-95816, 95819, 95822, 95829, 95955, 96360-96368, 96372, 96374-96377, 96523, 97597-97598, 97602, 99155, 99156, 99157, 99211-99223, 99231-99255, 99291-99292, 99304-99310, 99315-99316, 99334-99337, 99347-99350, 99374-99375, 99377-99378, 99446-99449, 99451-99452, 99495-99496, G0463, G0471

50360 0213T, 0216T, 0228T, 0230T, 11000-11006, 11042-11047, 12001-12007, 12011-12057, 13100-13133, 13151-13153, 35221, 35840, 36000, 36400-36410, 36420-36430, 36440, 36591-36592, 36600, 36640, 43752, 44602-44605, 44950, 44970, 49000-49010, 49421, 50200, 50220-50240, 50400, 50780, 51701-51703, 62320-62327, 64400, 64405-64408, 64415-64435, 64445-64454, 64461-64463, 64479-64505, 64510-64530, 69990, 92012-92014, 93000-93010, 93040-93042, 93318, 93355, 94002, 94200, 94250, 94680-94690, 94770, 95812-95816, 95819, 95822, 95829, 95955, 96360-96368, 96372, 96374-96377, 96523, 97597-97598, 97602, 99155, 99156, 99157, 99211-99223, 99231-99255, 99291-99292, 99304-99310, 99315-99316, 99334-99337, 99347-99350, 99374-99375, 99377-99378, 99446-99449, 99451-99452, 99495-99496, G0463, G0471

50365 0213T, 0216T, 0228T, 0230T, 11000-11006, 11042-11047, 12001-12007, 12011-12057, 13100-13133, 13151-13153, 36000, 36400-36410, 36420-36430, 36440, 36591-36592, 36600, 36640, 38100-38101, 38120, 43752, 44602-44605, 44950, 44970, 49000-49010, 50220-50240, 50340, 50541-50546, 50548, 50605, 50650, 50780, 51701-51703, 62320-62327, 64400, 64405-64408, 64415-64435, 64445-64454, 64461-64463, 64479-64505, 64510-64530, 69990, 92012-92014, 93000-93010, 93040-93042, 93318, 93355, 94002, 94200, 94250, 94680-94690, 94770, 95812-95816, 95819, 95822, 95829, 95955, 96360-96368, 96372, 96374-96377, 96523, 97597-97598, 97602, 99155, 99156, 99157, 99211-99223, 99231-99255, 99291-99292, 99304-99310, 99315-99316, 99334-99337, 99347-99350, 99374-99375, 99377-99378, 99446-99449, 99451-99452, 99495-99496, G0463, G0471

50370 0213T, 0216T, 0228T, 0230T, 11000-11006, 11042-11047, 12001-12007, 12011-12057, 13100-13133, 13151-13153, 36000, 36400-36410, 36420-36430, 36440, 36591-36592, 36600, 36640, 38100-38101, 38120, 43752, 44602-44605, 44950, 44970, 49000-49010, 50220-50240, 50340, 50541-50546, 50548, 50605, 51701-51703, 62320-62327, 64400, 64405-64408, 64415-64435, 64445-64454, 64461-64463, 64479-64505, 64510-64530, 69990, 92012-92014, 93000-93010, 93040-93042, 93318, 93355, 94002, 94200, 94250, 94680-94690, 94770, 95812-95816, 95819, 95822, 95829, 95955, 96360-96368, 96372, 96374-96377, 96523, 97597-97598, 97602, 99155, 99156, 99157, 99211-99223, 99231-99255, 99291-99292, 99304-99310, 99315-99316, 99334-99337, 99347-99350, 99374-99375, 99377-99378, 99446-99449, 99451-99452, 99495-99496, G0463, G0471

50380 0213T, 0216T, 0228T, 0230T, 12001-12007, 12011-12057, 13100-13133, 13151-13153, 35840, 36000, 36400-36410, 36420-36430, 36440, 36591-36592, 36600, 36640, 38100-38101, 38120, 43752, 44602-44605, 44950, 44970, 49000-49010, 50340, 50544, 50605, 50780, 51701-51703, 62320-62327, 64400, 64405-64408, 64415-64435, 64445-64454, 64461-64463, 64479-64505, 64510-64530, 69990, 92012-92014, 93000-93010, 93040-93042, 93318, 93355, 94002, 94200, 94250, 94680-94690, 94770, 95812-95816, 95819, 95822, 95829, 95955, 96360-96368, 96372, 96374-96377, 96523, 99155, 99156, 99157, 99211-99223, 99231-99255, 99291-99292, 99304-99310, 99315-99316, 99334-99337, 99347-99350, 99374-99375, 99377-99378, 99446-99449, 99451-99452, 99495-99496, G0463, G0471

50382 0213T, 0216T, 0228T, 0230T, 11000-11006, 11042-11047, 12001-12007, 12011-12057, 13100-13133, 13151-13153, 36000, 36400-36410, 36420-36430, 36440, 36591-36592, 36600, 36640, 43752, 50384-50387◆, 50390, 50430-50432, 50436-50437, 50688, 50693-50695, 51701-51703, 52332, 52356, 62320-62327, 64400, 64405-64408, 64415-64435, 64445-64454, 64461-64463, 64479-64505, 64510-64530, 69990, 76000, 76380, 76942, 76970, 76998, 77001-77002, 77012, 77021, 92012-92014, 93000-93010, 93040-93042, 93318, 93355, 94002, 94200, 94250, 94680-94690, 94770, 95812-95816, 95819, 95822, 95829, 95955, 96360-96368, 96372, 96374-96377, 96523, 97597-97598, 97602, 99155, 99156, 99157, 99211-99223, 99231-99255, 99291-99292, 99304-99310, 99315-99316, 99334-99337, 99347-99350, 99374-99375, 99377-99378, 99446-99449, 99451-99452, 99495-99496, G0463, G0471, J0670, J2001

50384 0213T, 0216T, 0228T, 0230T, 11000-11006, 11042-11047, 12001-12007, 12011-12057, 13100-13133, 13151-13153, 36000, 36400-36410, 36420-36430, 36440, 36591-36592, 36600, 36640, 43752, 50385-50387◆, 50390, 50430-50432, 50436, 50688, 50693-50695, 51701-51703, 52332, 52356, 62320-62327, 64400, 64405-64408, 64415-64435, 64445-64454, 64461-64463, 64479-64505, 64510-64530, 69990, 76000, 76380, 76942, 76970, 76998, 77001-77002, 77012, 77021, 92012-92014, 93000-93010, 93040-93042, 93318, 93355, 94002, 94200, 94250, 94680-94690, 94770, 95812-95816, 95819, 95822, 95829, 95955, 96360-96368, 96372, 96374-96377, 96523, 97597-97598, 97602, 99155, 99156, 99157, 99211-99223, 99231-99255, 99291-99292, 99304-99310, 99315-99316, 99334-99337, 99347-99350, 99374-99375, 99377-99378, 99446-99449, 99451-99452, 99495-99496, G0463, G0471, J0670, J2001

50385 0213T, 0216T, 0228T, 0230T, 11000-11006, 11042-11047, 12001-12007, 12011-12057, 13100-13133, 13151-13153, 36000, 36400-36410, 36420-36430, 36440, 36591-36592, 36600, 36640, 43752, 50386, 50693-50695, 52310◆, 52332, 52356, 62320-62327, 64400, 64405-64408, 64415-64435, 64445-64454, 64461-64463, 64479-64505, 64510-64530, 69990, 75984, 76000, 76942, 76970, 76998, 77001-77002, 92012-92014, 93000-93010, 93040-93042, 93318, 93355, 94002, 94200, 94250, 94680-94690, 94770, 95812-95816, 95819, 95822, 95829, 95955, 96360-96368, 96372, 96374-96377, 96523, 97597-97598, 97602, 99155, 99156, 99157, 99211-99223, 99231-99255, 99291-99292, 99304-99310, 99315-99316, 99334-99337, 99347-99350, 99374-99375, 99377-99378, 99446-99449, 99451-99452, 99495-99496, G0463

50386 0213T, 0216T, 0228T, 0230T, 11000-11006, 11042-11047, 12001-12007, 12011-12057, 13100-13133, 13151-13153, 36000, 36400-36410, 36420-36430, 36440, 36591-36592, 36600, 36640, 43752, 52310◆, 52332, 52356, 62320-62327, 64400, 64405-64408, 64415-64435, 64445-64454, 64461-64463, 64479-64505, 64510-64530, 69990, 75984, 76000, 76942, 76970, 76998, 77001-77002, 92012-92014, 93000-93010, 93040-93042, 93318, 93355, 94002, 94200, 94250, 94680-94690, 94770, 95812-95816, 95819, 95822, 95829, 95955, 96360-96368, 96372, 96374-96377, 96523, 97597-97598, 97602, 99155, 99156, 99157, 99211-99223, 99231-99255, 99291-99292, 99304-99310, 99315-99316, 99334-99337, 99347-99350, 99374-99375, 99377-99378, 99446-99449, 99451-99452, 99495-99496, G0463

50387 0213T, 0216T, 0228T, 0230T, 11000-11006, 11042-11047, 12001-12007, 12011-12057, 13100-13133, 13151-13153, 36000, 36400-36410, 36420-36430, 36440, 36591-36592, 36600, 36640, 43752, 50430-50433, 50435-50437, 50688◆, 50693-50695, 51701-51703, 62320-62327, 64400, 64405-64408, 64415-64435, 64445-64454, 64461-64463, 64479-64505, 64510-64530, 69990, 74485, 76000, 77001-77002, 92012-92014, 93000-93010, 93040-93042, 93318, 93355, 94002, 94200,

94250, 94680-94690, 94770, 95812-95816, 95819, 95822, 95829, 95955, 96360-96368, 96372, 96374-96377, 96523, 97597-97598, 97602, 99155, 99156, 99157, 99211-99223, 99231-99255, 99291-99292, 99304-99310, 99315-99316, 99334-99337, 99347-99350, 99374-99375, 99377-99378, 99446-99449, 99451-99452, 99495-99496, G0463, G0471, J0670, J2001

50389 0213T, 0216T, 0228T, 0230T, 11000-11006, 11042-11047, 12001-12007, 12011-12057, 13100-13133, 13151-13153, 36000, 36400-36410, 36420-36430, 36440, 36591-36592, 36600, 36640, 43752, 50430-50431, 50436-50437, 50693-50695, 51701-51703, 62320-62327, 64400, 64405-64408, 64415-64435, 64445-64454, 64461-64463, 64479-64505, 64510-64530, 69990, 76000, 77001-77002, 92012-92014, 93000-93010, 93040-93042, 93318, 93355, 94002, 94200, 94250, 94680-94690, 94770, 95812-95816, 95819, 95822, 95829, 95955, 96360-96368, 96372, 96374-96377, 96523, 97597-97598, 97602, 99155, 99156, 99157, 99211-99223, 99231-99255, 99291-99292, 99304-99310, 99315-99316, 99334-99337, 99347-99350, 99374-99375, 99377-99378, 99446-99449, 99451-99452, 99495-99496, G0463, G0471, J0670, J2001

50390 0213T, 0216T, 0228T, 0230T, 12001-12007, 12011-12057, 13100-13133, 13151-13153, 36000, 36400-36410, 36420-36430, 36440, 36591-36592, 36600, 36640, 43752, 51701-51703, 62320-62327, 64400, 64405-64408, 64415-64435, 64445-64454, 64461-64463, 64479-64505, 64510-64530, 69990, 76000, 76970, 76998, 77001, 92012-92014, 93000-93010, 93040-93042, 93318, 93355, 94002, 94200, 94250, 94680-94690, 94770, 95812-95816, 95819, 95822, 95829, 95955, 96360-96368, 96372, 96374-96377, 96523, 99155, 99156, 99157, 99211-99223, 99231-99255, 99291-99292, 99304-99310, 99315-99316, 99334-99337, 99347-99350, 99374-99375, 99377-99378, 99446-99449, 99451-99452, 99495-99496, G0463, G0471

50391 00860-00862, 0213T, 0216T, 0228T, 0230T, 12001-12007, 12011-12057, 13100-13133, 13151-13153, 36000, 36400-36410, 36420-36430, 36440, 36591-36592, 36600, 36640, 43752, 50390, 50432, 50436-50437, 50693-50695, 51701-51703, 62320-62327, 64400, 64405-64408, 64415-64435, 64445-64454, 64461-64463, 64479-64505, 64510-64530, 69990, 76000, 92012-92014, 93000-93010, 93040-93042, 93318, 93355, 94002, 94200, 94250, 94680-94690, 94770, 95812-95816, 95819, 95822, 95829, 95955, 96360-96368, 96372, 96374-96377, 96523, 99155, 99156, 99157, 99211-99223, 99231-99255, 99291-99292, 99304-99310, 99315-99316, 99334-99337, 99347-99350, 99374-99375, 99377-99378, 99446-99449, 99451-99452, 99495-99496, G0463, G0471

50396 0213T, 0216T, 0228T, 0230T, 12001-12007, 12011-12057, 13100-13133, 13151-13153, 36000, 36400-36410, 36420-36430, 36440, 36591-36592, 36600, 36640, 43752, 50436-50437, 51701-51703, 62320-62327, 64400, 64405-64408, 64415-64435, 64445-64454, 64461-64463, 64479-64505, 64510-64530, 69990, 76000, 76942, 76970, 76998, 77001-77002, 92012-92014, 93000-93010, 93040-93042, 93318, 93355, 94002, 94200, 94250, 94680-94690, 94770, 95812-95816, 95819, 95822, 95829, 95955, 96360-96368, 96372, 96374-96377, 96523, 99155, 99156, 99157, 99211-99223, 99231-99255, 99291-99292, 99304-99310, 99315-99316, 99334-99337, 99347-99350, 99374-99375, 99377-99378, 99446-99449, 99451-99452, 99495-99496, G0463, G0471

50400 0213T, 0216T, 0228T, 0230T, 11000-11006, 11042-11047, 12001-12007, 12011-12057, 13100-13133, 13151-13153, 36000, 36400-36410, 36420-36430, 36440, 36591-36592, 36600, 36640, 43752, 44602-44605, 44950, 44970, 49000-49010, 50544, 50605, 50715, 51701-51703, 52005, 62320-62327, 64400, 64405-64408, 64415-64435, 64445-64454, 64461-64463, 64479-64505, 64510-64530, 69990, 92012-92014, 93000-93010, 93040-93042, 93318, 93355, 94002, 94200, 94250, 94680-94690, 94770, 95812-95816, 95819, 95822, 95829, 95955,

50405 0213T, 0216T, 0228T, 0230T, 11000-11006, 11042-11047, 12001-12007, 12011-12057, 13100-13133, 13151-13153, 36000, 36400-36410, 36420-36430, 36440, 36591-36592, 36600, 36640, 43752, 44602-44605, 44950, 44970, 49000-49010, 50100, 50400, 50544, 50605, 50715, 51701-51703, 52005, 62320-62327, 64400, 64405-64408, 64415-64435, 64445-64454, 64461-64463, 64479-64505, 64510-64530, 69990, 92012-92014, 93000-93010, 93040-93042, 93318, 93355, 94002, 94200, 94250, 94680-94690, 94770, 95812-95816, 95819, 95822, 95829, 95955, 96360-96368, 96372, 96374-96377, 96523, 97597-97598, 97602, 99155, 99156, 99157, 99211-99223, 99231-99255, 99291-99292, 99304-99310, 99315-99316, 99334-99337, 99347-99350, 99374-99375, 99377-99378, 99446-99449, 99451-99452, 99495-99496, G0463, G0471

50430 0213T, 0216T, 0228T, 0230T, 12001-12007, 12011-12057, 13100-13133, 13151-13153, 36000, 36011, 36400-36410, 36420-36430, 36440, 36591-36592, 36600, 36640, 43752, 50431❖, 50436, 51701-51703, 62320-62327, 64400, 64405-64408, 64415-64435, 64445-64454, 64461-64463, 64479-64505, 64510-64530, 69990, 74425, 76000, 76942, 76970, 76998, 77001-77002, 92012-92014, 93000-93010, 93040-93042, 93318, 93355, 94002, 94200, 94250, 94680-94690, 94770, 95812-95816, 95819, 95822, 95829, 95955, 96360-96368, 96372, 96374-96377, 96523, 99155, 99156, 99157, 99211-99223, 99231-99255, 99291-99292, 99304-99310, 99315-99316, 99334-99337, 99347-99350, 99374-99375, 99377-99378, 99446-99449, 99451-99452, 99495-99496, G0463, G0471, J0670, J2001

50431 0213T, 0216T, 0228T, 0230T, 12001-12007, 12011-12057, 13100-13133, 13151-13153, 36000, 36011, 36400-36410, 36420-36430, 36440, 36591-36592, 36600, 36640, 43752, 51701-51703, 62320-62327, 64400, 64405-64408, 64415-64435, 64445-64454, 64461-64463, 64479-64505, 64510-64530, 69990, 74425, 76000, 76942, 76970, 76998, 77001-77002, 92012-92014, 93000-93010, 93040-93042, 93318, 93355, 94002, 94200, 94250, 94680-94690, 94770, 95812-95816, 95819, 95822, 95829, 95955, 96360-96368, 96372, 96374-96377, 96523, 99155, 99156, 99157, 99211-99223, 99231-99255, 99291-99292, 99304-99310, 99315-99316, 99334-99337, 99347-99350, 99374-99375, 99377-99378, 99446-99449, 99451-99452, 99495-99496, G0463, G0471

50432 0213T, 0216T, 0228T, 0230T, 12001-12007, 12011-12057, 13100-13133, 13151-13153, 36000, 36011, 36400-36410, 36420-36430, 36440, 36591-36592, 36600, 36640, 43752, 50390, 50430-50431, 50434-50437, 51701-51703, 62320-62327, 64400, 64405-64408, 64415-64435, 64445-64454, 64461-64463, 64479-64505, 64510-64530, 69990, 74425, 76000, 76380, 76942, 76970, 76998, 77001-77002, 77012, 77021, 92012-92014, 93000-93010, 93040-93042, 93318, 93355, 94002, 94200, 94250, 94680-94690, 94770, 95812-95816, 95819, 95822, 95829, 95955, 96360-96368, 96372, 96374-96377, 96523, 99155, 99156, 99157, 99211-99223, 99231-99255, 99291-99292, 99304-99310, 99315-99316, 99334-99337, 99347-99350, 99374-99375, 99377-99378, 99446-99449, 99451-99452, 99495-99496, G0463, G0471, J0670, J2001

50433 0213T, 0216T, 0228T, 0230T, 12001-12007, 12011-12057, 13100-13133, 13151-13153, 36000, 36011, 36400-36410, 36420-36430, 36440, 36591-36592, 36600, 36640, 43752, 50430-50432, 50436-50437, 50684, 51701-51703, 62320-62327, 64400, 64405-64408, 64415-64435, 64445-64454, 64461-64463, 64479-64505, 64510-64530, 69990, 74425, 76000, 76380, 76942, 76970, 76998, 77001-77002, 77012, 77021, 92012-92014, 93000-93010, 93040-93042, 93318, 94002, 94200, 94250, 94680-94690, 94770, 95812-95816, 95819, 95822, 95829, 95955,

CPT © 2020 American Medical Association. All Rights Reserved.

96360-96368, 96372, 96374-96377, 96523, 99155, 99156, 99157, 99211-99223, 99231-99255, 99291-99292, 99304-99310, 99315-99316, 99334-99337, 99347-99350, 99374-99375, 99377-99378, 99446-99449, 99451-99452, J0670, J2001

50434 0213T, 0216T, 0228T, 0230T, 12001-12007, 12011-12057, 13100-13133, 13151-13153, 36000, 36011, 36400-36410, 36420-36430, 36440, 36591-36592, 36600, 36640, 43752, 49185, 49424, 50387❖, 50430-50431, 50435-50436, 50684, 51701-51703, 62320-62327, 64400, 64405-64408, 64415-64435, 64445-64454, 64461-64463, 64479-64505, 64510-64530, 69990, 74425, 76000, 76380, 76942, 76970, 76998, 77001-77002, 77012, 77021, 92012-92014, 93000-93010, 93040-93042, 93318, 93355, 94002, 94200, 94250, 94680-94690, 94770, 95812-95816, 95819, 95822, 95829, 95955, 96360-96368, 96372, 96374-96377, 96523, 99155, 99156, 99157, 99211-99223, 99231-99255, 99291-99292, 99304-99310, 99315-99316, 99334-99337, 99347-99350, 99374-99375, 99377-99378, 99446-99449, 99451-99452, 99495-99496, G0463, G0471, J0670, J2001

50435 0213T, 0216T, 0228T, 0230T, 12001-12007, 12011-12057, 13100-13133, 13151-13153, 36000, 36011, 36400-36410, 36420-36430, 36440, 36591-36592, 36600, 36640, 43752, 49185, 49424, 50389, 50430-50431, 51701-51703, 62320-62327, 64400, 64405-64408, 64415-64435, 64445-64454, 64461-64463, 64479-64505, 64510-64530, 69990, 74425, 76000, 76380, 76942, 76970, 76998, 77001-77002, 77012, 77021, 92012-92014, 93000-93010, 93040-93042, 93318, 93355, 94002, 94200, 94250, 94680-94690, 94770, 95812-95816, 95819, 95822, 95829, 95955, 96360-96368, 96372, 96374-96377, 96523, 99155, 99156, 99157, 99211-99223, 99231-99255, 99291-99292, 99304-99310, 99315-99316, 99334-99337, 99347-99350, 99374-99375, 99377-99378, 99446-99449, 99451-99452, 99495-99496, G0463, G0471, J0670, J2001

50436 0213T, 0216T, 0228T, 0230T, 12001-12007, 12011-12057, 13100-13133, 13151-13153, 36000, 36400-36410, 36420-36430, 36440, 36591-36592, 36600, 36640, 43752, 50390, 50431, 50435, 51701-51703, 62320-62327, 64400, 64405-64408, 64415-64435, 64445-64454, 64461-64463, 64479-64505, 64510-64530, 69990, 74485, 76000, 76380, 76942, 76970, 76998, 77001-77002, 77012, 77021, 92012-92014, 93000-93010, 93040-93042, 93318, 93355, 94002, 94200, 94250, 94680-94690, 94770, 95812-95816, 95819, 95822, 95829, 95955, 96360-96368, 96372, 96374-96377, 96523, 99155, 99156, 99157, 99211-99223, 99231-99255, 99291-99292, 99304-99310, 99315-99316, 99334-99337, 99347-99350, 99374-99375, 99377-99378, 99446-99449, 99495-99496, G0463, G0471

50437 0213T, 0216T, 0228T, 0230T, 12001-12007, 12011-12057, 13100-13133, 13151-13153, 36000, 36400-36410, 36420-36430, 36440, 36591-36592, 36600, 36640, 43752, 50384, 50390, 50430-50431, 50434-50435, 51701-51703, 52334, 62320-62327, 64400, 64405-64408, 64415-64435, 64445-64454, 64461-64463, 64479-64505, 64510-64530, 69990, 74485, 76000, 76380, 76942, 76970, 76998, 77001-77002, 77012, 77021, 92012-92014, 93000-93010, 93040-93042, 93318, 93355, 94002, 94200, 94250, 94680-94690, 94770, 95812-95816, 95819, 95822, 95829, 95955, 96360-96368, 96372, 96374-96377, 96523, 99155, 99156, 99157, 99211-99223, 99231-99255, 99291-99292, 99304-99310, 99315-99316, 99334-99337, 99347-99350, 99374-99375, 99377-99378, 99446-99449, 99495-99496, G0463, G0471

50500 0213T, 0216T, 0228T, 0230T, 12001-12007, 12011-12057, 13100-13133, 13151-13153, 36000, 36400-36410, 36420-36430, 36440, 36591-36592, 36600, 36640, 43752, 44602-44605, 44950, 44970, 49000-49010, 51701-51703, 62320-62327, 64400, 64405-64408, 64415-64435, 64445-64454, 64461-64463, 64479-64505, 64510-64530, 69990,

92012-92014, 93000-93010, 93040-93042, 93318, 93355, 94002, 94200, 94250, 94680-94690, 94770, 95812-95816, 95819, 95822, 95829, 95955, 96360-96368, 96372, 96374-96377, 96523, 99155, 99156, 99157, 99211-99223, 99231-99255, 99291-99292, 99304-99310, 99315-99316, 99334-99337, 99347-99350, 99374-99375, 99377-99378, 99446-99449, 99451-99452, 99495-99496, G0463, G0471

50520 0213T, 0216T, 0228T, 0230T, 11000-11006, 11042-11047, 12001-12007, 12011-12057, 13100-13133, 13151-13153, 36000, 36400-36410, 36420-36430, 36440, 36591-36592, 36600, 36640, 43752, 44602-44605, 44950, 44970, 49000-49010, 50544, 51701-51703, 62320-62327, 64400, 64405-64408, 64415-64435, 64445-64454, 64461-64463, 64479-64505, 64510-64530, 69990, 92012-92014, 93000-93010, 93040-93042, 93318, 93355, 94002, 94200, 94250, 94680-94690, 94770, 95812-95816, 95819, 95822, 95829, 95955, 96360-96368, 96372, 96374-96377, 96523, 97597-97598, 97602, 99155, 99156, 99157, 99211-99223, 99231-99255, 99291-99292, 99304-99310, 99315-99316, 99334-99337, 99347-99350, 99374-99375, 99377-99378, 99446-99449, 99451-99452, 99495-99496, G0463, G0471

50525 0213T, 0216T, 0228T, 0230T, 11000-11006, 11042-11047, 12001-12007, 12011-12057, 13100-13133, 13151-13153, 36000, 36400-36410, 36420-36430, 36440, 36591-36592, 36600, 36640, 43752, 44602-44605, 44950, 44970, 49000-49010, 49320, 50520, 50526❖, 51701-51703, 62320-62327, 64400, 64405-64408, 64415-64435, 64445-64454, 64461-64463, 64479-64505, 64510-64530, 69990, 92012-92014, 93000-93010, 93040-93042, 93318, 93355, 94002, 94200, 94250, 94680-94690, 94770, 95812-95816, 95819, 95822, 95829, 95955, 96360-96368, 96372, 96374-96377, 96523, 97597-97598, 97602, 99155, 99156, 99157, 99211-99223, 99231-99255, 99291-99292, 99304-99310, 99315-99316, 99334-99337, 99347-99350, 99374-99375, 99377-99378, 99446-99449, 99451-99452, 99495-99496, G0463, G0471

50526 0213T, 0216T, 0228T, 0230T, 11000-11006, 11042-11047, 12001-12007, 12011-12057, 13100-13133, 13151-13153, 36000, 36400-36410, 36420-36430, 36440, 36591-36592, 36600, 36640, 43752, 49000-49010, 51701-51703, 62320-62327, 64400, 64405-64408, 64415-64435, 64445-64454, 64461-64463, 64479-64505, 64510-64530, 69990, 92012-92014, 93000-93010, 93040-93042, 93318, 93355, 94002, 94200, 94250, 94680-94690, 94770, 95812-95816, 95819, 95822, 95829, 95955, 96360-96368, 96372, 96374-96377, 96523, 97597-97598, 97602, 99155, 99156, 99157, 99211-99223, 99231-99255, 99291-99292, 99304-99310, 99315-99316, 99334-99337, 99347-99350, 99374-99375, 99377-99378, 99446-99449, 99451-99452, 99495-99496, G0463, G0471

50540 0213T, 0216T, 0228T, 0230T, 11000-11006, 11042-11047, 12001-12007, 12011-12057, 13100-13133, 13151-13153, 36000, 36400-36410, 36420-36430, 36440, 36591-36592, 36600, 36640, 43752, 44602-44605, 44950, 44970, 49000-49010, 50100, 50400-50405, 50544, 51701-51703, 62320-62327, 64400, 64405-64408, 64415-64435, 64445-64454, 64461-64463, 64479-64505, 64510-64530, 69990, 92012-92014, 93000-93010, 93040-93042, 93318, 93355, 94002, 94200, 94250, 94680-94690, 94770, 95812-95816, 95819, 95822, 95829, 95955, 96360-96368, 96372, 96374-96377, 96523, 97597-97598, 97602, 99155, 99156, 99157, 99211-99223, 99231-99255, 99291-99292, 99304-99310, 99315-99316, 99334-99337, 99347-99350, 99374-99375, 99377-99378, 99446-99449, 99451-99452, 99495-99496, G0463, G0471

50541 0213T, 0216T, 0228T, 0230T, 12001-12007, 12011-12057, 13100-13133, 13151-13153, 36000, 36400-36410, 36420-36430, 36440, 36591-36592, 36600, 36640, 43653, 43752, 44005, 44180, 44602-44605, 44950, 44970, 49082-49084, 49320, 49400, 50390, 50592-50593❖, 50715, 51701-51703, 58660, 62320-62327, 64400, 64405-64408, 64415-64435, 64445-64454, 64461-64463, 64479-64505, 64510-64530, 69990, 76000,

77001-77002, 92012-92014, 93000-93010, 93040-93042, 93318, 93355, 94002, 94200, 94250, 94680-94690, 94770, 95812-95816, 95819, 95822, 95829, 95955, 96360-96368, 96372, 96374-96377, 96523, 99155, 99156, 99157, 99211-99223, 99231-99255, 99291-99292, 99304-99310, 99315-99316, 99334-99337, 99347-99350, 99374-99375, 99377-99378, 99446-99449, 99451-99452, 99495-99496, G0463, G0471

50542 0213T, 0216T, 0228T, 0230T, 12001-12007, 12011-12057, 13100-13133, 13151-13153, 35840, 36000, 36400-36410, 36420-36430, 36440, 36591-36592, 36600, 36640, 43653, 43752, 44005, 44180, 44602-44605, 44950, 44970, 49082-49084, 49203, 49320, 49400, 50205♦, 50541, 50592-50593♦, 50715, 51701-51703, 58660, 60540-60545, 62320-62327, 64400, 64405-64408, 64415-64435, 64445-64454, 64461-64463, 64479-64505, 64510-64530, 69990, 76000, 76940, 76942, 76970, 76998, 77001-77002, 92012-92014, 93000-93010, 93040-93042, 93318, 93355, 94002, 94200, 94250, 94680-94690, 94770, 95812-95816, 95819, 95822, 95829, 95955, 96360-96368, 96372, 96374-96377, 96523, 99155, 99156, 99157, 99211-99223, 99231-99255, 99291-99292, 99304-99310, 99315-99316, 99334-99337, 99347-99350, 99374-99375, 99377-99378, 99446-99449, 99451-99452, 99495-99496, G0463, G0471

50543 0213T, 0216T, 0228T, 0230T, 11000-11006, 11042-11047, 12001-12007, 12011-12057, 13100-13133, 13151-13153, 35840, 36000, 36400-36410, 36420-36430, 36440, 36591-36592, 36600, 36640, 38100-38101, 38120, 43653, 43752, 44005, 44180, 44602-44605, 44950, 44970, 49082-49084, 49320-49321, 49400, 50205, 50541-50542, 50715, 51701-51703, 58660, 60540-60545, 60650, 62320-62327, 64400, 64405-64408, 64415-64435, 64445-64454, 64461-64463, 64479-64505, 64510-64530, 69990, 76000, 77001-77002, 92012-92014, 93000-93010, 93040-93042, 93318, 93355, 94002, 94200, 94250, 94680-94690, 94770, 95812-95816, 95819, 95822, 95829, 95955, 96360-96368, 96372, 96374-96377, 96523, 97597-97598, 97602, 99155, 99156, 99157, 99211-99223, 99231-99255, 99291-99292, 99304-99310, 99315-99316, 99334-99337, 99347-99350, 99374-99375, 99377-99378, 99446-99449, 99451-99452, 99495-99496, G0463, G0471

50544 0213T, 0216T, 0228T, 0230T, 11000-11006, 11042-11047, 12001-12007, 12011-12057, 13100-13133, 13151-13153, 36000, 36400-36410, 36420-36430, 36440, 36591-36592, 36600, 36640, 43653, 43752, 44005, 44180, 44602-44605, 44950, 44970, 49082-49084, 49320, 49400, 50390, 50715, 51701-51703, 58660, 62320-62327, 64400, 64405-64408, 64415-64435, 64445-64454, 64461-64463, 64479-64505, 64510-64530, 69990, 76000, 77001-77002, 92012-92014, 93000-93010, 93040-93042, 93318, 93355, 94002, 94200, 94250, 94680-94690, 94770, 95812-95816, 95819, 95822, 95829, 95955, 96360-96368, 96372, 96374-96377, 96523, 97597-97598, 97602, 99155, 99156, 99157, 99211-99223, 99231-99255, 99291-99292, 99304-99310, 99315-99316, 99334-99337, 99347-99350, 99374-99375, 99377-99378, 99446-99449, 99451-99452, 99495-99496, G0463, G0471

50545 0213T, 0216T, 0228T, 0230T, 11000-11006, 11042-11047, 12001-12007, 12011-12057, 13100-13133, 13151-13153, 35840, 36000, 36400-36410, 36420-36430, 36440, 36591-36592, 36600, 36640, 38100-38101, 38120, 38562-38570, 43653, 43752, 44005, 44180, 44602-44605, 44950, 44970, 49082-49084, 49320-49321, 49400, 49405-49406, 50020, 50040-50045, 50060-50100, 50205, 50240, 50390, 50541-50544, 50546-50548, 50605, 50650, 50715, 51701-51703, 58660, 60540-60545, 60650, 62320-62327, 64400, 64405-64408, 64415-64435, 64445-64454, 64461-64463, 64479-64505, 64510-64530, 69990, 76000, 77001-77002, 92012-92014, 93000-93010, 93040-93042, 93318, 93355, 94002, 94200, 94250, 94680-94690, 94770, 95812-95816, 95819, 95822, 95829, 95955, 96360-96368, 96372, 96374-96377, 96523, 97597-97598, 97602, 99155, 99156, 99157, 99211-99223, 99231-99255, 99291-99292,

99304-99310, 99315-99316, 99334-99337, 99347-99350, 99374-99375, 99377-99378, 99446-99449, 99451-99452, 99495-99496, G0463, G0471

50546 0213T, 0216T, 0228T, 0230T, 11000-11006, 11042-11047, 12001-12007, 12011-12057, 13100-13133, 13151-13153, 36000, 36400-36410, 36420-36430, 36440, 36591-36592, 36600, 36640, 38100-38101, 38120, 43653, 43752, 44005, 44180, 44602-44605, 44950, 44970, 49082-49084, 49320-49321, 49400, 49405-49406, 50020, 50040-50045, 50060-50100, 50205, 50240, 50390, 50542-50543, 50605, 50650, 50715, 51701-51703, 58660, 60540-60545, 60650, 62320-62327, 64400, 64405-64408, 64415-64435, 64445-64454, 64461-64463, 64479-64505, 64510-64530, 69990, 76000, 77001-77002, 92012-92014, 93000-93010, 93040-93042, 93318, 93355, 94002, 94200, 94250, 94680-94690, 94770, 95812-95816, 95819, 95822, 95829, 95955, 96360-96368, 96372, 96374-96377, 96523, 97597-97598, 97602, 99155, 99156, 99157, 99211-99223, 99231-99255, 99291-99292, 99304-99310, 99315-99316, 99334-99337, 99347-99350, 99374-99375, 99377-99378, 99446-99449, 99451-99452, 99495-99496, G0463, G0471

50547 0213T, 0216T, 0228T, 0230T, 11000-11006, 11042-11047, 12001-12007, 12011-12057, 13100-13133, 13151-13153, 36000, 36400-36410, 36420-36430, 36440, 36591-36592, 36600, 36640, 38100-38101, 38120, 43653, 43752, 44005, 44180, 44602-44605, 44950, 44970, 49082-49084, 49320-49321, 49400, 50542-50543, 50546♦, 50605, 50650, 50715, 51701-51703, 58660, 62320-62327, 64400, 64405-64408, 64415-64435, 64445-64454, 64461-64463, 64479-64505, 64510-64530, 69990, 76000, 77001-77002, 92012-92014, 93000-93010, 93040-93042, 93318, 93355, 94002, 94200, 94250, 94680-94690, 94770, 95812-95816, 95819, 95822, 95829, 95955, 96360-96368, 96372, 96374-96377, 96523, 97597-97598, 97602, 99155, 99156, 99157, 99211-99223, 99231-99255, 99291-99292, 99304-99310, 99315-99316, 99334-99337, 99347-99350, 99374-99375, 99377-99378, 99446-99449, 99451-99452, 99495-99496, G0463, G0471

50548 0213T, 0216T, 0228T, 0230T, 11000-11006, 11042-11047, 12001-12007, 12011-12057, 13100-13133, 13151-13153, 36000, 36400-36410, 36420-36430, 36440, 36591-36592, 36600, 36640, 38100-38101, 38120, 43653, 43752, 44005, 44180, 44602-44605, 44950, 44970, 49082-49084, 49320-49321, 49400, 49405-49406, 50020, 50040-50045, 50060-50100, 50205, 50240, 50390, 50542-50543, 50546, 50605, 50650-50660, 50715, 51701-51703, 58660, 60540-60545, 60650, 62320-62327, 64400, 64405-64408, 64415-64435, 64445-64454, 64461-64463, 64479-64505, 64510-64530, 69990, 76000, 77001-77002, 92012-92014, 93000-93010, 93040-93042, 93318, 93355, 94002, 94200, 94250, 94680-94690, 94770, 95812-95816, 95819, 95822, 95829, 95955, 96360-96368, 96372, 96374-96377, 96523, 97597-97598, 97602, 99155, 99156, 99157, 99211-99223, 99231-99255, 99291-99292, 99304-99310, 99315-99316, 99334-99337, 99347-99350, 99374-99375, 99377-99378, 99446-99449, 99451-99452, 99495-99496, G0463, G0471

50551 0213T, 0216T, 0228T, 0230T, 12001-12007, 12011-12057, 13100-13133, 13151-13153, 36000, 36400-36410, 36420-36430, 36440, 36591-36592, 36600, 36640, 43752, 50391, 50430-50431, 50436-50437, 50570-50576♦, 50580♦, 50684, 51701-51703, 62320-62327, 64400, 64405-64408, 64415-64435, 64445-64454, 64461-64463, 64479-64505, 64510-64530, 69990, 76000, 77001-77002, 92012-92014, 93000-93010, 93040-93042, 93318, 93355, 94002, 94200, 94250, 94680-94690, 94770, 95812-95816, 95819, 95822, 95829, 95955, 96360-96368, 96372, 96374-96377, 96523, 99155, 99156, 99157, 99211-99223, 99231-99255, 99291-99292, 99304-99310, 99315-99316, 99334-99337, 99347-99350, 99374-99375, 99377-99378, 99446-99449, 99451-99452, 99495-99496, G0463, G0471, J2001

CPT © 2020 American Medical Association. All Rights Reserved.

50553 0213T, 0216T, 0228T, 0230T, 12001-12007, 12011-12057, 13100-13133, 13151-13153, 36000, 36400-36410, 36420-36430, 36440, 36591-36592, 36600, 36640, 43752, 50432, 50436-50437, 50551, 50570-50576❖, 50580❖, 50684, 50706, 51701-51703, 62320-62327, 64400, 64405-64408, 64415-64435, 64445-64454, 64461-64463, 64479-64505, 64510-64530, 69990, 76000, 77001-77002, 92012-92014, 93000-93010, 93040-93042, 93318, 93355, 94002, 94200, 94250, 94680-94690, 94770, 95812-95816, 95819, 95822, 95829, 95955, 96360-96368, 96372, 96374-96377, 96523, 99155, 99156, 99157, 99211-99223, 99231-99255, 99291-99292, 99304-99310, 99315-99316, 99334-99337, 99347-99350, 99374-99375, 99377-99378, 99446-99449, 99451-99452, 99495-99496, G0463, G0471, J2001

50555 0213T, 0216T, 0228T, 0230T, 10005, 10007, 10009, 10011, 10021, 12001-12007, 12011-12057, 13100-13133, 13151-13153, 36000, 36400-36410, 36420-36430, 36440, 36591-36592, 36600, 36640, 43752, 50430-50432, 50436-50437, 50551, 50570-50575❖, 50580❖, 50606, 50684, 51701-51703, 62320-62327, 64400, 64405-64408, 64415-64435, 64445-64454, 64461-64463, 64479-64505, 64510-64530, 69990, 76000, 77001-77002, 92012-92014, 93000-93010, 93040-93042, 93318, 93355, 94002, 94200, 94250, 94680-94690, 94770, 95812-95816, 95819, 95822, 95829, 95955, 96360-96368, 96372, 96374-96377, 96523, 99155, 99156, 99157, 99211-99223, 99231-99255, 99291-99292, 99304-99310, 99315-99316, 99334-99337, 99347-99350, 99374-99375, 99377-99378, 99446-99449, 99451-99452, 99495-99496, G0463, G0471, J2001

50557 0213T, 0216T, 0228T, 0230T, 10005, 10007, 10009, 10011, 10021, 12001-12007, 12011-12057, 13100-13133, 13151-13153, 36000, 36400-36410, 36420-36430, 36440, 36591-36592, 36600, 36640, 43752, 50430-50432, 50436-50437, 50551, 50555, 50570-50576❖, 50580❖, 50684, 50955, 50974, 51701-51703, 62320-62327, 64400, 64405-64408, 64415-64435, 64445-64454, 64461-64463, 64479-64505, 64510-64530, 69990, 76000, 77001-77002, 92012-92014, 93000-93010, 93040-93042, 93318, 93355, 94002, 94200, 94250, 94680-94690, 94770, 95812-95816, 95819, 95822, 95829, 95955, 96360-96368, 96372, 96374-96377, 96523, 99155, 99156, 99157, 99211-99223, 99231-99255, 99291-99292, 99304-99310, 99315-99316, 99334-99337, 99347-99350, 99374-99375, 99377-99378, 99446-99449, 99451-99452, 99495-99496, G0463, G0471, J2001

50561 0213T, 0216T, 0228T, 0230T, 11000-11006, 11042-11047, 12001-12007, 12011-12057, 13100-13133, 13151-13153, 36000, 36400-36410, 36420-36430, 36440, 36591-36592, 36600, 36640, 43752, 50430-50432, 50436-50437, 50551, 50570-50576❖, 50580❖, 50684, 50961, 50980, 51701-51703, 52320-52325, 52330, 52352-52353, 62320-62327, 64400, 64405-64408, 64415-64435, 64445-64454, 64461-64463, 64479-64505, 64510-64530, 69990, 76000, 77001-77002, 92012-92014, 93000-93010, 93040-93042, 93318, 93355, 94002, 94200, 94250, 94680-94690, 94770, 95812-95816, 95819, 95822, 95829, 95955, 96360-96368, 96372, 96374-96377, 96523, 97597-97598, 97602, 99155, 99156, 99157, 99211-99223, 99231-99255, 99291-99292, 99304-99310, 99315-99316, 99334-99337, 99347-99350, 99374-99375, 99377-99378, 99446-99449, 99451-99452, 99495-99496, G0463, G0471, J2001

50562 0213T, 0216T, 0228T, 0230T, 11000-11006, 11042-11047, 12001-12007, 12011-12057, 13100-13133, 13151-13153, 36000, 36400-36410, 36420-36430, 36440, 36591-36592, 36600, 36640, 43752, 50430-50432, 50436-50437, 50551, 50555-50557, 50570-50572❖, 50684, 50955, 50974, 51701-51703, 62320-62327, 64400, 64405-64408, 64415-64435, 64445-64454, 64461-64463, 64479-64505, 64510-64530, 69990, 76000, 77001-77002, 92012-92014, 93000-93010, 93040-93042, 93318, 93355, 94002, 94200, 94250, 94680-94690, 94770, 95812-95816, 95819, 95822, 95829, 95955, 96360-96368, 96372, 96374-96377, 96523,

97597-97598, 97602, 99155, 99156, 99157, 99211-99223, 99231-99255, 99291-99292, 99304-99310, 99315-99316, 99334-99337, 99347-99350, 99374-99375, 99377-99378, 99446-99449, 99451-99452, 99495-99496, G0463, G0471

50570 0213T, 0216T, 0228T, 0230T, 11000-11006, 11042-11047, 12001-12007, 12011-12057, 13100-13133, 13151-13153, 36000, 36400-36410, 36420-36430, 36440, 36591-36592, 36600, 36640, 43752, 50391, 50430-50432, 50436-50437, 50684, 51701-51703, 62320-62327, 64400, 64405-64408, 64415-64435, 64445-64454, 64461-64463, 64479-64505, 64510-64530, 69990, 76000, 77001-77002, 92012-92014, 93000-93010, 93040-93042, 93318, 93355, 94002, 94200, 94250, 94680-94690, 94770, 95812-95816, 95819, 95822, 95829, 95955, 96360-96368, 96372, 96374-96377, 96523, 97597-97598, 97602, 99155, 99156, 99157, 99211-99223, 99231-99255, 99291-99292, 99304-99310, 99315-99316, 99334-99337, 99347-99350, 99374-99375, 99377-99378, 99446-99449, 99451-99452, 99495-99496, G0463, G0471

50572 0213T, 0216T, 0228T, 0230T, 11000-11006, 11042-11047, 12001-12007, 12011-12057, 13100-13133, 13151-13153, 36000, 36400-36410, 36420-36430, 36440, 36591-36592, 36600, 36640, 43752, 50432, 50436-50437, 50570, 50684, 50706, 51701-51703, 62320-62327, 64400, 64405-64408, 64415-64435, 64445-64454, 64461-64463, 64479-64505, 64510-64530, 69990, 76000, 77001-77002, 92012-92014, 93000-93010, 93040-93042, 93318, 93355, 94002, 94200, 94250, 94680-94690, 94770, 95812-95816, 95819, 95822, 95829, 95955, 96360-96368, 96372, 96374-96377, 96523, 97597-97598, 97602, 99155, 99156, 99157, 99211-99223, 99231-99255, 99291-99292, 99304-99310, 99315-99316, 99334-99337, 99347-99350, 99374-99375, 99377-99378, 99446-99449, 99451-99452, 99495-99496, G0463, G0471

50574 0213T, 0216T, 0228T, 0230T, 10005, 10007, 10009, 10011, 10021, 11000-11006, 11042-11047, 12001-12007, 12011-12057, 13100-13133, 13151-13153, 36000, 36400-36410, 36420-36430, 36440, 36591-36592, 36600, 36640, 43752, 50430-50432, 50436-50437, 50562-50570, 50606, 50684, 51701-51703, 62320-62327, 64400, 64405-64408, 64415-64435, 64445-64454, 64461-64463, 64479-64505, 64510-64530, 69990, 76000, 77001-77002, 92012-92014, 93000-93010, 93040-93042, 93318, 93355, 94002, 94200, 94250, 94680-94690, 94770, 95812-95816, 95819, 95822, 95829, 95955, 96360-96368, 96372, 96374-96377, 96523, 97597-97598, 97602, 99155, 99156, 99157, 99211-99223, 99231-99255, 99291-99292, 99304-99310, 99315-99316, 99334-99337, 99347-99350, 99374-99375, 99377-99378, 99446-99449, 99451-99452, 99495-99496, G0463, G0471

50575 0213T, 0216T, 0228T, 0230T, 11000-11006, 11042-11047, 12001-12007, 12011-12057, 13100-13133, 13151-13153, 36000, 36400-36410, 36420-36430, 36440, 36591-36592, 36600, 36640, 43752, 50382-50384, 50387, 50436-50437, 50562-50570, 50605, 50684, 50693-50695, 51701-51703, 62320-62327, 64400, 64405-64408, 64415-64435, 64445-64454, 64461-64463, 64479-64505, 64510-64530, 69990, 76000, 77001-77002, 92012-92014, 93000-93010, 93040-93042, 93318, 93355, 94002, 94200, 94250, 94680-94690, 94770, 95812-95816, 95819, 95822, 95829, 95955, 96360-96368, 96372, 96374-96377, 96523, 97597-97598, 97602, 99155, 99156, 99157, 99211-99223, 99231-99255, 99291-99292, 99304-99310, 99315-99316, 99334-99337, 99347-99350, 99374-99375, 99377-99378, 99446-99449, 99451-99452, 99495-99496, G0463, G0471

50576 0213T, 0216T, 0228T, 0230T, 10005, 10007, 10009, 10011, 10021, 11000-11006, 11042-11047, 12001-12007, 12011-12057, 13100-13133, 13151-13153, 36000, 36400-36410, 36420-36430, 36440, 36591-36592, 36600, 36640, 43752, 50432, 50436-50437, 50555, 50562-50570, 50574, 50684, 50955, 50974, 51701-51703, 62320-62327, 64400,

64405-64408, 64415-64435, 64445-64454, 64461-64463, 64479-64505, 64510-64530, 69990, 76000, 77001-77002, 92012-92014, 93000-93010, 93040-93042, 93318, 93355, 94002, 94200, 94250, 94680-94690, 94770, 95812-95816, 95819, 95822, 95829, 95955, 96360-96368, 96372, 96374-96377, 96523, 97597-97598, 97602, 99155, 99156, 99157, 99211-99223, 99231-99255, 99291-99292, 99304-99310, 99315-99316, 99334-99337, 99347-99350, 99374-99375, 99377-99378, 99446-99449, 99451-99452, 99495-99496, G0463, G0471

50580 0213T, 0216T, 0228T, 0230T, 11000-11006, 11042-11047, 12001-12007, 12011-12057, 13100-13133, 13151-13153, 36000, 36400-36410, 36420-36430, 36440, 36591-36592, 36600, 36640, 43752, 50432, 50436-50437, 50562-50570, 50684, 51701-51703, 62320-62327, 64400, 64405-64408, 64415-64435, 64445-64454, 64461-64463, 64479-64505, 64510-64530, 69990, 76000, 77001-77002, 92012-92014, 93000-93010, 93040-93042, 93318, 93355, 94002, 94200, 94250, 94680-94690, 94770, 95812-95816, 95819, 95822, 95829, 95955, 96360-96368, 96372, 96374-96377, 96523, 97597-97598, 97602, 99155, 99156, 99157, 99211-99223, 99231-99255, 99291-99292, 99304-99310, 99315-99316, 99334-99337, 99347-99350, 99374-99375, 99377-99378, 99446-99449, 99451-99452, 99495-99496, G0463, G0471

50590 0213T, 0216T, 0228T, 0230T, 12001-12007, 12011-12057, 13100-13133, 13151-13153, 36000, 36400-36410, 36420-36430, 36440, 36591-36592, 36600, 36640, 43752, 51701-51703, 52005, 52320-52325, 52330, 52351-52353✦, 52356✦, 62320-62327, 64400, 64405-64408, 64415-64435, 64445-64454, 64461-64463, 64479-64505, 64510-64530, 69990, 76000, 77001, 92012-92014, 93000-93010, 93040-93042, 93318, 93355, 94002, 94200, 94250, 94680-94690, 94770, 95812-95816, 95819, 95822, 95829, 95955, 96360-96368, 96372, 96374-96377, 96523, 99155, 99156, 99157, 99211-99223, 99231-99255, 99291-99292, 99304-99310, 99315-99316, 99334-99337, 99347-99350, 99374-99375, 99377-99378, 99446-99449, 99451-99452, 99495-99496, G0463, G0471

50592 0213T, 0216T, 0228T, 0230T, 12001-12007, 12011-12057, 13100-13133, 13151-13153, 36000, 36400-36410, 36420-36430, 36440, 36591-36592, 36600, 36640, 43752, 51701-51703, 62320-62327, 64400, 64405-64408, 64415-64435, 64445-64454, 64461-64463, 64479-64505, 64510-64530, 69990, 76000, 76380, 76942, 76970, 76998, 77001-77002, 77012, 77021, 92012-92014, 93000-93010, 93040-93042, 93318, 93355, 94002, 94200, 94250, 94680-94690, 94770, 95812-95816, 95819, 95822, 95829, 95955, 96360-96368, 96372, 96374-96377, 96523, 99155, 99156, 99157, 99211-99223, 99231-99255, 99291-99292, 99304-99310, 99315-99316, 99334-99337, 99347-99350, 99374-99375, 99377-99378, 99446-99449, 99451-99452, 99495-99496, G0463, G0471, J0670, J2001

50593 0213T, 0216T, 0228T, 0230T, 12001-12007, 12011-12057, 13100-13133, 13151-13153, 36000, 36400-36410, 36420-36430, 36440, 36591-36592, 36600, 36640, 43752, 50592✦, 62320-62327, 64400, 64405-64408, 64415-64435, 64445-64454, 64461-64463, 64479-64505, 64510-64530, 69990, 76000, 76380, 76942, 76970, 76998, 77001-77002, 77012, 77021, 92012-92014, 93000-93010, 93040-93042, 93318, 93355, 94002, 94200, 94250, 94680-94690, 94770, 95812-95816, 95819, 95822, 95829, 95955, 96360-96368, 96372, 96374-96377, 96523, 99155, 99156, 99157, 99211-99223, 99231-99255, 99291-99292, 99304-99310, 99315-99316, 99334-99337, 99347-99350, 99374-99375, 99377-99378, 99446-99449, 99451-99452, 99495-99496, G0463, J0670, J2001

50600 00910, 0213T, 0216T, 0228T, 0230T, 11000-11006, 11042-11047, 12001-12007, 12011-12057, 13100-13133, 13151-13153, 36000, 36400-36410, 36420-36430, 36440, 36591-36592, 36600, 36640, 43752, 44602-44605, 44950, 44970, 49000-49010, 50100, 50650, 51701-51703, 62320-62327, 64400, 64405-64408, 64415-64435, 64445-64454, 64461-64463, 64479-64505, 64510-64530, 69990, 92012-92014,

93000-93010, 93040-93042, 93318, 93355, 94002, 94200, 94250, 94680-94690, 94770, 95812-95816, 95819, 95822, 95829, 95955, 96360-96368, 96372, 96374-96377, 96523, 97597-97598, 97602, 99155, 99156, 99157, 99211-99223, 99231-99255, 99291-99292, 99304-99310, 99315-99316, 99334-99337, 99347-99350, 99374-99375, 99377-99378, 99446-99449, 99451-99452, 99495-99496, G0463, G0471

50605 00910, 0213T, 0216T, 0228T, 0230T, 11000-11006, 11042-11047, 12001-12007, 12011-12057, 13100-13133, 13151-13153, 36000, 36400-36410, 36420-36430, 36440, 36591-36592, 36600, 36640, 43752, 44602-44605, 44950, 44970, 49000-49010, 50100, 50382-50384, 50387, 50600, 50715, 51701-51703, 62320-62327, 64400, 64405-64408, 64415-64435, 64445-64454, 64461-64463, 64479-64505, 64510-64530, 69990, 92012-92014, 93000-93010, 93040-93042, 93318, 93355, 94002, 94200, 94250, 94680-94690, 94770, 95812-95816, 95819, 95822, 95829, 95955, 96360-96368, 96372, 96374-96377, 96523, 97597-97598, 97602, 99155, 99156, 99157, 99211-99223, 99231-99255, 99291-99292, 99304-99310, 99315-99316, 99334-99337, 99347-99350, 99374-99375, 99377-99378, 99446-99449, 99451-99452, 99495-99496, G0463, G0471

50606 0213T, 0216T, 0228T, 0230T, 10005, 10007, 10009, 10011, 10021, 12001-12007, 12011-12057, 13100-13133, 13151-13153, 36000, 36400-36410, 36420-36430, 36440, 36600, 36640, 43752, 51701-51703, 62320-62327, 64400, 64405-64408, 64415-64435, 64445-64454, 64461, 64463, 64479, 64483, 64486-64490, 64493, 64505, 64510-64530, 69990, 74425, 76000, 76380, 76942, 76970, 76998, 77002, 77012, 77021, 92012-92014, 93000-93010, 93040-93042, 93318, 94002, 94200, 94250, 94680-94690, 94770, 95812-95816, 95819, 95822, 95829, 95955, 96360, 96365, 96372, 96374-96377, 96523, 99155, 99156, 99157, 99211-99223, 99231-99255, 99291-99292, 99304-99310, 99315-99316, 99334-99337, 99347-99350, 99374-99375, 99377-99378

50610 00910, 0213T, 0216T, 0228T, 0230T, 11000-11006, 11042-11047, 12001-12007, 12011-12057, 13100-13133, 13151-13153, 36000, 36400-36410, 36420-36430, 36440, 36591-36592, 36600, 36640, 43752, 44602-44605, 44950, 44970, 49000-49010, 50600-50605, 50715, 50945, 51701-51703, 62320-62327, 64400, 64405-64408, 64415-64435, 64445-64454, 64461-64463, 64479-64505, 64510-64530, 69990, 92012-92014, 93000-93010, 93040-93042, 93318, 93355, 94002, 94200, 94250, 94680-94690, 94770, 95812-95816, 95819, 95822, 95829, 95955, 96360-96368, 96372, 96374-96377, 96523, 97597-97598, 97602, 99155, 99156, 99157, 99211-99223, 99231-99255, 99291-99292, 99304-99310, 99315-99316, 99334-99337, 99347-99350, 99374-99375, 99377-99378, 99446-99449, 99451-99452, 99495-99496, G0463, G0471

50620 00910, 0213T, 0216T, 0228T, 0230T, 11000-11006, 11042-11047, 12001-12007, 12011-12057, 13100-13133, 13151-13153, 36000, 36400-36410, 36420-36430, 36440, 36591-36592, 36600, 36640, 43752, 44602-44605, 44950, 44970, 49000-49010, 50600-50605, 50715, 50945, 51701-51703, 62320-62327, 64400, 64405-64408, 64415-64435, 64445-64454, 64461-64463, 64479-64505, 64510-64530, 69990, 92012-92014, 93000-93010, 93040-93042, 93318, 93355, 94002, 94200, 94250, 94680-94690, 94770, 95812-95816, 95819, 95822, 95829, 95955, 96360-96368, 96372, 96374-96377, 96523, 97597-97598, 97602, 99155, 99156, 99157, 99211-99223, 99231-99255, 99291-99292, 99304-99310, 99315-99316, 99334-99337, 99347-99350, 99374-99375, 99377-99378, 99446-99449, 99451-99452, 99495-99496, G0463, G0471

50630 00910, 0213T, 0216T, 0228T, 0230T, 11000-11006, 11042-11047, 12001-12007, 12011-12057, 13100-13133, 13151-13153, 36000, 36400-36410, 36420-36430, 36440, 36591-36592, 36600, 36640, 43752, 44602-44605, 44950, 44970, 49000-49010, 50600-50605, 50715, 50945, 51701-51703, 52000, 62320-62327, 64400, 64405-64408, 64415-64435, 64445-64454, 64461-64463, 64479-64505, 64510-64530, 69990,

CPT © 2020 American Medical Association. All Rights Reserved.

Coding Companion for Urology/Nephrology

92012-92014, 93000-93010, 93040-93042, 93318, 93355, 94002, 94200,
94250, 94680-94690, 94770, 95812-95816, 95819, 95822, 95829,
95955, 96360-96368, 96372, 96374-96377, 96523, 97597-97598, 97602,
99155, 99156, 99157, 99211-99223, 99231-99255, 99291-99292,
99304-99310, 99315-99316, 99334-99337, 99347-99350, 99374-99375,
99377-99378, 99446-99449, 99451-99452, 99495-99496, G0463, G0471

50650 00910, 0213T, 0216T, 0228T, 0230T, 11000-11006, 11042-11047,
12001-12007, 12011-12057, 13100-13133, 13151-13153, 36000,
36400-36410, 36420-36430, 36440, 36591-36592, 36600, 36640, 43752,
44950, 44970, 49010, 49320-49321, 50715, 51701-51703, 52000,
62320-62327, 64400, 64405-64408, 64415-64435, 64445-64454,
64461-64463, 64479-64505, 64510-64530, 69990, 92012-92014,
93000-93010, 93040-93042, 93318, 93355, 94002, 94200, 94250,
94680-94690, 94770, 95812-95816, 95819, 95822, 95829, 95955,
96360-96368, 96372, 96374-96377, 96523, 97597-97598, 97602, 99155,
99156, 99157, 99211-99223, 99231-99255, 99291-99292, 99304-99310,
99315-99316, 99334-99337, 99347-99350, 99374-99375, 99377-99378,
99446-99449, 99451-99452, 99495-99496, G0463, G0471

50660 00910, 0213T, 0216T, 0228T, 0230T, 11000-11006, 11042-11047,
12001-12007, 12011-12057, 13100-13133, 13151-13153, 36000,
36400-36410, 36420-36430, 36440, 36591-36592, 36600, 36640, 43752,
44602-44605, 44950, 44970, 49000-49010, 49320-49321, 50605, 50650,
50715, 51701-51703, 52000, 62320-62327, 64400, 64405-64408,
64415-64435, 64445-64454, 64461-64463, 64479-64505, 64510-64530,
69990, 92012-92014, 93000-93010, 93040-93042, 93318, 93355, 94002,
94200, 94250, 94680-94690, 94770, 95812-95816, 95819, 95822,
95829, 95955, 96360-96368, 96372, 96374-96377, 96523, 97597-97598,
97602, 99155, 99156, 99157, 99211-99223, 99231-99255, 99291-99292,
99304-99310, 99315-99316, 99334-99337, 99347-99350, 99374-99375,
99377-99378, 99446-99449, 99451-99452, 99495-99496, G0463, G0471

50684 00910, 0213T, 0216T, 0228T, 0230T, 12001-12007, 12011-12057,
13100-13133, 13151-13153, 36000, 36400-36410, 36420-36430, 36440,
36591-36592, 36600, 36640, 43752, 50436-50437, 50715, 51701-51703,
62320-62327, 64400, 64405-64408, 64415-64435, 64445-64454,
64461-64463, 64479-64505, 64510-64530, 69990, 76000, 77001,
92012-92014, 93000-93010, 93040-93042, 93318, 93355, 94002, 94200,
94250, 94680-94690, 94770, 95812-95816, 95819, 95822, 95829,
95955, 96360-96368, 96372, 96374-96377, 96523, 99155, 99156,
99157, 99211-99223, 99231-99255, 99291-99292, 99304-99310,
99315-99316, 99334-99337, 99347-99350, 99374-99375, 99377-99378,
99446-99449, 99451-99452, 99495-99496, G0463, G0471, J1644, J2001

50686 00910, 0213T, 0216T, 0228T, 0230T, 12001-12007, 12011-12057,
13100-13133, 13151-13153, 36000, 36400-36410, 36420-36430, 36440,
36591-36592, 36600, 36640, 43752, 50436-50437, 50715, 51701-51703,
62320-62327, 64400, 64405-64408, 64415-64435, 64445-64454,
64461-64463, 64479-64505, 64510-64530, 69990, 92012-92014,
93000-93010, 93040-93042, 93318, 93355, 94002, 94200, 94250,
94680-94690, 94770, 95812-95816, 95819, 95822, 95829, 95955,
96360-96368, 96372, 96374-96377, 96523, 99155, 99156, 99157,
99211-99223, 99231-99255, 99291-99292, 99304-99310, 99315-99316,
99334-99337, 99347-99350, 99374-99375, 99377-99378, 99446-99449,
99451-99452, 99495-99496, G0463, G0471

50688 00910, 0213T, 0216T, 0228T, 0230T, 12001-12007, 12011-12057,
13100-13133, 13151-13153, 36000, 36400-36410, 36420-36430, 36440,
36591-36592, 36600, 36640, 43752, 50693-50695, 50715, 51701-51703,
62320-62327, 64400, 64405-64408, 64415-64435, 64445-64454,
64461-64463, 64479-64505, 64510-64530, 69990, 74425, 76000,
77001-77002, 92012-92014, 93000-93010, 93040-93042, 93318, 93355,
94002, 94200, 94250, 94680-94690, 94770, 95812-95816, 95819,

95822, 95829, 95955, 96360-96368, 96372, 96374-96377, 96523,
99155, 99156, 99157, 99211-99223, 99231-99255, 99291-99292,
99304-99310, 99315-99316, 99334-99337, 99347-99350, 99374-99375,
99377-99378, 99446-99449, 99451-99452, 99495-99496, G0463, G0471

50690 00910, 0213T, 0216T, 0228T, 0230T, 12001-12007, 12011-12057,
13100-13133, 13151-13153, 36000, 36400-36410, 36420-36430, 36440,
36591-36592, 36600, 36640, 43752, 50715, 51701-51703, 62320-62327,
64400, 64405-64408, 64415-64435, 64445-64454, 64461-64463,
64479-64505, 64510-64530, 69990, 92012-92014, 93000-93010,
93040-93042, 93318, 93355, 94002, 94200, 94250, 94680-94690,
94770, 95812-95816, 95819, 95822, 95829, 95955, 96360-96368,
96372, 96374-96377, 96523, 99155, 99156, 99157, 99211-99223,
99231-99255, 99291-99292, 99304-99310, 99315-99316, 99334-99337,
99347-99350, 99374-99375, 99377-99378, 99446-99449, 99451-99452,
99495-99496, G0463, G0471, J1644, J2001

50693 0213T, 0216T, 0228T, 0230T, 12001-12007, 12011-12057, 13100-13133,
13151-13153, 36000, 36011, 36400-36410, 36420-36430, 36440,
36591-36592, 36600, 36640, 43752, 49185, 49424, 50390,
50430-50437, 50684, 51701-51703, 62320-62327, 64400, 64405-64408,
64415-64435, 64445-64454, 64461-64463, 64479-64505, 64510-64530,
69990, 74425, 76000, 76380, 76942, 76970, 76998, 77001-77002,
77012, 77021, 92012-92014, 93000-93010, 93040-93042, 93318, 93355,
94002, 94200, 94250, 94680-94690, 94770, 95812-95816, 95819,
95822, 95829, 95955, 96360-96368, 96372, 96374-96377, 96523,
99155, 99156, 99157, 99211-99223, 99231-99255, 99291-99292,
99304-99310, 99315-99316, 99334-99337, 99347-99350, 99374-99375,
99377-99378, 99446-99449, 99451-99452, 99495-99496, G0463,
G0471, J0670, J2001

50694 0213T, 0216T, 0228T, 0230T, 12001-12007, 12011-12057, 13100-13133,
13151-13153, 36000, 36011, 36400-36410, 36420-36430, 36440,
36591-36592, 36600, 36640, 43752, 49185, 49424, 50390,
50430-50437, 50684, 50693✦, 51701-51703, 62320-62327, 64400,
64405-64408, 64415-64435, 64445-64454, 64461-64463, 64479-64505,
64510-64530, 69990, 74425, 76000, 76380, 76942, 76970, 76998,
77001-77002, 77012, 77021, 92012-92014, 93000-93010, 93040-93042,
93318, 93355, 94002, 94200, 94250, 94680-94690, 94770,
95812-95816, 95819, 95822, 95829, 95955, 96360-96368, 96372,
96374-96377, 96523, 99155, 99156, 99157, 99211-99223, 99231-99255,
99291-99292, 99304-99310, 99315-99316, 99334-99337, 99347-99350,
99374-99375, 99377-99378, 99446-99449, 99451-99452, 99495-99496,
G0463, G0471, J0670, J2001

50695 0213T, 0216T, 0228T, 0230T, 12001-12007, 12011-12057, 13100-13133,
13151-13153, 36000, 36011, 36400-36410, 36420-36430, 36440,
36591-36592, 36600, 36640, 43752, 49185, 49424, 50390,
50430-50437, 50684, 50693-50694✦, 51701-51703, 62320-62327,
64400, 64405-64408, 64415-64435, 64445-64454, 64461-64463,
64479-64505, 64510-64530, 69990, 74425, 76000, 76380, 76942,
76970, 76998, 77001-77002, 77012, 77021, 92012-92014, 93000-93010,
93040-93042, 93318, 93355, 94002, 94200, 94250, 94680-94690,
94770, 95812-95816, 95819, 95822, 95829, 95955, 96360-96368,
96372, 96374-96377, 96523, 99155, 99156, 99157, 99211-99223,
99231-99255, 99291-99292, 99304-99310, 99315-99316, 99334-99337,
99347-99350, 99374-99375, 99377-99378, 99446-99449, 99451-99452,
99495-99496, G0463, G0471, J0670, J2001

50700 00910, 0213T, 0216T, 0228T, 0230T, 11000-11006, 11042-11047,
12001-12007, 12011-12057, 13100-13133, 13151-13153, 36000,
36400-36410, 36420-36430, 36440, 36591-36592, 36600, 36640, 43752,
44602-44605, 44850, 44950, 44970, 49000-49010, 50100, 50600-50605,
50715, 50722, 50900, 51701-51703, 62320-62327, 64400, 64405-64408,

64415-64435, 64445-64454, 64461-64463, 64479-64505, 64510-64530, 69990, 92012-92014, 93000-93010, 93040-93042, 93318, 93355, 94002, 94200, 94250, 94680-94690, 94770, 95812-95816, 95819, 95822, 95829, 95955, 96360-96368, 96372, 96374-96377, 96523, 97597-97598, 97602, 99155, 99156, 99157, 99211-99223, 99231-99255, 99291-99292, 99304-99310, 99315-99316, 99334-99337, 99347-99350, 99374-99375, 99377-99378, 99446-99449, 99451-99452, 99495-99496, G0463, G0471

50705 0213T, 0216T, 0228T, 0230T, 12001-12007, 12011-12057, 13100-13133, 13151-13153, 36000, 36400-36410, 36420-36430, 36440, 36600, 36640, 43752, 50436-50437, 51701-51703, 62320-62327, 64400, 64405-64408, 64415-64435, 64445-64454, 64461, 64463, 64479, 64483, 64486-64490, 64493, 64505, 64510-64530, 69990, 74425, 76000, 76380, 76942, 76970, 76998, 77002, 77012, 77021, 92012-92014, 93000-93010, 93040-93042, 93318, 94002, 94200, 94250, 94680-94690, 94770, 95812-95816, 95819, 95822, 95829, 95955, 96360, 96365, 96372, 96374-96377, 96523, 99155, 99156, 99157, 99211-99223, 99231-99255, 99291-99292, 99304-99310, 99315-99316, 99334-99337, 99347-99350, 99374-99375, 99377-99378

50706 0213T, 0216T, 0228T, 0230T, 12001-12007, 12011-12057, 13100-13133, 13151-13153, 36000, 36400-36410, 36420-36430, 36440, 36600, 36640, 43752, 50436-50437, 51701-51703, 62320-62327, 64400, 64405-64408, 64415-64435, 64445-64454, 64461, 64463, 64479, 64483, 64486-64490, 64493, 64505, 64510-64530, 69990, 74425, 74485, 76000, 76380, 76942, 76970, 76998, 77002, 77012, 77021, 92012-92014, 93000-93010, 93040-93042, 93318, 94002, 94200, 94250, 94680-94690, 94770, 95812-95816, 95819, 95822, 95829, 95955, 96360, 96365, 96372, 96374-96377, 96523, 99155, 99156, 99157, 99211-99223, 99231-99255, 99291-99292, 99304-99310, 99315-99316, 99334-99337, 99347-99350, 99374-99375, 99377-99378

50715 00910, 0213T, 0216T, 0228T, 0230T, 12001-12007, 12011-12057, 13100-13133, 13151-13153, 36000, 36400-36410, 36420-36430, 36440, 36591-36592, 36600, 36640, 43752, 44005, 44180, 44850, 44950, 44970, 49000-49010, 49203, 50100, 50600, 50900, 51100-51102, 51701-51703, 52005, 57423, 58570-58571, 62320-62327, 64400, 64405-64408, 64415-64435, 64445-64454, 64461-64463, 64479-64505, 64510-64530, 69990, 92012-92014, 93000-93010, 93040-93042, 93318, 93355, 94002, 94200, 94250, 94680-94690, 94770, 95812-95816, 95819, 95822, 95829, 95955, 96360-96368, 96372, 96374-96377, 96523, 99155, 99156, 99157, 99211-99223, 99231-99255, 99291-99292, 99304-99310, 99315-99316, 99334-99337, 99347-99350, 99374-99375, 99377-99378, 99446-99449, 99451-99452, 99495-99496, G0463, G0471

50722 00910, 0213T, 0216T, 0228T, 0230T, 12001-12007, 12011-12057, 13100-13133, 13151-13153, 36000, 36400-36410, 36420-36430, 36440, 36591-36592, 36600, 36640, 43752, 44602-44605, 44850, 44950, 44970, 49000-49010, 50600-50605, 50715, 50900, 51701-51703, 62320-62327, 64400, 64405-64408, 64415-64435, 64445-64454, 64461-64463, 64479-64505, 64510-64530, 69990, 92012-92014, 93000-93010, 93040-93042, 93318, 93355, 94002, 94200, 94250, 94680-94690, 94770, 95812-95816, 95819, 95822, 95829, 95955, 96360-96368, 96372, 96374-96377, 96523, 99155, 99156, 99157, 99211-99223, 99231-99255, 99291-99292, 99304-99310, 99315-99316, 99334-99337, 99347-99350, 99374-99375, 99377-99378, 99446-99449, 99451-99452, 99495-99496, G0463, G0471

50725 00910, 0213T, 0216T, 0228T, 0230T, 12001-12007, 12011-12057, 13100-13133, 13151-13153, 36000, 36400-36410, 36420-36430, 36440, 36591-36592, 36600, 36640, 43752, 44602-44605, 44850, 44950, 44970, 49000-49010, 50100, 50600-50605, 50715, 50900, 51701-51703, 62320-62327, 64400, 64405-64408, 64415-64435, 64445-64454, 64461-64463, 64479-64505, 64510-64530, 69990, 92012-92014,

93000-93010, 93040-93042, 93318, 93355, 94002, 94200, 94250, 94680-94690, 94770, 95812-95816, 95819, 95822, 95829, 95955, 96360-96368, 96372, 96374-96377, 96523, 99155, 99156, 99157, 99211-99223, 99231-99255, 99291-99292, 99304-99310, 99315-99316, 99334-99337, 99347-99350, 99374-99375, 99377-99378, 99446-99449, 99451-99452, 99495-99496, G0463, G0471

50727 00910, 0213T, 0216T, 0228T, 0230T, 11000-11006, 11042-11047, 12001-12007, 12011-12057, 13100-13133, 13151-13153, 36000, 36400-36410, 36420-36430, 36440, 36591-36592, 36600, 36640, 43752, 44602-44605, 44850, 44950, 44970, 49000-49010, 50605, 50715, 51701-51703, 53520, 62320-62327, 64400, 64405-64408, 64415-64435, 64445-64454, 64461-64463, 64479-64505, 64510-64530, 69990, 92012-92014, 93000-93010, 93040-93042, 93318, 93355, 94002, 94200, 94250, 94680-94690, 94770, 95812-95816, 95819, 95822, 95829, 95955, 96360-96368, 96372, 96374-96377, 96523, 97597-97598, 97602, 99155, 99156, 99157, 99211-99223, 99231-99255, 99291-99292, 99304-99310, 99315-99316, 99334-99337, 99347-99350, 99374-99375, 99377-99378, 99446-99449, 99451-99452, 99495-99496, G0463, G0471

50728 00910, 0213T, 0216T, 0228T, 0230T, 0437T, 11000-11006, 11042-11047, 12001-12007, 12011-12057, 13100-13133, 13151-13153, 15777, 36000, 36400-36410, 36420-36430, 36440, 36591-36592, 36600, 36640, 43752, 44602-44605, 44820-44850, 44950, 44970, 49000-49010, 49568, 50605, 50715, 50727, 51701-51703, 53520, 57267, 62320-62327, 64400, 64405-64408, 64415-64435, 64445-64454, 64461-64463, 64479-64505, 64510-64530, 69990, 92012-92014, 93000-93010, 93040-93042, 93318, 93355, 94002, 94200, 94250, 94680-94690, 94770, 95812-95816, 95819, 95822, 95829, 95955, 96360-96368, 96372, 96374-96377, 96523, 97597-97598, 97602, 99155, 99156, 99157, 99211-99223, 99231-99255, 99291-99292, 99304-99310, 99315-99316, 99334-99337, 99347-99350, 99374-99375, 99377-99378, 99446-99449, 99451-99452, 99495-99496, G0463, G0471

50740 00910, 0213T, 0216T, 0228T, 0230T, 12001-12007, 12011-12057, 13100-13133, 13151-13153, 36000, 36400-36410, 36420-36430, 36440, 36591-36592, 36600, 36640, 43752, 44602-44605, 44850, 44950, 44970, 49000-49010, 50100, 50605, 50650, 50782❖, 50800❖, 50860❖, 51701-51703, 62320-62327, 64400, 64405-64408, 64415-64435, 64445-64454, 64461-64463, 64479-64505, 64510-64530, 69990, 92012-92014, 93000-93010, 93040-93042, 93318, 93355, 94002, 94200, 94250, 94680-94690, 94770, 95812-95816, 95819, 95822, 95829, 95955, 96360-96368, 96372, 96374-96377, 96523, 99155, 99156, 99157, 99211-99223, 99231-99255, 99291-99292, 99304-99310, 99315-99316, 99334-99337, 99347-99350, 99374-99375, 99377-99378, 99446-99449, 99451-99452, 99495-99496, G0463, G0471

50750 00910, 0213T, 0216T, 0228T, 0230T, 12001-12007, 12011-12057, 13100-13133, 13151-13153, 36000, 36400-36410, 36420-36430, 36440, 36591-36592, 36600, 36640, 43752, 44602-44605, 44850, 44950, 44970, 49000-49010, 50605, 50650, 50740❖, 50760❖, 50780❖, 50782❖, 50800❖, 50860❖, 51701-51703, 62320-62327, 64400, 64405-64408, 64415-64435, 64445-64454, 64461-64463, 64479-64505, 64510-64530, 69990, 92012-92014, 93000-93010, 93040-93042, 93318, 93355, 94002, 94200, 94250, 94680-94690, 94770, 95812-95816, 95819, 95822, 95829, 95955, 96360-96368, 96372, 96374-96377, 96523, 99155, 99156, 99157, 99211-99223, 99231-99255, 99291-99292, 99304-99310, 99315-99316, 99334-99337, 99347-99350, 99374-99375, 99377-99378, 99446-99449, 99451-99452, 99495-99496, G0463, G0471

50760 00910, 0213T, 0216T, 0228T, 0230T, 12001-12007, 12011-12057, 13100-13133, 13151-13153, 36000, 36400-36410, 36420-36430, 36440, 36591-36592, 36600, 36640, 43752, 44602-44605, 44850, 44950, 44970, 49000-49010, 50605, 50650, 50740❖, 50782❖, 50800❖, 50860❖,

CPT © 2020 American Medical Association. All Rights Reserved.

51701-51703, 62320-62327, 64400, 64405-64408, 64415-64435,
64445-64454, 64461-64463, 64479-64505, 64510-64530, 69990,
92012-92014, 93000-93010, 93040-93042, 93318, 93355, 94002, 94200,
94250, 94680-94690, 94770, 95812-95816, 95819, 95822, 95829,
95955, 96360-96368, 96372, 96374-96377, 96523, 99155, 99156,
99157, 99211-99223, 99231-99255, 99291-99292, 99304-99310,
99315-99316, 99334-99337, 99347-99350, 99374-99375, 99377-99378,
99446-99449, 99451-99452, 99495-99496, G0463, G0471

50770 00910, 0213T, 0216T, 0228T, 0230T, 12001-12007, 12011-12057,
13100-13133, 13151-13153, 36000, 36400-36410, 36420-36430, 36440,
36591-36592, 36600, 36640, 43752, 44602-44605, 44850, 44950,
44970, 49000-49010, 50605, 50650, 50740-50760♦, 50780♦,
50782-50783♦, 50800♦, 50860♦, 51701-51703, 62320-62327, 64400,
64405-64408, 64415-64435, 64445-64454, 64461-64463, 64479-64505,
64510-64530, 69990, 92012-92014, 93000-93010, 93040-93042, 93318,
93355, 94002, 94200, 94250, 94680-94690, 94770, 95812-95816,
95819, 95822, 95829, 95955, 96360-96368, 96372, 96374-96377,
96523, 99155, 99156, 99157, 99211-99223, 99231-99255, 99291-99292,
99304-99310, 99315-99316, 99334-99337, 99347-99350, 99374-99375,
99377-99378, 99446-99449, 99451-99452, 99495-99496, G0463, G0471

50780 00910, 0213T, 0216T, 0228T, 0230T, 12001-12007, 12011-12057,
13100-13133, 13151-13153, 36000, 36400-36410, 36420-36430, 36440,
36591-36592, 36600, 36640, 43752, 44602-44605, 44850, 44950,
44970, 49000-49010, 50605, 50650, 50715, 50740♦, 50760♦,
50947-50948, 51701-51703, 52000, 62320-62327, 64400, 64405-64408,
64415-64435, 64445-64454, 64461-64463, 64479-64505, 64510-64530,
69990, 92012-92014, 93000-93010, 93040-93042, 93318, 93355, 94002,
94200, 94250, 94680-94690, 94770, 95812-95816, 95819, 95822,
95829, 95955, 96360-96368, 96372, 96374-96377, 96523, 99155,
99156, 99157, 99211-99223, 99231-99255, 99291-99292, 99304-99310,
99315-99316, 99334-99337, 99347-99350, 99374-99375, 99377-99378,
99446-99449, 99451-99452, 99495-99496, G0463, G0471

50782 00910, 0213T, 0216T, 0228T, 0230T, 12001-12007, 12011-12057,
13100-13133, 13151-13153, 36000, 36400-36410, 36420-36430, 36440,
36591-36592, 36600, 36640, 43752, 44602-44605, 44850, 44950,
44970, 49000-49010, 50605, 50650, 50715, 50780♦, 50785♦,
51701-51703, 51820, 52000, 62320-62327, 64400, 64405-64408,
64415-64435, 64445-64454, 64461-64463, 64479-64505, 64510-64530,
69990, 92012-92014, 93000-93010, 93040-93042, 93318, 93355, 94002,
94200, 94250, 94680-94690, 94770, 95812-95816, 95819, 95822,
95829, 95955, 96360-96368, 96372, 96374-96377, 96523, 99155,
99156, 99157, 99211-99223, 99231-99255, 99291-99292, 99304-99310,
99315-99316, 99334-99337, 99347-99350, 99374-99375, 99377-99378,
99446-99449, 99451-99452, 99495-99496, G0463, G0471

50783 00910, 0213T, 0216T, 0228T, 0230T, 12001-12007, 12011-12057,
13100-13133, 13151-13153, 36000, 36400-36410, 36420-36430, 36440,
36591-36592, 36600, 36640, 43752, 44602-44605, 44850, 44950,
44970, 49000-49010, 50605, 50650, 50715, 50740-50760♦, 50780♦,
50782♦, 50785♦, 51701-51703, 51820, 52000, 62320-62327, 64400,
64405-64408, 64415-64435, 64445-64454, 64461-64463, 64479-64505,
64510-64530, 69990, 92012-92014, 93000-93010, 93040-93042, 93318,
93355, 94002, 94200, 94250, 94680-94690, 94770, 95812-95816,
95819, 95822, 95829, 95955, 96360-96368, 96372, 96374-96377,
96523, 99155, 99156, 99157, 99211-99223, 99231-99255, 99291-99292,
99304-99310, 99315-99316, 99334-99337, 99347-99350, 99374-99375,
99377-99378, 99446-99449, 99451-99452, 99495-99496, G0463, G0471

50785 00910, 0213T, 0216T, 0228T, 0230T, 12001-12007, 12011-12057,
13100-13133, 13151-13153, 36000, 36400-36410, 36420-36430, 36440,
36591-36592, 36600, 36640, 43752, 44602-44605, 44850, 44950,

44970, 49000-49010, 49320, 50605, 50650, 50715, 50740-50780♦,
51701-51703, 51820, 52000, 62320-62327, 64400, 64405-64408,
64415-64435, 64445-64454, 64461-64463, 64479-64505, 64510-64530,
69990, 92012-92014, 93000-93010, 93040-93042, 93318, 93355, 94002,
94200, 94250, 94680-94690, 94770, 95812-95816, 95819, 95822,
95829, 95955, 96360-96368, 96372, 96374-96377, 96523, 99155,
99156, 99157, 99211-99223, 99231-99255, 99291-99292, 99304-99310,
99315-99316, 99334-99337, 99347-99350, 99374-99375, 99377-99378,
99446-99449, 99451-99452, 99495-99496, G0463, G0471

50800 00910, 0213T, 0216T, 0228T, 0230T, 12001-12007, 12011-12057,
13100-13133, 13151-13153, 36000, 36400-36410, 36420-36430, 36440,
36591-36592, 36600, 36640, 43752, 44005, 44180, 44602-44605,
44820-44850, 44950, 44970, 49000-49010, 49255, 49320, 50605,
50650, 50715, 50820♦, 50825♦, 50860♦, 51701-51703, 62320-62327,
64400, 64405-64408, 64415-64435, 64445-64454, 64461-64463,
64479-64505, 64510-64530, 69990, 92012-92014, 93000-93010,
93040-93042, 93318, 93355, 94002, 94200, 94250, 94680-94690,
94770, 95812-95816, 95819, 95822, 95829, 95955, 96360-96368,
96372, 96374-96377, 96523, 99155, 99156, 99157, 99211-99223,
99231-99255, 99291-99292, 99304-99310, 99315-99316, 99334-99337,
99347-99350, 99374-99375, 99377-99378, 99446-99449, 99451-99452,
99495-99496, G0463, G0471

50810 00910, 0213T, 0216T, 0228T, 0230T, 12001-12007, 12011-12057,
13100-13133, 13151-13153, 36000, 36400-36410, 36420-36430, 36440,
36591-36592, 36600, 36640, 43752, 44005, 44180, 44188♦, 44320,
44602-44605, 44820-44850, 44950, 44970, 49000-49010, 49255, 49320,
50605, 50650, 50715, 50740-50770♦, 50800, 50820♦, 50825♦,
51701-51703, 62320-62327, 64400, 64405-64408, 64415-64435,
64445-64454, 64461-64463, 64479-64505, 64510-64530, 69990,
92012-92014, 93000-93010, 93040-93042, 93318, 93355, 94002, 94200,
94250, 94680-94690, 94770, 95812-95816, 95819, 95822, 95829,
95955, 96360-96368, 96372, 96374-96377, 96523, 99155, 99156,
99157, 99211-99223, 99231-99255, 99291-99292, 99304-99310,
99315-99316, 99334-99337, 99347-99350, 99374-99375, 99377-99378,
99446-99449, 99451-99452, 99495-99496, G0463, G0471

50815 00910, 0213T, 0216T, 0228T, 0230T, 12001-12007, 12011-12057,
13100-13133, 13151-13153, 36000, 36400-36410, 36420-36430, 36440,
36591-36592, 36600, 36640, 43752, 44005, 44180, 44602-44605,
44820-44850, 44950, 44970, 49000-49010, 49255, 49320, 50605,
50650, 50715, 50740-50770♦, 50820♦, 50825♦, 51701-51703,
62320-62327, 64400, 64405-64408, 64415-64435, 64445-64454,
64461-64463, 64479-64505, 64510-64530, 69990, 92012-92014,
93000-93010, 93040-93042, 93318, 93355, 94002, 94200, 94250,
94680-94690, 94770, 95812-95816, 95819, 95822, 95829, 95955,
96360-96368, 96372, 96374-96377, 96523, 99155, 99156, 99157,
99211-99223, 99231-99255, 99291-99292, 99304-99310, 99315-99316,
99334-99337, 99347-99350, 99374-99375, 99377-99378, 99446-99449,
99451-99452, 99495-99496, G0463, G0471

50820 00910, 0213T, 0216T, 0228T, 0230T, 12001-12007, 12011-12057,
13100-13133, 13151-13153, 36000, 36400-36410, 36420-36430, 36440,
36591-36592, 36600, 36640, 43752, 44005, 44180, 44602-44605,
44820-44850, 44950, 44970, 49000-49010, 49255, 49320, 50605,
50650, 50715, 50740-50770♦, 50825♦, 51580-51585♦, 51701-51703,
62320-62327, 64400, 64405-64408, 64415-64435, 64445-64454,
64461-64463, 64479-64505, 64510-64530, 69990, 92012-92014,
93000-93010, 93040-93042, 93318, 93355, 94002, 94200, 94250,
94680-94690, 94770, 95812-95816, 95819, 95822, 95829, 95955,
96360-96368, 96372, 96374-96377, 96523, 99155, 99156, 99157,
99211-99223, 99231-99255, 99291-99292, 99304-99310, 99315-99316,

99334-99337, 99347-99350, 99374-99375, 99377-99378, 99446-99449, 99451-99452, 99495-99496, G0463, G0471

50825 00910, 0213T, 0216T, 0228T, 0230T, 11000-11006, 11042-11047, 12001-12007, 12011-12057, 13100-13133, 13151-13153, 36000, 36400-36410, 36420-36430, 36440, 36591-36592, 36600, 36640, 43752, 44005, 44180, 44602-44605, 44820-44850, 44950, 44970, 49000-49010, 49255, 49320, 50605, 50650, 50715, 50740-50770♦, 51701-51703, 62320-62327, 64400, 64405-64408, 64415-64435, 64445-64454, 64461-64463, 64479-64505, 64510-64530, 69990, 92012-92014, 93000-93010, 93040-93042, 93318, 93355, 94002, 94200, 94250, 94680-94690, 94770, 95812-95816, 95819, 95822, 95829, 95955, 96360-96368, 96372, 96374-96377, 96523, 97597-97598, 97602, 99155, 99156, 99157, 99211-99223, 99231-99255, 99291-99292, 99304-99310, 99315-99316, 99334-99337, 99347-99350, 99374-99375, 99377-99378, 99446-99449, 99451-99452, 99495-99496, G0463, G0471

50830 00910, 0213T, 0216T, 0228T, 0230T, 12001-12007, 12011-12057, 13100-13133, 13151-13153, 36000, 36400-36410, 36420-36430, 36440, 36591-36592, 36600, 36640, 43752, 44005, 44180, 44602-44605, 44820-44850, 44950, 44970, 49000-49010, 49255, 50605, 50650, 50715, 50780, 50782-50785, 50800, 50810-50815, 50860, 50947-50948♦, 51565, 51701-51703, 52000, 62320-62327, 64400, 64405-64408, 64415-64435, 64445-64454, 64461-64463, 64479-64505, 64510-64530, 69990, 92012-92014, 93000-93010, 93040-93042, 93318, 93355, 94002, 94200, 94250, 94680-94690, 94770, 95812-95816, 95819, 95822, 95829, 95955, 96360-96368, 96372, 96374-96377, 96523, 99155, 99156, 99157, 99211-99223, 99231-99255, 99291-99292, 99304-99310, 99315-99316, 99334-99337, 99347-99350, 99374-99375, 99377-99378, 99446-99449, 99451-99452, 99495-99496, G0463, G0471

50840 00910, 0213T, 0216T, 0228T, 0230T, 11000-11006, 11042-11047, 12001-12007, 12011-12057, 13100-13133, 13151-13153, 36000, 36400-36410, 36420-36430, 36440, 36591-36592, 36600, 36640, 43752, 44005, 44180, 44602-44605, 44820-44850, 44950, 44970, 49000-49010, 49255, 49320, 50605, 50650, 50715, 51701-51703, 62320-62327, 64400, 64405-64408, 64415-64435, 64445-64454, 64461-64463, 64479-64505, 64510-64530, 69990, 92012-92014, 93000-93010, 93040-93042, 93318, 93355, 94002, 94200, 94250, 94680-94690, 94770, 95812-95816, 95819, 95822, 95829, 95955, 96360-96368, 96372, 96374-96377, 96523, 97597-97598, 97602, 99155, 99156, 99157, 99211-99223, 99231-99255, 99291-99292, 99304-99310, 99315-99316, 99334-99337, 99347-99350, 99374-99375, 99377-99378, 99446-99449, 99451-99452, 99495-99496, G0463, G0471

50845 00910, 0213T, 0216T, 0228T, 0230T, 12001-12007, 12011-12057, 13100-13133, 13151-13153, 36000, 36400-36410, 36420-36430, 36440, 36591-36592, 36600, 36640, 43752, 44005, 44180, 44602-44605, 44820-44850, 44950, 44970, 49000-49010, 49255, 50650, 50715, 51701-51703, 62320-62327, 64400, 64405-64408, 64415-64435, 64445-64454, 64461-64463, 64479-64505, 64510-64530, 69990, 92012-92014, 93000-93010, 93040-93042, 93318, 93355, 94002, 94200, 94250, 94680-94690, 94770, 95812-95816, 95819, 95822, 95829, 95955, 96360-96368, 96372, 96374-96377, 96523, 99155, 99156, 99157, 99211-99223, 99231-99255, 99291-99292, 99304-99310, 99315-99316, 99334-99337, 99347-99350, 99374-99375, 99377-99378, 99446-99449, 99451-99452, 99495-99496, G0463, G0471

50860 00910, 0213T, 0216T, 0228T, 0230T, 12001-12007, 12011-12057, 13100-13133, 13151-13153, 36000, 36400-36410, 36420-36430, 36440, 36591-36592, 36600, 36640, 43752, 44602-44605, 44850, 44950, 44970, 49000-49010, 50605, 50650, 50715, 50810-50815♦, 50820♦, 50825♦, 51701-51703, 62320-62327, 64400, 64405-64408, 64415-64435, 64445-64454, 64461-64463, 64479-64505, 64510-64530,

69990, 92012-92014, 93000-93010, 93040-93042, 93318, 93355, 94002, 94200, 94250, 94680-94690, 94770, 95812-95816, 95819, 95822, 95829, 95955, 96360-96368, 96372, 96374-96377, 96523, 99155, 99156, 99157, 99211-99223, 99231-99255, 99291-99292, 99304-99310, 99315-99316, 99334-99337, 99347-99350, 99374-99375, 99377-99378, 99446-99449, 99451-99452, 99495-99496, G0463, G0471

50900 00910, 0213T, 0216T, 0228T, 0230T, 12001-12007, 12011-12057, 13100-13133, 13151-13153, 36000, 36400-36410, 36420-36430, 36440, 36591-36592, 36600, 36640, 43752, 44602-44605, 44850, 44950, 44970, 49000-49010, 50650, 51701-51703, 62320-62327, 64400, 64405-64408, 64415-64435, 64445-64454, 64461-64463, 64479-64505, 64510-64530, 69990, 92012-92014, 93000-93010, 93040-93042, 93318, 93355, 94002, 94200, 94250, 94680-94690, 94770, 95812-95816, 95819, 95822, 95829, 95955, 96360-96368, 96372, 96374-96377, 96523, 99155, 99156, 99157, 99211-99223, 99231-99255, 99291-99292, 99304-99310, 99315-99316, 99334-99337, 99347-99350, 99374-99375, 99377-99378, 99446-99449, 99451-99452, 99495-99496, G0463, G0471

50920 00910, 0213T, 0216T, 0228T, 0230T, 11000-11006, 11042-11047, 12001-12007, 12011-12057, 13100-13133, 13151-13153, 36000, 36400-36410, 36420-36430, 36440, 36591-36592, 36600, 36640, 43752, 44602-44605, 44850, 44950, 44970, 49000-49010, 50605, 50650, 50715, 50900, 51701-51703, 62320-62327, 64400, 64405-64408, 64415-64435, 64445-64454, 64461-64463, 64479-64505, 64510-64530, 69990, 92012-92014, 93000-93010, 93040-93042, 93318, 93355, 94002, 94200, 94250, 94680-94690, 94770, 95812-95816, 95819, 95822, 95829, 95955, 96360-96368, 96372, 96374-96377, 96523, 97597-97598, 97602, 99155, 99156, 99157, 99211-99223, 99231-99255, 99291-99292, 99304-99310, 99315-99316, 99334-99337, 99347-99350, 99374-99375, 99377-99378, 99446-99449, 99451-99452, 99495-99496, G0463, G0471

50930 00910, 0213T, 0216T, 0228T, 0230T, 11000-11006, 11042-11047, 12001-12007, 12011-12057, 13100-13133, 13151-13153, 36000, 36400-36410, 36420-36430, 36440, 36591-36592, 36600, 36640, 43752, 44005, 44180, 44602-44605, 44850, 44950, 44970, 49000-49010, 49255, 50605, 50650, 50715, 50900, 51701-51703, 62320-62327, 64400, 64405-64408, 64415-64435, 64445-64454, 64461-64463, 64479-64505, 64510-64530, 69990, 92012-92014, 93000-93010, 93040-93042, 93318, 93355, 94002, 94200, 94250, 94680-94690, 94770, 95812-95816, 95819, 95822, 95829, 95955, 96360-96368, 96372, 96374-96377, 96523, 97597-97598, 97602, 99155, 99156, 99157, 99211-99223, 99231-99255, 99291-99292, 99304-99310, 99315-99316, 99334-99337, 99347-99350, 99374-99375, 99377-99378, 99446-99449, 99451-99452, 99495-99496, G0463, G0471

50940 00910, 0213T, 0216T, 0228T, 0230T, 12001-12007, 12011-12057, 13100-13133, 13151-13153, 36000, 36400-36410, 36420-36430, 36440, 36591-36592, 36600, 36640, 43752, 44602-44605, 44850, 44950, 44970, 49000-49010, 50605, 50650, 50715, 50900, 51701-51703, 62320-62327, 64400, 64405-64408, 64415-64435, 64445-64454, 64461-64463, 64479-64505, 64510-64530, 69990, 92012-92014, 93000-93010, 93040-93042, 93318, 93355, 94002, 94200, 94250, 94680-94690, 94770, 95812-95816, 95819, 95822, 95829, 95955, 96360-96368, 96372, 96374-96377, 96523, 99155, 99156, 99157, 99211-99223, 99231-99255, 99291-99292, 99304-99310, 99315-99316, 99334-99337, 99347-99350, 99374-99375, 99377-99378, 99446-99449, 99451-99452, 99495-99496, G0463, G0471

50945 00910, 0213T, 0216T, 0228T, 0230T, 11000-11006, 11042-11047, 12001-12007, 12011-12057, 13100-13133, 13151-13153, 36000, 36400-36410, 36420-36430, 36440, 36591-36592, 36600, 36640, 43653, 43752, 44005, 44180, 44602-44605, 44950, 44970, 49082-49084, 49320, 49400, 50715, 51701-51703, 58660, 62320-62327, 64400,

CPT © 2020 American Medical Association. All Rights Reserved.

64405-64408, 64415-64435, 64445-64454, 64461-64463, 64479-64505, 64510-64530, 69990, 76000, 77001-77002, 92012-92014, 93000-93010, 93040-93042, 93318, 93355, 94002, 94200, 94250, 94680-94690, 94770, 95812-95816, 95819, 95822, 95829, 95955, 96360-96368, 96372, 96374-96377, 96523, 97597-97598, 97602, 99155, 99156, 99157, 99211-99223, 99231-99255, 99291-99292, 99304-99310, 99315-99316, 99334-99337, 99347-99350, 99374-99375, 99377-99378, 99446-99449, 99451-99452, 99495-99496, G0463, G0471

50947 00910, 0213T, 0216T, 0228T, 0230T, 12001-12007, 12011-12057, 13100-13133, 13151-13153, 35840, 36000, 36400-36410, 36420-36430, 36440, 36591-36592, 36600, 36640, 43653, 43752, 44005, 44180, 44602-44605, 44950, 44970, 49082-49084, 49320, 49400, 50382-50384, 50387, 50430-50431, 50605, 50650, 50684, 50715, 50782-50785◆, 51565, 51700-51703, 51820, 52000, 52310-52315, 52332, 52356, 53000-53025, 53660-53665, 58660, 62320-62327, 64400, 64405-64408, 64415-64435, 64445-64454, 64461-64463, 64479-64505, 64510-64530, 69990, 76000, 77001-77002, 92012-92014, 93000-93010, 93040-93042, 93318, 93355, 94002, 94200, 94250, 94680-94690, 94770, 95812-95816, 95819, 95822, 95829, 95955, 96360-96368, 96372, 96374-96377, 96523, 99155, 99156, 99157, 99211-99223, 99231-99255, 99291-99292, 99304-99310, 99315-99316, 99334-99337, 99347-99350, 99374-99375, 99377-99378, 99446-99449, 99451-99452, 99495-99496, G0463, G0471, P9612

50948 00910, 0213T, 0216T, 0228T, 0230T, 12001-12007, 12011-12057, 13100-13133, 13151-13153, 35840, 36000, 36400-36410, 36420-36430, 36440, 36591-36592, 36600, 36640, 43653, 43752, 44005, 44180, 44602-44605, 44950, 44970, 49082-49084, 49320, 49400, 50430-50431, 50605, 50650, 50684, 50715, 50782-50785◆, 51565, 51700-51703, 51820, 52000, 52332, 52356, 53660-53665, 58660, 62320-62327, 64400, 64405-64408, 64415-64435, 64445-64454, 64461-64463, 64479-64505, 64510-64530, 69990, 76000, 77001-77002, 92012-92014, 93000-93010, 93040-93042, 93318, 93355, 94002, 94200, 94250, 94680-94690, 94770, 95812-95816, 95819, 95822, 95829, 95955, 96360-96368, 96372, 96374-96377, 96523, 99155, 99156, 99157, 99211-99223, 99231-99255, 99291-99292, 99304-99310, 99315-99316, 99334-99337, 99347-99350, 99374-99375, 99377-99378, 99446-99449, 99451-99452, 99495-99496, G0463, G0471, P9612

50951 00910, 0213T, 0216T, 0228T, 0230T, 12001-12007, 12011-12057, 13100-13133, 13151-13153, 36000, 36400-36410, 36420-36430, 36440, 36591-36592, 36600, 36640, 43752, 50391, 50436-50437, 50684, 51701-51703, 62320-62327, 64400, 64405-64408, 64415-64435, 64445-64454, 64461-64463, 64479-64505, 64510-64530, 69990, 76000, 77001-77002, 92012-92014, 93000-93010, 93040-93042, 93318, 93355, 94002, 94200, 94250, 94680-94690, 94770, 95812-95816, 95819, 95822, 95829, 95955, 96360-96368, 96372, 96374-96377, 96523, 99155, 99156, 99157, 99211-99223, 99231-99255, 99291-99292, 99304-99310, 99315-99316, 99334-99337, 99347-99350, 99374-99375, 99377-99378, 99446-99449, 99451-99452, 99495-99496, G0463, G0471, J2001

50953 00910, 0213T, 0216T, 0228T, 0230T, 12001-12007, 12011-12057, 13100-13133, 13151-13153, 36000, 36400-36410, 36420-36430, 36440, 36591-36592, 36600, 36640, 43752, 50436-50437, 50684, 50706, 50951, 51701-51703, 62320-62327, 64400, 64405-64408, 64415-64435, 64445-64454, 64461-64463, 64479-64505, 64510-64530, 69990, 76000, 77001-77002, 92012-92014, 93000-93010, 93040-93042, 93318, 93355, 94002, 94200, 94250, 94680-94690, 94770, 95812-95816, 95819, 95822, 95829, 95955, 96360-96368, 96372, 96374-96377, 96523, 99155, 99156, 99157, 99211-99223, 99231-99255, 99291-99292, 99304-99310, 99315-99316, 99334-99337, 99347-99350, 99374-99375,

99377-99378, 99446-99449, 99451-99452, 99495-99496, G0463, G0471, J2001

50955 00910, 0213T, 0216T, 0228T, 0230T, 10005, 10007, 10009, 10011, 10021, 12001-12007, 12011-12057, 13100-13133, 13151-13153, 36000, 36400-36410, 36420-36430, 36440, 36591-36592, 36600, 36640, 43752, 50436-50437, 50606, 50684, 50715, 50951, 51701-51703, 62320-62327, 64400, 64405-64408, 64415-64435, 64445-64454, 64461-64463, 64479-64505, 64510-64530, 69990, 76000, 77001-77002, 92012-92014, 93000-93010, 93040-93042, 93318, 93355, 94002, 94200, 94250, 94680-94690, 94770, 95812-95816, 95819, 95822, 95829, 95955, 96360-96368, 96372, 96374-96377, 96523, 99155, 99156, 99157, 99211-99223, 99231-99255, 99291-99292, 99304-99310, 99315-99316, 99334-99337, 99347-99350, 99374-99375, 99377-99378, 99446-99449, 99451-99452, 99495-99496, G0463, G0471, J2001

50957 00910, 0213T, 0216T, 0228T, 0230T, 10005, 10007, 10009, 10011, 10021, 12001-12007, 12011-12057, 13100-13133, 13151-13153, 36000, 36400-36410, 36420-36430, 36440, 36591-36592, 36600, 36640, 43752, 50436-50437, 50684, 50715, 50951, 50955, 50974, 51701-51703, 62320-62327, 64400, 64405-64408, 64415-64435, 64445-64454, 64461-64463, 64479-64505, 64510-64530, 69990, 76000, 77001-77002, 92012-92014, 93000-93010, 93040-93042, 93318, 93355, 94002, 94200, 94250, 94680-94690, 94770, 95812-95816, 95819, 95822, 95829, 95955, 96360-96368, 96372, 96374-96377, 96523, 99155, 99156, 99157, 99211-99223, 99231-99255, 99291-99292, 99304-99310, 99315-99316, 99334-99337, 99347-99350, 99374-99375, 99377-99378, 99446-99449, 99451-99452, 99495-99496, G0463, G0471, J2001

50961 00910, 0213T, 0216T, 0228T, 0230T, 11000-11006, 11042-11047, 12001-12007, 12011-12057, 13100-13133, 13151-13153, 36000, 36400-36410, 36420-36430, 36440, 36591-36592, 36600, 36640, 43752, 50436-50437, 50684, 50715, 50951, 51701-51703, 52320, 52330, 62320-62327, 64400, 64405-64408, 64415-64435, 64445-64454, 64461-64463, 64479-64505, 64510-64530, 69990, 76000, 77001-77002, 92012-92014, 93000-93010, 93040-93042, 93318, 93355, 94002, 94200, 94250, 94680-94690, 94770, 95812-95816, 95819, 95822, 95829, 95955, 96360-96368, 96372, 96374-96377, 96523, 97597-97598, 97602, 99155, 99156, 99157, 99211-99223, 99231-99255, 99291-99292, 99304-99310, 99315-99316, 99334-99337, 99347-99350, 99374-99375, 99377-99378, 99446-99449, 99451-99452, 99495-99496, G0463, G0471, J2001

50970 00910, 0213T, 0216T, 0228T, 0230T, 11000-11006, 11042-11047, 12001-12007, 12011-12057, 13100-13133, 13151-13153, 36000, 36400-36410, 36420-36430, 36440, 36591-36592, 36600, 36640, 43752, 50391, 50684, 51701-51703, 62320-62327, 64400, 64405-64408, 64415-64435, 64445-64454, 64461-64463, 64479-64505, 64510-64530, 69990, 76000, 77001-77002, 92012-92014, 93000-93010, 93040-93042, 93318, 93355, 94002, 94200, 94250, 94680-94690, 94770, 95812-95816, 95819, 95822, 95829, 95955, 96360-96368, 96372, 96374-96377, 96523, 97597-97598, 97602, 99155, 99156, 99157, 99211-99223, 99231-99255, 99291-99292, 99304-99310, 99315-99316, 99334-99337, 99347-99350, 99374-99375, 99377-99378, 99446-99449, 99451-99452, 99495-99496, G0463, G0471

50972 00910, 0213T, 0216T, 0228T, 0230T, 11000-11006, 11042-11047, 12001-12007, 12011-12057, 13100-13133, 13151-13153, 36000, 36400-36410, 36420-36430, 36440, 36591-36592, 36600, 36640, 43752, 50684, 50706, 50970, 51701-51703, 62320-62327, 64400, 64405-64408, 64415-64435, 64445-64454, 64461-64463, 64479-64505, 64510-64530, 69990, 76000, 77001-77002, 92012-92014, 93000-93010, 93040-93042, 93318, 93355, 94002, 94200, 94250, 94680-94690, 94770, 95812-95816, 95819, 95822, 95829, 95955, 96360-96368, 96372,

96374-96377, 96523, 97597-97598, 97602, 99155, 99156, 99157, 99211-99223, 99231-99255, 99291-99292, 99304-99310, 99315-99316, 99334-99337, 99347-99350, 99374-99375, 99377-99378, 99446-99449, 99451-99452, 99495-99496, G0463, G0471

50974 00910, 0213T, 0216T, 0228T, 0230T, 10005, 10007, 10009, 10011, 10021, 11000-11006, 11042-11047, 12001-12007, 12011-12057, 13100-13133, 13151-13153, 36000, 36400-36410, 36420-36430, 36440, 36591-36592, 36600, 36640, 43752, 50606, 50684, 50715, 50970, 51701-51703, 62320-62327, 64400, 64405-64408, 64415-64435, 64445-64454, 64461-64463, 64479-64505, 64510-64530, 69990, 76000, 77001-77002, 92012-92014, 93000-93010, 93040-93042, 93318, 93355, 94002, 94200, 94250, 94680-94690, 94770, 95812-95816, 95819, 95822, 95829, 95955, 96360-96368, 96372, 96374-96377, 96523, 97597-97598, 97602, 99155, 99156, 99157, 99211-99223, 99231-99255, 99291-99292, 99304-99310, 99315-99316, 99334-99337, 99347-99350, 99374-99375, 99377-99378, 99446-99449, 99451-99452, 99495-99496, G0463, G0471

50976 00910, 0213T, 0216T, 0228T, 0230T, 10005, 10007, 10009, 10011, 10021, 11000-11006, 11042-11047, 12001-12007, 12011-12057, 13100-13133, 13151-13153, 36000, 36400-36410, 36420-36430, 36440, 36591-36592, 36600, 36640, 43752, 50684, 50715, 50955, 50970, 50974, 51701-51703, 62320-62327, 64400, 64405-64408, 64415-64435, 64445-64454, 64461-64463, 64479-64505, 64510-64530, 69990, 76000, 77001-77002, 92012-92014, 93000-93010, 93040-93042, 93318, 93355, 94002, 94200, 94250, 94680-94690, 94770, 95812-95816, 95819, 95822, 95829, 95955, 96360-96368, 96372, 96374-96377, 96523, 97597-97598, 97602, 99155, 99156, 99157, 99211-99223, 99231-99255, 99291-99292, 99304-99310, 99315-99316, 99334-99337, 99347-99350, 99374-99375, 99377-99378, 99446-99449, 99451-99452, 99495-99496, G0463, G0471

50980 00910, 0213T, 0216T, 0228T, 0230T, 11000-11006, 11042-11047, 12001-12007, 12011-12057, 13100-13133, 13151-13153, 36000, 36400-36410, 36420-36430, 36440, 36591-36592, 36600, 36640, 43752, 50684, 50715, 50961-50970, 51701-51703, 52320-52325, 52330, 52352, 62320-62327, 64400, 64405-64408, 64415-64435, 64445-64454, 64461-64463, 64479-64505, 64510-64530, 69990, 76000, 77001-77002, 92012-92014, 93000-93010, 93040-93042, 93318, 93355, 94002, 94200, 94250, 94680-94690, 94770, 95812-95816, 95819, 95822, 95829, 95955, 96360-96368, 96372, 96374-96377, 96523, 97597-97598, 97602, 99155, 99156, 99157, 99211-99223, 99231-99255, 99291-99292, 99304-99310, 99315-99316, 99334-99337, 99347-99350, 99374-99375, 99377-99378, 99446-99449, 99451-99452, 99495-99496, G0463, G0471

51020 00910, 0213T, 0216T, 0228T, 0230T, 11000-11006, 11042-11047, 12001-12007, 12011-12057, 13100-13133, 13151-13153, 36000, 36400-36410, 36420-36430, 36440, 36591-36592, 36600, 36640, 43752, 44602-44605, 44950, 44970, 49000-49002, 49320, 50715, 51045, 51100-51102, 51520-51525, 51701-51703, 52000, 62320-62327, 64400, 64405-64408, 64415-64435, 64445-64454, 64461-64463, 64479-64505, 64510-64530, 69990, 92012-92014, 93000-93010, 93040-93042, 93318, 93355, 94002, 94200, 94250, 94680-94690, 94770, 95812-95816, 95819, 95822, 95829, 95955, 96360-96368, 96372, 96374-96377, 96523, 97597-97598, 97602, 99155, 99156, 99157, 99211-99223, 99231-99255, 99291-99292, 99304-99310, 99315-99316, 99334-99337, 99347-99350, 99374-99375, 99377-99378, 99446-99449, 99451-99452, 99495-99496, G0463, G0471

51030 00910, 0213T, 0216T, 0228T, 0230T, 11000-11006, 11042-11047, 12001-12007, 12011-12057, 13100-13133, 13151-13153, 36000, 36400-36410, 36420-36430, 36440, 36591-36592, 36600, 36640, 43752, 44602-44605, 44950, 44970, 49000-49002, 49320, 50715, 51045,

51100-51102, 51520-51525, 51701-51703, 52000, 62320-62327, 64400, 64405-64408, 64415-64435, 64445-64454, 64461-64463, 64479-64505, 64510-64530, 69990, 92012-92014, 93000-93010, 93040-93042, 93318, 93355, 94002, 94200, 94250, 94680-94690, 94770, 95812-95816, 95819, 95822, 95829, 95955, 96360-96368, 96372, 96374-96377, 96523, 97597-97598, 97602, 99155, 99156, 99157, 99211-99223, 99231-99255, 99291-99292, 99304-99310, 99315-99316, 99334-99337, 99347-99350, 99374-99375, 99377-99378, 99446-99449, 99451-99452, 99495-99496, G0463, G0471

51040 00910, 0213T, 0216T, 0228T, 0230T, 11000-11006, 11042-11047, 12001-12007, 12011-12057, 13100-13133, 13151-13153, 36000, 36400-36410, 36420-36430, 36440, 36591-36592, 36600, 36640, 43752, 44602-44605, 44950, 44970, 49000-49002, 49320, 50715, 51045, 51100-51102, 51520-51525, 51570, 51701-51703, 52000, 52005, 52276, 52281, 62320-62327, 64400, 64405-64408, 64415-64435, 64445-64454, 64461-64463, 64479-64505, 64510-64530, 69990, 92012-92014, 93000-93010, 93040-93042, 93318, 93355, 94002, 94200, 94250, 94680-94690, 94770, 95812-95816, 95819, 95822, 95829, 95955, 96360-96368, 96372, 96374-96377, 96523, 97597-97598, 97602, 99155, 99156, 99157, 99211-99223, 99231-99255, 99291-99292, 99304-99310, 99315-99316, 99334-99337, 99347-99350, 99374-99375, 99377-99378, 99446-99449, 99451-99452, 99495-99496, G0463, G0471

51045 00910, 0213T, 0216T, 0228T, 0230T, 11000-11006, 11042-11047, 12001-12007, 12011-12057, 13100-13133, 13151-13153, 36000, 36400-36410, 36420-36430, 36440, 36591-36592, 36600, 36640, 43752, 44602-44605, 44950, 44970, 49000-49002, 49320, 50715, 51701-51703, 52000, 62320-62327, 64400, 64405-64408, 64415-64435, 64445-64454, 64461-64463, 64479-64505, 64510-64530, 69990, 92012-92014, 93000-93010, 93040-93042, 93318, 93355, 94002, 94200, 94250, 94680-94690, 94770, 95812-95816, 95819, 95822, 95829, 95955, 96360-96368, 96372, 96374-96377, 96523, 97597-97598, 97602, 99155, 99156, 99157, 99211-99223, 99231-99255, 99291-99292, 99304-99310, 99315-99316, 99334-99337, 99347-99350, 99374-99375, 99377-99378, 99446-99449, 99451-99452, 99495-99496, G0463, G0471

51050 00910, 0213T, 0216T, 0228T, 0230T, 11000-11006, 11042-11047, 12001-12007, 12011-12057, 13100-13133, 13151-13153, 36000, 36400-36410, 36420-36430, 36440, 36591-36592, 36600, 36640, 43752, 44602-44605, 44950, 44970, 49000-49002, 49320, 50715, 51045, 51520-51525, 51570, 51701-51703, 52000, 62320-62327, 64400, 64405-64408, 64415-64435, 64445-64454, 64461-64463, 64479-64505, 64510-64530, 69990, 92012-92014, 93000-93010, 93040-93042, 93318, 93355, 94002, 94200, 94250, 94680-94690, 94770, 95812-95816, 95819, 95822, 95829, 95955, 96360-96368, 96372, 96374-96377, 96523, 97597-97598, 97602, 99155, 99156, 99157, 99211-99223, 99231-99255, 99291-99292, 99304-99310, 99315-99316, 99334-99337, 99347-99350, 99374-99375, 99377-99378, 99446-99449, 99451-99452, 99495-99496, G0463, G0471

51060 00910, 0213T, 0216T, 0228T, 0230T, 11000-11006, 11042-11047, 12001-12007, 12011-12057, 13100-13133, 13151-13153, 36000, 36400-36410, 36420-36430, 36440, 36591-36592, 36600, 36640, 43752, 44602-44605, 44950, 44970, 49000-49002, 49320, 50715, 51045, 51520-51525, 51570, 51701-51703, 52000, 62320-62327, 64400, 64405-64408, 64415-64435, 64445-64454, 64461-64463, 64479-64505, 64510-64530, 69990, 92012-92014, 93000-93010, 93040-93042, 93318, 93355, 94002, 94200, 94250, 94680-94690, 94770, 95812-95816, 95819, 95822, 95829, 95955, 96360-96368, 96372, 96374-96377, 96523, 97597-97598, 97602, 99155, 99156, 99157, 99211-99223, 99231-99255, 99291-99292, 99304-99310, 99315-99316, 99334-99337, 99347-99350, 99374-99375, 99377-99378, 99446-99449, 99451-99452, 99495-99496, G0463, G0471

51065 00910, 0213T, 0216T, 0228T, 0230T, 11000-11006, 11042-11047, 12001-12007, 12011-12057, 13100-13133, 13151-13153, 36000, 36400-36410, 36420-36430, 36440, 36591-36592, 36600, 36640, 43752, 44602-44605, 44950, 44970, 49000-49002, 49320, 50715, 51045, 51520-51525, 51570, 51701-51703, 52000, 62320-62327, 64400, 64405-64408, 64415-64435, 64445-64454, 64461-64463, 64479-64505, 64510-64530, 69990, 92012-92014, 93000-93010, 93040-93042, 93318, 93355, 94002, 94200, 94250, 94680-94690, 94770, 95812-95816, 95819, 95822, 95829, 95955, 96360-96368, 96372, 96374-96377, 96523, 97597-97598, 97602, 99155, 99156, 99157, 99211-99223, 99231-99255, 99291-99292, 99304-99310, 99315-99316, 99334-99337, 99347-99350, 99374-99375, 99377-99378, 99446-99449, 99451-99452, 99495-99496, G0463, G0471

51080 00910, 0213T, 0216T, 0228T, 0230T, 12001-12007, 12011-12057, 13100-13133, 13151-13153, 36000, 36400-36410, 36420-36430, 36440, 36591-36592, 36600, 36640, 43752, 44602-44605, 44950, 44970, 49000-49002, 49320, 49406, 50715, 51045, 51570, 51701-51703, 52000, 62320-62327, 64400, 64405-64408, 64415-64435, 64445-64454, 64461-64463, 64479-64505, 64510-64530, 69990, 92012-92014, 93000-93010, 93040-93042, 93318, 93355, 94002, 94200, 94250, 94680-94690, 94770, 95812-95816, 95819, 95822, 95829, 95955, 96360-96368, 96372, 96374-96377, 96523, 99155, 99156, 99157, 99211-99223, 99231-99255, 99291-99292, 99304-99310, 99315-99316, 99334-99337, 99347-99350, 99374-99375, 99377-99378, 99446-99449, 99451-99452, 99495-99496, G0463, G0471

51100 00910, 0213T, 0216T, 0228T, 0230T, 12001-12007, 12011-12057, 13100-13133, 13151-13153, 36000, 36400-36410, 36420-36430, 36440, 36591-36592, 36600, 36640, 43752, 44970, 51701, 52000, 62320-62327, 64400, 64405-64408, 64415-64435, 64445-64454, 64461-64463, 64479-64505, 64510-64530, 69990, 92012-92014, 93000-93010, 93040-93042, 93318, 93355, 94002, 94200, 94250, 94680-94690, 94770, 95812-95816, 95819, 95822, 95829, 95955, 96360-96368, 96372, 96374-96377, 96523, 99155, 99156, 99157, 99211-99223, 99231-99255, 99291-99292, 99304-99310, 99315-99316, 99334-99337, 99347-99350, 99374-99375, 99377-99378, 99446-99449, 99451-99452, 99495-99496, G0463, J0670, J2001

51101 00910, 0213T, 0216T, 0228T, 0230T, 12001-12007, 12011-12057, 13100-13133, 13151-13153, 36000, 36400-36410, 36420-36430, 36440, 36591-36592, 36600, 36640, 43752, 44970, 51100, 51701, 52000, 62320-62327, 64400, 64405-64408, 64415-64435, 64445-64454, 64461-64463, 64479-64505, 64510-64530, 69990, 76000, 77001, 92012-92014, 93000-93010, 93040-93042, 93318, 93355, 94002, 94200, 94250, 94680-94690, 94770, 95812-95816, 95819, 95822, 95829, 95955, 96360-96368, 96372, 96374-96377, 96523, 99155, 99156, 99157, 99211-99223, 99231-99255, 99291-99292, 99304-99310, 99315-99316, 99334-99337, 99347-99350, 99374-99375, 99377-99378, 99446-99449, 99451-99452, 99495-99496, G0463, J0670, J2001

51102 00910, 0213T, 0216T, 0228T, 0230T, 11000-11006, 11042-11047, 12001-12007, 12011-12057, 13100-13133, 13151-13153, 36000, 36400-36410, 36420-36430, 36440, 36591-36592, 36600, 36640, 43752, 44970, 51100-51101✦, 51701-51702, 52000, 52281, 62320-62327, 64400, 64405-64408, 64415-64435, 64445-64454, 64461-64463, 64479-64505, 64510-64530, 69990, 76000, 77001, 92012-92014, 93000-93010, 93040-93042, 93318, 93355, 94002, 94200, 94250, 94680-94690, 94770, 95812-95816, 95819, 95822, 95829, 95955, 96360-96368, 96372, 96374-96377, 96523, 97597-97598, 97602, 99155, 99156, 99157, 99211-99223, 99231-99255, 99291-99292, 99304-99310, 99315-99316, 99334-99337, 99347-99350, 99374-99375, 99377-99378, 99446-99449, 99451-99452, 99495-99496, G0463, G0471, J0670, J2001

51500 00910, 0213T, 0216T, 0228T, 0230T, 0437T, 11000-11006, 11042-11047, 12001-12007, 12011-12057, 13100-13133, 13151-13153, 15777, 36000, 36400-36410, 36420-36430, 36440, 36591-36592, 36600, 36640, 43752, 44602-44605, 44950, 44970, 49000-49002, 49320, 49568, 49580, 49582-49587, 50715, 51045, 51570, 51701-51703, 52000, 57267, 62320-62327, 64400, 64405-64408, 64415-64435, 64445-64454, 64461-64463, 64479-64505, 64510-64530, 69990, 92012-92014, 93000-93010, 93040-93042, 93318, 93355, 94002, 94200, 94250, 94680-94690, 94770, 95812-95816, 95819, 95822, 95829, 95955, 96360-96368, 96372, 96374-96377, 96523, 97597-97598, 97602, 99155, 99156, 99157, 99211-99223, 99231-99255, 99291-99292, 99304-99310, 99315-99316, 99334-99337, 99347-99350, 99374-99375, 99377-99378, 99446-99449, 99451-99452, 99495-99496, G0463, G0471

51520 00910, 0213T, 0216T, 0228T, 0230T, 11000-11006, 11042-11047, 12001-12007, 12011-12057, 13100-13133, 13151-13153, 36000, 36400-36410, 36420-36430, 36440, 36591-36592, 36600, 36640, 43752, 44602-44605, 44950, 44970, 49000-49002, 49320, 50715, 51045, 51701-51703, 52000, 62320-62327, 64400, 64405-64408, 64415-64435, 64445-64454, 64461-64463, 64479-64505, 64510-64530, 69990, 92012-92014, 93000-93010, 93040-93042, 93318, 93355, 94002, 94200, 94250, 94680-94690, 94770, 95812-95816, 95819, 95822, 95829, 95955, 96360-96368, 96372, 96374-96377, 96523, 97597-97598, 97602, 99155, 99156, 99157, 99211-99223, 99231-99255, 99291-99292, 99304-99310, 99315-99316, 99334-99337, 99347-99350, 99374-99375, 99377-99378, 99446-99449, 99451-99452, 99495-99496, G0463, G0471

51525 00910, 0213T, 0216T, 0228T, 0230T, 11000-11006, 11042-11047, 12001-12007, 12011-12057, 13100-13133, 13151-13153, 36000, 36400-36410, 36420-36430, 36440, 36591-36592, 36600, 36640, 43752, 44602-44605, 44950, 44970, 49000-49002, 49320, 50715, 51045, 51520, 51701-51703, 52000, 62320-62327, 64400, 64405-64408, 64415-64435, 64445-64454, 64461-64463, 64479-64505, 64510-64530, 69990, 92012-92014, 93000-93010, 93040-93042, 93318, 93355, 94002, 94200, 94250, 94680-94690, 94770, 95812-95816, 95819, 95822, 95829, 95955, 96360-96368, 96372, 96374-96377, 96523, 97597-97598, 97602, 99155, 99156, 99157, 99211-99223, 99231-99255, 99291-99292, 99304-99310, 99315-99316, 99334-99337, 99347-99350, 99374-99375, 99377-99378, 99446-99449, 99451-99452, 99495-99496, G0463, G0471

51530 00910, 0213T, 0216T, 0228T, 0230T, 11000-11006, 11042-11047, 12001-12007, 12011-12057, 13100-13133, 13151-13153, 36000, 36400-36410, 36420-36430, 36440, 36591-36592, 36600, 36640, 43752, 44602-44605, 44950, 44970, 49000-49002, 49320, 50715, 51045, 51520-51525, 51570, 51701-51703, 52000, 62320-62327, 64400, 64405-64408, 64415-64435, 64445-64454, 64461-64463, 64479-64505, 64510-64530, 69990, 92012-92014, 93000-93010, 93040-93042, 93318, 93355, 94002, 94200, 94250, 94680-94690, 94770, 95812-95816, 95819, 95822, 95829, 95955, 96360-96368, 96372, 96374-96377, 96523, 97597-97598, 97602, 99155, 99156, 99157, 99211-99223, 99231-99255, 99291-99292, 99304-99310, 99315-99316, 99334-99337, 99347-99350, 99374-99375, 99377-99378, 99446-99449, 99451-99452, 99495-99496, G0463, G0471

51535 00910, 0213T, 0216T, 0228T, 0230T, 11000-11006, 11042-11047, 12001-12007, 12011-12057, 13100-13133, 13151-13153, 36000, 36400-36410, 36420-36430, 36440, 36591-36592, 36600, 36640, 43752, 44602-44605, 44950, 44970, 49000-49002, 49320, 50715, 51045, 51520-51525, 51570, 51701-51703, 52000, 62320-62327, 64400, 64405-64408, 64415-64435, 64445-64454, 64461-64463, 64479-64505, 64510-64530, 69990, 92012-92014, 93000-93010, 93040-93042, 93318, 93355, 94002, 94200, 94250, 94680-94690, 94770, 95812-95816, 95819, 95822, 95829, 95955, 96360-96368, 96372, 96374-96377, 96523, 97597-97598, 97602, 99155, 99156, 99157, 99211-99223,

99231-99255, 99291-99292, 99304-99310, 99315-99316, 99334-99337, 99347-99350, 99374-99375, 99377-99378, 99446-99449, 99451-99452, 99495-99496, G0463, G0471

51550 00910, 0213T, 0216T, 0228T, 0230T, 11000-11006, 11042-11047, 12001-12007, 12011-12057, 13100-13133, 13151-13153, 36000, 36400-36410, 36420-36430, 36440, 36591-36592, 36600, 36640, 43752, 44005, 44180, 44602-44605, 44850, 44950, 44970, 49000-49010, 49255, 49320-49321, 50650, 50715, 51045, 51520-51525, 51570, 51701-51703, 52000, 58662, 62320-62327, 64400, 64405-64408, 64415-64435, 64445-64454, 64461-64463, 64479-64505, 64510-64530, 69990, 92012-92014, 93000-93010, 93040-93042, 93318, 93355, 94002, 94200, 94250, 94680-94690, 94770, 95812-95816, 95819, 95822, 95829, 95955, 96360-96368, 96372, 96374-96377, 96523, 97597-97598, 97602, 99155, 99156, 99157, 99211-99223, 99231-99255, 99291-99292, 99304-99310, 99315-99316, 99334-99337, 99347-99350, 99374-99375, 99377-99378, 99446-99449, 99451-99452, 99495-99496, G0463, G0471

51555 00910, 0213T, 0216T, 0228T, 0230T, 11000-11006, 11042-11047, 12001-12007, 12011-12057, 13100-13133, 13151-13153, 36000, 36400-36410, 36420-36430, 36440, 36591-36592, 36600, 36640, 43752, 44005, 44180, 44602-44605, 44850, 44950, 44970, 49000-49010, 49255, 49320-49321, 50650, 50715, 51045, 51520-51525, 51550, 51570, 51701-51703, 52000, 58662, 62320-62327, 64400, 64405-64408, 64415-64435, 64445-64454, 64461-64463, 64479-64505, 64510-64530, 69990, 92012-92014, 93000-93010, 93040-93042, 93318, 93355, 94002, 94200, 94250, 94680-94690, 94770, 95812-95816, 95819, 95822, 95829, 95955, 96360-96368, 96372, 96374-96377, 96523, 97597-97598, 97602, 99155, 99156, 99157, 99211-99223, 99231-99255, 99291-99292, 99304-99310, 99315-99316, 99334-99337, 99347-99350, 99374-99375, 99377-99378, 99446-99449, 99451-99452, 99495-99496, G0463, G0471

51565 00910, 0213T, 0216T, 0228T, 0230T, 11000-11006, 11042-11047, 12001-12007, 12011-12057, 13100-13133, 13151-13153, 36000, 36400-36410, 36420-36430, 36440, 36591-36592, 36600, 36640, 43752, 44602-44605, 44850, 44950, 44970, 49000-49010, 49255, 49320-49321, 50605, 50650, 50715, 50780, 50782-50785, 51045, 51520-51525, 51550-51555, 51570, 51701-51703, 52000, 58662, 62320-62327, 64400, 64405-64408, 64415-64435, 64445-64454, 64461-64463, 64479-64505, 64510-64530, 69990, 92012-92014, 93000-93010, 93040-93042, 93318, 93355, 94002, 94200, 94250, 94680-94690, 94770, 95812-95816, 95819, 95822, 95829, 95955, 96360-96368, 96372, 96374-96377, 96523, 97597-97598, 97602, 99155, 99156, 99157, 99211-99223, 99231-99255, 99291-99292, 99304-99310, 99315-99316, 99334-99337, 99347-99350, 99374-99375, 99377-99378, 99446-99449, 99451-99452, 99495-99496, G0463, G0471

51570 00910, 0213T, 0216T, 0228T, 0230T, 11000-11006, 11042-11047, 12001-12007, 12011-12057, 13100-13133, 13151-13153, 36000, 36400-36410, 36420-36430, 36440, 36591-36592, 36600, 36640, 38573, 43752, 44602-44605, 44850, 44950, 44970, 49000-49010, 49255, 49320-49321, 50605, 50650, 50715, 50800, 50810, 50825, 51045, 51520-51525, 51701-51703, 52000, 52204, 58662, 62320-62327, 64400, 64405-64408, 64415-64435, 64445-64454, 64461-64463, 64479-64505, 64510-64530, 69990, 92012-92014, 93000-93010, 93040-93042, 93318, 93355, 94002, 94200, 94250, 94680-94690, 94770, 95812-95816, 95819, 95822, 95829, 95955, 96360-96368, 96372, 96374-96377, 96523, 97597-97598, 97602, 99155, 99156, 99157, 99211-99223, 99231-99255, 99291-99292, 99304-99310, 99315-99316, 99334-99337, 99347-99350, 99374-99375, 99377-99378, 99446-99449, 99451-99452, 99495-99496, G0463, G0471

51575 00910, 0213T, 0216T, 0228T, 0230T, 11000-11006, 11042-11047, 12001-12007, 12011-12057, 13100-13133, 13151-13153, 36000,

36400-36410, 36420-36430, 36440, 36591-36592, 36600, 36640, 38571-38573, 38770, 38780, 43752, 44005, 44180, 44602-44605, 44820-44850, 44950, 44970, 49000-49010, 49255, 49320-49321, 50605, 50650, 50715, 50800, 50810, 50825, 51045, 51520, 51550-51570, 51701-51703, 52000, 52204, 58662, 62320-62327, 64400, 64405-64408, 64415-64435, 64445-64454, 64461-64463, 64479-64505, 64510-64530, 69990, 92012-92014, 93000-93010, 93040-93042, 93318, 93355, 94002, 94200, 94250, 94680-94690, 94770, 95812-95816, 95819, 95822, 95829, 95955, 96360-96368, 96372, 96374-96377, 96523, 97597-97598, 97602, 99155, 99156, 99157, 99211-99223, 99231-99255, 99291-99292, 99304-99310, 99315-99316, 99334-99337, 99347-99350, 99374-99375, 99377-99378, 99446-99449, 99451-99452, 99495-99496, G0463, G0471

51580 00910, 0213T, 0216T, 0228T, 0230T, 11000-11006, 11042-11047, 12001-12007, 12011-12057, 13100-13133, 13151-13153, 36000, 36400-36410, 36420-36430, 36440, 36591-36592, 36600, 36640, 38573, 43752, 44005, 44180, 44602-44605, 44820-44850, 44950, 44970, 49000-49010, 49255, 49320-49321, 50605, 50650, 50715, 50800, 50810, 50825, 51045, 51520-51525, 51550-51575, 51701-51703, 52000, 52204, 58662, 62320-62327, 64400, 64405-64408, 64415-64435, 64445-64454, 64461-64463, 64479-64505, 64510-64530, 69990, 92012-92014, 93000-93010, 93040-93042, 93318, 93355, 94002, 94200, 94250, 94680-94690, 94770, 95812-95816, 95819, 95822, 95829, 95955, 96360-96368, 96372, 96374-96377, 96523, 97597-97598, 97602, 99155, 99156, 99157, 99211-99223, 99231-99255, 99291-99292, 99304-99310, 99315-99316, 99334-99337, 99347-99350, 99374-99375, 99377-99378, 99446-99449, 99451-99452, 99495-99496, G0463, G0471

51585 00910, 0213T, 0216T, 0228T, 0230T, 11000-11006, 11042-11047, 12001-12007, 12011-12057, 13100-13133, 13151-13153, 36000, 36400-36410, 36420-36430, 36440, 36591-36592, 36600, 36640, 38571-38573, 38770, 38780, 43752, 44005, 44180, 44602-44605, 44820-44850, 44950, 44970, 49000-49002, 49255, 49320-49321, 50605, 50650, 50715, 50800, 50810, 50825, 51045, 51525, 51550-51580, 51701-51703, 52000, 52204, 58662, 62320-62327, 64400, 64405-64408, 64415-64435, 64445-64454, 64461-64463, 64479-64505, 64510-64530, 69990, 92012-92014, 93000-93010, 93040-93042, 93318, 93355, 94002, 94200, 94250, 94680-94690, 94770, 95812-95816, 95819, 95822, 95829, 95955, 96360-96368, 96372, 96374-96377, 96523, 97597-97598, 97602, 99155, 99156, 99157, 99211-99223, 99231-99255, 99291-99292, 99304-99310, 99315-99316, 99334-99337, 99347-99350, 99374-99375, 99377-99378, 99446-99449, 99451-99452, 99495-99496, G0463, G0471

51590 00910, 0213T, 0216T, 0228T, 0230T, 11000-11006, 11042-11047, 12001-12007, 12011-12057, 13100-13133, 13151-13153, 36000, 36400-36410, 36420-36430, 36440, 36591-36592, 36600, 36640, 38573, 43752, 44005, 44180, 44602-44605, 44820-44850, 44950, 44970, 49000-49010, 49255, 49320-49321, 50605, 50650, 50715, 50800, 50810, 50820, 50825, 51045, 51520-51525, 51550-51585, 51701-51703, 52000, 52204, 58662, 62320-62327, 64400, 64405-64408, 64415-64435, 64445-64454, 64461-64463, 64479-64505, 64510-64530, 69990, 92012-92014, 93000-93010, 93040-93042, 93318, 93355, 94002, 94200, 94250, 94680-94690, 94770, 95812-95816, 95819, 95822, 95829, 95955, 96360-96368, 96372, 96374-96377, 96523, 97597-97598, 97602, 99155, 99156, 99157, 99211-99223, 99231-99255, 99291-99292, 99304-99310, 99315-99316, 99334-99337, 99347-99350, 99374-99375, 99377-99378, 99446-99449, 99451-99452, 99495-99496, G0463, G0471

51595 00910, 0213T, 0216T, 0228T, 0230T, 11000-11006, 11042-11047, 12001-12007, 12011-12057, 13100-13133, 13151-13153, 36000, 36400-36410, 36420-36430, 36440, 36591-36592, 36600, 36640, 38571-38573, 38770, 38780, 43752, 44005, 44130, 44180, 44602-44605, 44820-44850, 44950, 44970, 49000-49010, 49255, 49320-49321, 50605, 50650, 50715, 50800, 50810, 50820, 50825,

CPT © 2020 American Medical Association. All Rights Reserved.

Coding Companion for Urology/Nephrology

51045, 51525, 51550-51590, 51701-51703, 52000, 52204, 53210, 55842-55845, 58200, 58210, 58662, 62320-62327, 64400, 64405-64408, 64415-64435, 64445-64454, 64461-64463, 64479-64505, 64510-64530, 69990, 92012-92014, 93000-93010, 93040-93042, 93318, 93355, 94002, 94200, 94250, 94680-94690, 94770, 95812-95816, 95819, 95822, 95829, 95955, 96360-96368, 96372, 96374-96377, 96523, 97597-97598, 97602, 99155, 99156, 99157, 99211-99223, 99231-99255, 99291-99292, 99304-99310, 99315-99316, 99334-99337, 99347-99350, 99374-99375, 99377-99378, 99446-99449, 99451-99452, 99495-99496, G0463, G0471

51596 00910, 0213T, 0216T, 0228T, 0230T, 11000-11006, 11042-11047, 12001-12007, 12011-12057, 13100-13133, 13151-13153, 36000, 36400-36410, 36420-36430, 36440, 36591-36592, 36600, 36640, 43752, 44005, 44180, 44602-44605, 44820-44850, 44950, 44970, 49000-49010, 49255, 49320-49321, 50605, 50650, 50715, 50800, 50810, 50820, 50825, 51045, 51520-51525, 51550-51595, 51701-51703, 52000, 52204, 58662, 62320-62327, 64400, 64405-64408, 64415-64435, 64445-64454, 64461-64463, 64479-64505, 64510-64530, 69990, 92012-92014, 93000-93010, 93040-93042, 93318, 93355, 94002, 94200, 94250, 94680-94690, 94770, 95812-95816, 95819, 95822, 95829, 95955, 96360-96368, 96372, 96374-96377, 96523, 97597-97598, 97602, 99155, 99156, 99157, 99211-99223, 99231-99255, 99291-99292, 99304-99310, 99315-99316, 99334-99337, 99347-99350, 99374-99375, 99377-99378, 99446-99449, 99451-99452, 99495-99496, G0463, G0471

51597 00910, 0213T, 0216T, 0228T, 0230T, 11000-11006, 11042-11047, 12001-12007, 12011-12057, 13100-13133, 13151-13153, 36000, 36400-36410, 36420-36430, 36440, 36591-36592, 36600, 36640, 38562-38564, 38571-38573, 38770, 38780, 43752, 44005, 44140-44151, 44155-44158, 44180, 44188, 44320-44346, 44602-44605, 44620-44625, 44820-44850, 44950-44970, 45110-45135, 45160, 45171-45172, 45190, 45395-45397, 45505, 45540, 46080-46200, 46220-46280, 46285, 46600-46601, 46940-46942, 46947-46948, 49000-49010, 49020, 49040, 49082-49084, 49203-49205, 49255, 49320-49321, 49560-49566, 49570, 49580, 49582-49587, 50650, 50715, 50800, 50810, 50860, 51040-51045, 51520-51525, 51550-51596, 51701-51703, 52000, 52204, 55821-55845, 55866, 57106, 57410, 57530-57556, 58100, 58120-58200, 58210-58263, 58267-58280, 58290-58294, 58541-58544, 58548, 58558, 58570-58575, 58660, 58662, 58950-58958, 62320-62327, 64400, 64405-64408, 64415-64435, 64445-64454, 64461-64463, 64479-64505, 64510-64530, 69990, 92012-92014, 93000-93010, 93040-93042, 93318, 93355, 94002, 94200, 94250, 94680-94690, 94770, 95812-95816, 95819, 95822, 95829, 95955, 96360-96368, 96372, 96374-96377, 96523, 97597-97598, 97602, 99155, 99156, 99157, 99211-99223, 99231-99255, 99291-99292, 99304-99310, 99315-99316, 99334-99337, 99347-99350, 99374-99375, 99377-99378, 99446-99449, 99451-99452, 99495-99496, G0463, G0471, P9612

51600 00910, 0213T, 0216T, 0228T, 0230T, 12001-12007, 12011-12057, 13100-13133, 13151-13153, 36000, 36400-36410, 36420-36430, 36440, 36591-36592, 36600, 36640, 43752, 50715, 51700-51703, 62320-62327, 64400, 64405-64408, 64415-64435, 64445-64454, 64461-64463, 64479-64505, 64510-64530, 69990, 76000, 77001-77002, 92012-92014, 93000-93010, 93040-93042, 93318, 93355, 94002, 94200, 94250, 94680-94690, 94770, 95812-95816, 95819, 95822, 95829, 95955, 96360-96368, 96372, 96374-96377, 96523, 99155, 99156, 99157, 99211-99223, 99231-99255, 99291-99292, 99304-99310, 99315-99316, 99334-99337, 99347-99350, 99374-99375, 99377-99378, 99446-99449, 99451-99452, 99495-99496, G0463, G0471, J0670, J2001, P9612

51605 00910, 0213T, 0216T, 0228T, 0230T, 12001-12007, 12011-12057, 13100-13133, 13151-13153, 36000, 36400-36410, 36420-36430, 36440, 36591-36592, 36600, 36640, 43752, 50715, 51700-51703, 62320-62327, 64400, 64405-64408, 64415-64435, 64445-64454, 64461-64463,

---

64479-64505, 64510-64530, 69990, 76000, 77001-77002, 92012-92014, 93000-93010, 93040-93042, 93318, 93355, 94002, 94200, 94250, 94680-94690, 94770, 95812-95816, 95819, 95822, 95829, 95955, 96360-96368, 96372, 96374-96377, 96523, 99155, 99156, 99157, 99211-99223, 99231-99255, 99291-99292, 99304-99310, 99315-99316, 99334-99337, 99347-99350, 99374-99375, 99377-99378, 99446-99449, 99451-99452, 99495-99496, G0463, G0471, J0670, J1644, J2001, P9612

51610 00910, 0213T, 0216T, 0228T, 0230T, 12001-12007, 12011-12057, 13100-13133, 13151-13153, 36000, 36400-36410, 36420-36430, 36440, 36591-36592, 36600, 36640, 43752, 50715, 51600, 51700-51703, 62320-62327, 64400, 64405-64408, 64415-64435, 64445-64454, 64461-64463, 64479-64505, 64510-64530, 69990, 76000, 77001-77002, 92012-92014, 93000-93010, 93040-93042, 93318, 93355, 94002, 94200, 94250, 94680-94690, 94770, 95812-95816, 95819, 95822, 95829, 95955, 96360-96368, 96372, 96374-96377, 96523, 99155, 99156, 99157, 99211-99223, 99231-99255, 99291-99292, 99304-99310, 99315-99316, 99334-99337, 99347-99350, 99374-99375, 99377-99378, 99446-99449, 99451-99452, 99495-99496, G0463, G0471, J2001, P9612

51700 00910, 0213T, 0216T, 0228T, 0230T, 12001-12007, 12011-12057, 13100-13133, 13151-13153, 36000, 36400-36410, 36420-36430, 36440, 36591-36592, 36600, 36640, 43752, 50715, 51701-51702, 62320-62327, 64400, 64405-64408, 64415-64435, 64445-64454, 64461-64463, 64479-64505, 64510-64530, 69990, 92012-92014, 93000-93010, 93040-93042, 93318, 93355, 94002, 94200, 94250, 94680-94690, 94770, 95812-95816, 95819, 95822, 95829, 95955, 96360-96368, 96372, 96374-96377, 96523, 99155, 99156, 99157, 99211-99223, 99231-99255, 99291-99292, 99304-99310, 99315-99316, 99334-99337, 99347-99350, 99374-99375, 99377-99378, 99446-99449, 99451-99452, 99495-99496, G0463, G0471, J0670, J2001, P9612

51701 0543T-0544T, 0548T, 0567T-0574T, 0580T, 0581T, 0582T, 11000-11006, 11042-11047, 13102, 13122, 13133, 13153, 20560-20561, 36400-36406, 36420-36430, 36440, 36591-36592, 36600, 64480, 64484, 66987-66988, 69990, 92012-92014, 93000-93010, 93040-93042, 93318, 93355, 94002, 94200, 94250, 94680-94690, 94770, 95812-95816, 95819, 95822, 95829, 95955, 96360-96368, 96372, 96374-96377, 96523, 97597-97598, 97602, 99155, 99156, 99157, 99211-99223, 99231-99255, 99291-99292, 99304-99310, 99315-99316, 99334-99337, 99347-99350, 99374-99375, 99377-99378, 99446-99449, 99451-99452, 99495-99496, G0463, J0670, J2001, P9612-P9615❖

51702 0543T-0544T, 0548T, 0567T-0574T, 0580T, 0581T, 0582T, 11000-11006, 11042-11047, 13102, 13122, 13133, 13153, 20560-20561, 36400-36406, 36420-36430, 36440, 36591-36592, 36600, 51701, 64480, 64484, 66987-66988, 69990, 92012-92014, 93000-93010, 93040-93042, 93318, 93355, 94002, 94200, 94250, 94680-94690, 94770, 95812-95816, 95819, 95822, 95829, 95955, 96360-96368, 96372, 96374-96377, 96523, 97597-97598, 97602, 99155, 99156, 99157, 99211-99223, 99231-99255, 99291-99292, 99304-99310, 99315-99316, 99334-99337, 99347-99350, 99374-99375, 99377-99378, 99446-99449, 99451-99452, 99495-99496, G0463, J0670, J2001, P9612

51703 0543T-0544T, 0548T, 0567T-0574T, 0580T, 0581T, 0582T, 11000-11006, 11042-11047, 13102, 13122, 13133, 13153, 20560-20561, 20701, 36400-36406, 36420-36430, 36440, 36591-36592, 36600, 51700-51702, 53080, 64415, 64417, 64450, 64480, 64484-64489, 66987-66988, 69990, 92012-92014, 93000-93010, 93040-93042, 93318, 93355, 94002, 94200, 94250, 94680-94690, 94770, 95812-95816, 95819, 95822, 95829, 95955, 96360-96368, 96372, 96374-96377, 96523, 97597-97598, 97602, 99155, 99156, 99157, 99211-99223, 99231-99255, 99291-99292, 99304-99310, 99315-99316, 99334-99337, 99347-99350, 99374-99375,

99377-99378, 99446-99449, 99451-99452, 99495-99496, G0463, G0471, J0670, J2001, P9612

51705 00910, 0213T, 0216T, 0228T, 0230T, 12001-12007, 12011-12057, 13100-13133, 13151-13153, 36000, 36400-36410, 36420-36430, 36440, 36591-36592, 36600, 36640, 43752, 50715, 51700-51703, 52000, 62320-62327, 64400, 64405-64408, 64415-64435, 64445-64454, 64461-64463, 64479-64505, 64510-64530, 69990, 76000, 76942, 76970, 76998, 77001-77002, 92012-92014, 93000-93010, 93040-93042, 93318, 93355, 94002, 94200, 94250, 94680-94690, 94770, 95812-95816, 95819, 95822, 95829, 95955, 96360-96368, 96372, 96374-96377, 96523, 99155, 99156, 99157, 99211-99223, 99231-99255, 99291-99292, 99304-99310, 99315-99316, 99334-99337, 99347-99350, 99374-99375, 99377-99378, 99446-99449, 99451-99452, 99495-99496, G0463, G0471

51710 00910, 0213T, 0216T, 0228T, 0230T, 12001-12007, 12011-12057, 13100-13133, 13151-13153, 36000, 36400-36410, 36420-36430, 36440, 36591-36592, 36600, 36640, 43752, 50715, 51701-51705, 52000, 62320-62327, 64400, 64405-64408, 64415-64435, 64445-64454, 64461-64463, 64479-64505, 64510-64530, 69990, 76000, 76942, 76970, 76998, 77001-77002, 92012-92014, 93000-93010, 93040-93042, 93318, 93355, 94002, 94200, 94250, 94680-94690, 94770, 95812-95816, 95819, 95822, 95829, 95955, 96360-96368, 96372, 96374-96377, 96523, 99155, 99156, 99157, 99211-99223, 99231-99255, 99291-99292, 99304-99310, 99315-99316, 99334-99337, 99347-99350, 99374-99375, 99377-99378, 99446-99449, 99451-99452, 99495-99496, G0463, G0471

51715 00910, 0213T, 0216T, 0228T, 0230T, 0499T, 12001-12007, 12011-12057, 13100-13133, 13151-13153, 36000, 36400-36410, 36420-36430, 36440, 36591-36592, 36600, 36640, 43752, 50715, 51701-51703, 52000-52007, 52010-52224, 52281, 52283-52287, 52332, 52356, 53000-53025, 62320-62327, 64400, 64405-64408, 64415-64435, 64445-64454, 64461-64463, 64479-64505, 64510-64530, 69990, 92012-92014, 93000-93010, 93040-93042, 93318, 93355, 94002, 94200, 94250, 94680-94690, 94770, 95812-95816, 95819, 95822, 95829, 95955, 96360-96368, 96372, 96374-96377, 96523, 99155, 99156, 99157, 99211-99223, 99231-99255, 99291-99292, 99304-99310, 99315-99316, 99334-99337, 99347-99350, 99374-99375, 99377-99378, 99446-99449, 99451-99452, 99495-99496, G0463, G0471, J2001, P9612

51720 00910, 0213T, 0216T, 0228T, 0230T, 12001-12007, 12011-12057, 13100-13133, 13151-13153, 36000, 36400-36410, 36420-36430, 36440, 36591-36592, 36600, 36640, 43752, 50715, 51700-51703, 52000, 62320-62327, 64400, 64405-64408, 64415-64435, 64445-64454, 64461-64463, 64479-64505, 64510-64530, 69990, 92012-92014, 93000-93010, 93040-93042, 93318, 93355, 94002, 94200, 94250, 94680-94690, 94770, 95812-95816, 95819, 95822, 95829, 95955, 96360-96368, 96372, 96374-96377, 96523, 99155, 99156, 99157, 99211-99223, 99231-99255, 99291-99292, 99304-99310, 99315-99316, 99334-99337, 99347-99350, 99374-99375, 99377-99378, 99446-99449, 99451-99452, 99495-99496, G0463, G0471, J0670, J2001, P9612

51725 00910, 0213T, 0216T, 0228T, 0230T, 12001-12007, 12011-12057, 13100-13133, 13151-13153, 36000, 36400-36410, 36420-36430, 36440, 36591-36592, 36600, 36640, 43752, 50715, 51701-51703, 62320-62327, 64400, 64405-64408, 64415-64435, 64445-64454, 64461-64463, 64479-64505, 64510-64530, 69990, 92012-92014, 93000-93010, 93040-93042, 93318, 93355, 94002, 94200, 94250, 94680-94690, 94770, 95812-95816, 95819, 95822, 95829, 95955, 96360-96368, 96372, 96374-96377, 96523, 99155, 99156, 99157, 99211-99223, 99231-99255, 99291-99292, 99304-99310, 99315-99316, 99334-99337, 99347-99350, 99374-99375, 99377-99378, 99446-99449, 99451-99452, 99495-99496, G0463, G0471, P9612

51726 00910, 0228T, 0230T, 12001-12007, 12011-12057, 13100-13133, 13151-13153, 36000, 36400-36410, 36420-36430, 36440, 36591-36592, 36600, 36640, 43752, 50715, 51701-51703, 51725, 62320-62327, 64400, 64405-64408, 64415-64435, 64445-64454, 64461-64463, 64479-64505, 64510-64530, 69990, 92012-92014, 93000-93010, 93040-93042, 93318, 93355, 94002, 94200, 94250, 94680-94690, 94770, 95812-95816, 95819, 95822, 95829, 95955, 96360-96368, 96372, 96374-96377, 96523, 99155, 99156, 99157, 99211-99223, 99231-99255, 99291-99292, 99304-99310, 99315-99316, 99334-99337, 99347-99350, 99374-99375, 99377-99378, 99446-99449, 99451-99452, 99495-99496, G0463, G0471, P9612

51727 00910, 0213T, 0216T, 0228T, 0230T, 11000-11006, 11042-11047, 12001-12007, 12011-12057, 13100-13133, 13151-13153, 36000, 36400-36410, 36420-36430, 36440, 36591-36592, 36600, 36640, 43752, 50715, 51701-51703, 51725-51726, 62320-62327, 64400, 64405-64408, 64415-64435, 64445-64454, 64461-64463, 64479-64505, 64510-64530, 69990, 92012-92014, 93000-93010, 93040-93042, 93318, 93355, 94002, 94200, 94250, 94680-94690, 94770, 95812-95816, 95819, 95822, 95829, 95955, 96360-96368, 96372, 96374-96377, 96523, 97597-97598, 97602, 99155, 99156, 99157, 99211-99223, 99231-99255, 99291-99292, 99304-99310, 99315-99316, 99334-99337, 99347-99350, 99374-99375, 99377-99378, 99446-99449, 99451-99452, 99495-99496, G0463, G0471, J0670, J2001, P9612

51728 00910, 0213T, 0216T, 0228T, 0230T, 12001-12007, 12011-12057, 13100-13133, 13151-13153, 36000, 36400-36410, 36420-36430, 36440, 36591-36592, 36600, 36640, 43752, 50715, 51701-51703, 51725-51727, 62320-62327, 64400, 64405-64408, 64415-64435, 64445-64454, 64461-64463, 64479-64505, 64510-64530, 69990, 90901, 92012-92014, 93000-93010, 93040-93042, 93318, 93355, 94002, 94200, 94250, 94680-94690, 94770, 95812-95816, 95819, 95822, 95829, 95955, 96360-96368, 96372, 96374-96377, 96523, 99155, 99156, 99157, 99211-99223, 99231-99255, 99291-99292, 99304-99310, 99315-99316, 99334-99337, 99347-99350, 99374-99375, 99377-99378, 99446-99449, 99451-99452, 99495-99496, G0463, G0471, J0670, J2001, P9612

51729 00910, 0213T, 0216T, 0228T, 0230T, 11000-11006, 11042-11047, 12001-12007, 12011-12057, 13100-13133, 13151-13153, 36000, 36400-36410, 36420-36430, 36440, 36591-36592, 36600, 36640, 43752, 50715, 51701-51703, 51725-51728, 62320-62327, 64400, 64405-64408, 64415-64435, 64445-64454, 64461-64463, 64479-64505, 64510-64530, 69990, 90901, 92012-92014, 93000-93010, 93040-93042, 93318, 93355, 94002, 94200, 94250, 94680-94690, 94770, 95812-95816, 95819, 95822, 95829, 95955, 96360-96368, 96372, 96374-96377, 96523, 97597-97598, 97602, 99155, 99156, 99157, 99211-99223, 99231-99255, 99291-99292, 99304-99310, 99315-99316, 99334-99337, 99347-99350, 99374-99375, 99377-99378, 99446-99449, 99451-99452, 99495-99496, G0463, G0471, J0670, J2001, P9612

51736 00910, 0213T, 0216T, 0228T, 0230T, 36000, 36400-36410, 36420-36430, 36440, 36591-36592, 36600, 36640, 43752, 50715, 51701-51703, 61650, 62320-62327, 64400, 64405-64408, 64415-64435, 64445-64454, 64461, 64463, 64479, 64483, 64486-64490, 64493, 64505, 64510-64530, 69990, 93000-93010, 93040-93042, 93318, 93355, 94002, 94200, 94250, 94680-94690, 94770, 95812-95816, 95819, 95822, 95829, 95955, 96360, 96365, 96372, 96374-96377, 96523, 99155, 99156, 99157, G0471, P9612

51741 00910, 0213T, 0216T, 0228T, 0230T, 36000, 36400-36410, 36420-36430, 36440, 36591-36592, 36600, 36640, 43752, 50715, 51701-51703, 51736, 61650, 62320-62327, 64400, 64405-64408, 64415-64435, 64445-64454, 64461, 64463, 64479, 64483, 64486-64490, 64493, 64505, 64510-64530, 69990, 93000-93010, 93040-93042, 93318, 93355,

CPT © 2020 American Medical Association. All Rights Reserved.

Coding Companion for Urology/Nephrology

94002, 94200, 94250, 94680-94690, 94770, 95812-95816, 95819,
95822, 95829, 95955, 96360, 96365, 96372, 96374-96377, 96523,
99155, 99156, 99157, G0471, P9612

51784 00910, 0213T, 0216T, 0228T, 0230T, 0333T, 0464T, 12001-12007,
12011-12057, 13100-13133, 13151-13153, 36000, 36400-36410,
36420-36430, 36440, 36591-36592, 36600, 36640, 43752, 50715,
51701, 51703, 51785, 62320-62327, 64400, 64405-64408, 64415-64435,
64445-64454, 64461, 64463, 64479, 64483, 64486-64490, 64493,
64505, 64510-64530, 69990, 92012-92014, 92585, 93000-93010,
93040-93042, 93318, 93355, 94002, 94200, 94250, 94680-94690,
94770, 95812-95816, 95819, 95822, 95829, 95860-95861, 95867-95868,
95870, 95907-95913, 95925-95927, 95930-95933, 95937, 95940, 95955,
96360-96368, 96372, 96374-96377, 96523, 99155, 99156, 99157,
99211-99223, 99231-99255, 99291-99292, 99304-99310, 99315-99316,
99334-99337, 99347-99350, 99374-99375, 99377-99378, 99446-99449,
99451-99452, 99495-99496, G0453, G0463

51785 00910, 0213T, 0216T, 0228T, 0230T, 0333T, 0464T, 12001-12007,
12011-12057, 13100-13133, 13151-13153, 36000, 36400-36410,
36420-36430, 36440, 36591-36592, 36600, 36640, 43752, 50715,
51701-51703, 62320-62327, 64400, 64405-64408, 64415-64435,
64445-64454, 64461, 64463, 64479, 64483, 64486-64490, 64493,
64505, 64510-64530, 69990, 92012-92014, 92585, 93000-93010,
93040-93042, 93318, 93355, 94002, 94200, 94250, 94680-94690,
94770, 95812-95816, 95819, 95822, 95829, 95860-95861, 95867-95868,
95870, 95907-95913, 95925-95927, 95930-95933, 95937, 95940, 95955,
96360-96368, 96372, 96374-96377, 96523, 99155, 99156, 99157,
99211-99223, 99231-99255, 99291-99292, 99304-99310, 99315-99316,
99334-99337, 99347-99350, 99374-99375, 99377-99378, 99446-99449,
99451-99452, 99495-99496, G0453, G0463, G0471, P9612

51792 00910, 0213T, 0216T, 0228T, 0230T, 12001-12007, 12011-12057,
13100-13133, 13151-13153, 36000, 36400-36410, 36420-36430, 36440,
36591-36592, 36600, 36640, 43752, 50715, 51701-51703, 51784,
62320-62327, 64400, 64405-64408, 64415-64435, 64445-64454,
64461-64463, 64479-64505, 64510-64530, 69990, 92012-92014,
93000-93010, 93040-93042, 93318, 93355, 94002, 94200, 94250,
94680-94690, 94770, 95812-95816, 95819, 95822, 95829, 95870,
95955, 96360-96368, 96372, 96374-96377, 96523, 99155, 99156,
99157, 99211-99223, 99231-99255, 99291-99292, 99304-99310,
99315-99316, 99334-99337, 99347-99350, 99374-99375, 99377-99378,
99446-99449, 99451-99452, 99495-99496, G0463, G0471, P9612

51797 36591-36592, 96523

51798 0213T, 0216T, 36591-36592, 61650, 62324-62327, 64415, 64417,
64450, 64454, 64486-64490, 64493, 69990, 96523, 99211

51800 00910, 0213T, 0216T, 0228T, 0230T, 11000-11006, 11042-11047,
12001-12007, 12011-12057, 13100-13133, 13151-13153, 36000,
36400-36410, 36420-36430, 36440, 36591-36592, 36600, 36640, 43752,
44602-44605, 44950, 44970, 49000-49002, 49320, 50605, 50715,
51550, 51701-51703, 51860-51865, 52000, 53000-53025, 62320-62327,
64400, 64405-64408, 64415-64435, 64445-64454, 64461-64463,
64479-64505, 64510-64530, 69990, 92012-92014, 93000-93010,
93040-93042, 93318, 93355, 94002, 94200, 94250, 94680-94690,
94770, 95812-95816, 95819, 95822, 95829, 95955, 96360-96368,
96372, 96374-96377, 96523, 97597-97598, 97602, 99155, 99156,
99157, 99211-99223, 99231-99255, 99291-99292, 99304-99310,
99315-99316, 99334-99337, 99347-99350, 99374-99375, 99377-99378,
99446-99449, 99451-99452, 99495-99496, G0463, G0471

51820 00910, 0213T, 0216T, 0228T, 0230T, 11000-11006, 11042-11047,
12001-12007, 12011-12057, 13100-13133, 13151-13153, 36000,
36400-36410, 36420-36430, 36440, 36591-36592, 36600, 36640, 43752,

44602-44605, 44850, 44950, 44970, 49000-49010, 49320, 50605,
50715, 50780, 51701-51703, 51800, 51860-51865, 52000, 53000-53025,
62320-62327, 64400, 64405-64408, 64415-64435, 64445-64454,
64461-64463, 64479-64505, 64510-64530, 69990, 92012-92014,
93000-93010, 93040-93042, 93318, 93355, 94002, 94200, 94250,
94680-94690, 94770, 95812-95816, 95819, 95822, 95829, 95955,
96360-96368, 96372, 96374-96377, 96523, 97597-97598, 97602, 99155,
99156, 99157, 99211-99223, 99231-99255, 99291-99292, 99304-99310,
99315-99316, 99334-99337, 99347-99350, 99374-99375, 99377-99378,
99446-99449, 99451-99452, 99495-99496, G0463, G0471

51840 00910, 0213T, 0216T, 0228T, 0230T, 12001-12007, 12011-12057,
13100-13133, 13151-13153, 36000, 36400-36410, 36420-36430, 36440,
36591-36592, 36600, 36640, 43752, 44602-44605, 44950, 44970,
49000-49002, 49320, 50715, 51040, 51595✦, 51701-51703,
52000-52005, 53000-53025, 53660-53661, 62320-62327, 64400,
64405-64408, 64415-64435, 64445-64454, 64461-64463, 64479-64505,
64510-64530, 69990, 92012-92014, 93000-93010, 93040-93042, 93318,
93355, 94002, 94200, 94250, 94680-94690, 94770, 95812-95816,
95819, 95822, 95829, 95955, 96360-96368, 96372, 96374-96377,
96523, 99155, 99156, 99157, 99211-99223, 99231-99255, 99291-99292,
99304-99310, 99315-99316, 99334-99337, 99347-99350, 99374-99375,
99377-99378, 99446-99449, 99451-99452, 99495-99496, G0463, G0471

51841 00910, 0213T, 0216T, 0228T, 0230T, 12001-12007, 12011-12057,
13100-13133, 13151-13153, 36000, 36400-36410, 36420-36430, 36440,
36591-36592, 36600, 36640, 43752, 44602-44605, 44950, 44970,
49000-49002, 49320, 50715, 51595✦, 51701-51703, 51840,
52000-52001, 53000-53025, 57285✦, 62320-62327, 64400,
64405-64408, 64415-64435, 64445-64454, 64461-64463, 64479-64505,
64510-64530, 69990, 92012-92014, 93000-93010, 93040-93042, 93318,
93355, 94002, 94200, 94250, 94680-94690, 94770, 95812-95816,
95819, 95822, 95829, 95955, 96360-96368, 96372, 96374-96377,
96523, 99155, 99156, 99157, 99211-99223, 99231-99255, 99291-99292,
99304-99310, 99315-99316, 99334-99337, 99347-99350, 99374-99375,
99377-99378, 99446-99449, 99451-99452, 99495-99496, G0463, G0471

51845 00910, 0213T, 0216T, 0228T, 0230T, 12001-12007, 12011-12057,
13100-13133, 13151-13153, 36000, 36400-36410, 36420-36430, 36440,
36591-36592, 36600, 36640, 43752, 44602-44605, 44820-44850, 44950,
44970, 49000-49010, 49255, 49320, 50715, 51040, 51701-51703,
51840-51841✦, 52000-52005, 52281, 52332, 52356, 53660-53661,
57250, 57265, 57289, 62320-62327, 64400, 64405-64408, 64415-64435,
64445-64454, 64461-64463, 64479-64505, 64510-64530, 69990,
92012-92014, 93000-93010, 93040-93042, 93318, 93355, 94002, 94200,
94250, 94680-94690, 94770, 95812-95816, 95819, 95822, 95829,
95955, 96360-96368, 96372, 96374-96377, 96523, 99155, 99156,
99157, 99211-99223, 99231-99255, 99291-99292, 99304-99310,
99315-99316, 99334-99337, 99347-99350, 99374-99375, 99377-99378,
99446-99449, 99451-99452, 99495-99496, G0463, G0471

51860 00910, 0213T, 0216T, 0228T, 0230T, 12001-12007, 12011-12057,
13100-13133, 13151-13153, 36000, 36400-36410, 36420-36430, 36440,
36591-36592, 36600, 36640, 43752, 44602-44605, 44850, 44950,
44970, 49000-49010, 49255, 49320, 50715, 51701-51703, 52000,
62320-62327, 64400, 64405-64408, 64415-64435, 64445-64454,
64461-64463, 64479-64505, 64510-64530, 69990, 92012-92014,
93000-93010, 93040-93042, 93318, 93355, 94002, 94200, 94250,
94680-94690, 94770, 95812-95816, 95819, 95822, 95829, 95955,
96360-96368, 96372, 96374-96377, 96523, 99155, 99156, 99157,
99211-99223, 99231-99255, 99291-99292, 99304-99310, 99315-99316,
99334-99337, 99347-99350, 99374-99375, 99377-99378, 99446-99449,
99451-99452, 99495-99496, G0463, G0471

51865 00910, 0213T, 0216T, 0228T, 0230T, 12001-12007, 12011-12057, 13100-13133, 13151-13153, 36000, 36400-36410, 36420-36430, 36440, 36591-36592, 36600, 36640, 43752, 44005, 44180, 44602-44605, 44850, 44950, 44970, 49000-49010, 49255, 49320, 50715, 51040, 51701-51703, 51860, 52000, 62320-62327, 64400, 64405-64408, 64415-64435, 64445-64454, 64461-64463, 64479-64505, 64510-64530, 69990, 92012-92014, 93000-93010, 93040-93042, 93318, 93355, 94002, 94200, 94250, 94680-94690, 94770, 95812-95816, 95819, 95822, 95829, 95955, 96360-96368, 96372, 96374-96377, 96523, 99155, 99156, 99157, 99211-99223, 99231-99255, 99291-99292, 99304-99310, 99315-99316, 99334-99337, 99347-99350, 99374-99375, 99377-99378, 99446-99449, 99451-99452, 99495-99496, G0463, G0471

51880 00910, 0213T, 0216T, 0228T, 0230T, 11000-11006, 11042-11047, 12001-12007, 12011-12057, 13100-13133, 13151-13153, 36000, 36400-36410, 36420-36430, 36440, 36591-36592, 36600, 36640, 43752, 44950, 44970, 50715, 51701-51703, 52000, 62320-62327, 64400, 64405-64408, 64415-64435, 64445-64454, 64461-64463, 64479-64505, 64510-64530, 69990, 92012-92014, 93000-93010, 93040-93042, 93318, 93355, 94002, 94200, 94250, 94680-94690, 94770, 95812-95816, 95819, 95822, 95829, 95955, 96360-96368, 96372, 96374-96377, 96523, 97597-97598, 97602, 99155, 99156, 99157, 99211-99223, 99231-99255, 99291-99292, 99304-99310, 99315-99316, 99334-99337, 99347-99350, 99374-99375, 99377-99378, 99446-99449, 99451-99452, 99495-99496, G0463, G0471

51900 00910, 0213T, 0216T, 0228T, 0230T, 11000-11006, 11042-11047, 12001-12007, 12011-12057, 13100-13133, 13151-13153, 36000, 36400-36410, 36420-36430, 36440, 36591-36592, 36600, 36640, 43752, 44602-44605, 44850, 44950, 44970, 49000-49010, 49255, 49320, 50715, 51701-51703, 51860-51880, 52000, 62320-62327, 64400, 64405-64408, 64415-64435, 64445-64454, 64461-64463, 64479-64505, 64510-64530, 69990, 92012-92014, 93000-93010, 93040-93042, 93318, 93355, 94002, 94200, 94250, 94680-94690, 94770, 95812-95816, 95819, 95822, 95829, 95955, 96360-96368, 96372, 96374-96377, 96523, 97597-97598, 97602, 99155, 99156, 99157, 99211-99223, 99231-99255, 99291-99292, 99304-99310, 99315-99316, 99334-99337, 99347-99350, 99374-99375, 99377-99378, 99446-99449, 99451-99452, 99495-99496, G0463, G0471

51920 00910, 0213T, 0216T, 0228T, 0230T, 11000-11006, 11042-11047, 12001-12007, 12011-12057, 13100-13133, 13151-13153, 36000, 36400-36410, 36420-36430, 36440, 36591-36592, 36600, 36640, 43752, 44602-44605, 44850, 44950, 44970, 49000-49010, 49255, 49320, 50715, 51701-51703, 51860-51880, 52000, 62320-62327, 64400, 64405-64408, 64415-64435, 64445-64454, 64461-64463, 64479-64505, 64510-64530, 69990, 92012-92014, 93000-93010, 93040-93042, 93318, 93355, 94002, 94200, 94250, 94680-94690, 94770, 95812-95816, 95819, 95822, 95829, 95955, 96360-96368, 96372, 96374-96377, 96523, 97597-97598, 97602, 99155, 99156, 99157, 99211-99223, 99231-99255, 99291-99292, 99304-99310, 99315-99316, 99334-99337, 99347-99350, 99374-99375, 99377-99378, 99446-99449, 99451-99452, 99495-99496, G0463, G0471

51925 00910, 0213T, 0216T, 0228T, 0230T, 11000-11006, 11042-11047, 12001-12007, 12011-12057, 13100-13133, 13151-13153, 36000, 36400-36410, 36420-36430, 36440, 36591-36592, 36600, 36640, 43752, 44005, 44180, 44602-44605, 44850, 44950, 44970, 49000-49010, 49255, 49320-49321, 50715, 51701-51703, 51860-51880, 51920, 52000, 57505, 57530, 57550-57555♦, 57558, 58120-58140, 58146-58180, 58260-58263, 58267-58280, 58290-58294, 58545-58546, 58561, 62320-62327, 64400, 64405-64408, 64415-64435, 64445-64454, 64461-64463, 64479-64505, 64510-64530, 69990, 92012-92014, 93000-93010, 93040-93042, 93318, 93355, 94002, 94200, 94250,

94680-94690, 94770, 95812-95816, 95819, 95822, 95829, 95955, 96360-96368, 96372, 96374-96377, 96523, 97597-97598, 97602, 99155, 99156, 99157, 99211-99223, 99231-99255, 99291-99292, 99304-99310, 99315-99316, 99334-99337, 99347-99350, 99374-99375, 99377-99378, 99446-99449, 99451-99452, 99495-99496, G0463, G0471

51940 00910, 0213T, 0216T, 0228T, 0230T, 11000-11006, 11042-11047, 12001-12007, 12011-12057, 13100-13133, 13151-13153, 36000, 36400-36410, 36420-36430, 36440, 36591-36592, 36600, 36640, 43752, 44602-44605, 44850, 44950, 44970, 49000-49010, 49255, 50715, 51701-51703, 51880, 52000, 62320-62327, 64400, 64405-64408, 64415-64435, 64445-64454, 64461-64463, 64479-64505, 64510-64530, 69990, 92012-92014, 93000-93010, 93040-93042, 93318, 93355, 94002, 94200, 94250, 94680-94690, 94770, 95812-95816, 95819, 95822, 95829, 95955, 96360-96368, 96372, 96374-96377, 96523, 97597-97598, 97602, 99155, 99156, 99157, 99211-99223, 99231-99255, 99291-99292, 99304-99310, 99315-99316, 99334-99337, 99347-99350, 99374-99375, 99377-99378, 99446-99449, 99451-99452, 99495-99496, G0463, G0471

51960 00910, 0213T, 0216T, 0228T, 0230T, 11000-11006, 11042-11047, 12001-12007, 12011-12057, 13100-13133, 13151-13153, 36000, 36400-36410, 36420-36430, 36440, 36591-36592, 36600, 36640, 43752, 44005, 44180, 44602-44605, 44661, 44820-44850, 44950, 44970, 45800, 49000-49010, 49255, 49320, 50715, 51701-51703, 52000, 62320-62327, 64400, 64405-64408, 64415-64435, 64445-64454, 64461-64463, 64479-64505, 64510-64530, 69990, 92012-92014, 93000-93010, 93040-93042, 93318, 93355, 94002, 94200, 94250, 94680-94690, 94770, 95812-95816, 95819, 95822, 95829, 95955, 96360-96368, 96372, 96374-96377, 96523, 97597-97598, 97602, 99155, 99156, 99157, 99211-99223, 99231-99255, 99291-99292, 99304-99310, 99315-99316, 99334-99337, 99347-99350, 99374-99375, 99377-99378, 99446-99449, 99451-99452, 99495-99496, G0463, G0471

51980 00910, 0213T, 0216T, 0228T, 0230T, 12001-12007, 12011-12057, 13100-13133, 13151-13153, 36000, 36400-36410, 36420-36430, 36440, 36591-36592, 36600, 36640, 43752, 44602-44605, 44850, 44950, 44970, 49000-49002, 49320, 50715, 51701-51703, 51880, 52000, 62320-62327, 64400, 64405-64408, 64415-64435, 64445-64454, 64461-64463, 64479-64505, 64510-64530, 69990, 92012-92014, 93000-93010, 93040-93042, 93318, 93355, 94002, 94200, 94250, 94680-94690, 94770, 95812-95816, 95819, 95822, 95829, 95955, 96360-96368, 96372, 96374-96377, 96523, 99155, 99156, 99157, 99211-99223, 99231-99255, 99291-99292, 99304-99310, 99315-99316, 99334-99337, 99347-99350, 99374-99375, 99377-99378, 99446-99449, 99451-99452, 99495-99496, G0463, G0471

51990 00910, 0213T, 0216T, 0228T, 0230T, 12001-12007, 12011-12057, 13100-13133, 13151-13153, 36000, 36400-36410, 36420-36430, 36440, 36591-36592, 36600, 36640, 43653, 43752, 44005, 44180, 44602-44605, 44950, 44970, 49082-49084, 49320, 49400, 50715, 51701-51703, 51992♦, 52000, 57285, 58660, 62320-62327, 64400, 64405-64408, 64415-64435, 64445-64454, 64461-64463, 64479-64505, 64510-64530, 69990, 76000, 77001-77002, 92012-92014, 93000-93010, 93040-93042, 93318, 93355, 94002, 94200, 94250, 94680-94690, 94770, 95812-95816, 95819, 95822, 95829, 95955, 96360-96368, 96372, 96374-96377, 96523, 99155, 99156, 99157, 99211-99223, 99231-99255, 99291-99292, 99304-99310, 99315-99316, 99334-99337, 99347-99350, 99374-99375, 99377-99378, 99446-99449, 99451-99452, 99495-99496, G0463, G0471

51992 00910, 0213T, 0216T, 0228T, 0230T, 12001-12007, 12011-12057, 13100-13133, 13151-13153, 36000, 36400-36410, 36420-36430, 36440, 36591-36592, 36600, 36640, 43653, 43752, 44005, 44180, 44602-44605, 44950, 44970, 49082-49084, 49320, 49400, 50715,

CCI Edits

51701-51703, 52000, 53000-53025, 58660, 62320-62327, 64400, 64405-64408, 64415-64435, 64445-64454, 64461-64463, 64479-64505, 64510-64530, 69990, 76000, 77001-77002, 92012-92014, 93000-93010, 93040-93042, 93318, 93355, 94002, 94200, 94250, 94680-94690, 94770, 95812-95816, 95819, 95822, 95829, 95955, 96360-96368, 96372, 96374-96377, 96523, 99155, 99156, 99157, 99211-99223, 99231-99255, 99291-99292, 99304-99310, 99315-99316, 99334-99337, 99347-99350, 99374-99375, 99377-99378, 99446-99449, 99451-99452, 99495-99496, G0463, G0471

52000 00910, 00916, 0213T, 0216T, 0228T, 0230T, 0548T, 0582T, 12001-12007, 12011-12057, 13100-13133, 13151-13153, 36000, 36400-36410, 36420-36430, 36440, 36591-36592, 36600, 36640, 43752, 51700-51703, 53000-53025, 53600-53621, 53660-53665, 57410, 62320-62327, 64400, 64405-64408, 64415-64435, 64445-64454, 64461-64463, 64479-64505, 64510-64530, 69990, 76000, 77001-77002, 92012-92014, 93000-93010, 93040-93042, 93318, 93355, 94002, 94200, 94250, 94680-94690, 94770, 95812-95816, 95819, 95822, 95829, 95955, 96360-96368, 96372, 96374-96377, 96523, 99155, 99156, 99157, 99211-99223, 99231-99255, 99291-99292, 99304-99310, 99315-99316, 99334-99337, 99347-99350, 99374-99375, 99377-99378, 99446-99449, 99451-99452, 99495-99496, C9738, G0463, G0471, J2001, P9612

52001 00910, 00916, 0213T, 0216T, 0228T, 0230T, 12001-12007, 12011-12057, 13100-13133, 13151-13153, 36000, 36400-36410, 36420-36430, 36440, 36591-36592, 36600, 36640, 43752, 51700-51703, 52000, 52281, 53000-53025, 53600-53621, 53660-53661, 57410, 62320-62327, 64400, 64405-64408, 64415-64435, 64445-64454, 64461-64463, 64479-64505, 64510-64530, 76000, 77001-77002, 92012-92014, 93000-93010, 93040-93042, 93318, 93355, 94002, 94200, 94250, 94680-94690, 94770, 95812-95816, 95819, 95822, 95829, 95955, 96360-96368, 96372, 96374-96377, 96523, 99155, 99156, 99157, 99211-99223, 99231-99255, 99291-99292, 99304-99310, 99315-99316, 99334-99337, 99347-99350, 99374-99375, 99377-99378, 99446-99449, 99451-99452, 99495-99496, G0463, G0471, P9612

52005 00910, 00916, 0213T, 0216T, 0228T, 0230T, 12001-12007, 12011-12057, 13100-13133, 13151-13153, 36000, 36400-36410, 36420-36430, 36440, 36591-36592, 36600, 36640, 43752, 50684, 51600, 51610-51703, 52000-52001, 52265♦, 52310-52315, 53000-53025, 53600-53621, 53660-53665, 57410, 62320-62327, 64400, 64405-64408, 64415-64435, 64445-64454, 64461-64463, 64479-64505, 64510-64530, 69990, 76000, 77001-77002, 92012-92014, 93000-93010, 93040-93042, 93318, 93355, 94002, 94200, 94250, 94680-94690, 94770, 95812-95816, 95819, 95822, 95829, 95955, 96360-96368, 96372, 96374-96377, 96523, 99155, 99156, 99157, 99211-99223, 99231-99255, 99291-99292, 99304-99310, 99315-99316, 99334-99337, 99347-99350, 99374-99375, 99377-99378, 99446-99449, 99451-99452, 99495-99496, G0463, G0471, P9612

52007 00910, 00916, 0213T, 0216T, 0228T, 0230T, 10005, 10007, 10009, 10011, 10021, 12001-12007, 12011-12057, 13100-13133, 13151-13153, 36000, 36400-36410, 36420-36430, 36440, 36591-36592, 36600, 36640, 43752, 50606, 50684, 51700-51703, 52000-52005, 52204, 52281, 52310-52315, 53000-53025, 53600-53621, 53660-53665, 57410, 62320-62327, 64400, 64405-64408, 64415-64435, 64445-64454, 64461-64463, 64479-64505, 64510-64530, 69990, 76000, 77001-77002, 92012-92014, 93000-93010, 93040-93042, 93318, 93355, 94002, 94200, 94250, 94680-94690, 94770, 95812-95816, 95819, 95822, 95829, 95955, 96360-96368, 96372, 96374-96377, 96523, 99155, 99156, 99157, 99211-99223, 99231-99255, 99291-99292, 99304-99310, 99315-99316, 99334-99337, 99347-99350, 99374-99375, 99377-99378, 99446-99449, 99451-99452, 99495-99496, G0463, G0471, P9612

52010 00910, 00916, 0213T, 0216T, 0228T, 0230T, 12001-12007, 12011-12057, 13100-13133, 13151-13153, 36000, 36400-36410, 36420-36430, 36440, 36591-36592, 36600, 36640, 43752, 51701-51703, 52000-52001, 52250♦, 52281, 52310-52315, 53000-53025, 53600-53621, 53660-53665, 57410, 62320-62327, 64400, 64405-64408, 64415-64435, 64445-64454, 64461-64463, 64479-64505, 64510-64530, 69990, 76000, 77001-77002, 92012-92014, 93000-93010, 93040-93042, 93318, 93355, 94002, 94200, 94250, 94680-94690, 94770, 95812-95816, 95819, 95822, 95829, 95955, 96360-96368, 96372, 96374-96377, 96523, 99155, 99156, 99157, 99211-99223, 99231-99255, 99291-99292, 99304-99310, 99315-99316, 99334-99337, 99347-99350, 99374-99375, 99377-99378, 99446-99449, 99451-99452, 99495-99496, G0463, G0471, J2001, P9612

52204 00910, 00916, 0213T, 0216T, 0228T, 0230T, 10005, 10007, 10009, 10011, 10021, 12001-12007, 12011-12057, 13100-13133, 13151-13153, 36000, 36400-36410, 36420-36430, 36440, 36591-36592, 36600, 36640, 43752, 51700-51703, 52000-52005, 52310-52315, 53000-53025, 53600-53621, 53660-53665, 57410, 62320-62327, 64400, 64405-64408, 64415-64435, 64445-64454, 64461-64463, 64479-64505, 64510-64530, 69990, 76000, 77001-77002, 92012-92014, 93000-93010, 93040-93042, 93318, 93355, 94002, 94200, 94250, 94680-94690, 94770, 95812-95816, 95819, 95822, 95829, 95955, 96360-96368, 96372, 96374-96377, 96523, 99155, 99156, 99157, 99211-99223, 99231-99255, 99291-99292, 99304-99310, 99315-99316, 99334-99337, 99347-99350, 99374-99375, 99377-99378, 99446-99449, 99451-99452, 99495-99496, G0463, G0471, P9612

52214 00910-00912, 00916, 0213T, 0216T, 0228T, 0230T, 12001-12007, 12011-12057, 13100-13133, 13151-13153, 36000, 36400-36410, 36420-36430, 36440, 36591-36592, 36600, 36640, 43752, 51701-51703, 52000-52005, 52204, 52224, 52250-52265, 52281, 52310-52315, 52500♦, 53000-53025, 53600-53621, 53660-53665, 57410, 62320-62327, 64400, 64405-64408, 64415-64435, 64445-64454, 64461-64463, 64479-64505, 64510-64530, 69990, 76000, 77001-77002, 92012-92014, 93000-93010, 93040-93042, 93318, 93355, 94002, 94200, 94250, 94680-94690, 94770, 95812-95816, 95819, 95822, 95829, 95955, 96360-96368, 96372, 96374-96377, 96523, 99155, 99156, 99157, 99211-99223, 99231-99255, 99291-99292, 99304-99310, 99315-99316, 99334-99337, 99347-99350, 99374-99375, 99377-99378, 99446-99449, 99451-99452, 99495-99496, G0463, G0471, J0670, J2001, P9612

52224 00910-00912, 00916, 0213T, 0216T, 0228T, 0230T, 10005, 10007, 10009, 10011, 10021, 12001-12007, 12011-12057, 13100-13133, 13151-13153, 36000, 36400-36410, 36420-36430, 36440, 36591-36592, 36600, 36640, 43752, 51701-51703, 51720, 52000-52005, 52204, 52260, 52281, 52310-52315, 53000-53025, 53600-53621, 53660-53665, 57410, 62320-62327, 64400, 64405-64408, 64415-64435, 64445-64454, 64461-64463, 64479-64505, 64510-64530, 69990, 76000, 77001-77002, 92012-92014, 93000-93010, 93040-93042, 93318, 93355, 94002, 94200, 94250, 94680-94690, 94770, 95812-95816, 95819, 95822, 95829, 95955, 96360-96368, 96372, 96374-96377, 96523, 99155, 99156, 99157, 99211-99223, 99231-99255, 99291-99292, 99304-99310, 99315-99316, 99334-99337, 99347-99350, 99374-99375, 99377-99378, 99446-99449, 99451-99452, 99495-99496, G0463, G0471, J0670, J2001, P9612

52234 00910-00912, 00916, 0213T, 0216T, 0228T, 0230T, 11000-11006, 11042-11047, 12001-12007, 12011-12057, 13100-13133, 13151-13153, 36000, 36400-36410, 36420-36430, 36440, 36591-36592, 36600, 36640, 43752, 51700-51703, 51720, 52000-52005, 52204-52224, 52276, 52281, 52310-52315, 52332, 52356, 53000-53025, 53600-53621, 53660-53665, 57410, 62320-62327, 64400, 64405-64408, 64415-64435, 64445-64454,

CCI Edits

64461-64463, 64479-64505, 64510-64530, 69990, 76000, 77001-77002, 92012-92014, 93000-93010, 93040-93042, 93318, 93355, 94002, 94200, 94250, 94680-94690, 94770, 95812-95816, 95819, 95822, 95829, 95955, 96360-96368, 96372, 96374-96377, 96523, 97597-97598, 97602, 99155, 99156, 99157, 99211-99223, 99231-99255, 99291-99292, 99304-99310, 99315-99316, 99334-99337, 99347-99350, 99374-99375, 99377-99378, 99446-99449, 99451-99452, 99495-99496, G0463, G0471, P9612

52235 00910-00912, 00916, 0213T, 0216T, 0228T, 0230T, 11000-11006, 11042-11047, 12001-12007, 12011-12057, 13100-13133, 13151-13153, 36000, 36400-36410, 36420-36430, 36440, 36591-36592, 36600, 36640, 43752, 51700-51703, 51720, 52000-52005, 52204-52234, 52276, 52281, 52310-52315, 52332, 53000-53025, 53600-53621, 53660-53665, 57410, 62320-62327, 64400, 64405-64408, 64415-64435, 64445-64454, 64461-64463, 64479-64505, 64510-64530, 69990, 76000, 77001-77002, 92012-92014, 93000-93010, 93040-93042, 93318, 93355, 94002, 94200, 94250, 94680-94690, 94770, 95812-95816, 95819, 95822, 95829, 95955, 96360-96368, 96372, 96374-96377, 96523, 97597-97598, 97602, 99155, 99156, 99157, 99211-99223, 99231-99255, 99291-99292, 99304-99310, 99315-99316, 99334-99337, 99347-99350, 99374-99375, 99377-99378, 99446-99449, 99451-99452, 99495-99496, G0463, G0471, P9612

52240 00910-00912, 00916, 0213T, 0216T, 0228T, 0230T, 11000-11006, 11042-11047, 12001-12007, 12011-12057, 13100-13133, 13151-13153, 36000, 36400-36410, 36420-36430, 36440, 36591-36592, 36600, 36640, 43752, 51700-51703, 51720, 52000-52005, 52204-52235, 52276, 52281, 52310-52317, 52332, 52356-52400, 53000-53025, 53600-53621, 53660-53665, 57410, 62320-62327, 64400, 64405-64408, 64415-64435, 64445-64454, 64461-64463, 64479-64505, 64510-64530, 69990, 76000, 77001-77002, 92012-92014, 93000-93010, 93040-93042, 93318, 93355, 94002, 94200, 94250, 94680-94690, 94770, 95812-95816, 95819, 95822, 95829, 95955, 96360-96368, 96372, 96374-96377, 96523, 97597-97598, 97602, 99155, 99156, 99157, 99211-99223, 99231-99255, 99291-99292, 99304-99310, 99315-99316, 99334-99337, 99347-99350, 99374-99375, 99377-99378, 99446-99449, 99451-99452, 99495-99496, G0463, G0471, P9612

52250 00910, 00916, 0213T, 0216T, 0228T, 0230T, 10005, 10007, 10009, 10011, 10021, 11000-11006, 11042-11047, 12001-12007, 12011-12057, 13100-13133, 13151-13153, 36000, 36400-36410, 36420-36430, 36440, 36591-36592, 36600, 36640, 43752, 51701-51703, 52000-52001, 52204, 52224-52240✦, 52281, 52310-52315, 53000-53025, 53600-53621, 53660-53665, 57410, 62320-62327, 64400, 64405-64408, 64415-64435, 64445-64454, 64461-64463, 64479-64505, 64510-64530, 69990, 76000, 77001-77002, 92012-92014, 93000-93010, 93040-93042, 93318, 93355, 94002, 94200, 94250, 94680-94690, 94770, 95812-95816, 95819, 95822, 95829, 95955, 96360-96368, 96372, 96374-96377, 96523, 97597-97598, 97602, 99155, 99156, 99157, 99211-99223, 99231-99255, 99291-99292, 99304-99310, 99315-99316, 99334-99337, 99347-99350, 99374-99375, 99377-99378, 99446-99449, 99451-99452, 99495-99496, G0463, G0471, P9612

52260 00910, 00916, 0213T, 0216T, 0228T, 0230T, 12001-12007, 12011-12057, 13100-13133, 13151-13153, 36000, 36400-36410, 36420-36430, 36440, 36591-36592, 36600, 36640, 43752, 50715, 51701-51703, 52000-52005, 52204, 52281, 52310-52315, 53000-53025, 53600-53621, 53660-53665, 57410, 62320-62327, 64400, 64405-64408, 64415-64435, 64445-64454, 64461-64463, 64479-64505, 64510-64530, 69990, 76000, 77001-77002, 92012-92014, 93000-93010, 93040-93042, 93318, 93355, 94002, 94200, 94250, 94680-94690, 94770, 95812-95816, 95819, 95822, 95829, 95955, 96360-96368, 96372, 96374-96377, 96523, 99151✦, 99152✦, 99153✦, 99155, 99156, 99157, 99211-99223, 99231-99255,

99291-99292, 99304-99310, 99315-99316, 99334-99337, 99347-99350, 99374-99375, 99377-99378, 99446-99449, 99451-99452, 99495-99496, G0463, G0471, P9612

52265 00910, 00916, 0213T, 0216T, 0228T, 0230T, 12001-12007, 12011-12057, 13100-13133, 13151-13153, 36000, 36400-36410, 36420-36430, 36440, 36591-36592, 36600, 36640, 43752, 51701-51703, 52000-52001, 52204, 52260✦, 52281, 52310-52315, 53000-53025, 53600-53621, 53660-53665, 57410, 62320-62327, 64400, 64405-64408, 64415-64435, 64445-64454, 64461-64463, 64479-64505, 64510-64530, 69990, 76000, 77001-77002, 92012-92014, 93000-93010, 93040-93042, 93318, 93355, 94002, 94200, 94250, 94680-94690, 94770, 95812-95816, 95819, 95822, 95829, 95955, 96360-96368, 96372, 96374-96377, 96523, 99155, 99156, 99157, 99211-99223, 99231-99255, 99291-99292, 99304-99310, 99315-99316, 99334-99337, 99347-99350, 99374-99375, 99377-99378, 99446-99449, 99451-99452, 99495-99496, G0463, G0471, J2001, P9612

52270 00910, 00916, 0213T, 0216T, 0228T, 0230T, 11000-11006, 11042-11047, 12001-12007, 12011-12057, 13100-13133, 13151-13153, 36000, 36400-36410, 36420-36430, 36440, 36591-36592, 36600, 36640, 43752, 51701-51703, 52000-52001, 52281, 52310-52315, 53000-53025, 53600-53621, 53660-53665, 57410, 62320-62327, 64400, 64405-64408, 64415-64435, 64445-64454, 64461-64463, 64479-64505, 64510-64530, 69990, 76000, 77001-77002, 92012-92014, 93000-93010, 93040-93042, 93318, 93355, 94002, 94200, 94250, 94680-94690, 94770, 95812-95816, 95819, 95822, 95829, 95955, 96360-96368, 96372, 96374-96377, 96523, 97597-97598, 97602, 99155, 99156, 99157, 99211-99223, 99231-99255, 99291-99292, 99304-99310, 99315-99316, 99334-99337, 99347-99350, 99374-99375, 99377-99378, 99446-99449, 99451-99452, 99495-99496, G0463, G0471, J2001, P9612

52275 00910, 00916, 0213T, 0216T, 0228T, 0230T, 11000-11006, 11042-11047, 12001-12007, 12011-12057, 13100-13133, 13151-13153, 36000, 36400-36410, 36420-36430, 36440, 36591-36592, 36600, 36640, 43752, 51701-51703, 52000-52001, 52270, 52276, 52281, 52310-52315, 53000-53025, 53600-53621, 53660-53665, 57410, 62320-62327, 64400, 64405-64408, 64415-64435, 64445-64454, 64461-64463, 64479-64505, 64510-64530, 69990, 76000, 77001-77002, 92012-92014, 93000-93010, 93040-93042, 93318, 93355, 94002, 94200, 94250, 94680-94690, 94770, 95812-95816, 95819, 95822, 95829, 95955, 96360-96368, 96372, 96374-96377, 96523, 97597-97598, 97602, 99155, 99156, 99157, 99211-99223, 99231-99255, 99291-99292, 99304-99310, 99315-99316, 99334-99337, 99347-99350, 99374-99375, 99377-99378, 99446-99449, 99451-99452, 99495-99496, G0463, G0471, J2001, P9612

52276 00910, 00916, 0213T, 0216T, 0228T, 0230T, 11000-11006, 11042-11047, 12001-12007, 12011-12057, 13100-13133, 13151-13153, 36000, 36400-36410, 36420-36430, 36440, 36591-36592, 36600, 36640, 43752, 51102, 51700-51703, 52000-52001, 52204, 52270, 52281, 52310-52315, 53000-53025, 53600-53621, 53660-53665, 57410, 62320-62327, 64400, 64405-64408, 64415-64435, 64445-64454, 64461-64463, 64479-64505, 64510-64530, 69990, 76000, 77001-77002, 92012-92014, 93000-93010, 93040-93042, 93318, 93355, 94002, 94200, 94250, 94680-94690, 94770, 95812-95816, 95819, 95822, 95829, 95955, 96360-96368, 96372, 96374-96377, 96523, 97597-97598, 97602, 99155, 99156, 99157, 99211-99223, 99231-99255, 99291-99292, 99304-99310, 99315-99316, 99334-99337, 99347-99350, 99374-99375, 99377-99378, 99446-99449, 99451-99452, 99495-99496, G0463, G0471, J2001, P9612

52277 00910, 00916, 0213T, 0216T, 0228T, 0230T, 11000-11006, 11042-11047, 12001-12007, 12011-12057, 13100-13133, 13151-13153, 36000, 36400-36410, 36420-36430, 36440, 36591-36592, 36600, 36640, 43752, 51701-51703, 52000-52001, 52281, 52301, 52310-52315, 53000-53025,

CPT © 2020 American Medical Association. All Rights Reserved.
Coding Companion for Urology/Nephrology

53600-53621, 53660-53665, 57410, 62320-62327, 64400, 64405-64408, 64415-64435, 64445-64454, 64461-64463, 64479-64505, 64510-64530, 69990, 76000, 77001-77002, 92012-92014, 93000-93010, 93040-93042, 93318, 93355, 94002, 94200, 94250, 94680-94690, 94770, 95812-95816, 95819, 95822, 95829, 95955, 96360-96368, 96372, 96374-96377, 96523, 97597-97598, 97602, 99155, 99156, 99157, 99211-99223, 99231-99255, 99291-99292, 99304-99310, 99315-99316, 99334-99337, 99347-99350, 99374-99375, 99377-99378, 99446-99449, 99451-99452, 99495-99496, G0463, G0471, P9612

52281 00910, 00916, 0213T, 0216T, 0228T, 0230T, 11000-11006, 11042-11047, 12001-12007, 12011-12057, 13100-13133, 13151-13153, 36000, 36400-36410, 36420-36430, 36440, 36591-36592, 36600, 36640, 43752, 51600-51703, 51720, 52000, 52005, 52204, 52283, 52287, 52310, 53000-53025, 53600-53621, 53660-53665, 57410, 62320-62327, 64400, 64405-64408, 64415-64435, 64445-64454, 64461-64463, 64479-64505, 64510-64530, 69990, 76000, 77001-77002, 92012-92014, 93000-93010, 93040-93042, 93318, 93355, 94002, 94200, 94250, 94680-94690, 94770, 95812-95816, 95819, 95822, 95829, 95955, 96360-96368, 96372, 96374-96377, 96523, 97597-97598, 97602, 99155, 99156, 99157, 99211-99223, 99231-99255, 99291-99292, 99304-99310, 99315-99316, 99334-99337, 99347-99350, 99374-99375, 99377-99378, 99446-99449, 99451-99452, 99495-99496, G0463, G0471, P9612

52282 00910, 00916, 0213T, 0216T, 0228T, 0230T, 11000-11006, 11042-11047, 12001-12007, 12011-12057, 13100-13133, 13151-13153, 36000, 36400-36410, 36420-36430, 36440, 36591-36592, 36600, 36640, 43752, 51701-51703, 52000-52001, 52281, 52310-52315, 52441❖, 53000-53025, 53600-53621, 53660-53665, 53855❖, 57410, 62320-62327, 64400, 64405-64408, 64415-64435, 64445-64454, 64461-64463, 64479-64505, 64510-64530, 69990, 76000, 77001-77002, 92012-92014, 93000-93010, 93040-93042, 93318, 93355, 94002, 94200, 94250, 94680-94690, 94770, 95812-95816, 95819, 95822, 95829, 95955, 96360-96368, 96372, 96374-96377, 96523, 97597-97598, 97602, 99155, 99156, 99157, 99211-99223, 99231-99255, 99291-99292, 99304-99310, 99315-99316, 99334-99337, 99347-99350, 99374-99375, 99377-99378, 99446-99449, 99451-99452, 99495-99496, G0463, G0471, J2001, P9612

52283 00910, 00916, 0213T, 0216T, 0228T, 0230T, 12001-12007, 12011-12057, 13100-13133, 13151-13153, 36000, 36400-36410, 36420-36430, 36440, 36591-36592, 36600, 36640, 43752, 51701-51703, 52000-52001, 52310-52315, 53000-53025, 53600-53621, 53660-53665, 57410, 62320-62327, 64400, 64405-64408, 64415-64435, 64445-64454, 64461-64463, 64479-64505, 64510-64530, 69990, 76000, 77001-77002, 92012-92014, 93000-93010, 93040-93042, 93318, 93355, 94002, 94200, 94250, 94680-94690, 94770, 95812-95816, 95819, 95822, 95829, 95955, 96360-96368, 96372, 96374-96377, 96523, 99155, 99156, 99157, 99211-99223, 99231-99255, 99291-99292, 99304-99310, 99315-99316, 99334-99337, 99347-99350, 99374-99375, 99377-99378, 99446-99449, 99451-99452, 99495-99496, G0463, G0471, J2001, P9612

52285 00910, 00916, 0213T, 0216T, 0228T, 0230T, 11000-11006, 11042-11047, 12001-12007, 12011-12057, 13100-13133, 13151-13153, 36000, 36400-36410, 36420-36430, 36440, 36591-36592, 36600, 36640, 43752, 51701-51703, 52000-52005, 52214, 52270, 52276, 52281, 52310-52315, 53000-53025, 53600-53621, 53660-53665, 57410, 62320-62327, 64400, 64405-64408, 64415-64435, 64445-64454, 64461-64463, 64479-64505, 64510-64530, 69990, 76000, 77001-77002, 92012-92014, 93000-93010, 93040-93042, 93318, 93355, 94002, 94200, 94250, 94680-94690, 94770, 95812-95816, 95819, 95822, 95829, 95955, 96360-96368, 96372, 96374-96377, 96523, 97597-97598, 97602, 99155, 99156, 99157, 99211-99223, 99231-99255, 99291-99292, 99304-99310,

99315-99316, 99334-99337, 99347-99350, 99374-99375, 99377-99378, 99446-99449, 99451-99452, 99495-99496, G0463, G0471, J2001, P9612

52287 00910, 00916, 0213T, 0216T, 0228T, 0230T, 12001-12007, 12011-12057, 13100-13133, 13151-13153, 36000, 36400-36410, 36420-36430, 36440, 36591-36592, 36600, 36640, 43752, 51701-51703, 52000-52001, 52310-52315, 53000-53025, 53600-53621, 53660-53665, 57410, 62320-62327, 64400, 64405-64408, 64415-64435, 64445-64454, 64461-64463, 64479-64505, 64510-64530, 69990, 76000, 77001-77002, 92012-92014, 93000-93010, 93040-93042, 93318, 93355, 94002, 94200, 94250, 94680-94690, 94770, 95812-95816, 95819, 95822, 95829, 95955, 96360-96368, 96372, 96374-96377, 96523, 99155, 99156, 99157, 99211-99223, 99231-99255, 99291-99292, 99304-99310, 99315-99316, 99334-99337, 99347-99350, 99374-99375, 99377-99378, 99446-99449, 99451-99452, 99495-99496, G0463, G0471, J0670, J2001, P9612

52290 00910, 00916, 0213T, 0216T, 0228T, 0230T, 11000-11006, 11042-11047, 12001-12007, 12011-12057, 13100-13133, 13151-13153, 36000, 36400-36410, 36420-36430, 36440, 36591-36592, 36600, 36640, 43752, 51701-51703, 52000-52001, 52281, 52310-52315, 53000-53025, 53600-53621, 53660-53665, 57410, 62320-62327, 64400, 64405-64408, 64415-64435, 64445-64454, 64461-64463, 64479-64505, 64510-64530, 69990, 76000, 77001-77002, 92012-92014, 93000-93010, 93040-93042, 93318, 93355, 94002, 94200, 94250, 94680-94690, 94770, 95812-95816, 95819, 95822, 95829, 95955, 96360-96368, 96372, 96374-96377, 96523, 97597-97598, 97602, 99155, 99156, 99157, 99211-99223, 99231-99255, 99291-99292, 99304-99310, 99315-99316, 99334-99337, 99347-99350, 99374-99375, 99377-99378, 99446-99449, 99451-99452, 99495-99496, G0463, G0471, P9612

52300 00910, 00916, 0213T, 0216T, 0228T, 0230T, 11000-11006, 11042-11047, 12001-12007, 12011-12057, 13100-13133, 13151-13153, 36000, 36400-36410, 36420-36430, 36440, 36591-36592, 36600, 36640, 43752, 51701-51703, 52000-52001, 52281, 52290, 52310-52315, 53000-53025, 53600-53621, 53660-53665, 57410, 62320-62327, 64400, 64405-64408, 64415-64435, 64445-64454, 64461-64463, 64479-64505, 64510-64530, 69990, 76000, 77001-77002, 92012-92014, 93000-93010, 93040-93042, 93318, 93355, 94002, 94200, 94250, 94680-94690, 94770, 95812-95816, 95819, 95822, 95829, 95955, 96360-96368, 96372, 96374-96377, 96523, 97597-97598, 97602, 99155, 99156, 99157, 99211-99223, 99231-99255, 99291-99292, 99304-99310, 99315-99316, 99334-99337, 99347-99350, 99374-99375, 99377-99378, 99446-99449, 99451-99452, 99495-99496, G0463, G0471, P9612

52301 00910, 00916, 0213T, 0216T, 0228T, 0230T, 11000-11006, 11042-11047, 12001-12007, 12011-12057, 13100-13133, 13151-13153, 36000, 36400-36410, 36420-36430, 36440, 36591-36592, 36600, 36640, 43752, 51701-51703, 52000-52001, 52204, 52270-52276, 52281, 52290-52300, 52305-52315, 52332, 52356, 53000-53025, 53200, 53600-53621, 53660-53665, 57410, 62320-62327, 64400, 64405-64408, 64415-64435, 64445-64454, 64461-64463, 64479-64505, 64510-64530, 69990, 76000, 77001-77002, 92012-92014, 93000-93010, 93040-93042, 93318, 93355, 94002, 94200, 94250, 94680-94690, 94770, 95812-95816, 95819, 95822, 95829, 95955, 96360-96368, 96372, 96374-96377, 96523, 97597-97598, 97602, 99155, 99156, 99157, 99211-99223, 99231-99255, 99291-99292, 99304-99310, 99315-99316, 99334-99337, 99347-99350, 99374-99375, 99377-99378, 99446-99449, 99451-99452, 99495-99496, G0463, G0471, P9612

52305 00910, 00916, 0213T, 0216T, 0228T, 0230T, 11000-11006, 11042-11047, 12001-12007, 12011-12057, 13100-13133, 13151-13153, 36000, 36400-36410, 36420-36430, 36440, 36591-36592, 36600, 36640, 43752, 51701-51703, 52000-52001, 52281, 52310-52315, 53000-53025,

53600-53621, 53660-53665, 57410, 62320-62327, 64400, 64405-64408, 64415-64435, 64445-64454, 64461-64463, 64479-64505, 64510-64530, 69990, 76000, 77001-77002, 92012-92014, 93000-93010, 93040-93042, 93318, 93355, 94002, 94200, 94250, 94680-94690, 94770, 95812-95816, 95819, 95822, 95829, 95955, 96360-96368, 96372, 96374-96377, 96523, 97597-97598, 97602, 99155, 99156, 99157, 99211-99223, 99231-99255, 99291-99292, 99304-99310, 99315-99316, 99334-99337, 99347-99350, 99374-99375, 99377-99378, 99446-99449, 99451-99452, 99495-99496, G0463, G0471, P9612

52310 00910, 00916-00918, 0213T, 0216T, 0228T, 0230T, 11000-11006, 11042-11047, 12001-12007, 12011-12057, 13100-13133, 13151-13153, 20102, 36000, 36400-36410, 36420-36430, 36440, 36591-36592, 36600, 36640, 43752, 49013-49014, 50715, 51700-51703, 52000-52001, 53000-53025, 53600-53621, 53660-53665, 57410, 62320-62327, 64400, 64405-64408, 64415-64435, 64445-64454, 64461-64463, 64479-64505, 64510-64530, 69990, 76000, 77001-77002, 92012-92014, 93000-93010, 93040-93042, 93318, 93355, 94002, 94200, 94250, 94680-94690, 94770, 95812-95816, 95819, 95822, 95829, 95955, 96360-96368, 96372, 96374-96377, 96523, 97597-97598, 97602, 99155, 99156, 99157, 99211-99223, 99231-99255, 99291-99292, 99304-99310, 99315-99316, 99334-99337, 99347-99350, 99374-99375, 99377-99378, 99446-99449, 99451-99452, 99495-99496, G0463, G0471, J2001, P9612

52315 00910, 00916-00918, 0213T, 0216T, 0228T, 0230T, 11000-11006, 11042-11047, 12001-12007, 12011-12057, 13100-13133, 13151-13153, 20102, 36000, 36400-36410, 36420-36430, 36440, 36591-36592, 36600, 36640, 43752, 49013-49014, 50385-50386♦, 50715, 51701-51703, 52000-52001, 52281, 52310, 53000-53025, 53600-53621, 53660-53665, 57410, 62320-62327, 64400, 64405-64408, 64415-64435, 64445-64454, 64461-64463, 64479-64505, 64510-64530, 69990, 76000, 77001-77002, 92012-92014, 93000-93010, 93040-93042, 93318, 93355, 94002, 94200, 94250, 94680-94690, 94770, 95812-95816, 95819, 95822, 95829, 95955, 96360-96368, 96372, 96374-96377, 96523, 97597-97598, 97602, 99155, 99156, 99157, 99211-99223, 99231-99255, 99291-99292, 99304-99310, 99315-99316, 99334-99337, 99347-99350, 99374-99375, 99377-99378, 99446-99449, 99451-99452, 99495-99496, G0463, G0471, J2001, P9612

52317 00910, 00916-00918, 0213T, 0216T, 0228T, 0230T, 11000-11006, 11042-11047, 12001-12007, 12011-12057, 13100-13133, 13151-13153, 36000, 36400-36410, 36420-36430, 36440, 36591-36592, 36600, 36640, 43752, 51701-51703, 52000, 52204, 52276, 52281, 52310-52315, 53000-53025, 53600-53621, 53660-53665, 57410, 62320-62327, 64400, 64405-64408, 64415-64435, 64445-64454, 64461-64463, 64479-64505, 64510-64530, 69990, 76000, 77001-77002, 92012-92014, 93000-93010, 93040-93042, 93318, 93355, 94002, 94200, 94250, 94680-94690, 94770, 95812-95816, 95819, 95822, 95829, 95955, 96360-96368, 96372, 96374-96377, 96523, 97597-97598, 97602, 99155, 99156, 99157, 99211-99223, 99231-99255, 99291-99292, 99304-99310, 99315-99316, 99334-99337, 99347-99350, 99374-99375, 99377-99378, 99446-99449, 99451-99452, 99495-99496, G0463, G0471, J2001, P9612

52318 00910, 00916-00918, 0213T, 0216T, 0228T, 0230T, 11000-11006, 11042-11047, 12001-12007, 12011-12057, 13100-13133, 13151-13153, 36000, 36400-36410, 36420-36430, 36440, 36591-36592, 36600, 36640, 43752, 51701-51703, 52000, 52005, 52204, 52281, 52310-52317, 53000-53025, 53600-53621, 53660-53665, 57410, 62320-62327, 64400, 64405-64408, 64415-64435, 64445-64454, 64461-64463, 64479-64505, 64510-64530, 69990, 76000, 77001-77002, 92012-92014, 93000-93010, 93040-93042, 93318, 93355, 94002, 94200, 94250, 94680-94690, 94770, 95812-95816, 95819, 95822, 95829, 95955, 96360-96368, 96372, 96374-96377, 96523, 97597-97598, 97602, 99155, 99156, 99157, 99211-99223, 99231-99255, 99291-99292, 99304-99310,

99315-99316, 99334-99337, 99347-99350, 99374-99375, 99377-99378, 99446-99449, 99451-99452, 99495-99496, G0463, G0471, P9612

52320 00910, 00916-00918, 0213T, 0216T, 0228T, 0230T, 11000-11006, 11042-11047, 12001-12007, 12011-12057, 13100-13133, 13151-13153, 36000, 36400-36410, 36420-36430, 36440, 36591-36592, 36600, 36640, 43752, 50715, 50945, 51701-51703, 52000-52007, 52204, 52281, 52310-52318, 53000-53025, 53600-53621, 53660-53665, 57410, 62320-62327, 64400, 64405-64408, 64415-64435, 64445-64454, 64461-64463, 64479-64505, 64510-64530, 69990, 76000, 77001-77002, 92012-92014, 93000-93010, 93040-93042, 93318, 93355, 94002, 94200, 94250, 94680-94690, 94770, 95812-95816, 95819, 95822, 95829, 95955, 96360-96368, 96372, 96374-96377, 96523, 97597-97598, 97602, 99155, 99156, 99157, 99211-99223, 99231-99255, 99291-99292, 99304-99310, 99315-99316, 99334-99337, 99347-99350, 99374-99375, 99377-99378, 99446-99449, 99451-99452, 99495-99496, G0463, G0471, P9612

52325 00910, 00916-00918, 0213T, 0216T, 0228T, 0230T, 12001-12007, 12011-12057, 13100-13133, 13151-13153, 36000, 36400-36410, 36420-36430, 36440, 36591-36592, 36600, 36640, 43752, 50715, 50945, 50961, 51701-51703, 52000-52007, 52281, 52310-52320, 53000-53025, 53600-53621, 53660-53665, 57410, 62320-62327, 64400, 64405-64408, 64415-64435, 64445-64454, 64461-64463, 64479-64505, 64510-64530, 69990, 76000, 77001-77002, 92012-92014, 93000-93010, 93040-93042, 93318, 93355, 94002, 94200, 94250, 94680-94690, 94770, 95812-95816, 95819, 95822, 95829, 95955, 96360-96368, 96372, 96374-96377, 96523, 99155, 99156, 99157, 99211-99223, 99231-99255, 99291-99292, 99304-99310, 99315-99316, 99334-99337, 99347-99350, 99374-99375, 99377-99378, 99446-99449, 99451-99452, 99495-99496, G0463, G0471, P9612

52327 00910, 00916-00918, 0213T, 0216T, 0228T, 0230T, 12001-12007, 12011-12057, 13100-13133, 13151-13153, 36000, 36400-36410, 36420-36430, 36440, 36591-36592, 36600, 36640, 43752, 50715, 51701-51703, 52000-52007, 52281, 52310-52315, 53000-53025, 53600-53621, 53660-53665, 57410, 62320-62327, 64400, 64405-64408, 64415-64435, 64445-64454, 64461-64463, 64479-64505, 64510-64530, 69990, 76000, 77001-77002, 92012-92014, 93000-93010, 93040-93042, 93318, 93355, 94002, 94200, 94250, 94680-94690, 94770, 95812-95816, 95819, 95822, 95829, 95955, 96360-96368, 96372, 96374-96377, 96523, 99155, 99156, 99157, 99211-99223, 99231-99255, 99291-99292, 99304-99310, 99315-99316, 99334-99337, 99347-99350, 99374-99375, 99377-99378, 99446-99449, 99451-99452, 99495-99496, G0463, G0471, P9612

52330 00910, 00916-00918, 0213T, 0216T, 0228T, 0230T, 11000-11006, 11042-11047, 12001-12007, 12011-12057, 13100-13133, 13151-13153, 36000, 36400-36410, 36420-36430, 36440, 36591-36592, 36600, 36640, 43752, 50715, 51701-51703, 52000-52007, 52281, 52310-52315, 52320-52325, 53000-53025, 53600-53621, 53660-53665, 57410, 62320-62327, 64400, 64405-64408, 64415-64435, 64445-64454, 64461-64463, 64479-64505, 64510-64530, 69990, 76000, 77001-77002, 92012-92014, 93000-93010, 93040-93042, 93318, 93355, 94002, 94200, 94250, 94680-94690, 94770, 95812-95816, 95819, 95822, 95829, 95955, 96360-96368, 96372, 96374-96377, 96523, 97597-97598, 97602, 99155, 99156, 99157, 99211-99223, 99231-99255, 99291-99292, 99304-99310, 99315-99316, 99334-99337, 99347-99350, 99374-99375, 99377-99378, 99446-99449, 99451-99452, 99495-99496, G0463, G0471, J2001, P9612

52332 00910, 00916, 0213T, 0216T, 0228T, 0230T, 11000-11006, 11042-11047, 12001-12007, 12011-12057, 13100-13133, 13151-13153, 36000, 36400-36410, 36420-36430, 36440, 36591-36592, 36600, 36640, 43752,

50387, 50430-50431, 50684, 50693-50695, 50715, 51700-51703, 52000-52007, 52204, 52281, 52310-52315, 53000-53025, 53600-53621, 53660-53665, 57410, 62320-62327, 64400, 64405-64408, 64415-64435, 64445-64454, 64461-64463, 64479-64505, 64510-64530, 69990, 76000, 77001-77002, 92012-92014, 93000-93010, 93040-93042, 93318, 93355, 94002, 94200, 94250, 94680-94690, 94770, 95812-95816, 95819, 95822, 95829, 95955, 96360-96368, 96372, 96374-96377, 96523, 97597-97598, 97602, 99155, 99156, 99157, 99211-99223, 99231-99255, 99291-99292, 99304-99310, 99315-99316, 99334-99337, 99347-99350, 99374-99375, 99377-99378, 99446-99449, 99451-99452, 99495-99496, G0463, G0471, J2001, P9612

52334 00910, 00916, 0213T, 0216T, 0228T, 0230T, 11000-11006, 11042-11047, 12001-12007, 12011-12057, 13100-13133, 13151-13153, 36000, 36400-36410, 36420-36430, 36440, 36591-36592, 36600, 36640, 43752, 50436, 50715, 51701-51703, 52000-52007, 52281, 52310-52315, 52351, 53000-53025, 53600-53621, 53660-53665, 57410, 62320-62327, 64400, 64405-64408, 64415-64435, 64445-64454, 64461-64463, 64479-64505, 64510-64530, 69990, 76000, 77001-77002, 92012-92014, 93000-93010, 93040-93042, 93318, 93355, 94002, 94200, 94250, 94680-94690, 94770, 95812-95816, 95819, 95822, 95829, 95955, 96360-96368, 96372, 96374-96377, 96523, 97597-97598, 97602, 99155, 99156, 99157, 99211-99223, 99231-99255, 99291-99292, 99304-99310, 99315-99316, 99334-99337, 99347-99350, 99374-99375, 99377-99378, 99446-99449, 99451-99452, 99495-99496, G0463, G0471, P9612

52341 00910, 00916, 0213T, 0216T, 0228T, 0230T, 12001-12007, 12011-12057, 13100-13133, 13151-13153, 36000, 36400-36410, 36420-36430, 36440, 36591-36592, 36600, 36640, 43752, 50706-50715, 50953✦, 50972✦, 51701-51703, 52000-52007, 52204, 52281, 52310-52315, 52351, 53000-53025, 53600-53621, 53660-53665, 57410, 62320-62327, 64400, 64405-64408, 64415-64435, 64445-64454, 64461-64463, 64479-64505, 64510-64530, 69990, 76000, 77001-77002, 92012-92014, 93000-93010, 93040-93042, 93318, 93355, 94002, 94200, 94250, 94680-94690, 94770, 95812-95816, 95819, 95822, 95829, 95955, 96360-96368, 96372, 96374-96377, 96523, 99155, 99156, 99157, 99211-99223, 99231-99255, 99291-99292, 99304-99310, 99315-99316, 99334-99337, 99347-99350, 99374-99375, 99377-99378, 99446-99449, 99451-99452, 99495-99496, G0463, G0471, P9612

52342 00910, 00916, 0213T, 0216T, 0228T, 0230T, 12001-12007, 12011-12057, 13100-13133, 13151-13153, 36000, 36400-36410, 36420-36430, 36440, 36591-36592, 36600, 36640, 43752, 50706-50715, 50953✦, 50972✦, 51701-51703, 52000-52007, 52204, 52281, 52310-52315, 52351, 53000-53025, 53600-53621, 53660-53665, 57410, 62320-62327, 64400, 64405-64408, 64415-64435, 64445-64454, 64461-64463, 64479-64505, 64510-64530, 69990, 76000, 77001-77002, 92012-92014, 93000-93010, 93040-93042, 93318, 93355, 94002, 94200, 94250, 94680-94690, 94770, 95812-95816, 95819, 95822, 95829, 95955, 96360-96368, 96372, 96374-96377, 96523, 99155, 99156, 99157, 99211-99223, 99231-99255, 99291-99292, 99304-99310, 99315-99316, 99334-99337, 99347-99350, 99374-99375, 99377-99378, 99446-99449, 99451-99452, 99495-99496, G0463, G0471, P9612

52343 00910, 00916, 0213T, 0216T, 0228T, 0230T, 12001-12007, 12011-12057, 13100-13133, 13151-13153, 36000, 36400-36410, 36420-36430, 36440, 36591-36592, 36600, 36640, 43752, 50706-50715, 50953✦, 50972✦, 51701-51703, 52000-52007, 52204, 52281, 52310-52315, 52351, 53000-53025, 53600-53621, 53660-53665, 57410, 62320-62327, 64400, 64405-64408, 64415-64435, 64445-64454, 64461-64463, 64479-64505, 64510-64530, 69990, 76000, 77001-77002, 92012-92014, 93000-93010, 93040-93042, 93318, 93355, 94002, 94200, 94250, 94680-94690, 94770, 95812-95816, 95819, 95822, 95829, 95955, 96360-96368, 96372, 96374-96377, 96523, 99155, 99156, 99157, 99211-99223,

52344 00910, 00916, 0213T, 0216T, 0228T, 0230T, 12001-12007, 12011-12057, 13100-13133, 13151-13153, 36000, 36400-36410, 36420-36430, 36440, 36591-36592, 36600, 36640, 43752, 50706-50715, 50953✦, 50972✦, 51701-51703, 52000-52007, 52204, 52281, 52310-52315, 52341, 52351, 53000-53025, 53600-53621, 53660-53665, 57410, 62320-62327, 64400, 64405-64408, 64415-64435, 64445-64454, 64461-64463, 64479-64505, 64510-64530, 69990, 76000, 77001-77002, 92012-92014, 93000-93010, 93040-93042, 93318, 93355, 94002, 94200, 94250, 94680-94690, 94770, 95812-95816, 95819, 95822, 95829, 95955, 96360-96368, 96372, 96374-96377, 96523, 99155, 99156, 99157, 99211-99223, 99231-99255, 99291-99292, 99304-99310, 99315-99316, 99334-99337, 99347-99350, 99374-99375, 99377-99378, 99446-99449, 99451-99452, 99495-99496, G0463, G0471, P9612

52345 00910, 00916, 0213T, 0216T, 0228T, 0230T, 12001-12007, 12011-12057, 13100-13133, 13151-13153, 36000, 36400-36410, 36420-36430, 36440, 36591-36592, 36600, 36640, 43752, 50706-50715, 50953✦, 50972✦, 51701-51703, 52000-52007, 52204, 52281, 52310-52315, 52342, 52351, 53000-53025, 53600-53621, 53660-53665, 57410, 62320-62327, 64400, 64405-64408, 64415-64435, 64445-64454, 64461-64463, 64479-64505, 64510-64530, 69990, 76000, 77001-77002, 92012-92014, 93000-93010, 93040-93042, 93318, 93355, 94002, 94200, 94250, 94680-94690, 94770, 95812-95816, 95819, 95822, 95829, 95955, 96360-96368, 96372, 96374-96377, 96523, 99155, 99156, 99157, 99211-99223, 99231-99255, 99291-99292, 99304-99310, 99315-99316, 99334-99337, 99347-99350, 99374-99375, 99377-99378, 99446-99449, 99451-99452, 99495-99496, G0463, G0471, P9612

52346 00910, 00916, 0213T, 0216T, 0228T, 0230T, 12001-12007, 12011-12057, 13100-13133, 13151-13153, 36000, 36400-36410, 36420-36430, 36440, 36591-36592, 36600, 36640, 43752, 50706-50715, 50953✦, 50972✦, 51701-51703, 52000-52007, 52204, 52281, 52310-52315, 52343, 52351, 53000-53025, 53600-53621, 53660-53665, 57410, 62320-62327, 64400, 64405-64408, 64415-64435, 64445-64454, 64461-64463, 64479-64505, 64510-64530, 69990, 76000, 77001-77002, 92012-92014, 93000-93010, 93040-93042, 93318, 93355, 94002, 94200, 94250, 94680-94690, 94770, 95812-95816, 95819, 95822, 95829, 95955, 96360-96368, 96372, 96374-96377, 96523, 99155, 99156, 99157, 99211-99223, 99231-99255, 99291-99292, 99304-99310, 99315-99316, 99334-99337, 99347-99350, 99374-99375, 99377-99378, 99446-99449, 99451-99452, 99495-99496, G0463, G0471, P9612

52351 00910, 00916, 0213T, 0216T, 0228T, 0230T, 12001-12007, 12011-12057, 13100-13133, 13151-13153, 36000, 36400-36410, 36420-36430, 36440, 36591-36592, 36600, 36640, 43752, 51701-51703, 52000-52007, 52204, 52281, 52310-52315, 53000-53025, 53600-53621, 53660-53665, 57410, 62320-62327, 64400, 64405-64408, 64415-64435, 64445-64454, 64461-64463, 64479-64505, 64510-64530, 69990, 76000, 77001-77002, 92012-92014, 93000-93010, 93040-93042, 93318, 93355, 94002, 94200, 94250, 94680-94690, 94770, 95812-95816, 95819, 95822, 95829, 95955, 96360-96368, 96372, 96374-96377, 96523, 99155, 99156, 99157, 99211-99223, 99231-99255, 99291-99292, 99304-99310, 99315-99316, 99334-99337, 99347-99350, 99374-99375, 99377-99378, 99446-99449, 99451-99452, 99495-99496, G0463, G0471, P9612

52352 00910, 00916-00918, 0213T, 0216T, 0228T, 0230T, 11000-11006, 11042-11047, 12001-12007, 12011-12057, 13100-13133, 13151-13153, 36000, 36400-36410, 36420-36430, 36440, 36591-36592, 36600, 36640, 43752, 50945, 50961, 51700-51703, 52000-52007, 52235, 52281, 52310-52325, 52330, 52341-52346, 52351, 53000-53025, 53600-53621,

53660-53665, 57410, 62320-62327, 64400, 64405-64408, 64415-64435, 64445-64454, 64461-64463, 64479-64505, 64510-64530, 69990, 76000, 77001-77002, 92012-92014, 93000-93010, 93040-93042, 93318, 93355, 94002, 94200, 94250, 94680-94690, 94770, 95812-95816, 95819, 95822, 95829, 95955, 96360-96368, 96372, 96374-96377, 96523, 97597-97598, 97602, 99155, 99156, 99157, 99211-99223, 99231-99255, 99291-99292, 99304-99310, 99315-99316, 99334-99337, 99347-99350, 99374-99375, 99377-99378, 99446-99449, 99451-99452, 99495-99496, G0463, G0471, P9612

52353 00910, 00916-00918, 0213T, 0216T, 0228T, 0230T, 12001-12007, 12011-12057, 13100-13133, 13151-13153, 36000, 36400-36410, 36420-36430, 36440, 36591-36592, 36600, 36640, 43752, 50945, 50961, 50980, 51700-51703, 52000-52007, 52235, 52281, 52310-52325, 52330-52332, 52341-52346, 52351-52352, 53000-53025, 53600-53621, 53660-53665, 57410, 62320-62327, 64400, 64405-64408, 64415-64435, 64445-64454, 64461-64463, 64479-64505, 64510-64530, 69990, 76000, 77001-77002, 92012-92014, 93000-93010, 93040-93042, 93318, 93355, 94002, 94200, 94250, 94680-94690, 94770, 95812-95816, 95819, 95822, 95829, 95955, 96360-96368, 96372, 96374-96377, 96523, 99155, 99156, 99157, 99211-99223, 99231-99255, 99291-99292, 99304-99310, 99315-99316, 99334-99337, 99347-99350, 99374-99375, 99377-99378, 99446-99449, 99451-99452, 99495-99496, G0463, G0471, P9612

52354 00910-00912, 00916, 0213T, 0216T, 0228T, 0230T, 10005, 10007, 10009, 10011, 10021, 12001-12007, 12011-12057, 13100-13133, 13151-13153, 36000, 36400-36410, 36420-36430, 36440, 36591-36592, 36600, 36640, 43752, 50606❖, 51701-51703, 52000-52007, 52204, 52234-52240, 52281, 52301, 52310-52315, 52341-52346, 52351, 53000-53025, 53600-53621, 53660-53665, 57410, 62320-62327, 64400, 64405-64408, 64415-64435, 64445-64454, 64461-64463, 64479-64505, 64510-64530, 69990, 76000, 77001-77002, 92012-92014, 93000-93010, 93040-93042, 93318, 93355, 94002, 94200, 94250, 94680-94690, 94770, 95812-95816, 95819, 95822, 95829, 95955, 96360-96368, 96372, 96374-96377, 96523, 99155, 99156, 99157, 99211-99223, 99231-99255, 99291-99292, 99304-99310, 99315-99316, 99334-99337, 99347-99350, 99374-99375, 99377-99378, 99446-99449, 99451-99452, 99495-99496, G0463, G0471, P9612

52355 00910-00912, 00916, 0213T, 0216T, 0228T, 0230T, 11000-11006, 11042-11047, 12001-12007, 12011-12057, 13100-13133, 13151-13153, 36000, 36400-36410, 36420-36430, 36440, 36591-36592, 36600, 36640, 43752, 51701-51703, 52000-52007, 52204, 52224, 52281, 52310-52315, 52341-52346, 52351, 52354, 53000-53025, 53600-53621, 53660-53665, 57410, 62320-62327, 64400, 64405-64408, 64415-64435, 64445-64454, 64461-64463, 64479-64505, 64510-64530, 69990, 76000, 77001-77002, 92012-92014, 93000-93010, 93040-93042, 93318, 93355, 94002, 94200, 94250, 94680-94690, 94770, 95812-95816, 95819, 95822, 95829, 95955, 96360-96368, 96372, 96374-96377, 96523, 97597-97598, 97602, 99155, 99156, 99157, 99211-99223, 99231-99255, 99291-99292, 99304-99310, 99315-99316, 99334-99337, 99347-99350, 99374-99375, 99377-99378, 99446-99449, 99451-99452, 99495-99496, G0463, G0471, P9612

52356 00910, 00916-00918, 0213T, 0216T, 0228T, 0230T, 11000-11006, 11042-11047, 12001-12007, 12011-12057, 13100-13133, 13151-13153, 36000, 36400-36410, 36420-36430, 36440, 36591-36592, 36600, 36640, 43752, 50387, 50430-50431, 50561, 50684, 50715, 50945, 50961, 50980, 51700-51703, 52000-52007, 52204, 52235, 52281, 52310-52325, 52330-52332, 52341-52346, 52351-52353, 53000-53025, 53600-53621, 53660-53665, 57410, 62320-62327, 64400, 64405-64408, 64415-64435, 64445-64454, 64461-64463, 64479-64505, 64510-64530, 69990, 76000, 77001-77002, 92012-92014, 93000-93010, 93040-93042, 93318, 93355,

94002, 94200, 94250, 94680-94690, 94770, 95812-95816, 95819, 95822, 95829, 95955, 96360-96368, 96372, 96374-96377, 96523, 97597-97598, 97602, 99155, 99156, 99157, 99211-99223, 99231-99255, 99291-99292, 99304-99310, 99315-99316, 99334-99337, 99347-99350, 99374-99375, 99377-99378, 99446-99449, 99451-99452, G0463, G0471, J2001, P9612

52400 00910, 00916, 0213T, 0216T, 0228T, 0230T, 0499T, 11000-11006, 11042-11047, 12001-12007, 12011-12057, 13100-13133, 13151-13153, 36000, 36400-36410, 36420-36430, 36440, 36591-36592, 36600, 36640, 43752, 51701-51703, 52000-52001, 52270-52276, 52281, 52283, 52287, 52310-52315, 52441, 52500❖, 52630, 53000-53025, 53600-53621, 53660-53661, 53855, 57410, 62320-62327, 64400, 64405-64408, 64415-64435, 64445-64454, 64461-64463, 64479-64505, 64510-64530, 69990, 76000, 77001-77002, 92012-92014, 93000-93010, 93040-93042, 93318, 93355, 94002, 94200, 94250, 94680-94690, 94770, 95812-95816, 95819, 95822, 95829, 95955, 96360-96368, 96372, 96374-96377, 96523, 97597-97598, 97602, 99155, 99156, 99157, 99211-99223, 99231-99255, 99291-99292, 99304-99310, 99315-99316, 99334-99337, 99347-99350, 99374-99375, 99377-99378, 99446-99449, 99451-99452, 99495-99496, G0463, G0471, P9612

52402 00910, 00916, 0213T, 0216T, 0228T, 0230T, 11000-11006, 11042-11047, 12001-12007, 12011-12057, 13100-13133, 13151-13153, 36000, 36400-36410, 36420-36430, 36440, 36591-36592, 36600, 36640, 43752, 51701-51703, 52000-52001, 52010, 52281, 52310-52315, 52441, 53000-53025, 53080, 53600-53621, 53660-53665, 53855, 62320-62327, 64400, 64405-64408, 64415-64435, 64445-64454, 64461-64463, 64479-64505, 64510-64530, 69990, 76000, 77001-77002, 92012-92014, 93000-93010, 93040-93042, 93318, 93355, 94002, 94200, 94250, 94680-94690, 94770, 95812-95816, 95819, 95822, 95829, 95955, 96360-96368, 96372, 96374-96377, 96523, 97597-97598, 97602, 99155, 99156, 99157, 99211-99223, 99231-99255, 99291-99292, 99304-99310, 99315-99316, 99334-99337, 99347-99350, 99374-99375, 99377-99378, 99446-99449, 99451-99452, 99495-99496, G0463, G0471, P9612

52441 00910, 00916, 0213T, 0216T, 0228T, 0230T, 11000-11006, 11042-11047, 12001-12007, 12011-12057, 13100-13133, 13151-13153, 36000, 36400-36410, 36420-36430, 36440, 36591-36592, 36600, 36640, 43752, 51701-51703, 52000-52001, 52281, 52310-52315, 53000-53025, 53080, 53520-53621, 53660-53665, 53855❖, 57410, 62320-62327, 64400, 64405-64408, 64415-64435, 64445-64454, 64461-64463, 64479-64505, 64510-64530, 69990, 76000, 77001-77002, 92012-92014, 93000-93010, 93040-93042, 93318, 93355, 94002, 94200, 94250, 94680-94690, 94770, 95812-95816, 95819, 95822, 95829, 95955, 96360-96368, 96372, 96374-96377, 96523, 97597-97598, 97602, 99155, 99156, 99157, 99211-99223, 99231-99255, 99291-99292, 99304-99310, 99315-99316, 99334-99337, 99347-99350, 99374-99375, 99377-99378, 99446-99449, 99451-99452, 99495-99496, C9739-C9740❖, G0463, G0471, J0670, J2001, P9612

52442 00910, 00916, 0213T, 0216T, 0228T, 0230T, 11000-11006, 11042-11047, 12001-12007, 12011-12057, 13100-13133, 13151-13153, 36000, 36400-36410, 36420-36430, 36440, 36591-36592, 36600, 36640, 43752, 51701-51703, 52000-52001, 52281, 52310-52315, 53000-53025, 53080, 53520-53621, 53660-53665, 57410, 61650, 62320-62327, 64400, 64405-64408, 64415-64435, 64445-64454, 64461, 64463, 64479, 64483, 64486-64490, 64493, 64505, 64510-64530, 69990, 76000, 77001-77002, 92012-92014, 93000-93010, 93040-93042, 93318, 93355, 94002, 94200, 94250, 94680-94690, 94770, 95812-95816, 95819, 95822, 95829, 95955, 96360, 96365, 96372, 96374-96377, 96523, 97597-97598, 97602, 99155, 99156, 99157, 99211-99223, 99231-99255, 99291-99292, 99304-99310, 99315-99316, 99334-99337, 99347-99350, 99374-99375,

CPT © 2020 American Medical Association. All Rights Reserved.

Coding Companion for Urology/Nephrology

99377-99378, 99446-99449, 99451-99452, 99495-99496, G0463, G0471, J0670, J2001, P9612

52450 00910, 00914-00916, 0213T, 0216T, 0228T, 0230T, 0421T✦, 12001-12007, 12011-12057, 13100-13133, 13151-13153, 36000, 36400-36410, 36420-36430, 36440, 36591-36592, 36600, 36640, 43752, 51701-51703, 52000-52001, 52281, 52441, 52500, 52647-52648✦, 53000-53025, 53600-53621, 53855, 62320-62327, 64400, 64405-64408, 64415-64435, 64445-64454, 64461-64463, 64479-64505, 64510-64530, 69990, 76000, 77001-77002, 92012-92014, 93000-93010, 93040-93042, 93318, 93355, 94002, 94200, 94250, 94680-94690, 94770, 95812-95816, 95819, 95822, 95829, 95955, 96360-96368, 96372, 96374-96377, 96523, 99155, 99156, 99157, 99211-99223, 99231-99255, 99291-99292, 99304-99310, 99315-99316, 99334-99337, 99347-99350, 99374-99375, 99377-99378, 99446-99449, 99451-99452, 99495-99496, G0463, G0471, P9612

52500 00910-00916, 0213T, 0216T, 0228T, 0230T, 11000-11006, 11042-11047, 12001-12007, 12011-12057, 13100-13133, 13151-13153, 36000, 36400-36410, 36420-36430, 36440, 36591-36592, 36600, 36640, 43752, 51701-51703, 52000-52001, 52281, 52441, 53000-53025, 53600-53621, 53855, 62320-62327, 64400, 64405-64408, 64415-64435, 64445-64454, 64461-64463, 64479-64505, 64510-64530, 69990, 76000, 77001-77002, 92012-92014, 93000-93010, 93040-93042, 93318, 93355, 94002, 94200, 94250, 94680-94690, 94770, 95812-95816, 95819, 95822, 95829, 95955, 96360-96368, 96372, 96374-96377, 96523, 97597-97598, 97602, 99155, 99156, 99157, 99211-99223, 99231-99255, 99291-99292, 99304-99310, 99315-99316, 99334-99337, 99347-99350, 99374-99375, 99377-99378, 99446-99449, 99451-99452, 99495-99496, G0463, G0471, P9612

52601 00910, 00914-00916, 0213T, 0216T, 0228T, 0230T, 0421T✦, 0499T, 0582T✦, 11000-11006, 11042-11047, 12001-12007, 12011-12057, 13100-13133, 13151-13153, 36000, 36400-36410, 36420-36430, 36440, 36591-36592, 36600, 36640, 43752, 51040, 51102, 51700-51703, 52000-52005, 52204-52224, 52270-52276, 52281, 52283, 52287, 52310-52315, 52400, 52441, 52450-52500, 52630-52648✦, 53000-53025, 53600-53621, 53850-53852✦, 53854-53855, 55000, 55250, 55700-55706✦, 55873✦, 62320-62327, 64400, 64405-64408, 64415-64435, 64445-64454, 64461-64463, 64479-64505, 64510-64530, 69990, 76000, 77001-77002, 92012-92014, 93000-93010, 93040-93042, 93318, 93355, 94002, 94200, 94250, 94680-94690, 94770, 95812-95816, 95819, 95822, 95829, 95955, 96360-96368, 96372, 96374-96377, 96523, 97597-97598, 97602, 99155, 99156, 99157, 99211-99223, 99231-99255, 99291-99292, 99304-99310, 99315-99316, 99334-99337, 99347-99350, 99374-99375, 99377-99378, 99446-99449, 99451-99452, 99495-99496, G0463, G0471, P9612

52630 00910, 00914-00916, 0213T, 0216T, 0228T, 0230T, 0582T✦, 11000-11006, 11042-11047, 12001-12007, 12011-12057, 13100-13133, 13151-13153, 36000, 36400-36410, 36420-36430, 36440, 36591-36592, 36600, 36640, 43752, 51102, 51700-51703, 52000-52005, 52204-52224, 52270-52276, 52281, 52310-52315, 52441, 52450-52500✦, 52640✦, 53000-53025, 53600-53621, 53854-53855, 55250, 55700-55706, 55873✦, 62320-62327, 64400, 64405-64408, 64415-64435, 64445-64454, 64461-64463, 64479-64505, 64510-64530, 76000, 77001-77002, 92012-92014, 93000-93010, 93040-93042, 93318, 93355, 94002, 94200, 94250, 94680-94690, 94770, 95812-95816, 95819, 95822, 95829, 95955, 96360-96368, 96372, 96374-96377, 96523, 97597-97598, 97602, 99155, 99156, 99157, 99211-99223, 99231-99255, 99291-99292, 99304-99310, 99315-99316, 99334-99337, 99347-99350, 99374-99375, 99377-99378, 99446-99449, 99451-99452, 99495-99496, G0463, G0471, P9612

52640 00910, 00914-00916, 0213T, 0216T, 0228T, 0230T, 0421T✦, 0499T, 11000-11006, 11042-11047, 12001-12007, 12011-12057, 13100-13133, 13151-13153, 36000, 36400-36410, 36420-36430, 36440, 36591-36592, 36600, 36640, 43752, 51701-51703, 52000-52001, 52276, 52281, 52283, 52287, 52441, 52450-52500✦, 53000-53025, 53600-53621, 53855, 55873✦, 62320-62327, 64400, 64405-64408, 64415-64435, 64445-64454, 64461-64463, 64479-64505, 64510-64530, 69990, 76000, 77001-77002, 92012-92014, 93000-93010, 93040-93042, 93318, 93355, 94002, 94200, 94250, 94680-94690, 94770, 95812-95816, 95819, 95822, 95829, 95955, 96360-96368, 96372, 96374-96377, 96523, 97597-97598, 97602, 99155, 99156, 99157, 99211-99223, 99231-99255, 99291-99292, 99304-99310, 99315-99316, 99334-99337, 99347-99350, 99374-99375, 99377-99378, 99446-99449, 99451-99452, 99495-99496, G0463, G0471, P9612

52647 00910, 00914-00916, 0213T, 0216T, 0228T, 0230T, 0421T✦, 0499T, 0582T✦, 11000-11006, 11042-11047, 12001-12007, 12011-12057, 13100-13133, 13151-13153, 36000, 36400-36410, 36420-36430, 36440, 36591-36592, 36600, 36640, 43752, 51040, 51102, 51700-51703, 52000-52005, 52204-52240, 52270-52276, 52281, 52283, 52287, 52305-52315, 52400, 52441, 52500, 52630-52640✦, 52700, 53000-53025, 53600-53621, 53660-53665, 53850-53852✦, 53854-53855, 55000, 55200-55250, 55700-55706✦, 55873✦, 62320-62327, 64400, 64405-64408, 64415-64435, 64445-64454, 64461-64463, 64479-64505, 64510-64530, 69990, 76000, 77001-77002, 92012-92014, 93000-93010, 93040-93042, 93318, 93355, 94002, 94200, 94250, 94680-94690, 94770, 95812-95816, 95819, 95822, 95829, 95955, 96360-96368, 96372, 96374-96377, 96523, 97597-97598, 97602, 99155, 99156, 99157, 99211-99223, 99231-99255, 99291-99292, 99304-99310, 99315-99316, 99334-99337, 99347-99350, 99374-99375, 99377-99378, 99446-99449, 99451-99452, 99495-99496, G0463, G0471, J2001, P9612

52648 00910, 00914-00916, 0213T, 0216T, 0228T, 0230T, 0421T✦, 0499T, 0582T✦, 11000-11006, 11042-11047, 12001-12007, 12011-12057, 13100-13133, 13151-13153, 36000, 36400-36410, 36420-36430, 36440, 36591-36592, 36600, 36640, 43752, 51040, 51700-51703, 52000-52005, 52204-52240, 52270-52276, 52281, 52283, 52287, 52305-52315, 52400, 52441, 52500, 52630-52647✦, 52700, 53000-53025, 53600-53621, 53660-53665, 53850-53852✦, 53854-53855, 55000, 55200-55250, 55700-55706✦, 55873✦, 62320-62327, 64400, 64405-64408, 64415-64435, 64445-64454, 64461-64463, 64479-64505, 64510-64530, 69990, 76000, 77001-77002, 92012-92014, 93000-93010, 93040-93042, 93318, 93355, 94002, 94200, 94250, 94680-94690, 94770, 95812-95816, 95819, 95822, 95829, 95955, 96360-96368, 96372, 96374-96377, 96523, 97597-97598, 97602, 99155, 99156, 99157, 99211-99223, 99231-99255, 99291-99292, 99304-99310, 99315-99316, 99334-99337, 99347-99350, 99374-99375, 99377-99378, 99446-99449, 99451-99452, 99495-99496, G0463, G0471, P9612

52649 00910, 00914-00916, 0213T, 0216T, 0228T, 0230T, 0421T, 0499T, 11000-11006, 11042-11047, 12001-12007, 12011-12057, 13100-13133, 13151-13153, 36000, 36400-36410, 36420-36430, 36440, 36591-36592, 36600, 36640, 43752, 51040, 51102, 51700-51703, 52000-52005, 52204-52240, 52270-52276, 52281, 52283, 52287, 52305-52315, 52400, 52441, 52450-52500, 52601, 52630-52648, 52700, 53000-53025, 53600-53621, 53660-53665, 53855, 55000, 55200-55250, 55700-55706✦, 62320-62327, 64400, 64405-64408, 64415-64435, 64445-64454, 64461-64463, 64479-64505, 64510-64530, 69990, 76000, 77001-77002, 92012-92014, 93000-93010, 93040-93042, 93318, 93355, 94002, 94200, 94250, 94680-94690, 94770, 95812-95816, 95819, 95822, 95829, 95955, 96360-96368, 96372, 96374-96377, 96523, 97597-97598, 97602, 99155, 99156, 99157, 99211-99223, 99231-99255,

99291-99292, 99304-99310, 99315-99316, 99334-99337, 99347-99350, 99374-99375, 99377-99378, 99446-99449, 99451-99452, 99495-99496, G0463, G0471, P9612

52700 00910, 00914-00916, 0213T, 0216T, 0228T, 0230T, 12001-12007, 12011-12057, 13100-13133, 13151-13153, 36000, 36400-36410, 36420-36430, 36440, 36591-36592, 36600, 36640, 43752, 51701-51703, 52000-52001, 52281, 52441, 53000-53025, 53600-53621, 53855, 62320-62327, 64400, 64405-64408, 64415-64435, 64445-64454, 64461-64463, 64479-64505, 64510-64530, 69990, 76000, 77001-77002, 92012-92014, 93000-93010, 93040-93042, 93318, 93355, 94002, 94200, 94250, 94680-94690, 94770, 95812-95816, 95819, 95822, 95829, 95955, 96360-96368, 96372, 96374-96377, 96523, 99155, 99156, 99157, 99211-99223, 99231-99255, 99291-99292, 99304-99310, 99315-99316, 99334-99337, 99347-99350, 99374-99375, 99377-99378, 99446-99449, 99451-99452, 99495-99496, G0463, G0471, P9612

53000 0213T, 0216T, 0228T, 0230T, 11000-11006, 11042-11047, 12001-12007, 12011-12057, 13100-13133, 13151-13153, 36000, 36400-36410, 36420-36430, 36440, 36591-36592, 36600, 36640, 43752, 51701-51703, 62320-62327, 64400, 64405-64408, 64415-64435, 64445-64454, 64461-64463, 64479-64505, 64510-64530, 69990, 92012-92014, 93000-93010, 93040-93042, 93318, 93355, 94002, 94200, 94250, 94680-94690, 94770, 95812-95816, 95819, 95822, 95829, 95955, 96360-96368, 96372, 96374-96377, 96523, 97597-97598, 97602, 99155, 99156, 99157, 99211-99223, 99231-99255, 99291-99292, 99304-99310, 99315-99316, 99334-99337, 99347-99350, 99374-99375, 99377-99378, 99446-99449, 99451-99452, 99495-99496, G0463, G0471, J2001

53010 0213T, 0216T, 0228T, 0230T, 11000-11006, 11042-11047, 12001-12007, 12011-12057, 13100-13133, 13151-13153, 36000, 36400-36410, 36420-36430, 36440, 36591-36592, 36600, 36640, 43752, 51701-51703, 53000, 53020-53025, 62320-62327, 64400, 64405-64408, 64415-64435, 64445-64454, 64461-64463, 64479-64505, 64510-64530, 69990, 92012-92014, 93000-93010, 93040-93042, 93318, 93355, 94002, 94200, 94250, 94680-94690, 94770, 95812-95816, 95819, 95822, 95829, 95955, 96360-96368, 96372, 96374-96377, 96523, 97597-97598, 97602, 99155, 99156, 99157, 99211-99223, 99231-99255, 99291-99292, 99304-99310, 99315-99316, 99334-99337, 99347-99350, 99374-99375, 99377-99378, 99446-99449, 99451-99452, 99495-99496, G0463, G0471

53020 0213T, 0216T, 0228T, 0230T, 11000-11006, 11042-11047, 12001-12007, 12011-12057, 13100-13133, 13151-13153, 36000, 36400-36410, 36420-36430, 36440, 36591-36592, 36600, 36640, 43752, 51701, 51703, 53000, 62320-62327, 64400, 64405-64408, 64415-64435, 64445-64454, 64461-64463, 64479-64505, 64510-64530, 69990, 92012-92014, 93000-93010, 93040-93042, 93318, 93355, 94002, 94200, 94250, 94680-94690, 94770, 95812-95816, 95819, 95822, 95829, 95955, 96360-96368, 96372, 96374-96377, 96523, 97597-97598, 97602, 99155, 99156, 99157, 99211-99223, 99231-99255, 99291-99292, 99304-99310, 99315-99316, 99334-99337, 99347-99350, 99374-99375, 99377-99378, 99446-99449, 99451-99452, 99495-99496, G0463, J0670, J2001

53025 0213T, 0216T, 0228T, 0230T, 11000-11006, 11042-11047, 12001-12007, 12011-12057, 13100-13133, 13151-13153, 36000, 36400-36410, 36420-36430, 36440, 36591-36592, 36600, 36640, 43752, 51701, 51703, 53000, 53020, 62320-62327, 64400, 64405-64408, 64415-64435, 64445-64454, 64461-64463, 64479-64505, 64510-64530, 69990, 92012-92014, 93000-93010, 93040-93042, 93318, 93355, 94002, 94200, 94250, 94680-94690, 94770, 95812-95816, 95819, 95822, 95829, 95955, 96360-96368, 96372, 96374-96377, 96523, 97597-97598, 97602, 99155, 99156, 99157, 99211-99223, 99231-99255, 99291-99292, 99304-99310, 99315-99316, 99334-99337, 99347-99350, 99374-99375,

99377-99378, 99446-99449, 99451-99452, 99495-99496, G0463, J0670, J2001

53040 0213T, 0216T, 0228T, 0230T, 12001-12007, 12011-12057, 13100-13133, 13151-13153, 36000, 36400-36410, 36420-36430, 36440, 36591-36592, 36600, 36640, 43752, 51701-51703, 53000-53025, 53060-53080, 53265, 62320-62327, 64400, 64405-64408, 64415-64435, 64445-64454, 64461-64463, 64479-64505, 64510-64530, 69990, 92012-92014, 93000-93010, 93040-93042, 93318, 93355, 94002, 94200, 94250, 94680-94690, 94770, 95812-95816, 95819, 95822, 95829, 95955, 96360-96368, 96372, 96374-96377, 96523, 99155, 99156, 99157, 99211-99223, 99231-99255, 99291-99292, 99304-99310, 99315-99316, 99334-99337, 99347-99350, 99374-99375, 99377-99378, 99446-99449, 99451-99452, 99495-99496, G0463, G0471, J2001

53060 0213T, 0216T, 0228T, 0230T, 12001-12007, 12011-12057, 13100-13133, 13151-13153, 36000, 36400-36410, 36420-36430, 36440, 36591-36592, 36600, 36640, 43752, 51701-51703, 53000-53025, 53080, 53270◆, 62320-62327, 64400, 64405-64408, 64415-64435, 64445-64454, 64461-64463, 64479-64505, 64510-64530, 69990, 92012-92014, 93000-93010, 93040-93042, 93318, 93355, 94002, 94200, 94250, 94680-94690, 94770, 95812-95816, 95819, 95822, 95829, 95955, 96360-96368, 96372, 96374-96377, 96523, 99155, 99156, 99157, 99211-99223, 99231-99255, 99291-99292, 99304-99310, 99315-99316, 99334-99337, 99347-99350, 99374-99375, 99377-99378, 99446-99449, 99451-99452, 99495-99496, G0463, G0471, J2001

53080 0213T, 0216T, 0228T, 0230T, 12001-12007, 12011-12057, 13100-13133, 13151-13153, 36000, 36400-36410, 36420-36430, 36440, 36591-36592, 36600, 36640, 43752, 51701-51702, 53000-53025, 62320-62327, 64400, 64405-64408, 64415-64435, 64445-64454, 64461-64463, 64479-64505, 64510-64530, 69990, 92012-92014, 93000-93010, 93040-93042, 93318, 93355, 94002, 94200, 94250, 94680-94690, 94770, 95812-95816, 95819, 95822, 95829, 95955, 96360-96368, 96372, 96374-96377, 96523, 99155, 99156, 99157, 99211-99223, 99231-99255, 99291-99292, 99304-99310, 99315-99316, 99334-99337, 99347-99350, 99374-99375, 99377-99378, 99446-99449, 99451-99452, 99495-99496, G0463, G0471

53085 0213T, 0216T, 0228T, 0230T, 12001-12007, 12011-12057, 13100-13133, 13151-13153, 36000, 36400-36410, 36420-36430, 36440, 36591-36592, 36600, 36640, 43752, 51701-51703, 53000-53025, 53080, 62320-62327, 64400, 64405-64408, 64415-64435, 64445-64454, 64461-64463, 64479-64505, 64510-64530, 69990, 92012-92014, 93000-93010, 93040-93042, 93318, 93355, 94002, 94200, 94250, 94680-94690, 94770, 95812-95816, 95819, 95822, 95829, 95955, 96360-96368, 96372, 96374-96377, 96523, 99155, 99156, 99157, 99211-99223, 99231-99255, 99291-99292, 99304-99310, 99315-99316, 99334-99337, 99347-99350, 99374-99375, 99377-99378, 99446-99449, 99451-99452, 99495-99496, G0463, G0471

53200 0213T, 0216T, 0228T, 0230T, 10005, 10007, 10009, 10011, 10021, 12001-12007, 12011-12057, 13100-13133, 13151-13153, 36000, 36400-36410, 36420-36430, 36440, 36591-36592, 36600, 36640, 43752, 51701-51703, 52000, 53000-53025, 62320-62327, 64400, 64405-64408, 64415-64435, 64445-64454, 64461-64463, 64479-64505, 64510-64530, 69990, 92012-92014, 93000-93010, 93040-93042, 93318, 93355, 94002, 94200, 94250, 94680-94690, 94770, 95812-95816, 95819, 95822, 95829, 95955, 96360-96368, 96372, 96374-96377, 96523, 99155, 99156, 99157, 99211-99223, 99231-99255, 99291-99292, 99304-99310, 99315-99316, 99334-99337, 99347-99350, 99374-99375, 99377-99378, 99446-99449, 99451-99452, 99495-99496, G0463, G0471, J2001

53210 0213T, 0216T, 0228T, 0230T, 11000-11006, 11042-11047, 12001-12007, 12011-12057, 13100-13133, 13151-13153, 36000, 36400-36410, 36420-36430, 36440, 36591-36592, 36600, 36640, 43752, 51701-51703,

CPT © 2020 American Medical Association. All Rights Reserved.

Coding Companion for Urology/Nephrology

52000, 52301, 53000-53025, 53080, 53200, 53220, 53250-53275, 62320-62327, 64400, 64405-64408, 64415-64435, 64445-64454, 64461-64463, 64479-64505, 64510-64530, 69990, 92012-92014, 93000-93010, 93040-93042, 93318, 93355, 94002, 94200, 94250, 94680-94690, 94770, 95812-95816, 95819, 95822, 95829, 95955, 96360-96368, 96372, 96374-96377, 96523, 97597-97598, 97602, 99155, 99156, 99157, 99211-99223, 99231-99255, 99291-99292, 99304-99310, 99315-99316, 99334-99337, 99347-99350, 99374-99375, 99377-99378, 99446-99449, 99451-99452, 99495-99496, G0463, G0471

53215 0213T, 0216T, 0228T, 0230T, 11000-11006, 11042-11047, 12001-12007, 12011-12057, 13100-13133, 13151-13153, 36000, 36400-36410, 36420-36430, 36440, 36591-36592, 36600, 36640, 43752, 51701-51703, 52000, 52301, 53000-53025, 53080, 53200-53210, 53220, 53235, 53250-53275, 62320-62327, 64400, 64405-64408, 64415-64435, 64445-64454, 64461-64463, 64479-64505, 64510-64530, 69990, 92012-92014, 93000-93010, 93040-93042, 93318, 93355, 94002, 94200, 94250, 94680-94690, 94770, 95812-95816, 95819, 95822, 95829, 95955, 96360-96368, 96372, 96374-96377, 96523, 97597-97598, 97602, 99155, 99156, 99157, 99211-99223, 99231-99255, 99291-99292, 99304-99310, 99315-99316, 99334-99337, 99347-99350, 99374-99375, 99377-99378, 99446-99449, 99451-99452, 99495-99496, G0463, G0471

53220 0213T, 0216T, 0228T, 0230T, 11000-11006, 11042-11047, 12001-12007, 12011-12057, 13100-13133, 13151-13153, 36000, 36400-36410, 36420-36430, 36440, 36591-36592, 36600, 36640, 43752, 51701-51703, 52000, 52301, 53000-53025, 53080, 56740, 62320-62327, 64400, 64405-64408, 64415-64435, 64445-64454, 64461-64463, 64479-64505, 64510-64530, 69990, 92012-92014, 93000-93010, 93040-93042, 93318, 93355, 94002, 94200, 94250, 94680-94690, 94770, 95812-95816, 95819, 95822, 95829, 95955, 96360-96368, 96372, 96374-96377, 96523, 97597-97598, 97602, 99155, 99156, 99157, 99211-99223, 99231-99255, 99291-99292, 99304-99310, 99315-99316, 99334-99337, 99347-99350, 99374-99375, 99377-99378, 99446-99449, 99451-99452, 99495-99496, G0463, G0471

53230 0213T, 0216T, 0228T, 0230T, 11000-11006, 11042-11047, 12001-12007, 12011-12057, 13100-13133, 13151-13153, 36000, 36400-36410, 36420-36430, 36440, 36591-36592, 36600, 36640, 43752, 51701-51703, 52000, 52301, 53000-53025, 62320-62327, 64400, 64405-64408, 64415-64435, 64445-64454, 64461-64463, 64479-64505, 64510-64530, 69990, 92012-92014, 93000-93010, 93040-93042, 93318, 93355, 94002, 94200, 94250, 94680-94690, 94770, 95812-95816, 95819, 95822, 95829, 95955, 96360-96368, 96372, 96374-96377, 96523, 97597-97598, 97602, 99155, 99156, 99157, 99211-99223, 99231-99255, 99291-99292, 99304-99310, 99315-99316, 99334-99337, 99347-99350, 99374-99375, 99377-99378, 99446-99449, 99451-99452, 99495-99496, G0463, G0471

53235 0213T, 0216T, 0228T, 0230T, 11000-11006, 11042-11047, 12001-12007, 12011-12057, 13100-13133, 13151-13153, 36000, 36400-36410, 36420-36430, 36440, 36591-36592, 36600, 36640, 43752, 51701-51703, 52000, 52301, 53000-53025, 53080, 53230✦, 62320-62327, 64400, 64405-64408, 64415-64435, 64445-64454, 64461-64463, 64479-64505, 64510-64530, 69990, 92012-92014, 93000-93010, 93040-93042, 93318, 93355, 94002, 94200, 94250, 94680-94690, 94770, 95812-95816, 95819, 95822, 95829, 95955, 96360-96368, 96372, 96374-96377, 96523, 97597-97598, 97602, 99155, 99156, 99157, 99211-99223, 99231-99255, 99291-99292, 99304-99310, 99315-99316, 99334-99337, 99347-99350, 99374-99375, 99377-99378, 99446-99449, 99451-99452, 99495-99496, G0463, G0471

53240 0213T, 0216T, 0228T, 0230T, 12001-12007, 12011-12057, 13100-13133, 13151-13153, 36000, 36400-36410, 36420-36430, 36440, 36591-36592, 36600, 36640, 43752, 51701-51703, 52000, 52301, 53000-53025,

53250 0213T, 0216T, 0228T, 0230T, 11000-11006, 11042-11047, 12001-12007, 12011-12057, 13100-13133, 13151-13153, 36000, 36400-36410, 36420-36430, 36440, 36591-36592, 36600, 36640, 43752, 51701-51703, 52000, 53000-53040, 53080, 53230, 62320-62327, 64400, 64405-64408, 64415-64435, 64445-64454, 64461-64463, 64479-64505, 64510-64530, 69990, 92012-92014, 93000-93010, 93040-93042, 93318, 93355, 94002, 94200, 94250, 94680-94690, 94770, 95812-95816, 95819, 95822, 95829, 95955, 96360-96368, 96372, 96374-96377, 96523, 97597-97598, 97602, 99155, 99156, 99157, 99211-99223, 99231-99255, 99291-99292, 99304-99310, 99315-99316, 99334-99337, 99347-99350, 99374-99375, 99377-99378, 99446-99449, 99451-99452, 99495-99496, G0463, G0471

53260 0213T, 0216T, 0228T, 0230T, 11000-11006, 11042-11047, 12001-12007, 12011-12057, 13100-13133, 13151-13153, 36000, 36400-36410, 36420-36430, 36440, 36591-36592, 36600, 36640, 43752, 51701-51703, 52000, 53000-53025, 53080, 53230, 62320-62327, 64400, 64405-64408, 64415-64435, 64445-64454, 64461-64463, 64479-64505, 64510-64530, 69990, 92012-92014, 93000-93010, 93040-93042, 93318, 93355, 94002, 94200, 94250, 94680-94690, 94770, 95812-95816, 95819, 95822, 95829, 95955, 96360-96368, 96372, 96374-96377, 96523, 97597-97598, 97602, 99155, 99156, 99157, 99211-99223, 99231-99255, 99291-99292, 99304-99310, 99315-99316, 99334-99337, 99347-99350, 99374-99375, 99377-99378, 99446-99449, 99451-99452, 99495-99496, G0463, G0471, J2001

53265 0213T, 0216T, 0228T, 0230T, 11000-11006, 11042-11047, 12001-12007, 12011-12057, 13100-13133, 13151-13153, 36000, 36400-36410, 36420-36430, 36440, 36591-36592, 36600, 36640, 43752, 51701-51703, 52000, 53000-53025, 53080, 53230, 62320-62327, 64400, 64405-64408, 64415-64435, 64445-64454, 64461-64463, 64479-64505, 64510-64530, 69990, 92012-92014, 93000-93010, 93040-93042, 93318, 93355, 94002, 94200, 94250, 94680-94690, 94770, 95812-95816, 95819, 95822, 95829, 95955, 96360-96368, 96372, 96374-96377, 96523, 97597-97598, 97602, 99155, 99156, 99157, 99211-99223, 99231-99255, 99291-99292, 99304-99310, 99315-99316, 99334-99337, 99347-99350, 99374-99375, 99377-99378, 99446-99449, 99451-99452, 99495-99496, G0463, G0471, J0670, J2001

53270 0213T, 0216T, 0228T, 0230T, 11000-11006, 11042-11047, 12001-12007, 12011-12057, 13100-13133, 13151-13153, 36000, 36400-36410, 36420-36430, 36440, 36591-36592, 36600, 36640, 43752, 51701-51703, 52000, 53000-53025, 53080, 53230, 62320-62327, 64400, 64405-64408, 64415-64435, 64445-64454, 64461-64463, 64479-64505, 64510-64530, 69990, 92012-92014, 93000-93010, 93040-93042, 93318, 93355, 94002, 94200, 94250, 94680-94690, 94770, 95812-95816, 95819, 95822, 95829, 95955, 96360-96368, 96372, 96374-96377, 96523, 97597-97598, 97602, 99155, 99156, 99157, 99211-99223, 99231-99255, 99291-99292, 99304-99310, 99315-99316, 99334-99337, 99347-99350, 99374-99375, 99377-99378, 99446-99449, 99451-99452, 99495-99496, G0463, G0471, J2001

53275 0213T, 0216T, 0228T, 0230T, 11000-11006, 11042-11047, 12001-12007, 12011-12057, 13100-13133, 13151-13153, 36000, 36400-36410, 36420-36430, 36440, 36591-36592, 36600, 36640, 43752, 51701-51703, 52000, 53000-53025, 53080, 53230, 62320-62327, 64400, 64405-64408,

CPT © 2020 American Medical Association. All Rights Reserved.

64415-64435, 64445-64454, 64461-64463, 64479-64505, 64510-64530, 69990, 92012-92014, 93000-93010, 93040-93042, 93318, 93355, 94002, 94200, 94250, 94680-94690, 94770, 95812-95816, 95819, 95822, 95829, 95955, 96360-96368, 96372, 96374-96377, 96523, 97597-97598, 97602, 99155, 99156, 99157, 99211-99223, 99231-99255, 99291-99292, 99304-99310, 99315-99316, 99334-99337, 99347-99350, 99374-99375, 99377-99378, 99446-99449, 99451-99452, 99495-99496, G0463, G0471

53400 0213T, 0216T, 0228T, 0230T, 11000-11006, 11042-11047, 12001-12007, 12011-12057, 13100-13133, 13151-13153, 36000, 36400-36410, 36420-36430, 36440, 36591-36592, 36600, 36640, 43752, 51701-51703, 52000, 52301, 53000-53025, 53080, 53405♦, 53502-53520, 62320-62327, 64400, 64405-64408, 64415-64435, 64445-64454, 64461-64463, 64479-64505, 64510-64530, 69990, 92012-92014, 93000-93010, 93040-93042, 93318, 93355, 94002, 94200, 94250, 94680-94690, 94770, 95812-95816, 95819, 95822, 95829, 95955, 96360-96368, 96372, 96374-96377, 96523, 97597-97598, 97602, 99155, 99156, 99157, 99211-99223, 99231-99255, 99291-99292, 99304-99310, 99315-99316, 99334-99337, 99347-99350, 99374-99375, 99377-99378, 99446-99449, 99451-99452, 99495-99496, G0463, G0471

53405 0213T, 0216T, 0228T, 0230T, 11000-11006, 11042-11047, 12001-12007, 12011-12057, 13100-13133, 13151-13153, 36000, 36400-36410, 36420-36430, 36440, 36591-36592, 36600, 36640, 43752, 51701-51703, 52000, 52301, 53000-53025, 53080, 53502-53520, 62320-62327, 64400, 64405-64408, 64415-64435, 64445-64454, 64461-64463, 64479-64505, 64510-64530, 69990, 92012-92014, 93000-93010, 93040-93042, 93318, 93355, 94002, 94200, 94250, 94680-94690, 94770, 95812-95816, 95819, 95822, 95829, 95955, 96360-96368, 96372, 96374-96377, 96523, 97597-97598, 97602, 99155, 99156, 99157, 99211-99223, 99231-99255, 99291-99292, 99304-99310, 99315-99316, 99334-99337, 99347-99350, 99374-99375, 99377-99378, 99446-99449, 99451-99452, 99495-99496, G0463, G0471

53410 0213T, 0216T, 0228T, 0230T, 11000-11006, 11042-11047, 12001-12007, 12011-12057, 13100-13133, 13151-13153, 36000, 36400-36410, 36420-36430, 36440, 36591-36592, 36600, 36640, 43752, 51701-51703, 51990-51992, 52000, 52301, 53000-53025, 53080, 53502-53520, 62320-62327, 64400, 64405-64408, 64415-64435, 64445-64454, 64461-64463, 64479-64505, 64510-64530, 69990, 92012-92014, 93000-93010, 93040-93042, 93318, 93355, 94002, 94200, 94250, 94680-94690, 94770, 95812-95816, 95819, 95822, 95829, 95955, 96360-96368, 96372, 96374-96377, 96523, 97597-97598, 97602, 99155, 99156, 99157, 99211-99223, 99231-99255, 99291-99292, 99304-99310, 99315-99316, 99334-99337, 99347-99350, 99374-99375, 99377-99378, 99446-99449, 99451-99452, 99495-99496, G0463, G0471

53415 0213T, 0216T, 0228T, 0230T, 11000-11006, 11042-11047, 12001-12007, 12011-12057, 13100-13133, 13151-13153, 36000, 36400-36410, 36420-36430, 36440, 36591-36592, 36600, 36640, 43752, 51701-51703, 51990-51992, 52000, 52301, 52640, 53000-53025, 53080, 53502-53520, 62320-62327, 64400, 64405-64408, 64415-64435, 64445-64454, 64461-64463, 64479-64505, 64510-64530, 69990, 92012-92014, 93000-93010, 93040-93042, 93318, 93355, 94002, 94200, 94250, 94680-94690, 94770, 95812-95816, 95819, 95822, 95829, 95955, 96360-96368, 96372, 96374-96377, 96523, 97597-97598, 97602, 99155, 99156, 99157, 99211-99223, 99231-99255, 99291-99292, 99304-99310, 99315-99316, 99334-99337, 99347-99350, 99374-99375, 99377-99378, 99446-99449, 99451-99452, 99495-99496, G0463, G0471

53420 0213T, 0216T, 0228T, 0230T, 11000-11006, 11042-11047, 12001-12007, 12011-12057, 13100-13133, 13151-13153, 36000, 36400-36410, 36420-36430, 36440, 36591-36592, 36600, 36640, 43752, 51701-51703, 51990-51992, 52000, 52301, 52640, 53000-53025, 53080, 53425♦,

53502-53520, 62320-62327, 64400, 64405-64408, 64415-64435, 64445-64454, 64461-64463, 64479-64505, 64510-64530, 69990, 92012-92014, 93000-93010, 93040-93042, 93318, 93355, 94002, 94200, 94250, 94680-94690, 94770, 95812-95816, 95819, 95822, 95829, 95955, 96360-96368, 96372, 96374-96377, 96523, 97597-97598, 97602, 99155, 99156, 99157, 99211-99223, 99231-99255, 99291-99292, 99304-99310, 99315-99316, 99334-99337, 99347-99350, 99374-99375, 99377-99378, 99446-99449, 99451-99452, 99495-99496, G0463, G0471

53425 0213T, 0216T, 0228T, 0230T, 11000-11006, 11042-11047, 12001-12007, 12011-12057, 13100-13133, 13151-13153, 36000, 36400-36410, 36420-36430, 36440, 36591-36592, 36600, 36640, 43752, 51701-51703, 51990-51992, 52000, 52301, 52640, 53000-53025, 53080, 53502-53520, 62320-62327, 64400, 64405-64408, 64415-64435, 64445-64454, 64461-64463, 64479-64505, 64510-64530, 69990, 92012-92014, 93000-93010, 93040-93042, 93318, 93355, 94002, 94200, 94250, 94680-94690, 94770, 95812-95816, 95819, 95822, 95829, 95955, 96360-96368, 96372, 96374-96377, 96523, 97597-97598, 97602, 99155, 99156, 99157, 99211-99223, 99231-99255, 99291-99292, 99304-99310, 99315-99316, 99334-99337, 99347-99350, 99374-99375, 99377-99378, 99446-99449, 99451-99452, 99495-99496, G0463, G0471

53430 0213T, 0216T, 0228T, 0230T, 11000-11006, 11042-11047, 12001-12007, 12011-12057, 13100-13133, 13151-13153, 36000, 36400-36410, 36420-36430, 36440, 36591-36592, 36600, 36640, 43752, 51701-51703, 51990-51992, 52000, 52301, 53000-53025, 53080, 53502-53520, 53860♦, 62320-62327, 64400, 64405-64408, 64415-64435, 64445-64454, 64461-64463, 64479-64505, 64510-64530, 69990, 92012-92014, 93000-93010, 93040-93042, 93318, 93355, 94002, 94200, 94250, 94680-94690, 94770, 95812-95816, 95819, 95822, 95829, 95955, 96360-96368, 96372, 96374-96377, 96523, 97597-97598, 97602, 99155, 99156, 99157, 99211-99223, 99231-99255, 99291-99292, 99304-99310, 99315-99316, 99334-99337, 99347-99350, 99374-99375, 99377-99378, 99446-99449, 99451-99452, 99495-99496, G0463, G0471

53431 0213T, 0216T, 0228T, 0230T, 11000-11006, 11042-11047, 12001-12007, 12011-12057, 13100-13133, 13151-13153, 36000, 36400-36410, 36420-36430, 36440, 36591-36592, 36600, 36640, 43752, 51701-51703, 51990-51992, 52000, 52301, 53000-53025, 53080, 53502-53520, 53860♦, 62320-62327, 64400, 64405-64408, 64415-64435, 64445-64454, 64461-64463, 64479-64505, 64510-64530, 69990, 92012-92014, 93000-93010, 93040-93042, 93318, 93355, 94002, 94200, 94250, 94680-94690, 94770, 95812-95816, 95819, 95822, 95829, 95955, 96360-96368, 96372, 96374-96377, 96523, 97597-97598, 97602, 99155, 99156, 99157, 99211-99223, 99231-99255, 99291-99292, 99304-99310, 99315-99316, 99334-99337, 99347-99350, 99374-99375, 99377-99378, 99446-99449, 99451-99452, 99495-99496, G0463, G0471

53440 0213T, 0216T, 0228T, 0230T, 12001-12007, 12011-12057, 13100-13133, 13151-13153, 36000, 36400-36410, 36420-36430, 36440, 36591-36592, 36600, 36640, 43752, 51701-51703, 51990-51992, 52000, 52301, 53000-53025, 53080, 53444, 62320-62327, 64400, 64405-64408, 64415-64435, 64445-64454, 64461-64463, 64479-64505, 64510-64530, 69990, 92012-92014, 93000-93010, 93040-93042, 93318, 93355, 94002, 94200, 94250, 94680-94690, 94770, 95812-95816, 95819, 95822, 95829, 95955, 96360-96368, 96372, 96374-96377, 96523, 99155, 99156, 99157, 99211-99223, 99231-99255, 99291-99292, 99304-99310, 99315-99316, 99334-99337, 99347-99350, 99374-99375, 99377-99378, 99446-99449, 99451-99452, 99495-99496, G0463, G0471

53442 0213T, 0216T, 0228T, 0230T, 11000-11006, 11042-11047, 12001-12007, 12011-12057, 13100-13133, 13151-13153, 36000, 36400-36410, 36420-36430, 36440, 36591-36592, 36600, 36640, 43752, 51701-51703, 52000, 52301, 53000-53025, 53440♦, 62320-62327, 64400,

CPT © 2020 American Medical Association. All Rights Reserved.

64405-64408, 64415-64435, 64445-64454, 64461-64463, 64479-64505,
64510-64530, 69990, 92012-92014, 93000-93010, 93040-93042, 93318,
93355, 94002, 94200, 94250, 94680-94690, 94770, 95812-95816,
95819, 95822, 95829, 95955, 96360-96368, 96372, 96374-96377,
96523, 97597-97598, 97602, 99155, 99156, 99157, 99211-99223,
99231-99255, 99291-99292, 99304-99310, 99315-99316, 99334-99337,
99347-99350, 99374-99375, 99377-99378, 99446-99449, 99451-99452,
99495-99496, G0463, G0471

53444 0213T, 0216T, 0228T, 0230T, 0550T, 11000-11006, 11042-11047,
12001-12007, 12011-12057, 13100-13133, 13151-13153, 36000,
36400-36410, 36420-36430, 36440, 36591-36592, 36600, 36640, 43752,
51701-51703, 52000, 53000-53025, 53446, 53449, 62320-62327, 64400,
64405-64408, 64415-64435, 64445-64454, 64461-64463, 64479-64505,
64510-64530, 69990, 92012-92014, 93000-93010, 93040-93042, 93318,
93355, 94002, 94200, 94250, 94680-94690, 94770, 95812-95816,
95819, 95822, 95829, 95955, 96360-96368, 96372, 96374-96377,
96523, 97597-97598, 97602, 99155, 99156, 99157, 99211-99223,
99231-99255, 99291-99292, 99304-99310, 99315-99316, 99334-99337,
99347-99350, 99374-99375, 99377-99378, 99446-99449, 99451-99452,
99495-99496, G0463, G0471

53445 0213T, 0216T, 0228T, 0230T, 11000-11006, 11042-11047, 12001-12007,
12011-12057, 13100-13133, 13151-13153, 36000, 36400-36410,
36420-36430, 36440, 36591-36592, 36600, 36640, 43752, 51701-51703,
51990-51992, 52000, 52301, 53000-53025, 53080, 53444, 62320-62327,
64400, 64405-64408, 64415-64435, 64445-64454, 64461-64463,
64479-64505, 64510-64530, 69990, 92012-92014, 93000-93010,
93040-93042, 93318, 93355, 94002, 94200, 94250, 94680-94690,
94770, 95812-95816, 95819, 95822, 95955, 96360-96368,
96372, 96374-96377, 96523, 97597-97598, 97602, 99155, 99156,
99157, 99211-99223, 99231-99255, 99291-99292, 99304-99310,
99315-99316, 99334-99337, 99347-99350, 99374-99375, 99377-99378,
99446-99449, 99451-99452, 99495-99496, G0463, G0471

53446 0213T, 0216T, 0228T, 0230T, 0548T-0549T, 11000-11006, 11042-11047,
12001-12007, 12011-12057, 13100-13133, 13151-13153, 36000,
36400-36410, 36420-36430, 36440, 36591-36592, 36600, 36640, 43752,
51701-51703, 52000, 53000-53025, 53080, 53445, 62320-62327, 64400,
64405-64408, 64415-64435, 64445-64454, 64461-64463, 64479-64505,
64510-64530, 69990, 92012-92014, 93000-93010, 93040-93042, 93318,
93355, 94002, 94200, 94250, 94680-94690, 94770, 95812-95816,
95819, 95822, 95829, 95955, 96360-96368, 96372, 96374-96377,
96523, 97597-97598, 97602, 99155, 99156, 99157, 99211-99223,
99231-99255, 99291-99292, 99304-99310, 99315-99316, 99334-99337,
99347-99350, 99374-99375, 99377-99378, 99446-99449, 99451-99452,
99495-99496, G0463, G0471

53447 0213T, 0216T, 0228T, 0230T, 0548T-0549T, 0550T, 11000-11006,
11042-11047, 12001-12007, 12011-12057, 13100-13133, 13151-13153,
36000, 36400-36410, 36420-36430, 36440, 36591-36592, 36600, 36640,
43752, 51701-51703, 52000, 52301, 53000-53025, 53080, 53440,
53444-53446, 53448-53449, 62320-62327, 64400, 64405-64408,
64415-64435, 64445-64454, 64461-64463, 64479-64505, 64510-64530,
69990, 92012-92014, 93000-93010, 93040-93042, 93318, 93355, 94002,
94200, 94250, 94680-94690, 94770, 95812-95816, 95819, 95822,
95829, 95955, 96360-96368, 96372, 96374-96377, 96523, 97597-97598,
97602, 99155, 99156, 99157, 99211-99223, 99231-99255, 99291-99292,
99304-99310, 99315-99316, 99334-99337, 99347-99350, 99374-99375,
99377-99378, 99446-99449, 99451-99452, 99495-99496, G0463, G0471

53448 0213T, 0216T, 0228T, 0230T, 0548T-0549T, 0550T, 11000-11006,
11042-11047, 12001-12007, 12011-12057, 13100-13133, 13151-13153,
36000, 36400-36410, 36420-36430, 36440, 36591-36592, 36600, 36640,

43752, 51701-51703, 52000, 53000-53025, 53080, 53440, 53444-53446,
53449, 62320-62327, 64400, 64405-64408, 64415-64435, 64445-64454,
64461-64463, 64479-64505, 64510-64530, 69990, 92012-92014,
93000-93010, 93040-93042, 93318, 93355, 94002, 94200, 94250,
94680-94690, 94770, 95812-95816, 95819, 95822, 95829, 95955,
96360-96368, 96372, 96374-96377, 96523, 97597-97598, 97602, 99155,
99156, 99157, 99211-99223, 99231-99255, 99291-99292, 99304-99310,
99315-99316, 99334-99337, 99347-99350, 99374-99375, 99377-99378,
99446-99449, 99451-99452, 99495-99496, G0463, G0471

53449 0213T, 0216T, 0228T, 0230T, 12001-12007, 12011-12057, 13100-13133,
13151-13153, 36000, 36400-36410, 36420-36430, 36440, 36591-36592,
36600, 36640, 43752, 51701-51703, 52000, 52301, 53000-53025,
53080, 62320-62327, 64400, 64405-64408, 64415-64435, 64445-64454,
64461-64463, 64479-64505, 64510-64530, 69990, 92012-92014,
93000-93010, 93040-93042, 93318, 93355, 94002, 94200, 94250,
94680-94690, 94770, 95812-95816, 95819, 95822, 95829, 95955,
96360-96368, 96372, 96374-96377, 96523, 99155, 99156, 99157,
99211-99223, 99231-99255, 99291-99292, 99304-99310, 99315-99316,
99334-99337, 99347-99350, 99374-99375, 99377-99378, 99446-99449,
99451-99452, 99495-99496, G0463, G0471

53450 0213T, 0216T, 0228T, 0230T, 11000-11006, 11042-11047, 12001-12007,
12011-12057, 13100-13133, 13151-13153, 36000, 36400-36410,
36420-36430, 36440, 36591-36592, 36600, 36640, 43752, 51701-51703,
52000, 52301, 53000-53025, 53080, 53502-53520, 62320-62327, 64400,
64405-64408, 64415-64435, 64445-64454, 64461-64463, 64479-64505,
64510-64530, 69990, 92012-92014, 93000-93010, 93040-93042, 93318,
93355, 94002, 94200, 94250, 94680-94690, 94770, 95812-95816,
95819, 95822, 95829, 95955, 96360-96368, 96372, 96374-96377,
96523, 97597-97598, 97602, 99155, 99156, 99157, 99211-99223,
99231-99255, 99291-99292, 99304-99310, 99315-99316, 99334-99337,
99347-99350, 99374-99375, 99377-99378, 99446-99449, 99451-99452,
99495-99496, G0463, G0471

53460 0213T, 0216T, 0228T, 0230T, 11000-11006, 11042-11047, 12001-12007,
12011-12057, 13100-13133, 13151-13153, 36000, 36400-36410,
36420-36430, 36440, 36591-36592, 36600, 36640, 43752, 51701-51703,
52000, 52301, 53000-53025, 53080, 53502-53520, 62320-62327, 64400,
64405-64408, 64415-64435, 64445-64454, 64461-64463, 64479-64505,
64510-64530, 69990, 92012-92014, 93000-93010, 93040-93042, 93318,
93355, 94002, 94200, 94250, 94680-94690, 94770, 95812-95816,
95819, 95822, 95829, 95955, 96360-96368, 96372, 96374-96377,
96523, 97597-97598, 97602, 99155, 99156, 99157, 99211-99223,
99231-99255, 99291-99292, 99304-99310, 99315-99316, 99334-99337,
99347-99350, 99374-99375, 99377-99378, 99446-99449, 99451-99452,
99495-99496, G0463, G0471

53500 00910, 0213T, 0216T, 0228T, 0230T, 12001-12007, 12011-12057,
13100-13133, 13151-13153, 36000, 36400-36410, 36420-36430, 36440,
36591-36592, 36600, 36640, 43752, 51700-51703, 52000, 52310-52315,
53000-53025, 53080, 53502-53510, 53520-53621, 53660-53665,
62320-62327, 64400, 64405-64408, 64415-64435, 64445-64454,
64461-64463, 64479-64505, 64510-64530, 69990, 92012-92014,
93000-93010, 93040-93042, 93318, 93355, 94002, 94200, 94250,
94680-94690, 94770, 95812-95816, 95819, 95822, 95829, 95955,
96360-96368, 96372, 96374-96377, 96523, 99155, 99156, 99157,
99211-99223, 99231-99255, 99291-99292, 99304-99310, 99315-99316,
99334-99337, 99347-99350, 99374-99375, 99377-99378, 99446-99449,
99451-99452, 99495-99496, G0463, G0471

53502 0213T, 0216T, 0228T, 0230T, 12001-12007, 12011-12057, 13100-13133,
13151-13153, 36000, 36400-36410, 36420-36430, 36440, 36591-36592,
36600, 36640, 43752, 51701-51703, 52000, 52301, 53000-53025,

53080, 62320-62327, 64400, 64405-64408, 64415-64435, 64445-64454, 64461-64463, 64479-64505, 64510-64530, 69990, 92012-92014, 93000-93010, 93040-93042, 93318, 93355, 94002, 94200, 94250, 94680-94690, 94770, 95812-95816, 95819, 95822, 95829, 95955, 96360-96368, 96372, 96374-96377, 96523, 99155, 99156, 99157, 99211-99223, 99231-99255, 99291-99292, 99304-99310, 99315-99316, 99334-99337, 99347-99350, 99374-99375, 99377-99378, 99446-99449, 99451-99452, 99495-99496, G0463, G0471

53505 0213T, 0216T, 0228T, 0230T, 12001-12007, 12011-12057, 13100-13133, 13151-13153, 36000, 36400-36410, 36420-36430, 36440, 36591-36592, 36600, 36640, 43752, 51701-51703, 52000, 52301, 53000-53025, 53080, 53502❖, 62320-62327, 64400, 64405-64408, 64415-64435, 64445-64454, 64461-64463, 64479-64505, 64510-64530, 69990, 92012-92014, 93000-93010, 93040-93042, 93318, 93355, 94002, 94200, 94250, 94680-94690, 94770, 95812-95816, 95819, 95822, 95829, 95955, 96360-96368, 96372, 96374-96377, 96523, 99155, 99156, 99157, 99211-99223, 99231-99255, 99291-99292, 99304-99310, 99315-99316, 99334-99337, 99347-99350, 99374-99375, 99377-99378, 99446-99449, 99451-99452, 99495-99496, G0463, G0471

53510 0213T, 0216T, 0228T, 0230T, 12001-12007, 12011-12057, 13100-13133, 13151-13153, 36000, 36400-36410, 36420-36430, 36440, 36591-36592, 36600, 36640, 43752, 51701-51703, 52000, 52301, 53000-53025, 53080, 62320-62327, 64400, 64405-64408, 64415-64435, 64445-64454, 64461-64463, 64479-64505, 64510-64530, 69990, 92012-92014, 93000-93010, 93040-93042, 93318, 93355, 94002, 94200, 94250, 94680-94690, 94770, 95812-95816, 95819, 95822, 95829, 95955, 96360-96368, 96372, 96374-96377, 96523, 99155, 99156, 99157, 99211-99223, 99231-99255, 99291-99292, 99304-99310, 99315-99316, 99334-99337, 99347-99350, 99374-99375, 99377-99378, 99446-99449, 99451-99452, 99495-99496, G0463, G0471

53515 0213T, 0216T, 0228T, 0230T, 12001-12007, 12011-12057, 13100-13133, 13151-13153, 36000, 36400-36410, 36420-36430, 36440, 36591-36592, 36600, 36640, 43752, 51701-51703, 52000, 52301, 53000-53025, 53080, 53500, 62320-62327, 64400, 64405-64408, 64415-64435, 64445-64454, 64461-64463, 64479-64505, 64510-64530, 69990, 92012-92014, 93000-93010, 93040-93042, 93318, 93355, 94002, 94200, 94250, 94680-94690, 94770, 95812-95816, 95819, 95822, 95829, 95955, 96360-96368, 96372, 96374-96377, 96523, 99155, 99156, 99157, 99211-99223, 99231-99255, 99291-99292, 99304-99310, 99315-99316, 99334-99337, 99347-99350, 99374-99375, 99377-99378, 99446-99449, 99451-99452, 99495-99496, G0463, G0471

53520 0213T, 0216T, 0228T, 0230T, 11000-11006, 11042-11047, 12001-12007, 12011-12057, 13100-13133, 13151-13153, 36000, 36400-36410, 36420-36430, 36440, 36591-36592, 36600, 36640, 43752, 51701-51703, 52000, 52301, 53000-53025, 53080, 62320-62327, 64400, 64405-64408, 64415-64435, 64445-64454, 64461-64463, 64479-64505, 64510-64530, 69990, 92012-92014, 93000-93010, 93040-93042, 93318, 93355, 94002, 94200, 94250, 94680-94690, 94770, 95812-95816, 95819, 95822, 95829, 95955, 96360-96368, 96372, 96374-96377, 96523, 97597-97598, 97602, 99155, 99156, 99157, 99211-99223, 99231-99255, 99291-99292, 99304-99310, 99315-99316, 99334-99337, 99347-99350, 99374-99375, 99377-99378, 99446-99449, 99451-99452, 99495-99496, G0463, G0471

53600 0213T, 0216T, 0228T, 0230T, 12001-12007, 12011-12057, 13100-13133, 13151-13153, 36000, 36400-36410, 36420-36430, 36440, 36591-36592, 36600, 36640, 43752, 51701-51703, 53000-53025, 53601❖, 53660-53665, 62320-62327, 64400, 64405-64408, 64415-64435, 64445-64454, 64461-64463, 64479-64505, 64510-64530, 69990, 92012-92014, 93000-93010, 93040-93042, 93318, 93355, 94002, 94200, 94250, 94680-94690, 94770, 95812-95816, 95819, 95822, 95829,

95955, 96360-96368, 96372, 96374-96377, 96523, 99155, 99156, 99157, 99211-99223, 99231-99255, 99291-99292, 99304-99310, 99315-99316, 99334-99337, 99347-99350, 99374-99375, 99377-99378, 99446-99449, 99451-99452, 99495-99496, G0463, G0471, J0670, J2001, P9612

53601 0213T, 0216T, 0228T, 0230T, 12001-12007, 12011-12057, 13100-13133, 13151-13153, 36000, 36400-36410, 36420-36430, 36440, 36591-36592, 36600, 36640, 43752, 51701-51703, 53000-53025, 53660-53665, 62320-62327, 64400, 64405-64408, 64415-64435, 64445-64454, 64461-64463, 64479-64505, 64510-64530, 69990, 92012-92014, 93000-93010, 93040-93042, 93318, 93355, 94002, 94200, 94250, 94680-94690, 94770, 95812-95816, 95819, 95822, 95829, 95955, 96360-96368, 96372, 96374-96377, 96523, 99155, 99156, 99157, 99211-99223, 99231-99255, 99291-99292, 99304-99310, 99315-99316, 99334-99337, 99347-99350, 99374-99375, 99377-99378, 99446-99449, 99451-99452, 99495-99496, G0463, G0471, J0670, J2001, P9612

53605 0213T, 0216T, 0228T, 0230T, 12001-12007, 12011-12057, 13100-13133, 13151-13153, 36000, 36400-36410, 36420-36430, 36440, 36591-36592, 36600, 36640, 43752, 51701-51703, 53000-53025, 53600-53601❖, 53660-53665, 62320-62327, 64400, 64405-64408, 64415-64435, 64445-64454, 64461-64463, 64479-64505, 64510-64530, 69990, 92012-92014, 93000-93010, 93040-93042, 93318, 93355, 94002, 94200, 94250, 94680-94690, 94770, 95812-95816, 95819, 95822, 95829, 95955, 96360-96368, 96372, 96374-96377, 96523, 99151❖, 99152❖, 99153❖, 99155, 99156, 99157, 99211-99223, 99231-99255, 99291-99292, 99304-99310, 99315-99316, 99334-99337, 99347-99350, 99374-99375, 99377-99378, 99446-99449, 99451-99452, 99495-99496, G0463, G0471

53620 0213T, 0216T, 0228T, 0230T, 12001-12007, 12011-12057, 13100-13133, 13151-13153, 36000, 36400-36410, 36420-36430, 36440, 36591-36592, 36600, 36640, 43752, 51701-51703, 53000-53025, 53600-53605❖, 53621❖, 53660-53665, 62320-62327, 64400, 64405-64408, 64415-64435, 64445-64454, 64461-64463, 64479-64505, 64510-64530, 69990, 92012-92014, 93000-93010, 93040-93042, 93318, 93355, 94002, 94200, 94250, 94680-94690, 94770, 95812-95816, 95819, 95822, 95829, 95955, 96360-96368, 96372, 96374-96377, 96523, 99155, 99156, 99157, 99211-99223, 99231-99255, 99291-99292, 99304-99310, 99315-99316, 99334-99337, 99347-99350, 99374-99375, 99377-99378, 99446-99449, 99451-99452, 99495-99496, G0463, G0471, J0670, J2001

53621 0213T, 0216T, 0228T, 0230T, 12001-12007, 12011-12057, 13100-13133, 13151-13153, 36000, 36400-36410, 36420-36430, 36440, 36591-36592, 36600, 36640, 43752, 51701-51703, 53000-53025, 53600-53605❖, 62320-62327, 64400, 64405-64408, 64415-64435, 64445-64454, 64461-64463, 64479-64505, 64510-64530, 69990, 92012-92014, 93000-93010, 93040-93042, 93318, 93355, 94002, 94200, 94250, 94680-94690, 94770, 95812-95816, 95819, 95822, 95829, 95955, 96360-96368, 96372, 96374-96377, 96523, 99155, 99156, 99157, 99211-99223, 99231-99255, 99291-99292, 99304-99310, 99315-99316, 99334-99337, 99347-99350, 99374-99375, 99377-99378, 99446-99449, 99451-99452, 99495-99496, G0463, G0471, J0670, J2001

53660 0213T, 0216T, 0228T, 0230T, 0421T, 12001-12007, 12011-12057, 13100-13133, 13151-13153, 36000, 36400-36410, 36420-36430, 36440, 36591-36592, 36600, 36640, 43752, 51701-51703, 53000-53025, 53080, 53661❖, 62320-62327, 64400, 64405-64408, 64415-64435, 64445-64454, 64461-64463, 64479-64505, 64510-64530, 69990, 92012-92014, 93000-93010, 93040-93042, 93318, 93355, 94002, 94200, 94250, 94680-94690, 94770, 95812-95816, 95819, 95822, 95829, 95955, 96360-96368, 96372, 96374-96377, 96523, 99155, 99156, 99157, 99211-99223, 99231-99255, 99291-99292, 99304-99310,

CPT © 2020 American Medical Association. All Rights Reserved.

99315-99316, 99334-99337, 99347-99350, 99374-99375, 99377-99378, 99446-99449, 99451-99452, 99495-99496, G0463, G0471, J0670, J2001, P9612

53661 0213T, 0216T, 0228T, 0230T, 0421T, 12001-12007, 12011-12057, 13100-13133, 13151-13153, 36000, 36400-36410, 36420-36430, 36440, 36591-36592, 36600, 36640, 43752, 51700-51703, 53000-53025, 53080, 62320-62327, 64400, 64405-64408, 64415-64435, 64445-64454, 64461-64463, 64479-64505, 64510-64530, 69990, 92012-92014, 93000-93010, 93040-93042, 93318, 93355, 94002, 94200, 94250, 94680-94690, 94770, 95812-95816, 95819, 95822, 95829, 95955, 96360-96368, 96372, 96374-96377, 96523, 99155, 99156, 99157, 99211-99223, 99231-99255, 99291-99292, 99304-99310, 99315-99316, 99334-99337, 99347-99350, 99374-99375, 99377-99378, 99446-99449, 99451-99452, 99495-99496, G0463, G0471, J0670, J2001, P9612

53665 0213T, 0216T, 0228T, 0230T, 0421T, 12001-12007, 12011-12057, 13100-13133, 13151-13153, 36000, 36400-36410, 36420-36430, 36440, 36591-36592, 36600, 36640, 43752, 51701-51703, 53000-53025, 53080, 53660-53661✦, 62320-62327, 64400, 64405-64408, 64415-64435, 64445-64454, 64461-64463, 64479-64505, 64510-64530, 69990, 92012-92014, 93000-93010, 93040-93042, 93318, 93355, 94002, 94200, 94250, 94680-94690, 94770, 95812-95816, 95819, 95822, 95829, 95955, 96360-96368, 96372, 96374-96377, 96523, 99151✦, 99152✦, 99153✦, 99155, 99156, 99157, 99211-99223, 99231-99255, 99291-99292, 99304-99310, 99315-99316, 99334-99337, 99347-99350, 99374-99375, 99377-99378, 99446-99449, 99451-99452, 99495-99496, G0463, G0471

53850 0213T, 0216T, 0228T, 0230T, 0421T✦, 12001-12007, 12011-12057, 13100-13133, 13151-13153, 36000, 36400-36410, 36420-36430, 36440, 36591-36592, 36600, 36640, 43752, 51700-51703, 52000-52005, 52276, 52281, 52441, 52630-52640✦, 53000-53025, 53600-53621, 53855, 55700, 55706✦, 55873✦, 62320-62327, 64400, 64405-64408, 64415-64435, 64445-64454, 64461-64463, 64479-64505, 64510-64530, 69990, 76872-76873, 92012-92014, 93000-93010, 93040-93042, 93318, 93355, 94002, 94200, 94250, 94680-94690, 94770, 95812-95816, 95819, 95822, 95829, 95955, 96360-96368, 96372, 96374-96377, 96523, 99155, 99156, 99157, 99211-99223, 99231-99255, 99291-99292, 99304-99310, 99315-99316, 99334-99337, 99347-99350, 99374-99375, 99377-99378, 99446-99449, 99451-99452, 99495-99496, G0463, G0471, J0670, J2001, P9612

53852 0213T, 0216T, 0228T, 0230T, 0421T✦, 12001-12007, 12011-12057, 13100-13133, 13151-13153, 36000, 36400-36410, 36420-36430, 36440, 36591-36592, 36600, 36640, 43752, 51102, 51700-51703, 52000-52001, 52281, 52441, 52500, 52630-52640✦, 53000-53025, 53600-53621, 53850✦, 53855, 55700, 55706✦, 55873✦, 62320-62327, 64400, 64405-64408, 64415-64435, 64445-64454, 64461-64463, 64479-64505, 64510-64530, 69990, 76872-76873, 92012-92014, 93000-93010, 93040-93042, 93318, 93355, 94002, 94200, 94250, 94680-94690, 94770, 95812-95816, 95819, 95822, 95829, 95955, 96360-96368, 96372, 96374-96377, 96523, 99155, 99156, 99157, 99211-99223, 99231-99255, 99291-99292, 99304-99310, 99315-99316, 99334-99337, 99347-99350, 99374-99375, 99377-99378, 99446-99449, 99451-99452, 99495-99496, G0463, G0471, J0670, J2001, P9612

53854 0213T, 0216T, 0228T, 0230T, 0421T✦, 12001-12007, 12011-12057, 13100-13133, 13151-13153, 36000, 36400-36410, 36420-36430, 36440, 36591-36592, 36600, 36640, 43752, 51102, 51700-51703, 52000-52001, 52281, 52441, 52500, 52640✦, 53000-53025, 53600-53621, 53850-53852✦, 53855, 55700, 62320-62327, 64400, 64405-64408, 64415-64435, 64445-64454, 64461-64463, 64479-64505, 64510-64530, 69990, 76872-76873, 92012-92014, 93000-93010, 93040-93042, 93318,

93355, 94002, 94200, 94250, 94680-94690, 94770, 95812-95816, 95819, 95822, 95829, 95955, 96360-96368, 96372, 96374-96377, 96523, 99155, 99156, 99157, 99211-99223, 99231-99255, 99291-99292, 99304-99310, 99315-99316, 99334-99337, 99347-99350, 99374-99375, 99377-99378, 99446-99449, 99495-99496, G0463, G0471, J0670, J2001, P9612

53855 0213T, 0216T, 0228T, 0230T, 11000-11006, 11042-11047, 12001-12007, 12011-12057, 13100-13133, 13151-13153, 36000, 36400-36410, 36420-36430, 36440, 36591-36592, 36600, 36640, 43752, 51701-51703, 52000, 52442✦, 53000-53025, 53080, 53520-53621, 53660-53665, 62320-62327, 64400, 64405-64408, 64415-64435, 64445-64454, 64461-64463, 64479-64505, 64510-64530, 69990, 92012-92014, 93000-93010, 93040-93042, 93318, 93355, 94002, 94200, 94250, 94680-94690, 94770, 95812-95816, 95819, 95822, 95829, 95955, 96360-96368, 96372, 96374-96377, 96523, 97597-97598, 97602, 99155, 99156, 99157, 99211-99223, 99231-99255, 99291-99292, 99304-99310, 99315-99316, 99334-99337, 99347-99350, 99374-99375, 99377-99378, 99446-99449, 99451-99452, 99495-99496, G0463, G0471, J0670, J2001

53860 12001-12007, 12011-12057, 13100-13133, 13151-13153, 36000, 36400-36410, 36420-36430, 36440, 36591-36592, 36600, 36640, 43752, 51102, 51700-51703, 52000-52001, 52281, 52285✦, 52310-52315, 52500, 53000-53025, 53080, 53660-53665, 62320-62327, 64400, 64405-64408, 64415-64435, 64445-64454, 64461-64463, 64479-64505, 64510-64530, 69990, 92012-92014, 93000-93010, 93040-93042, 93318, 93355, 94002, 94200, 94250, 94680-94690, 94770, 95812-95816, 95819, 95822, 95829, 95955, 96360-96368, 96372, 96374-96377, 96523, 99155, 99156, 99157, 99211-99223, 99231-99255, 99291-99292, 99304-99310, 99315-99316, 99334-99337, 99347-99350, 99374-99375, 99377-99378, 99446-99449, 99451-99452, 99495-99496, G0463, G0471, J0670, J2001, P9612

54000 0213T, 0216T, 0228T, 0230T, 12001-12007, 12011-12057, 13100-13133, 13151-13153, 36000, 36400-36410, 36420-36430, 36440, 36591-36592, 36600, 36640, 43752, 51701-51703, 62320-62327, 64400, 64405-64408, 64415-64435, 64445-64454, 64461-64463, 64479-64505, 64510-64530, 69990, 92012-92014, 93000-93010, 93040-93042, 93318, 93355, 94002, 94200, 94250, 94680-94690, 94770, 95812-95816, 95819, 95822, 95829, 95955, 96360-96368, 96372, 96374-96377, 96523, 99155, 99156, 99157, 99211-99223, 99231-99255, 99291-99292, 99304-99310, 99315-99316, 99334-99337, 99347-99350, 99374-99375, 99377-99378, 99446-99449, 99451-99452, 99495-99496, G0463, G0471, J2001

54001 0213T, 0216T, 0228T, 0230T, 12001-12007, 12011-12057, 13100-13133, 13151-13153, 36000, 36400-36410, 36420-36430, 36440, 36591-36592, 36600, 36640, 43752, 51701-51703, 62320-62327, 64400, 64405-64408, 64415-64435, 64445-64454, 64461-64463, 64479-64505, 64510-64530, 69990, 92012-92014, 93000-93010, 93040-93042, 93318, 93355, 94002, 94200, 94250, 94680-94690, 94770, 95812-95816, 95819, 95822, 95829, 95955, 96360-96368, 96372, 96374-96377, 96523, 99155, 99156, 99157, 99211-99223, 99231-99255, 99291-99292, 99304-99310, 99315-99316, 99334-99337, 99347-99350, 99374-99375, 99377-99378, 99446-99449, 99451-99452, 99495-99496, G0463, G0471, J0670, J2001

54015 0213T, 0216T, 0228T, 0230T, 12001-12007, 12011-12057, 13100-13133, 13151-13153, 36000, 36400-36410, 36420-36430, 36440, 36591-36592, 36600, 36640, 43752, 51701-51703, 54001, 54450, 62320-62327, 64400, 64405-64408, 64415-64435, 64445-64454, 64461-64463, 64479-64505, 64510-64530, 69990, 92012-92014, 93000-93010, 93040-93042, 93318, 93355, 94002, 94200, 94250, 94680-94690, 94770, 95812-95816, 95819, 95822, 95829, 95955, 96360-96368, 96372, 96374-96377, 96523, 99155, 99156, 99157, 99211-99223, 99231-99255, 99291-99292, 99304-99310, 99315-99316, 99334-99337,

CCI Edits

99347-99350, 99374-99375, 99377-99378, 99446-99449, 99451-99452, 99495-99496, G0463, G0471, J2001

54050 0213T, 0216T, 0228T, 0230T, 12001-12007, 12011-12057, 13100-13133, 13151-13153, 36000, 36400-36410, 36420-36430, 36440, 36591-36592, 36600, 36640, 43752, 51701-51703, 54060♦, 62320-62327, 64400, 64405-64408, 64415-64435, 64445-64454, 64461-64463, 64479-64505, 64510-64530, 69990, 92012-92014, 93000-93010, 93040-93042, 93318, 93355, 94002, 94200, 94250, 94680-94690, 94770, 95812-95816, 95819, 95822, 95829, 95955, 96360-96368, 96372, 96374-96377, 96523, 99155, 99156, 99157, 99211-99223, 99231-99255, 99291-99292, 99304-99310, 99315-99316, 99334-99337, 99347-99350, 99374-99375, 99377-99378, 99446-99449, 99451-99452, 99495-99496, G0463, G0471

54055 0213T, 0216T, 0228T, 0230T, 12001-12007, 12011-12057, 13100-13133, 13151-13153, 36000, 36400-36410, 36420-36430, 36440, 36591-36592, 36600, 36640, 43752, 51701-51703, 54060♦, 62320-62327, 64400, 64405-64408, 64415-64435, 64445-64454, 64461-64463, 64479-64505, 64510-64530, 69990, 92012-92014, 93000-93010, 93040-93042, 93318, 93355, 94002, 94200, 94250, 94680-94690, 94770, 95812-95816, 95819, 95822, 95829, 95955, 96360-96368, 96372, 96374-96377, 96523, 99155, 99156, 99157, 99211-99223, 99231-99255, 99291-99292, 99304-99310, 99315-99316, 99334-99337, 99347-99350, 99374-99375, 99377-99378, 99446-99449, 99451-99452, 99495-99496, G0463, G0471

54056 0213T, 0216T, 0228T, 0230T, 12001-12007, 12011-12057, 13100-13133, 13151-13153, 36000, 36400-36410, 36420-36430, 36440, 36591-36592, 36600, 36640, 43752, 51701-51703, 54050-54055♦, 54060♦, 62320-62327, 64400, 64405-64408, 64415-64435, 64445-64454, 64461-64463, 64479-64505, 64510-64530, 69990, 92012-92014, 93000-93010, 93040-93042, 93318, 93355, 94002, 94200, 94250, 94680-94690, 94770, 95812-95816, 95819, 95822, 95829, 95955, 96360-96368, 96372, 96374-96377, 96523, 99155, 99156, 99157, 99211-99223, 99231-99255, 99291-99292, 99304-99310, 99315-99316, 99334-99337, 99347-99350, 99374-99375, 99377-99378, 99446-99449, 99451-99452, 99495-99496, G0463, G0471, J0670, J2001

54057 0213T, 0216T, 0228T, 0230T, 12001-12007, 12011-12057, 13100-13133, 13151-13153, 36000, 36400-36410, 36420-36430, 36440, 36591-36592, 36600, 36640, 43752, 51701-51703, 54050-54056♦, 54060♦, 62320-62327, 64400, 64405-64408, 64415-64435, 64445-64454, 64461-64463, 64479-64505, 64510-64530, 69990, 92012-92014, 93000-93010, 93040-93042, 93318, 93355, 94002, 94200, 94250, 94680-94690, 94770, 95812-95816, 95819, 95822, 95829, 95955, 96360-96368, 96372, 96374-96377, 96523, 99155, 99156, 99157, 99211-99223, 99231-99255, 99291-99292, 99304-99310, 99315-99316, 99334-99337, 99347-99350, 99374-99375, 99377-99378, 99446-99449, 99451-99452, 99495-99496, G0463, G0471, J0670, J2001

54060 0213T, 0216T, 0228T, 0230T, 11000-11006, 11042-11047, 12001-12007, 12011-12057, 13100-13133, 13151-13153, 36000, 36400-36410, 36420-36430, 36440, 36591-36592, 36600, 36640, 43752, 51701-51703, 62320-62327, 64400, 64405-64408, 64415-64435, 64445-64454, 64461-64463, 64479-64505, 64510-64530, 69990, 92012-92014, 93000-93010, 93040-93042, 93318, 93355, 94002, 94200, 94250, 94680-94690, 94770, 95812-95816, 95819, 95822, 95829, 95955, 96360-96368, 96372, 96374-96377, 96523, 97597-97598, 97602, 99155, 99156, 99157, 99211-99223, 99231-99255, 99291-99292, 99304-99310, 99315-99316, 99334-99337, 99347-99350, 99374-99375, 99377-99378, 99446-99449, 99451-99452, 99495-99496, G0463, G0471, J0670, J2001

54065 0213T, 0216T, 0228T, 0230T, 12001-12007, 12011-12057, 13100-13133, 13151-13153, 36000, 36400-36410, 36420-36430, 36440, 36591-36592, 36600, 36640, 43752, 51701-51703, 54050-54060, 62320-62327, 64400, 64405-64408, 64415-64435, 64445-64454, 64461-64463, 64479-64505,

64510-64530, 69990, 92012-92014, 93000-93010, 93040-93042, 93318, 93355, 94002, 94200, 94250, 94680-94690, 94770, 95812-95816, 95819, 95822, 95829, 95955, 96360-96368, 96372, 96374-96377, 96523, 99155, 99156, 99157, 99211-99223, 99231-99255, 99291-99292, 99304-99310, 99315-99316, 99334-99337, 99347-99350, 99374-99375, 99377-99378, 99446-99449, 99451-99452, 99495-99496, G0463, G0471, J0670, J2001

54100 0213T, 0216T, 0228T, 0230T, 10005, 10007, 10009, 10011, 10021, 11102-11107♦, 12001-12007, 12011-12057, 13100-13133, 13151-13153, 36000, 36400-36410, 36420-36430, 36440, 36591-36592, 36600, 36640, 43752, 51701, 51703, 54001, 62320-62327, 64400, 64405-64408, 64415-64435, 64445-64454, 64461-64463, 64479-64505, 64510-64530, 69990, 92012-92014, 93000-93010, 93040-93042, 93318, 93355, 94002, 94200, 94250, 94680-94690, 94770, 95812-95816, 95819, 95822, 95829, 95955, 96360-96368, 96372, 96374-96377, 96523, 99155, 99156, 99157, 99211-99223, 99231-99255, 99291-99292, 99304-99310, 99315-99316, 99334-99337, 99347-99350, 99374-99375, 99377-99378, 99446-99449, 99451-99452, 99495-99496, G0463, J0670, J2001

54105 0213T, 0216T, 0228T, 0230T, 10005, 10007, 10009, 10011, 10021, 12001-12007, 12011-12057, 13100-13133, 13151-13153, 36000, 36400-36410, 36420-36430, 36440, 36591-36592, 36600, 36640, 43752, 51701-51703, 54100, 62320-62327, 64400, 64405-64408, 64415-64435, 64445-64454, 64461-64463, 64479-64505, 64510-64530, 69990, 92012-92014, 93000-93010, 93040-93042, 93318, 93355, 94002, 94200, 94250, 94680-94690, 94770, 95812-95816, 95819, 95822, 95829, 95955, 96360-96368, 96372, 96374-96377, 96523, 99155, 99156, 99157, 99211-99223, 99231-99255, 99291-99292, 99304-99310, 99315-99316, 99334-99337, 99347-99350, 99374-99375, 99377-99378, 99446-99449, 99451-99452, 99495-99496, G0463, G0471, J0670, J2001

54110 0213T, 0216T, 0228T, 0230T, 11000-11006, 11042-11047, 12001-12007, 12011-12057, 13100-13133, 13151-13153, 36000, 36400-36410, 36420-36430, 36440, 36591-36592, 36600, 36640, 43752, 51701-51703, 54100-54105, 54200-54205, 62320-62327, 64400, 64405-64408, 64415-64435, 64445-64454, 64461-64463, 64479-64505, 64510-64530, 69990, 92012-92014, 93000-93010, 93040-93042, 93318, 93355, 94002, 94200, 94250, 94680-94690, 94770, 95812-95816, 95819, 95822, 95829, 95955, 96360-96368, 96372, 96374-96377, 96523, 97597-97598, 97602, 99155, 99156, 99157, 99211-99223, 99231-99255, 99291-99292, 99304-99310, 99315-99316, 99334-99337, 99347-99350, 99374-99375, 99377-99378, 99446-99449, 99451-99452, 99495-99496, G0463, G0471

54111 0213T, 0216T, 0228T, 0230T, 11000-11006, 11042-11047, 12001-12007, 12011-12057, 13100-13133, 13151-13153, 36000, 36400-36410, 36420-36430, 36440, 36591-36592, 36600, 36640, 43752, 51701-51703, 54100-54110, 54112-54115, 54200-54205, 62320-62327, 64400, 64405-64408, 64415-64435, 64445-64454, 64461-64463, 64479-64505, 64510-64530, 69990, 92012-92014, 93000-93010, 93040-93042, 93318, 93355, 94002, 94200, 94250, 94680-94690, 94770, 95812-95816, 95819, 95822, 95829, 95955, 96360-96368, 96372, 96374-96377, 96523, 97597-97598, 97602, 99155, 99156, 99157, 99211-99223, 99231-99255, 99291-99292, 99304-99310, 99315-99316, 99334-99337, 99347-99350, 99374-99375, 99377-99378, 99446-99449, 99451-99452, 99495-99496, G0463, G0471

54112 0213T, 0216T, 0228T, 0230T, 11000-11006, 11042-11047, 12001-12007, 12011-12057, 13100-13133, 13151-13153, 36000, 36400-36410, 36420-36430, 36440, 36591-36592, 36600, 36640, 43752, 51701-51703, 54100-54110, 54115, 54200-54205, 62320-62327, 64400, 64405-64408, 64415-64435, 64445-64454, 64461-64463, 64479-64505, 64510-64530, 69990, 92012-92014, 93000-93010, 93040-93042, 93318, 93355, 94002,

CPT © 2020 American Medical Association. All Rights Reserved.

94200, 94250, 94680-94690, 94770, 95812-95816, 95819, 95822,
95829, 95955, 96360-96368, 96372, 96374-96377, 96523, 97597-97598,
97602, 99155, 99156, 99157, 99211-99223, 99231-99255, 99291-99292,
99304-99310, 99315-99316, 99334-99337, 99347-99350, 99374-99375,
99377-99378, 99446-99449, 99451-99452, 99495-99496, G0463, G0471

54115 0213T, 0216T, 0228T, 0230T, 11000-11006, 11042-11047, 12001-12007,
12011-12057, 13100-13133, 13151-13153, 36000, 36400-36410,
36420-36430, 36440, 36591-36592, 36600, 36640, 43752, 51701-51703,
54100, 54110◆, 62320-62327, 64400, 64405-64408, 64415-64435,
64445-64454, 64461-64463, 64479-64505, 64510-64530, 69990,
92012-92014, 93000-93010, 93040-93042, 93318, 93355, 94002, 94200,
94250, 94680-94690, 94770, 95812-95816, 95819, 95822, 95829,
95955, 96360-96368, 96372, 96374-96377, 96523, 97597-97598, 97602,
99155, 99156, 99157, 99211-99223, 99231-99255, 99291-99292,
99304-99310, 99315-99316, 99334-99337, 99347-99350, 99374-99375,
99377-99378, 99446-99449, 99451-99452, 99495-99496, G0463,
G0471, J0670, J2001

54120 0213T, 0216T, 0228T, 0230T, 12001-12007, 12011-12057, 13100-13133,
13151-13153, 36000, 36400-36410, 36420-36430, 36440, 36591-36592,
36600, 36640, 43752, 51701-51703, 54100-54115, 62320-62327, 64400,
64405-64408, 64415-64435, 64445-64454, 64461-64463, 64479-64505,
64510-64530, 69990, 92012-92014, 93000-93010, 93040-93042, 93318,
93355, 94002, 94200, 94250, 94680-94690, 94770, 95812-95816,
95819, 95822, 95829, 95955, 96360-96368, 96372, 96374-96377,
96523, 99155, 99156, 99157, 99211-99223, 99231-99255, 99291-99292,
99304-99310, 99315-99316, 99334-99337, 99347-99350, 99374-99375,
99377-99378, 99446-99449, 99451-99452, 99495-99496, G0463, G0471

54125 0213T, 0216T, 0228T, 0230T, 12001-12007, 12011-12057, 13100-13133,
13151-13153, 36000, 36400-36410, 36420-36430, 36440, 36591-36592,
36600, 36640, 43752, 51701-51703, 54100-54120, 62320-62327, 64400,
64405-64408, 64415-64435, 64445-64454, 64461-64463, 64479-64505,
64510-64530, 69990, 92012-92014, 93000-93010, 93040-93042, 93318,
93355, 94002, 94200, 94250, 94680-94690, 94770, 95812-95816,
95819, 95822, 95829, 95955, 96360-96368, 96372, 96374-96377,
96523, 99155, 99156, 99157, 99211-99223, 99231-99255, 99291-99292,
99304-99310, 99315-99316, 99334-99337, 99347-99350, 99374-99375,
99377-99378, 99446-99449, 99451-99452, 99495-99496, G0463, G0471

54130 0213T, 0216T, 0228T, 0230T, 11000-11006, 11042-11047, 12001-12007,
12011-12057, 13100-13133, 13151-13153, 36000, 36400-36410,
36420-36430, 36440, 36591-36592, 36600, 36640, 38531, 38760,
43752, 51701-51703, 54100-54105, 62320-62327, 64400, 64405-64408,
64415-64435, 64445-64454, 64461-64463, 64479-64505, 64510-64530,
69990, 92012-92014, 93000-93010, 93040-93042, 93318, 93355, 94002,
94200, 94250, 94680-94690, 94770, 95812-95816, 95819, 95822,
95829, 95955, 96360-96368, 96372, 96374-96377, 96523, 97597-97598,
97602, 99155, 99156, 99157, 99211-99223, 99231-99255, 99291-99292,
99304-99310, 99315-99316, 99334-99337, 99347-99350, 99374-99375,
99377-99378, 99446-99449, 99451-99452, 99495-99496, G0463, G0471

54135 0213T, 0216T, 0228T, 0230T, 11000-11006, 11042-11047, 12001-12007,
12011-12057, 13100-13133, 13151-13153, 36000, 36400-36410,
36420-36430, 36440, 36591-36592, 36600, 36640, 38531, 38571-38573,
38765, 43752, 51701-51703, 52000, 54100-54105, 62320-62327, 64400,
64405-64408, 64415-64435, 64445-64454, 64461-64463, 64479-64505,
64510-64530, 69990, 92012-92014, 93000-93010, 93040-93042, 93318,
93355, 94002, 94200, 94250, 94680-94690, 94770, 95812-95816,
95819, 95822, 95829, 95955, 96360-96368, 96372, 96374-96377,
96523, 97597-97598, 97602, 99155, 99156, 99157, 99211-99223,
99231-99255, 99291-99292, 99304-99310, 99315-99316, 99334-99337,

99347-99350, 99374-99375, 99377-99378, 99446-99449, 99451-99452,
99495-99496, G0463, G0471

54150 0213T, 0216T, 0228T, 0230T, 12001-12007, 12011-12057, 13100-13133,
13151-13153, 36000, 36400-36410, 36420-36430, 36440, 36591-36592,
36600, 36640, 43752, 51701-51703, 54000-54001, 54100, 54162-54164,
62320-62327, 64400, 64405-64408, 64415-64435, 64445-64454,
64461-64463, 64479-64505, 64510-64530, 69990, 92012-92014,
93000-93010, 93040-93042, 93318, 93355, 94002, 94200, 94250,
94680-94690, 94770, 95812-95816, 95819, 95822, 95829, 95955,
96360-96368, 96372, 96374-96377, 96523, 99155, 99156, 99157,
99211-99223, 99231-99255, 99291-99292, 99304-99310, 99315-99316,
99334-99337, 99347-99350, 99374-99375, 99377-99378, 99446-99449,
99451-99452, 99495-99496, G0463, G0471, J0670, J2001

54160 0213T, 0216T, 0228T, 0230T, 11000-11006, 11042-11047, 12001-12007,
12011-12057, 13100-13133, 13151-13153, 36000, 36400-36410,
36420-36430, 36440, 36591-36592, 36600, 36640, 43752, 51701-51703,
54000-54001, 54100, 54162-54164, 62320-62327, 64400, 64405-64408,
64415-64435, 64445-64454, 64461-64463, 64479-64505, 64510-64530,
92012-92014, 93000-93010, 93040-93042, 93318, 93355, 94002, 94200,
94250, 94680-94690, 94770, 95812-95816, 95819, 95822, 95829,
95955, 96360-96368, 96372, 96374-96377, 96523, 97597-97598, 97602,
99155, 99156, 99157, 99211-99223, 99231-99255, 99291-99292,
99304-99310, 99315-99316, 99334-99337, 99347-99350, 99374-99375,
99377-99378, 99446-99449, 99451-99452, 99495-99496, G0463,
G0471, J2001

54161 0213T, 0216T, 0228T, 0230T, 11000-11006, 11042-11047, 12001-12007,
12011-12057, 13100-13133, 13151-13153, 36000, 36400-36410,
36420-36430, 36440, 36591-36592, 36600, 36640, 43752, 51701-51703,
54000-54001, 54100, 54162-54164, 54450, 62320-62327, 64400,
64405-64408, 64415-64435, 64445-64454, 64461-64463, 64479-64505,
64510-64530, 69990, 92012-92014, 93000-93010, 93040-93042, 93318,
93355, 94002, 94200, 94250, 94680-94690, 94770, 95812-95816,
95819, 95822, 95829, 95955, 96360-96368, 96372, 96374-96377,
96523, 97597-97598, 97602, 99155, 99156, 99157, 99211-99223,
99231-99255, 99291-99292, 99304-99310, 99315-99316, 99334-99337,
99347-99350, 99374-99375, 99377-99378, 99446-99449, 99451-99452,
99495-99496, G0463, G0471

54162 0213T, 0216T, 0228T, 0230T, 11000-11006, 11042-11047, 12001-12007,
12011-12057, 13100-13133, 13151-13153, 36000, 36400-36410,
36420-36430, 36440, 36591-36592, 36600, 36640, 43752, 51701-51703,
54000-54001, 54100, 54164, 62320-62327, 64400, 64405-64408,
64415-64435, 64445-64454, 64461-64463, 64479-64505, 64510-64530,
69990, 92012-92014, 93000-93010, 93040-93042, 93318, 93355, 94002,
94200, 94250, 94680-94690, 94770, 95812-95816, 95819, 95822,
95829, 95955, 96360-96368, 96372, 96374-96377, 96523, 97597-97598,
97602, 99155, 99156, 99157, 99211-99223, 99231-99255, 99291-99292,
99304-99310, 99315-99316, 99334-99337, 99347-99350, 99374-99375,
99377-99378, 99446-99449, 99451-99452, 99495-99496, G0463, G0471

54163 0213T, 0216T, 0228T, 0230T, 12001-12007, 12011-12057, 13100-13133,
13151-13153, 36000, 36400-36410, 36420-36430, 36440, 36591-36592,
36600, 36640, 43752, 51701-51703, 54000-54001, 54100, 54162,
54164, 62320-62327, 64400, 64405-64408, 64415-64435, 64445-64454,
64461-64463, 64479-64505, 64510-64530, 69990, 92012-92014,
93000-93010, 93040-93042, 93318, 93355, 94002, 94200, 94250,
94680-94690, 94770, 95812-95816, 95819, 95822, 95829, 95955,
96360-96368, 96372, 96374-96377, 96523, 99155, 99156, 99157,
99211-99223, 99231-99255, 99291-99292, 99304-99310, 99315-99316,
99334-99337, 99347-99350, 99374-99375, 99377-99378, 99446-99449,
99451-99452, 99495-99496, G0463, G0471

54164 0213T, 0216T, 0228T, 0230T, 11000-11006, 11042-11047, 12001-12007, 12011-12057, 13100-13133, 13151-13153, 36000, 36400-36410, 36420-36430, 36440, 36591-36592, 36600, 36640, 43752, 51701-51703, 54000-54001, 54100, 62320-62327, 64400, 64405-64408, 64415-64435, 64445-64454, 64461-64463, 64479-64505, 64510-64530, 69990, 92012-92014, 93000-93010, 93040-93042, 93318, 93355, 94002, 94200, 94250, 94680-94690, 94770, 95812-95816, 95819, 95822, 95829, 95955, 96360-96368, 96372, 96374-96377, 96523, 97597-97598, 97602, 99155, 99156, 99157, 99211-99223, 99231-99255, 99291-99292, 99304-99310, 99315-99316, 99334-99337, 99347-99350, 99374-99375, 99377-99378, 99446-99449, 99451-99452, 99495-99496, G0463, G0471

54200 0213T, 0216T, 0228T, 0230T, 12001-12007, 12011-12057, 13100-13133, 13151-13153, 36000, 36400-36410, 36420-36430, 36440, 36591-36592, 36600, 36640, 43752, 51701-51703, 62320-62327, 64400, 64405-64408, 64415-64435, 64445-64454, 64461-64463, 64479-64505, 64510-64530, 69990, 92012-92014, 93000-93010, 93040-93042, 93318, 93355, 94002, 94200, 94250, 94680-94690, 94770, 95812-95816, 95819, 95822, 95829, 95955, 96360-96368, 96372, 96374-96377, 96523, 99155, 99156, 99157, 99211-99223, 99231-99255, 99291-99292, 99304-99310, 99315-99316, 99334-99337, 99347-99350, 99374-99375, 99377-99378, 99446-99449, 99451-99452, 99495-99496, G0463, G0471, J0670, J2001

54205 0213T, 0216T, 0228T, 0230T, 12001-12007, 12011-12057, 13100-13133, 13151-13153, 36000, 36400-36410, 36420-36430, 36440, 36591-36592, 36600, 36640, 43752, 51701-51703, 54200, 62320-62327, 64400, 64405-64408, 64415-64435, 64445-64454, 64461-64463, 64479-64505, 64510-64530, 69990, 92012-92014, 93000-93010, 93040-93042, 93318, 93355, 94002, 94200, 94250, 94680-94690, 94770, 95812-95816, 95819, 95822, 95829, 95955, 96360-96368, 96372, 96374-96377, 96523, 99155, 99156, 99157, 99211-99223, 99231-99255, 99291-99292, 99304-99310, 99315-99316, 99334-99337, 99347-99350, 99374-99375, 99377-99378, 99446-99449, 99451-99452, 99495-99496, G0463, G0471

54220 0213T, 0216T, 0228T, 0230T, 12001-12007, 12011-12057, 13100-13133, 13151-13153, 36000, 36400-36410, 36420-36430, 36440, 36591-36592, 36600, 36640, 43752, 51701-51703, 62320-62327, 64400, 64405-64408, 64415-64435, 64445-64454, 64461-64463, 64479-64505, 64510-64530, 69990, 92012-92014, 93000-93010, 93040-93042, 93318, 93355, 94002, 94200, 94250, 94680-94690, 94770, 95812-95816, 95819, 95822, 95829, 95955, 96360-96368, 96372, 96374-96377, 96523, 99155, 99156, 99157, 99211-99223, 99231-99255, 99291-99292, 99304-99310, 99315-99316, 99334-99337, 99347-99350, 99374-99375, 99377-99378, 99446-99449, 99451-99452, 99495-99496, G0463, G0471, J0670, J2001

54230 0213T, 0216T, 0228T, 0230T, 12001-12007, 12011-12057, 13100-13133, 13151-13153, 36000, 36400-36410, 36420-36430, 36440, 36591-36592, 36600, 36640, 43752, 51701-51703, 62320-62327, 64400, 64405-64408, 64415-64435, 64445-64454, 64461-64463, 64479-64505, 64510-64530, 69990, 76000, 77001-77002, 92012-92014, 93000-93010, 93040-93042, 93318, 93355, 94002, 94200, 94250, 94680-94690, 94770, 95812-95816, 95819, 95822, 95829, 95955, 96360-96368, 96372, 96374-96377, 96523, 99155, 99156, 99157, 99211-99223, 99231-99255, 99291-99292, 99304-99310, 99315-99316, 99334-99337, 99347-99350, 99374-99375, 99377-99378, 99446-99449, 99451-99452, 99495-99496, G0463, G0471

54231 0213T, 0216T, 0228T, 0230T, 12001-12007, 12011-12057, 13100-13133, 13151-13153, 36000, 36400-36410, 36420-36430, 36440, 36591-36592, 36600, 36640, 43752, 51701-51703, 54235-54240, 62320-62327, 64400, 64405-64408, 64415-64435, 64445-64454, 64461-64463, 64479-64505, 64510-64530, 69990, 92012-92014, 93000-93010, 93040-93042, 93318, 93355, 94002, 94200, 94250, 94680-94690, 94770, 95812-95816, 95819, 95822, 95829, 95955, 96360-96368, 96372, 96374-96377,

96523, 99155, 99156, 99157, 99211-99223, 99231-99255, 99291-99292, 99304-99310, 99315-99316, 99334-99337, 99347-99350, 99374-99375, 99377-99378, 99446-99449, 99451-99452, 99495-99496, G0463, G0471, J2001

54235 0213T, 0216T, 0228T, 0230T, 12001-12007, 12011-12057, 13100-13133, 13151-13153, 36000, 36400-36410, 36420-36430, 36440, 36591-36592, 36600, 36640, 43752, 51701-51703, 62320-62327, 64400, 64405-64408, 64415-64435, 64445-64454, 64461-64463, 64479-64505, 64510-64530, 69990, 92012-92014, 93000-93010, 93040-93042, 93318, 93355, 94002, 94200, 94250, 94680-94690, 94770, 95812-95816, 95819, 95822, 95829, 95955, 96360-96368, 96372, 96374-96377, 96523, 99155, 99156, 99157, 99211-99223, 99231-99255, 99291-99292, 99304-99310, 99315-99316, 99334-99337, 99347-99350, 99374-99375, 99377-99378, 99446-99449, 99451-99452, 99495-99496, G0463, G0471

54240 0213T, 0216T, 0228T, 0230T, 12001-12007, 12011-12057, 13100-13133, 13151-13153, 36000, 36400-36410, 36420-36430, 36440, 36591-36592, 36600, 36640, 43752, 51701-51703, 62320-62327, 64400, 64405-64408, 64415-64435, 64445-64454, 64461-64463, 64479-64505, 64510-64530, 69990, 92012-92014, 93000-93010, 93040-93042, 93318, 93355, 94002, 94200, 94250, 94680-94690, 94770, 95812-95816, 95819, 95822, 95829, 95955, 96360-96368, 96372, 96374-96377, 96523, 99155, 99156, 99157, 99211-99223, 99231-99255, 99291-99292, 99304-99310, 99315-99316, 99334-99337, 99347-99350, 99374-99375, 99377-99378, 99446-99449, 99451-99452, 99495-99496, G0463, G0471

54250 0213T, 0216T, 0228T, 0230T, 12001-12007, 12011-12057, 13100-13133, 13151-13153, 36000, 36400-36410, 36420-36430, 36440, 36591-36592, 36600, 36640, 43752, 51701-51703, 62320-62327, 64400, 64405-64408, 64415-64435, 64445-64454, 64461-64463, 64479-64505, 64510-64530, 69990, 92012-92014, 93000-93010, 93040-93042, 93318, 93355, 94002, 94200, 94250, 94680-94690, 94770, 95812-95816, 95819, 95822, 95829, 95955, 96360-96368, 96372, 96374-96377, 96523, 99155, 99156, 99157, 99211-99223, 99231-99255, 99291-99292, 99304-99310, 99315-99316, 99334-99337, 99347-99350, 99374-99375, 99377-99378, 99446-99449, 99451-99452, 99495-99496, G0463, G0471

54300 0213T, 0216T, 0228T, 0230T, 12001-12007, 12011-12057, 13100-13133, 13151-13153, 36000, 36400-36410, 36420-36430, 36440, 36591-36592, 36600, 36640, 43752, 51701-51703, 53000-53025, 62320-62327, 64400, 64405-64408, 64415-64435, 64445-64454, 64461-64463, 64479-64505, 64510-64530, 69990, 92012-92014, 93000-93010, 93040-93042, 93318, 93355, 94002, 94200, 94250, 94680-94690, 94770, 95812-95816, 95819, 95822, 95829, 95955, 96360-96368, 96372, 96374-96377, 96523, 99155, 99156, 99157, 99211-99223, 99231-99255, 99291-99292, 99304-99310, 99315-99316, 99334-99337, 99347-99350, 99374-99375, 99377-99378, 99446-99449, 99451-99452, 99495-99496, G0463, G0471

54304 0213T, 0216T, 0228T, 0230T, 12001-12007, 12011-12057, 13100-13133, 13151-13153, 36000, 36400-36410, 36420-36430, 36440, 36591-36592, 36600, 36640, 43752, 51701-51703, 54300, 62320-62327, 64400, 64405-64408, 64415-64435, 64445-64454, 64461-64463, 64479-64505, 64510-64530, 69990, 92012-92014, 93000-93010, 93040-93042, 93318, 93355, 94002, 94200, 94250, 94680-94690, 94770, 95812-95816, 95819, 95822, 95829, 95955, 96360-96368, 96372, 96374-96377, 96523, 99155, 99156, 99157, 99211-99223, 99231-99255, 99291-99292, 99304-99310, 99315-99316, 99334-99337, 99347-99350, 99374-99375, 99377-99378, 99446-99449, 99451-99452, 99495-99496, G0463, G0471

54308 0213T, 0216T, 0228T, 0230T, 11000-11006, 11042-11047, 12001-12007, 12011-12057, 13100-13133, 13151-13153, 36000, 36400-36410, 36420-36430, 36440, 36591-36592, 36600, 36640, 43752, 51701-51703, 52000, 53000-53025, 54312✦, 62320-62327, 64400, 64405-64408, 64415-64435, 64445-64454, 64461-64463, 64479-64505, 64510-64530,

CPT © 2020 American Medical Association. All Rights Reserved.

Coding Companion for Urology/Nephrology

69990, 92012-92014, 93000-93010, 93040-93042, 93318, 93355, 94002, 94200, 94250, 94680-94690, 94770, 95812-95816, 95819, 95822, 95829, 95955, 96360-96368, 96372, 96374-96377, 96523, 97597-97598, 97602, 99155, 99156, 99157, 99211-99223, 99231-99255, 99291-99292, 99304-99310, 99315-99316, 99334-99337, 99347-99350, 99374-99375, 99377-99378, 99446-99449, 99451-99452, 99495-99496, G0463, G0471

54312 0213T, 0216T, 0228T, 0230T, 11000-11006, 11042-11047, 12001-12007, 12011-12057, 13100-13133, 13151-13153, 36000, 36400-36410, 36420-36430, 36440, 36591-36592, 36600, 36640, 43752, 51701-51703, 52000, 53000-53025, 62320-62327, 64400, 64405-64408, 64415-64435, 64445-64454, 64461-64463, 64479-64505, 64510-64530, 69990, 92012-92014, 93000-93010, 93040-93042, 93318, 93355, 94002, 94200, 94250, 94680-94690, 94770, 95812-95816, 95819, 95822, 95829, 95955, 96360-96368, 96372, 96374-96377, 96523, 97597-97598, 97602, 99155, 99156, 99157, 99211-99223, 99231-99255, 99291-99292, 99304-99310, 99315-99316, 99334-99337, 99347-99350, 99374-99375, 99377-99378, 99446-99449, 99451-99452, 99495-99496, G0463, G0471

54316 0213T, 0216T, 0228T, 0230T, 11000-11006, 11042-11047, 12001-12007, 12011-12057, 13100-13133, 13151-13153, 36000, 36400-36410, 36420-36430, 36440, 36591-36592, 36600, 36640, 43752, 51701-51703, 52000, 53000-53025, 62320-62327, 64400, 64405-64408, 64415-64435, 64445-64454, 64461-64463, 64479-64505, 64510-64530, 69990, 92012-92014, 93000-93010, 93040-93042, 93318, 93355, 94002, 94200, 94250, 94680-94690, 94770, 95812-95816, 95819, 95822, 95829, 95955, 96360-96368, 96372, 96374-96377, 96523, 97597-97598, 97602, 99155, 99156, 99157, 99211-99223, 99231-99255, 99291-99292, 99304-99310, 99315-99316, 99334-99337, 99347-99350, 99374-99375, 99377-99378, 99446-99449, 99451-99452, 99495-99496, G0463, G0471

54318 0213T, 0216T, 0228T, 0230T, 11000-11006, 11042-11047, 12001-12007, 12011-12057, 13100-13133, 13151-13153, 36000, 36400-36410, 36420-36430, 36440, 36591-36592, 36600, 36640, 43752, 51701-51703, 52000, 53000-53025, 62320-62327, 64400, 64405-64408, 64415-64435, 64445-64454, 64461-64463, 64479-64505, 64510-64530, 69990, 92012-92014, 93000-93010, 93040-93042, 93318, 93355, 94002, 94200, 94250, 94680-94690, 94770, 95812-95816, 95819, 95822, 95829, 95955, 96360-96368, 96372, 96374-96377, 96523, 97597-97598, 97602, 99155, 99156, 99157, 99211-99223, 99231-99255, 99291-99292, 99304-99310, 99315-99316, 99334-99337, 99347-99350, 99374-99375, 99377-99378, 99446-99449, 99451-99452, 99495-99496, G0463, G0471

54322 0213T, 0216T, 0228T, 0230T, 12001-12007, 12011-12057, 13100-13133, 13151-13153, 36000, 36400-36410, 36420-36430, 36440, 36591-36592, 36600, 36640, 43752, 51701-51703, 53000-53025, 62320-62327, 64400, 64405-64408, 64415-64435, 64445-64454, 64461-64463, 64479-64505, 64510-64530, 69990, 92012-92014, 93000-93010, 93040-93042, 93318, 93355, 94002, 94200, 94250, 94680-94690, 94770, 95812-95816, 95819, 95822, 95829, 95955, 96360-96368, 96372, 96374-96377, 96523, 99155, 99156, 99157, 99211-99223, 99231-99255, 99291-99292, 99304-99310, 99315-99316, 99334-99337, 99347-99350, 99374-99375, 99377-99378, 99446-99449, 99451-99452, 99495-99496, G0463, G0471

54324 0213T, 0216T, 0228T, 0230T, 11000-11006, 11042-11047, 12001-12007, 12011-12057, 13100-13133, 13151-13153, 36000, 36400-36410, 36420-36430, 36440, 36591-36592, 36600, 36640, 43752, 51701-51703, 52000, 53000-53025, 62320-62327, 64400, 64405-64408, 64415-64435, 64445-64454, 64461-64463, 64479-64505, 64510-64530, 69990, 92012-92014, 93000-93010, 93040-93042, 93318, 93355, 94002, 94200, 94250, 94680-94690, 94770, 95812-95816, 95819, 95822, 95829, 95955, 96360-96368, 96372, 96374-96377, 96523, 97597-97598, 97602, 99155, 99156, 99157, 99211-99223, 99231-99255, 99291-99292,

54326 0213T, 0216T, 0228T, 0230T, 11000-11006, 11042-11047, 12001-12007, 12011-12057, 13100-13133, 13151-13153, 36000, 36400-36410, 36420-36430, 36440, 36591-36592, 36600, 36640, 43752, 51701-51703, 52000, 53000-53025, 54324, 62320-62327, 64400, 64405-64408, 64415-64435, 64445-64454, 64461-64463, 64479-64505, 64510-64530, 69990, 92012-92014, 93000-93010, 93040-93042, 93318, 93355, 94002, 94200, 94250, 94680-94690, 94770, 95812-95816, 95819, 95822, 95829, 95955, 96360-96368, 96372, 96374-96377, 96523, 97597-97598, 97602, 99155, 99156, 99157, 99211-99223, 99231-99255, 99291-99292, 99304-99310, 99315-99316, 99334-99337, 99347-99350, 99374-99375, 99377-99378, 99446-99449, 99451-99452, 99495-99496, G0463, G0471

54328 0213T, 0216T, 0228T, 0230T, 11000-11006, 11042-11047, 12001-12007, 12011-12057, 13100-13133, 13151-13153, 36000, 36400-36410, 36420-36430, 36440, 36591-36592, 36600, 36640, 43752, 51701-51703, 52000, 53000-53025, 54326♦, 62320-62327, 64400, 64405-64408, 64415-64435, 64445-64454, 64461-64463, 64479-64505, 64510-64530, 69990, 92012-92014, 93000-93010, 93040-93042, 93318, 93355, 94002, 94200, 94250, 94680-94690, 94770, 95812-95816, 95819, 95822, 95829, 95955, 96360-96368, 96372, 96374-96377, 96523, 97597-97598, 97602, 99155, 99156, 99157, 99211-99223, 99231-99255, 99291-99292, 99304-99310, 99315-99316, 99334-99337, 99347-99350, 99374-99375, 99377-99378, 99446-99449, 99451-99452, 99495-99496, G0463, G0471

54332 0213T, 0216T, 0228T, 0230T, 11000-11006, 11042-11047, 12001-12007, 12011-12057, 13100-13133, 13151-13153, 36000, 36400-36410, 36420-36430, 36440, 36591-36592, 36600, 36640, 43752, 51701-51703, 52000, 53000-53025, 54352♦, 62320-62327, 64400, 64405-64408, 64415-64435, 64445-64454, 64461-64463, 64479-64505, 64510-64530, 69990, 92012-92014, 93000-93010, 93040-93042, 93318, 93355, 94002, 94200, 94250, 94680-94690, 94770, 95812-95816, 95819, 95822, 95829, 95955, 96360-96368, 96372, 96374-96377, 96523, 97597-97598, 97602, 99155, 99156, 99157, 99211-99223, 99231-99255, 99291-99292, 99304-99310, 99315-99316, 99334-99337, 99347-99350, 99374-99375, 99377-99378, 99446-99449, 99451-99452, 99495-99496, G0463, G0471

54336 0213T, 0216T, 0228T, 0230T, 11000-11006, 11042-11047, 12001-12007, 12011-12057, 13100-13133, 13151-13153, 36000, 36400-36410, 36420-36430, 36440, 36591-36592, 36600, 36640, 43752, 51701-51703, 52000, 53000-53025, 62320-62327, 64400, 64405-64408, 64415-64435, 64445-64454, 64461-64463, 64479-64505, 64510-64530, 69990, 92012-92014, 93000-93010, 93040-93042, 93318, 93355, 94002, 94200, 94250, 94680-94690, 94770, 95812-95816, 95819, 95822, 95829, 95955, 96360-96368, 96372, 96374-96377, 96523, 97597-97598, 97602, 99155, 99156, 99157, 99211-99223, 99231-99255, 99291-99292, 99304-99310, 99315-99316, 99334-99337, 99347-99350, 99374-99375, 99377-99378, 99446-99449, 99451-99452, 99495-99496, G0463, G0471

54340 0213T, 0216T, 0228T, 0230T, 11000-11006, 11042-11047, 12001-12007, 12011-12057, 13100-13133, 13151-13153, 36000, 36400-36410, 36420-36430, 36440, 36591-36592, 36600, 36640, 43752, 51701-51703, 53000-53025, 62320-62327, 64400, 64405-64408, 64415-64435, 64445-64454, 64461-64463, 64479-64505, 64510-64530, 69990, 92012-92014, 93000-93010, 93040-93042, 93318, 93355, 94002, 94200, 94250, 94680-94690, 94770, 95812-95816, 95819, 95822, 95829, 95955, 96360-96368, 96372, 96374-96377, 96523, 97597-97598, 97602, 99155, 99156, 99157, 99211-99223, 99231-99255, 99291-99292, 99304-99310, 99315-99316, 99334-99337, 99347-99350, 99374-99375, 99377-99378, 99446-99449, 99451-99452, 99495-99496, G0463, G0471

54344 0213T, 0216T, 0228T, 0230T, 11000-11006, 11042-11047, 12001-12007, 12011-12057, 13100-13133, 13151-13153, 36000, 36400-36410,

CPT © 2020 American Medical Association. All Rights Reserved.

© 2020 Optum360, LLC

36420-36430, 36440, 36591-36592, 36600, 36640, 43752, 51701-51703, 52000, 53000-53025, 62320-62327, 64400, 64405-64408, 64415-64435, 64445-64454, 64461-64463, 64479-64505, 64510-64530, 69990, 92012-92014, 93000-93010, 93040-93042, 93318, 93355, 94002, 94200, 94250, 94680-94690, 94770, 95812-95816, 95819, 95822, 95829, 95955, 96360-96368, 96372, 96374-96377, 96523, 97597-97598, 97602, 99155, 99156, 99157, 99211-99223, 99231-99255, 99291-99292, 99304-99310, 99315-99316, 99334-99337, 99347-99350, 99374-99375, 99377-99378, 99446-99449, 99451-99452, 99495-99496, G0463, G0471

54348 0213T, 0216T, 0228T, 0230T, 11000-11006, 11042-11047, 12001-12007, 12011-12057, 13100-13133, 13151-13153, 36000, 36400-36410, 36420-36430, 36440, 36591-36592, 36600, 36640, 43752, 51701-51703, 52000, 53000-53025, 62320-62327, 64400, 64405-64408, 64415-64435, 64445-64454, 64461-64463, 64479-64505, 64510-64530, 69990, 92012-92014, 93000-93010, 93040-93042, 93318, 93355, 94002, 94200, 94250, 94680-94690, 94770, 95812-95816, 95819, 95822, 95829, 95955, 96360-96368, 96372, 96374-96377, 96523, 97597-97598, 97602, 99155, 99156, 99157, 99211-99223, 99231-99255, 99291-99292, 99304-99310, 99315-99316, 99334-99337, 99347-99350, 99374-99375, 99377-99378, 99446-99449, 99451-99452, 99495-99496, G0463, G0471

54352 0213T, 0216T, 0228T, 0230T, 11000-11006, 11042-11047, 12001-12007, 12011-12057, 13100-13133, 13151-13153, 36000, 36400-36410, 36420-36430, 36440, 36591-36592, 36600, 36640, 43752, 51701-51703, 52000, 53000-53025, 62320-62327, 64400, 64405-64408, 64415-64435, 64445-64454, 64461-64463, 64479-64505, 64510-64530, 69990, 92012-92014, 93000-93010, 93040-93042, 93318, 93355, 94002, 94200, 94250, 94680-94690, 94770, 95812-95816, 95819, 95822, 95829, 95955, 96360-96368, 96372, 96374-96377, 96523, 97597-97598, 97602, 99155, 99156, 99157, 99211-99223, 99231-99255, 99291-99292, 99304-99310, 99315-99316, 99334-99337, 99347-99350, 99374-99375, 99377-99378, 99446-99449, 99451-99452, 99495-99496, G0463, G0471

54360 0213T, 0216T, 0228T, 0230T, 12001-12007, 12011-12057, 13100-13133, 13151-13153, 36000, 36400-36410, 36420-36430, 36440, 36591-36592, 36600, 36640, 43752, 51701-51703, 54437❖, 54440❖, 62320-62327, 64400, 64405-64408, 64415-64435, 64445-64454, 64461-64463, 64479-64505, 64510-64530, 69990, 92012-92014, 93000-93010, 93040-93042, 93318, 93355, 94002, 94200, 94250, 94680-94690, 94770, 95812-95816, 95819, 95822, 95829, 95955, 96360-96368, 96372, 96374-96377, 96523, 99155, 99156, 99157, 99211-99223, 99231-99255, 99291-99292, 99304-99310, 99315-99316, 99334-99337, 99347-99350, 99374-99375, 99377-99378, 99446-99449, 99451-99452, 99495-99496, G0463, G0471

54380 0213T, 0216T, 0228T, 0230T, 12001-12007, 12011-12057, 13100-13133, 13151-13153, 36000, 36400-36410, 36420-36430, 36440, 36591-36592, 36600, 36640, 43752, 51701-51703, 53000-53025, 54110-54112, 54200-54205, 62320-62327, 64400, 64405-64408, 64415-64435, 64445-64454, 64461-64463, 64479-64505, 64510-64530, 69990, 92012-92014, 93000-93010, 93040-93042, 93318, 93355, 94002, 94200, 94250, 94680-94690, 94770, 95812-95816, 95819, 95822, 95829, 95955, 96360-96368, 96372, 96374-96377, 96523, 99155, 99156, 99157, 99211-99223, 99231-99255, 99291-99292, 99304-99310, 99315-99316, 99334-99337, 99347-99350, 99374-99375, 99377-99378, 99446-99449, 99451-99452, 99495-99496, G0463, G0471

54385 0213T, 0216T, 0228T, 0230T, 12001-12007, 12011-12057, 13100-13133, 13151-13153, 36000, 36400-36410, 36420-36430, 36440, 36591-36592, 36600, 36640, 43752, 51701-51703, 53000-53025, 54380, 62320-62327, 64400, 64405-64408, 64415-64435, 64445-64454, 64461-64463, 64479-64505, 64510-64530, 69990, 92012-92014, 93000-93010, 93040-93042, 93318, 93355, 94002, 94200, 94250, 94680-94690,

94770, 95812-95816, 95819, 95822, 95829, 95955, 96360-96368, 96372, 96374-96377, 96523, 99155, 99156, 99157, 99211-99223, 99231-99255, 99291-99292, 99304-99310, 99315-99316, 99334-99337, 99347-99350, 99374-99375, 99377-99378, 99446-99449, 99451-99452, 99495-99496, G0463, G0471

54390 0213T, 0216T, 0228T, 0230T, 12001-12007, 12011-12057, 13100-13133, 13151-13153, 36000, 36400-36410, 36420-36430, 36440, 36591-36592, 36600, 36640, 43752, 51701-51703, 51940, 52000, 53000-53025, 54380, 62320-62327, 64400, 64405-64408, 64415-64435, 64445-64454, 64461-64463, 64479-64505, 64510-64530, 69990, 92012-92014, 93000-93010, 93040-93042, 93318, 93355, 94002, 94200, 94250, 94680-94690, 94770, 95812-95816, 95819, 95822, 95829, 95955, 96360-96368, 96372, 96374-96377, 96523, 99155, 99156, 99157, 99211-99223, 99231-99255, 99291-99292, 99304-99310, 99315-99316, 99334-99337, 99347-99350, 99374-99375, 99377-99378, 99446-99449, 99451-99452, 99495-99496, G0463, G0471

54400 0213T, 0216T, 0228T, 0230T, 12001-12007, 12011-12057, 13100-13133, 13151-13153, 36000, 36400-36410, 36420-36430, 36440, 36591-36592, 36600, 36640, 43752, 51701-51703, 54161, 54401❖, 54405❖, 62320-62327, 64400, 64405-64408, 64415-64435, 64445-64454, 64461-64463, 64479-64505, 64510-64530, 69990, 92012-92014, 93000-93010, 93040-93042, 93318, 93355, 94002, 94200, 94250, 94680-94690, 94770, 95812-95816, 95819, 95822, 95829, 95955, 96360-96368, 96372, 96374-96377, 96523, 99155, 99156, 99157, 99211-99223, 99231-99255, 99291-99292, 99304-99310, 99315-99316, 99334-99337, 99347-99350, 99374-99375, 99377-99378, 99446-99449, 99451-99452, 99495-99496, G0463, G0471

54401 0213T, 0216T, 0228T, 0230T, 12001-12007, 12011-12057, 13100-13133, 13151-13153, 36000, 36400-36410, 36420-36430, 36440, 36591-36592, 36600, 36640, 43752, 51701-51703, 54405❖, 62320-62327, 64400, 64405-64408, 64415-64435, 64445-64454, 64461-64463, 64479-64505, 64510-64530, 69990, 92012-92014, 93000-93010, 93040-93042, 93318, 93355, 94002, 94200, 94250, 94680-94690, 94770, 95812-95816, 95819, 95822, 95829, 95955, 96360-96368, 96372, 96374-96377, 96523, 99155, 99156, 99157, 99211-99223, 99231-99255, 99291-99292, 99304-99310, 99315-99316, 99334-99337, 99347-99350, 99374-99375, 99377-99378, 99446-99449, 99451-99452, 99495-99496, G0463, G0471

54405 0213T, 0216T, 0228T, 0230T, 12001-12007, 12011-12057, 13100-13133, 13151-13153, 36000, 36400-36410, 36420-36430, 36440, 36591-36592, 36600, 36640, 43752, 49000-49010, 51701-51703, 54110, 54161, 54408, 62270, 62320-62328, 64400, 64405-64408, 64415-64435, 64445-64454, 64461-64463, 64479-64505, 64510-64530, 69990, 92012-92014, 93000-93010, 93040-93042, 93318, 93355, 94002, 94200, 94250, 94680-94690, 94770, 95812-95816, 95819, 95822, 95829, 95955, 96360-96368, 96372, 96374-96377, 96523, 99155, 99156, 99157, 99211-99223, 99231-99255, 99291-99292, 99304-99310, 99315-99316, 99334-99337, 99347-99350, 99374-99375, 99377-99378, 99446-99449, 99451-99452, 99495-99496, G0463, G0471, P9612

54406 0213T, 0216T, 0228T, 0230T, 12001-12007, 12011-12057, 13100-13133, 13151-13153, 36000, 36400-36410, 36420-36430, 36440, 36591-36592, 36600, 36640, 43752, 51701-51703, 54405, 54416, 62320-62327, 64400, 64405-64408, 64415-64435, 64445-64454, 64461-64463, 64479-64505, 64510-64530, 69990, 92012-92014, 93000-93010, 93040-93042, 93318, 93355, 94002, 94200, 94250, 94680-94690, 94770, 95812-95816, 95819, 95822, 95829, 95955, 96360-96368, 96372, 96374-96377, 96523, 99155, 99156, 99157, 99211-99223, 99231-99255, 99291-99292, 99304-99310, 99315-99316, 99334-99337, 99347-99350, 99374-99375, 99377-99378, 99446-99449, 99451-99452, 99495-99496, G0463, G0471

CPT © 2020 American Medical Association. All Rights Reserved.

Coding Companion for Urology/Nephrology

54408 0213T, 0216T, 0228T, 0230T, 12001-12007, 12011-12057, 13100-13133, 13151-13153, 36000, 36400-36410, 36420-36430, 36440, 36591-36592, 36600, 36640, 43752, 51701-51703, 54400-54401, 54406, 54416, 62320-62327, 64400, 64405-64408, 64415-64435, 64445-64454, 64461-64463, 64479-64505, 64510-64530, 69990, 92012-92014, 93000-93010, 93040-93042, 93318, 93355, 94002, 94200, 94250, 94680-94690, 94770, 95812-95816, 95819, 95822, 95829, 95955, 96360-96368, 96372, 96374-96377, 96523, 99155, 99156, 99157, 99211-99223, 99231-99255, 99291-99292, 99304-99310, 99315-99316, 99334-99337, 99347-99350, 99374-99375, 99377-99378, 99446-99449, 99451-99452, 99495-99496, G0463, G0471

54410 0213T, 0216T, 0228T, 0230T, 12001-12007, 12011-12057, 13100-13133, 13151-13153, 36000, 36400-36410, 36420-36430, 36440, 36591-36592, 36600, 36640, 43752, 51701-51703, 54400-54401, 54405-54406, 54408, 54411-54417, 62320-62327, 64400, 64405-64408, 64415-64435, 64445-64454, 64461-64463, 64479-64505, 64510-64530, 69990, 92012-92014, 93000-93010, 93040-93042, 93318, 93355, 94002, 94200, 94250, 94680-94690, 94770, 95812-95816, 95819, 95822, 95829, 95955, 96360-96368, 96372, 96374-96377, 96523, 99155, 99156, 99157, 99211-99223, 99231-99255, 99291-99292, 99304-99310, 99315-99316, 99334-99337, 99347-99350, 99374-99375, 99377-99378, 99446-99449, 99451-99452, 99495-99496, G0463, G0471

54411 0213T, 0216T, 0228T, 0230T, 11000-11006, 11042-11047, 12001-12007, 12011-12057, 13100-13133, 13151-13153, 36000, 36400-36410, 36420-36430, 36440, 36591-36592, 36600, 36640, 43752, 51701-51703, 54400-54401, 54405-54406, 54408, 54415-54417, 62320-62327, 64400, 64405-64408, 64415-64435, 64445-64454, 64461-64463, 64479-64505, 64510-64530, 69990, 92012-92014, 93000-93010, 93040-93042, 93318, 93355, 94002, 94200, 94250, 94680-94690, 94770, 95812-95816, 95819, 95822, 95829, 95955, 96360-96368, 96372, 96374-96377, 96523, 97597-97598, 97602, 99155, 99156, 99157, 99211-99223, 99231-99255, 99291-99292, 99304-99310, 99315-99316, 99334-99337, 99347-99350, 99374-99375, 99377-99378, 99446-99449, 99451-99452, 99495-99496, G0463, G0471

54415 0213T, 0216T, 0228T, 0230T, 12001-12007, 12011-12057, 13100-13133, 13151-13153, 36000, 36400-36410, 36420-36430, 36440, 36591-36592, 36600, 36640, 43752, 51701-51703, 54400-54401, 62320-62327, 64400, 64405-64408, 64415-64435, 64445-64454, 64461-64463, 64479-64505, 64510-64530, 69990, 92012-92014, 93000-93010, 93040-93042, 93318, 93355, 94002, 94200, 94250, 94680-94690, 94770, 95812-95816, 95819, 95822, 95829, 95955, 96360-96368, 96372, 96374-96377, 96523, 99155, 99156, 99157, 99211-99223, 99231-99255, 99291-99292, 99304-99310, 99315-99316, 99334-99337, 99347-99350, 99374-99375, 99377-99378, 99446-99449, 99451-99452, 99495-99496, G0463, G0471

54416 0213T, 0216T, 0228T, 0230T, 12001-12007, 12011-12057, 13100-13133, 13151-13153, 36000, 36400-36410, 36420-36430, 36440, 36591-36592, 36600, 36640, 43752, 51701-51703, 54400-54401, 54405, 54415, 54417❖, 62320-62327, 64400, 64405-64408, 64415-64435, 64445-64454, 64461-64463, 64479-64505, 64510-64530, 69990, 92012-92014, 93000-93010, 93040-93042, 93318, 93355, 94002, 94200, 94250, 94680-94690, 94770, 95812-95816, 95819, 95822, 95829, 95955, 96360-96368, 96372, 96374-96377, 96523, 99155, 99156, 99157, 99211-99223, 99231-99255, 99291-99292, 99304-99310, 99315-99316, 99334-99337, 99347-99350, 99374-99375, 99377-99378, 99446-99449, 99451-99452, 99495-99496, G0463, G0471

54417 0213T, 0216T, 0228T, 0230T, 11000-11006, 11042-11047, 12001-12007, 12011-12057, 13100-13133, 13151-13153, 36000, 36400-36410, 36420-36430, 36440, 36591-36592, 36600, 36640, 43752, 51701-51703, 54400-54401, 54405-54406, 54408, 54415, 62320-62327, 64400,

54420 0213T, 0216T, 0228T, 0230T, 12001-12007, 12011-12057, 13100-13133, 13151-13153, 36000, 36400-36410, 36420-36430, 36440, 36591-36592, 36600, 36640, 43752, 51701-51703, 54430-54435, 62320-62327, 64400, 64405-64408, 64415-64435, 64445-64454, 64461-64463, 64479-64505, 64510-64530, 69990, 92012-92014, 93000-93010, 93040-93042, 93318, 93355, 94002, 94200, 94250, 94680-94690, 94770, 95812-95816, 95819, 95822, 95829, 95955, 96360-96368, 96372, 96374-96377, 96523, 99155, 99156, 99157, 99211-99223, 99231-99255, 99291-99292, 99304-99310, 99315-99316, 99334-99337, 99347-99350, 99374-99375, 99377-99378, 99446-99449, 99451-99452, 99495-99496, G0463, G0471

54430 0213T, 0216T, 0228T, 0230T, 12001-12007, 12011-12057, 13100-13133, 13151-13153, 36000, 36400-36410, 36420-36430, 36440, 36591-36592, 36600, 36640, 43752, 51701-51703, 62320-62327, 64400, 64405-64408, 64415-64435, 64445-64454, 64461-64463, 64479-64505, 64510-64530, 69990, 92012-92014, 93000-93010, 93040-93042, 93318, 93355, 94002, 94200, 94250, 94680-94690, 94770, 95812-95816, 95819, 95822, 95829, 95955, 96360-96368, 96372, 96374-96377, 96523, 99155, 99156, 99157, 99211-99223, 99231-99255, 99291-99292, 99304-99310, 99315-99316, 99334-99337, 99347-99350, 99374-99375, 99377-99378, 99446-99449, 99451-99452, 99495-99496, G0463, G0471

54435 0213T, 0216T, 0228T, 0230T, 10005, 10007, 10009, 10011, 10021, 12001-12007, 12011-12057, 13100-13133, 13151-13153, 36000, 36400-36410, 36420-36430, 36440, 36591-36592, 36600, 36640, 43752, 51701-51703, 54430❖, 62320-62327, 64400, 64405-64408, 64415-64435, 64445-64454, 64461-64463, 64479-64505, 64510-64530, 69990, 92012-92014, 93000-93010, 93040-93042, 93318, 93355, 94002, 94200, 94250, 94680-94690, 94770, 95812-95816, 95819, 95822, 95829, 95955, 96360-96368, 96372, 96374-96377, 96523, 99155, 99156, 99157, 99211-99223, 99231-99255, 99291-99292, 99304-99310, 99315-99316, 99334-99337, 99347-99350, 99374-99375, 99377-99378, 99446-99449, 99451-99452, 99495-99496, G0463, G0471

54437 0213T, 0216T, 0228T, 0230T, 12001-12007, 12011-12057, 13100-13133, 13151-13153, 36000, 36400-36410, 36420-36430, 36440, 36591-36592, 36600, 36640, 43752, 51701-51703, 54440❖, 62320-62327, 64400, 64405-64408, 64415-64435, 64445-64454, 64461-64463, 64479-64505, 64510-64530, 69990, 92012-92014, 93000-93010, 93040-93042, 93318, 93355, 94002, 94200, 94250, 94680-94690, 94770, 95812-95816, 95819, 95822, 95829, 95955, 96360-96368, 96372, 96374-96377, 96523, 99155, 99156, 99157, 99211-99223, 99231-99255, 99291-99292, 99304-99310, 99315-99316, 99334-99337, 99347-99350, 99374-99375, 99377-99378, 99446-99449, 99451-99452, 99495-99496, G0463, G0471

54438 0213T, 0216T, 0228T, 0230T, 12001-12007, 12011-12057, 13100-13133, 13151-13153, 36000, 36400-36410, 36420-36430, 36440, 36591-36592, 36600, 36640, 43752, 51701-51703, 53410-53415, 54360❖, 54437❖, 54440❖, 62320-62327, 64400, 64405-64408, 64415-64435, 64445-64454, 64461-64463, 64479-64505, 64510-64530, 69990, 92012-92014, 93000-93010, 93040-93042, 93318, 93355, 94002, 94200, 94250, 94680-94690, 94770, 95812-95816, 95819, 95822, 95829, 95955, 96360-96368, 96372, 96374-96377, 96523, 99155, 99156, 99157, 99211-99223, 99231-99255, 99291-99292, 99304-99310,

CPT © 2020 American Medical Association. All Rights Reserved.

© 2020 Optum360, LLC

99315-99316, 99334-99337, 99347-99350, 99374-99375, 99377-99378, 99446-99449, 99451-99452, 99495-99496, G0463, G0471

54440 0213T, 0216T, 0228T, 0230T, 12001-12007, 12011-12057, 13100-13133, 13151-13153, 36000, 36400-36410, 36420-36430, 36440, 36591-36592, 36600, 36640, 43752, 51701-51703, 62320-62327, 64400, 64405-64408, 64415-64435, 64445-64454, 64461-64463, 64479-64505, 64510-64530, 69990, 92012-92014, 93000-93010, 93040-93042, 93318, 93355, 94002, 94200, 94250, 94680-94690, 94770, 95812-95816, 95819, 95822, 95829, 95955, 96360-96368, 96372, 96374-96377, 96523, 99155, 99156, 99157, 99211-99223, 99231-99255, 99291-99292, 99304-99310, 99315-99316, 99334-99337, 99347-99350, 99374-99375, 99377-99378, 99446-99449, 99451-99452, 99495-99496, G0463, G0471

54450 0213T, 0216T, 0228T, 0230T, 12001-12007, 12011-12057, 13100-13133, 13151-13153, 36000, 36400-36410, 36420-36430, 36440, 36591-36592, 36600, 36640, 43752, 51701-51703, 54000-54001, 62320-62327, 64400, 64405-64408, 64415-64435, 64445-64454, 64461-64463, 64479-64505, 64510-64530, 69990, 92012-92014, 93000-93010, 93040-93042, 93318, 93355, 94002, 94200, 94250, 94680-94690, 94770, 95812-95816, 95819, 95822, 95829, 95955, 96360-96368, 96372, 96374-96377, 96523, 99155, 99156, 99157, 99211-99223, 99231-99255, 99291-99292, 99304-99310, 99315-99316, 99334-99337, 99347-99350, 99374-99375, 99377-99378, 99446-99449, 99451-99452, 99495-99496, G0463, G0471

54500 0213T, 0216T, 0228T, 0230T, 10005, 10007, 10009, 10011, 10021, 12001-12007, 12011-12057, 13100-13133, 13151-13153, 36000, 36400-36410, 36420-36430, 36440, 36591-36592, 36600, 36640, 43752, 51701-51703, 54660, 62320-62327, 64400, 64405-64408, 64415-64435, 64445-64454, 64461-64463, 64479-64505, 64510-64530, 69990, 92012-92014, 93000-93010, 93040-93042, 93318, 93355, 94002, 94200, 94250, 94680-94690, 94770, 95812-95816, 95819, 95822, 95829, 95955, 96360-96368, 96372, 96374-96377, 96523, 99155, 99156, 99157, 99211-99223, 99231-99255, 99291-99292, 99304-99310, 99315-99316, 99334-99337, 99347-99350, 99374-99375, 99377-99378, 99446-99449, 99451-99452, 99495-99496, G0463, G0471

54505 0213T, 0216T, 0228T, 0230T, 10005, 10007, 10009, 10011, 10021, 12001-12007, 12011-12057, 13100-13133, 13151-13153, 36000, 36400-36410, 36420-36430, 36440, 36591-36592, 36600, 36640, 43752, 51701-51703, 62320-62327, 64400, 64405-64408, 64415-64435, 64445-64454, 64461-64463, 64479-64505, 64510-64530, 69990, 92012-92014, 93000-93010, 93040-93042, 93318, 93355, 94002, 94200, 94250, 94680-94690, 94770, 95812-95816, 95819, 95822, 95829, 95955, 96360-96368, 96372, 96374-96377, 96523, 99155, 99156, 99157, 99211-99223, 99231-99255, 99291-99292, 99304-99310, 99315-99316, 99334-99337, 99347-99350, 99374-99375, 99377-99378, 99446-99449, 99451-99452, 99495-99496, G0463, G0471

54512 0213T, 0216T, 0228T, 0230T, 12001-12007, 12011-12057, 13100-13133, 13151-13153, 36000, 36400-36410, 36420-36430, 36440, 36591-36592, 36600, 36640, 43752, 51701-51703, 54500-54505, 54620, 54660, 54700, 55110, 62320-62327, 64400, 64405-64408, 64415-64435, 64445-64454, 64461-64463, 64479-64505, 64510-64530, 69990, 92012-92014, 93000-93010, 93040-93042, 93318, 93355, 94002, 94200, 94250, 94680-94690, 94770, 95812-95816, 95819, 95822, 95829, 95955, 96360-96368, 96372, 96374-96377, 96523, 99155, 99156, 99157, 99211-99223, 99231-99255, 99291-99292, 99304-99310, 99315-99316, 99334-99337, 99347-99350, 99374-99375, 99377-99378, 99446-99449, 99451-99452, 99495-99496, G0463, G0471

54520 0213T, 0216T, 0228T, 0230T, 12001-12007, 12011-12057, 13100-13133, 13151-13153, 36000, 36400-36410, 36420-36430, 36440, 36591-36592, 36600, 36640, 43752, 49000-49010, 51701-51703, 54500-54505, 54512, 54522, 54660, 54690, 55040-55041, 55110, 62320-62327, 64400,

54522 0213T, 0216T, 0228T, 0230T, 11000-11006, 11042-11047, 12001-12007, 12011-12057, 13100-13133, 13151-13153, 36000, 36400-36410, 36420-36430, 36440, 36591-36592, 36600, 36640, 43752, 51701-51703, 54500-54505, 54512, 54620, 54660, 55110, 62320-62327, 64400, 64405-64408, 64415-64435, 64445-64454, 64461-64463, 64479-64505, 64510-64530, 69990, 92012-92014, 93000-93010, 93040-93042, 93318, 93355, 94002, 94200, 94250, 94680-94690, 94770, 95812-95816, 95819, 95822, 95829, 95955, 96360-96368, 96372, 96374-96377, 96523, 97597-97598, 97602, 99155, 99156, 99157, 99211-99223, 99231-99255, 99291-99292, 99304-99310, 99315-99316, 99334-99337, 99347-99350, 99374-99375, 99377-99378, 99446-99449, 99451-99452, 99495-99496, G0463, G0471

54530 0213T, 0216T, 0228T, 0230T, 11000-11006, 11042-11047, 12001-12007, 12011-12057, 13100-13133, 13151-13153, 36000, 36400-36410, 36420-36430, 36440, 36591-36592, 36600, 36640, 43752, 51701-51703, 54505, 54512-54520, 54522, 54535✦, 54620, 54660, 54690, 55110, 62320-62327, 64400, 64405-64408, 64415-64435, 64445-64454, 64461-64463, 64479-64505, 64510-64530, 69990, 92012-92014, 93000-93010, 93040-93042, 93318, 93355, 94002, 94200, 94250, 94680-94690, 94770, 95812-95816, 95819, 95822, 95829, 95955, 96360-96368, 96372, 96374-96377, 96523, 97597-97598, 97602, 99155, 99156, 99157, 99211-99223, 99231-99255, 99291-99292, 99304-99310, 99315-99316, 99334-99337, 99347-99350, 99374-99375, 99377-99378, 99446-99449, 99451-99452, 99495-99496, G0463, G0471

54535 0213T, 0216T, 0228T, 0230T, 11000-11006, 11042-11047, 12001-12007, 12011-12057, 13100-13133, 13151-13153, 36000, 36400-36410, 36420-36430, 36440, 36591-36592, 36600, 36640, 43752, 44005, 44180, 44820-44850, 44950, 44970, 49000-49010, 49255, 49320-49321, 51701-51703, 54500-54505, 54512, 54522, 54620, 54660, 54690, 55110, 62320-62327, 64400, 64405-64408, 64415-64435, 64445-64454, 64461-64463, 64479-64505, 64510-64530, 69990, 92012-92014, 93000-93010, 93040-93042, 93318, 93355, 94002, 94200, 94250, 94680-94690, 94770, 95812-95816, 95819, 95822, 95829, 95955, 96360-96368, 96372, 96374-96377, 96523, 97597-97598, 97602, 99155, 99156, 99157, 99211-99223, 99231-99255, 99291-99292, 99304-99310, 99315-99316, 99334-99337, 99347-99350, 99374-99375, 99377-99378, 99446-99449, 99451-99452, 99495-99496, G0463, G0471

54550 0213T, 0216T, 0228T, 0230T, 12001-12007, 12011-12057, 13100-13133, 13151-13153, 36000, 36400-36410, 36420-36430, 36440, 36591-36592, 36600, 36640, 43752, 51701-51703, 54500-54505, 54560✦, 54660, 55110, 62320-62327, 64400, 64405-64408, 64415-64435, 64445-64454, 64461-64463, 64479-64505, 64510-64530, 69990, 92012-92014, 93000-93010, 93040-93042, 93318, 93355, 94002, 94200, 94250, 94680-94690, 94770, 95812-95816, 95819, 95822, 95829, 95955, 96360-96368, 96372, 96374-96377, 96523, 99155, 99156, 99157, 99211-99223, 99231-99255, 99291-99292, 99304-99310, 99315-99316, 99334-99337, 99347-99350, 99374-99375, 99377-99378, 99446-99449, 99451-99452, 99495-99496, G0463, G0471

54560 0213T, 0216T, 0228T, 0230T, 12001-12007, 12011-12057, 13100-13133, 13151-13153, 36000, 36400-36410, 36420-36430, 36440, 36591-36592, 36600, 36640, 43752, 44005, 44180, 44602-44605, 44820-44850, 44950, 44970, 49000-49010, 49255, 49320, 51701-51703, 54500-54505,

54620,62320-62327,64400,64405-64408,64415-64435,64445-64454,
64461-64463,64479-64505,64510-64530,69990,92012-92014,
93000-93010,93040-93042,93318,93355,94002,94200,94250,
94680-94690,94770,95812-95816,95819,95822,95829,95955,
96360-96368,96372,96374-96377,96523,99155,99156,99157,
99211-99223,99231-99255,99291-99292,99304-99310,99315-99316,
99334-99337,99347-99350,99374-99375,99377-99378,99446-99449,
99451-99452,99495-99496,G0463,G0471

54600   0213T,0216T,0228T,0230T,12001-12007,12011-12057,13100-13133,
13151-13153,36000,36400-36410,36420-36430,36440,36591-36592,
36600,36640,43752,51701-51703,54500-54505,54620,55110,
62320-62327,64400,64405-64408,64415-64435,64445-64454,
64461-64463,64479-64505,64510-64530,69990,92012-92014,
93000-93010,93040-93042,93318,93355,94002,94200,94250,
94680-94690,94770,95812-95816,95819,95822,95829,95955,
96360-96368,96372,96374-96377,96523,99155,99156,99157,
99211-99223,99231-99255,99291-99292,99304-99310,99315-99316,
99334-99337,99347-99350,99374-99375,99377-99378,99446-99449,
99451-99452,99495-99496,G0463,G0471

54620   0213T,0216T,0228T,0230T,12001-12007,12011-12057,13100-13133,
13151-13153,36000,36400-36410,36420-36430,36440,36591-36592,
36600,36640,43752,51701-51703,54505,55110,62320-62327,
64400,64405-64408,64415-64435,64445-64454,64461-64463,
64479-64505,64510-64530,69990,92012-92014,93000-93010,
93040-93042,93318,93355,94002,94200,94250,94680-94690,
94770,95812-95816,95819,95822,95829,95955,96360-96368,
96372,96374-96377,96523,99155,99156,99157,99211-99223,
99231-99255,99291-99292,99304-99310,99315-99316,99334-99337,
99347-99350,99374-99375,99377-99378,99446-99449,99451-99452,
99495-99496,G0463,G0471

54640   0213T,0216T,0228T,0230T,0437T,12001-12007,12011-12057,
13100-13133,13151-13153,15777,36000,36400-36410,36420-36430,
36440,36591-36592,36600,36640,43752,49568,51701-51703,
54500-54505,54512,54550,54650♦,54692,55110,57267,
62320-62327,64400,64405-64408,64415-64435,64445-64454,
64461-64463,64479-64505,64510-64530,69990,92012-92014,
93000-93010,93040-93042,93318,93355,94002,94200,94250,
94680-94690,94770,95812-95816,95819,95822,95829,95955,
96360-96368,96372,96374-96377,96523,99155,99156,99157,
99211-99223,99231-99255,99291-99292,99304-99310,99315-99316,
99334-99337,99347-99350,99374-99375,99377-99378,99446-99449,
99451-99452,99495-99496,G0463,G0471

54650   0213T,0216T,0228T,0230T,12001-12007,12011-12057,13100-13133,
13151-13153,36000,36400-36410,36420-36430,36440,36591-36592,
36600,36640,43752,44005,44180,44602-44605,44820-44850,
44950,44970,49000-49010,49255,49320,51701-51703,54500-54505,
54512,54560,54692,55110,62320-62327,64400,64405-64408,
64415-64435,64445-64454,64461-64463,64479-64505,64510-64530,
69990,92012-92014,93000-93010,93040-93042,93318,93355,94002,
94200,94250,94680-94690,94770,95812-95816,95819,95822,
95829,95955,96360-96368,96372,96374-96377,96523,99155,
99156,99157,99211-99223,99231-99255,99291-99292,99304-99310,
99315-99316,99334-99337,99347-99350,99374-99375,99377-99378,
99446-99449,99451-99452,99495-99496,G0463,G0471

54660   0213T,0216T,0228T,0230T,12001-12007,12011-12057,13100-13133,
13151-13153,36000,36400-36410,36420-36430,36440,36591-36592,
36600,36640,43752,51701-51703,54505,55110,62320-62327,
64400,64405-64408,64415-64435,64445-64454,64461-64463,
64479-64505,64510-64530,69990,92012-92014,93000-93010,

54670   0213T,0216T,0228T,0230T,12001-12007,12011-12057,13100-13133,
13151-13153,36000,36400-36410,36420-36430,36440,36591-36592,
36600,36640,43752,51701-51703,54500-54505,54620,55110,
62320-62327,64400,64405-64408,64415-64435,64445-64454,
64461-64463,64479-64505,64510-64530,69990,92012-92014,
93000-93010,93040-93042,93318,93355,94002,94200,94250,
94680-94690,94770,95812-95816,95819,95822,95829,95955,
96360-96368,96372,96374-96377,96523,99155,99156,99157,
99211-99223,99231-99255,99291-99292,99304-99310,99315-99316,
99334-99337,99347-99350,99374-99375,99377-99378,99446-99449,
99451-99452,99495-99496,G0463,G0471

54680   0213T,0216T,0228T,0230T,12001-12007,12011-12057,13100-13133,
13151-13153,36000,36400-36410,36420-36430,36440,36591-36592,
36600,36640,43752,51701-51703,54500-54505,54620,54670,
55110,62320-62327,64400,64405-64408,64415-64435,64445-64454,
64461-64463,64479-64505,64510-64530,69990,92012-92014,
93000-93010,93040-93042,93318,93355,94002,94200,94250,
94680-94690,94770,95812-95816,95819,95822,95829,95955,
96360-96368,96372,96374-96377,96523,99155,99156,99157,
99211-99223,99231-99255,99291-99292,99304-99310,99315-99316,
99334-99337,99347-99350,99374-99375,99377-99378,99446-99449,
99451-99452,99495-99496,G0463,G0471

54690   0213T,0216T,0228T,0230T,11000-11006,11042-11047,12001-12007,
12011-12057,13100-13133,13151-13153,36000,36400-36410,
36420-36430,36440,36591-36592,36600,36640,43653,43752,
44005,44180,44602-44605,44950,44970,49082-49084,49320-49321,
49400,50715,51701-51703,54512,54522,55110,62320-62327,
64400,64405-64408,64415-64435,64445-64454,64461-64463,
64479-64505,64510-64530,69990,76000,77001-77002,92012-92014,
93000-93010,93040-93042,93318,93355,94002,94200,94250,
94680-94690,94770,95812-95816,95819,95822,95829,95955,
96360-96368,96372,96374-96377,96523,97597-97598,97602,99155,
99156,99157,99211-99223,99231-99255,99291-99292,99304-99310,
99315-99316,99334-99337,99347-99350,99374-99375,99377-99378,
99446-99449,99451-99452,99495-99496,G0463,G0471

54692   0213T,0216T,0228T,0230T,12001-12007,12011-12057,13100-13133,
13151-13153,36000,36400-36410,36420-36430,36440,36591-36592,
36600,36640,43653,43752,44005,44180,44602-44605,44950,
44970,49082-49084,49320,49400,50715,51701-51703,55110,
58660,62320-62327,64400,64405-64408,64415-64435,64445-64454,
64461-64463,64479-64505,64510-64530,69990,76000,77001-77002,
92012-92014,93000-93010,93040-93042,93318,93355,94002,94200,
94250,94680-94690,94770,95812-95816,95819,95822,95829,
95955,96360-96368,96372,96374-96377,96523,99155,99156,
99157,99211-99223,99231-99255,99291-99292,99304-99310,
99315-99316,99334-99337,99347-99350,99374-99375,99377-99378,
99446-99449,99451-99452,99495-99496,G0463,G0471

54700   0213T,0216T,0228T,0230T,12001-12007,12011-12057,13100-13133,
13151-13153,36000,36400-36410,36420-36430,36440,36591-36592,
36600,36640,43752,51701-51703,54500-54505,55100-55110,
62320-62327,64400,64405-64408,64415-64435,64445-64454,
64461-64463,64479-64505,64510-64530,69990,92012-92014,
93000-93010,93040-93042,93318,93355,94002,94200,94250,

94680-94690, 94770, 95812-95816, 95819, 95822, 95829, 95955, 96360-96368, 96372, 96374-96377, 96523, 99155, 99156, 99157, 99211-99223, 99231-99255, 99291-99292, 99304-99310, 99315-99316, 99334-99337, 99347-99350, 99374-99375, 99377-99378, 99446-99449, 99451-99452, 99495-99496, G0463, G0471, J2001

54800 0213T, 0216T, 0228T, 0230T, 10005, 10007, 10009, 10011, 10021, 12001-12007, 12011-12057, 13100-13133, 13151-13153, 36000, 36400-36410, 36420-36430, 36440, 36591-36592, 36600, 36640, 43752, 51701-51703, 54500-54505, 62320-62327, 64400, 64405-64408, 64415-64435, 64445-64454, 64461-64463, 64479-64505, 64510-64530, 69990, 92012-92014, 93000-93010, 93040-93042, 93318, 93355, 94002, 94200, 94250, 94680-94690, 94770, 95812-95816, 95819, 95822, 95829, 95955, 96360-96368, 96372, 96374-96377, 96523, 99155, 99156, 99157, 99211-99223, 99231-99255, 99291-99292, 99304-99310, 99315-99316, 99334-99337, 99347-99350, 99374-99375, 99377-99378, 99446-99449, 99451-99452, 99495-99496, G0463, G0471

54830 0213T, 0216T, 0228T, 0230T, 11000-11006, 11042-11047, 12001-12007, 12011-12057, 13100-13133, 13151-13153, 36000, 36400-36410, 36420-36430, 36440, 36591-36592, 36600, 36640, 43752, 51701-51703, 54500-54505, 55110, 62320-62327, 64400, 64405-64408, 64415-64435, 64445-64454, 64461-64463, 64479-64505, 64510-64530, 69990, 92012-92014, 93000-93010, 93040-93042, 93318, 93355, 94002, 94200, 94250, 94680-94690, 94770, 95812-95816, 95819, 95822, 95829, 95955, 96360-96368, 96372, 96374-96377, 96523, 97597-97598, 97602, 99155, 99156, 99157, 99211-99223, 99231-99255, 99291-99292, 99304-99310, 99315-99316, 99334-99337, 99347-99350, 99374-99375, 99377-99378, 99446-99449, 99451-99452, 99495-99496, G0463, G0471

54840 0213T, 0216T, 0228T, 0230T, 11000-11006, 11042-11047, 12001-12007, 12011-12057, 13100-13133, 13151-13153, 36000, 36400-36410, 36420-36430, 36440, 36591-36592, 36600, 36640, 43752, 51701-51703, 54500-54505, 55110, 62320-62327, 64400, 64405-64408, 64415-64435, 64445-64454, 64461-64463, 64479-64505, 64510-64530, 69990, 92012-92014, 93000-93010, 93040-93042, 93318, 93355, 94002, 94200, 94250, 94680-94690, 94770, 95812-95816, 95819, 95822, 95829, 95955, 96360-96368, 96372, 96374-96377, 96523, 97597-97598, 97602, 99155, 99156, 99157, 99211-99223, 99231-99255, 99291-99292, 99304-99310, 99315-99316, 99334-99337, 99347-99350, 99374-99375, 99377-99378, 99446-99449, 99451-99452, 99495-99496, G0463, G0471

54860 0213T, 0216T, 0228T, 0230T, 11000-11006, 11042-11047, 12001-12007, 12011-12057, 13100-13133, 13151-13153, 36000, 36400-36410, 36420-36430, 36440, 36591-36592, 36600, 36640, 43752, 51701-51703, 54500-54505, 55110, 62320-62327, 64400, 64405-64408, 64415-64435, 64445-64454, 64461-64463, 64479-64505, 64510-64530, 69990, 92012-92014, 93000-93010, 93040-93042, 93318, 93355, 94002, 94200, 94250, 94680-94690, 94770, 95812-95816, 95819, 95822, 95829, 95955, 96360-96368, 96372, 96374-96377, 96523, 97597-97598, 97602, 99155, 99156, 99157, 99211-99223, 99231-99255, 99291-99292, 99304-99310, 99315-99316, 99334-99337, 99347-99350, 99374-99375, 99377-99378, 99446-99449, 99451-99452, 99495-99496, G0463, G0471

54861 0213T, 0216T, 0228T, 0230T, 11000-11006, 11042-11047, 12001-12007, 12011-12057, 13100-13133, 13151-13153, 36000, 36400-36410, 36420-36430, 36440, 36591-36592, 36600, 36640, 43752, 51701-51703, 54500-54505, 54860, 55110, 62320-62327, 64400, 64405-64408, 64415-64435, 64445-64454, 64461-64463, 64479-64505, 64510-64530, 69990, 92012-92014, 93000-93010, 93040-93042, 93318, 93355, 94002, 94200, 94250, 94680-94690, 94770, 95812-95816, 95819, 95822, 95829, 95955, 96360-96368, 96372, 96374-96377, 96523, 97597-97598, 97602, 99155, 99156, 99157, 99211-99223, 99231-99255, 99291-99292,

54865 0213T, 0216T, 0228T, 0230T, 10005, 10007, 10009, 10011, 10021, 12001-12007, 12011-12057, 13100-13133, 13151-13153, 36000, 36400-36410, 36420-36430, 36440, 36591-36592, 36600, 36640, 43752, 51701-51703, 54500-54505, 55110, 62320-62327, 64400, 64405-64408, 64415-64435, 64445-64454, 64461-64463, 64479-64505, 64510-64530, 69990, 92012-92014, 93000-93010, 93040-93042, 93318, 93355, 94002, 94200, 94250, 94680-94690, 94770, 95812-95816, 95819, 95822, 95829, 95955, 96360-96368, 96372, 96374-96377, 96523, 99155, 99156, 99157, 99211-99223, 99231-99255, 99291-99292, 99304-99310, 99315-99316, 99334-99337, 99347-99350, 99374-99375, 99377-99378, 99446-99449, 99451-99452, 99495-99496, G0463, G0471

54900 0213T, 0216T, 0228T, 0230T, 12001-12007, 12011-12057, 13100-13133, 13151-13153, 36000, 36400-36410, 36420-36430, 36440, 36591-36592, 36600, 36640, 43752, 51701-51703, 54500-54505, 55110, 62320-62327, 64400, 64405-64408, 64415-64435, 64445-64454, 64461-64463, 64479-64505, 64510-64530, 69990, 92012-92014, 93000-93010, 93040-93042, 93318, 93355, 94002, 94200, 94250, 94680-94690, 94770, 95812-95816, 95819, 95822, 95829, 95955, 96360-96368, 96372, 96374-96377, 96523, 99155, 99156, 99157, 99211-99223, 99231-99255, 99291-99292, 99304-99310, 99315-99316, 99334-99337, 99347-99350, 99374-99375, 99377-99378, 99446-99449, 99451-99452, 99495-99496, G0463, G0471

54901 0213T, 0216T, 0228T, 0230T, 12001-12007, 12011-12057, 13100-13133, 13151-13153, 36000, 36400-36410, 36420-36430, 36440, 36591-36592, 36600, 36640, 43752, 51701-51703, 54500-54505, 54900, 55110, 62320-62327, 64400, 64405-64408, 64415-64435, 64445-64454, 64461-64463, 64479-64505, 64510-64530, 69990, 92012-92014, 93000-93010, 93040-93042, 93318, 93355, 94002, 94200, 94250, 94680-94690, 94770, 95812-95816, 95819, 95822, 95829, 95955, 96360-96368, 96372, 96374-96377, 96523, 99155, 99156, 99157, 99211-99223, 99231-99255, 99291-99292, 99304-99310, 99315-99316, 99334-99337, 99347-99350, 99374-99375, 99377-99378, 99446-99449, 99451-99452, 99495-99496, G0463, G0471

55000 0213T, 0216T, 0228T, 0230T, 12001-12007, 12011-12057, 13100-13133, 13151-13153, 36000, 36400-36410, 36420-36430, 36440, 36591-36592, 36600, 36640, 43752, 51701-51703, 54500-54505, 55110, 62320-62327, 64400, 64405-64408, 64415-64435, 64445-64454, 64461-64463, 64479-64505, 64510-64530, 69990, 92012-92014, 93000-93010, 93040-93042, 93318, 93355, 94002, 94200, 94250, 94680-94690, 94770, 95812-95816, 95819, 95822, 95829, 95955, 96360-96368, 96372, 96374-96377, 96523, 99155, 99156, 99157, 99211-99223, 99231-99255, 99291-99292, 99304-99310, 99315-99316, 99334-99337, 99347-99350, 99374-99375, 99377-99378, 99446-99449, 99451-99452, 99495-99496, G0463, G0471, J0670, J2001

55040 0213T, 0216T, 0228T, 0230T, 11000-11006, 11042-11047, 12001-12007, 12011-12057, 13100-13133, 13151-13153, 36000, 36400-36410, 36420-36430, 36440, 36591-36592, 36600, 36640, 43752, 51701-51703, 54500-54505, 54840, 55110, 62320-62327, 64400, 64405-64408, 64415-64435, 64445-64454, 64461-64463, 64479-64505, 64510-64530, 69990, 92012-92014, 93000-93010, 93040-93042, 93318, 93355, 94002, 94200, 94250, 94680-94690, 94770, 95812-95816, 95819, 95822, 95829, 95955, 96360-96368, 96372, 96374-96377, 96523, 97597-97598, 97602, 99155, 99156, 99157, 99211-99223, 99231-99255, 99291-99292, 99304-99310, 99315-99316, 99334-99337, 99347-99350, 99374-99375, 99377-99378, 99446-99449, 99451-99452, 99495-99496, G0463, G0471

55041 0213T, 0216T, 0228T, 0230T, 11000-11006, 11042-11047, 12001-12007, 12011-12057, 13100-13133, 13151-13153, 36000, 36400-36410,

CPT © 2020 American Medical Association. All Rights Reserved.

Coding Companion for Urology/Nephrology

36420-36430, 36440, 36591-36592, 36600, 36640, 43752, 51701-51703, 54500-54505, 55040, 55110, 62320-62327, 64400, 64405-64408, 64415-64435, 64445-64454, 64461-64463, 64479-64505, 64510-64530, 69990, 92012-92014, 93000-93010, 93040-93042, 93318, 93355, 94002, 94200, 94250, 94680-94690, 94770, 95812-95816, 95819, 95822, 95829, 95955, 96360-96368, 96372, 96374-96377, 96523, 97597-97598, 97602, 99155, 99156, 99157, 99211-99223, 99231-99255, 99291-99292, 99304-99310, 99315-99316, 99334-99337, 99347-99350, 99374-99375, 99377-99378, 99446-99449, 99451-99452, 99495-99496, G0463, G0471

55060 0213T, 0216T, 0228T, 0230T, 12001-12007, 12011-12057, 13100-13133, 13151-13153, 36000, 36400-36410, 36420-36430, 36440, 36591-36592, 36600, 36640, 43752, 49010, 51701-51703, 55110, 62320-62327, 64400, 64405-64408, 64415-64435, 64445-64454, 64461-64463, 64479-64505, 64510-64530, 69990, 92012-92014, 93000-93010, 93040-93042, 93318, 93355, 94002, 94200, 94250, 94680-94690, 94770, 95812-95816, 95819, 95822, 95829, 95955, 96360-96368, 96372, 96374-96377, 96523, 99155, 99156, 99157, 99211-99223, 99231-99255, 99291-99292, 99304-99310, 99315-99316, 99334-99337, 99347-99350, 99374-99375, 99377-99378, 99446-99449, 99451-99452, 99495-99496, G0463, G0471

55100 0213T, 0216T, 0228T, 0230T, 12001-12007, 12011-12057, 13100-13133, 13151-13153, 36000, 36400-36410, 36420-36430, 36440, 36591-36592, 36600, 36640, 43752, 51701-51703, 54500-54505, 55110, 62320-62327, 64400, 64405-64408, 64415-64435, 64445-64454, 64461-64463, 64479-64505, 64510-64530, 69990, 92012-92014, 93000-93010, 93040-93042, 93318, 93355, 94002, 94200, 94250, 94680-94690, 94770, 95812-95816, 95819, 95822, 95829, 95955, 96360-96368, 96372, 96374-96377, 96523, 99155, 99156, 99157, 99211-99223, 99231-99255, 99291-99292, 99304-99310, 99315-99316, 99334-99337, 99347-99350, 99374-99375, 99377-99378, 99446-99449, 99451-99452, 99495-99496, G0463, G0471, J0670, J2001

55110 0213T, 0216T, 0228T, 0230T, 12001-12007, 12011-12057, 13100-13133, 13151-13153, 36000, 36400-36410, 36420-36430, 36440, 36591-36592, 36600, 36640, 43752, 51701-51703, 54500-54505, 62320-62327, 64400, 64405-64408, 64415-64435, 64445-64454, 64461-64463, 64479-64505, 64510-64530, 69990, 92012-92014, 93000-93010, 93040-93042, 93318, 93355, 94002, 94200, 94250, 94680-94690, 94770, 95812-95816, 95819, 95822, 95829, 95955, 96360-96368, 96372, 96374-96377, 96523, 99155, 99156, 99157, 99211-99223, 99231-99255, 99291-99292, 99304-99310, 99315-99316, 99334-99337, 99347-99350, 99374-99375, 99377-99378, 99446-99449, 99451-99452, 99495-99496, G0463, G0471

55120 0213T, 0216T, 0228T, 0230T, 11000-11006, 11042-11047, 12001-12007, 12011-12057, 13100-13133, 13151-13153, 36000, 36400-36410, 36420-36430, 36440, 36591-36592, 36600, 36640, 43752, 51701-51703, 54500-54505, 55100-55110, 62320-62327, 64400, 64405-64408, 64415-64435, 64445-64454, 64461-64463, 64479-64505, 64510-64530, 69990, 92012-92014, 93000-93010, 93040-93042, 93318, 93355, 94002, 94200, 94250, 94680-94690, 94770, 95812-95816, 95819, 95822, 95829, 95955, 96360-96368, 96372, 96374-96377, 96523, 97597-97598, 97602, 99155, 99156, 99157, 99211-99223, 99231-99255, 99291-99292, 99304-99310, 99315-99316, 99334-99337, 99347-99350, 99374-99375, 99377-99378, 99446-99449, 99451-99452, 99495-99496, G0463, G0471, J2001

55150 0213T, 0216T, 0228T, 0230T, 11000-11006, 11042-11047, 12001-12007, 12011-12057, 13100-13133, 13151-13153, 36000, 36400-36410, 36420-36430, 36440, 36591-36592, 36600, 36640, 43752, 51701-51703, 54500-54505, 55110, 55180✦, 62320-62327, 64400, 64405-64408, 64415-64435, 64445-64454, 64461-64463, 64479-64505, 64510-64530, 69990, 92012-92014, 93000-93010, 93040-93042, 93318, 93355, 94002,

94200, 94250, 94680-94690, 94770, 95812-95816, 95819, 95822, 95829, 95955, 96360-96368, 96372, 96374-96377, 96523, 97597-97598, 97602, 99155, 99156, 99157, 99211-99223, 99231-99255, 99291-99292, 99304-99310, 99315-99316, 99334-99337, 99347-99350, 99374-99375, 99377-99378, 99446-99449, 99451-99452, 99495-99496, G0463, G0471

55175 0213T, 0216T, 0228T, 0230T, 11000-11006, 11042-11047, 12001-12007, 12011-12057, 13100-13133, 13151-13153, 36000, 36400-36410, 36420-36430, 36440, 36591-36592, 36600, 36640, 43752, 51701-51703, 55110, 55150✦, 62320-62327, 64400, 64405-64408, 64415-64435, 64445-64454, 64461-64463, 64479-64505, 64510-64530, 69990, 92012-92014, 93000-93010, 93040-93042, 93318, 93355, 94002, 94200, 94250, 94680-94690, 94770, 95812-95816, 95819, 95822, 95829, 95955, 96360-96368, 96372, 96374-96377, 96523, 97597-97598, 97602, 99155, 99156, 99157, 99211-99223, 99231-99255, 99291-99292, 99304-99310, 99315-99316, 99334-99337, 99347-99350, 99374-99375, 99377-99378, 99446-99449, 99451-99452, 99495-99496, G0463, G0471

55180 0213T, 0216T, 0228T, 0230T, 11000-11006, 11042-11047, 12001-12007, 12011-12057, 13100-13133, 13151-13153, 36000, 36400-36410, 36420-36430, 36440, 36591-36592, 36600, 36640, 43752, 51701-51703, 55110, 55175, 62320-62327, 64400, 64405-64408, 64415-64435, 64445-64454, 64461-64463, 64479-64505, 64510-64530, 69990, 92012-92014, 93000-93010, 93040-93042, 93318, 93355, 94002, 94200, 94250, 94680-94690, 94770, 95812-95816, 95819, 95822, 95829, 95955, 96360-96368, 96372, 96374-96377, 96523, 97597-97598, 97602, 99155, 99156, 99157, 99211-99223, 99231-99255, 99291-99292, 99304-99310, 99315-99316, 99334-99337, 99347-99350, 99374-99375, 99377-99378, 99446-99449, 99451-99452, 99495-99496, G0463, G0471

55200 00921, 0213T, 0216T, 0228T, 0230T, 11000-11006, 11042-11047, 12001-12007, 12011-12057, 13100-13133, 13151-13153, 36000, 36400-36410, 36420-36430, 36440, 36591-36592, 36600, 36640, 43752, 51701-51703, 62320-62327, 64400, 64405-64408, 64415-64435, 64445-64454, 64461-64463, 64479-64505, 64510-64530, 69990, 92012-92014, 93000-93010, 93040-93042, 93318, 93355, 94002, 94200, 94250, 94680-94690, 94770, 95812-95816, 95819, 95822, 95829, 95955, 96360-96368, 96372, 96374-96377, 96523, 97597-97598, 97602, 99155, 99156, 99157, 99211-99223, 99231-99255, 99291-99292, 99304-99310, 99315-99316, 99334-99337, 99347-99350, 99374-99375, 99377-99378, 99446-99449, 99451-99452, 99495-99496, G0463, G0471, J0670, J2001

55250 00921, 0213T, 0216T, 0228T, 0230T, 11000-11006, 11042-11047, 12001-12007, 12011-12057, 13100-13133, 13151-13153, 36000, 36400-36410, 36420-36430, 36440, 36591-36592, 36600, 36640, 43752, 51701-51703, 54500-54505, 55200, 62320-62327, 64400, 64405-64408, 64415-64435, 64445-64454, 64461-64463, 64479-64505, 64510-64530, 69990, 92012-92014, 93000-93010, 93040-93042, 93318, 93355, 94002, 94200, 94250, 94680-94690, 94770, 95812-95816, 95819, 95822, 95829, 95955, 96360-96368, 96372, 96374-96377, 96523, 97597-97598, 97602, 99155, 99156, 99157, 99211-99223, 99231-99255, 99291-99292, 99304-99310, 99315-99316, 99334-99337, 99347-99350, 99374-99375, 99377-99378, 99446-99449, 99451-99452, 99495-99496, G0463, G0471, J0670, J2001

55300 0213T, 0216T, 0228T, 0230T, 11000-11006, 11042-11047, 12001-12007, 12011-12057, 13100-13133, 13151-13153, 36000, 36400-36410, 36420-36430, 36440, 36591-36592, 36600, 36640, 43752, 51701-51703, 55200-55250, 62320-62327, 64400, 64405-64408, 64415-64435, 64445-64454, 64461-64463, 64479-64505, 64510-64530, 69990, 76000, 76942, 76970, 76998, 77001-77002, 92012-92014, 93000-93010, 93040-93042, 93318, 93355, 94002, 94200, 94250, 94680-94690, 94770, 95812-95816, 95819, 95822, 95829, 95955, 96360-96368,

CCI Edits

96372, 96374-96377, 96523, 97597-97598, 97602, 99155, 99156,
99157, 99211-99223, 99231-99255, 99291-99292, 99304-99310,
99315-99316, 99334-99337, 99347-99350, 99374-99375, 99377-99378,
99446-99449, 99451-99452, 99495-99496, G0463, G0471

55400 0213T, 0216T, 0228T, 0230T, 12001-12007, 12011-12057, 13100-13133,
13151-13153, 36000, 36400-36410, 36420-36430, 36440, 36591-36592,
36600, 36640, 43752, 51701-51703, 55200-55250, 62320-62327, 64400,
64405-64408, 64415-64435, 64445-64454, 64461-64463, 64479-64505,
64510-64530, 69990, 92012-92014, 93000-93010, 93040-93042, 93318,
93355, 94002, 94200, 94250, 94680-94690, 94770, 95812-95816,
95819, 95822, 95829, 95955, 96360-96368, 96372, 96374-96377,
96523, 99155, 99156, 99157, 99211-99223, 99231-99255, 99291-99292,
99304-99310, 99315-99316, 99334-99337, 99347-99350, 99374-99375,
99377-99378, 99446-99449, 99451-99452, 99495-99496, G0463, G0471

55500 0213T, 0216T, 0228T, 0230T, 11000-11006, 11042-11047, 12001-12007,
12011-12057, 13100-13133, 13151-13153, 36000, 36400-36410,
36420-36430, 36440, 36591-36592, 36600, 36640, 43752, 51701-51703,
62320-62327, 64400, 64405-64408, 64415-64435, 64445-64454,
64461-64463, 64479-64505, 64510-64530, 69990, 92012-92014,
93000-93010, 93040-93042, 93318, 93355, 94002, 94200, 94250,
94680-94690, 94770, 95812-95816, 95819, 95822, 95829, 95955,
96360-96368, 96372, 96374-96377, 96523, 97597-97598, 97602, 99155,
99156, 99157, 99211-99223, 99231-99255, 99291-99292, 99304-99310,
99315-99316, 99334-99337, 99347-99350, 99374-99375, 99377-99378,
99446-99449, 99451-99452, 99495-99496, G0463, G0471

55520 0213T, 0216T, 0228T, 0230T, 11000-11006, 11042-11047, 12001-12007,
12011-12057, 13100-13133, 13151-13153, 36000, 36400-36410,
36420-36430, 36440, 36591-36592, 36600, 36640, 43752, 49000-49002,
51701-51703, 55500, 62320-62327, 64400, 64405-64408, 64415-64435,
64445-64454, 64461-64463, 64479-64505, 64510-64530, 69990,
92012-92014, 93000-93010, 93040-93042, 93318, 93355, 94002, 94200,
94250, 94680-94690, 94770, 95812-95816, 95819, 95822, 95829,
95955, 96360-96368, 96372, 96374-96377, 96523, 97597-97598, 97602,
99155, 99156, 99157, 99211-99223, 99231-99255, 99291-99292,
99304-99310, 99315-99316, 99334-99337, 99347-99350, 99374-99375,
99377-99378, 99446-99449, 99451-99452, 99495-99496, G0463, G0471

55530 0213T, 0216T, 0228T, 0230T, 11000-11006, 11042-11047, 12001-12007,
12011-12057, 13100-13133, 13151-13153, 36000, 36400-36410,
36420-36430, 36440, 36591-36592, 36600, 36640, 43752, 51701-51703,
55500-55520, 55550, 62320-62327, 64400, 64405-64408, 64415-64435,
64445-64454, 64461-64463, 64479-64505, 64510-64530, 69990,
92012-92014, 93000-93010, 93040-93042, 93318, 93355, 94002, 94200,
94250, 94680-94690, 94770, 95812-95816, 95819, 95822, 95829,
95955, 96360-96368, 96372, 96374-96377, 96523, 97597-97598, 97602,
99155, 99156, 99157, 99211-99223, 99231-99255, 99291-99292,
99304-99310, 99315-99316, 99334-99337, 99347-99350, 99374-99375,
99377-99378, 99446-99449, 99451-99452, 99495-99496, G0463, G0471

55535 0213T, 0216T, 0228T, 0230T, 11000-11006, 11042-11047, 12001-12007,
12011-12057, 13100-13133, 13151-13153, 36000, 36400-36410,
36420-36430, 36440, 36591-36592, 36600, 36640, 43752, 44602-44605,
44950, 44970, 49000-49002, 49320, 51701-51703, 55500, 55550,
62320-62327, 64400, 64405-64408, 64415-64435, 64445-64454,
64461-64463, 64479-64505, 64510-64530, 69990, 92012-92014,
93000-93010, 93040-93042, 93318, 93355, 94002, 94200, 94250,
94680-94690, 94770, 95812-95816, 95819, 95822, 95829, 95955,
96360-96368, 96372, 96374-96377, 96523, 97597-97598, 97602, 99155,
99156, 99157, 99211-99223, 99231-99255, 99291-99292, 99304-99310,
99315-99316, 99334-99337, 99347-99350, 99374-99375, 99377-99378,
99446-99449, 99451-99452, 99495-99496, G0463, G0471

55540 0213T, 0216T, 0228T, 0230T, 0437T, 11000-11006, 11042-11047,
12001-12007, 12011-12057, 13100-13133, 13151-13153, 15777, 36000,
36400-36410, 36420-36430, 36440, 36591-36592, 36600, 36640, 43752,
49491-49495, 49500-49507, 49520-49525, 49568, 49650-49651,
51701-51703, 55500-55530, 55550, 57267, 62320-62327, 64400,
64405-64408, 64415-64435, 64445-64454, 64461-64463, 64479-64505,
64510-64530, 69990, 92012-92014, 93000-93010, 93040-93042, 93318,
93355, 94002, 94200, 94250, 94680-94690, 94770, 95812-95816,
95819, 95822, 95829, 95955, 96360-96368, 96372, 96374-96377,
96523, 97597-97598, 97602, 99155, 99156, 99157, 99211-99223,
99231-99255, 99291-99292, 99304-99310, 99315-99316, 99334-99337,
99347-99350, 99374-99375, 99377-99378, 99446-99449, 99451-99452,
99495-99496, G0463, G0471

55550 0213T, 0216T, 0228T, 0230T, 12001-12007, 12011-12057, 13100-13133,
13151-13153, 36000, 36400-36410, 36420-36430, 36440, 36591-36592,
36600, 36640, 43653, 43752, 44005, 44180, 44602-44605, 44950,
44970, 49082-49084, 49320, 49400, 50715, 51701-51703, 62320-62327,
64400, 64405-64408, 64415-64435, 64445-64454, 64461-64463,
64479-64505, 64510-64530, 69990, 76000, 77001-77002, 92012-92014,
93000-93010, 93040-93042, 93318, 93355, 94002, 94200, 94250,
94680-94690, 94770, 95812-95816, 95819, 95822, 95829, 95955,
96360-96368, 96372, 96374-96377, 96523, 99155, 99156, 99157,
99211-99223, 99231-99255, 99291-99292, 99304-99310, 99315-99316,
99334-99337, 99347-99350, 99374-99375, 99377-99378, 99446-99449,
99451-99452, 99495-99496, G0463, G0471

55600 0213T, 0216T, 0228T, 0230T, 11000-11006, 11042-11047, 12001-12007,
12011-12057, 13100-13133, 13151-13153, 36000, 36400-36410,
36420-36430, 36440, 36591-36592, 36600, 36640, 43752, 44602-44605,
44950, 44970, 49000-49002, 49320, 51701-51703, 62320-62327, 64400,
64405-64408, 64415-64435, 64445-64454, 64461-64463, 64479-64505,
64510-64530, 69990, 92012-92014, 93000-93010, 93040-93042, 93318,
93355, 94002, 94200, 94250, 94680-94690, 94770, 95812-95816,
95819, 95822, 95829, 95955, 96360-96368, 96372, 96374-96377,
96523, 97597-97598, 97602, 99155, 99156, 99157, 99211-99223,
99231-99255, 99291-99292, 99304-99310, 99315-99316, 99334-99337,
99347-99350, 99374-99375, 99377-99378, 99446-99449, 99451-99452,
99495-99496, G0463, G0471

55605 0213T, 0216T, 0228T, 0230T, 11000-11006, 11042-11047, 12001-12007,
12011-12057, 13100-13133, 13151-13153, 36000, 36400-36410,
36420-36430, 36440, 36591-36592, 36600, 36640, 43752, 44602-44605,
44950, 44970, 49000-49002, 49320, 51701-51703, 55600, 62320-62327,
64400, 64405-64408, 64415-64435, 64445-64454, 64461-64463,
64479-64505, 64510-64530, 69990, 92012-92014, 93000-93010,
93040-93042, 93318, 93355, 94002, 94200, 94250, 94680-94690,
94770, 95812-95816, 95819, 95822, 95829, 95955, 96360-96368,
96372, 96374-96377, 96523, 97597-97598, 97602, 99155, 99156,
99157, 99211-99223, 99231-99255, 99291-99292, 99304-99310,
99315-99316, 99334-99337, 99347-99350, 99374-99375, 99377-99378,
99446-99449, 99451-99452, 99495-99496, G0463, G0471

55650 0213T, 0216T, 0228T, 0230T, 11000-11006, 11042-11047, 12001-12007,
12011-12057, 13100-13133, 13151-13153, 36000, 36400-36410,
36420-36430, 36440, 36591-36592, 36600, 36640, 43752, 44602-44605,
44950, 44970, 49000-49002, 49320, 51701-51703, 55600, 55605,
62320-62327, 64400, 64405-64408, 64415-64435, 64445-64454,
64461-64463, 64479-64505, 64510-64530, 69990, 92012-92014,
93000-93010, 93040-93042, 93318, 93355, 94002, 94200, 94250,
94680-94690, 94770, 95812-95816, 95819, 95822, 95829, 95955,
96360-96368, 96372, 96374-96377, 96523, 97597-97598, 97602, 99155,
99156, 99157, 99211-99223, 99231-99255, 99291-99292, 99304-99310,

CPT © 2020 American Medical Association. All Rights Reserved.

Coding Companion for Urology/Nephrology

99315-99316, 99334-99337, 99347-99350, 99374-99375, 99377-99378, 99446-99449, 99451-99452, 99495-99496, G0463, G0471

55680 0213T, 0216T, 0228T, 0230T, 11000-11006, 11042-11047, 12001-12007, 12011-12057, 13100-13133, 13151-13153, 36000, 36400-36410, 36420-36430, 36440, 36591-36592, 36600, 36640, 43752, 44602-44605, 44950, 44970, 49000-49002, 49320, 51701-51703, 62320-62327, 64400, 64405-64408, 64415-64435, 64445-64454, 64461-64463, 64479-64505, 64510-64530, 69990, 92012-92014, 93000-93010, 93040-93042, 93318, 93355, 94002, 94200, 94250, 94680-94690, 94770, 95812-95816, 95819, 95822, 95829, 95955, 96360-96368, 96372, 96374-96377, 96523, 97597-97598, 97602, 99155, 99156, 99157, 99211-99223, 99231-99255, 99291-99292, 99304-99310, 99315-99316, 99334-99337, 99347-99350, 99374-99375, 99377-99378, 99446-99449, 99451-99452, 99495-99496, G0463, G0471

55700 0213T, 0216T, 0228T, 0230T, 10005, 10007, 10009, 10011, 10021, 12001-12007, 12011-12057, 13100-13133, 13151-13153, 36000, 36400-36410, 36420-36430, 36440, 36591-36592, 36600, 36640, 43752, 44950, 44970, 51701, 51703, 55873❖, 62320-62327, 64400, 64405-64408, 64415-64435, 64445-64454, 64461-64463, 64479-64505, 64510-64530, 69990, 76000, 77001, 92012-92014, 93000-93010, 93040-93042, 93318, 93355, 94002, 94200, 94250, 94680-94690, 94770, 95812-95816, 95819, 95822, 95829, 95955, 96360-96368, 96372, 96374-96377, 96523, 99155, 99156, 99157, 99211-99223, 99231-99255, 99291-99292, 99304-99310, 99315-99316, 99334-99337, 99347-99350, 99374-99375, 99377-99378, 99446-99449, 99451-99452, 99495-99496, G0463, J0670, J2001

55705 0213T, 0216T, 0228T, 0230T, 10005, 10007, 10009, 10011, 10021, 12001-12007, 12011-12057, 13100-13133, 13151-13153, 36000, 36400-36410, 36420-36430, 36440, 36591-36592, 36600, 36640, 43752, 44950, 44970, 51701-51703, 55700, 55873❖, 62320-62327, 64400, 64405-64408, 64415-64435, 64445-64454, 64461-64463, 64479-64505, 64510-64530, 69990, 92012-92014, 93000-93010, 93040-93042, 93318, 93355, 94002, 94200, 94250, 94680-94690, 94770, 95812-95816, 95819, 95822, 95829, 95955, 96360-96368, 96372, 96374-96377, 96523, 99155, 99156, 99157, 99211-99223, 99231-99255, 99291-99292, 99304-99310, 99315-99316, 99334-99337, 99347-99350, 99374-99375, 99377-99378, 99446-99449, 99451-99452, 99495-99496, G0463, G0471

55706 0213T, 0216T, 0421T❖, 0582T❖, 10005, 10007, 10009, 10011, 10021, 12001-12007, 12011-12057, 13100-13133, 13151-13153, 36000, 36400-36410, 36420-36430, 36440, 36591-36592, 36600, 36640, 43752, 51701-51703, 53854❖, 55700-55705❖, 62320-62327, 64400, 64405-64408, 64415-64435, 64445-64454, 64461-64463, 64479-64505, 64510-64530, 69990, 76000, 76942, 76970, 76998, 77001-77002, 92012-92014, 93000-93010, 93040-93042, 93318, 93355, 94002, 94200, 94250, 94680-94690, 94770, 95812-95816, 95819, 95822, 95829, 95955, 96360-96368, 96372, 96374-96377, 96523, 99155, 99156, 99157, 99211-99223, 99231-99255, 99291-99292, 99304-99310, 99315-99316, 99334-99337, 99347-99350, 99374-99375, 99377-99378, 99446-99449, 99451-99452, 99495-99496, G0463, G0471

55720 0213T, 0216T, 0228T, 0230T, 11000-11006, 11042-11047, 12001-12007, 12011-12057, 13100-13133, 13151-13153, 36000, 36400-36410, 36420-36430, 36440, 36591-36592, 36600, 36640, 43752, 44005, 44180, 44820-44850, 44950, 44970, 49000-49010, 49255, 51701-51703, 52000, 62320-62327, 64400, 64405-64408, 64415-64435, 64445-64454, 64461-64463, 64479-64505, 64510-64530, 69990, 92012-92014, 93000-93010, 93040-93042, 93318, 93355, 94002, 94200, 94250, 94680-94690, 94770, 95812-95816, 95819, 95822, 95829, 95955, 96360-96368, 96372, 96374-96377, 96523, 97597-97598, 97602, 99155, 99156, 99157, 99211-99223, 99231-99255, 99291-99292, 99304-99310,

99315-99316, 99334-99337, 99347-99350, 99374-99375, 99377-99378, 99446-99449, 99451-99452, 99495-99496, G0463, G0471

55725 0213T, 0216T, 0228T, 0230T, 11000-11006, 11042-11047, 12001-12007, 12011-12057, 13100-13133, 13151-13153, 36000, 36400-36410, 36420-36430, 36440, 36591-36592, 36600, 36640, 43752, 44005, 44180, 44820-44850, 44950, 44970, 49000-49010, 49255, 51701-51703, 52000, 55720, 62320-62327, 64400, 64405-64408, 64415-64435, 64445-64454, 64461-64463, 64479-64505, 64510-64530, 69990, 92012-92014, 93000-93010, 93040-93042, 93318, 93355, 94002, 94200, 94250, 94680-94690, 94770, 95812-95816, 95819, 95822, 95829, 95955, 96360-96368, 96372, 96374-96377, 96523, 97597-97598, 97602, 99155, 99156, 99157, 99211-99223, 99231-99255, 99291-99292, 99304-99310, 99315-99316, 99334-99337, 99347-99350, 99374-99375, 99377-99378, 99446-99449, 99451-99452, 99495-99496, G0463, G0471

55801 0213T, 0216T, 0228T, 0230T, 0421T❖, 0582T❖, 11000-11006, 11042-11047, 12001-12007, 12011-12057, 13100-13133, 13151-13153, 36000, 36400-36410, 36420-36430, 36440, 36591-36592, 36600, 36640, 43752, 44950, 44970, 51701-51703, 51800, 52000, 52601❖, 52630-52648❖, 53020, 53850-53852❖, 53854❖, 55250, 55650, 55706❖, 55821-55831❖, 55875-55876, 62320-62327, 64400, 64405-64408, 64415-64435, 64445-64454, 64461-64463, 64479-64505, 64510-64530, 69990, 92012-92014, 93000-93010, 93040-93042, 93318, 93355, 94002, 94200, 94250, 94680-94690, 94770, 95812-95816, 95819, 95822, 95829, 95955, 96360-96368, 96372, 96374-96377, 96523, 97597-97598, 97602, 99155, 99156, 99157, 99211-99223, 99231-99255, 99291-99292, 99304-99310, 99315-99316, 99334-99337, 99347-99350, 99374-99375, 99377-99378, 99446-99449, 99451-99452, 99495-99496, G0463, G0471

55810 0213T, 0216T, 0228T, 0230T, 0421T❖, 0582T❖, 11000-11006, 11042-11047, 12001-12007, 12011-12057, 13100-13133, 13151-13153, 36000, 36400-36410, 36420-36430, 36440, 36591-36592, 36600, 36640, 38573, 43752, 44950, 44970, 51701-51703, 51800, 52000, 52601❖, 52630-52648❖, 53850-53852❖, 53854❖, 55650, 55706❖, 55801, 55821-55831❖, 55875-55876, 62320-62327, 64400, 64405-64408, 64415-64435, 64445-64454, 64461-64463, 64479-64505, 64510-64530, 69990, 92012-92014, 93000-93010, 93040-93042, 93318, 93355, 94002, 94200, 94250, 94680-94690, 94770, 95812-95816, 95819, 95822, 95829, 95955, 96360-96368, 96372, 96374-96377, 96523, 97597-97598, 97602, 99155, 99156, 99157, 99211-99223, 99231-99255, 99291-99292, 99304-99310, 99315-99316, 99334-99337, 99347-99350, 99374-99375, 99377-99378, 99446-99449, 99451-99452, 99495-99496, G0463, G0471

55812 0213T, 0216T, 0228T, 0230T, 0421T❖, 0582T❖, 10005, 10007, 10009, 10011, 10021, 11000-11006, 11042-11047, 12001-12007, 12011-12057, 13100-13133, 13151-13153, 36000, 36400-36410, 36420-36430, 36440, 36591-36592, 36600, 36640, 38562, 38573, 43752, 44950, 44970, 49000-49002, 51701-51703, 51800, 52000, 52601❖, 52630-52648❖, 53850-53852❖, 53854❖, 55650, 55706❖, 55801-55810, 55821-55842❖, 55873, 55875-55876, 62320-62327, 64400, 64405-64408, 64415-64435, 64445-64454, 64461-64463, 64479-64505, 64510-64530, 69990, 92012-92014, 93000-93010, 93040-93042, 93318, 93355, 94002, 94200, 94250, 94680-94690, 94770, 95812-95816, 95819, 95822, 95829, 95955, 96360-96368, 96372, 96374-96377, 96523, 97597-97598, 97602, 99155, 99156, 99157, 99211-99223, 99231-99255, 99291-99292, 99304-99310, 99315-99316, 99334-99337, 99347-99350, 99374-99375, 99377-99378, 99446-99449, 99451-99452, 99495-99496, G0463, G0471

55815 0213T, 0216T, 0228T, 0230T, 0421T❖, 0582T❖, 11000-11006, 11042-11047, 12001-12007, 12011-12057, 13100-13133, 13151-13153, 36000, 36400-36410, 36420-36430, 36440, 36591-36592, 36600, 36640, 38562, 38571-38573, 38770, 38780, 43752, 44005, 44180, 44602-44605, 44820-44850, 44950, 44970, 49000-49010, 49255,

CCI Edits

49320-49321, 51701-51703, 51800, 52000, 52601❖, 52630-52648❖,
53850-53852❖, 53854❖, 55650, 55706❖, 55801-55812, 55821-55845❖,
55866, 55873, 55875-55876, 62320-62327, 64400, 64405-64408,
64415-64435, 64445-64454, 64461-64463, 64479-64505, 64510-64530,
69990, 92012-92014, 93000-93010, 93040-93042, 93318, 93355, 94002,
94200, 94250, 94680-94690, 94770, 95812-95816, 95819, 95822,
95829, 95955, 96360-96368, 96372, 96374-96377, 96523, 97597-97598,
97602, 99155, 99156, 99157, 99211-99223, 99231-99255, 99291-99292,
99304-99310, 99315-99316, 99334-99337, 99347-99350, 99374-99375,
99377-99378, 99446-99449, 99451-99452, 99495-99496, G0463, G0471

55821 0213T, 0216T, 0228T, 0230T, 0421T❖, 0582T❖, 11000-11006,
11042-11047, 12001-12007, 12011-12057, 13100-13133, 13151-13153,
35840, 36000, 36400-36410, 36420-36430, 36440, 36591-36592, 36600,
36640, 43752, 44005, 44180, 44602-44605, 44820-44850, 44950,
44970, 49000-49010, 49255, 49320-49321, 51040, 51050, 51102,
51700-51703, 51800, 52000, 52281, 52601❖, 52630-52648❖, 53020,
53600, 53850-53852❖, 53854❖, 55250, 55650, 55706❖, 55873❖,
55875-55876, 62320-62327, 64400, 64405-64408, 64415-64435,
64445-64454, 64461-64463, 64479-64505, 64510-64530, 69990,
92012-92014, 93000-93010, 93040-93042, 93318, 93355, 94002, 94200,
94250, 94680-94690, 94770, 95812-95816, 95819, 95822, 95829,
95955, 96360-96368, 96372, 96374-96377, 96523, 97597-97598, 97602,
99155, 99156, 99157, 99211-99223, 99231-99255, 99291-99292,
99304-99310, 99315-99316, 99334-99337, 99347-99350, 99374-99375,
99377-99378, 99446-99449, 99451-99452, 99495-99496, G0463, G0471

55831 0213T, 0216T, 0228T, 0230T, 0421T❖, 0582T❖, 11000-11006,
11042-11047, 12001-12007, 12011-12057, 13100-13133, 13151-13153,
36000, 36400-36410, 36420-36430, 36440, 36591-36592, 36600, 36640,
43752, 44005, 44180, 44602-44605, 44820-44850, 44950, 44970,
49000-49010, 49255, 49320-49321, 51040, 51050, 51102, 51700-51703,
51800, 52000, 52281, 52601❖, 52630-52648❖, 53020, 53600,
53850-53852❖, 53854❖, 55250, 55650, 55706❖, 55821❖, 55873❖,
55875-55876, 62320-62327, 64400, 64405-64408, 64415-64435,
64445-64454, 64461-64463, 64479-64505, 64510-64530, 69990,
92012-92014, 93000-93010, 93040-93042, 93318, 93355, 94002, 94200,
94250, 94680-94690, 94770, 95812-95816, 95819, 95822, 95829,
95955, 96360-96368, 96372, 96374-96377, 96523, 97597-97598, 97602,
99155, 99156, 99157, 99211-99223, 99231-99255, 99291-99292,
99304-99310, 99315-99316, 99334-99337, 99347-99350, 99374-99375,
99377-99378, 99446-99449, 99451-99452, 99495-99496, G0463, G0471

55840 0213T, 0216T, 0228T, 0230T, 0421T❖, 0582T❖, 11000-11006,
11042-11047, 12001-12007, 12011-12057, 13100-13133, 13151-13153,
36000, 36400-36410, 36420-36430, 36440, 36591-36592, 36600, 36640,
38573, 43752, 44005, 44180, 44602-44605, 44820-44850, 44950,
44970, 49000-49010, 49255, 51701-51703, 51800, 52000, 52601❖,
52630-52648❖, 53850-53852❖, 53854❖, 55650, 55706❖, 55801-55810❖,
55821-55831❖, 55875-55876, 62320-62327, 64400, 64405-64408,
64415-64435, 64445-64454, 64461-64463, 64479-64505, 64510-64530,
69990, 92012-92014, 93000-93010, 93040-93042, 93318, 93355, 94002,
94200, 94250, 94680-94690, 94770, 95812-95816, 95819, 95822,
95829, 95955, 96360-96368, 96372, 96374-96377, 96523, 97597-97598,
97602, 99155, 99156, 99157, 99211-99223, 99231-99255, 99291-99292,
99304-99310, 99315-99316, 99334-99337, 99347-99350, 99374-99375,
99377-99378, 99446-99449, 99451-99452, 99495-99496, G0463, G0471

55842 0213T, 0216T, 0228T, 0230T, 0421T❖, 0582T❖, 10005, 10007, 10009,
10011, 10021, 11000-11006, 11042-11047, 12001-12007, 12011-12057,
13100-13133, 13151-13153, 36000, 36400-36410, 36420-36430, 36440,
36591-36592, 36600, 36640, 38562, 38573, 43752, 44005, 44180,
44602-44605, 44820-44850, 44950, 44970, 49000-49010, 49255, 49320,
51701-51703, 51800, 52000, 52601❖, 52630-52648❖, 53850-53852❖,

53854❖, 55650, 55706❖, 55801-55810❖, 55821-55840, 55873,
55875-55876, 62320-62327, 64400, 64405-64408, 64415-64435,
64445-64454, 64461-64463, 64479-64505, 64510-64530, 69990,
92012-92014, 93000-93010, 93040-93042, 93318, 93355, 94002, 94200,
94250, 94680-94690, 94770, 95812-95816, 95819, 95822, 95829,
95955, 96360-96368, 96372, 96374-96377, 96523, 97597-97598, 97602,
99155, 99156, 99157, 99211-99223, 99231-99255, 99291-99292,
99304-99310, 99315-99316, 99334-99337, 99347-99350, 99374-99375,
99377-99378, 99446-99449, 99451-99452, 99495-99496, G0463, G0471

55845 0213T, 0216T, 0228T, 0230T, 0421T❖, 0582T❖, 11000-11006,
11042-11047, 12001-12007, 12011-12057, 13100-13133, 13151-13153,
27070, 36000, 36400-36410, 36420-36430, 36440, 36591-36592, 36600,
36640, 38562, 38571-38573, 38770, 38780, 43752, 44005, 44180,
44602-44605, 44820-44850, 44950, 44970, 49000-49010, 49255,
49320-49321, 51040, 51050, 51102, 51550, 51700-51703, 51800,
52000, 52601❖, 52630-52648❖, 53020, 53620, 53850-53852❖, 53854❖,
55250, 55650, 55706❖, 55801-55812❖, 55821-55842, 55866, 55873,
55875-55876, 62320-62327, 64400, 64405-64408, 64415-64435,
64445-64454, 64461-64463, 64479-64505, 64510-64530, 69990,
92012-92014, 93000-93010, 93040-93042, 93318, 93355, 94002, 94200,
94250, 94680-94690, 94770, 95812-95816, 95819, 95822, 95829,
95955, 96360-96368, 96372, 96374-96377, 96523, 97597-97598, 97602,
99155, 99156, 99157, 99211-99223, 99231-99255, 99291-99292,
99304-99310, 99315-99316, 99334-99337, 99347-99350, 99374-99375,
99377-99378, 99446-99449, 99451-99452, 99495-99496, G0463, G0471

55860 0213T, 0216T, 0228T, 0230T, 11000-11006, 11042-11047, 12001-12007,
12011-12057, 13100-13133, 13151-13153, 36000, 36400-36410,
36420-36430, 36440, 36591-36592, 36600, 36640, 43752, 44602-44605,
44950, 44970, 49000-49002, 49320, 51701-51703, 55873❖, 55875,
62320-62327, 64400, 64405-64408, 64415-64435, 64445-64454,
64461-64463, 64479-64505, 64510-64530, 69990, 92012-92014,
93000-93010, 93040-93042, 93318, 93355, 94002, 94200, 94250,
94680-94690, 94770, 95812-95816, 95819, 95822, 95829, 95955,
96360-96368, 96372, 96374-96377, 96523, 97597-97598, 97602, 99155,
99156, 99157, 99211-99223, 99231-99255, 99291-99292, 99304-99310,
99315-99316, 99334-99337, 99347-99350, 99374-99375, 99377-99378,
99446-99449, 99451-99452, 99495-99496, G0463, G0471

55862 0213T, 0216T, 0228T, 0230T, 10005, 10007, 10009, 10011, 10021,
11000-11006, 11042-11047, 12001-12007, 12011-12057, 13100-13133,
13151-13153, 36000, 36400-36410, 36420-36430, 36440, 36591-36592,
36600, 36640, 38562, 43752, 44602-44605, 44950, 44970,
49000-49002, 49320-49321, 51701-51703, 55860, 55875, 62320-62327,
64400, 64405-64408, 64415-64435, 64445-64454, 64461-64463,
64479-64505, 64510-64530, 69990, 92012-92014, 93000-93010,
93040-93042, 93318, 93355, 94002, 94200, 94250, 94680-94690,
94770, 95812-95816, 95819, 95822, 95829, 95955, 96360-96368,
96372, 96374-96377, 96523, 97597-97598, 97602, 99155, 99156,
99157, 99211-99223, 99231-99255, 99291-99292, 99304-99310,
99315-99316, 99334-99337, 99347-99350, 99374-99375, 99377-99378,
99446-99449, 99451-99452, 99495-99496, G0463, G0471

55865 0213T, 0216T, 0228T, 0230T, 11000-11006, 11042-11047, 12001-12007,
12011-12057, 13100-13133, 13151-13153, 36000, 36400-36410,
36420-36430, 36440, 36591-36592, 36600, 36640, 38562, 38571-38573,
38770, 38780, 43752, 44005, 44180, 44602-44605, 44820-44850,
44950, 44970, 49000-49010, 49255, 49320-49321, 51701-51703, 52000,
55860-55862, 55873, 62320-62327, 64400, 64405-64408, 64415-64435,
64445-64454, 64461-64463, 64479-64505, 64510-64530, 69990,
92012-92014, 93000-93010, 93040-93042, 93318, 93355, 94002, 94200,
94250, 94680-94690, 94770, 95812-95816, 95819, 95822, 95829,
95955, 96360-96368, 96372, 96374-96377, 96523, 97597-97598, 97602,

CPT © 2020 American Medical Association. All Rights Reserved.

55866 0213T, 0216T, 0228T, 0230T, 0421T❖, 11000-11006, 11042-11047, 12001-12007, 12011-12057, 13100-13133, 13151-13153, 35840, 36000, 36400-36410, 36420-36430, 36440, 36591-36592, 36600, 36640, 43653, 43752, 44005, 44180, 44602-44605, 44950, 44970, 49082-49084, 49320-49321, 49400, 50715, 51701-51703, 51800, 52000, 52601❖, 52630-52649❖, 55700-55706❖, 55801-55812, 55821-55842, 55860-55865❖, 55873❖, 55875-55876, 58660, 62320-62327, 64400, 64405-64408, 64415-64435, 64445-64454, 64461-64463, 64479-64505, 64510-64530, 69990, 76000, 77001-77002, 92012-92014, 93000-93010, 93040-93042, 93318, 93355, 94002, 94200, 94250, 94680-94690, 94770, 95812-95816, 95819, 95822, 95829, 95955, 96360-96368, 96372, 96374-96377, 96523, 97597-97598, 97602, 99155, 99156, 99157, 99211-99223, 99231-99255, 99291-99292, 99304-99310, 99315-99316, 99334-99337, 99347-99350, 99374-99375, 99377-99378, 99446-99449, 99451-99452, 99495-99496, G0463, G0471

55870 0213T, 0216T, 0228T, 0230T, 12001-12007, 12011-12057, 13100-13133, 13151-13153, 36000, 36400-36410, 36420-36430, 36440, 36591-36592, 36600, 36640, 43752, 51701, 51703, 62320-62327, 64400, 64405-64408, 64415-64435, 64445-64454, 64461-64463, 64479-64505, 64510-64530, 69990, 92012-92014, 93000-93010, 93040-93042, 93318, 93355, 94002, 94200, 94250, 94680-94690, 94770, 95812-95816, 95819, 95822, 95829, 95955, 96360-96368, 96372, 96374-96377, 96523, 99155, 99156, 99157, 99211-99223, 99231-99255, 99291-99292, 99304-99310, 99315-99316, 99334-99337, 99347-99350, 99374-99375, 99377-99378, 99446-99449, 99451-99452, 99495-99496, G0463

55873 0213T, 0216T, 0228T, 0230T, 0421T❖, 0582T❖, 12001-12007, 12011-12057, 13100-13133, 13151-13153, 35840, 36000, 36400-36410, 36420-36430, 36440, 36591-36592, 36600, 36640, 43752, 44005, 44820-44850, 49000, 49010, 49255, 51040, 51050, 51102, 51700-51703, 52000, 52270-52275, 52281, 52450-52500, 52649❖, 52700, 53020, 53080, 53600-53621, 53660-53665, 53854❖, 55250, 55706❖, 55801-55810❖, 55840❖, 55862, 55875-55876, 62320-62327, 64400, 64405-64408, 64415-64435, 64445-64454, 64461-64463, 64479-64505, 64510-64530, 69990, 76380, 76872, 76940, 76970, 76998, 77013, 77022, 92012-92014, 93000-93010, 93040-93042, 93318, 93355, 94002, 94200, 94250, 94680-94690, 94770, 95812-95816, 95819, 95822, 95829, 95955, 96360-96368, 96372, 96374-96377, 96523, 99155, 99156, 99157, 99211-99223, 99231-99255, 99291-99292, 99304-99310, 99315-99316, 99334-99337, 99347-99350, 99374-99375, 99377-99378, 99446-99449, 99451-99452, 99495-99496, G0463, G0471, J0670, J2001

55874 0213T, 0216T, 0228T, 0230T, 12001-12007, 12011-12057, 13100-13133, 13151-13153, 36000, 36400-36410, 36420-36430, 36440, 36591-36592, 36600, 36640, 43752, 51701-51703, 62320-62327, 64400, 64405-64408, 64415-64435, 64445-64454, 64461-64463, 64479-64505, 64510-64530, 69990, 76000, 76942, 76970, 76998, 77002-77003, 77012, 77021, 92012-92014, 93000-93010, 93040-93042, 93318, 94002, 94200, 94250, 94680-94690, 94770, 95812-95816, 95819, 95822, 95829, 95955, 96360-96368, 96372, 96374-96377, 96523, 99155, 99156, 99157, 99211-99223, 99231-99255, 99291-99292, 99304-99310, 99315-99316, 99334-99337, 99347-99350, 99374-99375, 99377-99378

55875 00860, 0213T, 0216T, 0228T, 0230T, 10035-10036❖, 12001-12007, 12011-12057, 13100-13133, 13151-13153, 36000, 36400-36410, 36420-36430, 36440, 36591-36592, 36600, 36640, 43752, 51701-51703, 52000, 52250, 55920❖, 62320-62327, 64400, 64405-64408, 64415-64435, 64445-64454, 64461-64463, 64479-64505, 64510-64530,

69990, 76942, 76970, 76998, 92012-92014, 93000-93010, 93040-93042, 93318, 93355, 94002, 94200, 94250, 94680-94690, 94770, 95812-95816, 95819, 95822, 95829, 95955, 96360-96368, 96372, 96374-96377, 96523, 99155, 99156, 99157, 99211-99223, 99231-99255, 99291-99292, 99304-99310, 99315-99316, 99334-99337, 99347-99350, 99374-99375, 99377-99378, 99446-99449, 99451-99452, 99495-99496, G0463, G0471, P9612

55876 00860, 0213T, 0216T, 0228T, 0230T, 10035-10036❖, 12001-12007, 12011-12057, 13100-13133, 13151-13153, 36000, 36400-36410, 36420-36430, 36440, 36591-36592, 36600, 36640, 43752, 49327❖, 49411-49412❖, 51701-51703, 62320-62327, 64400, 64405-64408, 64415-64435, 64445-64454, 64461-64463, 64479-64505, 64510-64530, 69990, 76000, 76970, 76998, 92012-92014, 93000-93010, 93040-93042, 93318, 93355, 94002, 94200, 94250, 94680-94690, 94770, 95812-95816, 95819, 95822, 95829, 95955, 96360-96368, 96372, 96374-96377, 96523, 99155, 99156, 99157, 99211-99223, 99231-99255, 99291-99292, 99304-99310, 99315-99316, 99334-99337, 99347-99350, 99374-99375, 99377-99378, 99446-99449, 99451-99452, 99495-99496, G0463, G0471, J0670, J2001

55880 No CCI edits apply to this code.

55920 0213T, 0216T, 0228T, 0230T, 0347T❖, 10035-10036❖, 12001-12007, 12011-12057, 13100-13133, 13151-13153, 20555❖, 36000, 36400-36410, 36420-36430, 36440, 36591-36592, 36600, 36640, 43752, 57155-57156, 58346, 62320-62327, 64400, 64405-64408, 64415-64435, 64445-64454, 64461-64463, 64479-64505, 64510-64530, 69990, 92012-92014, 93000-93010, 93040-93042, 93318, 93355, 94002, 94200, 94250, 94680-94690, 94770, 95812-95816, 95819, 95822, 95829, 95955, 96360-96368, 96372, 96374-96377, 96523, 99155, 99156, 99157, 99211-99223, 99231-99255, 99291-99292, 99304-99310, 99315-99316, 99334-99337, 99347-99350, 99374-99375, 99377-99378, 99446-99449, 99451-99452, 99495-99496, G0463

55970 36591-36592, 96523

55980 36591-36592, 96523

57220 00940, 0213T, 0216T, 0228T, 0230T, 12001-12007, 12011-12057, 13100-13133, 13151-13153, 36000, 36400-36410, 36420-36430, 36440, 36591-36592, 36600, 36640, 43752, 44950, 44970, 45560, 50715, 51701-51703, 52000, 53000-53025, 53200, 56810, 57000, 57061, 57065-57105, 57150, 57180, 57210, 57268, 57410, 57420, 57452, 57500, 57800, 58100, 62320-62327, 64400, 64405-64408, 64415-64435, 64445-64454, 64461-64463, 64479-64505, 64510-64530, 69990, 92012-92014, 93000-93010, 93040-93042, 93318, 93355, 94002, 94200, 94250, 94680-94690, 94770, 95812-95816, 95819, 95822, 95829, 95955, 96360-96368, 96372, 96374-96377, 96523, 99155, 99156, 99157, 99211-99223, 99231-99255, 99291-99292, 99304-99310, 99315-99316, 99334-99337, 99347-99350, 99374-99375, 99377-99378, 99446-99449, 99451-99452, 99495-99496, G0463, G0471, P9612

57230 00940, 0213T, 0216T, 0228T, 0230T, 12001-12007, 12011-12057, 13100-13133, 13151-13153, 36000, 36400-36410, 36420-36430, 36440, 36591-36592, 36600, 36640, 43752, 44950, 44970, 45560, 50715, 51701-51703, 52000, 53000-53025, 53200, 53275, 53450-53460, 56810, 57100-57105, 57150, 57180, 57220, 57268, 57410, 57420, 57452, 57500, 57800, 58100, 62320-62327, 64400, 64405-64408, 64415-64435, 64445-64454, 64461-64463, 64479-64505, 64510-64530, 69990, 92012-92014, 93000-93010, 93040-93042, 93318, 93355, 94002, 94200, 94250, 94680-94690, 94770, 95812-95816, 95819, 95822, 95829, 95955, 96360-96368, 96372, 96374-96377, 96523, 99155, 99156, 99157, 99211-99223, 99231-99255, 99291-99292, 99304-99310, 99315-99316, 99334-99337, 99347-99350, 99374-99375, 99377-99378, 99446-99449, 99451-99452, 99495-99496, G0463, G0471, P9612

57240 00940, 0213T, 0216T, 0228T, 0230T, 0437T, 12001-12007, 12011-12057, 13100-13133, 13151-13153, 15777, 36000, 36400-36410, 36420-36430, 36440, 36591-36592, 36600, 36640, 43752, 44950, 44970, 49568, 50715, 51701-51703, 52000, 53000-53025, 56810, 57000, 57065-57106, 57150, 57180-57200, 57220-57230, 57250, 57285, 57410, 57420, 57452, 57500, 57800, 58100, 62320-62327, 64400, 64405-64408, 64415-64435, 64445-64454, 64461-64463, 64479-64505, 64510-64530, 69990, 92012-92014, 93000-93010, 93040-93042, 93318, 93355, 94002, 94200, 94250, 94680-94690, 94770, 95812-95816, 95819, 95822, 95829, 95955, 96360-96368, 96372, 96374-96377, 96523, 99155, 99156, 99157, 99211-99223, 99231-99255, 99291-99292, 99304-99310, 99315-99316, 99334-99337, 99347-99350, 99374-99375, 99377-99378, 99446-99449, 99451-99452, 99495-99496, G0463, G0471, P9612

57260 00940, 0213T, 0216T, 0228T, 0230T, 0437T, 12001-12007, 12011-12057, 13100-13133, 13151-13153, 15777, 36000, 36400-36410, 36420-36430, 36440, 36591-36592, 36600, 36640, 43752, 44950, 44970, 45560, 49568, 50715, 51701-51703, 52000, 53620, 53660, 56800, 56810, 57000, 57061, 57100-57106, 57120, 57150, 57180, 57210-57250, 57268-57270, 57285, 57410, 57420, 57452, 57500, 57800, 58100, 62320-62327, 64400, 64405-64408, 64415-64435, 64445-64454, 64461-64463, 64479-64505, 64510-64530, 69990, 92012-92014, 93000-93010, 93040-93042, 93318, 93355, 94002, 94200, 94250, 94680-94690, 94770, 95812-95816, 95819, 95822, 95829, 95955, 96360-96368, 96372, 96374-96377, 96523, 99155, 99156, 99157, 99211-99223, 99231-99255, 99291-99292, 99304-99310, 99315-99316, 99334-99337, 99347-99350, 99374-99375, 99377-99378, 99446-99449, 99451-99452, 99495-99496, G0463, G0471, P9612

57265 00940, 0213T, 0216T, 0228T, 0230T, 0437T, 12001-12007, 12011-12057, 13100-13133, 13151-13153, 15777, 36000, 36400-36410, 36420-36430, 36440, 36591-36592, 36600, 36640, 43752, 44950, 44970, 45560, 49407, 49568, 50715, 51701-51703, 52000, 56800, 56810, 57000, 57061, 57100-57106, 57150, 57180, 57210-57260, 57268-57270, 57284-57285, 57410, 57420, 57452, 57500, 57800, 58100, 58800, 62320-62327, 64400, 64405-64408, 64415-64435, 64445-64454, 64461-64463, 64479-64505, 64510-64530, 69990, 92012-92014, 93000-93010, 93040-93042, 93318, 93355, 94002, 94200, 94250, 94680-94690, 94770, 95812-95816, 95819, 95822, 95829, 95955, 96360-96368, 96372, 96374-96377, 96523, 99155, 99156, 99157, 99211-99223, 99231-99255, 99291-99292, 99304-99310, 99315-99316, 99334-99337, 99347-99350, 99374-99375, 99377-99378, 99446-99449, 99451-99452, 99495-99496, G0463, G0471, P9612

57267 0437T♦, 11000-11001, 11042-11047, 15777♦, 36591-36592, 56810, 57000, 57100-57105, 57150, 57180, 57210, 96523, 97597-97598, 97602

57284 00940, 0213T, 0216T, 0228T, 0230T, 12001-12007, 12011-12057, 13100-13133, 13151-13153, 36000, 36400-36410, 36420-36430, 36440, 36591-36592, 36600, 36640, 43653, 43752, 44005, 44180, 44602-44605, 44820-44850, 44950, 44970, 49000-49010, 49255, 49320, 49570, 50715, 51701-51703, 51715, 51840-51841, 51990, 52000, 57100, 57240, 57260, 57268-57270, 57285♦, 57410, 57420, 57423, 57452, 57500, 57800, 58100, 58660, 62320-62327, 64400, 64405-64408, 64415-64435, 64445-64454, 64461-64463, 64479-64505, 64510-64530, 69990, 92012-92014, 93000-93010, 93040-93042, 93318, 93355, 94002, 94200, 94250, 94680-94690, 94770, 95812-95816, 95819, 95822, 95829, 95955, 96360-96368, 96372, 96374-96377, 96523, 99155, 99156, 99157, 99211-99223, 99231-99255, 99291-99292, 99304-99310, 99315-99316, 99334-99337, 99347-99350, 99374-99375, 99377-99378, 99446-99449, 99451-99452, 99495-99496, G0463, G0471, P9612

57285 00940, 0213T, 0216T, 0228T, 0230T, 0437T, 12001-12007, 12011-12057, 13100-13133, 13151-13153, 15777, 36000, 36400-36410, 36420-36430, 36440, 36591-36592, 36600, 36640, 43752, 49568, 51701-51703, 51840♦, 52000, 56810, 57020, 57100, 57150, 57180, 57268, 57400-57420, 57423, 57452, 57500, 57530, 57800, 58100, 62320-62327, 64400, 64405-64408, 64415-64435, 64445-64454, 64461-64463, 64479-64505, 64510-64530, 69990, 92012-92014, 93000-93010, 93040-93042, 93318, 93355, 94002, 94200, 94250, 94680-94690, 94770, 95812-95816, 95819, 95822, 95829, 95955, 96360-96368, 96372, 96374-96377, 96523, 99155, 99156, 99157, 99211-99223, 99231-99255, 99291-99292, 99304-99310, 99315-99316, 99334-99337, 99347-99350, 99374-99375, 99377-99378, 99446-99449, 99451-99452, 99495-99496, G0463, G0471, P9612

57287 00940, 0213T, 0216T, 0228T, 0230T, 11000-11006, 11042-11047, 12001-12007, 12011-12057, 13100-13133, 13151-13153, 36000, 36400-36410, 36420-36430, 36440, 36591-36592, 36600, 36640, 43752, 44950, 44970, 50715, 51701-51703, 51992♦, 52000, 53000-53025, 57000, 57020, 57100, 57150, 57180, 57220, 57268, 57288-57289, 57410, 57420, 57452, 57500, 57800, 58100, 58267♦, 58293♦, 62320-62327, 64400, 64405-64408, 64415-64435, 64445-64454, 64461-64463, 64479-64505, 64510-64530, 69990, 92012-92014, 93000-93010, 93040-93042, 93318, 93355, 94002, 94200, 94250, 94680-94690, 94770, 95812-95816, 95819, 95822, 95829, 95955, 96360-96368, 96372, 96374-96377, 96523, 97597-97598, 97602, 99155, 99156, 99157, 99211-99223, 99231-99255, 99291-99292, 99304-99310, 99315-99316, 99334-99337, 99347-99350, 99374-99375, 99377-99378, 99446-99449, 99451-99452, 99495-99496, G0463, G0471, P9612

57288 00940, 0213T, 0216T, 0228T, 0230T, 12001-12007, 12011-12057, 13100-13133, 13151-13153, 36000, 36400-36410, 36420-36430, 36440, 36591-36592, 36600, 36640, 43752, 44950, 44970, 50715, 51701-51703, 51992, 52000, 53000-53025, 56810, 57000, 57100, 57150, 57180, 57220, 57267-57268, 57289, 57410, 57420, 57452, 57500, 57800, 58100, 58267♦, 58293♦, 62320-62327, 64400, 64405-64408, 64415-64435, 64445-64454, 64461-64463, 64479-64505, 64510-64530, 92012-92014, 93000-93010, 93040-93042, 93318, 93355, 94002, 94200, 94250, 94680-94690, 94770, 95812-95816, 95819, 95822, 95829, 95955, 96360-96368, 96372, 96374-96377, 96523, 99155, 99156, 99157, 99211-99223, 99231-99255, 99291-99292, 99304-99310, 99315-99316, 99334-99337, 99347-99350, 99374-99375, 99377-99378, 99446-99449, 99451-99452, 99495-99496, G0463, G0471, P9612

57289 00940, 0213T, 0216T, 0228T, 0230T, 12001-12007, 12011-12057, 13100-13133, 13151-13153, 36000, 36400-36410, 36420-36430, 36440, 36591-36592, 36600, 36640, 43752, 44950, 44970, 50715, 51701-51703, 51840♦, 52000, 56810, 57000, 57100, 57150, 57180-57200, 57230-57240, 57260, 57268, 57410, 57420, 57452, 57500, 57800, 58100, 62320-62327, 64400, 64405-64408, 64415-64435, 64445-64454, 64461-64463, 64479-64505, 64510-64530, 69990, 92012-92014, 93000-93010, 93040-93042, 93318, 93355, 94002, 94200, 94250, 94680-94690, 94770, 95812-95816, 95819, 95822, 95829, 95955, 96360-96368, 96372, 96374-96377, 96523, 99155, 99156, 99157, 99211-99223, 99231-99255, 99291-99292, 99304-99310, 99315-99316, 99334-99337, 99347-99350, 99374-99375, 99377-99378, 99446-99449, 99451-99452, 99495-99496, G0463, G0471, P9612

57423 0213T, 0216T, 0228T, 0230T, 12001-12007, 12011-12057, 13100-13133, 13151-13153, 36000, 36400-36410, 36420-36430, 36440, 36591-36592, 36600, 36640, 43752, 44180, 44602-44605, 49082-49084, 49320, 49400, 51701-51703, 51840-51841, 51990, 52000, 57180, 57240, 57260-57265, 57410, 58660, 62320-62327, 64400, 64405-64408, 64415-64435, 64445-64454, 64461-64463, 64479-64505, 64510-64530,

© 2020 Optum360, LLC

CPT © 2020 American Medical Association. All Rights Reserved.

69990, 76000, 77001-77002, 92012-92014, 93000-93010, 93040-93042, 93318, 93355, 94002, 94200, 94250, 94680-94690, 94770, 95812-95816, 95819, 95822, 95829, 95955, 96360-96368, 96372, 96374-96377, 96523, 99155, 99156, 99157, 99211-99223, 99231-99255, 99291-99292, 99304-99310, 99315-99316, 99334-99337, 99347-99350, 99374-99375, 99377-99378, 99446-99449, 99451-99452, 99495-99496, G0463, G0471

76700 36591-36592, 51701-51702, 76705, 76942, 76970, 76981-76983✦, 76998, 96523, G0471

76705 36591-36592, 51701-51702, 76942, 76970, 76983✦, 76998, 96523, G0471

76770 36591-36592, 51701-51702, 51798, 76706✦, 76775, 76942, 76970, 76981-76983✦, 76998, 96523, G0471

76775 36591-36592, 51701-51702, 76857, 76942, 76970, 76983✦, 76998, 96523, G0471

76776 36591-36592, 76706, 76775, 76942, 76970, 76981-76983✦, 76998, 96523

76870 36591-36592, 76942, 76970, 76981-76983✦, 76998, 96523

76872 0582T, 36591-36592, 46600, 51701-51702, 51798, 76873, 76942, 76970, 76981-76983✦, 76998, 96523, 99446-99449, 99451-99452, G0471, J0670, J2001

76873 36591-36592, 46600, 51701-51702, 51798, 55873✦, 76942, 76970, 76981-76983✦, 76998, 96523, 99446-99449, 99451-99452, G0471

76981 0567T✦, 36591-36592, 76511-76529✦, 76604✦, 76642✦, 76705-76706✦, 76775✦, 76857✦, 76881-76882✦, 76970✦, 76982-76983, 91200, 96523

76982 0567T✦, 36591-36592, 76511-76512✦, 76514-76529✦, 76604✦, 76642✦, 76705-76706✦, 76775✦, 76857✦, 76881-76882✦, 76970✦, 96523

76983 0567T✦, 36591-36592, 76514-76519✦, 76857✦, 76882✦, 91200, 96523

80047 80048, 80051, 82330, 82374, 82435, 82565, 82947, 84132, 84295, 84520, 96523

80048 80051, 82310, 82374, 82435, 82565, 82947, 84132, 84295, 84520, 96523

80050 96523

80051 82374, 82435, 84132, 84295, 96523

80053 80047-80048, 80051, 80069, 80076, 82040, 82247, 82310, 82374, 82435, 82565, 82947, 84075, 84132, 84155, 84295, 84450, 84460, 84520, 96523

80069 80047-80048, 80051, 80076, 82040, 82310, 82374, 82435, 82565, 82947, 84100, 84132, 84295, 84520, 96523

80158 96523

81000 81002, 81015, 96523

81001 81000✦, 81002-81003, 81007, 81015✦, 96523

81002 81007✦, 81015✦, 96523

81003 81000, 81002✦, 81007✦, 81015✦, 96523

81005 81000, 81002-81003✦, 81007✦, 81015✦, 96523

81007 81000✦, 81015✦, 87086, 87088, 96523

81015 96523

82565 96523

82948 82950✦, 82952✦, 96523

83516 83518, 96523

83518 96523

84152 96523

84153 96523

84154 96523

84402 96523

84403 80500-80502, 96523

84410 84402✦, 96523

85004 85008, 96523

85007 85004, 96523

85008 85007✦, 96523

85009 85004, 96523

85013 88738✦, 96523

85014 85013✦, 88738✦, 96523

85018 85008✦, 88738✦, 96523

85025 85004, 85007-85009, 85013-85018, 85027, 85032-85041, 85048-85049, 88738, 96523, G0306-G0307

85027 85004, 85008, 85013-85018, 85032-85041, 85048-85049, 88738, 96523, G0307

85032 85008, 96523

85041 85032, 96523

85044 96523

85045 85044, 96523

85046 85044-85045, 96523

85048 85008, 85032, 96523

85049 85008, 85032, 96523

87081 87040-87045✦, 87075✦, 87084✦, 87088✦, 88387-88388, 96523

87084 87040-87045✦, 87070✦, 87075✦, 88387-88388, 96523

87086 87070-87071, 87073-87075, 87081, 87084✦, 88387-88388, 96523

87088 87070-87071, 87073-87075, 87084✦, 88387-88388, 96523

87880 80500-80502, 87650-87652✦, 96523

90460 0591T-0593T, 36591-36592, 90471, 90473, 96160-96161, 96372, 96377, 96523, 99201-99215, 99241-99245, 99281-99285, 99381-99412, 99483, 99497, G0008-G0010, G0442-G0445, G0463

90461 0591T-0593T, 36591-36592, 96160-96161, 96523, 99201-99215, 99241-99245, 99281-99285, 99381-99412, 99483, 99497, G0442-G0445, G0463

90473 0591T-0593T, 36591-36592, 96160-96161, 96523, 99201-99215, 99241-99245, 99281-99285, 99381-99412, 99483, 99497, G0008✦, G0442-G0445, G0463

90474 0591T-0593T, 36591-36592, 96160-96161, 96523, 99201-99215, 99241-99245, 99281-99285, 99381-99412, 99483, 99497, G0442-G0445, G0463

90935 12001-12007, 12011-12057, 13100-13133, 13151-13153, 36000, 36400-36410, 36420-36430, 36440, 36591-36592, 36600, 36901-36909, 43752, 51701-51703, 62320-62327, 64400, 64405-64408, 64415-64435, 64445-64454, 64461-64463, 64479-64505, 64510-64530, 90997✦, 92012-92014, 93000-93010, 93040-93042, 93318, 93355, 94002, 94200, 94250, 94680-94690, 94770, 95812-95816, 95819, 95822, 95829, 95955, 96360-96368, 96372, 96374-96377, 96523, 97802-97804, 99155, 99156, 99157, 99201-99255, 99281-99285, 99291-99292, 99304-99310, 99315-99318, 99324-99328, 99334-99337, 99341-99350, 99354-99360, 99374-99375, 99377-99378, 99415-99416, 99446-99449, 99451-99452, 99455-99456, 99460-99472, 99475-99480, 99483, 99485, 99495-99497, G0270-G0271, G0380-G0384, G0406-G0408, G0425-G0427, G0463, G0471, G0491-G0492✦, G0508-G0509

90937 11000-11006, 11042-11047, 12001-12007, 12011-12057, 13100-13133, 13151-13153, 36000, 36400-36410, 36420-36430, 36440, 36591-36592, 36600, 36901-36909, 43752, 51701-51703, 62320-62327, 64400, 64405-64408, 64415-64435, 64445-64454, 64461-64463, 64479-64505, 64510-64530, 90935♦, 90945♦, 92012-92014, 93000-93010, 93040-93042, 93318, 93355, 94002, 94200, 94250, 94680-94690, 94770, 95812-95816, 95819, 95822, 95829, 95955, 96360-96368, 96372, 96374-96377, 96523, 97597-97598, 97602, 97802-97804, 99155, 99156, 99157, 99201-99255, 99281-99285, 99291-99292, 99304-99310, 99315-99318, 99324-99328, 99334-99337, 99341-99350, 99354-99360, 99374-99375, 99377-99378, 99415-99416, 99446-99449, 99451-99452, 99455-99456, 99460-99472, 99475-99480, 99483, 99485, 99495-99497, G0270-G0271, G0380-G0384, G0406-G0408, G0425-G0427, G0463, G0471, G0491-G0492♦, G0508-G0509

90940 36000, 36410, 36591-36592, 96360, 96365, 96372, 96374-96377, 96523, 97802-97804, G0270-G0271

90945 0213T, 0216T, 0228T, 0230T, 11000-11006, 11042-11047, 12001-12007, 12011-12057, 13100-13133, 13151-13153, 36000, 36400-36410, 36420-36430, 36440, 36591-36592, 36600, 36640, 36901-36909, 43752, 51701-51703, 62320-62327, 64400, 64405-64408, 64415-64435, 64445-64454, 64461-64463, 64479-64505, 64510-64530, 90935♦, 92012-92014, 93000-93010, 93040-93042, 93318, 93355, 94002, 94200, 94250, 94680-94690, 94770, 95812-95816, 95819, 95822, 95829, 95955, 96360-96368, 96372, 96374-96377, 96523, 97597-97598, 97602, 97802-97804, 99155, 99156, 99157, 99201-99255, 99281-99285, 99291-99292, 99304-99310, 99315-99318, 99324-99328, 99334-99337, 99341-99350, 99354-99359, 99374-99375, 99377-99378, 99415-99416, 99446-99449, 99451-99452, 99455-99456, 99460-99472, 99475-99480, 99483, 99485, 99495-99497, G0270-G0271, G0380-G0384, G0406-G0408, G0425-G0427, G0463, G0471, G0491-G0492♦, G0508-G0509

90947 0213T, 0216T, 0228T, 0230T, 11000-11006, 11042-11047, 12001-12007, 12011-12057, 13100-13133, 13151-13153, 36000, 36400-36410, 36420-36430, 36440, 36591-36592, 36600, 36640, 36901-36909, 43752, 51701-51703, 62320-62327, 64400, 64405-64408, 64415-64435, 64445-64454, 64461-64463, 64479-64505, 64510-64530, 90935-90937♦, 90945♦, 92012-92014, 93000-93010, 93040-93042, 93318, 93355, 94002, 94200, 94250, 94680-94690, 94770, 95812-95816, 95819, 95822, 95829, 95955, 96360-96368, 96372, 96374-96377, 96523, 97597-97598, 97602, 97802-97804, 99155, 99156, 99157, 99201-99255, 99281-99285, 99291-99292, 99304-99310, 99315-99318, 99324-99328, 99334-99337, 99341-99350, 99354-99359, 99374-99375, 99377-99378, 99415-99416, 99446-99449, 99451-99452, 99455-99456, 99460-99472, 99475-99480, 99483, 99485, 99495-99497, G0270-G0271, G0380-G0384, G0406-G0408, G0425-G0427, G0463, G0471, G0491-G0492♦, G0508-G0509

90951 0405T, 0591T-0593T, 36591-36592, 90952♦, 90953♦, 90954♦, 90955♦, 90956♦, 90957♦, 90958♦, 90959-90965♦, 90966♦, 90967, 90968, 90969, 90970, 96160-96161, 96523, 97802-97804, 99201-99220, 99224-99226, 99234-99255, 99281-99288, 99291-99292, 99304-99310, 99315-99318, 99324-99328, 99334-99350, 99354-99360, 99366-99368, 99374-99375, 99377-99416, 99421-99423, 99441-99443, 99450, 99455-99456, 99460-99472, 99475-99480, 99483-99484, 99487, 99489-99497, G0270-G0271, G0442-G0445, G0463, G0506, G0511-G0512

90952 0405T, 0591T-0593T, 36591-36592, 90953♦, 96160-96161, 96523, 97802-97804, 99201-99220, 99224-99226, 99234-99255, 99281-99288, 99291-99292, 99304-99310, 99315-99318, 99324-99328, 99334-99350, 99354-99360, 99366-99368, 99374-99375, 99377-99416, 99421-99423, 99441-99443, 99450, 99455-99456, 99460-99472, 99475-99480,

99483-99484, 99487, 99489-99497, G0270-G0271, G0442-G0445, G0463, G0506, G0511-G0512

90953 0405T, 0591T-0593T, 36591-36592, 96160-96161, 96523, 97802-97804, 99201-99220, 99224-99226, 99234-99255, 99281-99288, 99291-99292, 99304-99310, 99315-99318, 99324-99328, 99334-99350, 99354-99360, 99366-99368, 99374-99375, 99377-99416, 99421-99423, 99441-99443, 99450, 99455-99456, 99460-99472, 99475-99480, 99483-99484, 99487, 99489-99497, G0270-G0271, G0442-G0445, G0463, G0506, G0511-G0512

90954 0405T, 0591T-0593T, 36591-36592, 90952♦, 90953♦, 90955♦, 90956♦, 90957♦, 90958♦, 90959-90965♦, 90966♦, 90967, 90968, 90969, 90970, 96160-96161, 96523, 97802-97804, 99201-99220, 99224-99226, 99234-99255, 99281-99288, 99291-99292, 99304-99310, 99315-99318, 99324-99328, 99334-99350, 99354-99360, 99366-99368, 99374-99375, 99377-99416, 99421-99423, 99441-99443, 99450, 99455-99456, 99460-99472, 99475-99480, 99483-99484, 99487, 99489-99497, G0270-G0271, G0442-G0445, G0463, G0506, G0511-G0512

90955 0405T, 0591T-0593T, 36591-36592, 90952♦, 90953♦, 90956♦, 90958♦, 90959-90962♦, 90965♦, 90966♦, 90967, 90968, 90969, 90970, 96160-96161, 96523, 97802-97804, 99201-99220, 99224-99226, 99234-99255, 99281-99288, 99291-99292, 99304-99310, 99315-99318, 99324-99328, 99334-99350, 99354-99360, 99366-99368, 99374-99375, 99377-99416, 99421-99423, 99441-99443, 99450, 99455-99456, 99460-99472, 99475-99480, 99483-99484, 99487, 99489-99497, G0270-G0271, G0442-G0445, G0463, G0506, G0511-G0512

90956 0405T, 0591T-0593T, 36591-36592, 90952♦, 90953♦, 90959-90962♦, 90966♦, 90967, 90968, 90969, 90970, 96160-96161, 96523, 97802-97804, 99201-99220, 99224-99226, 99234-99255, 99281-99288, 99291-99292, 99304-99310, 99315-99318, 99324-99328, 99334-99350, 99354-99360, 99366-99368, 99374-99375, 99377-99416, 99421-99423, 99441-99443, 99450, 99455-99456, 99460-99472, 99475-99480, 99483-99484, 99487, 99489-99497, G0270-G0271, G0442-G0445, G0463, G0506, G0511-G0512

90957 0405T, 0591T-0593T, 36591-36592, 90952♦, 90953♦, 90955♦, 90956♦, 90958♦, 90959-90965♦, 90966♦, 90967, 90968, 90969, 90970, 96160-96161, 96523, 97802-97804, 99201-99220, 99224-99226, 99234-99255, 99281-99288, 99291-99292, 99304-99310, 99315-99318, 99324-99328, 99334-99350, 99354-99360, 99366-99368, 99374-99375, 99377-99416, 99421-99423, 99441-99443, 99450, 99455-99456, 99460-99472, 99475-99480, 99483-99484, 99487, 99489-99497, G0270-G0271, G0442-G0445, G0463, G0506, G0511-G0512

90958 0405T, 0591T-0593T, 36591-36592, 90952♦, 90953♦, 90956♦, 90959-90962♦, 90965♦, 90966♦, 90967, 90968, 90969, 90970, 96160-96161, 96523, 97802-97804, 99201-99220, 99224-99226, 99234-99255, 99281-99288, 99291-99292, 99304-99310, 99315-99318, 99324-99328, 99334-99350, 99354-99360, 99366-99368, 99374-99375, 99377-99416, 99421-99423, 99441-99443, 99450, 99455-99456, 99460-99472, 99475-99480, 99483-99484, 99487, 99489-99497, G0270-G0271, G0442-G0445, G0463, G0506, G0511-G0512

90959 0405T, 0591T-0593T, 36591-36592, 90952♦, 90953♦, 90961-90962♦, 90966♦, 90967, 90968, 90969, 90970, 96160-96161, 96523, 97802-97804, 99201-99220, 99224-99226, 99234-99255, 99281-99288, 99291-99292, 99304-99310, 99315-99318, 99324-99328, 99334-99350, 99354-99360, 99366-99368, 99374-99375, 99377-99416, 99421-99423, 99441-99443, 99450, 99455-99456, 99460-99472, 99475-99480, 99483-99484, 99487, 99489-99497, G0270-G0271, G0442-G0445, G0463, G0506, G0511-G0512

CPT © 2020 American Medical Association. All Rights Reserved.

Coding Companion for Urology/Nephrology

90960 0405T, 0591T-0593T, 36591-36592, 90952◆, 90953◆, 90959◆, 90961-90962◆, 90966◆, 90967, 90968, 90969, 90970, 96160-96161, 96523, 97802-97804, 99201-99220, 99224-99226, 99234-99255, 99281-99288, 99291-99292, 99304-99310, 99315-99318, 99324-99328, 99334-99350, 99354-99360, 99366-99368, 99374-99375, 99377-99416, 99421-99423, 99441-99443, 99450, 99455-99456, 99460-99472, 99475-99480, 99483-99484, 99487, 99489-99497, G0270-G0271, G0442-G0445, G0463, G0506, G0511-G0512

90961 0405T, 0591T-0593T, 36591-36592, 90952◆, 90953◆, 90962◆, 90966◆, 90967, 90968, 90969, 90970, 96160-96161, 96523, 97802-97804, 99201-99220, 99224-99226, 99234-99255, 99281-99288, 99291-99292, 99304-99310, 99315-99318, 99324-99328, 99334-99350, 99354-99360, 99366-99368, 99374-99375, 99377-99416, 99421-99423, 99441-99443, 99450, 99455-99456, 99460-99472, 99475-99480, 99483-99484, 99487, 99489-99497, G0270-G0271, G0442-G0445, G0463, G0506, G0511-G0512

90962 0405T, 0591T-0593T, 36591-36592, 90952◆, 90953◆, 90967, 90968, 90969, 90970, 96160-96161, 96523, 97802-97804, 99201-99220, 99224-99226, 99234-99255, 99281-99288, 99291-99292, 99304-99310, 99315-99318, 99324-99328, 99334-99350, 99354-99360, 99366-99368, 99374-99375, 99377-99416, 99421-99423, 99441-99443, 99450, 99455-99456, 99460-99472, 99475-99480, 99483-99484, 99487, 99489-99497, G0270-G0271, G0442-G0445, G0463, G0506, G0511-G0512

90963 0405T, 0591T-0593T, 36591-36592, 90952◆, 90953◆, 90955◆, 90956◆, 90958◆, 90959-90962◆, 90964-90965◆, 90966◆, 90967, 90968, 90969, 90970, 96160-96161, 96523, 97802-97804, 99201-99255, 99281-99288, 99291-99292, 99304-99310, 99315-99318, 99324-99328, 99334-99350, 99354-99360, 99366-99368, 99374-99375, 99377-99416, 99421-99423, 99441-99443, 99450, 99455-99456, 99460-99472, 99475-99480, 99483-99484, 99487, 99489-99497, G0270-G0271, G0442-G0445, G0463, G0506, G0511-G0512

90964 0405T, 0591T-0593T, 36591-36592, 90952◆, 90953◆, 90955◆, 90956◆, 90958◆, 90959-90962◆, 90965◆, 90966◆, 90967, 90968, 90969, 90970, 96160-96161, 96523, 97802-97804, 99201-99255, 99281-99288, 99291-99292, 99304-99310, 99315-99318, 99324-99328, 99334-99350, 99354-99360, 99366-99368, 99374-99375, 99377-99416, 99421-99423, 99441-99443, 99450, 99455-99456, 99460-99472, 99475-99480, 99483-99484, 99487, 99489-99497, G0270-G0271, G0442-G0445, G0463, G0506, G0511-G0512

90965 0405T, 0591T-0593T, 36591-36592, 90952◆, 90953◆, 90956◆, 90959-90962◆, 90966◆, 90967, 90968, 90969, 90970, 96160-96161, 96523, 97802-97804, 99201-99255, 99281-99288, 99291-99292, 99304-99310, 99315-99318, 99324-99328, 99334-99350, 99354-99360, 99366-99368, 99374-99375, 99377-99416, 99421-99423, 99441-99443, 99450, 99455-99456, 99460-99472, 99475-99480, 99483-99484, 99487, 99489-99497, G0270-G0271, G0442-G0445, G0463, G0506, G0511-G0512

90966 0405T, 0591T-0593T, 36591-36592, 90952◆, 90953◆, 90962◆, 90967, 90968, 90969, 90970, 96160-96161, 96523, 97802-97804, 99201-99255, 99281-99288, 99291-99292, 99304-99310, 99315-99318, 99324-99328, 99334-99350, 99354-99360, 99366-99368, 99374-99375, 99377-99416, 99421-99423, 99441-99443, 99450, 99455-99456, 99460-99472, 99475-99480, 99483-99484, 99487, 99489-99497, G0270-G0271, G0442-G0445, G0463, G0506, G0511-G0512

90967 0405T, 0591T-0593T, 36591-36592, 90952, 90953, 96160-96161, 96523, 97802-97804, 99201-99255, 99281-99288, 99291-99292, 99304-99310, 99315-99318, 99324-99328, 99334-99350, 99354-99360, 99366-99368, 99374-99375, 99377-99416, 99421-99423, 99441-99443, 99450,

99455-99456, 99460-99472, 99475-99480, 99483-99484, 99487, 99489-99497, G0270-G0271, G0442-G0445, G0463, G0506, G0511-G0512

90968 0405T, 0591T-0593T, 36591-36592, 90952, 90953, 96160-96161, 96523, 97802-97804, 99201-99255, 99281-99288, 99291-99292, 99304-99310, 99315-99318, 99324-99328, 99334-99350, 99354-99360, 99366-99368, 99374-99375, 99377-99416, 99421-99423, 99441-99443, 99450, 99455-99456, 99460-99472, 99475-99480, 99483-99484, 99487, 99489-99497, G0270-G0271, G0442-G0445, G0463, G0506, G0511-G0512

90969 0405T, 0591T-0593T, 36591-36592, 90952, 90953, 96160-96161, 96523, 97802-97804, 99201-99255, 99281-99288, 99291-99292, 99304-99310, 99315-99318, 99324-99328, 99334-99350, 99354-99360, 99366-99368, 99374-99375, 99377-99416, 99421-99423, 99441-99443, 99450, 99455-99456, 99460-99472, 99475-99480, 99483-99484, 99487, 99489-99497, G0270-G0271, G0442-G0445, G0463, G0506, G0511-G0512

90970 0405T, 0591T-0593T, 36591-36592, 90952, 90953, 96160-96161, 96523, 97802-97804, 99201-99255, 99281-99288, 99291-99292, 99304-99310, 99315-99318, 99324-99328, 99334-99350, 99354-99360, 99366-99368, 99374-99375, 99377-99416, 99421-99423, 99441-99443, 99450, 99455-99456, 99460-99472, 99475-99480, 99483-99484, 99487, 99489-99497, G0270-G0271, G0442-G0445, G0463, G0506, G0511-G0512

90989 36591-36592, 96523, 97802-97804, G0270-G0271

90993 36591-36592, 96523, 97802-97804, G0270-G0271

90997 12001-12007, 12011-12057, 13100-13133, 13151-13153, 36000, 36400-36410, 36420-36430, 36440, 36591-36592, 36600, 36640, 43752, 51701-51703, 62320-62327, 64400, 64405-64408, 64415-64435, 64445-64454, 64461-64463, 64479-64505, 64510-64530, 90937◆, 92012-92014, 93000-93010, 93040-93042, 93318, 93355, 94002, 94200, 94250, 94680-94690, 94770, 95812-95816, 95819, 95822, 95829, 95955, 96360-96368, 96372, 96374-96377, 96523, 99155, 99156, 99157, 99211-99223, 99231-99255, 99291-99292, 99304-99310, 99315-99316, 99334-99337, 99347-99350, 99374-99375, 99377-99378, 99446-99449, 99451-99452, 99495-99496, G0463, G0471

93975 36591-36592, 76700-76776, 76856, 76970, 76998, 93976-93979, 96523

93976 36591-36592, 76700-76776, 76970, 76998, 93978-93979, 96523

93980 36591-36592, 76970, 76998, 93981, 96523

93981 36591-36592, 76856◆, 76970, 76998, 96523

93985 36591-36592, 76881-76882, 76937, 76970, 76998◆, 93922-93931, 93970-93971, 93986-93990, 96523

93986 36591-36592, 76881-76882, 76937, 76970, 76998◆, 93922-93924, 93926, 93931, 93971, 96523

93990 36591-36592, 76970, 76998, 90940, 93925-93931, 93970-93971, 93986, 96523

95990 36591-36592, 62367-62368, 96523, A4220

95991 36591-36592, 62367-62368, 95990◆, 96523, A4220

96360 0543T-0544T, 0548T, 0567T-0574T, 0580T, 0581T, 0582T, 36000, 36410, 36425, 36591-36592, 64450, 66987-66988, 96372, 96374, 96377, 96523, 99201-99215, 99354-99355, 99358-99359, 99455-99456, 99483, 99497, E0781, G0463

96361 0543T-0544T, 0548T, 0567T-0574T, 0580T, 0581T, 0582T, 36591-36592, 66987-66988, 96523, 99354-99355, 99358-99359, E0781

96365 0543T-0544T, 0567T-0574T, 0580T, 0581T, 0582T, 36000, 36410, 36425, 36591-36592, 64450, 66987-66988, 96360, 96372, 96374, 96377,

CCI Edits

96523, 99201-99215, 99354-99355, 99358-99359, 99455-99456, 99483, 99497, E0781, G0463, J1642-J1644

96366 0543T-0544T, 0567T-0574T, 0580T, 0581T, 0582T, 36591-36592, 66987-66988, 96523, 99354-99355, 99358-99359, E0781

96367 0543T-0544T, 0567T-0574T, 0580T, 0581T, 0582T, 36591-36592, 66987-66988, 96523, 99354-99355, 99358-99359, E0781

96368 0543T-0544T, 0567T-0574T, 0580T, 0581T, 0582T, 36591-36592, 66987-66988, 96523, 99354-99355, 99358-99359

96372 0543T-0544T, 0567T-0574T, 0580T, 0581T, 0582T, 36591-36592, 66987-66988, 96523, 99201-99215, 99354-99355, 99358-99359, 99455-99456, 99483, 99497, G0463

96373 36591-36592, 96523, 99201-99215, 99354-99355, 99358-99359, 99455-99456, 99483, 99497, G0463

96374 0543T-0544T, 0567T-0574T, 0580T, 0581T, 0582T, 36000, 36591-36592, 66987-66988, 96372, 96377, 96523, 99201-99215, 99354-99355, 99358-99359, 99455-99456, 99483, 99497, G0463

96375 0543T-0544T, 0567T-0574T, 0580T, 0581T, 0582T, 36000, 36591-36592, 66987-66988, 96523, 99354-99355, 99358-99359

96376 36000, 36591-36592, 66987, 96523, 99354-99355, 99358-99359

98960 0592T, 36591-36592, 96523

98961 0593T, 36591-36592, 96523

98962 0593T, 36591-36592, 96523

99051 36591-36592, 96523

99053 36591-36592, 96523

99060 36591-36592, 96523

99202 0362T, 0373T, 0469T, 36591-36592, 43752, 80500-80502, 90863, 90940, 92002-92014, 92227-92228, 92531-92532, 93561-93562, 93792, 93793, 94002-94004, 94660-94662, 95851-95852, 96020, 96105, 96116, 96125, 96130, 96132, 96136, 96138, 96146, 96156-96159, 96164-96168, 96523, 97151, 97153-97158, 97169-97172, 97802-97804, 99091, 99172-99173, 99174, 99177, 99201, 99211-99215, 99408-99409, 99421-99423, 99446-99449, 99463✦, 99474, 99605-99606, G0102, G0117-G0118, G0245-G0246, G0248, G0250, G0270-G0271, G0396-G0397, G0406-G0408✦, G0425-G0427✦, G0442-G0447, G0459, G0473, G0508-G0509✦, G2011

99203 0362T, 0373T, 0469T, 36591-36592, 43752, 80500-80502, 90863, 90940, 92002-92014, 92227-92228, 92531-92532, 93561-93562, 93792, 93793, 94002-94004, 94660-94662, 95851-95852, 96020, 96105, 96116, 96125, 96130, 96132, 96136, 96138, 96146, 96156-96159, 96164-96168, 96523, 97151, 97153-97158, 97169-97172, 97802-97804, 99091, 99172-99173, 99174, 99177, 99201-99202, 99211-99215, 99408-99409, 99421-99423, 99446-99449, 99463✦, 99474, 99605-99606, G0102, G0117-G0118, G0245-G0246, G0248, G0250, G0270-G0271, G0396-G0397, G0406-G0408✦, G0425-G0427✦, G0442-G0447, G0459, G0473, G0508-G0509✦, G2011

99204 0362T, 0373T, 0469T, 36591-36592, 43752, 80500-80502, 90863, 90940, 92002-92014, 92227-92228, 92531-92532, 93561-93562, 93792, 93793, 94002-94004, 94660-94662, 95851-95852, 96020, 96105, 96116, 96125, 96130, 96132, 96136, 96138, 96146, 96156-96159, 96164-96168, 96523, 97151, 97153-97158, 97169-97172, 97802-97804, 99091, 99172-99173, 99174, 99177, 99201-99203, 99211-99215, 99408-99409, 99421-99423, 99446-99449, 99463✦, 99474, 99605-99606, G0102, G0117-G0118, G0245-G0246, G0248, G0250, G0270-G0271, G0396-G0397, G0406-G0408✦, G0425-G0427✦, G0442-G0447, G0459, G0473, G0508-G0509✦, G2011

99205 0362T, 0373T, 0469T, 36591-36592, 43752, 80500-80502, 90863, 90940, 92002-92014, 92227-92228, 92531-92532, 93561-93562, 93792, 93793, 94002-94004, 94660-94662, 95851-95852, 96020, 96105, 96116, 96125, 96130, 96132, 96136, 96138, 96146, 96156-96159, 96164-96168, 96523, 97151, 97153-97158, 97169-97172, 97802-97804, 99091, 99172-99173, 99174, 99177, 99201-99204, 99211-99215, 99408-99409, 99421-99423, 99446-99449, 99463✦, 99474, 99605-99606, G0102, G0117-G0118, G0245-G0246, G0248, G0250, G0270-G0271, G0396-G0397, G0406-G0408✦, G0425-G0427✦, G0442-G0447, G0459, G0473, G0508-G0509✦, G2011

99211 0362T, 0373T, 0469T, 0543T-0544T, 0567T-0574T, 0580T, 0581T, 0582T, 36591-36592, 43752, 80500-80502, 90863, 90940, 92002-92014, 92227-92228, 92531-92532, 93561-93562, 93792, 93793, 94002-94004, 94660-94662, 95851-95852, 96020, 96105, 96116, 96125, 96130, 96132, 96136, 96138, 96146, 96156-96159, 96164-96168, 96523, 97151, 97153-97158, 97169-97172, 97802-97804, 99091, 99172-99173, 99174, 99177, 99408-99409, 99446-99449, 99474, 99605-99606, G0102, G0117-G0118, G0245-G0246, G0248, G0250, G0270-G0271, G0396-G0397, G0406-G0408✦, G0425-G0427✦, G0442-G0447, G0459, G0473, G0508-G0509✦, G2011

99212 0362T, 0373T, 0469T, 0543T-0544T, 0567T-0574T, 0580T, 0581T, 0582T, 20560-20561, 36591-36592, 43752, 80500-80502, 90863, 90940, 92002-92014, 92227-92228, 92531-92532, 93561-93562, 93792, 93793, 94002-94004, 94660-94662, 95851-95852, 96020, 96105, 96116, 96125, 96130, 96132, 96136, 96138, 96146, 96156-96159, 96164-96168, 96523, 97151, 97153-97158, 97169-97172, 97802-97804, 99091, 99172-99173, 99174, 99177, 99211, 99408-99409, 99421, 99446-99449, 99474, 99605-99606, G0102, G0117-G0118, G0245-G0246, G0248, G0250, G0270-G0271, G0396-G0397, G0406-G0408✦, G0425-G0427✦, G0442-G0447, G0459, G0473, G0508-G0509✦, G2011

99213 0362T, 0373T, 0469T, 0543T-0544T, 0567T-0574T, 0580T, 0581T, 0582T, 20560-20561, 36591-36592, 43752, 80500-80502, 90863, 90940, 92002-92014, 92227-92228, 92531-92532, 93561-93562, 93792, 93793, 94002-94004, 94660-94662, 95851-95852, 96020, 96105, 96116, 96125, 96130, 96132, 96136, 96138, 96146, 96156-96159, 96164-96168, 96523, 97151, 97153-97158, 97169-97172, 97802-97804, 99091, 99172-99173, 99174, 99177, 99211-99212, 99408-99409, 99421-99423, 99446-99449, 99463✦, 99474, 99605-99606, G0102, G0117-G0118, G0245-G0246, G0248, G0250, G0270-G0271, G0396-G0397, G0406-G0408✦, G0425-G0427✦, G0442-G0447, G0459, G0473, G0508-G0509✦, G2011

99214 0362T, 0373T, 0469T, 0543T-0544T, 0567T-0574T, 0580T, 0581T, 0582T, 20560-20561, 20700-20701, 36591-36592, 43752, 80500-80502, 90863, 90940, 92002-92014, 92227-92228, 92531-92532, 93561-93562, 93792, 93793, 94002-94004, 94660-94662, 95851-95852, 96020, 96105, 96116, 96125, 96130, 96132, 96136, 96138, 96146, 96156-96159, 96164-96168, 96523, 97151, 97153-97158, 97169-97172, 97802-97804, 99091, 99172-99173, 99174, 99177, 99211-99213, 99408-99409, 99421-99423, 99446-99449, 99463✦, 99474, 99605-99606, G0102, G0117-G0118, G0245-G0246, G0248, G0250, G0270-G0271, G0396-G0397, G0406-G0408✦, G0425-G0427✦, G0442-G0447, G0459, G0473, G0508-G0509✦, G2011

99215 0362T, 0373T, 0469T, 0543T-0544T, 0567T-0574T, 0580T, 0581T, 0582T, 20560-20561, 20700-20701, 36591-36592, 43752, 62329, 80500-80502, 90863, 90940, 92002-92014, 92227-92228, 92531-92532, 93561-93562, 93792, 93793, 94002-94004, 94660-94662, 95851-95852, 96020, 96105, 96116, 96125, 96130, 96132, 96136, 96138, 96146, 96156-96159, 96164-96168, 96523, 97151, 97153-97158, 97169-97172, 97802-97804, 99091, 99172-99173, 99174, 99177, 99211-99214, 99408-99409,

99421-99423, 99446-99449, 99463✦, 99474, 99605-99606, G0102, G0117-G0118, G0245-G0246, G0248, G0250, G0270-G0271, G0396-G0397, G0406-G0408✦, G0425-G0427✦, G0442-G0447, G0459, G0473, G0508-G0509✦, G2011

99217 0362T, 0373T, 0469T, 0543T-0544T, 0567T-0574T, 0580T, 0581T, 0582T, 20560-20561, 20701, 36591-36592, 43752, 90863, 90940, 92002-92014, 92227-92228, 92531-92532, 93792, 93793, 94002-94004, 94644, 94660-94662, 95851-95852, 96020, 96105, 96116, 96125-96130, 96132, 96136, 96138, 96146, 96156-96159, 96164-96168, 96360, 96365, 96369, 96372-96374, 96377, 96401-96406, 96409, 96413, 96416, 96420-96422, 96425-96440, 96446-96450, 96523, 97151, 97153-97158, 97169-97172, 97802-97804, 99091, 99172-99173, 99174, 99177, 99281-99285, 99408-99409, 99446-99449, 99451-99452, 99474, 99605-99606, G0102, G0245-G0246, G0250, G0270-G0271, G0396-G0397, G0442-G0447, G0459, G0473, G0498, G2011

99218 0362T, 0373T, 0469T, 0543T-0544T, 0567T-0574T, 0580T, 0581T, 0582T, 0591T-0593T, 20560-20561, 20700-20701, 36591-36592, 43752, 90863, 90940, 92002-92014, 92227-92228, 92531-92532, 93792, 93793, 94002-94004, 94644, 94660-94662, 95851-95852, 96020, 96105, 96116, 96125-96130, 96132, 96136, 96138, 96146, 96156-96159, 96164-96168, 96360, 96365, 96369, 96372-96374, 96377, 96401-96406, 96409, 96413, 96416, 96420-96422, 96425-96440, 96446-96450, 96523, 97151, 97153-97158, 97169-97172, 97802-97804, 99091, 99172-99173, 99174, 99177, 99201-99217, 99224-99226, 99238-99239, 99281-99285, 99307-99310, 99315-99318, 99324-99328, 99334-99337, 99341-99350, 99381-99404, 99408-99412, 99446-99449, 99451-99452, 99474, 99483, 99497, 99605-99606, G0102, G0245-G0246, G0250, G0270-G0271, G0380-G0384, G0396-G0397, G0442-G0447, G0459, G0463, G0473, G0498, G2011

99219 0362T, 0373T, 0469T, 0543T-0544T, 0567T-0574T, 0580T, 0581T, 0582T, 0591T-0593T, 15772, 15774, 20560-20561, 20700-20701, 36591-36592, 43752, 90863, 90940, 92002-92014, 92227-92228, 92531-92532, 93792, 93793, 94002-94004, 94644, 94660-94662, 95851-95852, 96020, 96105, 96116, 96125-96130, 96132, 96136, 96138, 96146, 96156-96159, 96164-96168, 96360, 96365, 96369, 96372-96374, 96377, 96401-96406, 96409, 96413, 96416, 96420-96422, 96425-96440, 96446-96450, 96523, 97151, 97153-97158, 97169-97172, 97802-97804, 99091, 99172-99173, 99174, 99177, 99201-99218, 99224-99226, 99238-99239, 99281-99285, 99307-99310, 99315-99318, 99324-99328, 99334-99337, 99341-99350, 99381-99404, 99408-99412, 99446-99449, 99451-99452, 99463✦, 99474, 99483, 99497, 99605-99606, G0102, G0245-G0246, G0250, G0270-G0271, G0380-G0384, G0396-G0397, G0442-G0447, G0459, G0463, G0473, G0498, G2011

99220 0362T, 0373T, 0469T, 0543T-0544T, 0567T-0574T, 0580T, 0581T, 0582T, 0591T-0593T, 15772, 15774, 20560-20561, 20700-20701, 36591-36592, 43752, 62329, 90863, 90940, 92002-92014, 92227-92228, 92531-92532, 93792, 93793, 94002-94004, 94644, 94660-94662, 95851-95852, 96020, 96105, 96116, 96125-96130, 96132, 96136, 96138, 96146, 96156-96159, 96164-96168, 96360, 96365, 96369, 96372-96374, 96377, 96401-96406, 96409, 96413, 96416, 96420-96422, 96425-96440, 96446-96450, 96523, 97151, 97153-97158, 97169-97172, 97802-97804, 99091, 99172-99173, 99174, 99177, 99201-99219, 99224-99226, 99238-99239, 99281-99285, 99307-99310, 99315-99318, 99324-99328, 99334-99337, 99341-99350, 99381-99404, 99408-99412, 99446-99449, 99451-99452, 99463✦, 99474, 99483, 99497, 99605-99606, G0102, G0245-G0246, G0250, G0270-G0271, G0380-G0384, G0396-G0397, G0442-G0447, G0459, G0463, G0473, G0498, G2011

99221 0362T, 0373T, 0469T, 0543T-0544T, 0567T-0574T, 0580T, 0581T, 0582T, 0591T-0593T, 20560-20561, 20700-20701, 36591-36592, 43752,

80500-80502, 90863, 90940, 92002-92014, 92227-92228, 92531-92532, 93792, 93793, 94002-94004, 94644, 94660-94662, 95851-95852, 96020, 96105, 96116, 96125-96130, 96132, 96136, 96138, 96146, 96156-96159, 96164-96168, 96360, 96365, 96369, 96372-96374, 96377, 96401-96406, 96409, 96413, 96416, 96420-96422, 96425-96440, 96446-96450, 96523, 97151, 97153-97158, 97169-97172, 97802-97804, 99091, 99172-99173, 99174, 99177, 99184, 99201-99220, 99224-99233, 99238-99239, 99281-99285, 99304-99310, 99315-99318, 99324-99328, 99334-99337, 99341-99350, 99381-99404, 99408-99412, 99446-99449, 99451-99452, 99460, 99462-99463✦, 99474, 99483, 99497, 99605-99606, G0102, G0245-G0246, G0250, G0270-G0271, G0380-G0384, G0396-G0397, G0406-G0408, G0424-G0427, G0442-G0447, G0459, G0463, G0473, G0498, G0508-G0509, G2011

99222 0362T, 0373T, 0469T, 0543T-0544T, 0567T-0574T, 0580T, 0581T, 0582T, 0591T-0593T, 15774, 20560-20561, 20700-20701, 36591-36592, 43752, 62329, 80500-80502, 90863, 90940, 92002-92014, 92227-92228, 92531-92532, 93792, 93793, 94002-94004, 94644, 94660-94662, 95851-95852, 96020, 96105, 96116, 96125-96130, 96132, 96136, 96138, 96146, 96156-96159, 96164-96168, 96360, 96365, 96369, 96372-96374, 96377, 96401-96406, 96409, 96413, 96416, 96420-96422, 96425-96440, 96446-96450, 96523, 97151, 97153-97158, 97169-97172, 97802-97804, 99091, 99172-99173, 99174, 99177, 99184, 99201-99221, 99224-99233, 99238-99239, 99281-99285, 99304-99310, 99315-99318, 99324-99328, 99334-99337, 99341-99350, 99381-99404, 99408-99412, 99446-99449, 99451-99452, 99460, 99462-99463✦, 99474, 99479-99480, 99483, 99497, 99605-99606, G0102, G0245-G0246, G0250, G0270-G0271, G0380-G0384, G0396-G0397, G0406-G0408, G0424-G0427, G0442-G0447, G0459, G0463, G0473, G0498, G0508-G0509, G2011

99223 0362T, 0373T, 0469T, 0543T-0544T, 0567T-0574T, 0580T, 0581T, 0582T, 0591T-0593T, 15772, 15774, 20560-20561, 20700-20701, 36591-36592, 43752, 62329, 80500-80502, 90863, 90940, 92002-92014, 92227-92228, 92531-92532, 93792, 93793, 94002-94004, 94644, 94660-94662, 95851-95852, 96020, 96105, 96116, 96125-96130, 96132, 96136, 96138, 96146, 96156-96159, 96164-96168, 96360, 96365, 96369, 96372-96374, 96377, 96401-96406, 96409, 96413, 96416, 96420-96422, 96425-96440, 96446-96450, 96523, 97151, 97153-97158, 97169-97172, 97802-97804, 99091, 99172-99173, 99174, 99177, 99184, 99201-99222, 99224-99233, 99238-99239, 99281-99285, 99304-99310, 99315-99318, 99324-99328, 99334-99337, 99341-99350, 99381-99404, 99408-99412, 99446-99449, 99451-99452, 99460-99463✦, 99474, 99478-99480, 99483, 99497, 99605-99606, G0102, G0245-G0246, G0250, G0270-G0271, G0380-G0384, G0396-G0397, G0406-G0408, G0424-G0427, G0442-G0447, G0459, G0463, G0473, G0498, G0508-G0509, G2011

99224 0362T, 0373T, 0469T, 36591-36592, 43752, 90863, 90940, 92002-92014, 92227-92228, 92531-92532, 93792, 93793, 94002-94004, 94644, 94660-94662, 95851-95852, 96020, 96116, 96127, 96156-96159, 96164-96168, 96360, 96365, 96369, 96372-96374, 96377, 96401-96406, 96409, 96413, 96416, 96420-96422, 96425-96440, 96446-96450, 96523, 97151, 97153-97158, 97169-97172, 97802-97804, 99091, 99172-99173, 99174, 99177, 99201-99217, 99281-99285, 99307-99310, 99318, 99324-99328, 99334-99337, 99341-99350, 99408-99409, 99446-99449, 99451-99452, 99460-99462, 99474, 99483, 99497, 99605-99606, G0102, G0245-G0246, G0250, G0270-G0271, G0380-G0384, G0396-G0397, G0442-G0447, G0459, G0463, G0473, G0498, G2011

99225 0362T, 0373T, 0469T, 36591-36592, 43752, 90863, 90940, 92002-92014, 92227-92228, 92531-92532, 93792, 93793, 94002-94004, 94644, 94660-94662, 95851-95852, 96020, 96116, 96127, 96360, 96365, 96369, 96372-96374, 96377, 96401-96406, 96409, 96413, 96416,

96420-96422, 96425-96440, 96446-96450, 96523, 97151, 97153-97158, 97802-97804, 99091, 99172-99173, 99174, 99177, 99201-99217, 99224, 99281-99285, 99307-99310, 99318, 99324-99328, 99334-99337, 99341-99350, 99408-99409, 99446-99449, 99451-99452, 99460-99462, 99483, 99497, 99605-99606, G0102, G0245-G0246, G0250, G0270-G0271, G0380-G0384, G0396-G0397, G0442-G0447, G0459, G0463, G0473, G0498, G2011

99226 0362T, 0373T, 0469T, 36591-36592, 43752, 90863, 90940, 92002-92014, 92227-92228, 92531-92532, 93792, 93793, 94002-94004, 94644, 94660-94662, 95851-95852, 96020, 96116, 96127, 96360, 96365, 96369, 96372-96374, 96377, 96401-96406, 96409, 96413, 96416, 96420-96422, 96425-96440, 96446-96450, 96523, 97151, 97153-97158, 97802-97804, 99091, 99172-99173, 99174, 99177, 99201-99217, 99224-99225, 99281-99285, 99307-99310, 99318, 99324-99328, 99334-99337, 99341-99350, 99408-99409, 99446-99449, 99451-99452, 99460-99462, 99483, 99497, 99605-99606, G0102, G0245-G0246, G0250, G0270-G0271, G0380-G0384, G0396-G0397, G0442-G0447, G0459, G0463, G0473, G0498, G2011

99231 0362T, 0373T, 0469T, 0543T-0544T, 0567T-0574T, 0580T, 0581T, 0582T, 20560-20561, 36591-36592, 43752, 80500-80502, 90863, 90940, 92002-92014, 92227-92228, 92531-92532, 93792, 93793, 94002-94004, 94644, 94660-94662, 95851-95852, 96020, 96105, 96116, 96125-96130, 96132, 96136, 96138, 96146, 96156-96159, 96164-96168, 96360, 96365, 96369, 96372-96374, 96377, 96401-96406, 96409, 96413, 96416, 96420-96422, 96425-96440, 96446-96450, 96523, 97151, 97153-97158, 97169-97172, 97802-97804, 99091, 99172-99173, 99174, 99177, 99184, 99281-99285, 99408-99409, 99446-99449, 99451-99452, 99474, 99605-99606, G0102, G0245-G0246, G0250, G0270-G0271, G0380-G0384, G0396-G0397, G0406-G0408, G0425-G0427, G0442-G0447, G0459, G0473, G0498, G0508-G0509, G2011

99232 0362T, 0373T, 0469T, 0543T-0544T, 0567T-0574T, 0580T, 0581T, 0582T, 20560-20561, 20701, 36591-36592, 43752, 80500-80502, 90863, 90940, 92002-92014, 92227-92228, 92531-92532, 93792, 93793, 94002-94004, 94644, 94660-94662, 95851-95852, 96020, 96105, 96116, 96125-96130, 96132, 96136, 96138, 96146, 96156-96159, 96164-96168, 96360, 96365, 96369, 96372-96374, 96377, 96401-96406, 96409, 96413, 96416, 96420-96422, 96425-96440, 96446-96450, 96523, 97151, 97153-97158, 97169-97172, 97802-97804, 99091, 99172-99173, 99174, 99177, 99184, 99231, 99281-99285, 99408-99409, 99446-99449, 99451-99452, 99462, 99474, 99605-99606, G0102, G0245-G0246, G0250, G0270-G0271, G0380-G0384, G0396-G0397, G0406-G0408, G0425-G0427, G0442-G0447, G0459, G0473, G0498, G0508-G0509, G2011

99233 0362T, 0373T, 0469T, 0543T-0544T, 0567T-0574T, 0580T, 0581T, 0582T, 20560-20561, 20700-20701, 36591-36592, 43752, 80500-80502, 90863, 90940, 92002-92014, 92227-92228, 92531-92532, 93792, 93793, 94002-94004, 94644, 94660-94662, 95851-95852, 96020, 96105, 96116, 96125-96130, 96132, 96136, 96138, 96146, 96156-96159, 96164-96168, 96360, 96365, 96369, 96372-96374, 96377, 96401-96406, 96409, 96413, 96416, 96420-96422, 96425-96440, 96446-96450, 96523, 97151, 97153-97158, 97169-97172, 97802-97804, 99091, 99172-99173, 99174, 99177, 99184, 99231-99232, 99281-99285, 99408-99409, 99446-99449, 99451-99452, 99460, 99462-99463✦, 99474, 99605-99606, G0102, G0245-G0246, G0250, G0270-G0271, G0380-G0384, G0396-G0397, G0406-G0408, G0425-G0427, G0442-G0447, G0459, G0473, G0498, G0508-G0509, G2011

99234 0362T, 0373T, 0469T, 0543T-0544T, 0567T-0574T, 0580T, 0581T, 0582T, 15772, 15774, 20560-20561, 20700-20701, 36591-36592, 43752, 62329, 80500-80502, 90863, 90940, 92002-92014, 92227-92228, 92531-92532,

93792, 93793, 94002-94004, 94644, 94660-94662, 95851-95852, 96020, 96105, 96116, 96125-96130, 96132, 96136, 96138, 96146, 96156-96159, 96164-96168, 96360, 96365, 96369, 96372-96374, 96377, 96401-96406, 96409, 96413, 96416, 96420-96422, 96425-96440, 96446-96450, 96523, 97151, 97153-97158, 97169-97172, 97802-97804, 99091, 99172-99173, 99174, 99177, 99201-99233, 99238-99239, 99281-99285, 99307-99310, 99318, 99324-99328, 99334-99337, 99341-99350, 99408-99409, 99446-99449, 99451-99452, 99474, 99483, 99497, 99605-99606, G0102, G0245-G0246, G0250, G0270-G0271, G0380-G0384, G0396-G0397, G0406-G0408, G0425-G0427, G0442-G0447, G0459, G0463, G0473, G0498, G0508-G0509, G2011

99235 0362T, 0373T, 0469T, 0543T-0544T, 0567T-0574T, 0580T, 0581T, 0582T, 15772, 15774, 20560-20561, 20700-20701, 36591-36592, 43752, 62329, 80500-80502, 90863, 90940, 92002-92014, 92227-92228, 92531-92532, 93792, 93793, 94002-94004, 94644, 94660-94662, 95851-95852, 96020, 96105, 96116, 96125-96130, 96132, 96136, 96138, 96146, 96156-96159, 96164-96168, 96360, 96365, 96369, 96372-96374, 96377, 96401-96406, 96409, 96413, 96416, 96420-96422, 96425-96440, 96446-96450, 96523, 97151, 97153-97158, 97169-97172, 97802-97804, 99091, 99172-99173, 99174, 99177, 99201-99234, 99238-99239, 99281-99285, 99307-99310, 99318, 99324-99328, 99334-99337, 99341-99350, 99408-99409, 99446-99449, 99451-99452, 99474, 99483, 99497, 99605-99606, G0102, G0245-G0246, G0250, G0270-G0271, G0380-G0384, G0396-G0397, G0406-G0408, G0425-G0427, G0442-G0447, G0459, G0463, G0473, G0498, G0508-G0509, G2011

99236 0362T, 0373T, 0469T, 0543T-0544T, 0567T-0574T, 0580T, 0581T, 0582T, 15772, 15774, 20560-20561, 20700-20701, 36591-36592, 43752, 62329, 80500-80502, 90863, 90940, 92002-92014, 92227-92228, 92531-92532, 93792, 93793, 94002-94004, 94644, 94660-94662, 95851-95852, 96020, 96105, 96116, 96125-96130, 96132, 96136, 96138, 96146, 96156-96159, 96164-96168, 96360, 96365, 96369, 96372-96374, 96377, 96401-96406, 96409, 96413, 96416, 96420-96422, 96425-96440, 96446-96450, 96523, 97151, 97153-97158, 97169-97172, 97802-97804, 99091, 99172-99173, 99174, 99177, 99201-99235, 99238-99239, 99281-99285, 99307-99310, 99318, 99324-99328, 99334-99337, 99341-99350, 99408-99409, 99446-99449, 99451-99452, 99474, 99483, 99497, 99605-99606, G0102, G0245-G0246, G0250, G0270-G0271, G0380-G0384, G0396-G0397, G0406-G0408, G0425-G0427, G0442-G0447, G0459, G0463, G0473, G0498, G0508-G0509, G2011

99238 0362T, 0373T, 0469T, 0543T-0544T, 0567T-0574T, 0580T, 0581T, 0582T, 20560-20561, 20701, 36591-36592, 43752, 80500-80502, 90863, 90940, 92002-92014, 92227-92228, 92531-92532, 93792, 93793, 94002-94004, 94644, 94660-94662, 95851-95852, 96020, 96105, 96116, 96125-96130, 96132, 96136, 96138, 96146, 96156-96159, 96164-96168, 96360, 96365, 96369, 96372-96374, 96377, 96401-96406, 96409, 96413, 96416, 96420-96422, 96425-96440, 96446-96450, 96523, 97151, 97153-97158, 97169-97172, 97802-97804, 99091, 99172-99173, 99174, 99177, 99201-99217✦, 99231-99233, 99281-99285, 99408-99409, 99446-99449, 99451-99452, 99474, 99483, 99605-99606, G0102, G0245-G0246, G0250, G0270-G0271, G0380-G0384, G0396-G0397, G0442-G0447, G0459, G0463, G0473, G0498, G2011

99239 0362T, 0373T, 0469T, 0543T-0544T, 0567T-0574T, 0580T, 0581T, 0582T, 20560-20561, 20700-20701, 36591-36592, 43752, 80500-80502, 90863, 90940, 92002-92014, 92227-92228, 92531-92532, 93792, 93793, 94002-94004, 94644, 94660-94662, 95851-95852, 96020, 96105, 96116, 96125-96130, 96132, 96136, 96138, 96146, 96156-96159, 96164-96168, 96360, 96365, 96369, 96372-96374, 96377, 96401-96406, 96409, 96413, 96416, 96420-96422, 96425-96440, 96446-96450, 96523, 97151, 97153-97158, 97169-97172, 97802-97804, 99091, 99172-99173, 99174, 99177, 99201-99217✦, 99231-99233, 99238, 99281-99285,

CPT © 2020 American Medical Association. All Rights Reserved.

99408-99409, 99446-99449, 99451-99452, 99474, 99483, 99605-99606,
G0102, G0245-G0246, G0250, G0270-G0271, G0380-G0384,
G0396-G0397, G0442-G0447, G0459, G0463, G0473, G0498, G2011

99241 0362T, 0373T, 0469T, 0543T-0544T, 0567T-0574T, 0580T, 0581T, 0582T,
20560-20561, 36591-36592, 90863, 93792, 93793, 94002-94004,
94660-94662, 96523, 97151, 97153-97158, 99091, 99172-99173, 99174,
99177, 99421-99422, 99446-99449, 99451-99452, 99474,
G0406-G0408♦, G0425-G0427♦, G0459♦, G0473, G0508-G0509♦

99242 0362T, 0373T, 0469T, 0543T-0544T, 0567T-0574T, 0580T, 0581T, 0582T,
20560-20561, 20701, 36591-36592, 90863, 93792, 93793, 94002-94004,
94660-94662, 96523, 97151, 97153-97158, 99091, 99172-99173, 99174,
99177, 99421-99423, 99446-99449, 99451-99452, 99474,
G0406-G0408♦, G0425-G0427♦, G0459♦, G0473, G0508-G0509♦

99243 0362T, 0373T, 0469T, 0543T-0544T, 0567T-0574T, 0580T, 0581T, 0582T,
20560-20561, 20700-20701, 36591-36592, 90863, 93792, 93793,
94002-94004, 94660-94662, 96523, 97151, 97153-97158, 99091,
99172-99173, 99174, 99177, 99421-99423, 99446-99449, 99451-99452,
99474, G0406-G0408♦, G0425-G0427♦, G0459♦, G0473, G0508-G0509♦

99244 0362T, 0373T, 0469T, 0543T-0544T, 0567T-0574T, 0580T, 0581T, 0582T,
15774, 20560-20561, 20700-20701, 36591-36592, 62329, 90863, 93792,
93793, 94002-94004, 94660-94662, 96523, 97151, 97153-97158, 99091,
99172-99173, 99174, 99177, 99421-99423, 99446-99449, 99451-99452,
99474, G0406-G0408♦, G0425-G0427♦, G0459♦, G0473, G0508-G0509♦

99245 0362T, 0373T, 0469T, 0543T-0544T, 0567T-0574T, 0580T, 0581T, 0582T,
15774, 20560-20561, 20700-20701, 36591-36592, 62329, 90863, 93792,
93793, 94002-94004, 94660-94662, 96523, 97151, 97153-97158, 99091,
99172-99173, 99174, 99177, 99421-99423, 99446-99449, 99451-99452,
99474, G0406-G0408♦, G0425-G0427♦, G0459♦, G0473, G0508-G0509♦

99251 0362T, 0373T, 0469T, 0543T-0544T, 0567T-0574T, 0580T, 0581T, 0582T,
20560-20561, 20701, 36591-36592, 90863, 93792, 93793, 94002-94004,
94660-94662, 96127, 96523, 97151, 97153-97158, 99091, 99172-99173,
99174, 99177, 99241-99245, 99446-99449, 99451-99452, 99474,
G0406-G0408♦, G0425-G0427♦, G0459♦, G0473, G0508-G0509♦

99252 0362T, 0373T, 0469T, 0543T-0544T, 0567T-0574T, 0580T, 0581T, 0582T,
20560-20561, 20701, 36591-36592, 90863, 93792, 93793, 94002-94004,
94660-94662, 96127, 96523, 97151, 97153-97158, 99091, 99172-99173,
99174, 99177, 99241-99245, 99446-99449, 99451-99452, 99474,
G0406-G0408♦, G0425-G0427♦, G0459♦, G0473, G0508-G0509♦

99253 0362T, 0373T, 0469T, 0543T-0544T, 0567T-0574T, 0580T, 0581T, 0582T,
20560-20561, 20700-20701, 36591-36592, 62329, 90863, 93792, 93793,
94002-94004, 94660-94662, 96127, 96523, 97151, 97153-97158, 99091,
99172-99173, 99174, 99177, 99241-99245, 99446-99449, 99451-99452,
99474, G0406-G0408♦, G0425-G0427♦, G0459♦, G0473, G0508-G0509♦

99254 0362T, 0373T, 0469T, 0543T-0544T, 0567T-0574T, 0580T, 0581T, 0582T,
20560-20561, 20700-20701, 36591-36592, 62329, 90863, 93792, 93793,
94002-94004, 94660-94662, 96127, 96523, 97151, 97153-97158, 99091,
99172-99173, 99174, 99177, 99241-99245, 99446-99449, 99451-99452,
99474, G0406-G0408♦, G0425-G0427♦, G0459♦, G0473, G0508-G0509♦

99255 0362T, 0373T, 0469T, 0543T-0544T, 0567T-0574T, 0580T, 0581T, 0582T,
20560-20561, 20700-20701, 36591-36592, 62329, 90863, 93792, 93793,
94002-94004, 94660-94662, 96127, 96523, 97151, 97153-97158, 99091,
99172-99173, 99174, 99177, 99241-99245, 99446-99449, 99451-99452,
99474, G0406-G0408♦, G0425-G0427♦, G0459♦, G0473, G0508-G0509♦

99281 0362T, 0373T, 0469T, 36591-36592, 43752, 90863, 90940, 92002-92014,
92227-92228, 92531-92532, 93792, 93793, 94002-94004, 94660-94662,
95851-95852, 96020, 96105, 96116, 96125-96130, 96132, 96136,
96138, 96146, 96156-96159, 96164-96168, 96360, 96365, 96369,
96372-96374, 96377, 96401-96406, 96409, 96413, 96416, 96420-96422,

96425-96440, 96446-96450, 96523, 97151, 97153-97172, 97802-97804,
99091, 99172-99173, 99174, 99177, 99408-99409, 99446-99449,
99451-99452, 99474, 99605-99606, G0102, G0245-G0246,
G0270-G0271, G0380♦, G0382-G0384♦, G0396-G0397, G0406-G0408♦,
G0425-G0427♦, G0442-G0447, G0459, G0473, G0498, G0508-G0509♦,
G2011

99282 0362T, 0373T, 0469T, 36591-36592, 43752, 90863, 90940, 92002-92014,
92227-92228, 92531-92532, 93792, 93793, 94002-94004, 94660-94662,
95851-95852, 96020, 96105, 96116, 96125-96130, 96132, 96136,
96138, 96146, 96156-96159, 96164-96168, 96360, 96365, 96369,
96372-96374, 96377, 96401-96406, 96409, 96413, 96416, 96420-96422,
96425-96440, 96446-96450, 96523, 97151, 97153-97172, 97802-97804,
99091, 99172-99173, 99174, 99177, 99281, 99408-99409, 99446-99449,
99451-99452, 99474, 99605-99606, G0102, G0245-G0246,
G0270-G0271, G0380-G0384♦, G0396-G0397, G0406-G0408,
G0425-G0427, G0442-G0447, G0459, G0473, G0498, G0508-G0509,
G2011

99283 0362T, 0373T, 0469T, 36591-36592, 43752, 90863, 90940, 92002-92014,
92227-92228, 92531-92532, 93792, 93793, 94002-94004, 94660-94662,
95851-95852, 96020, 96105, 96116, 96125-96130, 96132, 96136,
96138, 96146, 96156-96159, 96164-96168, 96360, 96365, 96369,
96372-96374, 96377, 96401-96406, 96409, 96413, 96416, 96420-96422,
96425-96440, 96446-96450, 96523, 97151, 97153-97172, 97802-97804,
99091, 99172-99173, 99174, 99177, 99281-99282, 99408-99409,
99446-99449, 99451-99452, 99474, 99605-99606, G0102,
G0245-G0246, G0270-G0271, G0380-G0384♦, G0396-G0397,
G0406-G0408, G0425-G0427, G0442-G0447, G0459, G0473, G0498,
G0508-G0509, G2011

99284 0362T, 0373T, 0469T, 36591-36592, 43752, 90863, 90940, 92002-92014,
92227-92228, 92531-92532, 93792, 93793, 94002-94004, 94660-94662,
95851-95852, 96020, 96105, 96116, 96125-96130, 96132, 96136,
96138, 96146, 96156-96159, 96164-96168, 96360, 96365, 96369,
96372-96374, 96377, 96401-96406, 96409, 96413, 96416, 96420-96422,
96425-96440, 96446-96450, 96523, 97151, 97153-97172, 97802-97804,
99091, 99172-99173, 99174, 99177, 99281-99283, 99408-99409,
99446-99449, 99451-99452, 99463♦, 99474, 99605-99606, G0102,
G0245-G0246, G0270-G0271, G0380-G0384♦, G0396-G0397,
G0406-G0408, G0425-G0427, G0442-G0447, G0459, G0473, G0498,
G0508-G0509, G2011

99285 0362T, 0373T, 0469T, 36591-36592, 43752, 90863, 90940, 92002-92014,
92227-92228, 92531-92532, 93792, 93793, 94002-94004, 94660-94662,
95851-95852, 96020, 96105, 96116, 96125-96130, 96132, 96136,
96138, 96146, 96156-96159, 96164-96168, 96360, 96365, 96369,
96372-96374, 96377, 96401-96406, 96409, 96413, 96416, 96420-96422,
96425-96440, 96446-96450, 96523, 97151, 97153-97172, 97802-97804,
99091, 99172-99173, 99174, 99177, 99281-99284, 99408-99409,
99446-99449, 99451-99452, 99463♦, 99474, 99605-99606, G0102,
G0245-G0246, G0270-G0271, G0380-G0384♦, G0396-G0397,
G0406-G0408, G0425-G0427, G0442-G0447, G0459, G0473, G0498,
G0508-G0509, G2011

99291 0362T, 0373T, 0469T, 0543T-0544T, 0567T-0574T, 0580T, 0581T, 0582T,
15772, 15774, 20560-20561, 20700-20701, 36000, 36410-36415,
36591-36592, 36600, 43752-43753, 62329, 71045-71047, 80500-80502,
90846-90849, 90940, 92002-92014, 92227-92228, 92531-92532,
92953-92960, 93040-93042, 93318, 93355, 93561-93562, 93701, 93792,
93793, 94002-94004, 94375-94450, 94610, 94644, 94660-94662,
94760-94762, 94780-94781, 95851-95852, 96020, 96105, 96116,
96125-96130, 96132, 96136, 96138, 96146, 96156-96159, 96164-96168,
96360, 96365, 96369, 96372-96374, 96377, 96401-96406, 96409,

96413, 96416, 96420-96422, 96425-96440, 96446-96450, 96523, 97151,
97153-97158, 97169-97172, 97802-97804, 99091, 99172-99173, 99174,
99177, 99281-99285, 99408-99409, 99446-99449, 99451-99452,
99460-99462, 99474, 99477-99480, 99497-99498, 99605-99606, G0102,
G0245-G0246, G0250, G0270-G0271, G0380-G0384, G0396-G0397,
G0442-G0447, G0459, G0471, G0473, G0498, G0508-G0509, G2011

99292 0362T, 0373T, 0469T, 0543T-0544T, 0567T-0574T, 0580T, 0581T, 0582T,
20560-20561, 20700-20701, 36000, 36410, 36591-36592, 36600,
43752-43753, 62329, 71045-71047, 80500-80502, 90846-90849, 90940,
92002-92014, 92953-92960, 93040-93042, 93318, 93355, 93561-93562,
93792, 93793, 94002-94004, 94375-94450, 94660-94662, 94760-94762,
94780-94781, 95851-95852, 96020, 96116, 96127, 96156-96159,
96164-96168, 96523, 97151, 97153-97158, 97169-97172, 97802-97804,
99091, 99172-99173, 99174, 99177, 99281-99285, 99408-99409,
99446-99449, 99451-99452, 99474, 99497-99498, G0102,
G0245-G0246, G0250, G0270-G0271, G0396-G0397, G0442-G0447,
G0459, G0473, G2011

99304 0362T, 0373T, 0469T, 0567T-0574T, 0580T, 0581T, 0582T, 20560-20561,
20700-20701, 36591-36592, 43752, 80500-80502, 90863, 90940,
92002-92014, 92227-92228, 92531-92532, 93040-93042, 93792, 93793,
94002-94004, 94660-94662, 95851-95852, 96020, 96105, 96116,
96125-96130, 96132, 96136, 96138, 96146, 96156-96159, 96164-96168,
96360, 96365, 96369, 96372-96374, 96377, 96401-96406, 96409,
96413, 96416, 96420-96422, 96425-96440, 96446-96450, 96523, 97151,
97153-97158, 97169-97172, 97802-97804, 99091, 99172-99173, 99174,
99177, 99201-99215, 99218-99220, 99224-99233, 99281-99285,
99307-99310♦, 99315-99318, 99324-99328, 99334-99337,
99341-99350, 99354-99355, 99358-99359, 99408-99409, 99415-99416,
99446-99449, 99451-99452, 99455-99456, 99474, 99483, 99605-99606,
G0102, G0117-G0118, G0245-G0246, G0248, G0250, G0270-G0271,
G0380-G0384, G0396-G0397, G0406-G0408, G0424-G0427,
G0442-G0447, G0459, G0463, G0473, G0498, G0508-G0509, G2011

99305 0362T, 0373T, 0469T, 0567T-0574T, 0580T, 0581T, 0582T, 20560-20561,
20700-20701, 36591-36592, 43752, 62329, 80500-80502, 90863, 90940,
92002-92014, 92227-92228, 92531-92532, 93040-93042, 93792, 93793,
94002-94004, 94660-94662, 95851-95852, 96020, 96105, 96116,
96125-96130, 96132, 96136, 96138, 96146, 96156-96159, 96164-96168,
96360, 96365, 96369, 96372-96374, 96377, 96401-96406, 96409,
96413, 96416, 96420-96422, 96425-96440, 96446-96450, 96523, 97151,
97153-97158, 97169-97172, 97802-97804, 99091, 99172-99173, 99174,
99177, 99201-99215, 99218-99220, 99224-99233, 99281-99285,
99304♦, 99307-99310♦, 99315-99318, 99324-99328, 99334-99337,
99341-99350, 99354-99355, 99358-99359, 99408-99409, 99415-99416,
99446-99449, 99451-99452, 99455-99456, 99474, 99483, 99605-99606,
G0102, G0117-G0118, G0245-G0246, G0248, G0250, G0270-G0271,
G0380-G0384, G0396-G0397, G0406-G0408, G0424-G0427,
G0442-G0447, G0459, G0463, G0473, G0498, G0508-G0509, G2011

99306 0362T, 0373T, 0469T, 0567T-0574T, 0580T, 0581T, 0582T, 15774,
20560-20561, 20700-20701, 36591-36592, 43752, 62329, 80500-80502,
90863, 90940, 92002-92014, 92227-92228, 92531-92532, 93040-93042,
93792, 93793, 94002-94004, 94660-94662, 95851-95852, 96020, 96105,
96116, 96125-96130, 96132, 96136, 96138, 96146, 96156-96159,
96164-96168, 96360, 96365, 96369, 96372-96374, 96377, 96401-96406,
96409, 96413, 96416, 96420-96422, 96425-96440, 96446-96450, 96523,
97151, 97153-97158, 97169-97172, 97802-97804, 99091, 99172-99173,
99174, 99177, 99201-99215, 99218-99220, 99224-99233, 99281-99285,
99304-99305♦, 99307-99310♦, 99315-99318, 99324-99328,
99334-99337, 99341-99350, 99354-99355, 99358-99359, 99408-99409,
99415-99416, 99446-99449, 99451-99452, 99455-99456, 99474, 99483,
99605-99606, G0102, G0117-G0118, G0245-G0246, G0248, G0250,

G0270-G0271, G0380-G0384, G0396-G0397, G0406-G0408,
G0424-G0427, G0442-G0447, G0459, G0463, G0473, G0498,
G0508-G0509, G2011

99307 0362T, 0373T, 0469T, 0567T-0574T, 0580T, 0581T, 0582T, 20560-20561,
36591-36592, 43752, 80500-80502, 90863, 90940, 92002-92014,
92227-92228, 92531-92532, 93040-93042, 93792, 93793, 94002-94004,
94660-94662, 95851-95852, 96020, 96105, 96116, 96125-96130, 96132,
96136, 96138, 96146, 96156-96159, 96164-96168, 96360, 96365,
96369, 96372-96374, 96377, 96401-96406, 96409, 96413, 96416,
96420-96422, 96425-96440, 96446-96450, 96523, 97151, 97153-97158,
97169-97172, 97802-97804, 99091, 99172-99173, 99174, 99177,
99354-99355, 99358-99359, 99408-99409, 99415-99416, 99446-99449,
99451-99452, 99474, 99605-99606, G0102, G0117-G0118,
G0245-G0246, G0248, G0250, G0270-G0271, G0396-G0397,
G0406-G0408, G0425-G0427, G0442-G0447, G0459, G0473, G0498,
G0508-G0509, G2011

99308 0362T, 0373T, 0469T, 0567T-0574T, 0580T, 0581T, 0582T, 20560-20561,
20701, 36591-36592, 43752, 80500-80502, 90863, 90940, 92002-92014,
92227-92228, 92531-92532, 93040-93042, 93792, 93793, 94002-94004,
94660-94662, 95851-95852, 96020, 96105, 96116, 96125-96130, 96132,
96136, 96138, 96146, 96156-96159, 96164-96168, 96360, 96365,
96369, 96372-96374, 96377, 96401-96406, 96409, 96413, 96416,
96420-96422, 96425-96440, 96446-96450, 96523, 97151, 97153-97158,
97169-97172, 97802-97804, 99091, 99172-99173, 99174, 99177,
99307♦, 99354-99355, 99358-99359, 99408-99409, 99415-99416,
99446-99449, 99451-99452, 99474, 99605-99606, G0102,
G0117-G0118, G0245-G0246, G0248, G0250, G0270-G0271,
G0396-G0397, G0406-G0408, G0425-G0427, G0442-G0447, G0459,
G0473, G0498, G0508-G0509, G2011

99309 0362T, 0373T, 0469T, 0567T-0574T, 0580T, 0581T, 0582T, 20560-20561,
20700-20701, 36591-36592, 43752, 80500-80502, 90863, 90940,
92002-92014, 92227-92228, 92531-92532, 93040-93042, 93532, 93792,
93793, 94002-94004, 94660-94662, 95851-95852, 96020, 96105, 96116,
96125-96130, 96132, 96136, 96138, 96146, 96156-96159, 96164-96168,
96360, 96365, 96369, 96372-96374, 96377, 96401-96406, 96409,
96413, 96416, 96420-96422, 96425-96440, 96446-96450, 96523, 97151,
97153-97158, 97169-97172, 97802-97804, 99091, 99172-99173, 99174,
99177, 99307-99308♦, 99315♦, 99318, 99354-99355, 99358-99359,
99408-99409, 99415-99416, 99446-99449, 99451-99452, 99474,
99605-99606, G0102, G0117-G0118, G0245-G0246, G0248, G0250,
G0270-G0271, G0396-G0397, G0406-G0408, G0425-G0427,
G0442-G0447, G0459, G0473, G0498, G0508-G0509, G2011

99310 0362T, 0373T, 0469T, 0567T-0574T, 0580T, 0581T, 0582T, 20560-20561,
20700-20701, 36591-36592, 43752, 62329, 80500-80502, 90863, 90940,
92002-92014, 92227-92228, 92531-92532, 93040-93042, 93792, 93793,
94002-94004, 94660-94662, 95851-95852, 96020, 96105, 96116,
96125-96130, 96132, 96136, 96138, 96146, 96156-96159, 96164-96168,
96360, 96365, 96369, 96372-96374, 96377, 96401-96406, 96409,
96413, 96416, 96420-96422, 96425-96440, 96446-96450, 96523, 97151,
97153-97158, 97169-97172, 97802-97804, 99091, 99172-99173, 99174,
99177, 99307-99309♦, 99315-99318, 99354-99355, 99358-99359,
99408-99409, 99415-99416, 99446-99449, 99451-99452, 99474,
99605-99606, G0102, G0117-G0118, G0245-G0246, G0248, G0250,
G0270-G0271, G0396-G0397, G0406-G0408, G0425-G0427,
G0442-G0447, G0459, G0473, G0498, G0508-G0509, G2011

99315 0362T, 0373T, 0469T, 0567T-0574T, 0580T, 0581T, 0582T, 20560-20561,
20701, 36591-36592, 43752, 90863, 90940, 92002-92014, 92227-92228,
92531-92532, 93792, 93793, 94002-94004, 94660-94662, 95851-95852,
96020, 96105, 96116, 96125-96130, 96132, 96136, 96138, 96146,

96156-96159, 96164-96168, 96360, 96365, 96369, 96372-96374, 96377, 96401-96406, 96409, 96413, 96416, 96420-96422, 96425-96440, 96446-96450, 96523, 97151, 97153-97158, 97169-97172, 97802-97804, 99091, 99172-99173, 99174, 99177, 99307-99308♦, 99354-99359, 99408-99409, 99415-99416, 99446-99449, 99451-99452, 99474, 99605-99606, G0102, G0117-G0118, G0245-G0246, G0248, G0250, G0270-G0271, G0396-G0397, G0442-G0447, G0459, G0473, G0498, G2011

99316 0362T, 0373T, 0469T, 0567T-0574T, 0580T, 0581T, 0582T, 20560-20561, 20700-20701, 36591-36592, 43752, 90863, 90940, 92002-92014, 92227-92228, 92531-92532, 93792, 93793, 94002-94004, 94660-94662, 95851-95852, 96020, 96105, 96116, 96125-96130, 96132, 96136, 96138, 96146, 96156-96159, 96164-96168, 96360, 96365, 96369, 96372-96374, 96377, 96401-96406, 96409, 96413, 96416, 96420-96422, 96425-96440, 96446-96450, 96523, 97151, 97153-97158, 97169-97172, 97802-97804, 99091, 99172-99173, 99174, 99177, 99307-99309♦, 99315♦, 99318, 99354-99359, 99408-99409, 99415-99416, 99446-99449, 99451-99452, 99474, 99605-99606, G0102, G0117-G0118, G0245-G0246, G0248, G0250, G0270-G0271, G0396-G0397, G0442-G0447, G0459, G0473, G0498, G2011

99318 0362T, 0373T, 0469T, 36591-36592, 43752, 80500-80502, 90863, 90940, 92002-92014, 92227-92228, 92531-92532, 93040-93042, 93792, 93793, 94002-94004, 94660-94662, 95851-95852, 96020, 96105, 96116, 96125-96130, 96132, 96136, 96138, 96146, 96156-96159, 96164-96168, 96360, 96365, 96369, 96372-96374, 96377, 96401-96406, 96409, 96413, 96416, 96420-96422, 96425-96440, 96446-96450, 96523, 97151, 97153-97158, 97169-97172, 97802-97804, 99091, 99172-99173, 99174, 99177, 99307-99308, 99315, 99354-99355, 99358-99359, 99408-99409, 99415-99416, 99446-99449, 99451-99452, 99463♦, 99474, 99605-99606, G0102, G0117-G0118, G0245-G0246, G0248, G0250, G0270-G0271, G0396-G0397, G0442-G0447, G0459, G0473, G0498, G2011

99324 0362T, 0373T, 0469T, 36591-36592, 43752, 80500-80502, 90863, 92002-92014, 92227-92228, 92531-92532, 93040-93042, 93561-93562, 93792, 93793, 94002-94004, 94660-94662, 95851-95852, 96020, 96105, 96116, 96125, 96130, 96132, 96136, 96138, 96146, 96156-96159, 96164-96168, 96360, 96365, 96369, 96372-96374, 96377, 96401-96406, 96409, 96413, 96416, 96420-96422, 96425-96440, 96446-96450, 96523, 97151, 97153-97158, 97169-97172, 97802-97804, 99091, 99172-99173, 99174, 99177, 99408-99409, 99446-99449, 99451-99452, 99474, 99605-99606, G0102, G0117-G0118, G0179-G0180, G0245-G0246, G0248, G0250, G0270-G0271, G0396-G0397, G0442-G0447, G0459, G0473, G0498, G2011

99325 0362T, 0373T, 0469T, 36591-36592, 43752, 80500-80502, 90863, 92002-92014, 92227-92228, 92531-92532, 93040-93042, 93561-93562, 93792, 93793, 94002-94004, 94660-94662, 95851-95852, 96020, 96105, 96116, 96125, 96130, 96132, 96136, 96138, 96146, 96156-96159, 96164-96168, 96360, 96365, 96369, 96372-96374, 96377, 96401-96406, 96409, 96413, 96416, 96420-96422, 96425-96440, 96446-96450, 96523, 97151, 97153-97158, 97169-97172, 97802-97804, 99091, 99172-99173, 99174, 99177, 99324, 99408-99409, 99446-99449, 99451-99452, 99463♦, 99474, 99605-99606, G0102, G0117-G0118, G0179-G0180, G0245-G0246, G0248, G0250, G0270-G0271, G0396-G0397, G0442-G0447, G0459, G0473, G0498, G2011

99326 0362T, 0373T, 0469T, 36591-36592, 43752, 80500-80502, 90863, 92002-92014, 92227-92228, 92531-92532, 93040-93042, 93561-93562, 93792, 93793, 94002-94004, 94660-94662, 95851-95852, 96020, 96105, 96116, 96125, 96130, 96132, 96136, 96138, 96146, 96156-96159, 96164-96168, 96360, 96365, 96369, 96372-96374, 96377, 96401-96406,

96409, 96413, 96416, 96420-96422, 96425-96440, 96446-96450, 96523, 97151, 97153-97158, 97169-97172, 97802-97804, 99091, 99172-99173, 99174, 99177, 99324-99325, 99408-99409, 99446-99449, 99451-99452, 99463♦, 99474, 99605-99606, G0102, G0117-G0118, G0179-G0180, G0245-G0246, G0248, G0250, G0270-G0271, G0396-G0397, G0442-G0447, G0459, G0473, G0498, G2011

99327 0362T, 0373T, 0469T, 36591-36592, 43752, 80500-80502, 90863, 92002-92014, 92227-92228, 92531-92532, 93040-93042, 93561-93562, 93792, 93793, 94002-94004, 94660-94662, 95851-95852, 96020, 96105, 96116, 96125, 96130, 96132, 96136, 96138, 96146, 96156-96159, 96164-96168, 96360, 96365, 96369, 96372-96374, 96377, 96401-96406, 96409, 96413, 96416, 96420-96422, 96425-96440, 96446-96450, 96523, 97151, 97153-97158, 97169-97172, 97802-97804, 99091, 99172-99173, 99174, 99177, 99324-99326, 99408-99409, 99446-99449, 99451-99452, 99463♦, 99474, 99605-99606, G0102, G0117-G0118, G0179-G0180, G0245-G0246, G0248, G0250, G0270-G0271, G0396-G0397, G0442-G0447, G0459, G0473, G0498, G2011

99328 0362T, 0373T, 0469T, 36591-36592, 43752, 80500-80502, 90863, 92002-92014, 92227-92228, 92531-92532, 93040-93042, 93561-93562, 93792, 93793, 94002-94004, 94660-94662, 95851-95852, 96020, 96105, 96116, 96125, 96130, 96132, 96136, 96138, 96146, 96156-96159, 96164-96168, 96360, 96365, 96369, 96372-96374, 96377, 96401-96406, 96409, 96413, 96416, 96420-96422, 96425-96440, 96446-96450, 96523, 97151, 97153-97158, 97169-97172, 97802-97804, 99091, 99172-99173, 99174, 99177, 99324-99327, 99408-99409, 99446-99449, 99451-99452, 99463♦, 99474, 99605-99606, G0102, G0117-G0118, G0179-G0180, G0245-G0246, G0248, G0250, G0270-G0271, G0396-G0397, G0442-G0447, G0459, G0473, G0498, G2011

99334 0362T, 0373T, 0469T, 0567T-0574T, 0580T, 0581T, 0582T, 20560-20561, 36591-36592, 43752, 80500-80502, 90863, 92002-92014, 92227-92228, 92531-92532, 93040-93042, 93561-93562, 93792, 93793, 94002-94004, 94660-94662, 95851-95852, 96020, 96105, 96116, 96125, 96130, 96132, 96136, 96138, 96146, 96156-96159, 96164-96168, 96360, 96365, 96369, 96372-96374, 96377, 96401-96406, 96409, 96413, 96416, 96420-96422, 96425-96440, 96446-96450, 96523, 97151, 97153-97158, 97169-97172, 97802-97804, 99091, 99172-99173, 99174, 99177, 99408-99409, 99446-99449, 99451-99452, 99474, 99605-99606, G0102, G0117-G0118, G0179-G0180, G0245-G0246, G0248, G0250, G0270-G0271, G0396-G0397, G0442-G0447, G0459, G0473, G0498, G2011

99335 0362T, 0373T, 0469T, 0566T-0574T, 0580T, 0581T, 0582T, 20560-20561, 20700-20701, 36591-36592, 43752, 80500-80502, 90863, 92002-92014, 92227-92228, 92531-92532, 93040-93042, 93561-93562, 93792, 93793, 94002-94004, 94660-94662, 95851-95852, 96020, 96105, 96116, 96125, 96130, 96132, 96136, 96138, 96146, 96156-96159, 96164-96168, 96360, 96365, 96369, 96372-96374, 96377, 96401-96406, 96409, 96413, 96416, 96420-96422, 96425-96440, 96446-96450, 96523, 97151, 97153-97158, 97169-97172, 97802-97804, 99091, 99172-99173, 99174, 99177, 99334, 99408-99409, 99446-99449, 99451-99452, 99463♦, 99474, 99605-99606, G0102, G0117-G0118, G0179-G0180, G0245-G0246, G0248, G0250, G0270-G0271, G0396-G0397, G0442-G0447, G0459, G0473, G0498, G2011

99336 0362T, 0373T, 0469T, 0566T-0574T, 0580T, 0581T, 0582T, 15774, 20560-20561, 20700-20701, 36591-36592, 43752, 62329, 80500-80502, 90863, 92002-92014, 92227-92228, 92531-92532, 93040-93042, 93561-93562, 93792, 93793, 94002-94004, 94660-94662, 95851-95852, 96020, 96105, 96116, 96125, 96130, 96132, 96136, 96138, 96146, 96156-96159, 96164-96168, 96360, 96365, 96369, 96372-96374, 96377, 96401-96406, 96409, 96413, 96416, 96420-96422, 96425-96440,

96446-96450, 96523, 97151, 97153-97158, 97169-97172, 97802-97804, 99091, 99172-99173, 99174, 99177, 99334-99335, 99408-99409, 99446-99449, 99451-99452, 99463♦, 99474, 99605-99606, G0102, G0117-G0118, G0179-G0180, G0245-G0246, G0248, G0250, G0270-G0271, G0396-G0397, G0442-G0447, G0459, G0473, G0498, G2011

99337 0362T, 0373T, 0469T, 0566T-0574T, 0580T, 0581T, 0582T, 15772, 15774, 20560-20561, 20700-20701, 36591-36592, 43752, 62329, 80500-80502, 90863, 92002-92014, 92227-92228, 92531-92532, 93040-93042, 93561-93562, 93792, 93793, 94002-94004, 94660-94662, 95851-95852, 96020, 96105, 96116, 96125, 96130, 96132, 96136, 96138, 96146, 96156-96159, 96164-96168, 96360, 96365, 96369, 96372-96374, 96377, 96401-96406, 96409, 96413, 96416, 96420-96422, 96425-96440, 96446-96450, 96523, 97151, 97153-97158, 97169-97172, 97802-97804, 99091, 99172-99173, 99174, 99177, 99334-99336, 99408-99409, 99446-99449, 99451-99452, 99463♦, 99474, 99605-99606, G0102, G0117-G0118, G0179-G0180, G0245-G0246, G0248, G0250, G0270-G0271, G0396-G0397, G0442-G0447, G0459, G0473, G0498, G2011

99341 0362T, 0373T, 0469T, 36591-36592, 43752, 80500-80502, 90863, 92002-92014, 92227-92228, 92531-92532, 93040-93042, 93561-93562, 93792, 93793, 94002-94004, 94660-94662, 95851-95852, 96020, 96105, 96116, 96125, 96130, 96132, 96136, 96138, 96146, 96156-96159, 96164-96168, 96360, 96365, 96369, 96372-96374, 96377, 96401-96406, 96409, 96413, 96416, 96420-96422, 96425-96440, 96446-96450, 96523, 97151, 97153-97158, 97169-97172, 97802-97804, 99091, 99172-99173, 99174, 99177, 99408-99409, 99446-99449, 99451-99452, 99474, 99605-99606, G0102, G0117-G0118, G0179-G0180, G0245-G0246, G0248, G0250, G0270-G0271, G0396-G0397, G0442-G0447, G0459, G0473, G0498, G2011

99342 0362T, 0373T, 0469T, 36591-36592, 43752, 80500-80502, 90863, 92002-92014, 92227-92228, 92531-92532, 93040-93042, 93561-93562, 93792, 93793, 94002-94004, 94660-94662, 95851-95852, 96020, 96105, 96116, 96125, 96130, 96132, 96136, 96138, 96146, 96156-96159, 96164-96168, 96360, 96365, 96369, 96372-96374, 96377, 96401-96406, 96409, 96413, 96416, 96420-96422, 96425-96440, 96446-96450, 96523, 97151, 97153-97158, 97169-97172, 97802-97804, 99091, 99172-99173, 99174, 99177, 99341, 99408-99409, 99446-99449, 99451-99452, 99463♦, 99474, 99605-99606, G0102, G0117-G0118, G0179-G0180, G0245-G0246, G0248, G0250, G0270-G0271, G0396-G0397, G0442-G0447, G0459, G0473, G0498, G2011

99343 0362T, 0373T, 0469T, 36591-36592, 43752, 80500-80502, 90863, 92002-92014, 92227-92228, 92531-92532, 93040-93042, 93561-93562, 93792, 93793, 94002-94004, 94660-94662, 95851-95852, 96020, 96105, 96116, 96125, 96130, 96132, 96136, 96138, 96146, 96156-96159, 96164-96168, 96360, 96365, 96369, 96372-96374, 96377, 96401-96406, 96409, 96413, 96416, 96420-96422, 96425-96440, 96446-96450, 96523, 97151, 97153-97158, 97169-97172, 97802-97804, 99091, 99172-99173, 99174, 99177, 99341-99342, 99408-99409, 99446-99449, 99451-99452, 99463♦, 99474, 99605-99606, G0102, G0117-G0118, G0179-G0180, G0245-G0246, G0248, G0250, G0270-G0271, G0396-G0397, G0442-G0447, G0459, G0473, G0498, G2011

99344 0362T, 0373T, 0469T, 36591-36592, 43752, 80500-80502, 90863, 92002-92014, 92227-92228, 92531-92532, 93561-93562, 93792, 93793, 94002-94004, 94660-94662, 95851-95852, 96020, 96105, 96116, 96125, 96130, 96132, 96136, 96138, 96146, 96156-96159, 96164-96168, 96360, 96365, 96369, 96372-96374, 96377, 96401-96406, 96409, 96413, 96416, 96420-96422, 96425-96440, 96446-96450, 96523, 97151, 97153-97158, 97169-97172, 97802-97804, 99091, 99172-99173, 99174,

99177, 99341-99343, 99408-99409, 99446-99449, 99451-99452, 99474, 99605-99606, G0102, G0117-G0118, G0179-G0180, G0245-G0246, G0248, G0250, G0270-G0271, G0396-G0397, G0442-G0447, G0459, G0473, G0498, G2011

99345 0362T, 0373T, 0469T, 36591-36592, 43752, 80500-80502, 90863, 92002-92014, 92227-92228, 92531-92532, 93561-93562, 93792, 93793, 94002-94004, 94660-94662, 95851-95852, 96020, 96105, 96116, 96125, 96130, 96132, 96136, 96138, 96146, 96156-96159, 96164-96168, 96360, 96365, 96369, 96372-96374, 96377, 96401-96406, 96409, 96413, 96416, 96420-96422, 96425-96440, 96446-96450, 96523, 97151, 97153-97158, 97169-97172, 97802-97804, 99091, 99172-99173, 99174, 99177, 99341-99344, 99408-99409, 99446-99449, 99451-99452, 99474, 99605-99606, G0102, G0117-G0118, G0179-G0180, G0245-G0246, G0248, G0250, G0270-G0271, G0396-G0397, G0442-G0447, G0459, G0473, G0498, G2011

99347 0362T, 0373T, 0469T, 0566T-0574T, 0580T, 0581T, 0582T, 20560-20561, 36591-36592, 43752, 80500-80502, 90863, 92002-92014, 92227-92228, 92531-92532, 93040-93042, 93561-93562, 93792, 93793, 94002-94004, 94660-94662, 95851-95852, 96020, 96105, 96116, 96125, 96130, 96132, 96136, 96138, 96146, 96156-96159, 96164-96168, 96360, 96365, 96369, 96372-96374, 96377, 96401-96406, 96409, 96413, 96416, 96420-96422, 96425-96440, 96446-96450, 96523, 97151, 97153-97158, 97169-97172, 97802-97804, 99091, 99172-99173, 99174, 99177, 99408-99409, 99446-99449, 99451-99452, 99474, 99605-99606, G0102, G0117-G0118, G0179-G0180, G0245-G0246, G0248, G0250, G0270-G0271, G0396-G0397, G0442-G0447, G0459, G0473, G0498, G2011

99348 0362T, 0373T, 0469T, 0566T-0574T, 0580T, 0581T, 0582T, 20560-20561, 20700-20701, 36591-36592, 43752, 80500-80502, 90863, 92002-92014, 92227-92228, 92531-92532, 93040-93042, 93561-93562, 93792, 93793, 94002-94004, 94660-94662, 95851-95852, 96020, 96105, 96116, 96125, 96130, 96132, 96136, 96138, 96146, 96156-96159, 96164-96168, 96360, 96365, 96369, 96372-96374, 96377, 96401-96406, 96409, 96413, 96416, 96420-96422, 96425-96440, 96446-96450, 96523, 97151, 97153-97158, 97169-97172, 97802-97804, 99091, 99172-99173, 99174, 99177, 99347, 99408-99409, 99446-99449, 99451-99452, 99463♦, 99474, 99605-99606, G0102, G0117-G0118, G0179-G0180, G0245-G0246, G0248, G0250, G0270-G0271, G0396-G0397, G0442-G0447, G0459, G0473, G0498, G2011

99349 0362T, 0373T, 0469T, 0566T-0574T, 0580T, 0581T, 0582T, 20560-20561, 20700-20701, 36591-36592, 43752, 62329, 80500-80502, 90863, 92002-92014, 92227-92228, 92531-92532, 93040-93042, 93561-93562, 93792, 93793, 94002-94004, 94660-94662, 95851-95852, 96020, 96105, 96116, 96125, 96130, 96132, 96136, 96138, 96146, 96156-96159, 96164-96168, 96360, 96365, 96369, 96372-96374, 96377, 96401-96406, 96409, 96413, 96416, 96420-96422, 96425-96440, 96446-96450, 96523, 97151, 97153-97158, 97169-97172, 97802-97804, 99091, 99172-99173, 99174, 99177, 99347-99348, 99408-99409, 99446-99449, 99451-99452, 99463♦, 99474, 99605-99606, G0102, G0117-G0118, G0179-G0180, G0245-G0246, G0248, G0250, G0270-G0271, G0396-G0397, G0442-G0447, G0459, G0473, G0498, G2011

99350 0362T, 0373T, 0469T, 0566T-0574T, 0580T, 0581T, 0582T, 15772, 15774, 20560-20561, 20700-20701, 36591-36592, 43752, 62329, 80500-80502, 90863, 92002-92014, 92227-92228, 92531-92532, 93561-93562, 93792, 93793, 94002-94004, 94660-94662, 95851-95852, 96020, 96105, 96116, 96125, 96130, 96132, 96136, 96138, 96146, 96156-96159, 96164-96168, 96360, 96365, 96369, 96372-96374, 96377, 96401-96406, 96409, 96413, 96416, 96420-96422, 96425-96440, 96446-96450, 96523, 97151, 97153-97158, 97169-97172, 97802-97804, 99091, 99172-99173,

99174, 99177, 99347-99349, 99408-99409, 99446-99449, 99451-99452, 99474, 99605-99606, G0102, G0117-G0118, G0179-G0180, G0245-G0246, G0248, G0250, G0270-G0271, G0396-G0397, G0442-G0447, G0459, G0473, G0498, G2011

99354 0362T, 0373T, 0469T, 36591-36592, 43752, 90940, 92531-92532, 93561-93562, 93792, 93793, 94002-94004, 94660-94662, 96020, 96105, 96116, 96125, 96130, 96132, 96136, 96138, 96146, 96156-96159, 96164-96168, 96523, 97151, 97153-97158, 99091, 99172-99173, 99174, 99177, 99408-99409, 99415-99416, 99446-99449, 99451-99452, 99463❖, 99474, G0102, G0396-G0397, G0406-G0408❖, G0425-G0427❖, G0442-G0447, G0459❖, G0473, G0508-G0509❖, G2011

99355 0362T, 0373T, 0469T, 36591-36592, 43752, 92531-92532, 93561-93562, 93792, 93793, 94002-94004, 94660-94662, 96020, 96105, 96116, 96125, 96130, 96132, 96136, 96138, 96146, 96156-96159, 96164-96168, 96523, 97151, 97153-97158, 99091, 99172-99173, 99174, 99177, 99408-99409, 99415-99416, 99446-99449, 99451-99452, 99463❖, 99474, G0102, G0396-G0397, G0406-G0408❖, G0425-G0427❖, G0442-G0447, G0459❖, G0473, G0508-G0509❖, G2011

99356 0362T, 0373T, 0469T, 36591-36592, 43752, 90940, 92531-92532, 93792, 93793, 94002-94004, 94660-94662, 96020, 96105, 96116, 96125-96130, 96132, 96136, 96138, 96146, 96156-96159, 96164-96168, 96523, 97151, 97153-97158, 99091, 99172-99173, 99174, 99177, 99408-99409, 99446-99449, 99451-99452, 99463❖, 99474, G0102, G0396-G0397, G0442-G0447, G0473, G2011

99357 0362T, 0373T, 0469T, 36591-36592, 43752, 92531-92532, 93792, 93793, 94002-94004, 94660-94662, 96020, 96105, 96116, 96125-96130, 96132, 96136, 96138, 96146, 96156-96159, 96164-96168, 96523, 97151, 97153-97158, 99091, 99172-99173, 99174, 99177, 99408-99409, 99446-99449, 99451-99452, 99463❖, 99474, G0102, G0396-G0397, G0442-G0447, G0473, G2011

99358 0362T, 0373T, 0469T, 36591-36592, 43752, 90940, 92531-92532, 93561-93562, 93792, 93793, 94002-94004, 94660-94662, 96020, 96105, 96116, 96125-96130, 96132, 96136, 96138, 96146, 96156-96159, 96164-96168, 97151, 97153-97158, 98970-98972, 99091, 99172-99173, 99174, 99177, 99339-99340, 99366-99368, 99374-99375, 99377-99380, 99415-99416, 99421-99423, 99446-99449, 99452, 99474, G0102, G0396-G0397, G0406-G0408❖, G0425-G0427❖, G0442-G0447, G0459❖, G0473, G2011, G2061-G2063

99359 0362T, 0373T, 0469T, 36591-36592, 43752, 92531-92532, 93561-93562, 93792, 93793, 94002-94004, 94660-94662, 96020, 96105, 96116, 96125-96130, 96132, 96136, 96138, 96146, 96156-96159, 96164-96168, 97151, 97153-97158, 98970-98972, 99091, 99172-99173, 99174, 99177, 99339-99340, 99366-99368, 99374-99375, 99377-99380, 99415-99416, 99421-99423, 99446-99449, 99452, 99474, G0102, G0396-G0397, G0406-G0408❖, G0425-G0427❖, G0442-G0447, G0459❖, G0473, G2011, G2061-G2063

99406 0362T, 0373T, 0469T, 36591-36592, 92531-92532, 93792, 93793, 94002-94004, 94660-94662, 96105, 96125-96130, 96132, 96136, 96138, 96146, 96164-96165, 96170, 96523, 97151, 97153-97158, 99091, 99172-99173, 99174, 99177, 99408-99409, 99446-99449, 99451-99452, 99474, G0396-G0397, G0406-G0408❖, G0425-G0427❖, G0442-G0444, G0459❖, G0508-G0509❖, G2011

99407 0362T, 0373T, 0469T, 36591-36592, 92531-92532, 93792, 93793, 94002-94004, 94660-94662, 96105, 96125-96130, 96132, 96136, 96138, 96146, 96159, 96164-96165, 96523, 97151, 97153-97158, 99091, 99172-99173, 99174, 99177, 99406, 99408-99409, 99446-99449, 99451-99452, 99474, G0396-G0397, G0406-G0408❖, G0425-G0427❖, G0442-G0444, G0459❖, G0508-G0509❖, G2011

99408 0362T, 0373T, 0469T, 36591-36592, 93792, 93793, 94002-94004, 94660-94662, 96159, 96164-96165, 96168-96171, 96523, 97151, 97153-97158, 99091, 99172-99173, 99174, 99177, 99358-99359, 99446-99449, 99451-99452, 99474, G0406-G0408❖, G0425-G0427❖, G0444, G0459❖, G0508-G0509❖

99409 0362T, 0373T, 0469T, 36591-36592, 93792, 93793, 94002-94004, 94660-94662, 96159, 96164-96165, 96168-96171, 96523, 97151, 97153-97158, 99091, 99172-99173, 99174, 99177, 99358-99359, 99408, 99446-99449, 99451-99452, 99474, G0406-G0408❖, G0425-G0427❖, G0444, G0459❖, G0508-G0509❖

99415 0362T, 0373T, 0469T, 36591-36592, 43752, 90940, 92531-92532, 93561-93562, 93792, 93793, 94002-94004, 94660-94662, 96020, 96105, 96116, 96125, 96130, 96132, 96136, 96138, 96146, 96156-96159, 96164-96168, 96523, 97151, 97153-97158, 99091, 99172-99173, 99174, 99177, 99408-99409, 99446-99449, 99451-99452, G0102, G0396-G0397, G0442-G0447, G0473, G2011

99416 0362T, 0373T, 0469T, 36591-36592, 43752, 92531-92532, 93561-93562, 93792, 93793, 94002-94004, 94660-94662, 96020, 96105, 96116, 96125, 96130, 96132, 96136, 96138, 96146, 96156-96159, 96164-96168, 96523, 97151, 97153-97158, 99091, 99172-99173, 99174, 99177, 99408-99409, 99446-99449, 99451-99452, G0102, G0396-G0397, G0442-G0447, G0473, G2011

99417 No CCI edits apply to this code.

99421 0362T, 0373T, 0469T, 36591-36592, 93792, 93793, 94002-94004, 94660-94662, 96127, 96523, 97151, 97153-97158, 98966, 98970-98972, 99172-99173, 99174, 99177, 99211, 99441, 99474, G0250, G0378-G0379, G2061-G2063, Q3014

99422 0362T, 0373T, 0469T, 36591-36592, 93792, 93793, 94002-94004, 94660-94662, 96127, 96523, 97151, 97153-97158, 98966-98967, 98970-98972, 99172-99173, 99174, 99177, 99201, 99211-99212, 99421, 99441-99442, 99446, 99474, G0250, G0378-G0379, G2061-G2063, Q3014

99423 0362T, 0373T, 0469T, 36591-36592, 93792, 93793, 94002-94004, 94660-94662, 96127, 96523, 97151, 97153-97158, 98966-98968, 98970-98972, 99172-99173, 99174, 99177, 99201, 99211-99212, 99241, 99421-99422, 99441-99443, 99446-99447, 99451-99452, 99474, 99490, G0250, G0378-G0379, G0406, G2061-G2063, Q3014

99439 No CCI edits apply to this code.

99441 0362T, 0373T, 0469T, 36591-36592, 93792, 93793, 94002-94004, 94660-94662, 96127, 96523, 97151, 97153-97158, 98970-98972, 99091, 99172-99173, 99174, 99177, 99474, G0250, G2061-G2063

99442 0362T, 0373T, 0469T, 36591-36592, 93792, 93793, 94002-94004, 94660-94662, 96127, 96523, 97151, 97153-97158, 98970-98972, 99091, 99172-99173, 99174, 99177, 99421, 99474, G0250, G2061-G2063

99443 0362T, 0373T, 0469T, 36591-36592, 93792, 93793, 94002-94004, 94660-94662, 96127, 96523, 97151, 97153-97158, 98970-98972, 99091, 99172-99173, 99174, 99177, 99421-99422, 99446-99447, 99474, G0250, G2061-G2063

99487 0362T, 0373T, 0405T, 0469T, 0488T, 36591-36592, 93792, 93793, 94002-94004, 94660-94662, 96127, 96523, 97151, 97153-97158, 98960-98968, 98970-98972, 99071, 99078-99080, 99091, 99172-99173, 99174, 99177, 99339-99340, 99358-99359, 99366-99368, 99374-99375, 99377-99380, 99421-99423, 99441-99443, 99490-99491, 99495-99496, 99605-99607, G0506, G0511

99489 0362T, 0373T, 0469T, 0488T, 36591-36592, 93792, 93793, 94002-94004, 94660-94662, 96127, 96523, 97151, 97153-97158, 98960-98968, 99071, 99078-99080, 99091, 99172-99173, 99174, 99177, 99339-99340,

99358-99359, 99366-99368, 99374-99375, 99377-99380, 99421-99423, 99441-99443, 99474, 99495-99496, 99605-99607

99490 0362T, 0373T, 0405T✦, 0469T, 0488T, 36591-36592, 93792, 93793, 94002-94004, 94660-94662, 96127, 96523, 97151-97158, 98960-98968, 98970-98972, 99071, 99078-99080, 99091, 99172-99173, 99174, 99177, 99339-99340, 99358-99359, 99366-99368, 99374-99375, 99377-99380, 99421-99422, 99441-99443, 99473-99474, 99495-99496, 99605-99607

99491 0362T, 0373T, 0405T✦, 0469T, 0488T, 36591-36592, 93792, 93793, 94002-94004, 94660-94662, 96127, 96523, 97151-97154, 97156-97158, 98960-98968, 98970-98972, 99071, 99078-99080, 99091, 99172-99173, 99174, 99177, 99358-99359, 99366-99368, 99374-99375, 99377-99380, 99421-99423, 99441-99443, 99473-99474, 99489-99490, 99495-99496, 99605-99607

99495 0362T, 0373T, 0469T, 0488T, 36591-36592, 93792, 93793, 94002-94004, 94660-94662, 96127, 96523, 97151, 97153-97158, 98960-98968, 98970-98972, 99071, 99078-99080, 99091, 99172-99173, 99174, 99177, 99339-99340, 99358-99359, 99366-99368, 99374-99375, 99377-99380, 99421-99423, 99441-99443, 99473-99474, 99492-99493✦, 99605-99607, G0175, G0181-G0182, G0406-G0408✦, G0425-G0427✦, G0459✦, G0508-G0509✦, G0512✦

99496 0362T, 0373T, 0469T, 0488T, 36591-36592, 93792, 93793, 94002-94004, 94660-94662, 96127, 96523, 97151, 97153-97158, 98960-98968, 98970-98972, 99071, 99078-99080, 99091, 99172-99173, 99174, 99177, 99339-99340, 99358-99359, 99366-99368, 99374-99375, 99377-99380, 99421-99423, 99441-99443, 99473-99474, 99495✦, 99605-99607, G0175, G0181-G0182, G0406-G0408✦, G0425-G0427✦, G0459✦, G0508-G0509✦

99497 0362T, 0373T, 0469T, 11719✦, 36591-36592, 43752, 80500-80502, 90863, 90940, 92002-92014, 92227-92228, 92531-92532, 93561-93562, 93792, 93793, 94002-94004, 94660-94662, 95851-95852, 96020, 96105, 96116, 96125, 96130, 96132, 96136, 96138, 96146, 96156-96159, 96164-96171, 96523, 97151, 97153-97158, 97169-97172, 97802-97804, 99091, 99172-99173, 99174, 99177, 99408-99409, 99446-99449, 99451-99452, 99474, 99605-99606, G0102, G0117-G0118, G0245-G0246, G0248, G0250, G0270-G0271, G0337✦, G0396-G0397, G0442-G0447, G0459, G0473, G2011

99498 0469T, 36591-36592, 93792, 93793, 94002-94004, 94660-94662, 96523, 99091, 99172-99173, 99174, 99177, 99474

99512 36591-36592, 96523

99601 36591-36592, 96523

99602 36591-36592, 96523

G0102 36591-36592, 96523, 99446-99449, 99451-99452, 99463

G0168 0213T, 0216T, 0228T, 0230T, 11000-11006, 11042-11047, 11900-11901, 13102, 13122, 13133, 13153, 36000, 36400-36410, 36420-36430, 36440, 36591-36592, 36600, 36640, 43752, 51701-51703, 62320-62327, 64400, 64405-64408, 64415-64435, 64445-64454, 64461-64463, 64479-64505, 64510-64530, 92012-92014, 93000-93010, 93040-93042, 93318, 93355, 94002, 94200, 94250, 94680-94690, 94770, 95812-95816, 95819, 95822, 95829, 95955, 96360-96368, 96372, 96374-96377, 96523, 97597-97598, 97602, 99155, 99156, 99157, 99211-99223, 99231-99255, 99291-99292, 99304-99310, 99315-99316, 99334-99337, 99347-99350, 99374-99375, 99377-99378, 99446-99449, 99451-99452, 99495-99496, G0463, G0471, J0670, J2001

G0420 36591-36592, 96523, G0421

G0421 36591-36592, 96523

CPT Index

A

Abdomen, Abdominal
Abscess, 49020
  Open
    Peritoneal, 49020
    Peritonitis, Localized, 49020
    Retroperitoneal, 49060
Biopsy
  Open, 49000
  Percutaneous, 49180
Cannula/Catheter
  Insertion, 49421
  Removal, 49422
Catheter
  Removal, 49422
Celiotomy, 49000
Cyst
  Sclerotherapy, 49185
Delivery
  Peritoneal Abscess
    Open, 49020
    Peritonitis, Localized, 49020
Drainage, 49020
  Fluid, 49082-49083
  Retroperitoneal
    Open, 49060
Exploration, 49000-49010, 49020, 49060, 49082-49084
  Blood Vessel, 35840
Incision, 49000-49010, 49020, 49060, 49082-49084
Injection
  Air, 49400
  Contrast Material, 49400
Insertion
  Catheter, 49324, 49418, 49421
Intraperitoneal
  Catheter Exit Site, 49436
  Catheter Insertion, 49324, 49418, 49421, 49435
  Catheter Removal, 49422
  Catheter Revision, 49325
Laparoscopy, 49320-49321, 49324-49325, 49327
Laparotomy
  Exploration, 49000-49002
  Hemorrhage Control, 49002
  Reopening, 49002
  with Biopsy, 49000
Needle Biopsy
  Mass, 49180
Paracentesis, 49082-49083
Peritoneal Abscess, 49020
Peritoneal Lavage, 49084
Placement Guidance Devices, 49412
Radical Resection, 51597
Ultrasound, 76700-76705
Wall
  Debridement
    Infected, 11005-11006
  Removal
    Mesh, 11008
    Prosthesis, 11008
Ablation
Cryosurgical
  Renal Mass, 50250
  Renal Tumor
    Percutaneous, 50593
Prostate, 55873
  High Intensity-focused Ultrasound (HIFU)
    Transrectal, 55880
  High-energy Water Vapor Thermotherapy, 0582T
  Transurethral Waterjet, 0421T
Radiofrequency
  Renal Tumor(s), 50592
Renal
  Cyst, 50541
  Mass, 50542
    Radiofrequency, 50592

Ablation — *continued*
Renal — *continued*
  Tumor, 50593
    Cryotherapy
      Percutaneous, 50593
Abscess
Abdomen
  Drainage, 49020
    Peritoneal
      Open, 49020
      Peritonitis, Localized, 49020
    Retroperitoneal
      Open, 49060
Bladder
  Incision and Drainage, 51080
Epididymis
  Incision and Drainage, 54700
Kidney
  Incision and Drainage
    Open, 50020
Lymphocele
  Sclerotherapy, 49185
Paraurethral Gland
  Incision and Drainage, 53060
Perirenal or Renal
  Drainage, 50020
Peritoneum
  Incision and Drainage
    Open, 49020
Prostate
  Incision and Drainage, 55720-55725
    Prostatotomy, 55720-55725
    Transurethral, 52700
Retroperitoneal, 49060
  Drainage
    Open, 49060
Scrotum
  Incision and Drainage, 54700, 55100
Skene's Gland
  Incision and Drainage, 53060
Soft Tissue
  Catheter Drainage, 10030
Testis
  Incision and Drainage, 54700
Urethra
  Incision and Drainage, 53040
Visceral, 49405
Adhesion, Adhesions
Penile
  Lysis
    Post–Circumcision, 54162
Preputial
  Lysis, 54450
Urethral
  Lysis, 53500
Adjustment
Transperineal Periurethral Balloon, 0551T
Administration
Immunization
  with Counseling, 90460-90461
  without Counseling, 90473-90474
Injection
  Intramuscular Antibiotic, 96372
  Therapeutic, Diagnostic, Prophylactic
    Intra–arterial, 96373
    Intramuscular, 96372
    Intravenous, 96374-96376
    Subcutaneous, 96372
Advance Care Planning, 99497-99498
Advance Directives, 99497-99498
Advanced Life Support
Emergency Department Services, 99281-99285
After Hours Medical Services, 99051-99053, 99060
Alcohol
Abuse Screening and Intervention, 99408-99409
Allogeneic Donor
Backbench Preparation
  Kidney, 50323-50329

Allogeneic Transplantation
Backbench Preparation
  Kidney, 50323-50329
Allograft Preparation
Kidney, 50323-50329
Renal, 50323-50329
Alloplastic Dressing
Burns, 15002, 15004-15005
Allotransplantation
Renal, 50360-50365
Removal, 50370
Amputation
Penis
  Partial, 54120
  Radical, 54130-54135
  Total, 54125
Anastomosis
Arteriovenous Fistula
  Direct, 36821
  Revision, 36832-36833
    with Thrombectomy, 36833
    without Thrombectomy, 36832
  with Graft, 36825-36830, 36832
  with Thrombectomy, 36831
Epididymis
  to Vas Deferens
    Bilateral, 54901
    Unilateral, 54900
Intestines
  Cystectomy, 51590
  Enterocystoplasty, 51960
Ureter
  to Bladder, 50780-50785
  to Colon, 50810-50815
    Removal, 50830
  to Intestine, 50800, 50820-50825
    Removal, 50830
  to Kidney, 50727-50750
  to Ureter, 50725-50728, 50760-50770
Anatomic
Guide, 3D Printed, 0561T-0562T
Model, 3D Printed, 0559T-0560T
ANC, 85048
Anesthesia
Cystourethroscopy
  Local, 52265
  Spinal, 52260
Anorectovaginoplasty, 46744-46746
Antibiotic Administration
Injection, 96372-96376
Antibody Identification
Immunoassay, 83516-83518
Antigen Detection
Immunoassay
  Direct Optical (Visual), 87880
    Streptococcus, Group A, 87880
Antigen
Prostate Specific
  Complexed, 84152
  Free, 84154
  Total, 84153
Anus
Repair
  Cloacal Anomaly, 46744-46746
Sphincter
  Electromyography, 51784-51785
  Needle, 51785
Aorta
Ultrasound, 76770-76775
AP, [51797]
Appendico-Vesicostomy, 50845
Arteriovenous Anastomosis, 36818-36821
Arteriovenous Fistula
Cannulization
  Vein, 36815
Creation, 36825-36830
Revision
  Hemodialysis Graft or Fistula
    with Thrombectomy, 36833
    without Thrombectomy, 36832
Arteriovenous Shunt
Thomas Shunt, 36835

Artery
Cannulization
  to Vein, 36810-36821
Revision
  Hemodialysis Graft or Fistula
    Open without Revision, 36831
    Revision
      with Thrombectomy, 36833
      without Thrombectomy, 36832
  Thrombectomy
    Hemodialysis Graft or Fistula, 36831
Aspiration
Bladder, 51100-51102
Cyst
  Fine Needle, 10021 [10004, 10005, 10006, 10007, 10008, 10009, 10010, 10011, 10012]
  Kidney, 50390
  Pelvis, 50390
Fine Needle, 10021 [10004, 10005, 10006, 10007, 10008, 10009, 10010, 10011, 10012]
Hydrocele
  Tunica Vaginalis, 55000
Tunica Vaginalis
  Hydrocele, 55000
Assessment
Online
  Physician, [99421, 99422, 99423]
Telephone
  Physician, 99441-99443
Autotransplantation
Renal, 50380
AV Fistula (Arteriovenous Fistula)
Cannulization
  Vein, 36815
Revision
  Hemodialysis Graft or Fistula
    with Thrombectomy, 36833
    without Thrombectomy, 36832
Thrombectomy
  Dialysis Graft
    without Revision, 36831
AVF, 36815
Axilla
Wound Repair, 13131-13133

B

Backbench Reconstruction Prior to Implant
Kidney, 50323-50329
Bacteria Culture
Screening, 87081
Urine, 87086-87088
Benedict Test for Urea, 81005
Bevan's Operation, 54640
Biopsy
Abdomen, 49000, 49321
  Mass, 49180
Bladder, 52354
  Cystourethroscope, 52204
  Cystourethroscopy, 52224, 52250
    with Fulguration, 52224
    with Insertion Transprostatic Implant, 52441-52442
    with Radioactive Substance, 52250
Brush
  Renal Pelvis, 52007
  Ureter, 52007
  with Cystourethroscopy, 52204
Epididymis, 54800, 54865
Fallopian Tube, 49321
Kidney, 50200-50205
  Endoluminal, Renal Pelvis, 50606
  Endoscopic, 50555-50557, 50574-50576, 52354
Lymph Nodes, 38500-38505, 38570
  Laparoscopic, 38570-38572
  Needle, 38505
  Open, 38500
    Superficial, 38500

Biopsy — *continued*

Lymph Nodes — *continued*
Prostate, 55812, 55842, 55862
Needle
Abdomen
Mass, 49180
Omentum, 49321
Ovary, 49321
Penis, 54100
Cutaneous, 54100
Deep Structures, 54105
Peritoneum
Endoscopic, 49321
Prostate, 55700-55706
Lymph Nodes, 55812, 55842, 55862
Renal Pelvis, 50606
Retroperitoneal Area, 49010, 49180
Testis, 54500-54505
Ureter, 52354
Endoluminal, 50606
Endoscopic, 50955-50957, 50974-50976
Urethra, 52204, 52250, 52354, 53200
with Cystourethroscopy, 52354

Bladder

Abscess
Incision and Drainage, 51080
Anastomosis
Ureter to Bladder, 50780-50782
with Intestine, 51960
Aspiration, 51100-51102
Biopsy, 52204
by Cystourethroscopy, 52204
Catheterization, 51045, 51102, 51701-51703
Change Tube, 51705-51710
Chemodenervation, 52287
Creation/Stoma, 51980
Cuff, 50234-50236, 50650
Cyst
Urachal
Excision, 51500
Cystometrogram (CMG), 51725-51729
Cystostomy Tube, 51705-51710
Cystourethroscopy, 52000
Biopsy, 52204, 52224, 52250, 52354
Catheterization, 52005, 52010
Destruction, 52214-52224, 52400
Dilation, 52260-52265
Urethra, 52281
Diverticulum, 52305
Evacuation
Clot, 52001
Excision
Tumor, 52234-52240, 52355
Exploration, 52351
Fulguration, 52214-52250, 52400
Injection, 52283
Insertion of Stent, 52332-52334
Lithotripsy, 52353
Radiotracer, 52250
Removal
Calculus, 52310-52315, 52352
Foreign Body, 52310-52315
Sphincter Surgery, 52277
Tumor
Excision, 52355
Ureter Surgery, 52290-52300
Urethral Syndrome, 52285
with Urethrotomy, 52270-52276
Destruction
Endoscopic, 52214-52240, 52354
Dilation
Ureter, 52260-52265
Diverticulum
Excision, 51525
Incision, 52305
Resection, 52305
Excision
Partial, 51550-51565
Total, 51570, 51580, 51590-51597
with Nodes, 51575, 51585, 51595
Transurethral of Neck, 52640
Tumor, 52234-52240
Fulguration, 52214, 52250, 52400
Tumor(s), 52224-52240

Bladder — *continued*

Incision
Catheter or Stent, 51045
with
Cryosurgery, 51030
Destruction, 51020-51030
Fulguration, 51020
Insertion Radioactive, 51020
Radiotracer, 51020
Incision and Drainage, 51040
Injection
Radiologic, 51600-51610
Insertion
Stent, 51045, 52282, 52334
Instillation
Anticarcinogenics, 51720
Drugs, 51720
Interstitial Cystitis, 52260-52265
with Cystourethroscopy, 52005, 52010
Irrigation, 51700, 52005, 52010
Clot, 52001
Lesion
Destruction, 51030
Neck
Endoscopy
Injection of Implant Material, 51715
Excision, 51520
Remodeling for Incontinence, 53860
Radiotracer, 51020, 52250
Reconstruction
Radiofrequency Micro-Remodeling, 53860
with Intestines, 51960
with Urethra, 51800-51820
Removal
Calculus, 51050, 51065, 52310-52315, 52352
Foreign Body, 52310-52315
Litholapaxy, 52317-52318
Lithotripsy, 51065, 52353
Urethral Stent, 52310-52315
Repair
Diverticulum, 52305
Exstrophy, 51940
Fistula, 44660-44661, 51880-51925
Neck, 51845
Wound, 51860-51865
Resection, 52500
Sphincter Surgery, 52277
Suspension, 51990
Suture
Fistula, 44660-44661, 51880-51925
Wound, 51860-51865
Tumor
Excision, 51530
Fulguration, 52234-52240
Resection, 52234-52240
Ureterocele, 51535
Urethrotomy, 52270-52276
Urinary Incontinence Procedures
Laparoscopy, 51990-51992
Radiofrequency Micro-Remodeling, 53860
Sling Operation, 51992
Urethral Suspension, 51990
Uroflowmetry, 51736-51741
Voiding Pressure Studies, 51727-51729 [51797]

Blood Pressure
Monitoring, 24 hour, 93975-93976, 93980-93990

Blood Vessel(s)
Exploration
Abdomen, 35840
Kidney
Repair, 50100
Repair
Kidney, 50100
Shunt Creation
Direct, 36821
Thomas Shunt, 36835
with Graft, 36825-36830
with Transposition, 36818-36820
Shunt Revision
with Graft, 36832

Blood

Cell Count
Automated, 85049
Blood Smear, 85007-85008
Complete Blood Count (CBC), 85025-85027
Differential WBC Count, 85004-85007, 85009
Hematocrit, 85014
Hemoglobin, 85018
Hemogram
Added Indices, 85025-85027
Automated, 85025-85027
Manual, 85032
Microhematocrit, 85013
Red Blood Cells, 85032-85041
Reticulocyte, 85044-85046
White Blood Cell, 85032, 85048
Flow Check
Graft, 90940
Hemoglobin
Concentration, 85046
Platelet
Automated Count, 85049
Count, 85008
Manual Count, 85032
Reticulocyte, 85046
Smear, 85060
Microscopic Examination, 85007-85008
Peripheral, 85060
Test(s)
Panels
Electrolyte, 80051
General Health Panel, 80050
Metabolic Panel, Basic
Basic, 80047-80048
Comprehensive, 80053
Ionized Calcium, 80047
Total Calcium, 80048
Renal Function, 80069

Boarding Home Care, 99324-99337
Bottle Type Procedure, 55060
Boyce Operation, 50040-50045
Brachytherapy
Placement of Device
Genitalia, 55920
Pelvis, 55920
Planning
Prostate Volume Study, 76873
Brain
Infusion, 95990-95991
Bricker Operation
Intestines Anastomosis, 50820
Browne's Operation, 54324
Bulbourethral Gland
Excision, 53250
Burch Operation, 51840-51841
Burns
Escharotomy, 15002-15005

C

Calcium
Deposits
Removal, Calculi–Stone
Bladder, 51050, 52310-52318
Kidney, 50060-50081, 50130, 50561, 50580
Ureter, 50610-50630, 50961, 50980, 51060-51065, 52320-52330
Urethra, 52310-52315
Ionized
Panel, 80047
Total
Panel, 80048
Calculus
Destruction
Kidney
Extracorporeal Shock Wave Lithotripsy, 50590
Ureter
Lithotripsy, 52353 [52356]
Removal
Bladder, 51050, 52310-52318, 52352

Calculus — *continued*

Removal — *continued*
Kidney, 50060-50081, 50130, 50561, 50580, 52352
Ureter, 50610-50630, 50945, 50961, 50980, 51060-51065, 52310-52315, 52320-52325, 52352
Urethra, 52310-52315, 52352
Calycoplasty, 50405
Camey Enterocystoplasty, 50825
Cannulation
Arteriovenous, 36810-36815
Vas Deferens, 55200
Vein to Vein, 36800
Cannulization
Arteriovenous (AV), 36810-36815
Declotting, 36593, 36860-36861
External
Declotting, 36860-36861
Vas Deferens, 55200
Vein to Vein, 36800
CAPD, 90945-90947
Case Management Services
Telephone Calls
Physician, 99441-99443
Catheter
Bladder, 51701-51703
Irrigation, 51700
Cystourethroscopy, 52320-52353 [52356]
Declotting, 36593, 36861
Drainage
Peritoneal, 49406-49407
Retroperitoneal, 49406-49407
Exchange
Nephrostomy, [50435]
Intraperitoneal
Tunneled
Laparoscopic, 49324
Open, 49421
Percutaneous, 49418
Placement
Nephrostomy, Percutaneous, [50432]
Nephroureteral, [50433, 50434]
Removal
Nephroureteral, Accessible, 50387
Peritoneum, 49422
Repair
Intraperitoneal, 49325
Replacement
Nephroureteral, Accessible, 50387
Ureteral
Manometric Studies, 50396, 50686
Ureterography, 50684
Ureteropyelography, 50684
Catheterization
Abdomen, 49324, 49418, 49421
Bladder, 51045, 51102
Cystourethroscopy
Ejaculatory Duct, 52010
Ureteral, 52005
with Insertion Transprostatic Implant, 52441-52442
Dialysis, 49418, 49421
Interstitial Radioelement Application
Genitalia, 55920
Pelvic Organs, 55920
Prostate, 55875
Intraperitoneal Tunneled, 49324, 49421
Ureter
Endoscopic, 50553, 50572, 50953, 50972, 52005
Injection, 50684
Manometric Studies, 50396, 50686
Cauterization
Intrarenal Stricture, 52343, 52346
Prostate Resection, 52601
Skin Lesion
Malignant, 17270-17276
Ureteral Stricture, 52341, 52344
Ureteropelvic Junction Stricture, 52342, 52345
Urethral Caruncle, 53265
Cavernosography
Corpora, 54230
Cavernosometry, 54231
CBC (Complete Blood Count), 85025-85027

Cecil Repair, 54318
Celiotomy, 49000
Cell
  Count
    Bacterial Colony, 87086
Change
  Stent
    Ureteral, 50688
  Tube
    Ureterostomy, 50688
Cheek
  Wound Repair, 13131-13133
Chemistry Tests
  Organ or Disease Oriented Panel
    Electrolyte, 80051
    General Health Panel, 80050
    Metabolic
      Basic, 80047-80048
        Calcium
          Ionized, 80047
          Total, 80048
      Comprehensive, 80053
Chemodenervation
  Bladder, 52287
Chemosurgery
  Destruction
    Malignant Lesion, 17270-17276
Chemotherapy
  Bladder Instillation, 51720
  Home Infusion Procedures, 99601-99602
  Kidney Instillation, 50391
  Peritoneal Cavity
    Catheterization, 49418
  Pump Services
    Maintenance, 95990-95991
  Ureteral Instillation, 50391
Chin
  Wound Repair, 13131-13133
Chloride
  Panels
    Basic Metabolic, 80047-80048
    Comprehensive Metabolic, 80053
    Electrolyte, 80051
    Renal Function, 80069
Cimino Type Procedure, 36821
Circumcision
  Adhesions, 54162
  Incomplete, 54163
  Repair, 54163
  Surgical Excision
    28 Days or Less, 54160
    Older Than 28 Days, 54161
  with Clamp or Other Device, 54150
Closure
  Cystostomy, 51880
  Fistula
    Enterovesical, 44660-44661
    Kidney, 50520-50526
    Ureter, 50920-50930
    Urethra, 53400-53405
    Vesicouterine, 51920-51925
    Vesicovaginal, 51900
  Skin
    Abdomen
      Simple, 12001-12007
      Superficial, 12001-12007
    Back
      Simple, 12001-12007
      Superficial, 12001-12007
    Chest
      Simple, 12001-12007
      Superficial, 12001-12007
    External
      Genitalia
        Intermediate, 12041-12047
        Layered, 12041-12047
        Simple, 12001-12007
        Superficial, 12001-12007
    Genitalia
      Complex, 13131-13133
      External
        Intermediate, 12041-12047
        Layered, 12041-12047
        Simple, 12001-12007
        Superficial, 12001-12007

Closure — *continued*
  Skin — *continued*
    Trunk
      Simple, 12001-12007
      Superficial, 12001-12007
Clot, 50230
CMG (Cystometrogram), 51725-51729
Collection and Processing
  Brushings
    Abdomen, 49320
    Omentum, 49320
    Peritoneum, 49320
  Specimen
    Capillary, 36416
    Ear, 36416
    Vein, 36415
    Venous Blood, 36415
  Washings
    Abdomen, 49320
    Omentum, 49320
    Peritoneum, 49320
Colon–Sigmoid
  Reconstruction Bladder Using Sigmoid, 50810
Colon
  Reconstruction
    Bladder from, 50810
  Repair
    Fistula, 44660-44661
  Suture
    Fistula, 44660-44661
Colostomy
  Abdominal
    with Creation Sigmoid Bladder, 50810
  Abdominoperineal, 51597
  Perineal, 50810
  with Pelvic Exenteration, 51597
Colporrhaphy
  Anterior, 57240, 57289
    with Insertion of Mesh, 57267
    with Insertion of Prosthesis, 57267
  Anteroposterior, 57260-57265
    with Enterocele Repair, 57265
    with Insertion of Mesh, 57267
    with Insertion of Prosthesis, 57267
  Posterior
    with Insertion of Mesh, 57267
    with Insertion of Prosthesis, 57267
Commissurotomy
  Anterior Prostate, Transurethral, 0619T
Complete Blood Count, 85025-85027
Complex Chronic Care Management Services, 99487-99489 [99439, 99490, 99491]
Condyloma
  Destruction
    Penis, 54050-54065
Congenital Kidney Abnormality
  Nephrolithotomy, 50070
  Pyeloplasty, 50405
  Pyelotomy, 50135
Construction
  Bladder from Sigmoid Colon, 50810
  Neobladder, 51596
Consultation
  Initial Inpatient
    New or Established Patient, 99251-99255
  Office and/or Other Outpatient
    New or Established Patient, 99241-99245
Contracture
  Bladder Neck Resection, 52640
Contrast Material
  Injection
    Central Venous Access Device, 36598
  Peritoneal
    Tunneled Catheter Insertion, 49418
  Peritoneal Cavity, 49400
  Urethrocystography, 51605
Corpora Cavernosa
  Corpora Cavernosography
    Injection, 54230
  Corpus Spongiosum Shunt, 54430
  Dynamic Cavernosometry, 54231
  Glans Penis Fistulization, 54435

Corpora Cavernosa — *continued*
  Injection
    Peyronie Disease, 54200-54205
    Pharmacologic Agent, 54235
  Irrigation
    Priapism, 54220
  Peyronie Disease, 54200-54205
  Priapism, 54220, 54430
  Repair
    Corporeal Tear, 54437
    Saphenous Vein Shunt, 54420
Corpora Cavernosography
  Injection, 54230
Counseling and /or Risk Factor Reduction Intervention – Preventive Medicine, Individual Counseling
  Behavior Change Interventions, 99406-99409
Counseling
  Smoking and Tobacco Use Cessation, 99406-99407
Cowper's Gland
  Excision, 53250
CR, 82565
Creatinine
  Blood, 82565
Creation
  Arteriovenous
    Fistula, 36825-36830
  Catheter Exit Site, 49436
  Recipient Site, 15002-15005
  Sigmoid Bladder, 50810
  Stoma
    Bladder, 51980
    Kidney, [50436, 50437]
    Renal Pelvis, [50436, 50437]
    Ureter, 50860
CRIT, 85013
Critical Care Services
  Evaluation and Management, 99291-99292
Cryofixation
  for Transplantation, 50300-50320, 50547
Cryopreservation
  for Transplantation, 50300-50320, 50547
Cryosurgery, 17270-17276
  Lesion
    Bladder, 51030, 52224
      Tumor(s), 52234-52240
    Kidney, 50250
    Penis, 54056, 54065
    Skin
      Malignant, 17270-17276
    Urethra, 52224
  Prostate, 52214, 55873
  Tumor
    Bladder, 52234-52240
Cryotherapy
  Ablation
    Renal Tumor, 50593
  Renal Tumor, 50593
Culture
  Bacteria
    Screening, 87081
    Urine, 87086-87088
  Pathogen
    by Kit, 87084
    Screening Only, 87081
Curettement
  Skin Lesion, 17270
    Malignant, 17270-17274
Cyclosporine
  Assay, 80158
Cyst
  Bladder
    Excision, 51500
  Drainage
    Image-guided by catheter, 10030
  Kidney
    Ablation, 50541
    Aspiration, 50390
    Excision, 50280-50290
    Injection, 50390
  Mullerian Duct
    Excision, 55680
  Pelvis
    Aspiration, 50390

Cyst — *continued*
  Pelvis — *continued*
    Injection, 50390
  Seminal Vesicles
    Excision, 55680
  Skene's Gland
    Destruction, 53270
    Drainage, 53060
  Urachal
    Bladder
      Excision, 51500
Cystectomy
  Complete, 51570
    with Bilateral Pelvic Lymphadenectomy, 51575, 51585, 51595
    with Continent Diversion, 51596
    with Ureteroileal Conduit, 51590
    with Ureterosigmoidostomy, 51580
  Partial, 51550
    Complicated, 51555
    Reimplantation of Ureters, 51565
    Simple, 51550
Cystitis
  Interstitial, 52260-52265
Cystography
  Injection, 52281
  Radiologic, 51600
Cystolithotomy, 51050
Cystometrogram, 51725-51729
Cystoplasty, 51800
Cystorrhaphy, 51860-51865
Cystoscopy, 52000
  with Ureteroneocystostomy, 50947
Cystostomy
  Change Tube, 51705-51710
  Closure, 51880
  Destruction Intravesical Lesion, 51030
  with Drainage, 51040
  with Fulguration, 51020
  with Insertion
    Radioactive Material, 51020
  with Urethrectomy
    Female, 53210
    Male, 53215
Cystotomy
  Excision
    Bladder Diverticulum, 51525
    Bladder Tumor, 51530
    Diverticulum, 51525
    Repair of Ureterocele, 51535
    Vesical Neck, 51520
  Repair Ureterocele, 51535
  with Calculus Basket Extraction, 51065
  with Destruction Intravesical Lesion, 51030
  with Drainage, 51040
  with Fulguration, 51020
  with Insertion
    Radioactive Material, 51020
    Urethral Catheter, 51045
  with Removal Calculus, 51050, 51065
Cystourethrogram, Retrograde, 51610
Cystourethropexy, 51840-51841
Cystourethroplasty, 51800-51820
  Radiofrequency Micro-Remodeling, 53860
Cystourethroscopy, 52000, 52320-52355, 52601, 52647-52648, 53500 [52356]
  Biopsy, 52204, 52224, 52250, 52354
  Brush, 52007
  Calibration and/or Dilation Urethral Stricture or Stenosis, 52281, 52630, 52647-52649
  Catheterization
    Ejaculatory Duct, 52010
    Ureteral, 52005
  Chemodenervation of Bladder, 52287
  Destruction
    Lesion, 52400
  Dilation
    Bladder, 52260-52265
    Intrarenal Stricture, 52343, 52346
    Ureter, 52341-52342, 52344-52345
    Urethra, 52281, 52285
  Evacuation
    Clot, 52001
  Examination, 52000
  Female Urethral Syndrome, 52285

CPT Index

Cystourethroscopy — *continued*
  Incision
    Bladder Neck, 52285
    Congenital Obstructive Mucosal Folds, 52400
    Diverticulum, 52305
    Ejaculatory Duct, 52402
    Urethral Valves, 52400
  Injection
    for Cystography, 52281
    Implant Material, 52327
  Insertion
    Indwelling Urethral Stent, 52282, 52332
    Radioactive Substance, 52250
    Ureteral Guide Wire, 52334
    Urethral Stent, 52282
  Instillation, 52005, 52010
  Irrigation, 52005, 52010
  Lithotripsy, 52353
    with Ureteral Stent, [52356]
  Lysis
    Urethra, 53500
    Urethrovaginal Septal Fibrosis, 52285
  Manipulation of Ureteral Calculus, 52330, 52352
  Meatotomy
    Ureteral, 52290
    Urethral, 52281, 52285, 52630, 52647-52649
  Removal
    Calculus, 52310-52315, 52320-52325, 52352
    Foreign Body, 52310-52315
    Urethral Stent, 52310-52315
  Resection
    Congenital Obstructive Mucosal Folds, 52400
    Diverticulum, 52305
    Ejaculatory Duct, 52402
    External Sphincter, 52277
    Prostate, 52601-52630
    Tumor, 52234-52240, 52355
    Ureterocele(s), 52300-52301
    Urethral Valves, 52400
  Treatment
    Lesion(s), 52224
    Ureteral Stricture, 52341
  Urethral Syndrome, 52285
  Vasectomy
    Transurethral, 52402, 52630, 52647-52649
  Vasotomy
    Transurethral, 52402
  with Direct Vision Internal Urethrotomy, 52276
  with Duct Radiography, 52010
  with Ejaculatory Duct Catheterization, 52010
  with Fulguration, 52214, 52354
    Congenital Obstructive Mucosal Folds, 52400
    Lesion, 52224
    Polyps, 52285
    Tumor, 52234-52240
    Ureterocele(s), 52300-52301
    Urethral Valves, 52400
  with Internal Urethrotomy, 52630, 52647-52649
    Female, 52270, 52285
    Male, 52275
  with Prostate
    Insertion Transprostatic Implant, 52441-52442
    Laser Coagulation, 52647
    Laser Enucleation, 52649
    Laser Vaporization, 52648
  with Steroid Injection, 52283
  with Transurethral Anterior Prostate Commissurotomy, 0619T
  with Ureteropyelography, 52005
  with Ureteroscopy, 52351
  with Urethral Catheterization, 52005
  with Urethral Meatotomy, 52290-52300, 52305

D

Debridement
  Infected Inflatable Urethral/Bladder Neck Sphincter, 53448
  Infected Tissue, with Removal Penile Implant, 54411, 54417
  Muscle
    Infected, 11004-11008
  Necrotizing Soft Tissue, 11004-11008
  Skin
    Infected, 11004-11006
    Subcutaneous Tissue
      Infected, 11004-11008
Declotting
  Vascular Access Device, 36593
Dehiscence
  Suture
    Abdominal Wall
      Skin and Subcutaneous Tissue
        Complex, 13160
        Complicated, 13160
        Extensive, 13160
      Skin and Subcutaneous Tissue
        Simple, 12020
          with Packing, 12021
        Superficial, 12020
          with Packing, 12021
  Wound
    Abdominal Wall
      Skin and Subcutaneous Tissue
        Complex, 13160
        Complicated, 13160
        Extensive, 13160
      Skin and Subcutaneous Tissue
        Simple, 12020
          with Packing, 12021
        Superficial, 12020
          with Packing, 12021
Deligation
  Ureter, 50940
Destruction
  Bladder, 51020, 52214-52224, 52354
    Endoscopic, 52214
      Large Tumors, 52240
      Medium Tumors, 52235
      Minor Lesions, 52224
      Small Tumors, 52234
  Calculus
    Kidney, 50590
  Condyloma
    Penis, 54050-54065
  Kidney, 52354
    Endoscopic, 50557, 50576
  Lesion
    Bladder, 51030
    Penis
      Cryosurgery, 54056
      Electrodesiccation, 54055
      Extensive, 54065
      Laser Surgery, 54057
      Simple, 54050-54060
      Surgical Excision, 54060
    Prostate
      Thermotherapy, 53850-53852
        Microwave, 53850
        Radiofrequency, 53852
    Skin
      Malignant, 17270-17276
    Ureter, 52341-52342, 52344-52345
    Urethra, 52400, 53265
  Polyp
    Urethra, 53260
  Prostate
    Cryosurgical Ablation, 55873
    Microwave Thermotherapy, 53850
    Radiofrequency Thermotherapy, 53852-53854
  Skene's Gland, 53270
  Skin Lesion
    Malignant, 17270-17276
  Tumor
    Urethra, 53220
  Ureter
    Endoscopic, 50957, 50976
  Urethra, 52214-52224, 52354

Destruction — *continued*
  Urethra — *continued*
    Prolapse, 53275
    with Cystourethroscopy, 52354
Device
  Transperineal Periurethral Balloon, 0548T-0551T
Dialysis
  Arteriovenous Fistula
    Revision
      without Thrombectomy, 36832
      Thrombectomy, 36831
  Arteriovenous Shunt
    Revision
      with Thrombectomy, 36833
      Thrombectomy, 36831
  End-Stage Renal Disease, 90951-90953, 90963, 90967
  Hemodialysis, 90935-90937
    Blood Flow Study, 90940
  Hemoperfusion, 90997
  Patient Training
    Completed Course, 90989
    Per Session, 90993
  Peritoneal, 90945-90947
    Catheter Insertion, 49418, 49421
    Catheter Removal, 49422
    Home Infusion, 99601-99602
Differential Count
  White Blood Cell Count, 85007, 85009
Dilation
  Bladder
    Cystourethroscopy, 52260-52265
  Kidney, 50080-50081 [50436, 50437]
    Intrarenal Stricture, 52343, 52346
  Ureter, 50706, 52341-52342, 52344-52346 [50436, 50437]
    Endoscopic, 50553, 50572, 50575, 50953, 50972
  Urethra, 52260-52265
    Female Urethral Syndrome, 52285
    General, 53665
    Suppository and/or Instillation, 53660-53661
    with Prostate Resection, 52601-52630, 52647-52649
    with Prostatectomy, 55801, 55821
  Urethral
    Stenosis, 52281
    Stricture, 52281, 53600-53621
Discharge Services
  Hospital, 99238-99239
  Nursing Facility, 99315-99316
  Observation Care, 99217, 99234-99236
Dissection
  Donor Organs
    Kidney, 50323-50325
  Urethra, 54328-54336, 54348-54352
Diverticulum
  Repair
    Excision, 53230-53235
    Marsupialization, 53240
    Urethroplasty, 53400-53405
Domiciliary Services
  Discharge Services, 99315-99316
  Established Patient, 99334-99337
  New Patient, 99324-99328
Donor Procedures
  Backbench Preparation Prior to Transplantation
    Kidney, 50323-50329
  Kidney, 50300-50320
Doppler Echocardiography
  Hemodialysis Access, 93990
    Prior to Access Creation, 93985-93986
Doppler Scan
  Transplanted Kidney, 76776
Double–J Stent, 52332
  Cystourethroscopy, 52000, 52601, 52647-52648
Drainage
  Abdomen
    Abdominal Fluid, 49082-49083
    Paracentesis, 49082-49083
    Peritoneal, 49020
    Peritoneal Lavage, 49084

Drainage — *continued*
  Abdomen — *continued*
    Peritonitis, Localized, 49020
    Retroperitoneal, 49060
  Abscess
    Abdomen
      Peritoneal
        Open, 49020
      Peritonitis, localized, 49020
      Retroperitoneal
        Open, 49060
    Bladder
      Cystotomy or Cystostomy, 51040
      Incision and Drainage, 51080
    Epididymis
      Incision and Drainage, 54700
    Kidney
      Incision and Drainage
        Open, 50020
    Lymphocele, 49185
    Paraurethral Gland
      Incision and Drainage, 53060
    Pelvic
      Percutaneous, 49406
      Transrectal, 49407
      Transvaginal, 49407
    Perirenal or Renal
      Open, 50020
    Peritoneum
      Open, 49020
    Prostate
      Incision and Drainage
        Prostatotomy, 55720-55725
        Transurethral, 52700
    Renal, 50020
    Retroperitoneal
      Open, 49060
    Scrotum
      Incision and Drainage, 54700, 55100
    Skene's Gland
      Incision and Drainage, 53060
    Soft Tissue
      Image-Guided by Catheter, 10030
      Percutaneous, 10030
    Testis
      Incision and Drainage, 54700
    Urethra
      Incision and Drainage, 53040
    Visceral, 49405
  Cyst
    Skene's Gland, 53060
  Extraperitoneal Lymphocele
    Percutaneous, Sclerotherapy, 49185
  Fluid
    Abdominal, 49082-49083
    Peritoneal
      Percutaneous, 49406
      Transrectal, 49407
      Transvaginal, 49407
    Retroperitoneal
      Percutaneous, 49406
      Transrectal, 49407
      Transvaginal, 49407
    Visceral, 49405
  Kidney, 50040
  Lymphocele
    Percutaneous, Sclerotherapy, 49185
  Pelvis, 50125
  Penis, 54015
  Peritonitis, 49020
  Postoperative Wound Infection, 10180
  Seroma, 49185
  Skin, 10180
  Ureter, 50600, 53080-53085
  Urethra
    Extravasation, 53080-53085
Drug Assay
  Cyclosporine, 80158
  Therapeutic, 80158
Drug Delivery Implant
  Maintenance
    Brain, 95990-95991
    Epidural, 95990-95991
    Intrathecal, 95990-95991

Drug Delivery Implant — *continued*
  Maintenance — *continued*
    Intraventricular, 95990-95991
Drug Screen, 99408-99409
Drug
  Administration For
    Infusion
      Home Services, 99601-99602
      Intravenous, 96365-96368
    Infusion, 96365-96368
Duplex Scan
  Arterial Studies
    Penile, 93980-93981
    Visceral, 93975-93976
  Hemodialysis Access, 93990
    Prior to Access Creation, 93985-93986
  Venous Studies
    Penile, 93980-93981

E

Ear
  Collection of Blood From, 36416
Echography
  Abdomen, 76700-76705
  Kidney
    Transplant, 76776
  Prostate, 76872-76873
  Retroperitoneal, 76770-76775
  Scrotum, 76870
  Transrectal, 76872-76873
ED, 99281-99285
Education
  Patient
    Self-management by Nonphysician, 98960-98962
Elastography
  Ultrasound, Parenchyma, 76981-76983
Electro–Hydraulic Procedure, 52325
Electrocautery, 17270-17276
  Prostate Resection, 52601
  Ureteral Stricture, 52341-52346
Electrodesiccation, 17270-17276
  Lesion
    Penis, 54055
Electroejaculation, 55870
Electromyography
  Sphincter Muscles
    Anus, 51784-51785
      Needle, 51785
    Urethra, 51784-51785
      Needle, 51785
Electronic Analysis
  Drug Infusion Pump, 95990-95991
Electrosurgery
  Penile, 54065
  Skin Lesion, 17270-17276
Embolization
  Ureter, 50705
Emergency Department Services, 99281-99285
EMG (Electromyography, Needle), 51784-51785
End-Stage Renal Disease Services, 90951-90962, 90967-90970
  Home, 90963-90966
Endopyelotomy, 50575
Endoscopy
  Bladder
    Biopsy, 52204, 52250, 52354
    Catheterization, 52005, 52010
    Destruction, 52354
      Lesion, 52400
      Polyps, 52285
      with Fulguration, 52214
    Diagnostic, 52000
    Dilation, 52260-52265
    Evacuation
      Clot, 52001
    Excision
      Tumor, 52355
    Exploration, 52351
    Insertion
      Radioactive Substance, 52250
      Stent, 52282, 53855
    Instillation, 52010
    Irrigation, 52010
    Lesion, 52224-52240, 52400
    Litholapaxy, 52317-52318

Endoscopy — *continued*
  Bladder — *continued*
    Lithotripsy, 52353
    Neck, 51715
    Removal
      Calculus, 52310-52315, 52352
      Urethral Stent, 52310-52315
  Bladder Neck
    Injection of Implant Material, 51715
  Kidney
    Biopsy, 50555-50557, 50574-50576, 52354
    Catheterization, 50553, 50572
    Destruction, 50557, 50576, 52354
    Dilation
      Stricture, 52343, 52346
    Excision
      Tumor, 50562, 52355
    Exploration, 52351
    Lithotripsy, 52353
    Removal
      Calculus, 50561, 50580, 52352
      Foreign Body, 50561, 50580
    via Incision, 50562-50580
    via Stoma, 50551-50562
  Pelvis
    Destruction of Lesions, 52354
  Peritoneum
    Drainage Lymphocele, 54690
  Prostate
    Abscess Drainage, 52700
    Destruction, 52214
    Incision, 52450
    Laser, 52647
      Coagulation, 52647
      Enucleation, 52649
      Vaporization, 52647
    Resection
      Complete, 52601
      Obstructive Tissue, 52630
  Testis
    Removal, 54690
  Ureter
    Biopsy, 50955-50957, 50974-50976, 52007, 52354
    Catheterization, 50572, 50953, 50972, 52005
    Destruction, 50957, 50976, 52354
      Uterocele, 52300-52301
    Diagnostic, 52351
    Dilation, 50572, 50575, 50953
      Stricture, 52341-52342, 52344-52345
    Excision
      Tumor, 52355
    Exploration, 52351
    Incision, 52290
    Injection of Implant Material, 52327
    Insertion Guide Wire, 52334
    Lithotripsy, 52325, 52353
    Manipulation of Ureteral Calculus, 52330
    Placement
      Stent, 50947, 52332
    Removal
      Calculus, 50961, 50980, 52310-52315, 52320, 52352
      Foreign Body, 50961, 50980
    Resection, 52305, 52355
    via Incision, 50970-50980
    via Stoma, 50951-50961
    via Ureterotomy, 50970-50980
    With Endopyelotomy, 50575
  Urethra, 52000, 52010
    Biopsy, 52204, 52354
    Catheterization, 52005, 52010
    Destruction, 52214, 52354
      Congenital Posterior Valves, 52400
      Lesion, 52214-52240
      Polyps, 52285
    Evacuation
      Clot, 52001
    Excision
      Tumor, 52355
    Exploration, 52351

Endoscopy — *continued*
  Urethra — *continued*
    Incision, 52285
      Congenital Posterior Valves, 52400
      Ejaculatory Duct, 52402
      Internal, 52270-52276
      Meatotomy, 52281, 52285
    Injection
      for Cystography, 52281
      Implant Material, 51715
      Steroid, 52283
    Insertion
      Radioactive Substance, 52250
      Stent, 52282
    Lithotripsy, 52353
    Lysis Fibrosis, 52285
    Removal
      Stent, 52310
    Resection
      Congenital Posterior Valves, 52400
      Ejaculatory Duct, 52402
      Sphincter, 52277
    Vasectomy, 52402
    Vasotomy, 52402
Enterocele
  Repair
    with Colporrhaphy, 57265
Enterocystoplasty, 51960
  Camey, 50825
Enucleation
  Prostate, 52649
Epididymectomy
  Bilateral, 54861
  Unilateral, 54860
  with Excision Spermatocele, 54840
Epididymis
  Abscess
    Incision and Drainage, 54700
  Anastomosis
    to Vas Deferens
      Bilateral, 54901
      Unilateral, 54900
  Biopsy, 54800, 54865
  Excision
    Bilateral, 54861
    Unilateral, 54860
  Exploration
    Biopsy, 54865
  Hematoma
    Incision and Drainage, 54700
  Lesion
    Excision
      Local, 54830
      Spermatocele, 54840
  Needle Biopsy, 54800
  Repair, 54900-54901
  Spermatocele
    Excision, 54840
Epididymograms, 55300
Epididymovasostomy
  Bilateral, 54901
  Unilateral, 54900
Epispadias
  Penis
    Reconstruction, 54385
  Repair, 54380-54390
    with Exstrophy of Bladder, 54390
    with Incontinence, 54385
ER, 99281-99285
Escharotomy
  Graft Site, 15002-15005
ESRD, 90951-90961, 90967-90970
  Home, 90963-90966
Established Patient
  Critical Care, 99291-99292
  Domiciliary or Rest Home Visit, 99334-99337
  Emergency Department Services, 99281-99285
  Home Services, 99347-99350, 99601-99602
  Hospital Inpatient Services, 99221-99223, 99231-99239

Established Patient — *continued*
  Hospital Observation Services, 99217-99220, 99234-99236 [99224, 99225, 99226]
  Initial Inpatient Consultation, 99251-99255
  Nursing Facility, 99304-99318
  Office and/or Other Outpatient Consultations, 99241-99245
  Office Visit, 99211-99215
  Online Evaluation and Management Services
    Physician, [99421, 99422, 99423]
  Outpatient Visit, 99211-99215
  Prolonged Services, 99354-99359 [99415, 99416, 99417]
    with Patient Contact, 99354-99357
    without Patient Contact, 99358-99359
  Telephone Services, 99441-99443
Establishment
  Colostomy
    Abdominal, 50810
    Perineal, 50810
ESWL, 50590
Evacuation
  Hematoma
    Bladder/Urethra, 52001
Evaluation and Management
  Alcohol and/or Substance Abuse, 99408-99409
  Consultation, 99241-99255
  Critical Care, 99291-99292
  Domiciliary or Rest Home
    Established Patient, 99334-99337
    New Patient, 99324-99328
  Emergency Department, 99281-99285
  Home Services, 99341-99350
  Hospital, 99221-99223, 99231-99233
  Hospital Discharge, 99238-99239
  Hospital Services
    Initial, 99221-99223, 99231-99233
    Observation Care, 99217-99220
    Subsequent, 99231
  Internet Communication
    Physician, [99421, 99422, 99423]
  Nursing Facility, 99304-99318
    Annual Assessment, 99318
    Discharge, 99315-99316
    Initial Care, 99304-99306
    Subsequent Care, 99307-99310
  Observation Care, 99217-99220
  Office and Other Outpatient, 99202-99215
  Online Assessment
    Physician, [99421, 99422, 99423]
  Online Evaluation
    Physician, [99421, 99422, 99423]
  Preventive Services, 99406-99409
  Prolonged Services, 99356-99357
  Smoking and Tobacco Cessation Counseling, 99406-99407
  Telephone Assessment
    Physician, 99441-99443
Excision
  Bladder
    Diverticulum, 51525
    Neck, 51520
    Partial, 51550-51565
    Total, 51570, 51580, 51590-51597
      with Nodes, 51575, 51585, 51595
    Transurethral, 52640
    Tumor, 51530
  Bladder Neck Contracture, Postoperative, 52640
  Bulbourethral Gland, 53250
  Caruncle, Urethra, 53265
  Cowper's gland, 53250
  Cyst
    Bladder, 51500
    Kidney, 50280-50290
    Mullerian Duct, 55680
    Seminal Vesicle, 55680
    Urachal
      Bladder, 51500
  Epididymis
    Bilateral, 54861
    Unilateral, 54860

● New   ▲ Revised   + Add On AMA: CPT Assist [Resequenced]

CPT © 2020 American Medical Association. All Rights Reserved.

CPT © 2020 American Medical Association. All Rights Reserved.   ● New   ▲ Revised   + Add On   AMA: CPT Assist[Resequenced]   © 2020 Optum360, LLC

CPT Index

Kidney — *continued*
  Repair — *continued*
    Wound, 50500
  Solitary, 50405
  Suture
    Fistula, 50520-50526
    Horseshoe Kidney, 50540
  Transplantation
    Allograft Preparation, 50323-50329
    Donor Nephrectomy, 50300-50320, 50547
    Graft Implantation, 50360-50365
    Implantation of Graft, 50360
    Recipient Nephrectomy, 50340, 50365
    Reimplantation Kidney, 50380
    Removal Transplant Allograft, 50370
  Tumor
    Ablation
      Cryotherapy, 50250, 50593
    Ultrasound, 76770-76776
Kock Pouch
  Formation, 50825
Koop Inguinal Orchiopexy, 54640

L

Laparoscopy
  Abdominal, 49320-49321, 49324-49325, 49327
    Surgical, 49321, 49324-49325
  Biopsy, 49321
    Lymph Nodes, 38570
    Ovary, 49321
  Bladder
    Repair
      Sling Procedure, 51992
      Urethral Suspension, 51990
  Diagnostic, 49320
  Incontinence Repair, 51990-51992
  Kidney
    Ablation, 50541-50542
  Ligation
    Veins, Spermatic, 55500
  Lymphadenectomy, 38571-38573
  Lymphatic, 38570-38573
  Nephrectomy, 50545-50548
    Partial, 50543
  Orchiectomy, 54690
  Orchiopexy, 54692
  Ovary
    Biopsy, 49321
  Pelvis, 49320
  Placement Interstitial Device, 49327
  Prostatectomy, 55866
  Pyeloplasty, 50544
  Removal
    Testis, 54690
  Surgical, 38570-38572, 49321, 49324-49325, 49327, 50541, 50543, 50545, 50945-50948, 51992, 54690-54692, 55550, 55866
  Ureterolithotomy, 50945
  Ureteroneocystostomy, 50947-50948
  Urethral Suspension, 51990
Laparotomy, Exploratory, 49000-49002
Laparotomy
  Exploration, 49000-49002
  Hemorrhage Control, 49002
  with Biopsy, 49000
Laser Surgery
  Lesion
    Penis, 54057
    Skin, 17270-17276
  Prostate, 52647-52649
  Tumor
    Urethra and Bladder, 52234-52240
  Urethra and Bladder, 52214
Laser Treatment, 17270-17276
Lavage
  Peritoneal, 49084
Leadbetter Procedure, 53431
Lesion
  Bladder
    Destruction, 51030
  Destruction
    Ureter, 52341-52342, 52344-52345, 52354

Lesion — *continued*
  Epididymis
    Excision, 54830
  Excision
    Bladder, 52224
    Urethra, 52224, 53265
    Penis
      Destruction
        Any Method, 54065
        Cryosurgery, 54056
        Electrodesiccation, 54055
        Extensive, 54065
        Laser Surgery, 54057
        Simple, 54050-54060
        Surgical Excision, 54060
      Excision, 54060
        Penile Plaque, 54110-54112
    Resection, 52354
    Skin
      Destruction
        Malignant, 17270-17276
    Spermatic Cord
      Excision, 55520
    Testis
      Excision, 54512
Leukocyte Count, 85032, 85048
Ligation
  Vas Deferens, 55250
Litholapaxy, 52317-52318
Lithotripsy
  Bladder, 52353
  Kidney, 50590, 52353
  Ureter, 52353
  Urethra, 52353
  with Cystourethroscopy, 52353
Liver
  Ultrasound Scan (LUSS), 76705
Long Term Care Facility Visits
  Annual Assessment, 99318
  Discharge Services, 99315-99316
  Initial, 99304-99306
  Subsequent, 99307-99310
Lowsley's Operation, 54380
LUSS (Liver Ultrasound Scan), 76705
Lymph Node(s)
  Biopsy, 38500, 38570
    Needle, 38505
  Excision, 38500
    Abdominal, 38747
    Inguinofemoral, 38760-38765
    Laparoscopic, 38571-38573
    Limited, for Staging
      Para–Aortic, 38562
      Pelvic, 38562
      Retroperitoneal, 38564
    Pelvic, 38770
    Retroperitoneal Transabdominal, 38780
  Removal
    Abdominal, 38747
    Inguinofemoral, 38760-38765
    Pelvic, 38747, 38770
    Retroperitoneal Transabdominal, 38780
Lymphadenectomy
  Abdominal, 38747
  Bilateral Inguinofemoral, 54130
  Bilateral Pelvic, 51575, 51585, 51595, 54135, 55845, 55865
    Total, 38571-38573
  Gastric, 38747
  Inguinofemoral, 38760-38765
  Limited Pelvic, 55842, 55862
  Limited, for Staging
    Para–Aortic, 38562
    Pelvic, 38562
    Retroperitoneal, 38564
  Peripancreatic, 38747
  Portal, 38747
  Radical
    Groin Area, 38760-38765
    Pelvic, 54135, 55845
  Retroperitoneal Transabdominal, 38780
Lysis
  Adhesions
    Foreskin, 54450

Lysis — *continued*
  Adhesions — *continued*
    Penile
      Post–circumcision, 54162
    Ureter, 50715-50725
    Urethra, 53500

M

MAGPI Operation, 54322
Magpi Procedure, 54322
Manipulation
  Foreskin, 54450
Manometric Studies
  Kidney
    Pressure, 50396
  Ureter
    Pressure, 50686
  Ureterostomy, 50686
Marshall–Marchetti–Krantz Procedure, 51840-51841
Marsupialization
  Urethral Diverticulum, 53240
Mass
  Kidney
    Ablation, 50542
    Cryosurgery, 50250
Maydl Operation, 50810
Measurement
  Glomerular Filtration Rate (GFR), 0602T
Meatotomy, 53020-53025
  Contact Laser Vaporization with/without Transurethral Resection of Prostate, 52648
  with Cystourethroscopy, 52281
  Infant, 53025
  Non–contact Laser Coagulation Prostate, 52647
  Prostate
    Laser Coagulation, 52647
    Laser Vaporization, 52648
  Transurethral Electrosurgical Resection Prostate, 52601
  Ureter, 52290
  Urethral
    Cystourethroscopy, 52290-52305
Mesh Implantation
  Vagina, 57267
Mesh
  Insertion
    Pelvic Floor, 57267
  Removal
    Abdominal Infected, 11008
Metabolic Panel
  Calcium Ionized, 80047
  Calcium Total, 80048
  Comprehensive, 80053
Micro-Remodeling Female Bladder, 53860
Microbiology, 87081-87088, 87880
Millin-Read Operation, 57288
Mitrofanoff Operation, 50845
MMK, 51841
Model
  3D Printed, Anatomic, 0559T-0560T
Molluscum Contagiosum Destruction
  Penis, 54050-54060
Monitoring
  Glomerular Filtration Rate (GFR), 0603T
  Prolonged, with Physician Attendance, 99354-99359 [99415, 99416, 99417]
Mosenthal Test, 81002
Mucosa
  Urethra, Mucosal Advancement, 53450
Muscle(s)
  Debridement
    Infected, 11004-11006

N

Needle Biopsy
  Abdomen Mass, 49180
  Epididymis, 54800
  Kidney, 50200
  Lymph Node, 38505
  Prostate, 55700
  Retroperitoneal Mass, 49180
  Testis, 54500

Neobladder
  Construction, 51596
Nephrectomy
  Donor, 50300-50320, 50547
  Laparoscopic, 50545-50548
  Partial, 50240
    Laparoscopic, 50543
  Recipient, 50340
  with Ureters, 50220-50236, 50546, 50548
Nephrolithotomy, 50060-50075
Nephropexy, 50400-50405
Nephropyeloplasty, 50400-50405, 50544
Nephrorrhaphy, 50500
Nephrostogram, [50430, 50431]
Nephrostolithotomy
  Percutaneous, 50080-50081
Nephrostomy Tract
  Establishment, [50436, 50437]
Nephrostomy
  Change Tube, [50435]
    with Drainage, 50400
  Endoscopic, 50562-50570
    with Exploration, 50045
  Percutaneous, 52334
Nephrotomy, 50040-50045
  with Exploration, 50045
Neurology
  Central Motor
    Electromyography
      Needle, 51785
    Urethral Sphincter, 51785
  Diagnostic
    Anal Sphincter, 51785
New Patient
  Domiciliary or Rest Home Visit, 99324-99328
  Emergency Department Services, 99281-99285
  Home Services, 99341-99345
  Hospital Inpatient Services, 99221-99223, 99231-99239
  Hospital Observation Services, 99217-99220
  Initial Inpatient Consultations, 99251-99255
  Initial Office Visit, 99202-99205
  Office and/or Other Outpatient Consultations, 99241-99245
  Outpatient Visit, 99211-99215
Newborn Care
  Circumcision
    Clamp or Other Device, 54150
    Surgical Excision, 54160
  Prepuce Slitting, 54000
Nitrate Reduction Test
  Urinalysis, 81000-81015
Nocturnal Penile Rigidity Test, 54250
Nocturnal Penile Tumescence Test, 54250
Non–office Medical Services
  Emergency Care, 99060
Nursing Facility Services
  Annual Assessment, 99318
  Discharge Services, 99315-99316
  Initial, 99304-99306
  Subsequent Nursing Facility Care, 99307-99310
    New or Established Patient, 99307-99310
Nutrition Therapy
  Home Infusion, 99601-99602

O

Observation
  Discharge, 99217
  Initial, 99218-99220
  Same Date Admit/Discharge, 99234-99236
  Subsequent, [99224, 99225, 99226]
Obstruction
  Penis (Vein), 37790
Occlusion
  Penis
    Vein, 37790
  Ureteral, 50705
Office and/or Other Outpatient Visits
  Consultation, 99241-99245
  Established Patient, 99211-99215
  New Patient, 99202-99205

CPT Index

© 2020 Optum360, LLC

● New   ▲ Revised   + Add On   AMA: CPT Assist [Resequenced]

CPT © 2020 American Medical Association. All Rights Reserved.

CPT © 2020 American Medical Association. All Rights Reserved.

● New   ▲ Revised   + Add On   AMA: CPT Assist[Resequenced]

© 2020 Optum360, LLC

Stimulus Evoked Response, 51792
Stoma
Creation
Bladder, 51980
Kidney, 50551-50561
Ureter, 50860
Ureter
Endoscopy via, 50951-50961
Stone, Kidney
Removal, 50060-50081, 50130, 50561, 50580, 52352
Stone
Calculi
Bladder, 51050, 52310-52318, 52352
Kidney, 50060-50081, 50130, 50561, 50580, 52352
Ureter, 50610-50630, 50961, 50980, 51060-51065, 52320-52330, 52352
Urethra, 52310-52315, 52352
Streptococcus, Group A
Direct Optical Observation, 87880
Stricture
Ureter, 50706
Urethra
Dilation, 52281
Repair, 53400
STSG, 15120-15121
Subcutaneous Tissue
Repair
Complex, 13131-13133, 13160
Intermediate, 12041-12047
Simple, 12020-12021
Subcutaneous
Injection, 96372
Substance and/or Alcohol Abuse Screening and Intervention, 99408-99409
Suprapubic Prostatectomies, 55821
Surgeries
Laser
Bladder/Urethra, 52214-52240
Lesion
Penis, 54057
Skin, 17270-17276
Prostate, 52647-52648
Surgical
Diathermy
Lesions
Malignant, 17270-17276
Pneumoperitoneum, 49400
Suspension
Kidney, 50400-50405
Urethra, 51990, 57289
Vesical Neck, 51845
Suture
Bladder
Fistulization, 44660-44661, 51880-51925
Vesicouterine, 51920-51925
Vesicovaginal, 51900
Wound, 51860-51865
Colon
Fistula, 44660-44661
Intestines
Small
Fistula, 44660-44661
Kidney
Fistula, 50520-50526
Horseshoe, 50540
Wound, 50500
Testis
Injury, 54670
Suspension, 54620-54640
Ureter, 50900, 50940
Deligation, 50940
Fistula, 50920-50930
Urethra
Fistula, 53520
Stoma, 53520
to Bladder, 51840-51841
Wound, 53502-53515
Uterus
Fistula, 51920-51925
Vagina
Cystocele, 57240, 57260
Enterocele, 57265

Suture — *continued*
Vagina — *continued*
Fistula
Vesicovaginal, 51900
Rectocele, 57260
Vas Deferens, 55400
Wound
Skin
Complex, 13131-13133, 13160
Intermediate, 12041-12047
Simple, 12020-12021
Symphysiotomy
Horseshoe Kidney, 50540
Syndrome
Ovarian Vein
Ureterolysis, 50722
Urethral
Cystourethroscopy, 52285
System
Cardiovascular, 35840, 36415-36416, 36593, 36598, 36800-36821, 36825-36835, 36860-36861, 37788-37790
Digestive, 44660-44661, 46744-46746, 49000-49010, 49020, 49060, 49082-49185, 49320-49321, 49324-49325, 49327, 49400-49407, 49412-49418, 49421-49422, 49435-49436
Genital
Female, 57220-57240, 57260-57267, 57284-57289, 57423
Male, 54000-54692, 54700-55550, 55600-55880
Hemic/Lymphatic, 38500-38505, 38531, 38562-38573, 38747-38780
Integumentary, 10180, 11004-11008, 12001-12007, 12020-12021, 12041-12047, 13131-13133, 13160, 15002-15005, 15120-15121, 15240-15241, 17270-17276
Urinary, 50010-50405, 50500-50548, 50551-50948, 50951-51792, 51798-51992, 52000-52355, 52400-53860 [50430, 50431, 50432, 50433, 50434, 50435, 50436, 50437, 51797, 52356]

T

TAH, 51925
Telephone
Non-face-to-face
Physician, 99441-99443
Tenago Procedure, 53431
Testes
Undescended
Exploration, 54550-54560
Testicular Vein
Excision, 55530-55540
Ligation, 55530-55550
Testis
Abscess
Incision and Drainage, 54700
Biopsy, 54500-54505
Excision
Laparoscopic, 54690
Partial, 54522
Radical, 54530-54535
Simple, 54520
Hematoma
Incision and Drainage, 54700
Insertion
Prosthesis, 54660
Lesion
Excision, 54512
Needle Biopsy, 54500
Repair
Injury, 54670
Suspension, 54620-54640
Torsion, 54600
Suture
Injury, 54670
Suspension, 54620-54640
Transplantation
to Thigh, 54680
Tumor
Excision, 54530-54535
Undescended
Exploration, 54550-54560

Testosterone, 84402
Bioavailable, Direct, 84410
Total, 84403
Thermocoagulation, 17270-17276
Thermotherapy
Prostate, 53850-53852
High-Energy Water Vapor, 0582T
Microwave, 53850
Radiofrequency, 53852
Thrombectomy
Dialysis Graft
without Revision, 36831
Vena Caval, 50230
Thrombocyte (Platelet)
Automated Count, 85049
Count, 85008
Manual Count, 85032
Tissue
Culture
Skin Grafts, 15120-15121
Torek Procedure
Orchiopexy, 54650
Total
Cystectomy, 51570-51597
Transection
Blood Vessel
Kidney, 50100
Transitional Care Management, 99495-99496
Transperineal Periurethral Balloon Device, 0548T-0551T
Transperineal Placement
Biodegradable Material
Periprostatic, 55874
Transplantation
Backbench Preparation Prior to Transplantation
Kidney, 50323-50329
Renal
Allograft Preparation, 50323-50329
Allotransplantation, 50360
with Recipient Nephrectomy, 50365
Autotransplantation, 50380
Donor Nephrectomy, 50300-50320, 50547
Recipient Nephrectomy, 50340
Removal Transplanted Renal Allograft, 50370
Testis
to Thigh, 54680
Transureteroureterostomy, 50770
Transurethral
Fulguration
Postoperative Bleeding, 52214
Prostate
Ablation
Waterjet, 0421T
Anterior Commissurotomy, 0619T
Incision, 52450
Resection, 52601-52640
Thermotherapy, 53850-53852
High-Energy Water Vapor, 0582T
Microwave, 53850
Radiofrequency, 53852
Radiofrequency Micro-Remodeling
Female Bladder, 53860
TRUSP (Transrectal Ultrasound of Prostate), 76873
Tudor "Rabbit Ear"
Urethra, Repair
Diverticulum, 53240, 53400-53405
Fistula, 53400-53405, 53520
Sphincter, 57220
Stricture, 53400-53405
Urethrocele, 57230
Wound, 53502-53515
TULIP, 52647-52648
Tumor
Bladder, 52234-52240
Excision, 51530, 52355
Destruction
Urethra, 53220
Kidney
Excision, 52355
Prostate
Thermotherapy Ablation, 0582T

Tumor — *continued*
Resection
with Cystourethroscopy, 52355
Testis
Excision, 54530-54535
Ureter
Excision, 52355
Urethra, 52234-52240, 53220
Excision, 52355
TUMT (Transurethral Microwave Thermotherapy), 53850
TUNA, 53852
Tunica Vaginalis
Hydrocele
Aspiration, 55000
Excision, 55040-55041
Repair, 55060
TURP, 52601-52630

U

UCX (Urine Culture), 87086-87088
UFR, 51736-51741
Ulcerative, Cystitis, 52260-52265
Ultrasonic Fragmentation Ureteral Calculus, 52325
Ultrasound
Abdomen, 76700-76705
Bladder, 51798
Guidance
Cryosurgery, 55873
Kidney, 76770-76776
Prostate, 76872-76873
Rectal, 76872-76873
Retroperitoneal, 76770-76775
Scrotum, 76870
Undescended Testicle
Exploration, 54550-54560
UPP (Urethral Pressure Profile), 51727, 51729
Urachal Cyst
Bladder
Excision, 51500
Urecholine Supersensitivity Test
Cystometrogram, 51725-51726
Ureter
Anastomosis
to Bladder, 50780-50785
to Colon, 50810-50815
to Intestine, 50800, 50820-50825
to Kidney, 50740-50750
to Ureter, 50760-50770
Biopsy, 50606, 50955-50957, 50974-50976, 52007
Catheterization, 52005
Continent Diversion, 50825
Creation
Stoma, 50860
Destruction
Endoscopic, 50957, 50976
Dilation, 52341-52342, 52344-52345
Endoscopic, 50553, 50572, 50953, 50972
Endoscopy
Biopsy, 50955-50957, 50974-50976, 52007, 52354
Catheterization, 50953, 50972, 52005
Destruction, 50957, 50976, 52354
Endoscopic, 50957, 50976
Dilation, 52341-52342, 52344-52345
Excision
Tumor, 52355
Exploration, 52351
Injection of Implant Material, 52327
Insertion
Stent, 50947, 52332
Lithotripsy, 52353
with Indwelling Stent, [52356]
Manipulation of Ureteral Calculus, 52330
Removal
Calculus, 50961, 50980, 52320-52325, 52352
Foreign Body, 50961, 50980
Resection, 50970-50980, 52355
via Incision, 50970-50980
via Stoma, 50951-50961
Exploration, 50600

© 2020 Optum360, LLC   ● New   ▲ Revised   + Add On   AMA: CPT Assist [Resequenced]   CPT © 2020 American Medical Association. All Rights Reserved.

Coding Companion for Urology/Nephrology

CPT Index

Urethrostomy, 53000-53010
Urethrotomy, 53000-53010
  Direct Vision
    with Cystourethroscopy, 52276
  Internal, 52601, 52647 52648
    with Cystourethroscopy
      Female, 52270
      Male, 52275
Urinalysis, 81000-81015
  Automated, 81001, 81003
  Microscopic, 81015
  Qualitative, 81005
  Routine, 81002
  Screen, 81007
  Semiquantitative, 81005
  without Microscopy, 81002
Urinary Catheter Irrigation, 51700
Urinary Sphincter, Artificial
  Insertion, 53445
  Removal, 53446
    with Replacement, 53447-53448
  Repair, 53449
Urine
  Blood, 81000-81005
  Colony Count, 87086
  Tests, 81000-81015
Urodynamic Tests
  Bladder Capacity
    Ultrasound, 51798
  Cystometrogram, 51725-51729
  Electromyography Studies
    Needle, 51785
    Rectal, [51797]
  Residual Urine
    Ultrasound, 51798
  Stimulus Evoked Response, 51792
  Urethra Pressure Profile, [51797]
  Uroflowmetry, 51736-51741
  Voiding Pressure Studies
    Bladder, 51728-51729
    Intra–abdominal, [51797]
Uroflowmetry, 51736-51741
Urostomy, 50727-50728
Uterus
  Repair
    Fistula, 51920-51925

V

V–Flap Procedure
  One Stage Distal Hypospadias Repair, 54322
V–Y Operation, Bladder, Neck, 51845
Vagina
  Removal
    Sling
      Stress Incontinence, 57287
  Repair
    Cystocele, 57240, 57260
      Anterior, 57240
      Combined Anteroposterior,
        57260-57265
    Enterocele, 57265

Vagina — continued
  Repair — continued
    Fistula, 51900
      Vesicovaginal, 51900
    Incontinence, 57288
    Paravaginal Defect, 57284
    Pereyra Procedure, 57289
    Prolapse, 57284
    Prosthesis Insertion, 57267
    Rectocele
      Combined Anteroposterior,
        57260-57265
    Urethra Sphincter, 57220
  Revision
    Sling
      Stress Incontinence, 57287
  Suture
    Cystocele, 57240, 57260
    Enterocele, 57265
    Fistula, 51900
    Rectocele, 57260
Varicocele
  Spermatic Cord
    Excision, 55530-55540
Vas Deferens
  Anastomosis
    to Epididymis, 54900-54901
  Excision, 55250
  Incision, 55200
    for X–ray, 55300
  Ligation, 55250
  Repair
    Suture, 55400
Vascular Studies
  Hemodialysis Access, 93990
    Prior to Access Creation, 93985-93986
  Penile Vessels, 93980-93981
  Visceral Studies, 93975-93976
Vasectomy, 55250
  Laser Coagulation of Prostate, 52647
  Laser Vaporization of Prostate, 52648
  Reversal, 55400
  Transurethral
    Cystourethroscopic, 52402
  Transurethral Electrosurgical Resection of
    Prostate, 52601
  Transurethral Resection of Prostate, 52648
Vasoactive Drugs
  Injection
    Penis, 54231
Vasotomy, 55200, 55300
  Transurethral
    Cystourethroscopic, 52402
Vasovasorrhaphy, 55400
Vasovasostomy, 55400
VCU (Voiding Cystourethrogram), 51600
VCUG (Voiding Cystourethrogram), 51600
Vein
  Cannulization
    to Artery, 36810-36815
    to Vein, 36800
  External Cannula Declotting, 36860-36861

Vein — continued
  Spermatic
    Excision, 55530-55540
    Ligation, 55500
Vena Caval
  Thrombectomy, 50230
Venipuncture
  Routine, 36415
Venous Access Device
  Declotting, 36593
Vesicle, Seminal
  Excision, 55650
    Cyst, 55680
    Mullerian Duct, 55680
  Incision, 55600-55605
Vesico–Psoas Hitch, 50785
Vesicostomy
  Cutaneous, 51980
Vesicourethropexy, 51840-51841
Vesicovaginal Fistula
  Closure
    Abdominal Approach, 51900
Vesiculectomy, 55650
Vesiculogram, Seminal, 55300
Vesiculography, 55300
Vesiculotomy, 55600-55605
  Complicated, 55605
Vidal Procedure
  Varicocele, Spermatic Cord, Excision, 55530-55540
Visit, Home, 99341-99350
Visualization
  Ideal Conduit, 50690
Voiding
  EMG, 51784-51785
  Pressure Studies
    Abdominal, [51797]
    Bladder, 51728-51729 [51797]
    Rectum, [51797]
  Prosthesis
    Intraurethral Valve Pump, 0596T-0597T
VP, 51728-51729 [51797]

W

Walsh Modified Radical Prostatectomy, 55810
Water Wart
  Destruction
    Penis, 54050-54060
Waterjet Ablation
  Prostate, 0421T
WBC, 85007, 85009, 85025, 85048
Wellness Behavior
  Alcohol and/or Substance Abuse, 99408-99409
  Smoking and Tobacco Cessation Counseling, 99406-99407
White Blood Cell
  Count, 85032, 85048
  Differential, 85004-85007, 85009
Winter Procedure, 54435

Wound
  Dehiscence
    Repair
      Secondary
        Skin and Subcutaneous Tissue
          Complex, 13160
          Complicated, 13160
          Extensive, 13160
        Skin and Subcutaneous Tissue
          Simple, 12020
            with Packing, 12021
          Superficial, 12020
            with Packing, 12021
      Suture
        Secondary
          Skin and Subcutaneous Tissue
            Complex, 13160
            Complicated, 13160
            Extensive, 13160
        Skin and Subcutaneous Tissue
          Simple, 12020
            with Packing, 12021
          Superficial, 12020
            with Packing, 12021
  Infection
    Incision and Drainage
      Postoperative, 10180
  Repair
    Skin
      Complex, 13131-13133, 13160
      Intermediate, 12041-12047
      Simple, 12001-12007, 12020-12021
    Urethra, 53502-53515
    Secondary
      Skin and Subcutaneous Tissue
        Complex, 13160
        Complicated, 13160
        Extensive, 13160
        Simple, 12020
        Simple with Packing, 12021
        Superficial, 12020
          with Packing, 12021
  Suture
    Bladder, 51860-51865
    Kidney, 50500
    Urethra, 53502-53515

X

X–ray
  with Contrast
    Central Venous Access Device, 36598

Y

Y–Plasty, 51800

CPT Index

© 2020 Optum360, LLC

● New   ▲ Revised   + Add On   AMA: CPT Assist [Resequenced]

CPT © 2020 American Medical Association. All Rights Reserved.

544

Coding Companion for Urology/Nephrology